Third Edition

VETERINARY MICROBIOLOGY

Third Edition

VETERINARY MICROBIOLOGY

Editors

D. Scott McVey, DVM, PhD, DACVM

Research Leader, Supervisory Veterinary Medical Officer, and Professor of Immunology
USDA ARS CGAHR
Arthropod-Borne Animal Diseases Research Unit
Manhattan, KS

Melissa Kennedy, DVM, PhD, DACVM

Associate Professor and Director
Department of Biomedical and Diagnostic Sciences Department
College of Veterinary Medicine
University of Tennessee
Knoxville, TN

M.M. Chengappa, BVSc, MVSc, MS, PhD, DACVM

Department Head and University Distinguished Professor
Diagnostic Medicine Pathobiology
College of Veterinary Medicine
Kansas State University
Manhattan, KS

WILEY-BLACKWELL

A John Wiley & Sons, Inc., Publication

Editorial offices: 2121 State Avenue, Ames, Iowa 50014-8300, USA
The Atrium, Southern Gate, Chichester, West Sussex, PO19 8SQ, UK
9600 Garsington Road, Oxford, OX4 2DQ, UK

For details of our global editorial offices, for customer services and for information about how to apply for permission to reuse the copyright material in this book please see our website at www.wiley.com/wiley-blackwell.

Library of Congress Cataloging-in-Publication Data

Veterinary microbiology. – 3rd ed. / editors, D.S. McVey, Melissa Kennedy, M.M. Chengappa.
p. ; cm.
Includes bibliographical references and index.
ISBN 978-0-470-95949-7 (softback : alk. paper) – ISBN 978-1-118-65054-7 (eMobi) – ISBN 978-1-118-65056-1 (ePDF) – ISBN 978-1-118-65062-2 (ePub) – ISBN 978-1-118-65338-8 – ISBN 978-1-118-65340-1
I. McVey, D. Scott II. Kennedy, Melissa (Melissa Anne), 1959- III. Chengappa, M. M.
[DNLM: 1. Animal Population Groups–microbiology. 2. Veterinary Medicine. QW 70]
SF780.2
636.089′69041–dc23

2013002830

A catalogue record for this book is available from the British Library.

Wiley also publishes its books in a variety of electronic formats. Some content that appears in print may not be available in electronic books.

Cover design by Modern Alchemy LLC

Set in 9/11pt ITC Stone Serif by Aptara® Inc., New Delhi, India
Printed and bound in Malaysia by Vivar Printing Sdn Bhd
1 2013

Contents

Contributors

Udeni B.R. Balasuriya, BVSc, MS, PhD
Associate Professor of Virology
Department of Veterinary Science
University of Kentucky
Lexington, KY

Raul G. Barletta, PhD
Professor
School of Veterinary Medicine and Biomedical Sciences
University of Nebraska-Lincoln
Lincoln, NE

Brian Bellaire, PhD
Assistant Professor
Veterinary Microbiology and Preventative Medicine
College of Veterinary Medicine
Iowa State University
Ames, IA

Karen E. Beenken, PhD
Fellow
Department of Microbiology and Immunology
College of Medicine
University of Arkansas for Medical Sciences
Little Rock, AR

Deborah J. Briggs, MS, PhD
Professor of Virology
Diagnostic Medicine Pathobiology
College of Veterinary Medicine
Kansas State University
Manhattan, KS

Christopher C.L. Chase, DVM, MS, PhD, DACVM
Professor of Virology
Department of Veterinary and Biomedical Sciences
South Dakota State University
Brookings, SD

M.M. Chengappa, BVSc, MVSc, MS, PhD, DACVM
Department Head and University Distinguished Professor
Diagnostic Medicine Pathobiology
College of Veterinary Medicine
Kansas State University
Manhattan, KS

Bruno B. Chomel, MS, PhD
Professor
University of California
School of Veterinary Medicine
Department of Population Health and Reproduction
Davis, CA

Charles Czuprynski, PhD
Professor in Microbiology
Department of Pathobiological Sciences
School of Veterinary Medicine
University of Wisconsin
Madison, WI

Joshua B. Daniels, DVM, PhD, DACVM
Assistant Professor
Department of Veterinary Clinical Sciences
College of Veterinary Medicine
The Ohio State University
Columbus, OH

Gustavo A. Delhon, DVM, MS, PhD
Associate Professor
School of Veterinary Medicine and Biomedical Sciences
University of Nebraska-Lincoln
Lincoln, NE

Barbara Drolet, MS, PhD
Research Microbiologist
USDA ARS CGAHR
Arthropod-Borne Animal Diseases Research Unit
Manhattan, KS

Bradley W. Fenwick, DVM, MS, PhD, DACVM
Professor and Jefferson Science Fellow
University of Tennessee
Knoxville, TN

Timothy Frana, DVM, MS, MPH, PhD, DAVPM, DACVM
Associate Professor
Veterinary Diagnostic Laboratory
College of Veterinary Medicine
Iowa State University
Ames, IA

Frederick J. Fuller, MS, PhD
Professor of Virology
North Carolina State University
College of Veterinary Medicine
Raleigh, NC

Roman R. Ganta, MS, PhD
Professor
Diagnostic Medicine Pathobiology
College of Veterinary Medicine
Kansas State University
Manhattan, KS

Laurel J. Gershwin, DVM, PhD, DACVM
Professor of Immunology
University of California
College of Veterinary Medicine
Department of Pathology, Microbiology, and Immunology
Davis, CA

Seth P. Harris, DVM, PhD
Assistant Professor
School of Veterinary Medicine and Biomedical Sciences
University of Nebraska-Lincoln
Lincoln, NE

Richard A. Hesse, MS, PhD
Professor
Diagnostic Medicine Pathobiology
College of Veterinary Medicine
Kansas State University
Manhattan, KS

Douglas E. Hostetler, DVM, MS
Associate Professor
School of Veterinary Medicine and Biomedical Sciences
University of Nebraska-Lincoln
Lincoln, NE

Peter C. Iwen, MS, PhD, D(ABBM)
Professor of Pathology and Microbiology
Pathology and Microbiology
NE Public Health Laboratory
Nebraska Medical Center
Omaha, NE

Megan E. Jacob, MS, PhD
Assistant Professor of Clinical Microbiology
and Director, Clinical Microbiology Laboratory
North Carolina State University
College of Veterinary Medicine
Department of Population Health and Pathobiology
Raleigh, NC

Huchappa Jayappa, BVSc, MVSc, PhD
Associate Director
Merck Animal Health
Elkhorn, NE

Rickie W. Kasten, MS, PhD
Staff Research Associate
University of California
School of Veterinary Medicine
Department of Population Health and Reproduction
Davis, CA

Melissa Kennedy, DVM, PhD, DACVM
Associate Professor
College of Veterinary Medicine
Biomedical and Diagnostic Sciences
University of Tennessee
Knoxville, TN

Peter W. Krug, PhD
Research Molecular Biologist
USDA ARS PIADC
Foreign Animal Disease Research Unit
Greenport, NY

Rance B. LeFebvre, PhD
Professor and Associate Dean of Student Affairs
University of California
School of Veterinary Medicine
Department of Pathology, Microbiology, and Immunology
Davis, CA

Wenjun Ma, BVSc, MVSc, PhD
Assistant Professor
Diagnostic Medicine Pathobiology
Center of Excellence in Emerging and Zoonotic Diseases
College of Veterinary Medicine
Kansas State University
Manhattan, KS

Melissa L. Madsen, PhD
Research and Development Project Leader
CEVA Biomune
Olathe, KS

D. Scott McVey, DVM, PhD, DACVM
Research Leader, Supervisory Veterinary Medical Officer, and Professor of Immunology
USDA ARS CGAHR
Arthropod-Borne Animal Diseases Research Unit
Manhattan, KS

Rodney Moxley, DVM, PhD
Professor
School of Veterinary Medicine and Biomedical Sciences
University of Nebraska-Lincoln
Lincoln, NE

T.G. Nagaraja, MVSc, MS, PhD
University Distinguished Professor
Diagnostic Medicine Pathobiology
College of Veterinary Medicine
Kansas State University
Manhattan, KS

Sanjeev Narayanan, BVSc, MS, PhD, DACVM, DACVP
Associate Professor
Diagnostic Medicine Pathobiology
College of Veterinary Medicine
Kansas State University
Manhattan, KS

Jerome C. Neitfeld, DVM, MS, PhD
Professor
Diagnostic Medicine Pathobiology
College of Veterinary Medicine
Kansas State University
Manhattan, KS

Stefan Niewiesk, DVM, PhD, DECLAM
Associate Professor
Department of Veterinary Biosciences
College of Veterinary Medicine
The Ohio State University
Columbus, OH

Michael Oglesbee, DVM, PhD, DACVP
Professor and Chair
Department of Veterinary Biosciences
College of Veterinary Medicine
The Ohio State University
Columbus, OH

Steven Olsen, DVM, PhD, DACVM
Research Leader and Supervisory Veterinary Medical Officer
USDA ARS NADC
Infectious Bacterial Disease Unit
Ames, IA

Lisa M. Pohlman, DVM, MS, DACVP
Assistant Professor and Director, Clinical Pathology Laboratory
Diagnostic Medicine Pathobiology
College of Veterinary Medicine
Kansas State University
Manhattan, KS

John F. Prescott, MA, Vet MB, PhD
Professor
Department of Pathobiology
University of Guelph
Guelph, Ontario

Juergen A. Richt, DVM, PhD
Regents Distinguished Professor and KBA Eminent Scholar
Director of the Center of Excellence in Emerging and Zoonotic Diseases
Diagnostic Medicine Pathobiology
Center of Excellence in Emerging and Zoonotic Diseases
College of Veterinary Medicine
Kansas State University
Manhattan, KS

Luis L. Rodriguez, DVM, PhD
Research Leader and Supervisory Veterinary Medical Officer
USDA ARS PIADC
Foreign Animal Disease Research Unit
Greenport, NY

Raymond R. Rowland, MS, PhD
Professor
Diagnostic Medicine Pathobiology
College of Veterinary Medicine
Kansas State University
Manhattan, KS

Ronald D. Schultz, MS, PhD, Honorary DACVM
Professor and Chair
Department of Pathobiological Sciences
School of Veterinary Medicine
University of Wisconsin
Madison, WI

Mark S. Smeltzer, PhD
Professor
Department of Microbiology and Immunology
College of Medicine
University of Arkansas for Medical Sciences
Little Rock, AR

David J. Steffen, DVM, PhD, DACVP
Professor
School of Veterinary Medicine and Biomedical Sciences
University of Nebraska-Lincoln
Lincoln, NE

George C. Stewart, MS, PhD
Chair and McKee Professor of Microbial Pathogenesis
Department of Veterinary Pathobiology
University of Missouri
Columbia, MO

Erin L. Strait, DVM, PhD
Director, US Swine Biological R&D
Merck Animal Health
De Soto, KS

Dongseob Tark, DVM, PhD
Animal Plant Quarantine Agency, Manan-gu, Anyang-si
Gyeonggi-do, South Korea

Brian M. Thompson
MS, PhD
President and CEO
Elemental Enzymes, Inc.
Columbia, MO

Benjamin R. Trible, MS
Diagnostic Medicine Pathobiology
College of Veterinary Medicine
Kansas State University
Manhattan, KS

Rebecca P. Wilkes, DVM, PhD, DACVM
Research Assistant Professor
Diagnostic Sciences and Education
College of Veterinary Medicine
University of Tennessee
Knoxville, TN

William Wilson, MS, PhD
Research Microbiologist
USDA ARS CGAHR
Arthropod-Borne Animal Diseases Research Unit
Manhattan, KS

Amelia R. Woolums, DVM, MVSc, PhD, DACVIM, DACVM
Senior Teaching Fellow
College of Veterinary Medicine
University of Georgia
Athens, GA

Preface

This collection of chapters and supporting materials is intended to provide a very broad overview of veterinary microbiology and infectious diseases. The writings represent a combination of the biology of the organisms that cause or are associated with disease and the diseases themselves. The scope of this book is intended to be general to appeal both to beginning students of veterinary sciences and to seasoned veterinary practitioners and scientists. Like many textbooks, this book will hopefully be a strong starting place for the study of veterinary infectious diseases as well as a good reference text. The content emphasizes diseases that occur in North America, but many global, transboundary disease content is included.

The first section of the book is an introduction to infectious disease pathogenesis, diagnosis, and clinical management. These chapters are intended to provide a basis of understanding and discussion for later chapters describing specific organisms and diseases. The second section describes bacterial and fungal pathogens. This section covers a very diverse set of pathogens and many diseases, but yet the similarities of pathogenesis, virulence properties, and host responses among these organisms are striking. The third section of the book describes viral diseases and the viruses responsible. We have tried to emphasize the consequences of virus infections and the host responses. The last section of the book is a systematic approach of describing infection and disease of animals. In the spirit of one medicine, the chapters take a comparative approach to describing both differences and similarities of diseases across many affected species.

We have invited a group of outstanding microbiologists/experts to contribute to this book. We believe the contents are accurate and up-to-date. However, we welcome any comments or suggestions that you may have regarding the contents of this book.

D. Scott McVey, Melissa Kennedy, and
M.M. Chengappa

Acknowledgments

We wish to thank Drs Dwight C. Hirsh, N. James MacLachlan, and Richard L. Walker for allowing us to retain a significant portion of the second edition of the book. Also, we thank all of the chapter authors who contributed to the second edition, as we have retained some of their contributions in the revised edition. This book would not have been possible without the contributions of many outstanding research and diagnostic microbiologists. We also thank the respective institutional support for making the book possible. Finally, we would like to acknowledge John Wiley & Sons, Inc., and its staff for their guidance and support in completing the book. We also wish to thank Ms Brandy Nowakowski for assisting in the preparation of manuscripts.

About the Companion Website

This book is accompanied by a companion website:
www.wiley.com/go/mcvey/microbiology

The website includes:

- Review questions and answers
- Powerpoints of all figures from the book for downloading

PART I

Introduction

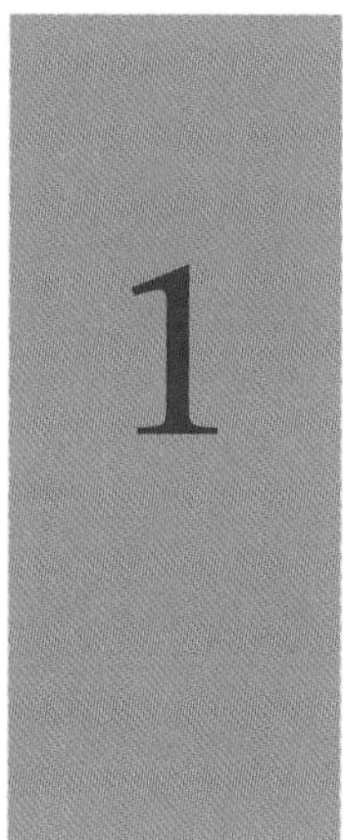

Pathogenicity and Virulence

D. SCOTT MCVEY AND CHARLES CZUPRYNSKI

Veterinary microbiology deals with microbial agents affecting animals. Such agents are categorized by their ecologic associations with animals: **parasites** live in permanent association with, and at the expense of, animal hosts; saprophytes normally inhabit the inanimate environment. Parasites that cause their host no discernible harm are called **commensals**. The term "symbiosis" usually refers to reciprocally beneficial associations of organisms. This arrangement is also called **mutualism**. Pathogenic organisms can be either parasites or saprophytes, and cause disease in one or more animal species. The process by which they establish themselves in a host individual is infection, but infection is not necessarily followed by clinical illness. The term "virulence" is sometimes used to express degrees of pathogenicity that may be related to the severity of clinical illness (Table 1.1).

Some Attributes of Host–Parasite Relationships

Many pathogenic microorganisms are host specific in that they parasitize only one or a few animal species. For example, the cause of equine strangles, *Streptococcus equi* subspecies *equi*, is essentially limited to infection of horses. Others—certain *Salmonella* serotypes, for example—have a broad host range. The basis for this difference in host specificity is often incompletely understood, but it may in part be related to the need for specific attachment devices between hosts (receptors) and parasites (adhesins).

Some agents infect several host species with varying effects. For example, the plague bacillus *Yersinia pestis* behaves as a commensal parasite in many small rodent species but causes fatal disease in rats and humans. Evolutionary pressure may have produced some of these differences. For instance, *Coccidioides immitis*, a saprophytic fungus that requires no living host, infects cattle and dogs with equal ease; yet it produces no clinical signs in cattle but frequently causes progressive fatal disease in dogs.

Potential pathogens also vary in their effects on different tissues in the same host. The *Escherichia coli* strains that are commensals in the intestine can cause severe disease in the urinary tract and peritoneal cavity. Some microorganisms that are commensals in one habitat may be pathogenic in the same, or some other, habitat that is pathologically altered or otherwise compromised. For example, oral streptococci, which occasionally enter the bloodstream, may colonize a damaged heart valve and initiate bacterial endocarditis. In the absence of such a lesion, however, the streptococci would not colonize and would be cleared uneventfully by the innate immune system. Similarly, the frequent translocation of intestinal bacteria across the intestinal mucosa, and into the vascular channels, normally leads to their clearance by innate and adaptive defense mechanisms. In immunodeficient hosts, however, such entrance may lead to fatal septicemia.

Commensalism is the stable form of parasitic existence. Gaining entrance into a novel host or tissue, or a change in host resistance, is a common way that commensal parasites are converted into active pathogens that ensure the survival of the microorganism. Active disease can jeopardize agent survival by killing the host or evoking an active immune response. Either outcome can deprive the agent of its habitat. Evolutionary selective pressure, therefore, tends to eliminate host–parasite relationships that threaten the survival of either partner. Less virulent strains of the pathogen, which permit survival of the host, tend to arise and thereby replace the more lethal strain. Evolutionary selection also favors establishment of a resistant host population by eliminating highly susceptible stock. The trend of host–agent adaptation is thus toward commensalism. Most agents causing serious disease have alternative modes of survival as commensals in tissues (e.g., *E. coli* in the intestine) or hosts not subject to disease (e.g., plague in small rodents) or in the inanimate environment (e.g., coccidioidomycosis). Some pathogens may cause chronic infections lasting months or years (tuberculosis and syphilis), during which time their dissemination to other hosts can occur and ensure their survival.

Veterinary Microbiology, Third Edition. Edited by D. Scott McVey, Melissa Kennedy and M.M. Chengappa.

Table 1.1. Degrees of Pathogenicity

Saprophytes	No disease—environmental bacteria
Commensal organisms	Colonize host tissue—no disease
Symbiotic species	Beneficial relationship for the host; colonize host tissue—mutually and parasitic microorganisms
Opportunistic parasites	Colonize host tissue (may usually be commensal) but cause disease with tissue damage or change in environment
Pathogenic microorganisms	Infection directly causes disease (although this may be host specific)

Criteria of Pathogenicity—Koch's Postulates

The presence of a microorganism in diseased individuals does not prove its pathogenic significance. To demonstrate the causal role of an agent in a disease, the following qualifications or "postulates" formulated by Robert Koch (1843–1910) should be satisfied:

1. The suspected agent is present in all cases of the disease.
2. The agent is isolated from such disease and propagated serially in pure culture, apart from its natural host.
3. Upon introduction into an experimental host, the isolate produces the original disease.
4. The agent can be reisolated from this experimental infection.

These postulates are ideals that cannot be completely satisfied in all cases of infectious diseases. The presence of some microorganisms cannot be demonstrated at the time of disease, especially in tissues affected by intoxication (e.g., tetanus and botulism). Other pathogens are difficult to isolate or die rapidly after isolation (e.g., *Leptospira* spp.). Still others, although clearly pathogenic, require undetermined accessory factors to cause disease (e.g., *Pasteurella*-related pneumonias). For some human viral pathogens (e.g., *Cytomegalovirus*), no experimental host is known. Finally, some agents (e.g., *Mycobacterium leprae*) cannot be grown in culture apart from their natural hosts.

Elements in the Production of an Infectious Disease

Effective transmission of a microbial agent occurs by ingestion; inhalation; or mucosal, cutaneous, or wound contamination. Airborne infection takes place largely via droplet nuclei, which are 0.1–5 mm in diameter. Particles of this size stay suspended in air and can be inhaled. Larger particles settle but can be resuspended in dust, which may also harbor infectious agents from nonrespiratory sources (e.g., skin squames, feces, and saliva). Arthropods may serve as mechanical carriers of pathogens (e.g., *Shigella* and *Dermatophilus*) or play an indispensable part in the life cycles of disease-producing agents (e.g., plague, ehrlichiosis, and viral encephalitides).

Attachment to host surfaces requires interaction between the agent's adhesins, which are usually proteins, and the host's receptors, which are most often protein or carbohydrate residues. Examples of bacterial adhesins are fimbrial proteins (*E. coli* and *Salmonella* spp.), P-1 protein of *Mycoplasma* (*Mycoplasma pneumoniae*), and afimbrial surface proteins (some streptococci). Examples of host receptor substances include fibronectin for some streptococci and staphylococci, mannose for many *E. coli* strains, and sialic acid for *M. pneumoniae*.

Attachment is inhibited by normal commensal floras that occupy or block available receptor sites or discourage colonization by excreting toxic metabolites, bacteriocins, and microcins. This "colonization resistance" is an important defense mechanism and may be assisted by host-determined antibacterial substances (e.g., defensins, lysozyme, lactoferrin, and organic acids) or by mucosal antibodies.

Penetration of an epithelial or mucosal host surface is a variable requirement among pathogens. Some agents, having reached a primary target cell population, penetrate no farther (e.g., enterotoxigenic *E. coli*). Others traverse surface membranes after inducing cytoskeletal rearrangements, resulting in "ruffles" that entrap adhered bacteria or passage between epithelial cells (e.g., *Salmonella* and *Yersinia*). Inhaled facultative intracellular parasites like *Mycobacterium tuberculosis* are ingested by pulmonary macrophages, in which they may multiply and travel via lymphatics to lymph nodes and other tissues. Percutaneous penetration occurs mostly through injuries, including arthropod bites. Dissemination within tissues or among adjacent tissues takes place by invasion, aided perhaps by bacterial enzymes such as collagenase and hyaluronidase, which are produced by many pathogens. Microorganisms are also spread via lymph and blood vessels, the bronchial tree, bile ducts, nerve trunks, and mobile phagocytes.

Except for the few foodborne pathogens that produce toxins in foodstuffs prior to ingestion, growth in or on host tissue is a prerequisite for all pathogenic organisms. In order to multiply to pathogenic levels, they must be able to circumvent host defense efforts. Pathogenic adaptations of various bacteria include firm attachment to prevent mechanical removal, avoidance of phagocytosis, and interference with phagocytic function by release of toxins or other components that prevent phagocytic digestion. Some bacteria digest or divert antibodies or deplete complement. Other pathogens alter the vascular supply to tissue, restricting defensive resources and impairing antimicrobial activity in the affected area.

When host defenses are significantly inhibited, microbial growth can proceed if nutritional supplies are adequate and the pH, temperature, and oxidation–reduction potential are appropriate. Iron is often a limiting nutrient. Microbial ability to appropriate iron from iron-binding host proteins (transferrin and lactoferrin) is an important factor in virulence. Gastric acidity accounts for the resistance of the stomach to most pathogenic bacteria, although expression of alternative sigma factors when bacteria are in stationary phase results in an RNA polymerase that transcribes genes whose products help the pathogen survive in an acidic environment (e.g., *Salmonella* and enterohemorrhagic *E. coli*). The higher body temperature of birds may explain their resistance to some diseases (e.g., anthrax and histoplasmosis), while requirements for an anaerobic environment account for the restriction of anaerobic growth to devitalized (i.e., nonoxygenated) tissues or tissues in which simultaneous aerobic growth has lowered the available oxygen.

Pathogenic Action

Microbial disease manifests itself either as direct damage to host structures and functions by exotoxins and other products of microbial growth, or as collateral damage due to host inflammatory or immune reactions triggered by the microbe or microbial components (endotoxin).

Direct Damage

Exotoxins are usually bacterial proteins, which are freely excreted into the environment. The differences between endotoxins and exotoxins are described in Table 1.2.

Two general types of exotoxins exist. One acts extracellularly or on cell membranes, attacking intercellular substances or cell surfaces by enzymatic or detergent-like mechanisms. Examples of these toxins include bacterial hemolysins, leukocidins, collagenases, and hyaluronidases, which may play an ancillary role in infections.

Another type of exotoxin consists of proteins or polypeptides that enter cells and enzymatically disrupt cellular processes. Many, but not all, of these usually consist of an A fragment, which has enzymatic activity, and a B fragment, which is responsible for binding the toxin to its target cell. Exotoxins are encoded chromosomally, on plasmids or on bacteriophages. In a manner similar to viruses, these toxins produce injury by destroying the cells in which they replicate or by altering cell function, appearance, and growth characteristics.

Table 1.2. Exo- and Endotoxins Compared

Exotoxins	Endotoxins
Often spontaneously diffusible	Cell-bound as part of the cell wall
Proteins or polypeptides	LPS (lipid A is a toxic component)
Produced by gram-positive and gram-negative bacteria	Limited to gram-negative bacteria
Produce a single, pharmacologically specific effect	Produce a range of effects, largely due to host-derived mediators
Each is distinct in structure and reactivity according to its bacterial species of origin	All similar in structure and effect regardless of bacterial species of origin
Lethal in minute amounts (mice = nanograms)	Lethal in larger amounts (mice = micrograms)
Labile to heat, chemicals, and storage	Very stable to heat, chemicals, and storage
Convertible to toxoids (nontoxic, immunogenic toxin-derivatives); elicit antitoxin production	Not convertible to toxoids

Endotoxins are lipopolysaccharides (LPS) that are part of the gram-negative cell wall and outer membrane. They consist of polysaccharide surface chains, which can act as an adhesin or virulence factors and are the somatic (O) antigens recognized by the immune response; a core polysaccharide; and lipid A, which is the toxic moiety. LPS may bind directly to leukocytes, or to LPS-binding protein (a plasma protein), which in turn transfers it to CD14. The CD14–LPS complex binds to receptor proteins (e.g., Toll-like receptor 4) on the surface of macrophages and other cells, triggering the release of proinflammatory cytokines. CD14–LPS complexes elicit the manifestations of endotoxemia, which includes fever, headache, hypotension, leukopenia, thrombocytopenia, intravascular coagulation, inflammation, endothelial damage, hemorrhage, fluid extravasation, and circulatory collapse. Many of these outcomes result from (1) activation of the complement cascade and (2) production of arachidonic acid metabolites (prostaglandins, leukotrienes, and thromboxanes). The manifestations of endotoxemia closely resemble the pathology associated with gram-negative septicemias. Although mediated by different bacterial components (lipoproteins) and host receptors (Toll-like receptor 2), most of these same manifestations can also be induced by the cell walls (peptidoglycans) of gram-positive bacteria.

Immune-Mediated Damage

Tissue damage due to immune reactions is considered elsewhere (see Chapter 2). Complement-mediated responses (such as inflammation) and reactions resembling immediate-type allergic phenomena can occur in response to endotoxins or to peptidoglycan without preceding sensitization.

Specific immune responses participate in the pathogenesis of many infections, particularly chronic granulomatous infections such as tuberculosis. Granulomas form as a result of cell-mediated hypersensitivity, which is initiated in the early stages of infection. Cell-mediated immune responses intensify inflammatory responses and tissue destruction upon subsequent encounters with the agent or its protein through the release of effector substances from T lymphocytes (e.g., cytokines and perforins). Immune mechanisms apparently contribute to anemias seen in anaplasmosis, and the hemotrophic mycoplasmas. The antibody response to hemoparasitism does not distinguish between the parasite and the host erythrocyte. Both are removed by phagocytosis.

Further Reading

Gyles CL (2011) Relevance in pathogenesis research. *Vet Microbiol*, **153** (1–2), 2–12. Epub April 22, 2011.

Hajishengallis G, Krauss JL, Liang S *et al.* (2012) Pathogenic microbes and community service through manipulation of innate immunity. *Adv Exp Med Biol*, **946**, 69–85.

Henderson B and Martin A (2011) Bacterial virulence in the moonlight: multitasking bacterial moonlighting proteins are virulence determinants in infectious disease. *Infect Immun*, **79** (9), 3476–3491. Epub June 6, 2011.

Høiby N, Ciofu O, Johansen HK *et al.* (2011) The clinical impact of bacterial biofilms. *Int J Oral Sci*, **3** (2), 55–65.

Hunt PW (2011) Molecular diagnosis of infections and resistance in veterinary and human parasites. *Vet Parasitol*, **180** (1–2), 12–46. Epub May 27, 2011.

Livorsi DJ, Stenehjem E, and Stephens DS (2011) Virulence factors of gram-negative bacteria in sepsis with a focus on *Neisseria meningitidis*. *Contrib Microbiol*, **17**, 31–47. Epub June 9, 2011.

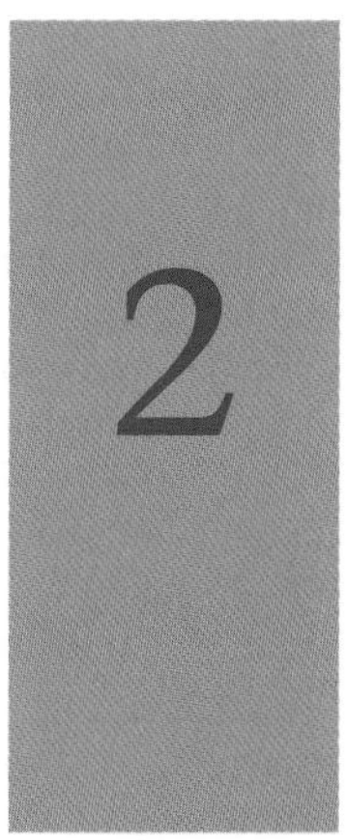

Immune Responses to Infectious Agents

LAUREL J. GERSHWIN

The ability of the host animal to respond to infection by pathogens is generated by a unique and connected series of cells and molecules produced by the immune system in response to pathogen invasion. The initial contact between sentinel cells and pathogens serves to alert antigen-presenting dendritic cells to the type of pathogen that has been encountered. This information determines how the dendritic cell responds: with the production of appropriate cytokines to simulate primarily humoral or cellular responses. The messengers in this system are cytokines, produced first by the sentinel cell, then by the differentiated dendritic cell and acting on the ultimate target cell, a T lymphocyte. Once the appropriate response has been induced, products of the adaptive immune system act to decrease the spread of the infectious agent within the body.

Innate Immunity

Detection of Pathogen-Associated Molecular Patterns (PAMPs) by Sentinel Cells and the Effects on Immune System Stimulation

When a pathogen enters a host, it encounters cells that line the portals of entry to the body—skin and mucous membranes. These sentinel cells display pattern recognition receptors that serve as ligands for various components of bacterial and viral organisms. Sentinel cells include mast cells, dendritic cells, Langerhans' cells, and macrophages. The receptors on the sentinel cells detect PAMPS, which vary by pathogens but consist of substances like bacterial lipopolysaccharide (LPS), flagellar protein, and viral proteins. Binding of the PAMPS to their ligands triggers sentinel cell activation and production of proinflammatory cytokines—interleukin 1 (IL-1), tumor necrosis factor α (TNFα), and IL-6. Among other functions, these cytokines trigger the "sickness behavior" that is associated with infection.

Toll-like receptors (TLRs) are pattern-recognition receptors that are present on sentinel cells and on a variety of other cells. Originally described in *Drosophila*, these molecules and their signaling pathways are important for detection of invading pathogens in fruit flies, mammals, and plants. There are 10 known TLRs in mammals. Each TLR recognizes a specific component of a pathogen. For example, TLR1, 2, and 6 recognize various microbial components. TLR2 recognizes lipoproteins, lipoteichoic acid from gram-positive bacteria, and lipoarabinomannan from mycobacteria. TLR3 recognizes double-stranded RNA and is, therefore, important in viral recognition. TLR4 has a role in transducing the signals of LPS from gram-negative bacteria. TLR5 is activated by flagellin, its specific ligand. Thus, TLR5 is important in the response to motile bacteria, but not to those that lack flagella. When the basolateral surface of the intestinal epithelium is exposed to flagellin, an inflammatory response occurs. This is the site of expression of the TLR5. TLR7 is activated by certain synthetic compounds that have antiviral activity. TLR9, a receptor expressed within the cell, recognizes bacterial CpG motifs in DNA.

Anatomic Features, Physiological Processes, and Normal Flora

There are a variety of anatomic structures and physiological processes that serve to prevent entry of pathogens into the host. The skin and mucous membrane form barriers, whose importance is most readily appreciated after the barrier has been breached. Infected skin wounds are one example. The protective role of desiccation is best illustrated by the horse that becomes infected with *Dermatophilus congolensis* after rain-soaked skin is debilitated sufficiently for the organism to gain access to the epidermal tissues. The condition called "Thrush" occurs when the desiccated state of the horny equine hoof is compromised after the horse stands for prolonged times in wet and muddy conditions. The importance of the mucociliary apparatus in protection of the respiratory tract can be appreciated by observation of the consequences of abnormal cilia lining the trachea. In cases of ciliary dyskinesis, the affected dog has recurrent bouts of pneumonia because the abnormal cilia fail to move the mucous blanket containing inhaled bacteria

Veterinary Microbiology, Third Edition. Edited by D. Scott McVey, Melissa Kennedy and M.M. Chengappa.

and other particles up and out of the animal. The alveolar macrophage is capable of removing material that makes its way into the lower airways and alveoli, and their exit from the body is facilitated by this mucociliary elevator.

The normal flora that is present in the gut plays an important role in prevention of colonization by more virulent organisms. These bacteria and fungi establish a unique relationship with the host, a relationship that begins as the microbiologically sterile fetus begins its journey down the birth canal. Acquisition of bacteria and fungi begins immediately, with infection (colonization) of all exposed surfaces, including mucosal surfaces (alimentary canal, upper respiratory tract, and distal genitourinary tract), with microorganisms from the birth canal and from the mother's immediate environment. The association of the microbe with the host is not haphazard but rather is an association that depends upon (1) receptors (usually in the form of carbohydrates that are part of glycoproteins on the surface of the host cell) and adhesins on the microbe cell surface, (2) the chemicals in the immediate environment of the microbe–host interaction, in part due to products secreted by competing microorganisms (e.g., microcins, bacteriocins, and volatile fatty acids) and in part due to products secreted by the host (e.g., acid environment of the stomach, defensins secreted by Paneth cells, the contents of bile in the upper small intestine, or the content of sebum on the skin), and (3) the availability of nutrient substances.

The establishment of the normal flora is a dynamic one, with replacement at various exposed locations with microbes more capable of living at a particular site (niche) than the ones preceding. In addition, the immune system appears to play some role, since it has been shown that members of the normal flora are very poorly immunogenic in the host from which the microbes are isolated. This suggests that immune responses to microbes attempting to colonize a particular location (niche) will result in the blockage of association between the adhesin (microbe) and the receptor (host). If a microbe cannot associate, then it will be replaced with one that will. This occurs until a strain of microbe is encountered that is more similar to the host than its predecessor, which is subsequently "accepted" as part of the normal flora of that particular animal. The result is an ecosystem composed of numerous species of bacteria and fungi that are associated with an abundance of niches, each of which is occupied with a particular species of microbe most suited to live at that location. This "occupation" results in a barrier to colonization (infection) by microbes that are not members of the normal flora, thus the term "colonization resistance." We notice a disruption of this effect when long-term antibiotic treatment removes a population of bacteria, leaving a space that can be occupied with other organisms; diarrhea is a common result of such long-term antibiotic therapy.

Antimicrobial Peptides and Their Role in Innate Immunity

Antimicrobial peptides (AMPs) have been found in a diverse array of organisms, including bacteria and *Xenopus* as well as mammals. In general, AMPs are about 30 amino acid residues and are cationic in nature. The cationic nature of these peptides helps them to get close to negatively charged cell membranes of pathogens and to ultimately integrate. The AMPs that are best characterized in mammals are defensins and cathelicidins. Defensins are configured as a β-pleated sheet and cathelicidins are in an α-helix configuration. Defensins are subdivided into three groups—α, β, and θ—depending on the distribution of cysteines and disulfide bonds. AMPs line up in multimeric units on the cell membrane to create pores that lead to osmotic fragility and cell rupture. In addition, defensins can stimulate production of proinflammatory cytokines. The major source of α-defensins is the neutrophilic leukocyte, although other cell types can also produce them. β-Defensins are produced by epithelial cells in the respiratory and gastrointestinal tracts as well as by epithelial cells in skin and other sites. Cathelicidins are made not only by neutrophils but also by epithelial cells, NK cells, and mast cells.

Effector Cells of the Innate Immune System

Neutrophil. The polymorphonuclear leukocyte, neutrophil, is a bone-marrow-derived end cell that normally comprises 30–70% of the total leukocytes in the peripheral blood of various species. The neutrophil is a granulocytic leukocyte and contains two types of granules: primary or azurophilic granules and secondary or specific granules. Neutrophils spend only about 12 h in circulation, and then go into the tissues where they survive for additional 2–3 days. Within the bone marrow, there is a large storage compartment for neutrophils. A bacterial infection within the body causes a rapid mobilization of this pool, and the neutrophils accumulate at the site of the infectious process. They are attracted by the chemotactic factors, C3a and C5a, which are generated subsequent to activation of the complement system. The process of neutrophil accumulation begins by adherence of the circulating neutrophils to the vascular endothelium (margination), extravasation into tissue spaces, and chemotaxis of the cells toward the focus of injury (Figure 2.1). Invading microorganisms are ingested by neutrophils in a process called phagocytosis (Figure 2.2A–C).

Phagocytosis of bacteria by neutrophils involves several steps. First, initial recognition and binding occur. This process is made more efficient by the presence of opsonins consisting of immunoglobulin and/or complement components. Opsonization coats the surface of a particle, neutralizing the net negative charges, which might otherwise cause the neutrophil and bacterial cell to repel each other (Figure 2.2C). In addition, on the cell membrane of the neutrophil, receptors are present for antibodies (Fc receptors) and for complements (CR). These receptors facilitate firm attachment of the opsonized bacterium to the neutrophil. Next, pseudopodia form around the organism and then fuse to form a phagocytic vacuole containing the organism. Some organisms are more readily engulfed than others. For example, the presence of a polysaccharide capsule causes an organism to be resistant to phagocytosis. After engulfment, lysosomal granules fuse with the phagosome membrane to form the phagolysosome. The eventual elimination of the engulfed organism occurs within this structure.

FIGURE 2.1. *Neutrophils respond to chemotactic signals by binding to endothelial cells with L-selectin molecules; firmer adhesion is accomplished by the binding of integrins to E-selectins. Once adhesion is accomplished, the neutrophil undergoes diapedesis between endothelial cells and then follows the chemotactic gradient to the source of infection. Once the cells arrive at the site of infection, the process of phagocytosis engulfs and destroys the bacteria. (Reproduced with permission from http://ap-projectstew.wikispaces.com/Chapter+15+The+Immune+System.)*

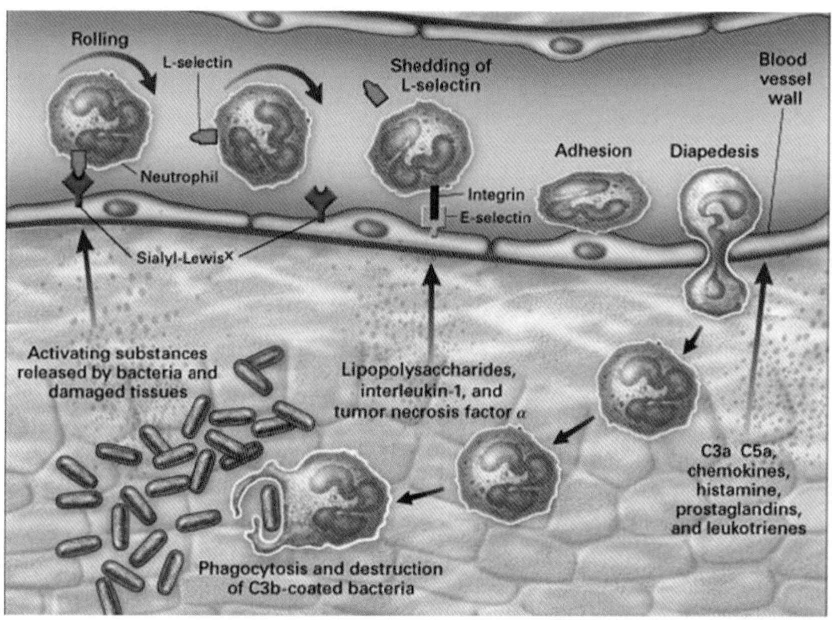

FIGURE 2.2. *(A) Neutrophils were incubated with* Staphylococcus aureus *in saline solution. Numbers of bacteria (small purple dots) engulfed are small. (B) Neutrophils were incubated with* S. aureus *in the presence of normal serum (contains some antibody and complement components). (C) Neutrophils were incubated with* S. aureus *in serum containing antibodies specific for* S. aureus. *This demonstrates the role of opsonization in enhancing phagocytosis.*

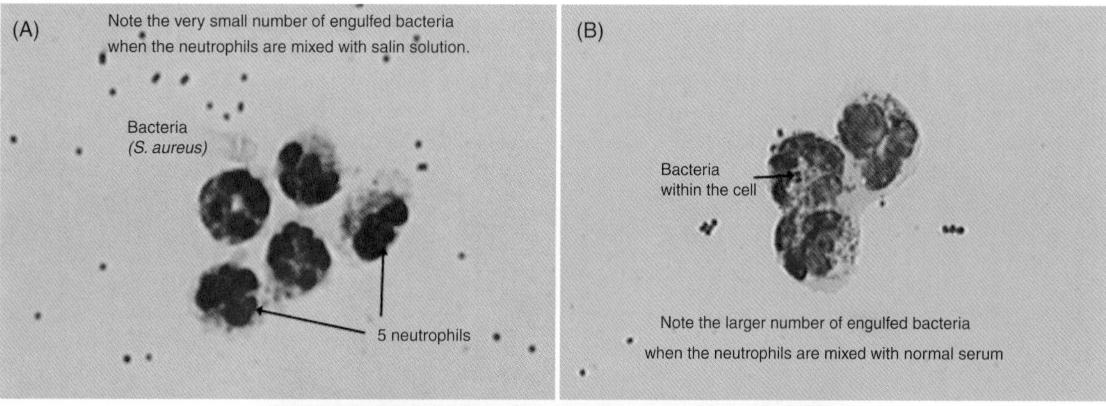

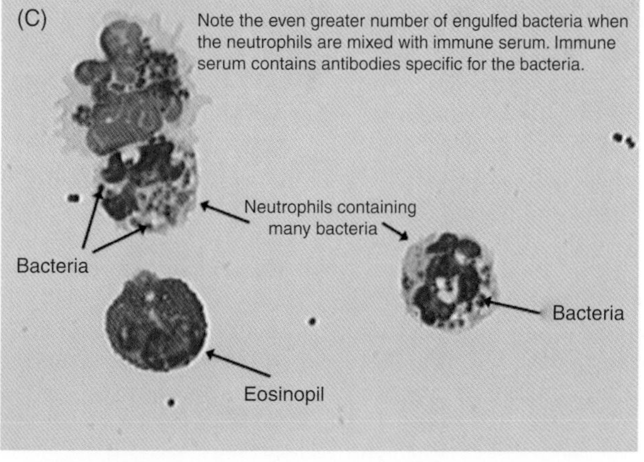

Bacterial killing is accomplished by a series of metabolic and enzymatic events. Metabolic activity increases within a neutrophil during phagocytosis. Oxygen consumption increases and light energy is emitted (chemiluminescence). This metabolic or respiratory burst involves oxidation of glucose by the hexose monophosphate shunt. Bactericidal products are generated. Superoxide radicals are produced and converted to H_2O_2 by superoxide dismutase. Hydrogen peroxide is toxic for bacteria that lack catalase. The enzyme myeloperoxidase, present in azurophil granules, catalyzes the oxidation of halide ions to hypohalite, which is also toxic to microorganisms. Thus, the myeloperoxidase–hydrogen-peroxide–halide system is efficient in bacterial killing. Susceptible organisms are killed within minutes. Inside the primary granules of neutrophils, enzymes released during degranulation act on proteins, lipids, carbohydrates, and nucleic acids to degrade the killed bacterial cells. Some of these enzymes are collagenase, elastase, acid phosphatase, phospholipase, lysozyme, hyaluronidase, acid ribonuclease, and deoxyribonuclease. Lysozyme can cleave glycosyl bonds in the bacterial cell wall, making the cell susceptible to lysis. Also, lysosomes contain cationic peptides (defensins), described above, that form lethal pores in bacteria as well as fungal cell walls.

Macrophage. The macrophage is a mononuclear cell derived from the bone marrow. For several days after release from the bone marrow, it circulates as a blood monocyte before going into the tissues, where it becomes a functional macrophage. Free macrophages are present in many parts of the body and are named accordingly, for example, alveolar macrophages (lung) and peritoneal macrophages. Fixed macrophages line sinus cavities that filter blood. These include the Kupffer cells (liver), Langerhans cells (skin), histiocytes (connective tissue), mesangial cells (kidneys), and sinus-lining cells of the spleen, lymph nodes, and bone marrow. Some of these macrophages are important in antigen processing for induction of an immune response (described later in this chapter).

The macrophage differs from the neutrophil in that it has a longer life span in tissue and can reuse phagolysosomes. In addition, macrophages stimulated by cytokines (e.g., interferon γ) or microbial products (e.g., LPS) result in activation of nitric oxide synthase that catalyzes the production of nitric oxide (NO) from L-arginine. NO is toxic to many bacteria, especially those residing within macrophages (e.g., *Salmonella* and *Listeria*). The macrophage is similar to the neutrophil in that toxic oxygen metabolites are generated for bacterial killing and the lysosomes contain potent hydrolytic enzymes and cationic peptides (defensins). While the neutrophil responds to a stimulus rapidly, the macrophage is not present until later in an infectious process, often after 8–12 h. In some instances, neutrophils may eliminate an organism before macrophages arrive in any great number. When tissue destruction has occurred as a result of an inflammatory response, macrophages are attracted to the area by products from dying neutrophils and bacteria. They phagocytose the debris and remove it. In some instances, macrophages may engulf particulate material that they are unable to digest. When this occurs, the macrophage may migrate to a mucosal surface such as the respiratory or gastrointestinal tract for elimination from the body.

Unlike the neutrophil, which is a cell of the innate immune system, the macrophage can serve as a link between innate and acquired immunity. After destruction of a pathogen, the macrophage can serve as an antigen-presenting cell by breaking the pathogen into peptides that are subsequently bound to major histocompatibility complex (MHC) class II molecules on the cell membrane (described under Section "Adaptive Immunity").

Some pathogens have developed mechanisms to elude immune defenses. A group of organisms, often referred to as the facultative intracellular bacteria, have developed such abilities. For example, bacteria in the *Mycobacterium* genus are able to prevent fusion of the lysosomes with the phagosome, thereby preventing the release of destructive enzymes into the vacuole and hence prevention of microbe killing. This accounts for the chronic and severe nature if infection with pathogens such as *Mycobacterium* species, *Brucella* species, *Nocardia*, and *Listeria*. Other bacteria that are not capable of surviving within phagosomes have polysaccharide capsules that make them less readily engulfed than their unencapsulated counterparts. Opsonizing antibody or complement components must be present to coat such organisms before phagocytes can engulf them. Thus, innate defenses often require the assistance of products of the acquired immune response.

Natural Killer Cell. Natural killer (NK) cells are a central and important component of the innate immune response to viruses and some bacteria. NK cells are a distinct lineage of lymphocytes that, unlike the T and B lymphocytes, do not have a specific receptor for antigens—i.e., they do not rearrange genes encoding membrane receptors. Yet, this cell type is able to recognize and target cells for destruction. NK cells comprise 5–20% of lymphocytes in the peripheral blood and more than 90% of lymphocytes in the placenta. Their function includes cell-mediated immunity, antibody-dependent cellular cytotoxicity (ADCC), production of interferon γ early in infection, and secretion of a variety of other cytokines. In the adult mammal, NK cells develop within the bone marrow from hematopoietic cell precursors. NK cells are responsive to several cytokines and they secrete cytokines, including interferon γ and TNFα. The NK cell response is coordinated and modulated by cytokines that include interferons α and β and IL-2, IL-12, IL-15, and IL-18. Recently, a variety of receptors have been identified on NK cells. These receptors allow the NK cell either to kill a target cell or to turn off the potential killing response. Inhibitory receptors expressed on NK cells include the killer immunoglobulin-like receptor. This receptor binds to MHC class I molecules on body cells and facilitates an inhibitory response through activation of intracellular tyrosine-based inhibitory motifs. This function prevents the powerful killing capacity of the NK cell from acting on normal body cells. In contrast, when a cell lacks MHC class I, the NK cell recognizes the absence and begins the process of killing that target cell.

The NK cell is particularly effective in eliminating tumor cells and cells infected with some viruses. A number of viruses (and some tumor cells) downregulate cellular MHC class I molecule synthesis. These viruses effectively evade the acquired T cytotoxic cell (CD8) response (detailed later in this chapter) by removing the MHC molecule that presents antigens to cytotoxic T cells. However, the NK cell targets these cells that display the "missing self" appearance. The mechanism for pathogen recognition uses activating and inhibitory receptors; normal cells that display MHC class I molecules (all nucleated cells) provide an inhibitory signal to the receptors of the NK cell. However, the absence of these molecules triggers activation and thus allows the NK cell to kill the target cell. NK cells are important in elimination of herpesviruses. For example, in human beings who lack NK cells, the diseases varicella zoster and cytomegalovirus infection (both herpesviruses) are often fatal, whereas the normal individual is able to successfully recover from these infections. The ultimate killing mechanism involves secretion of perforin molecules that are able to poke holes in the cell membrane, permitting caustic granzymes entry to the cytosol.

The early production of interferon γ by NK cells is helpful in initiating a T helper 1 type response (described later in this chapter) that activates macrophages for more efficient killing of some bacteria. Other killing mechanisms that are used by NK cells include ADCC. NK cells display the cell membrane receptor CD16, a low-affinity IgG receptor. By using this receptor to bind IgG, the NK cell is able to participate in ADCC, killing cells that are recognized by the attached immunoglobulin. In this way the NK cell collaborates with the acquired immune system to eliminate infected cells.

$\gamma\delta$ T Cell. T cells that display membrane receptors called $\gamma\delta$ chains ($\gamma\delta$ T cells) constitute a small percentage of the circulating pool of lymphocytes in nonruminant species. In ruminants, however, $\gamma\delta$ T cells may represent up to 30% of the circulating lymphocyte pool. In most species, $\gamma\delta$ T cells are present in the lamina propria underlying mucosal epithelia, strategically beneficial sites for cells involved in host defense.

Functional studies in mouse models and data from human beings have demonstrated a role for these cells in defense against mycobacterial pathogens. The role of $\gamma\delta$ T cells in innate defense against *Mycobacterium tuberculosis* appears to be most important early in the infection. Activation of these cells by *M. tuberculosis* antigens is dependent on accessory cells, such as alveolar macrophages, which provide costimulatory molecules. The ligands on the mycobacterium that stimulate the $\gamma\delta$ T cells have recently been shown to be small phosphate-containing molecules. The major effector function of $\gamma\delta$ T lymphocytes in defense against *M. tuberculosis* is in cytokine secretion and in cytotoxic effector cell function. These cells produce interferon γ, TNFα, and a small amount of IL-2.

$\gamma\delta$ T cells have a role in limiting viral replication in some viral diseases. In mouse models of influenza virus infection, these cells accumulate in the lung presumably to resolve the pneumonic process. In both mouse models and human patients, the role of $\gamma\delta$ T cells in resolution of herpes simplex virus type 1 infection has been demonstrated.

Recognition of viruses by TLR has been reported for some viruses. TLR4 binds to one of the major surface proteins on respiratory syncytial virus (RSV), an important pathogen of human children and bovine calves. In an experimental mouse model with mutated TLR4, RSV was found to be cleared less efficiently than from mice that had normal TLR4. Other viruses, such as mouse mammary tumor virus, have been shown to bind TLR4 to envelope proteins. In addition, signaling through TLR3 and TLR7 has been shown to induce synthesis of α and β interferons.

Other studies with TLR-mutant mice have demonstrated the importance of these receptors in resistance to bacterial infection. TLR4-mutant mice are highly susceptible to infection with the gram-negative bacteria, *Salmonella typhimurium*; whereas mice defective in TLR2 are highly sensitive to infection with gram-positive bacteria, *Streptococcus pneumoniae.*

Adaptive Immunity

The sentinel cells that are so important in alerting the host that PAMPS have been detected also serve to instruct the T helper cells in selection of the appropriate cytokines to produce for modulation of the immune response in the correct direction for optimum pathogen killing. For example, production of IL-12 by a dendritic cell can enhance the differentiation of T helper cells into T helper type 1 cells that make interferon γ, a cytokine that helps to arm macrophages for elimination of those bacteria that preferentially resist phagosome killing. In contrast, the PAMPS present on a heavily polysaccharide encapsulated bacteria such as *S. pneumoniae* would preferentially stimulate the dendritic cell to make IL-4, which stimulates B lymphocytes to develop into the plasma cells making opsonizing antibodies that are required for this pathogen to be effectively endocytosed and then killed.

The stimulation of the appropriate T helper cell requires not only the production of cytokines, but also the binding to antigenic peptides presented within the groove of the T cell receptor. In the primary immune response, the cell type that performs this antigen presentation function is the dendritic cell, sometimes referred to as a "professional antigen-presenting cell" because antigen capture, processing, and presentation constitute its primary role. The dendritic cell is the main antigen-presenting cell in a primary immune response. When an antigen is encountered in a host that has had previous contact with it, there are other cell types that can present the antigen to T lymphocytes. These include macrophages and B lymphocytes. It is important to note that all cells that present antigens to CD4+ T lymphocytes express the MHC class II molecule on their surface.

The process of antigen presentation occurs either by the extracellular (phagocytic) pathway or by the endocytic (cytosolic) pathway. Inactivated and killed organisms, once digested and processed in a phagosome, are bound to MHC class II molecules and are brought to the cell surface for presentation to CD4 T (helper) lymphocytes. This occurs after the antigen has been broken down into peptides in endosomes; fusion of the endosomes with other endosomes that contain newly synthesized MHC class II molecules brings them together so that then peptide containing endosomes can fuse with the MHC class II containing endosomes. The peptide replaces an invariant chain (II) CLIP (class II associated invariant peptide) molecule, which has served as a space holder, in the antigen-binding site of the MHC molecule. The MHC class II with the peptide in the groove is then transported to the cell surface to await recognition by a T cell receptor. Recognition of the antigenic peptide–MHC class II complex by a T cell with the same MHC class II is referred to as MHC restriction and is a characteristic of the acquired immune response. Production of IL-2 by the T cell occurs after binding with the antigenic peptide and costimulatory molecules. IL-2 is a T cell growth factor that facilitates clonal expansion of the participating T cell. These T cells, which are phenotypically CD4 and functionally called helper T cells, produce additional cytokines to influence the development of B cells, which are specific for the antigen. Under the influence of T cell-produced IL-4, B cells develop and mature into plasma cells secreting antibodies. Helper T cells predominantly produce IL-4 (T helper type 2 cells or T_{H2}), which facilitate production of IgG_1 and IgE.

The T helper cells mentioned above that have been stimulated by dendritic cells making IL-12 must also recognize the antigenic peptide on MHC class II. These cytokines are important in activation of macrophages for killing facultative intracellular bacteria and for supporting other cell-mediated responses. T helper type 1 cells produce interferon γ and IL-2, in addition to IL-12. As noted above, the initial production of IL-12 by the dendritic cell or NK cell can prejudice the T helper cell response toward T_{H1}. This response may be initiated through TLR binding to the dendritic cell.

Antigen presentation for intracellular pathogens follows the endocytic pathway through the cytosol. When a virus is replicating in the cytosol, viral proteins are processed and united with MHC class I molecules. The way in which this occurs is not like the process described for MHC class II presentation. Unused proteins are continually broken down in the cytosol; they are ubiquitinated and targeted to the proteosome in which further breakdown occurs to peptides that are between 8 and 15 amino acids in size. When a virus is replicating within the cytosol of a cell, the viral proteins have this same fate and are subsequently bound to transporter proteins (TAP1 and TAP2) for movement from the cytoplasm to the endosomes. There, they are further shortened and bound to MHC class I molecules. These peptide–MHC complexes are then sent to the surface of the cell where they are recognized by T cell receptors on the CD8 cytotoxic T cells. This is a very important point as it explains why a vaccine that is able to replicate in the cell is more likely to induce a cytotoxic T cell response than a killed vaccine. MHC class I recognition is required for cytotoxic T cell activation.

The ultimate result of antigen presentation to CD4 T lymphocytes is the development of an immune response. As stated above, the type of cytokine environment that has been created mediates this response. If the T_{H2} cytokines are present, and for most pathogens there are usually some, there will be a humoral (antibody) response. When the pathogen has skewed the T helper cell response toward T_{H1} cytokine production (this occurs with facultative intracellular bacterial and viral pathogens), cytokines are produced to activate macrophages and CD8 T cells to become more effective killers.

Humoral Immunity (Antibody Response)

The initial introduction of an antigen to a host followed by presentation of antigenic peptides to CD4 T cells results in stimulation of these cells to become T helper type 2 cells, secreting cytokines that assist B cells in differentiating into cells that become antibody-producing plasma cells. Production of IL-4 by these T_{H2} cells results in expansion of B cell clones specific to the different epitopes on the antigen. The B cells also recognize antigenic epitopes on the microbe and in addition develop binding of costimulatory molecules on the T cell. Then under the influence of T cell cytokines, these B cells differentiate into antibody-producing plasma cells.

The first antibody to be produced is IgM and it appears in the circulation 7–10 days after initiation of the immune response. Next, IgG appears but does not rise to very high titers in this primary immune response. Subsequent encounters with antigen result in a secondary or anamnestic response. In the secondary response, the kinetics of antibody appearance in the circulation is more rapid and the quantity of antibodies produced is greater. Most importantly, the isotype that predominates in the secondary response is predominantly IgG. The longer half-life of IgG facilitates the maintenance of an antibody titer higher for a longer duration (Figure 2.3). Often evaluation of the immune response (IgG vs. IgM) to a disease agent can yield important information as to the chronicity of the exposure. It is a well-accepted diagnostic procedure to obtain acute and convalescent serum samples to be evaluated for antibody titer and isotype. Generally, when a disease agent is responsible for clinical signs 2–3 weeks after the initial appearance of signs, the titer will have increased by at least fourfold if the agent was involved in the infectious process. In an initial exposure to a disease agent, IgM is the predominant isotype, while a second or tertiary exposure (or vaccination) will elicit mostly IgG.

FIGURE 2.3. *The initial antibody response is primarily IgM in a primary immune response; subsequent exposures to the same antigen elicit IgG as the predominant isotype.*

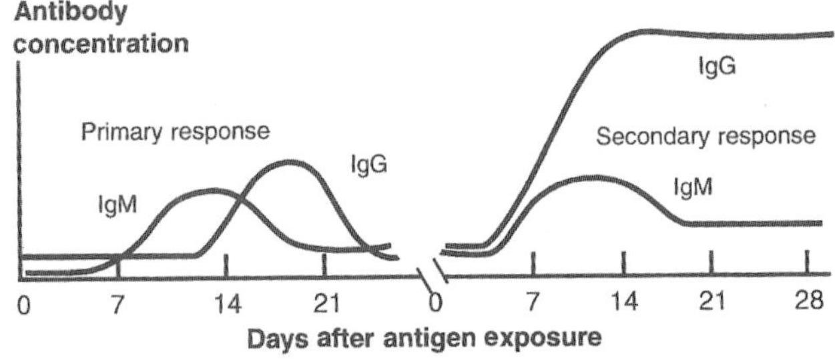

Effector Functions of Antibody

Antibodies can neutralize virus, bacteria, and soluble toxins. Some isotypes of an antibody (IgG and IgM) can lyse target cells after activating the complement cascade. Antibodies can facilitate phagocytosis by acting as opsonins to help phagocytes adhere to microbes. The antibody response that is important in defense against bacterial disease depends on the pathogenic mechanisms involved, the site of the infectious process, and the isotype of the antibody elicited. In a disease caused by an extracellular toxin, such as tetanus, antitoxin antibodies are important to neutralize and bind the toxin before it can bind to cellular sites and initiate clinical signs. This mechanism is important in diseases such as tetanus, anthrax, and botulism—all toxin-mediated diseases. In some instances, when a nonimmune host is at risk of developing a toxin-mediated disease, immediate administration of antitoxin (a solution containing antibodies to the toxin) is required to prevent the disease. In order to eliminate infectious agents, antibodies serve as opsonins as well as initiating the complement cascade (activation through the classical pathway). Opsonins lead to increased uptake by phagocytic cells, whereas complement activation leads to initiation of inflammation and generation of compounds that are detrimental to the infectious agent (e.g., membrane attack complex), as bacteria that have capsules are particularly resistant to engulfment by phagocytes unless they have opsonins present.

Generally, the IgE response is limited to parasitic infections and hypersensitivity reactions to various environmental allergens, such as pollens and grasses. Occasionally, IgE is elicited in response to vaccination against some bacterial and viral pathogens. When this occurs, very serious adverse responses, such as anaphylactic shock, can result. Often there is a hereditary predisposition toward IgE production, and these individuals are at increased risk of having such a vaccine reaction. For immunity to parasite infections, IgE may assist in the phenomenon of "self-cure," in which large numbers of nematodes are purged from the gut by mast cell mediator-induced smooth muscle contraction. Alternatively, some infestations are controlled by ADCC, in which IgE binds to eosinophils by low-affinity Fc receptors and facilitates release of major basic protein and other caustic enzymes on the parasite surface.

IgA is a very desirable response to infectious agents that affect mucosal surfaces. Since secretory IgA (SIgA) is protected by a secretory component from digestion in the gut by proteolytic enzymes, it is the most efficient antibody to be active in the environment of the gastrointestinal lumen. There, it can neutralize viruses and bacteria to prevent their respective attachment to cellular receptors. Similarly, SIgA is effective within the secretions of the respiratory tract. Before a virus or a bacterium can infect a cell, it must first bind to a cell surface protein that acts as a receptor for the infectious agent. Thus, binding of the infectious agent by an antibody can inhibit binding to the receptor, and thus lower the infectivity of the agent. For example, influenza virus expresses a hemagglutinin that binds to certain glycoproteins expressed on epithelial cells in the respiratory tract. Binding of antibodies to the hemagglutinin prevents entry of the virus into these cells, and disease is prevented.

Antibodies are most effective against viruses that undergo a viremic phase, when there are numerous virus particles in the extracellular environment. For example, viruses such as influenza viruses are neutralized by antibodies specific for the major surface antigens (hemagglutinin and neuraminidase). Other viruses, such as herpesvirus, remain closely associated with cells and do not present much opportunity for antibody-mediated inactivation. The IgA isotype is especially effective on mucosal surfaces and functions to neutralize viruses before entry into the body. SIgA is an extremely effective defense against respiratory and gastrointestinal viruses, as well as viruses that cause systemic disease but enter via the oral route. Virus neutralization occurs because the antibody binds to surface determinants of the virus and prevents the virus from binding to the cellular receptors to which it must attach in order to initiate the infectious process.

The relative importance of antibodies and cell-mediated immune response depends upon the pathogenesis of the disease. For example, bacteria that produce potent exotoxins, such as *Clostridium tetani*, require antibodies to neutralize the toxin. Heavily encapsulated bacteria, such as *Klebsiella pneumonia*, require opsonizing antibodies for effective removal of the bacteria and ultimate killing by phagocytes. In contrast, bacteria that are capable of living within phagocytes, such as *Listeria monocytogenes*, are not effectively killed by an antibody, and require the T_{H1} response for effective elimination. Similarly, viral infections that produce viremia, such as influenza, are handled well by an appropriate antibody response, compared with herpesviruses that are cell-associated and require a cell-mediated immune response for effective control.

Cell-Mediated Immunity

Cell-mediated immune responses mediated by T cells involve two different mechanisms: macrophage activation and cytotoxic T cell activity.

Killing of Facultative Intracellular Bacteria by Activated Macrophages

As previously mentioned, as a mechanism of immune evasion some bacteria have the ability to prevent phagosome–lysosome fusion. Bacteria in this category include *Brucella, Mycobacterium, Listeria, Salmonella*, and *Rhodococcus equi*. Infection by one of these organisms often results in death of the macrophage. In the presence of CD4 T lymphocytes that produce interferon γ, the macrophage is armed and able to circumvent the bacteria and to kill. The cytokine induces lysosomal fusion and increases macrophage bacteriocidal activity. Thus, macrophages are activated following the production of interferon γ by these T_{H1} cells, and the "arming" of macrophages results in destruction of the infectious agent that the macrophage previously had been unable to destroy.

Killing of Virus-Infected Cells by Cytotoxic T Cells

Pathogens, such as viruses, that live and grow inside of cells are best contained by elimination of the cell in which they are reproducing. As previously described, viral proteins made in the cytosol associate with MHC class I molecules for presentation to T cells. Cytotoxic T cells (CD8) recognize an antigenic peptide that is held in the groove formed by the chains of the MHC class I molecule on the cell surface. All nucleated cells have MHC class I on their surface and are, therefore, able to bind and present antigens from inside the cell in this manner. Recognition of the combination of MHC class I and the antigenic determinant by T cell receptors on the cytotoxic T cells stimulates release of perforins that make small pores in the cell membrane. This allows destructive enzymes called granzymes to enter the cytoplasm. In addition, TNFα is produced. Death of the cell can also be facilitated by the interaction of Fas–Fas ligand system, stimulating apoptosis. One CD8 T cell can repeatedly kill infected target cells, programming one to die, and then moving on to the next cell to kill it. The cytotoxic T cell is an efficient way to decrease viral progeny in an infected host.

Effector Cells Can Use Antibody to Bind Target Cells

ADCC occurs when an antibody binds to a cell that has receptors for the Fc portion of IgG or IgE. The Fc receptor for the γ chain is CD21 and the low-affinity IgE receptor is CD23. These molecules are present on several types of effector cells, including neutrophils, macrophages, NK cells, and eosinophils. The attachment of an antibody to a cell that previously had no receptor for antigens renders it antigen-specific and capable of binding antigens. Besides NK cells, eosinophils and macrophages can become involved in ADCC. ADCC is an effective method of killing cells infected with microorganisms (viral, bacterial, or fungal) as well as parasites. In the case of parasites, the eosinophil releases granules containing major basic protein, rendering the cuticle of the parasite permeable.

Evaluation of Immune Responses to Infectious Agents

The use of serological assays to evaluate exposure to or infection with bacterial and viral pathogens has been a mainstay for control of infectious diseases. In addition, for some infections, such as those with mycobacterial species, the *in vivo* skin testing for cell-mediated responses has been of even greater use. For determination of recent infection status, serum samples are obtained during acute illness and again 2–3 weeks later. These acute and convalescent samples are then assayed for antibody titer. When the titer has increased at least fourfold (two dilutions), seroconversion has occurred and the disease agent for which the titers are specific is confirmed as having stimulated a recent response.

Antibody-Based Serology

The current trend for immunodiagnosis utilizes the solid phase-binding assays, such as the enzyme-linked immunosorbent assay (ELISA). These assays are generally more sensitive than assays based on precipitin formation

FIGURE 2.4. *(A) Solid phase ELISA based detection of feline leukemia antigens in cat blood. Note the line indicating positive serum compared with the positive control line. (B) Microtiter well FeLV ELISA compares color in the test well with that in positive and negative wells.*

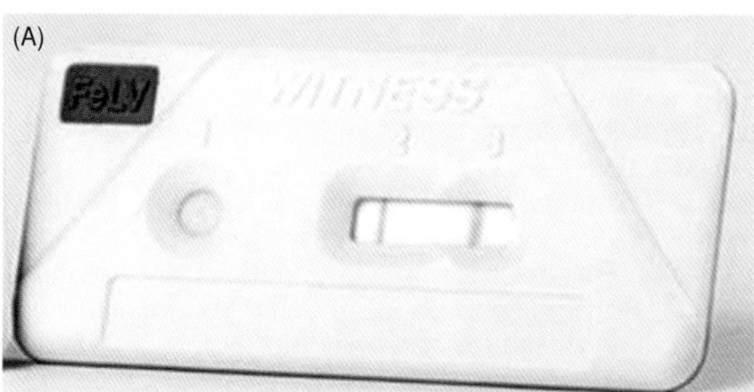

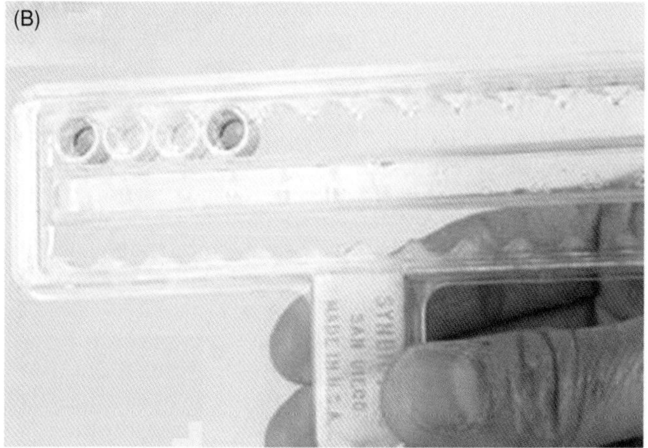

or complement fixation. Depending on the disease to be diagnosed, ELISA can be designed to detect antigens (as in feline leukemia virus (FeLV) and canine parvovirus infections) or antibodies (as in feline immunodeficiency virus). ELISA has the advantage that the format is easily adaptable to either a quick (positive or negative) readout or a titer determination. Numerous test kits are available for the veterinarian to evaluate the FeLV infection status of a cat. Some use a solid phase format (Figure 2.4A), while others use a well-based assay (Figure 2.4B).

When using antibodies as an indication of potential protection, it is important to remember that the ELISA detects binding antibodies, which is not always equivalent to effective neutralizing antibodies. The serum virus neutralization (SVN) assay uses serum as a source of antibodies, incubated with virus, which is then tested for ability to infect an appropriate cell culture. When a neutralizing antibody is present in a sample, it will prevent viral entry into the cells and subsequent cell infection and death. Thus, a high SVN titer is more meaningful than a high ELISA titer for prediction of protection (Figure 2.5).

For many years a gel diffusion test has been used for detection of antibodies to equine infectious anemia virus (Coggins test). Recently, several commercially available ELISA kits have become available. The comparison of these testing formats is a good illustration of differences in sensitivity, because the gel diffusion test is very much

FIGURE 2.5. *Virus neutralization assay: serum from an exposed patient is incubated with a virus and inoculated onto tissue-cultured cells. The focus of cytopathic effect (CPE) is evaluated for each serum dilution and compared with the control wells (virus + positive serum showing 100% neutralization of infectivity) and the virus only showing extent of CPE without antibody protection. The serum shows a protective titer through the 1:40 dilution.*

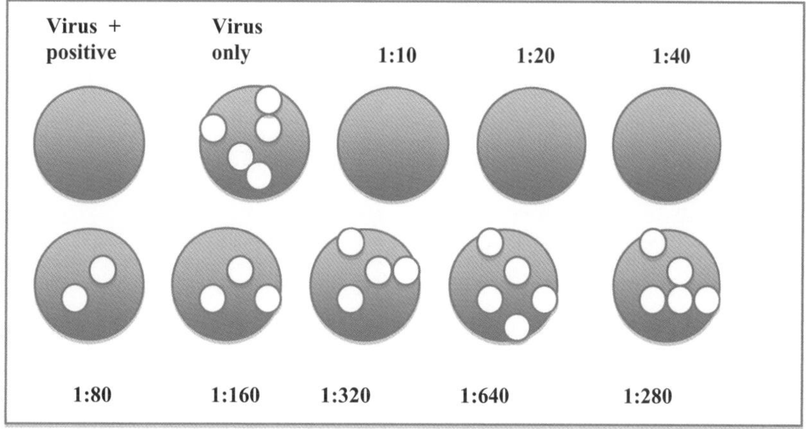

dependent on concentration of antigens and antibodies for a positive test result; whereas the ELISA, a primary binding assay, is more sensitive and less dependent on concentration effects. The ultimate effect is that a positive Coggins test, when read by an approved laboratory technician, is thought to be diagnostic, while a positive ELISA needs to be confirmed by a Coggins test, so as to prevent false-positive readings. The gel diffusion test can also be used for detection of antibodies against other pathogens, such as *Aspergillus fumigatus*, which stimulates a strong IgG/precipitating antibody response in infected dogs (Figure 2.6).

Indirect immunofluorescence is still used as a diagnostic test, and although the requirement for a microscope equipped for immunofluorescence limits the use outside of diagnostic laboratories, it is a sensitive assay for evaluation of antibody titers to a number of viral pathogens. Although detection of antibodies against feline coronavirus is not specific for the clinical syndrome of feline infectious peritonitis, an indirect immunofluorescence assay is sometimes used to determine the titer of antibodies in a feline infectious peritonitis suspect patient (Figure 2.7).

Direct immunofluorescence has been used for many years to detect the presence of virus in cells and in organ sections at necropsy. For example, a conjunctival swab from a canine distemper virus (CDV)-infected dog can be used to demonstrate the presence of virus (Figure 2.8). With the introduction of RT-PCR techniques, the application of this technique is less common than previously. For detection of pathogens in tissue, direct immunofluorescence has been replaced in many laboratories with immunohistochemical techniques, such as immunoperoxidase staining. The

FIGURE 2.6. *Detection of antibodies against* A. fumigatus: *the center well contains antigens. Sera are distributed clockwise with positive sera at 12 and 6 locations. The presence of a line of identity with positive controls indicates the presence of antibodies binding to the antigens in the center well.*

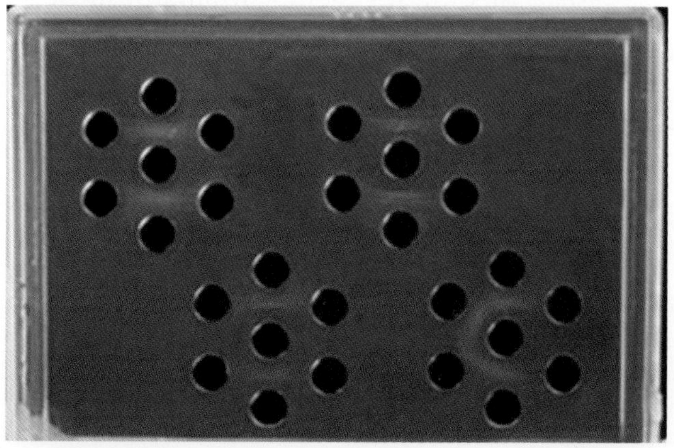

FIGURE 2.7. *Indirect immunofluorescence: showing antibodies specific for feline corona virus. Cells were infected with the feline corona virus and the fixed slide was incubated with dilutions of cat serum followed by fluroscein isothiocyanate (FITC) -conjugated rabbit antifeline IgG.*

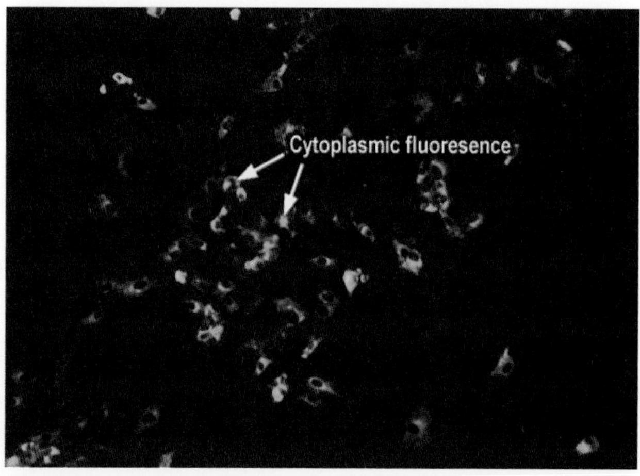

FIGURE 2.8. *Conjunctival epithelial cells infected with CDV are demonstrated by direct immunofluorescence using FITC-conjugated antibodies against CDV.*

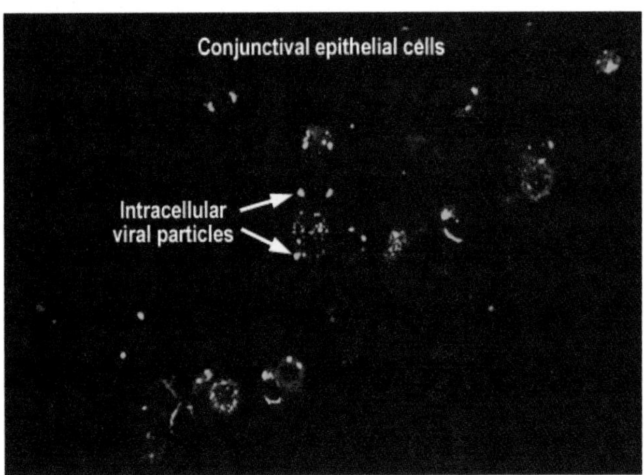

ability to perform the latter technique on fixed tissues makes it a more logical choice for necropsy specimens. For example, CDV is readily identified in lung tissue from an infected dog using anti-CDV sera conjugated with horseradish peroxidase (Figure 2.9).

For determination of antibody titers to those viruses that have hemagglutinins, the hemagglutination inhibition test is often used. For example, influenza virus will agglutinate red blood cells, but if preincubated with serum containing hemagglutinin-specific antibodies, the hemagglutination will not occur. The last dilution of serum that still inhibits the hemagglutination is the end point that determines the titer.

The principle of agglutination is a standard method for demonstrating antibody responses to bacteria. These assays depend upon the ability of antibodies to cross-link the cells to form a lattice of agglutinated cells as opposed to a pellet which would result from the settling of unagglutinated cells. *Brucella canis* antibody titers are often determined using the tube agglutination test, as seen in Figure 2.10. Soluble antigens can be made particulate for use in a passive agglutination test by covalently linking them to latex particles. Antibodies to *Toxoplasma gondii* are identified and tittered this method in a microtiter plate format (Figure 2.11).

FIGURE 2.9. *A necropsy specimen of the lung from a dog infected with CDV; immunoperoxidase staining shows the presence of viral antigens in lung cells.*

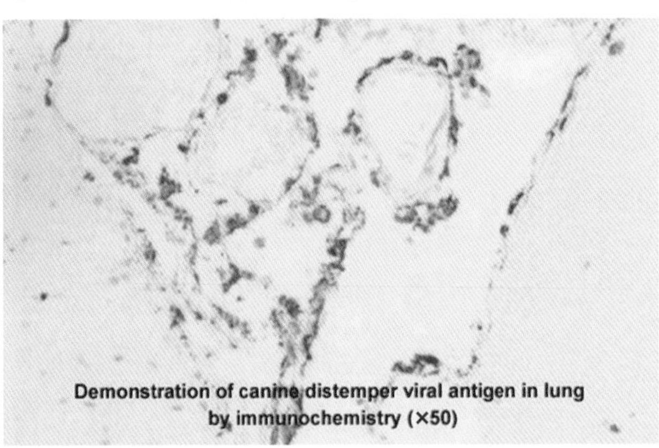

FIGURE 2.10. *Serial dilutions of patient serum are performed: 1 : 50, 1 : 100, 1 : 200, and so on; whole bacteria are added to each test tube. After incubation, tubes are evaluated for agglutination and a titer is determined.*

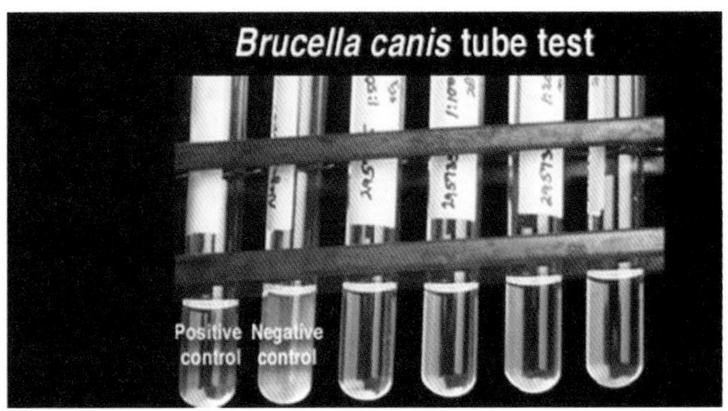

Cell-Mediated Immunity-Based Diagnostics

For those pathogens that induce a strong T helper 1 type immune response with production of associated cytokines (such as interferon γ), an intradermal skin test with antigens from the pathogens can often be used to demonstrate exposure or infection. Recently, *in vitro* correlates have been used for some diseases. *Mycobacterium bovis* infection can be diagnosed with intradermal injection of tuberculin. Within 48–72 h of antigen injection, erythema and induration at the site are apparent in infected patients. Infection with *Mycobacterium avium* subspecies pseudotuberculosis (Johnes disease agent) can be detected by *in vitro* incubation

FIGURE 2.11. *Latex agglutination test for* T. gondii. *Serum is serially twofold diluted from left to right starting with 1:16. PC indicates positive control; NC indicates negative control. Row C shows high-titer serum (2048). Row F shows a low-titer (64), and row E demonstrates a prozone with high-titer serum.*

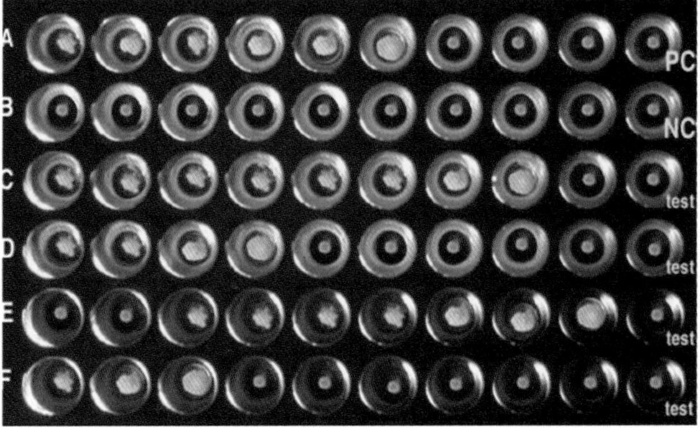

of patient lymphocytes with antigens and subsequent analysis of interferon γ levels in the culture supernatant. Infection by additional organisms that are among the group called facultative intracellular pathogens can be detected using similar testing strategies.

Evaluation of cytotoxic T cell responses has been problematic in domestic animal species and in humans; only in syngeneic mouse strains is it easy to evaluate virus-infected target cell killing by effector T lymphocytes. This is because MHC restriction (discussed above) requires that targets have the same MHC type as effectors; and that targets with noncompatible MHC will be attacked by heterologous T cells regardless of infection status. Nonetheless, there have been studies carried out in veterinary species in which autologous target cells were infected with virus and T cell killing evaluated using either dye or radioactive chromium incorporation as a readout.

Another way to examine T cell responses to pathogens is to perform *in vitro* cultivation of the animal's T lymphocytes with inactivated antigens of the pathogen. The culture supernatant is then assayed for production of cytokines by ELISA or Luminex assay, and the demonstration of Th1 cytokines is indicative of specific T cell responses. An older version of this type of assay is the lymphocyte stimulation test in which tritiated thymidine incorporation is measured as an indication of T cell activation by the antigen.

Summary

The immune system is composed of innate and acquired responses that recognize pathogens or their component parts and respond to induce the most effective response to that particular pathogen. Cytokines, cell receptors and ligands, and a variety of effector mechanisms are initiated depending on the need, as initially directed by the dendritic cells that first interact with the pathogen. We can detect these responses for diagnostic purposes and in some cases may be able to modulate the responses with targeted vaccines and adjuvants.

Further Reading

Cederlund A, Gudmundsson GH, and Agerberth B (2011) Antimicrobial peptides important in innate immunity. *FEBS J*, **278** (20), 3942–3951.

Marcenaro E, Carlomagno S, Pesce S *et al.* (2011) NK cells and their receptors during viral infections. *Immunotherapy*, **3** (9), 1075–1086.

Oliphant CJ, Barlow JL, and McKenzie AN (2011) Insights into the initiation of type 2 immune responses. *Immunology*, **134** (4), 378–385.

Zhang N and Bevan MJ (2011) CD8(+) T cells: foot soldiers of the immune system. *Immunity*, **35** (2), 161–168.

3 Laboratory Diagnosis

D. Scott McVey

Bacteria and Fungi

A key decision made early in the microbiological diagnostic workup is whether the patient's clinical signs indicate a possible infectious etiology. This decision is important because drugs used to treat conditions with noninfectious etiologies—corticosteroids, for example—are often contraindicated for treatment of conditions with an infectious one, for which antibiotics are appropriate.

One of the first major goals of the microbiology laboratory is to isolate or detect clinically significant microorganisms from an affected site and, if more than one type of microorganism is present, to isolate them in approximately the same ratio as occurs *in vivo*. Whether an isolate is "clinically significant" or not depends upon the circumstances of isolation. For example, the isolation of large numbers of a particular microorganism from a normally sterile site in the presence of an inflammatory cytology would be interpreted as significant.

Attention must be given to the site cultured as well as to the method of obtaining the sample for culture. The determination of significance is made a great deal easier if the sample is obtained from a normally sterile site. Obtaining a sample from the alimentary canal, and expecting meaningful answers, may be unrealistic unless one is looking for the presence or absence of a specific microorganism, for example, *Salmonella* or *Campylobacter*.

Sample Collection

Attention must be given to how the diagnostic specimens are collected; if not, interpretation of results may be difficult. Most infectious processes arise subsequent to the contamination of a compromised surface or site by microorganisms that are also a part of the flora occurring on a contiguous mucosal surface. In other words, microorganisms isolated from an affected site are often similar (if not identical) to those found as part of the normal flora of the patient.

Transport of Samples

The sooner the specimen is processed in the microbiology laboratory, the better. Realistically, the time between sample collection and processing may range from minutes to hours to days. Drying (all microorganisms) and exposure to a noxious atmosphere (oxygen for obligate anaerobes) are the major factors that compromise specimens and lead to inaccurate diagnosis. For this reason, it is important that the specimen be kept moist and, if conditions warrant (see below), air excluded. Moistness is maintained by placing the sample in a transport (holding) medium composed of a balanced salt solution usually in a gelled matrix. Because this medium does not contain any nutrient material, microorganisms in the sample multiply poorly if at all (and thereby relative numbers and ratios are preserved) but remain viable for some time, generally for at least 24–48 h. Swabs should always be placed in transport medium, regardless of the time elapsed between processing and collection. Fluids that may contain anaerobic bacteria (e.g., exudate from draining tracts, peritoneal and pleural effusions, abscess material) should be inoculated onto appropriate media immediately. If this material is contained in a syringe, then the air should be expelled and a sterile stopper placed over the needle. If a swab is used to collect the sample, it should be placed in an anaerobic transport medium. If a syringe full of sample cannot be processed immediately, the syringe should be emptied into an anaerobic transport medium and held at room temperature. It is best not to refrigerate samples suspected of containing anaerobes because some species do not tolerate reduced temperatures.

Demonstration of an Infectious Agent

The presence of an infectious agent is accomplished by examination of stained smears made from a portion of the clinical sample, culture techniques, molecular/immunological methods, or a combination of these methods.

Direct Smears. Information obtained from examination of a stained smear is valuable because it may be the first indication (and sometimes the only one) that an infectious agent is present. Also, what is seen (shape, staining characteristics) will help guide the choice of therapy 24 h before culture results are available. At least 104 microorganisms/ml or gram of material must be present in order to be readily detected microscopically.

Veterinary Microbiology, Third Edition. Edited by D. Scott McVey, Melissa Kennedy and M.M. Chengappa.

As is the case with a sample obtained from a normally sterile site, the presence of bacteria in bladder urine is a significant finding. However, interpretation of the results of analysis of urine samples obtained by catheter or by "catch" is difficult because of the confounding presence of flora flushed from the distal urethra. Finding bacteria by direct smear in concentrated (the preferred) or unconcentrated urine obtained by percutaneous aspiration of bladder urine is a significant finding. Demonstration of one bacteria cell per oil field in a drop of unconcentrated urine (which has been allowed to dry and then stained) represents about 10^5–10^6 bacteria/ml of urine.

Two types of stains are available, the gram stain and Romanovsky-type stains such as Wright's or Giemsa. Each type of stain has advantages and disadvantages. The gram stain is useful in that the shape and the gram-staining characteristics of the agent are seen. The disadvantage of the gram stain is that the cellular content of the sample is not readily discerned. On the other hand, a Romanovsky-type stain gives the observer a feeling for the cellular nature of the sample and whether or not there is an infectious agent present. Cytologic evaluation of the sample is very important in assessing the significance of the microorganism observed and subsequently isolated by culture.

Culture Techniques. Media are inoculated with a portion of the specimen. Inoculation should be performed in a semiquantitative fashion (especially samples of bladder urine obtained by catheter or catch).

Determination of the relative numbers of microorganisms in a sample greatly helps interpretation of significance. Colonies of microorganisms growing on all four quadrants of a petri plate indicate that there are large numbers of microorganisms in the sample. If a sample yielded one or two colonies growing on the plate, the significance of these colonies and thus the question as to the infectious etiology of the condition would be in doubt. Enrichment prior to plating of a sample obtained from a normally sterile site should usually not be unless necessary because one microorganism may replicate to numbers that equal many thousands in a very short period of time. Enrichment culture procedures lead to the proliferation of contaminating microorganisms.

Determination of clinical significance is aided by the cytology of the sample obtained from the affected site. Isolation (demonstration) of numerous microorganisms from a normally sterile site without the presence of inflammatory cells should be suspect. One exception to this rule is cryptococcal infection wherein the sample may contain a large number of yeast cells but very few inflammatory cells (the cryptococcal capsule is immunosuppressive). The isolation or demonstration of a "significant number" of microorganisms from a normally sterile site without evidence of an inflammatory response can be explained by contaminated collection devices; contamination of the collection device from a contiguous, normally nonsterile site; contamination of the medium inoculation device in the microbiology laboratory; or contamination of the medium before inoculation. Collection devices (e.g., catheters) sterilized by liquid disinfectants quite often become contaminated by microorganisms able to survive in such environments (*Pseudomonas*, for example).

Media plates may be streaked in any fashion as long as individual isolated colonies are produced after incubation. Assessing relative numbers is very subjective. Relative numbers of microorganisms may be reported by noting how much growth occurs on the surface of the plate. Obviously, growth of one colony (presumably from one bacterium) versus growth of colonies over the whole plate would be viewed differently with respect to clinical significance. Determination of the actual numbers of bacteria present is only important when analyzing urine obtained by "catch" or catheter because of the problem of contamination of the sample by bacteria in the distal urethra. In this instance, disposable calibrated loops containing 0.001 or 0.01 ml of urine are used to inoculate appropriate media. Greater than 10^5 bacteria/ml of urine obtained by catheter or "catch" is considered significant (i.e., the bacteria are more likely to be coming from the bladder rather than the distal urethra).

Aerobic Bacteria. The standard medium inoculated for the isolation of facultative microorganisms is a blood agar plate (usually sheep blood suspended in a growth medium in a semisolid matrix containing agarose). Many laboratories include a MacConkey agar plate as well. MacConkey agar is useful because enteric microorganisms (members of the family Enterobacteriaceae, e.g., *Escherichia coli*, *Klebsiella*, and *Enterobacter*) grow very well, as does the nonenteric *Pseudomonas*. Most other nonenteric gram-negative rods and all gram-positive microorganisms do not grow well on this medium. Assessing growth on MacConkey agar will facilitate detection of enteric organisms (Figure 3.1).

Anaerobic Bacteria. Anaerobic bacteria will grow on blood agar that is specially prepared to eliminate oxygen. After anaerobic plates are inoculated, they should be placed in a closed, anaerobic environment. Processing specimens for anaerobic culture is time-consuming and expensive. The most common sites that contain anaerobic bacteria are deep tissue wounds; draining tracts; abscesses; pleural, pericardial, and peritoneal effusions; pyometra; osteomyelitis; and pneumonic lungs. Anaerobic culture of sites that contain a population of anaerobic bacteria as part of the normal flora is often unrewarding (e.g., feces, vagina, distal urethra, and oral cavity) unless the diagnostician is looking for a specific species or type of anaerobic organism. Anaerobic culture of the urinary tract is not routinely performed because the recovery of these microorganisms from this site is extremely rare.

Molecular/Immunological Methods. Sometimes it is important to determine the presence or absence of a particular microorganism as quickly as possible so that appropriate control measures can be initiated. This is especially true when infectious agents are suspected that pose a threat to other animals, including human care givers (e.g., *Salmonella* and *Leptospira*). Likewise, some infectious agents take so long to isolate in culture that formulation of a rational therapeutic strategy is difficult (e.g., some fungal agents and *Mycobacterium*). Still others are hard to detect because

FIGURE 3.1. *Escherichia coli on blood agar plate (hemolytic, A) and MacConkey agar (B). Purple color indicates acid production (lactose fermentation).*

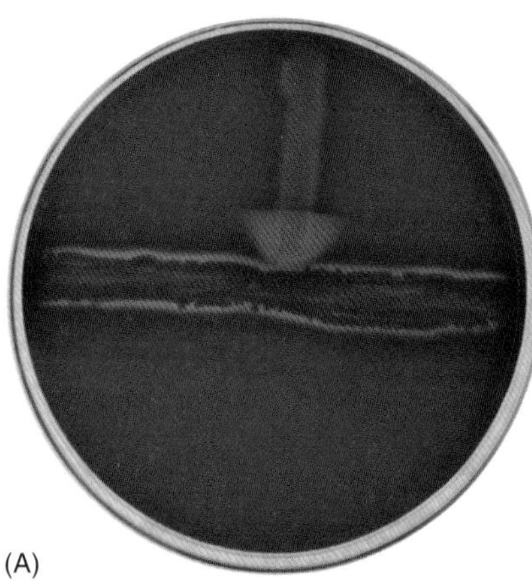

(A)

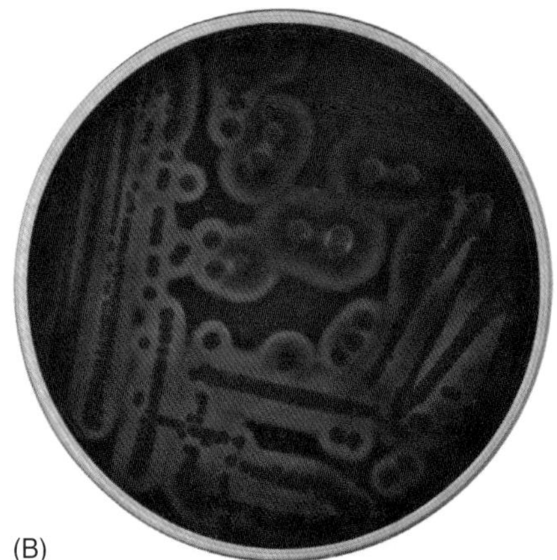

(B)

they are difficult to culture (e.g., *Leptospira* and rickettsiae) or have not been cultured in artificial media (e.g., *Clostridium piliformis* and *Mycobacterium leprae*). In these instances, other diagnostic techniques are available.

Immunologically based techniques make use of antibodies specific for the microorganism in question. These antibodies are usually immobilized on a solid support and are used to trap the agent. The presence of the trapped agent is then detected with a specific antibody that has been labeled in some way (usually with a color reagent). Some kits making use of this approach are commercially available (e.g., *Salmonella*). Molecular techniques utilizing DNA probes specific for a segment of DNA that is unique to the microorganism in question, or the polymerase chain reaction (PCR) using specific DNA primers, have been designed for a number of agents.

Virus

General Considerations

The diagnosis of viral diseases traditionally has been both tedious and time-consuming, but modern technologies such as the PCR have increased the utility of this approach. Prompt and accurate diagnosis of viral diseases is therefore essential to determine an effective course of disease prevention and control.

Proper methods of collecting and processing clinical specimens and a complete history are vital to the successful isolation of viruses. Tissues that are extensively autolyzed or poorly stored usually do not yield infectious viruses because of the susceptibility of most viruses to detrimental environmental conditions. Viral isolation and/or identification should be attempted in the following conditions:

1. During outbreaks of vesicular disease in livestock (e.g., foot-and-mouth disease in cattle, pigs, sheep, or goats).
2. During outbreaks of disease in large animal populations such as feedlots, poultry houses, or catteries where many animals are at risk and prompt, accurate diagnosis is critical to the institution of control methods (such as vaccination).
3. In instances of potentially zoonotic diseases such as rabies, West Nile fever, and equine encephalomyelitis, particularly when human exposure has occurred.
4. In determining the etiology of new disease, or in defining uncharacterized aspects of existing ones.

Tissues for virus isolation should be collected from recently dead animals whenever possible (Table 3.1). Collection of appropriate specimens during the acute phase of the disease, and inclusion of additional submissions from similarly affected animals, enhances the likelihood of isolating viruses. The following factors should be considered in selecting clinical specimens: (1) type of disease (e.g., respiratory—lung or trachea, or vesicular—vesicle or skin biopsy), (2) the age and species of the host, (3) the nature of the lesions in affected animals, and (4) the size of carcasses or tissues (able to be shipped on ice?). The following is a systematic approach for the rapid laboratory diagnosis of a viral-caused disease in animals:

1. Examination (gross and histologic) of the diseased animal/tissues as a presumptive diagnosis for a viral etiology.
2. Detection of viral-specific antibodies (ideally using acute and convalescent sera to demonstrate responding antibodies) during clinical disease.
3. Immunohistochemical staining of tissue sections with virus-specific antibodies to detect individual viral antigens in the tissue.
4. Examination of feces, plasma, or serum by immunoassays that detect specific viral antigens (e.g., the rotavirus in feces, feline leukemia virus in serum, and bovine respiratory syncytial virus in lung).
5. Examination of positive- or negative-stained specimens by electron microscopy to identify the morphology of viruses. This diagnostic procedure is limited by the concentration of viral particles required for detection (>105/ml).

Table 3.1. Suggested Specimens from Mammalian Species for Virus Isolation and Identification

Type of Illness or Infection	Common Name or Associated Virus	Other Infections	Clinical Specimens to Collect	Diagnostic Identification Tests
Respiratory	Adenovirus (bovine, porcine, canine)		Nasal and ocular secretions, feces, lung, brain, tonsil	VI (CPE), HA, CF, FA, VN
	Infectious canine hepatitis (adenovirus)		Spleen, liver, lymph nodes, kidney, blood	VI (CPE), HA, FA, VN
	Bovine viral diarrhea (mucosal disease) (pestivirus)	Genital, abortions, enteric	Nasal sections, oral lesions, lung, spleen, blood, mesenteric lymph nodes, intestinal mucosa, vaginal secretions, fetal tissues, unclotted blood	VI (CPE and virus interference), FA, VN
	Infectious bovine rhinotracheitis (herpesvirus)	Central nervous system (CNS), genital, abortions	Nasal and ocular secretions, lung, tracheal swab, tracheal segment, brain, vaginal secretions, serum, aborted fetus, liver, spleen, kidney	VI (CPE), FA, VN
	Feline rhinotracheitis (herpesvirus)		Nasal and pharyngeal secretions, conjunctival membranes, liver, lung, spleen, kidney, salivary gland, brain	VI (CPE and inclusions), FA
	Equine rhinopneumonitis (herpesvirus)	Genital, abortions	Placenta, fetus, lung, nasal secretions, lymph nodes	FA, VI (ECE and CPE), VN
	Influenza (equine, porcine) (orthomyxovirus)		Nasal and ocular secretions, lung, tracheal swab	VI
	Influenza (equine, porcine) (orthomyxovirus)		Nasal and ocular secretions, lung, tracheal swab	VI (ECE), HA, HI
	Parainfluenza (bovine, equine, porcine, ovine, canine) (paramyxovirus)		Nasal and ocular secretions, lung, tracheal swab	VI (ECE), HA, HI, VN
	Bovine respiratory syncytial virus (pneumovirus)		Trachea, lung, nasal secretions, clotted blood	VI (CPE), FA, ELISA
	Bovine herpesvirus 4 (Movar, DN599)	Abortions	Trachea, lung, nasal secretions, fetus, clotted blood	VI (CPE), FA, VN
	Reovirus (bovine, equine, canine, feline)		Feces, intestinal mucosa, nasal and pharyngeal secretions	VI, HA, HI
	African horse sickness (orbivirus)		Whole blood in anticoagulant, lesion material, nasal and pharyngeal secretions	VI (CPE), ELISA, FA, VN, EM
	Malignant catarrhal fever (herpesvirus)		Whole blood in anticoagulant, lymph nodes, spleen, lung	VI (CPE), ELISA, FA, VN, EM
	Pseudorabies (herpesvirus)	CNS, genital, abortions	Nasal secretions, tonsil, lung, brain (midbrain, pons, medulla), spinal cord (sheep and cattle), spleen (swine), vaginal secretion, serum	VI (CPE and rabbits), VN, ELISA, FA
	Canine herpesvirus		Kidney, liver, lung, spleen, nasal oropharyngeal, and vaginal secretions	VI (CPE and inclusions), FA, VN
	Porcine inclusion body rhinitis (cytomegalovirus)		Turbinate, nasal mucosa	EM, VI (CPE), FA, VN
	Equine rhinovirus		Nasal secretions, feces	VI (CPE), FN
	Maedi-Visna, ovine progressive pneumonia (retrovirus, lentivirus)	CNS	CSF, whole blood, salivary glands, lung, mediastinal lymph nodes, choroid plexus, spleen	VI (CPE), VN
	Bovine rhinovirus		Nasal secretions	VI (CPE), VN
	Rift Valley fever (bovine, ovine, phlebovirus)		Whole blood in anticoagulant, fetus, liver, spleen, kidney, brain	VI (CPE and mice), VN, CF, FA
Enteric	Bovine enterovirus		Feces, oropharyngeal swab	VI (CPE), VN
	Transmissible gastroenteritis (coronavirus)		Feces, nasal secretions, jejunum, ileum	VI (newborn pigs), FA, EM
	Neonatal diarrheas			
	1. Rotaviruses		Feces, small intestine	VI (CPE with trypsin), ELISA, FA, EM
	2. Parvoviruses	Abortion	Feces, intestinal mucosa, regional lymph nodes, brain, heart	VI (CPE), FA, EM, HA, HI, VN
	3. Coronaviruses		Feces, small intestine	VI (CPE with trypsin), FA, EM

(Continued)

Table 3.1. (*Continued*)

Type of Illness or Infection	Common Name or Associated Virus	Other Infections	Clinical Specimens to Collect	Diagnostic Identification Tests
	Piconavirus SMEDI (enterovirus)		Feces, intestine, brain, tonsil, liver	VI (CPE, VN, EM)
	Polioencephalitis (Teschen, Talfan), enterovirus)	CNS	Brain, intestine, feces	VI (CPE, VN)
	Rinderpest (morbillivirus)		Blood in anticoagulant, spleen, mesenteric lymph nodes	VI (CPE and cattle), AGID, CF, VN
	Peste des petits ruminants (morbillivirus)		Blood in anticoagulant, spleen, mesenteric lymph nodes	VI (CPE and goats), AGID
CNS	Rabies (lyssavirus)		Brain, salivary gland	VI (mice)
	Equine encephalomyelitis (VEE, EEE, WEE) (alphavirus)		Whole blood, brain, cerebrospinal fluid, nasal and pharyngeal secretions, pancreas	VI (ECE and mice), VN, CF
	Louping ill encephalomyelitis (flavivirus)		Whole blood, brain, cerebrospinal fluid	VI, ECE, and CPE
	Hemagglutinating encephalomyelitis virus (coronavirus)		Brain, spinal cord, tonsil, blood	VI

VI, virus isolation; CPE, cytopathic effect; HA, hemagglutinin; CF, complement fixation; FA, fluorescent antibody; VN, virus neutralization; ECE, embryonating chicken eggs; HI, hemagglutination inhibition; ELISA, enzyme-linked immunosorbent assay; EM, electron microscopy; AGID, agar gel immunodiffusion.

6. Isolation or amplification of infectious viruses in cell cultures and identification of the virus propagated from clinical submission. Alternatively, detection of virus-specific RNA or DNA may be an acceptable approach.

Many viral diseases do not kill the host, but the host may serve as a reservoir of viruses and disseminate the virus to other contact animals. Serologic assays can sometimes be used to determine which animals carry specific viruses and which animals may be susceptible to infection.

Isolation of a virus from an animal does not necessarily implicate that virus as the causative agent of any disease that is occurring in that animal. It is very important to confirm that the isolated virus produces a similar disease in the same or related species, which may even involve the inoculation of susceptible or nonimmune animals. When two or more viruses are isolated from a specimen, a clear interpretation of the role of each isolate in the disease process is also necessary. Finally, it must be remembered that vaccine strains of attenuated viruses can also be reisolated from vaccinated animals, and can be confused with true field strains.

Isolation of Virus from Clinical Specimens

Cultivation in Tissue Culture. Viruses are isolated from clinical specimens by inoculating susceptible primary or continuous cell cultures derived from the host or related species, embryonated eggs, or laboratory animals. Specimens submitted for viral isolation should be placed in virus transport media (e.g., a balanced salt solution containing antibiotics) in sealed containers for safety in handling. They should be clearly identified by appropriate labeling, and submitted on ice (4 °C) or frozen (−20 °C). Attention to aseptic technique during specimen collection procedures will improve the probability of successful virus isolation.

Specimens should be collected from live animals during acute phases of the disease. Depending on the specific disease process, excretions or secretions, swabs of body orifices or liquids (lymph or blood), and tissue collected by biopsy are all suitable specimens for viral isolation. In the laboratory, tissue specimens are processed as a 10% or 20% (w/v) homogenate in a balanced salt solution along with antibiotics. Heavily contaminated specimens may be filtered to remove other microorganisms. Virus isolation should be conducted in cell cultures free of contaminating agents such as the noncytopathic bovine viral diarrhea virus or *Mycoplasma*. The cell culture medium may contain low concentrations of broad-spectrum antibiotics.

To isolate the virus, tissue homogenates are placed onto cellular monolayers and absorbed 1 h or longer at 35–37 °C, and the inoculum is left on or removed and fresh media added. Inoculated and uninfected cell cultures are observed for 7–10 days. Viral cytopathic effect (CPE) in cells is usually evident between 24 h and 72 h for most cytopathic viruses (Figure 3.2). However, for most clinical material containing low concentrations of viruses, several (>3) blind cell passages are recommended.

After a virus has been demonstrated at limiting dilution to replicate in a cell by CPE or other parameters, the infectious virus is released from cells by three cycles of freeze–thaw or sonication, followed by centrifugation and storage to maintain maximum infectivity. Each virus isolated should be identified as to species of origin, morphologic type, passage level, and host cell used for propagation.

Embryonated Eggs. A number of mammalian viruses and many avian viral pathogens can be isolated in embryonating chicken eggs (ECEs). A key to successful viral isolation

FIGURE 3.2. *CPE (syncytial) on bovine fetal kidney cells by the herpesvirus of malignant catarrhal fever (×200).*

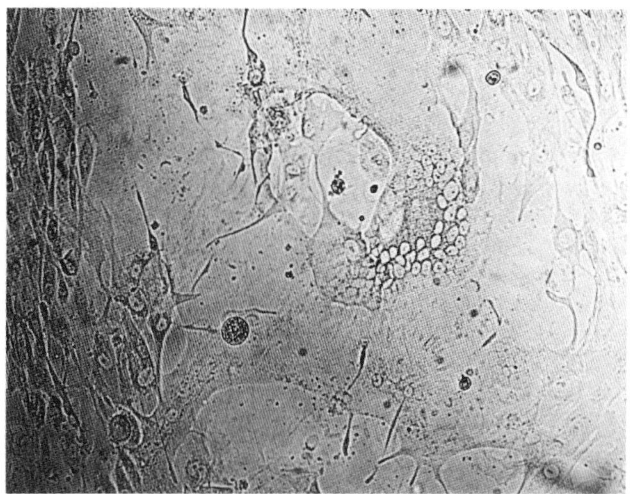

in ECEs is the route of inoculation (Figure 3.3). Candled ECE that die within 24 h after inoculation are considered traumatic deaths. Subsequent deaths of inoculated ECE are placed at 4 °C for several hours (to avoid hemorrhages) prior to collection of fluids or visual examination of the embryos and egg membranes. Embryos that are stunted, deformed, edematous, or hemorrhagic, and membranes that contain lesions (i.e., pocks) should be homogenized in a sterile balanced saline as a 10% (w/v) suspension and repassaged in ECEs or cell cultures.

FIGURE 3.3. *Inoculating an embryonated chicken egg (10–12 days old). For chorioallantoic membrane inoculation, a hole is first drilled through the egg shell and shell membrane; the shell over the air sac is then perforated, causing air to enter between the shell membrane and the chorioallantoic membrane, creating an artificial air sac, where the sample is deposited. The sample comes in contact with the chorionic epithelium. Yolk sac inoculation is usually carried out in younger (6 days old) embryos, in which the yolk sac is larger. (Courtesy of Dr. Bill Wilson, USDA ARS.)*

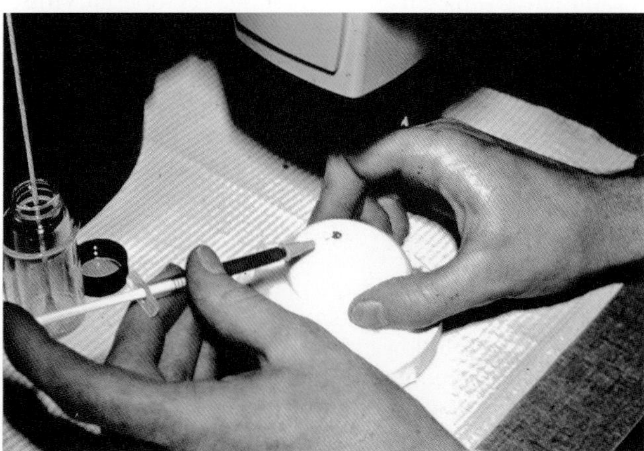

Animal Inoculation. The inoculation of susceptible laboratory animals remains a useful procedure for the identification procedure for the identification of some viral pathogens, particularly those that are highly fastidious and difficult to propagate in other systems.

Identification of Viruses or Viral Antigens in Clinical Specimens

Electron Microscopy. Electron microscopy (EM) can be used to rapidly identify the morphology and size of any virus present in a specimen or isolated in cell culture of ECEs. Tentative diagnosis of viral diseases can be made by EM on thin sections of affected tissues and cell-free homogenates of clinical specimens. The use of EM for diagnosis is limited, however, because the method is not very sensitive (>105 virus particles/ml are required to see a single viral particle on a 200-mesh grid), and viruses from different species have similar morphology and size.

Immune Electron Microscopy. Immune electron microscopy (IEM) enhances detection of viruses in tissues, cells, or fecal specimens by reacting specific immune sera with viruses. In IEM, a specific antibody to a virus, preferably polyclonal, is mixed with the virus for 1 h to produce antigen–antibody complexes. These immune complexes are centrifuged at 1000 × g onto Formvar-coated grids, then stained with 4% phosphotunstic acid (PTA), pH 7.0, and examined by EM. The reaction of viral fluids with specific acute or convalescent serum as viewed by EM determines if a virus is associated with a specific disease. This procedure has been used successfully for viruses associated with infectious diarrhea.

Immunofluorescence. Immunofluorescence is a visible fluorescence accentuated by ultraviolet light as a specific antibody covalently bound to a fluorochrome (e.g., fluorescein isothiocyanate and rhodamine) that combines with a fixed antigen. This technique provides a sensitive and rapid method for detecting and identifying specific viruses in either tissues or cell cultures (Figure 3.4). Immunofluorescence is detectable by either a direct or indirect procedure. The direct immunofluorescence test employs a virus-specific antibody labeled with fluorescein that combines with a specific viral antigen located in cells or tissues. The indirect test requires the use of a fluorescein-labeled antiserum to a virus-specific immunoglobulin.

Immunohistochemical staining uses the same approach, except that the virus-specific antibody is either directly or indirectly labeled with an enzyme. The presence of the enzyme is determined by addition of its substrate, and the reaction detected by a color change. The advantage of immunohistochemical staining over immunofluorescence is that a fluorescent microscope is not required, and the use of an enzyme-enhancement step greatly increases the sensitivity of the procedure.

Nucleic Acid Hybridization. Molecular hybridization techniques have led to the synthetic production of viral DNA probes that are highly specific for individual viruses. These probes are labeled with various detection systems

FIGURE 3.4. *Immunohistochemistry assay demonstrating the presence of Rify Valley fever virus in the liver of an infected mouse. A Rift Valley fever virus antigen-specific antibody reacts specifically to viral antigen in the tissue (red color). (Courtesy of Dr. Barbara Drolet, USDA ARS.)*

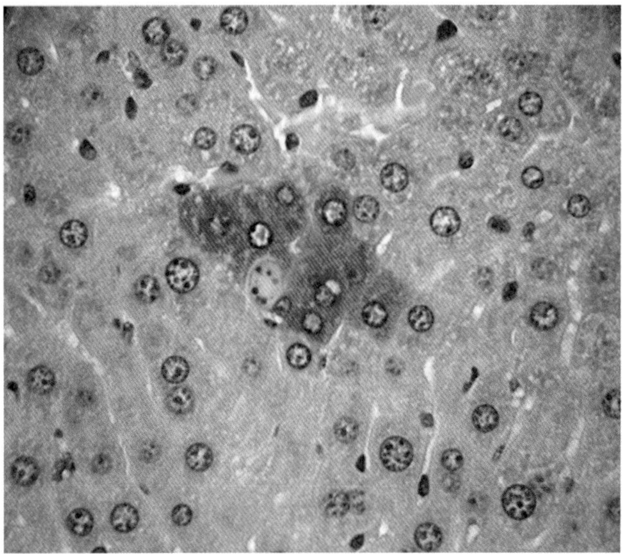

that allow identification of the presence of individual viruses, either in tissues or in extracts of them.

Polymerase Chain Reaction. The relatively recent development of the PCR has revolutionized the rapid diagnosis of many viral diseases. The importance of the procedure lies in its ability to amplify small amounts of viral DNA or RNA even from contaminated specimens, and on its ability to be conducted on a large scale so that vast numbers of samples can simultaneously be evaluated. Furthermore, technical developments such as real-time PCR allow the quantitation of template that is present in a sample, which is reflective of the viral load. The PCR assay is based on the cyclic synthesis of a DNA segment limited by two specific oligonucleotides that are used as primers to specifically amplify portions of the viral genome. Properly run, the PCR assay is both sensitive and specific, although the identification of viral nucleic acid does not prove that an infectious virus was present, so PCR-positive samples often should be subjected to traditional virus isolation procedures.

Enzyme-Linked Immunosorbent Assay for Antigen Detection. The enzyme-linked immunosorbent assay (ELISA) is a rapid, highly sensitive immunoassay adapted to measure viral antigens or antibodies (see Chapter 2). ELISAs have been developed for numerous avian viral pathogens (e.g., the avian laryngotracheitis virus, avian encephalitis, Newcastle disease virus, infectious bronchitis virus, and reovirus), and increasingly are being developed to detect viruses that infect other species of domestic animals.

Serologic Detection of Viruses

Most viruses usually elicit an immune response in the host; thus, the detection of a humoral (antibody) or cellular response is often used to determine prior infection of an animal with a viral pathogen. Serologic assays measure humoral immunity in animals, and assays for measuring cellular immunity to viruses are used infrequently in veterinary diagnostic medicine.

Viruses have certain antigens that are type- or group-specific and that in part determine the serologic assay used. Serologic diagnosis of virus infections typically requires the collection of paired samples: an acute (at or prior to the onset of clinical signs) and a convalescent serum (10–28 days later). A fourfold or greater rise in antibody titer (the reciprocal of the serum dilution) indicates recent or ongoing viral infection. Antibody titers in single serum samples are more difficult to interpret, although the presence of antibodies is indicative of prior exposure (or resulting from the passive transfer of maternal antibodies in young animals), which is especially important in chronic diseases with a carrier state like the bovine leukemia virus in cattle, equine infectious anemia, and the equine arteritis virus infection of stallions.

Serology can help to rapidly establish a diagnosis when viral isolation procedures are negative. Serology can also be used to definitively rule out the absence of specific viruses in a given disease outbreak, whereas a negative viral isolation cannot.

Serum Virus Neutralization Test. Most viruses produce a visible CPE in cell cultures. CPE is used to determine the presence of protective or virus-neutralizing antibodies in a serum. To quantify the amount of neutralizing antibodies, serum from an animal is serially diluted and mixed with a known amount of virus (generally 50–300 infectious doses of virus—TCID50) for 1 h at 37 °C prior to inoculation of a volume of the mixture into animals, ECEs, or cell cultures. The serum neutralization (SN) test is very specific and highly sensitive, but it is time-consuming and expensive. The SN can be used to confirm recent infection of animals if paired sera are evaluated.

Hemagglutination Inhibition Test. Viruses that possess a hemagglutinin (HA) protein will agglutinate erythrocytes, a fact that has been used to quantify the amount (titrate) of these viruses present in a sample. The hemagglutination inhibition (HI) test can be used to identify or type a virus through the inhibition of hemagglutination by virus-specific antiserum.

Hemadsorption Inhibition Test. The hemadsorption inhibition test is based on the ability of certain virus-infected cells (monolayers) to attract specific erythrocytes to their surface. The presence of hemadsorbing erythrocyte clusters on a cellular monolayer indicates that viral protein (hemagglutinin) has accumulated on the surface of the cell membrane. The hemadsorption phenomenon can be inhibited by pretreatment of virus-infected cells for 30 min, usually at ambient temperature with twofold dilutions of antisera followed by the addition of 0.05–0.5% erythrocytes. Antibody (Ab) can be quantified by comparing the observed washed virus-infected cell monolayers that contain adhered clumped erythrocytes on the surface of the cell (Ab negative) with the cell monolayers that contain free-floating erythrocytes (Ab positive).

Complement Fixation. Complement fixation (CF) tests employ the complement cascade in reactions with viral antigens that fix complement—usually from guinea pig serum—when combined with specific, anti-viral antibodies. Although CF has been used in early test tube assays to detect viruses (e.g., leukemia viruses), virus-infected cells, or virus-specific antibodies, the complexity of the assay and the time required have led to its replacement by simpler procedures.

Immunodiffusion. The immunodiffusion procedure is routinely used as a diagnostic tool to monitor the spread of specific viral pathogens in various animal diseases (e.g., bluetongue, equine infectious anemia, bovine leukosis, caprine arthritis, encephalitis, and infectious bursal disease). The basis of the test is the ability of certain soluble viral antigens to diffuse in a semisolid medium (agar) with the formation of a precipitin line with specific antisera.

Radioimmunoassay. The radioimmunoassay (RIA) is an exquisitely sensitive method for quantifying antigens or antibodies when one component is radio-labeled. Although RIA has an advantage for detecting minute amounts of antibodies, the need for a scintillation counter to measure radioactivity and very pure reagents limits use of this assay to appropriately equipped diagnostic laboratories.

ELISA for Antibody Detection. ELISAs are highly specific and sensitive immunoassays in which the specificity of the reaction can be enhanced by increasing the level of purification of the antigen or antibody employed. The ELISA can detect nanogram levels of IgG-, IgM-, and IgA-type antibodies. ELISAs can be made quantitative if appropriate standard curves are developed. Numerous commercially available assays for avian and mammalian viruses provide qualitative information on antibodies to various viruses, whereas others detect the viruses themselves in clinical specimens. The blocking ELISA evaluates the ability of a test serum to displace the binding of a virus protein-specific antibody to its antigen.

Western Immunoblot Assay. The Western immunoblot assay can detect antibodies to a full range of viral proteins as revealed on a strip of nitrocellulose paper as discrete bands by electrophoresis. When a serum sample is applied to the nitrocellulose strip, antibodies from animals infected with a specific virus bind to the specific viral proteins at the appropriate positions. These bands become dark and distinct when the nitrocellulose paper is treated with a reagent (Figure 3.5). Because it provides a full viral antibody profile of the serum sample, this test is the most specific viral diagnostic test currently available.

FIGURE 3.5. *Western immunoblot demonstrating antibody binding to specific protein antigens separated by gel electrophoresis chromatography. Baculovirus-expressed EHDV-2 or BTV-11 VP-7 from cell supernatant (S) or cell pellet (C). Membrane blotted with 1 : 2000 monoclonal antibody [EHDV(4F4.H1) or BTV(1AA4.E4)] and 1 : 4000 goat α-mouse HRP. (Courtesy of Dr. Chris Lehiy, USDA ARS.)*

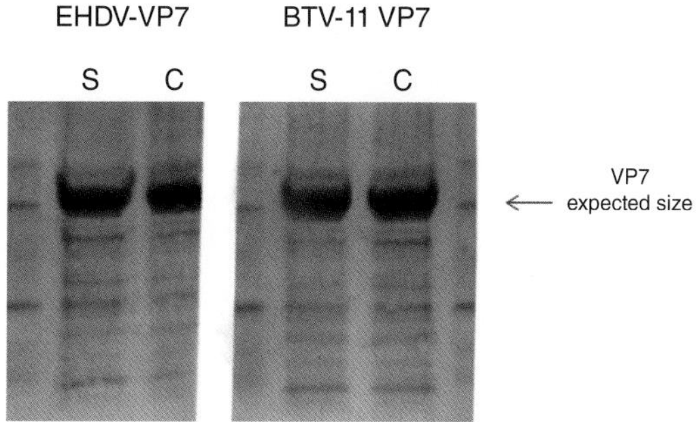

Further Reading

Coghe F, Orrù G, Pautasso M *et al.* (2011) The role of the laboratory in choosing antibiotics. *J Matern Fetal Neonatal Med*, **24** (Suppl 2), 18–20.

O'Brien TF and Stelling J (2011) Integrated multilevel surveillance of the World's infecting microbes and their resistance to antimicrobial agents. *Clin Microbiol Rev*, **24** (2), 281–295. doi:10.1128/CMR.00021-10.

Weinstein MP (2011) Diagnostic strategies and general topics, in *Manual of Clinical Microbiology*, vol. I. Section I, 10th edn (ed. JH Jorgensen), ASM Press.

Wilson D, Howell V, Toppozini C *et al.* (2011) Against all odds: diagnosing tuberculosis in South Africa. *J Infect Dis*, **204** (Suppl 4), S1102–S1109.

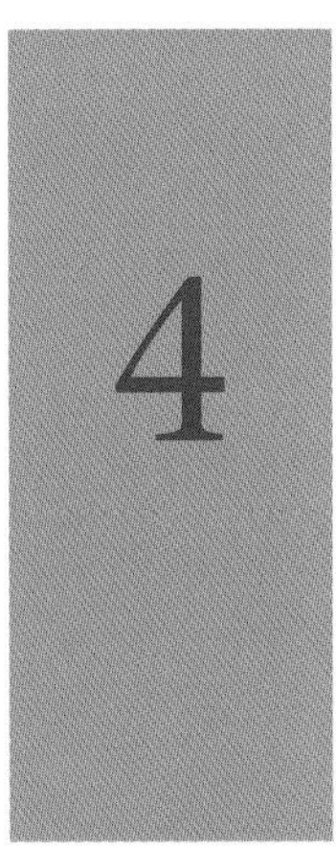

Antimicrobial Chemotherapy

John F. Prescott

Antimicrobial drugs exploit differences in structure or biochemical function between the host and parasite. Modern chemotherapy is traced to the work of Paul Ehrlich, who devoted his life to discovering agents that possessed selective toxicity. The first clinically successful broad-spectrum antibacterial drugs were the sulfonamides, developed in 1935 as a result of Ehrlich's work with synthetic dyes. It was, however, the discovery of penicillin by Fleming in 1928 and its later development by Chain and Florey in World War II that led to the subsequent discovery of further antibiotics, chemical substances produced by microorganisms that at low concentrations inhibited or killed other microorganisms. The chemical modification of many of the drugs discovered early in the antibiotic revolution led to the development of new and powerful antimicrobial drugs with properties distinct from their parents. Antibiotics and their derivatives have more importance as antimicrobial agents than do the fewer synthetic antibacterial drugs. By contrast, antiviral drugs are all chemically synthesized. The term antimicrobial will be used throughout to include both antibiotics and synthetic antimicrobial drugs. The therapeutic use of antimicrobial drugs in veterinary medicine has followed their use in human medicine because of the high cost of their development.

This chapter discusses systemic antibacterial and antifungal agents, and their use, as well as the important topic of antibiotic resistance.

Classification of Antimicrobial Drugs

Antimicrobial drugs can be classified in a number of ways, each of which has clinical importance:

1. *Spectrum of activity against class of microorganism*: Penicillins are narrow-spectrum because they inhibit only bacteria; sulfonamides, trimethoprim, and lincosamides are broader because they inhibit both bacteria and protozoa. Polyenes only inhibit fungi.
2. *Antibacterial activity*: Some antibiotics are narrow-spectrum in that they inhibit only gram-positive (bacitracin and vancomycin) or mainly gram-negative bacteria (polymyxin), whereas broad-spectrum drugs such as tetracyclines inhibit both gram-positive and gram-negative bacteria. Other drugs such as penicillin G or lincosamides are most active against gram-positive bacteria but will inhibit some gram-negatives.
3. *Bacteriostatic or bactericidal*: This distinction is an approximation that depends on drug concentrations and the organism involved. For example, penicillin is bactericidal at high concentrations and bacteriostatic at lower ones. The distinction between bactericidal and bacteriostatic is critical in certain circumstances, such as the treatment of meningitis or of septicemia in neutropenic patients.
4. *Pharmacodynamic activity*: Antibacterial action is concentration or time dependent (see Section "Design of drug dosage and pharmacodynamic properties" for the effect of this activity on dosing considerations).
5. *Mechanism of action*: Like pharmacodynamic activity, this is dependent on the drug class and is discussedlater. This is probably the most useful of the classifications, since it determines the previous four classification approaches.

Mechanism of Action of Antimicrobial Drugs

The marked structural and biochemical differences between eukaryotic and prokaryotic cells give greater opportunity for selective toxicity of antibacterial drugs compared to antifungal drugs because fungi, like mammalian cells, are eukaryotic. Developing selectively toxic antiviral drugs is particularly difficult because viral replication depends largely on the metabolic pathways of the host cell. This chapter mainly discusses antibacterial drugs.

The mechanisms of action of antibacterial drugs fall into four categories: (1) inhibition of cell wall synthesis, (2) damage to cell membrane function, (3) inhibition of nucleic acid synthesis or function, and (4) inhibition of protein synthesis (Figure 4.1).

Veterinary Microbiology, Third Edition. Edited by D. Scott McVey, Melissa Kennedy and M.M. Chengappa.

FIGURE 4.1. *Mechanisms of action of antibacterial drugs.*

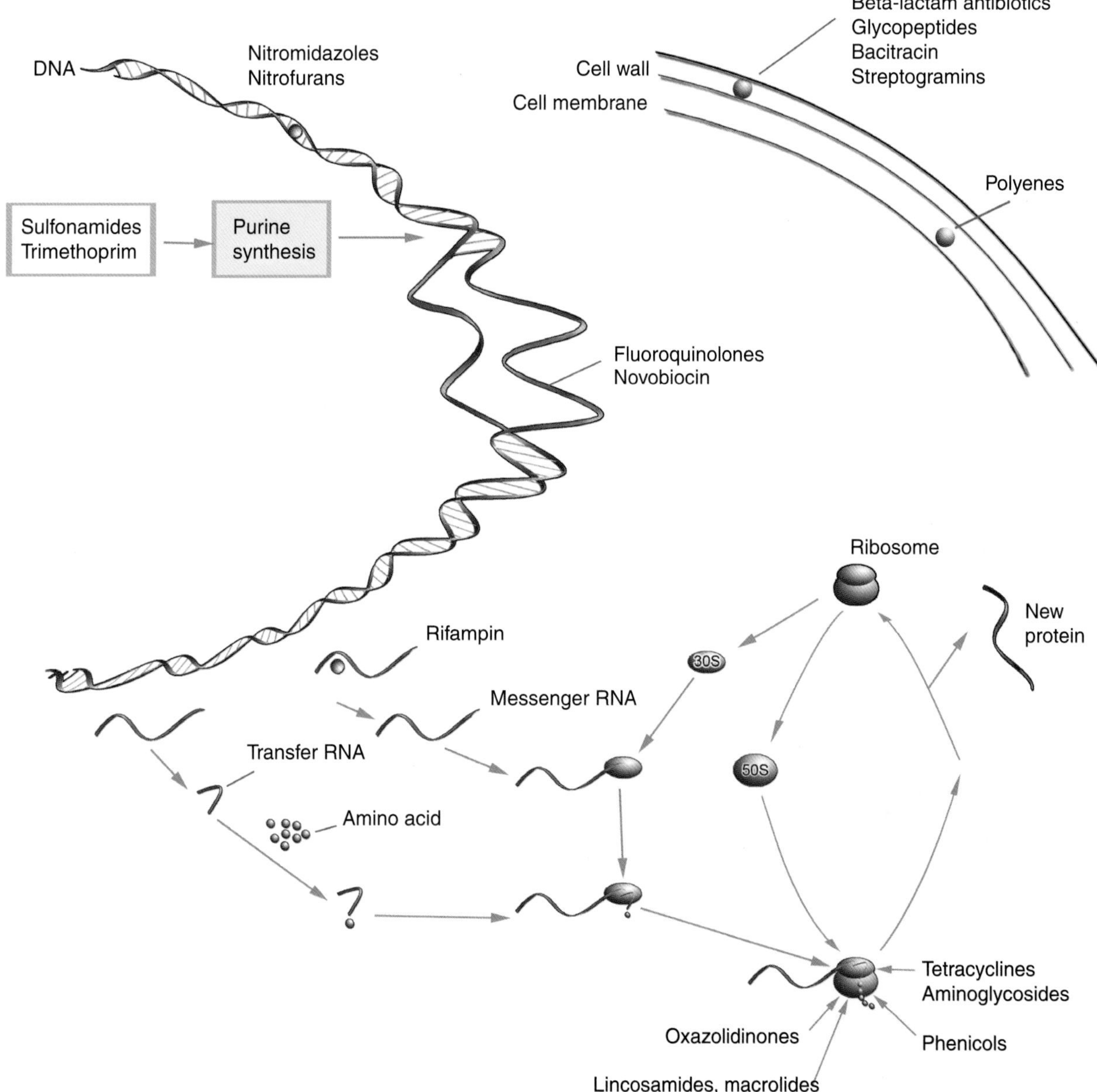

Inhibition of Cell Wall Synthesis

Antibiotics that interfere with cell wall synthesis include penicillins and cephalosporins (β-lactam antibiotics), bacitracin, and vancomycin. The bacterial cell wall is a thick envelope that gives shape to the cell. This tough wall outside the cell membrane is a major difference between bacteria and mammalian cells. In gram-positive bacteria, it consists largely of a thick layer of peptidoglycan, which gives the cell rigidity and maintains a high internal osmotic pressure of about 20 atmospheres. In gram-negative bacteria, this layer is thinner and the internal osmotic pressure is correspondingly lower. Peptidoglycan consists of a polysaccharide chain made up of a repeating disaccharide backbone of alternating *N*-acetylglucosamine-*N*-acetylmuramic acid in β-1,4 linkage, a tetra peptide attached to the *N*-acetylmuramic acid, and a peptide bridge from one tetrapeptide to another, so that the disaccharide backbone is cross-linked both within and between layers. The cross-linkage between transpeptides gives the cell wall remarkable strength. Several enzymes are involved in transpeptidation reactions.

The effect of β-lactam antibiotics (penicillins and cephalosporins) is to prevent the final cross-linking in the cell wall, inhibiting division and creating weak points. Among the targets of these drugs are penicillin-binding proteins (PBPs), of which there are three to eight in bacteria; many of these PBPs are transpeptidase enzymes. They are responsible for the formation and remodeling of the cell wall during growth and division. Different PBPs have different affinities for drugs, explaining the variation in the spectrum of action of different β-lactam antibiotics. Degradative mechanisms are also involved in cell wall production. These are carried out by autolysins, and some penicillins act partly by decreasing normal inhibition of the autolysins.

The action of β-lactam antibiotics is thus to block peptidoglycan synthesis, which severely weakens the cell wall, and to promote the action of the autolysins, which lyse the cell. β-Lactams are active only against actively growing cells. The greater activity of some β-lactams against gram-positive bacteria is the result of the greater quantity of peptidoglycan and higher osmotic pressure in gram-positive bacteria, the impermeability of some gram-negative bacteria because of their lipopolysaccharide and lipid exterior, and the presence of β-lactamase enzymes in many gram-negative organisms. The remarkable activity of some of the newest penicillins and cephalosporins against gram-negatives is the result not only of their improved ability to enter gram-negative cells and bind PBPs but also of their ability to resist a variety of β-lactamase enzymes normally found in the periplasmic space of gram-negative bacteria. More recently, β-lactamase-inhibiting drugs with no intrinsic antibacterial activity, such as clavulanic acid and sulbactam, have been combined with amoxicillin or ticarcillin to expand the spectrum of activity of these latter compounds by neutralizing enzymes that might otherwise degrade them.

Bacitracin and vancomycin inhibit the early stages in peptidoglycan synthesis. They are active only against gram-positive bacteria.

Penicillins. Sir Alexander Fleming's observation that colonies of staphylococci lysed on a plate that had become contaminated with a *Penicillium* fungus was the discovery that led to the development of antibiotics. In 1940, Chain, Florey, and their associates succeeded in producing therapeutic quantities of penicillin from *Penicillium notatum*. Almost a decade later, penicillin G became widely available for clinical use. In the years that followed, this antibiotic was found to have certain limitations: its relative instability to stomach acid, its susceptibility to inactivation by penicillinase, and its relative inactivity against most gram-negative bacteria. Isolation of the active moiety, 6-aminopenicillanic acid, in the penicillin molecule has resulted in the design and development of semisynthetic penicillins that overcome some of these limitations.

The development of the cephalosporin family, which shares with penicillin the β-lactam ring, has led to a remarkable array of drugs with improved ability to penetrate different gram-negative bacterial species and to resist β-lactamase enzymes. In recent years, other naturally occurring β-lactam antibiotics have been described that lack the bicyclic ring of the classical β-lactam penicillins and cephalosporins. Many of these new drugs have potent antibacterial activity and are highly resistant to β-lactamase enzymes.

Clinically important penicillins can be divided into six groups:

1. *Benzyl penicillins and its long-acting forms*: Injectable penicillins, highest activity against gram-positive organisms, but susceptible to acid hydrolysis and β-lactamase inactivation (e.g., penicillin G).
2. *Orally absorbed penicillins*: Spectrum similar to benzyl penicillins (e.g., penicillin V).
3. *Antistaphylococcal isoxazolyl penicillins*: Relatively resistant to staphylococcal β-lactamases (e.g., cloxacillin and methicillin).
4. *Extended-spectrum penicillins*: Aminopenicillins (e.g., amoxicillin and ampicillin).
5. *Antipseudomonal penicillins*: Carboxy- and ureido-penicillins (e.g., carbenicillin, piperacillin, and ticarcillin).
6. *β-Lactamase resistant penicillins*: Temocillin.

Antimicrobial Activity. Penicillin G is the most active of the penicillins against gram-positive aerobic bacteria such as non-β-lactamase-producing coagulase-positive staphylococci, β-hemolytic streptococci, *Bacillus anthracis* and other gram-positive rods, corynebacteria, *Erysipelothrix*, *Listeria*, and against most anaerobes. It is moderately active against the more fastidious gram-negative aerobes such as *Haemophilus*, *Pasteurella*, and some *Actinobacillus*, but it is inactive against members of the family Enterobacteriaceae, and the genera *Bordetella*, and *Pseudomonas*. The penicillinase-resistant isoxazolyl penicillins (oxacillin, cloxacillin, methicillin, and nafcillin) are resistant to coagulase-positive staphylococcal penicillinase, but are less active than penicillin G against other penicillin-sensitive gram-positive bacteria. Most gram-negative bacteria are resistant to them. Ampicillin and amoxicillin are slightly less active than penicillin G against gram-positive and anaerobic bacteria and are also inactivated by penicillinase produced by coagulase-positive staphylococci. They have considerably greater activity against gram-negative bacteria. They are ineffective against *Pseudomonas aeruginosa*. Carbenicillin and ticarcillin resemble ampicillin in spectrum of activity with the notable difference of having activity against *P. aeruginosa*. Temocillin is highly resistant to β-lactamases including extended-spectrum cephalosporinases, and has broad-activity against members of the family Enterobacteriaceae, including otherwise resistant isolates. *Mycoplasma* and mycobacteria are resistant to penicillins. Methicillin-resistant staphylococci are resistant to all β-lactam antibiotics.

Resistance. In gram-positive bacteria (particularly coagulase-positive staphylococci), resistance is mainly through production of extracellular β-lactamase (penicillinase) enzymes that break the β-lactam ring of most penicillins. Resistance in gram-negative bacteria results, in part, from a wide variety of β-lactamase enzymes and also from low bacterial permeability or lack of PBP receptors. Most or all gram-negative bacteria express low levels of species-specific chromosomally mediated β-lactamase enzymes within the periplasmic space, and these sometimes contribute to resistance.

Plasmid-mediated β-lactamase production is widespread among common gram-negative bacteria.

The enzymes are constitutively expressed and cause high-level resistance. The majority are penicillinases rather than cephalosporinases. The most widespread are TEM-type β-lactamases, which readily hydrolyze penicillin G and ampicillin rather than methicillin, cloxacillin, or carbenicillin. The less widespread OXA-type β-lactamases hydrolyze isoxazolyl penicillins (oxacillin, cloxacillin, and related compounds). SHV-type β-lactamases are found particularly in *Klebsiella pneumoniae* but may be found in other members of the family Enterobacteriaceae. In recent years, β-lactamases resistant to third-generation cephalosporins have emerged. These include AmpC hyperproducers (such as the CMY2 β-lactamase), as well as extended-spectrum β-lactamases (mostly TEM and SHV gene variants, but including PER, CTX-M, VEB, and other β-lactamase groups) and metallo-β-lactamases including the IMP, SPM, and VOM β-lactamases. These latter enzymes are not inhibited by clavulanic acid.

A major advance was the discovery of broad-spectrum inhibitors of β-lactamase (e.g., clavulanic acid and sulbactam). These drugs have weak antibacterial activity but show extraordinary synergism when administered with penicillin G, ampicillin, amoxicillin, or ticarcillin because they irreversibly bind the β-lactamase enzymes of resistant bacteria.

Absorption, Distribution, and Excretion. The penicillins are organic acids that are generally available as the sodium or potassium salt of the free acid. Apart from the isoxazolyl penicillins and penicillin V, acid hydrolysis limits the systemic availability of most penicillins from oral preparations. Both ampicillin and amoxicillin are relatively stable in acid.

The penicillins are predominantly ionized in the blood plasma, have relatively small apparent volumes of distribution, and have short half-lives (0.5–1.2 h) in all species of domestic animals. After absorption, penicillins are widely distributed in body fluids. Because of their high degree of ionization and low solubility in lipid, they attain only low intracellular concentrations and do not penetrate well into transcellular fluids. The relatively poor diffusibility of penicillins across cell membranes is reflected in their milk-to-plasma concentration ratios (0.3). The relatively low tissue levels attained may, however, be clinically effective because of the high sensitivity of susceptible bacteria to penicillins and their bactericidal action. Ampicillin and amoxicillin, in addition to having a wider spectrum of antimicrobial activity, penetrate cellular barriers more readily than penicillin G. Their somewhat longer half-lives might be attributed to enterohepatic circulation. Penetration to cerebrospinal fluid (CSF) is usually poor but is enhanced by inflammation. In addition, active removal of penicillin from CSF is diminished by inflammation. The penicillins are eliminated almost entirely by renal excretion, which results in very high levels in the urine. The renal excretion mechanisms include glomerular filtration and mainly proximal tubular secretion.

Adverse Effects. Penicillins are remarkably free of toxic effects, even at doses grossly in excess of those recommended. The major adverse effect is acute anaphylaxis; milder hypersensitivity reactions (urticaria, fever, angioneurotic edema) are more common. All penicillins are cross-sensitizing and cross-reacting. Anaphylactic reactions are less common after oral penicillin administration than after parenteral administration. Many of the acute toxicities reported in animals are the toxic effects of the potassium or procaine with which the penicillin is combined. The use of penicillin and ampicillin in guinea pigs invariably causes fatal *Clostridium difficile* colitis, and use of ampicillin in rabbits causes fatal *C. difficile* or *Clostridium spiroforme* colitis.

Cephalosporins. Cephalosporins are natural or semisynthetic products of the fungi *Cephalosporium* spp.; the related cephamycins are derived from the actinomycetes type of bacteria. The nucleus of the semisynthetic cephalosporins, 7-aminocephalosporanic acid, bears a close structural resemblance to that of the penicillins, which accounts for a common mechanism of action and other properties shared by these two classes of drugs. They are bactericidal. Like the penicillins, cephalosporins have short half-lives, and most are excreted unchanged in the urine. Attachment of various R groups to the cephalosporanic acid nucleus has resulted in compounds with low toxicity and high therapeutic activity. Though not an ideal description, the classification of cephalosporins as belonging to four generations relates to their increasing spectrum of activity against gram-negative bacteria because of improved penetration of cells and their progressive resistance to the β-lactamases of gram-negative bacteria.

Antimicrobial Activity. The first-generation cephalosporins (e.g., cephalothin, cephalexin, cephaloridine, and cefadroxil) have a similar spectrum of activity to ampicillin, with the notable difference that β-lactamase-producing staphylococci are susceptible. They are active against a variety of gram-positive bacteria such as coagulase-positive staphylococci, many streptococci (except enterococci), corynebacteria, and gram-positive anaerobes (*Clostridium*). Among gram-negative bacteria, *Haemophilus* and *Pasteurella* are susceptible, as are some *Escherichia coli*, *Klebsiella*, *Proteus*, and *Salmonella*. *Enterobacter* and *P. aeruginosa* are resistant. Many anaerobic bacteria, except members of the *Bacteroides fragilis* group, are susceptible. The second-generation cephalosporins (e.g., cefoxitin and cefuroxime) have increased resistance to gram-negative β-lactamases and thus broader activity against gram-negative bacteria as well as against bacteria susceptible to the first-generation drugs. They are active against some strains of *Enterobacter* and against cephalothin-resistant *E. coli*, *Klebsiella*, and *Proteus*. Some *B. fragilis* are susceptible. Like the first-generation cephalosporins, these drugs are not active against *P. aeruginosa* or *Serratia*. The third-generation cephalosporins (e.g., cefotaxime, ceftiofur, and cefoperazone) are characterized by reduced activity against gram-positive bacteria, modest activity against *P. aeruginosa*, and remarkable activity against members of the family Enterobacteriaceae. Some third-generation cephalosporins (e.g., ceftazidime) are highly active against *P. aeruginosa* at the expense of activity against members of the family Enterobacteriaceae. Fourth-generation cephalosporins (e.g., cefepime and cefpirome) have very broad-spectrum activity and are stable to hydrolysis by many β-lactamases.

Resistance. Methicillin-resistant coagulase-positive staphylococci are resistant to all generations of cephalosporins. Plasmid-mediated resistance to first-, second-, and third-generation drugs has been described in gram-negative bacteria. Emergence of resistance in *Enterobacter*, *Serratia*, and *P. aeruginosa* during treatment with third-generation drugs results from derepression of inducible, chromosomal β-lactamase enzymes, which in turn results in broad-spectrum resistance to β-lactam antibiotics. In addition, plasmid-mediated resistance to third-generation cephalosporins is increasingly reported. It can involve either TEM- or SHV-β-lactamases or other β-lactamase families including CTX-M1, which hydrolyses cefotaxime. These β-lactamases are inhibited by clavulanic acid. More recently, broad-spectrum cephalosporinases (cephamycinases), CMY-2 β-lactamases, have been recognized on plasmids of *E. coli* and *Salmonella*; these are not inhibited by clavulanic acid.

Absorption, Distribution, and Excretion. Cephalosporins are water-soluble drugs. Of the first-generation cephalosporins, cephalexin and cephadroxil are relatively acid-stable and sufficiently well absorbed from the intestine to be administered orally to dogs and cats, but not to herbivores. Other first-generation cephalosporins must be administered parenterally although they are often painful on intramuscular injection and irritating on intravenous injection. Second- and third-generation cephalosporins are sometimes available for oral use and could be given to dogs and cats by this route rather than parenterally. Following absorption from injection sites, cephalosporins are widely distributed into tissue and body fluids. Third-generation cephalosporins penetrate CSF moderately well, and because of their high activity against gram-negative bacteria have particular potential application in the treatment of meningitis.

Adverse Effects. Cephalosporins are relatively nontoxic antibiotics in humans. Allergic reactions occur in 5–10% of human patients who are hypersensitive to penicillin. Intravenous and intramuscular injections of some drugs are an irritant.

Other β-Lactam Antibiotics. Other naturally occurring β-lactam antibiotics discovered in recent years include the cephamycins, clavulanic acid, thienamycin, the monobactams (such as aztreonam), the carbapenems (such as imipenem), the PS-compounds, and the carpetimycins—all compounds with the basic β-lactam ring but without the bicyclic ring structure of the classical β-lactams. All are highly resistant to β-lactamases, and many possess potent antibacterial properties or are used in combination with earlier β-lactams (ampicillin, amoxicillin, ticarcillin) for their potent β-lactamase inhibitory effects (clavulanic acid, sulbactam, tazobactam). Carbapenems (biapenem, imipenem-cilastatin, meropenem) have exceptional activity against clinically important aerobic and anaerobic bacteria, with the greatest activity of all antimicrobials against gram-negative bacteria.

Damage to Cell Membrane Function

Antibiotics that damage cell membrane function include the polymyxins, monensin, and the antifungal polyenes (amphotericin, nystatin) and imidazoles (fluconazole, itraconazole, ketoconazole, miconazole), discussed under antifungal drugs. The cell membrane lies beneath the cell wall, enclosing the cytoplasm. It controls the passage of materials into or out of the cell. If its function is damaged, cellular contents (proteins, nucleotides, ions) can leak from the cell and result in cell damage and death.

Polymyxins. The structure of the polymyxins is such that they have well-defined separate hydrophilic and hydrophobic sectors. Polymyxins act by binding to membrane phospholipids, which results in structural disorganization, permeability damage, and cell lysis. The polymyxins are selectively toxic to gram-negative bacteria because of the presence of certain phospholipids in the cell membrane and because the outer surface of the outer membrane of gram-negative bacteria consists mainly of lipopolysaccharide. Parenteral use is associated with nephrotoxic, neurotoxic, and neuromuscular blocking effects. The major clinical applications are limited to the oral treatment of gram-negative bacterial infections, although these drugs are becoming again more commonly systemically in human patients, because of the absence of alternative treatments for multiresistant bacterial pathogens.

Inhibition of Nucleic Acid Function

Examples of drugs that inhibit nucleic acid function are nitroimidazoles, nitrofurans, nalidixic acid, the fluoroquinolones (ciprofloxacin, danofloxacin, difloxacin, enrofloxacin, orbifloxacin, sarafloxacin), novobiocin, rifampin, sulfonamides, trimethoprim, and 5-flucytosine. Because the mechanisms of nucleic acid synthesis, replication, and transcription are similar in all cells, drugs affecting nucleic acid function have poor selective toxicity. Most act by binding to DNA to inhibit its replication or transcription. Drugs with greater selective toxicity are the sulfonamides and trimethoprim, which inhibit the synthesis of folic acid.

Nitroimidazoles. Nitroimidazoles, such as metronidazole and dimetridazole, possess antiprotozoal and antibacterial properties. Activity within bacterial cells is due to the unidentified, reduced products of the drug, which are only seen in anaerobes or microaerophiles. Nitroimidazoles cause extensive DNA strand breakage either by inhibiting the DNA repair enzyme, DNase 1, or by forming complexes with the nucleotide bases that the enzyme does not recognize. Nitroimidazoles are bactericidal to anaerobic gram-negative and many gram-positive bacteria and are active against protozoa such as *Tritrichomonas fetus*, *Giardia lamblia*, and *Histomonas meleagridis*. Chromosomal resistance may cause slight increases in minimum inhibitory concentrations (MIC), but as is the case for nitrofurans, plasmid-encoded resistance is rare. Nitroimidazoles are generally well absorbed after oral administration, but parenteral injection is highly irritating. They are well distributed throughout body tissues and fluids, including brain and CSF. Excretion is through the urine. The most serious potential hazard is the controversial report of carcinogenicity in laboratory animals. For this reason, these drugs are not used in food animals.

Nitrofurans. Like the nitroimidazoles, the nitrofurans are antiprotozoal but have wider antibacterial activity; they are most active under anaerobic conditions. After entry into the cell, bacterial nitroreductases produce uncharacterized unstable reduction products, which differ with each type of nitrofuran. These products cause strand breakage in bacterial DNA. The nitrofurans are synthetic 5-nitrofuraldehyde derivatives with broad antimicrobial activity. Toxicity and low tissue concentrations limit their use to the local treatment of infections and to the treatment of urinary tract infections.

Fluoroquinolones. Fluoroquinolones (e.g., ciprofloxacin, danofloxacin, difloxacin, enrofloxacin, orbifloxacin, and sarafloxacin) are active against gram-negative bacteria. They cause selective inhibition of bacterial DNA synthesis by inhibiting DNA gyrase (topoisomerase II) and DNA topoisomerase IV. DNA gyrase is involved in packing (supercoiling) DNA into bacterial cells, whereas topoisomerase IV is involved in relaxing supercoiled DNA. Fluoroquinolones are bactericidal drugs. Nalidixic acid (a quinolone rarely used because of toxicity) is most active against gram-negative bacteria except *P. aeruginosa*, but the newer fluoroquinolone derivatives are broader spectrum and active against some gram-positive bacteria, including mycobacteria. Activity against *Mycoplasma* and rickettsia is also an important attribute of the newer fluoroquinolones. The fluoroquinolones are rapidly absorbed after oral administration and have half-lives varying from 4 to 12 h. They are widely distributed in tissues, and may be concentrated, for example, in the prostate. Penetration into CSF is about half that of serum, which makes these drugs useful to treat meningitis. They are being introduced rapidly into veterinary use, particularly for use against gram-negative bacteria and *Mycoplasma*. One significant drawback is the fairly rapid development of chromosomally mediated resistance, which in *Campylobacter jejuni* and *P. aeruginosa* can produce high-level resistance after single nucleotide mutations but is more gradual in other bacteria, usually as the result of cumulative rather than individual nucleotide mutations. Resistance can also result from decreased permeability of the cell wall as well as from acquisition or enhanced activity of an efflux pump that actively transports fluoroquinolones from the cell.

Rifampin. Rifampin, which has particular activity against gram-positive bacteria and mycobacteria, has remarkable selectivity of inhibition of bacterial DNA-dependent ribonucleic acid (RNA) polymerase. Rifampin prevents initiation of transcription. Resistance develops rapidly as the result of chromosomal mutation, so that this drug is rarely used on its own but rather is used in combination with other antimicrobial drugs.

Sulfonamides and Trimethoprim. Sulfonamides are synthetic drugs with broad antibacterial and antiprotozoal properties. They interfere with the biosynthesis of folic acid and prevent the formation of purine nucleotides. Sulfonamides are functional analogs of para-aminobenzoic acid (PABA) and compete with it for the same enzyme, tetrahydropteroate synthetase, forming nonfunctional folic acid analogs and inhibiting bacterial growth. Selective toxicity of sulfonamides occurs because mammalian cells have lost their ability to synthesize folic acid but rather absorb it from the intestine, whereas bacteria must synthesize it. In the bacterial cell, preformed folic acid is progressively exhausted by several bacterial divisions.

Other drugs affect folic acid synthesis by interfering with the enzyme dihydrofolate reductase. One example is trimethoprim, which is selectively toxic to bacteria rather than to mammalian cells because of greater affinity for the bacterial enzyme. The enzyme inhibits the conversion of dihydrofolate to tetrahydrofolate, producing with sulfonamides a sequential blockade of folic acid synthesis.

Sulfonamides. The sulfonamides constitute a series of weak organic acids that enter most tissues and body fluids. The degree of ionization and lipid solubility of the large number of individual sulfonamides influences absorption, determines capacity to penetrate cell membranes, and can affect the rate of elimination. Sulfonamides exert a bacteriostatic effect against both gram-positive and gram-negative bacteria and can also inhibit other microorganisms (some protozoa). They are available in a wide variety of preparations for either oral or parenteral use. They have largely been abandoned because of widespread resistance, difficulties in administration, and the existence of better alternatives. Certain individual sulfonamides are combined with trimethoprim in fixed ratio (5 : 1) combination preparations that have the advantage of both synergistic and bactericidal effects.

Individual sulfonamides are derivatives of sulfanilamide, which contains the structural prerequisites for antibacterial activity. The various derivatives differ in physicochemical and pharmacokinetic properties and in degree of antimicrobial activity. The sodium salts of sulfonamides are readily soluble in water, and parenteral preparations are available for intravenous administration. Certain sulfonamide molecules are designed for low solubility (e.g., phthalylsulfathiazole) so that they will be slowly absorbed; these are intended for use in the treatment of enteric infections.

Antimicrobial Activity. Sulfonamides are broad-spectrum antimicrobial drugs. They are active against aerobic gram-positive cocci and some rods and some gram-negative bacteria, including members of the family Enterobacteriaceae. Many anaerobes are sensitive.

Resistance. Resistance to sulfonamides in pathogenic and nonpathogenic bacteria isolated from animals is widespread. This situation reflects their extensive use in human and veterinary medicine for many years. Sulfonamide resistance may occur as a result of mutation causing overproduction of PABA or as a result of a structural change in the dihydrofolic acid-synthesizing enzyme with a lowered affinity for sulfonamides. Most often, sulfonamide resistance is plasmid mediated.

Absorption, Distribution, and Excretion. Most sulfonamides are rapidly absorbed from the gastrointestinal tract and distributed widely to all tissues and body fluids, including synovial and CSF. They are bound to plasma proteins to a variable extent. In addition to differences among sulfonamides in extent of binding, there is variation among species in binding of individual sulfonamides. Extensive (80%) protein binding serves to increase half-life. They enter CSF well.

Sulfonamides are eliminated by a combination of renal excretion and biotransformation processes in the liver. This combination of elimination processes contributes to the species variation in the half-life of individual sulfonamides. While a large number of sulfonamide preparations are available for use in veterinary medicine, many of these are different dosage forms of sulfamethazine. This sulfonamide is most widely used in the food-producing animals and can attain effective plasma concentrations (within the range 50–150 μg/ml) when administered either orally or parenterally. Due to their alkalinity, most parenteral preparations should only be administered by intravenous injection. Prolonged-release oral dosage forms of sulfamethazine are available.

Adverse Effects. The sulfonamides can produce a wide variety of side effects, some of which may have an allergic basis whereas others are due to direct toxicity. The more common adverse effects are urinary tract disturbances (crystalluria, hematuria, or even obstruction) and hematopoietic disorders (thrombocytopenia and leukopenia). Some adverse effects are associated with particular sulfonamides. Sulfadiazine and sulfasalazine given for long periods to dogs to control chronic hemorrhagic colitis have caused *keratoconjunctivitis sicca*.

Trimethoprim–Sulfonamide Combinations. Trimethoprim is combined with a variety of sulfonamides in a fixed ratio. The combination produces a bactericidal effect against a wide range of bacteria, with some important exceptions, and also inhibits certain other microorganisms. Veterinary preparations contain trimethoprim combined with sulfadiazine or sulfadoxine in the 1 : 5 ratio. Other antibacterial diaminopyrimidines combined with sulfonamides for use in animals include baquiloprim and ormetoprim.

Antimicrobial Activity. Trimethoprim-sulfonamide combinations have a generally broad-spectrum and usually bactericidal action against many gram-positive and gram-negative aerobic bacteria, including members of the family Enterobacteriaceae. The combination is active against a large proportion of anaerobic bacteria, at least under *in vitro* conditions. *Mycoplasma* and *P. aeruginosa* are resistant.

Synergism occurs when the microorganisms are sensitive to both drugs in the combination. When bacteria are resistant to sulfonamides, synergism may still be obtained in up to 40% of cases, even when bacteria are only moderately susceptible to trimethoprim. Because of differences between the trimethoprim and sulfonamide in distribution pattern and processes of elimination, the concentration ratios of the two drugs will differ considerably in tissues and urine from the ratio in the plasma. This variation is not important since the synergistic interaction occurs over a wide range of concentration ratios of the two drugs.

Resistance. Resistance to sulfonamides is due to structural alteration in the dihydrofolic acid synthesizing enzyme (dihydropteroate synthetase), whereas resistance to trimethoprim usually results from plasmid-encoded synthesis of a resistant dihydrofolate reductase enzyme. Bacterial resistance to the combination has progressively developed with use of these preparations in animals.

Absorption, Distribution, and Elimination. Trimethoprim is a lipid-soluble organic base that is approximately 60% bound to plasma proteins and 60% ionized in the plasma. This combination of physicochemical properties enables the drug to distribute widely, to penetrate cellular barriers by nonionic diffusion, and to attain effective concentrations in most body fluids and tissues, including brain and CSF. Hepatic metabolism is the principal process for elimination of trimethoprim. The half-life and fraction of the dose that is excreted unchanged in the urine vary widely among different species. The drug is well absorbed following oral administration in dogs, cats, and horses or from injection sites in these and other species.

Adverse Effects. Serious side effects are uncommon; those that do occur can usually be attributed to the sulfonamide component. Oral trimethoprim-sulfonamide has the advantage over other oral antimicrobials of causing little disturbance among the normal intestinal anaerobic microflora.

Inhibition of Protein Synthesis

Examples of drugs that inhibit protein synthesis are tetracyclines; aminoglycosides (amikacin, gentamicin, kanamycin, neomycin, streptomycin, tobramycin, and others); aminocyclitols (spectinomycin); chloramphenicol; lincosamides (clindamycin, lincomycin); and macrolides (azithromycin, clarithromycin, erythromycin, tylosin, tiamulin, and others). Because of the marked differences in ribosomal structure, composition, and function between prokaryotic and eukaryotic cells, many important antibacterial drugs selectively inhibit bacterial protein synthesis. Antibiotics affecting protein synthesis can be divided into those affecting the 30S ribosome (tetracyclines, aminoglycosides, aminocyclitols) and those affecting the 50S ribosome (chloramphenicol, macrolides, lincosamides).

Tetracyclines. Tetracyclines interfere with protein synthesis by inhibiting the binding of aminoacyl tRNA to the recognition site. The various tetracyclines have similar antimicrobial activity but differ in pharmacologic characteristics.

Antimicrobial Activity. Tetracyclines are broad-spectrum drugs active against gram-positive and gram-negative bacteria, including rickettsia and chlamydia, some mycoplasmas, and protozoa such as *Theileria*. Tetracyclines have good activity against many gram-positive bacteria, the more fastidious nonenteric bacteria such as *Actinobacillus, Bordetella, Brucella, Haemophilus*, some *Pasteurella*, and many anaerobic bacteria, but their activity against these bacteria and against members of the family Enterobacteriaceae are limited by acquired resistance. *P. aeruginosa* is resistant, except in urinary tract infections where, because of their high concentrations, tetracyclines may be drugs of choice.

Resistance. Widespread resistance to the tetracyclines has considerably reduced their usefulness, which is largely limited to intracellular bacterial pathogens of different types. Such resistance is high level and usually plasmid- and transposon-mediated. Cross-resistance between tetracyclines is complete.

Adverse Effects. Tetracyclines are generally safe antibiotics with a reasonably high therapeutic index. The main adverse effects are associated with their severely irritant nature, with disturbances in gastrointestinal flora, with their ability to bind calcium (cardiovascular effects, teeth or bone deposition), and with the toxic effects of degradation products on liver and kidney cells. Their use in horses has largely been abandoned because of a tendency to produce broad-spectrum suppression of the normal intestinal flora and fatal superinfection with *Salmonella* or *C. difficile*.

Chloramphenicol and Florfenicol. Chloramphenicol and florfenicol are broad-spectrum, generally bacteriostatic drugs that bind the 50S ribosome, distorting the region and inhibiting the peptidyl transferase reaction. They are stable, lipid-soluble, neutral compounds.

Antimicrobial Activity. Chloramphenicol and florfenicol are active against gram-positive and gram-negative bacteria, including chlamydia and rickettsia, and some mycoplasmas. Most gram-positive and many gram-negative pathogenic aerobic and anaerobic bacteria are susceptible, though resistance is increasing in members of the family Enterobacteriaceae. Florfenicol is less active against members of the family Enterobacteriaceae but has high activity against *Haemophilus, Mannheimia haemolytica*, and *Pasteurella*. The drugs are generally bacteriostatic.

Resistance. Most resistance is the result of plasmid-encoded acetylase enzymes.

Absorption, Distribution, and Excretion. In dogs, cats, and preruminants, chloramphenicol is well absorbed from the intestine; in ruminants the drug is inactivated after oral administration. Because of its low molecular weight, lipid solubility, and modest plasma protein binding, the drug is well distributed in most tissues and fluids, including the CSF and aqueous humor. The half-life of chloramphenicol varies widely in animals from a low of 1 h in horses to 5 or 6 h in cats. In neonates, the half-life is considerably longer. The drug is mainly eliminated by glucuronide conjugation in the liver.

Adverse Effects. The fatal aplastic anemia seen in 1 in 25 000–40 000 humans treated with chloramphenicol does not occur in animals, although prolonged high dosing may cause reversible abnormalities in bone marrow activity. The potential for nondose-related fatal aplastic anemia in humans has led to its prohibition for use in food animals in most countries because of fear of the presence of drug residues in meat products. Florfenicol does not have this effect and so has selective use for food animals.

Aminoglycosides

The aminoglycosides are bactericidal. The mode of action of streptomycin is best understood. Streptomycin has a variety of complex effects in the bacterial cell: (a) it binds to a specific receptor protein in the 30S ribosomal subunit, distorting the codon–anticodon interactions at the recognition site and causing misreading of the genetic code so that faulty proteins are produced; (b) it binds to "initiating" ribosomes to prevent the formation of 70S ribosomes; and (c) it inhibits the elongation reaction of protein synthesis. The other aminoglycosides act similarly to streptomycin in causing mistranslation of the genetic code and in irreversible inhibition of initiation, although the extent and type often differ. They have multiple binding sites on the ribosome, whereas streptomycin has only one, and can also inhibit the translocation step in protein synthesis. Spectinomycin is a bacteriostatic aminocyclitol antibiotic that is believed to inhibit polypeptide chain elongation at the translocation step.

The aminoglycoside antibiotics are polar organic bases. Their polarity largely accounts for the similar pharmacokinetic properties that are shared by all members of the group. Chemically, they consist of a hexose nucleus to which amino sugars are attached by glycosidic linkages. All are potentially ototoxic and nephrotoxic. The newer aminoglycosides are more resistant to plasmid-mediated enzymatic degradation and are less toxic than the older compounds. Amikacin > tobramycin > gentamicin > neomycin = kanamycin > streptomycin in potency, spectrum of activity, and stability to plasmid-mediated resistance. This activity mirrors the chronology of introduction of the drugs, with streptomycin being the oldest of the aminoglycosides.

Antimicrobial Activity. Aminoglycosides are particularly active against gram-negative bacteria as well as against mycobacteria and some *Mycoplasma*. Anaerobic bacteria are usually resistant. As a general rule, gram-positive bacteria are resistant to older drugs (streptomycin, neomycin) but may be inhibited by newer drugs (gentamicin, amikacin). A particularly useful property is the activity of newer aminoglycosides against *P. aeruginosa*. Their bactericidal action on aerobic gram-negative bacilli is markedly influenced by pH; they are most active in an alkaline environment.

Increased local acidity secondary to tissue damage may account for the failure of an aminoglycoside to kill usually susceptible microorganisms at infection sites or in abscess cavities. Combinations of aminoglycosides with penicillins are often synergistic; the concurrent administration of the newer β-lactam antibiotics with gentamicin or tobramycin has been used to treat serious gram-negative infections, for example, those caused by *P. aeruginosa*.

Resistance. Most clinically important resistance is caused by a variety of plasmid-specified degradative enzymes located in the periplasmic space. Certain of these enzymes inactivate only the older aminoglycosides (streptomycin, or neomycin and kanamycin), but others are broader spectrum. The remarkable property of amikacin is its resistance to many of the enzymes that inactivate other aminoglycosides. Plasmid-mediated and transposon-based resistance to streptomycin is widespread and commonly linked to sulfonamides, tetracyclines, and ampicillin. Chromosomal resistance to streptomycin, but not to the other aminoglycosides, develops fairly readily during treatment.

Absorption, Distribution, and Excretion. Aminoglycosides are poorly absorbed from the gastrointestinal tract, bind to a low extent to plasma proteins, and have limited capacity to enter cells and to penetrate cellular barriers. They do not readily attain therapeutic concentrations in transcellular fluids, particularly cerebrospinal and ocular fluid. Poor diffusibility is because of their low degree of lipid solubility. Their apparent volumes of distribution are relatively small, and their half-lives are short (2 h) in domestic animals. Even though these drugs have a small volume of distribution, selective binding to renal tissue (kidney cortex) occurs. Elimination takes place entirely by renal excretion (glomerular filtration), and unchanged drug is rapidly excreted in the urine. Impaired renal function decreases their rate of excretion and makes adjustment of the maintenance dosage necessary to prevent accumulation with attendant toxicity.

Major changes have taken place in recommendations for intramuscular dosage with aminoglycosides, which has moved from three times daily to a single daily dosage. This has the effect of increasing therapeutic efficacy, since antibacterial activity depends on both peak concentrations and total concentration, and of reducing toxicity, since the nephrotoxic effects depend on a threshold effect, concentrations above which have no further action. This dramatically changed understanding of aminoglycoside dosage may increase the use of the less toxic members.

Adverse Effects. All aminoglycosides can cause varying degrees of ototoxicity and nephrotoxicity. The tendency to produce vestibular or cochlear damage varies with the drug: neomycin is the most likely to cause cochlear damage and streptomycin to cause vestibular damage. Nephrotoxicity (acute tubular necrosis) occurs in association with prolonged therapy and excessive trough concentrations of the aminoglycoside (particularly gentamicin) in plasma. The aminoglycosides can produce neuromuscular blockage of the nondepolarizing type, which causes flaccid paralysis and apnea. This is most likely to occur in association with anesthesia.

Aminocyclitols. Spectinomycin is an aminocyclitol antibiotic with a spectrum of activity and mechanism of action similar to that of kanamycin but without the toxic effects of the aminoglycosides. It is normally bacteriostatic and is not particularly active on a weight basis. Its activity against gram-negative bacteria is unpredictable because of naturally resistant strains. Chromosomal resistance develops readily but does not cross-react with aminoglycosides. Plasmid resistance is uncommon but often extends to streptomycin. The drug has most of the pharmacokinetic properties of aminoglycosides but appears to penetrate CSF better. It has been used in agricultural practice to treat salmonellosis and mycoplasma infections.

Macrolides. Macrolide antibiotics are bacteriostatic with activity particularly against gram-positive bacteria and *Mycoplasma*. They bind to 50S ribosome in competition with chloramphenicol and inhibit the translocation step of protein synthesis. The precise mechanism of action is unknown. Macrolide antibiotics (azithromycin, clarithromycin, erythromycin, tylosin, tiamulin, tulathromycin, and spiramycin) have action and pharmacokinetic properties similar to the lincosamides. Like the lincosamides they are lipid soluble, basic drugs that are concentrated in tissue compared to serum and penetrate cells well.

Antimicrobial Activity. Erythromycin has an antibacterial spectrum similar to penicillin G, but it includes activity against penicillinase-producing coagulase-positive staphylococci, *Campylobacter*, *Leptospira*, *Bordetella*, rickettsia, chlamydia, some *Mycoplasma*, and atypical mycobacteria. It may be bactericidal at high concentrations. Tylosin and spiramycin are less active than erythromycin against bacteria but more active against a broad range of *Mycoplasma*. Tiamulin has better activity than the other macrolides against anaerobes, including *Brachyspira hyodysenteriae*, and is distinguished for its remarkable activity against mycoplasmas. Azithromycin and clarithromycin are particularly active against nontuberculous mycobacteria. The activity of these two drugs against a variety of intracellular bacteria depends not only on their intrinsic activity but also on the often remarkable concentration of the drugs in cells, including macrophages. Azithromycin may concentrate 200–500-fold inside macrophages compared to its serum concentrations.

Resistance. One-step chromosomal resistance to erythromycin develops fairly readily, even during treatment, but is generally unstable. Plasmid-mediated resistance is common. Cross-resistance between erythromycin and lincosamides and other macrolides is common. There is little information about resistance of veterinary pathogens to tylosin. Development of resistance to tiamulin appears to be relatively uncommon; organisms resistant to tiamulin show one-way cross-resistance with other macrolides.

Absorption, Distribution, and Excretion. Erythromycin stearate and estolate are well absorbed after oral administration, but the base is not. Intramuscular injection of erythromycin is very irritating. The absorption of tylosin from the intestine varies with the formulation. Tiamulin is well absorbed. These drugs are well distributed through body tissues and fluids, except the CSF. Tissue concentrations often exceed serum concentrations, notably for azithromycin and clarithromycin, which are, therefore, often dosed once a day or less frequently. In the case of spiramycin, such tissue concentration is extreme and is associated with tissue binding. A large proportion of these drugs is degraded in the body, but some is excreted through the kidney and the liver.

Adverse Effects. Macrolides are generally safe drugs though painful on injection. Their potential for causing irreversible diarrhea in adult horses means that they should be avoided in this species. The drugs should not be given orally to ruminants because of their potential for disturbing the rumen flora.

Lincosamides. Lincomycin and clindamycin have antibacterial activity mainly against gram-positive aerobic bacteria and against anaerobic bacteria. The drugs bind the 50S ribosomal subunits at binding sites that overlap with those of chloramphenicol and the macrolides. They inhibit the peptidyl transferase reaction. The lincosamides, lincomycin and clindamycin, are products of an actinomycete with activity and mechanism of action similar to that of the macrolides. Lincomycin is most commonly used in veterinary medicine, although it is less active on a weight basis than clindamycin. Lincosamides are active against gram-positive aerobic and all anaerobic bacteria, and against mycoplasmas, but most gram-negative aerobes are resistant. Clindamycin is more active than lincomycin against anaerobes and may be bactericidal.

Chromosomal stepwise resistance develops fairly readily, and plasmid-mediated resistance is common. Cross-resistance between lincosamides is complete and commonly occurs also with macrolides. Lincomycin is readily absorbed after oral or intramuscular administration. Food delays and reduces absorption. The absorption of different clindamycin compounds is variable. The lincosamides are widely distributed in body tissues and fluids, including the prostate and milk, but CSF concentrations are low. They penetrate intracellularly because of their lipophilic properties. Most excretion is through the liver. The major adverse effect of lincosamides is their ability to cause fatal *C. difficile* typhlocolitis in horses, rabbits, guinea pigs, and hamsters. In rabbits, fatal diarrhea may also result from proliferation of *C. spiroforme*. Oral lincosamides at low concentrations produce severe ruminal disturbances in adult ruminants.

Antimicrobial Susceptibility and Drug Dosage Prediction

The use of antimicrobial drugs in treating infections depends on the relation of the quantitative susceptibility of the microorganism to tissue concentrations of drug. The antimicrobial susceptibility of many veterinary pathogens is predictable and clinical experience has established effective dosages for infections caused by these organisms. In many bacteria, however, the presence of various mechanisms for acquiring resistance means that susceptibility to a particular antibacterial drug may need to be tested.

Antimicrobial Susceptibility Testing

There are two general methods for antimicrobial susceptibility testing *in vitro*: the dilution method and the diffusion method. The dilution method gives quantitative information on drug susceptibility while the diffusion method gives qualitative (or at best semiquantitative) information. The tests must be performed under standardized conditions. The description of a bacterium as susceptible or resistant to an antimicrobial drug depends ultimately on clinical success or failure of treatment. Quantitative information on susceptibility is obtained in the laboratory under artificial circumstances, which cannot easily take into account host defenses, the dynamics of drug disposition, or the dynamics of interaction of a varying drug concentration with a bacterium in the host environment. Nevertheless, infections caused by bacteria classified as resistant in susceptibility tests rarely respond successfully to treatment, except under exceptional circumstances. Infections caused by bacteria classified as susceptible can be predicted to do so, depending, however, on the clinical circumstances, the nature of the infection, appropriate dosage, and a variety of other factors, some of which are discussed later.

Dilution Antimicrobial Tests. Antimicrobial drugs of known potency are prepared in doubling dilutions of concentrations similar to those achievable in the tissues of patients given usual drug dosages. The highest dilution at which there is no visible bacterial growth following inoculation and incubation is the MIC, which is usually less than the minimum bactericidal concentration (MBC) for drugs (Table 4.1).

Table 4.1. Minimum Concentration of Tetracycline Inhibitory to Selected Veterinary Pathogens

	Minimum Inhibitory Concentration (μg/ml)	
	MIC_{50}[a]	MIC_{90}[a]
Bordetella bronchiseptica	2	2
Brucella canis	0.25	0.25
Corynebacterium pseudotuberculosis	0.25	0.25
Escherichia coli	4.0	64.0
Klebsiella pneumoniae	2.0	64.0
Mycoplasma canis	4.0	8.0
Pasteurella multocida	0.5	0.5

[a]Highest MIC_{50} of 50% of isolates tested, MIC_{90} of 90% of isolates tested. The MIC of different organisms varies with strain and species.

The advantage of determining quantitative susceptibility of an organism is that this information can be related to knowledge of drug concentrations in particular tissues in the prediction of appropriate drug dosage. In medical practice, MIC results are usually interpreted by the system of categories suggested by the US Clinical Laboratory Standards Institute (CLSI). These interpretative guidelines take into account the inherent susceptibility of the organism to each drug, the pharmacokinetic and pharmacodynamic properties of the particular drug, dosage, site of infection, and drug toxicity. These categories are (1) susceptible, meaning that the infecting organism is usually inhibited by concentrations of a particular antibiotic attained in tissues by usual dosage; (2) intermediately susceptible, meaning that the infecting organism is inhibited by blood or tissue concentrations achieved with maximum dosage; and (3) resistant, meaning that it is resistant to normally achievable and tolerated concentrations of antimicrobial drugs. A fourth category, flexible, has been introduced by the CLSI Subcommittee on Veterinary Antimicrobial Susceptibility Testing. This indicates the availability in the United States of the US Food and Drug Administration flexible label, which allows veterinarians to adjust the dose, within a given range, based on the MIC of the pathogen.

Diffusion Antimicrobial Tests. A standard concentration of a pure culture of the pathogen is placed on appropriate agar and individual filter paper discs containing known concentrations of individual antibiotics are placed on the agar, which is incubated for 18 h at 35 °C. The zone of inhibition around each disc is measured and the measurement is referred to a chart that classifies the organism as being susceptible, resistant, or intermediately susceptible to the particular antibiotic in each disc. Standards for performing these tests are defined. Under standard conditions, there is a linear inverse relationship between the diameter of the zone of growth inhibition and MIC. The interpretation of zone diameters as susceptible, resistant, or intermediate relates to serum drug concentrations of antibiotics in different animal species commonly achievable under standard dosage regimens. From these drug concentrations, MIC breakpoints have been selected and extrapolated to zone diameters in providing the interpretative standards. A specialized modified diffusion system is the E test, which is a modified diffusion concentration gradient strip system that gives quantitative results.

Design of Drug Dosage and Pharmacodynamic Properties

Pharmacokinetic descriptions of drug disposition in different animal species, when combined with quantitative susceptibility (MIC) data and knowledge of the pharmacodynamic properties of the antimicrobial, allow prediction of reasonable drug dosage in animals.

Pharmacokinetic properties include the route of administration, rate of absorption, rate of distribution, volume of distribution, and route and rate of elimination. Pharmacodynamic properties include concentration versus time in the tissue and other body fluids, as well as at the site of infection, toxicologic effect, and antimicrobial effect at the site of infection. The pharmacodynamic effects at the site of infection include the MIC, MBC, concentration-dependent killing effect, postantibiotic effect, sub-MIC effect, postantibiotic leukocyte enhancement effect, as well as first exposure effect. For the "concentration-dependent" antimicrobials (aminoglycosides, fluoroquinolones), killing is a function of antimicrobial concentration relative to MIC, a function that may persist long after drug concentrations are below MIC. For these drugs, the total amount of the drug above MIC ("area under the curve") is also important. By contrast, for the "time-dependent" antimicrobials (β-lactams, chloramphenicol, lincosamides, macrolides, tetracyclines, trimethoprim-sulfonamides), bacterial inhibition is a function of the time that tissue concentrations exceed MIC; these drugs, therefore, have to be dosed to maintain concentrations at the site of infection above MIC. For these drugs, the total amount of drug above MIC is not important since no additional killing occurs with increased concentrations (and indeed for some drugs killing may actually decrease at high concentrations). The maximum interval of drug dosing should preclude resumption of bacterial growth.

Factors Affecting Tissue Drug Concentrations

Dosage. The dosage regimen is made up of the size of the dose, which is limited by drug toxicity, and the dosage interval, which is determined by the half-life of the drug. The dosage interval required to maintain therapeutic tissue concentrations by intravenous dosing should not exceed twice the half-life for most antibiotics, but giving drugs by other routes lengthens the dosage interval.

Routes of Administration. Antibacterial drugs can be administered by a wide variety of routes—for example, intravenous, intramuscular, oral, subcutaneous, intramammary, intrauterine, or respiratory:

1. Intravenous injection of a drug gives immediate high serum drug concentrations, which rapidly decline as the drug is distributed. Intravenous dosing may be the only way to exceed the MIC of some pathogens, but frequent dosing by this route is generally impractical in veterinary medicine.
2. Intramuscular injection is commonly used in veterinary medicine because it gives good serum concentrations within 1–2 h of administration. The major advantage is that intramuscular injection gives the highest serum concentration of all routes other than intravenous, although subcutaneous injection is a reasonable alternative. Drug formulation can be prepared to give slow release of the drug after intramuscular injection and thus prolong dosage intervals to reduce handling of animals.
3. The oral administration of antimicrobial drugs is limited to monogastric and preruminant animals and to young foals. The oral dose is generally several times greater than the parenteral dose because the drug is less well absorbed. Although the oral route is often the easiest way to administer drugs, it is not always the most reliable. Some drugs (aminoglycosides, polymyxins) are not absorbed from the

intestine, others are destroyed by stomach acidity (benzyl penicillin), and absorption may be impaired by food (as occurs with ampicillin, tetracyclines, lincomycin). Administration of antibiotics in water is nevertheless a particularly simple, convenient, and inexpensive way to treat livestock because it involves little if any handling of animals and avoids the expense of mixing antibiotics in feed.

4. Infections of the udder, female genital tract, external ear canal, and skin are commonly treated by local application of antibiotics. High drug concentrations are obtained without systemic toxic effects. The concentration of free drug in the serum largely determines the concentration in tissue fluids, since penetration of drugs into interstitial fluids in most tissues of the body is through pores in capillary endothelium.

Physicochemical Properties of the Drug. These characteristics largely determine the extent of the distribution of a drug in the body. Most antimicrobial drugs distribute well in extravascular tissue fluids, principally the interstitial fluid. They penetrate capillary endothelium through pores that admit molecules with a molecular weight of less than about 1000. Passage across biological membranes such as into tissue cells or across nonfenestrated capillary endothelium depends on drug ionization, lipid solubility, molecular weight, and the amount of free drug present. Lipid-soluble and nonionized drugs such as the macrolides and chloramphenicol distribute well and even concentrate in tissue, whereas ionized and weakly lipid-soluble drugs such as penicillins and aminoglycosides distribute poorly. These physicochemical differences largely determine the pharmacokinetic characteristics of the drugs; thus, aminoglycosides and penicillins have small apparent volumes of distribution and short half-lives after intravenous injection and are eliminated through the urinary tract, whereas macrolides and tetracyclines have large apparent volumes of distribution and longer half-lives and are eliminated in part through the liver. Penetration of special sites in the body such as the central nervous system, eye, and prostate (which among other differences lack capillary pores) is only by low molecular weight, lipid-soluble, nonionized drugs.

Protein Binding of Drug. In general, serum protein binding of drugs up to 90% is of little clinical importance. Aminoglycosides and polymyxin bind extensively to intracellular constituents and thus are inactivated by pus.

Excretion Mechanisms. These determine the concentration of drugs in the organs of excretion. Remarkably high concentrations of drugs may be achieved in urine or bile.

Physiological Barriers. Anatomic-physiologic barriers in the brain, CSF, eye, and mammary gland reduce the entry of drugs from the blood. Inflammation reduces but does not abolish these barriers.

Duration of Treatment. Although it is axiomatic that a drug must be present for adequate time at the site of infection, the variables affecting time of treatment have not been defined. The response of different types of infection to antibiotics varies, and clinical experience with different types of infection is important in assessing response to treatment. In general, if no response to treatment is observed after 2 days, diagnosis and treatment should be reassessed. Treatment should be continued for 48 h after symptoms have resolved, depending on the severity of infection. For serious infections, treatment should last 7–10 days. Some uncomplicated infections, such as cystitis in women, have been successfully treated with single doses of antibiotics.

Use of Antibacterial Combinations. Combinations of drugs sometimes have dramatic success where individual drugs fail. An outstanding early historical example was the use of penicillin-streptomycin combinations in enterococcal endocarditis in humans. However, early studies of the outcome of combination treatment of pneumococcal meningitis in humans showed the serious clinical effects of mixing bacteriostatic and bactericidal drugs. The importance of antagonistic interactions between drugs is greatest in those infections or patients where immune defenses are poor (meningitis, endocarditis, or chronic osteomyelitis), or where immunodeficiencies are present, and where a bactericidal action is needed. If a bacteriostatic drug is mixed with a bactericidal drug, then the former may neutralize the latter, which may be crucial for clearance of infection from certain sites or infections (meningitis, endocarditis, chronic osteomyelitis). In other patients or diseases, because of the complexity of the host-bacterial–antimicrobial interaction, it is harder to detect either synergistic or antagonistic effects clinically, and it is likely that antagonistic effects of drugs are "laboratory artifacts" with no clinical meaning.

A drug combination is additive if the combined effect of several drugs is the sum of their independent activities measured separately, synergistic if the combined effect is significantly greater than their independent effects, and antagonistic if it is significantly less than their independent effects. Synergism and antagonism are not absolute characteristics; such interactions are often difficult to predict, vary with bacterial species and strains, and may occur only over a narrow range of concentrations. No single *in vitro* method detects all such interactions. The methods used to determine *in vitro* interactions are generally time-consuming and are not often available in the laboratory.

Antimicrobial combinations are frequently synergistic if they involve the following mechanisms: (1) sequential inhibition of successive steps in metabolism (e.g., trimethoprim-sulfonamide combination); (2) sequential inhibition of cell wall synthesis (e.g., vancomycin-penicillin and mecillinam-ampicillin); (3) facilitation of drug entry of one antibiotic by another (e.g., β-lactam-aminoglycoside and polymyxin-sulfonamide); (4) inhibition of inactivating enzymes (e.g., ampicillin-clavulanic acid); and (5) prevention of emergence of resistant populations (e.g., erythromycin-rifampin combination against *Rhodococcus equi*).

As suggested earlier, to some extent, antagonism between antibiotic combinations is a laboratory artifact that depends on the method of measurement and is thus, with some exceptions, unimportant clinically. The antagonistic effects of some combinations are, however, detected clinically. Antagonism may occur if antimicrobial combinations involve the following mechanisms: (1) inhibition of bactericidal activity (e.g., bacteriostatic and bactericidal drugs used to treat meningitis where, depending on the time-dose relation, bactericidal effects are prevented); (2) competition for drug binding sites (e.g., macrolide-chloramphenicol combinations, which are of unclear clinical significance); (3) inhibition of cell permeability mechanisms (e.g., chloramphenicol or tetracycline-aminoglycoside combinations, which are of unclear clinical significance); and (4) derepression of resistance enzymes (e.g., new third-generation cephalosporin antibiotics with older β-lactam drugs).

Antifungal Chemotherapy

The susceptibility of fungi to different drugs is often, but not always, predictable. Fungal drug susceptibility testing is technically complex and simple methods paralleling the disk diffusion antibacterial susceptibility test are not generally available.

Antifungal Agents for Topical Use

Many chemicals have antifungal properties and are used for topical treatment of fungal infections of the skin and sometimes of the mucosal surfaces. These include phenolic antiseptics such as hexachlorophene; iodides; quaternary ammonium antiseptics; 8-hydroxyquinoline; salicylamide; propionic, salicylic, and undecanoic acids; and chlorphenesin. Among the more effective topical broad-spectrum antifungal drugs are natamycin (a polyene antimicrobial), clotrimazole (an imidazole compound), nystatin (a polyene antimicrobial), and ketoconazole and miconazole (some of which are briefly described in Section "Antifungal Agents for Systemic Use").

Antifungal Agents for Systemic Use

Historically, the major antifungal drug for systemic use, amphotericin B, had the disadvantages of toxicity and intravenous administration, but it did have the advantage of fungicidal activity. The development of the imidazoles (ketoconazole, itraconazole, and fluconazole) was a major advance in systemic fungal therapy because of their oral administration, relative lack of toxicity, and effectiveness.

Griseofulvin. Griseofulvin is a fungistatic antimicrobial that inhibits mitosis and is active only against dermatophytes (ringworm fungi). Resistance in some dermatophytes has been reported to develop during treatment. Griseofulvin is effective against ringworm fungi only if administered orally. The drug is incorporated into keratin in the basal cells of the epidermis and reaches the superficial dead and parasitized keratinized epithelium through progressive maturation of the basal cells.

Amphotericin. Amphotericin B is a polyene antimicrobial, like nystatin, which binds ergosterol, the principal sterol of the fungal membrane, causing leakage of the cell contents. It is a broad-spectrum, generally fungicidal antimicrobial. It is active against *Blastomyces dermatitidis*, *Candida* spp., *Coccidioides immitis*, *Cryptococcus neoformans*, *Histoplasma capsulatum*, and *Sporothrix schenckii*. Strains of filamentous fungi, though commonly susceptible, vary from extreme susceptibility to resistance. Amphotericin B must be administered intravenously. Renal toxicity is an inevitable side effect of such treatment and must be monitored; the effect is reversible if the drug is stopped. Amphotericin is still an important drug available for treating systemic mycoses caused by dimorphic fungi and by yeasts. The drug is given by slow intravenous injection, usually every other day over 6–10 weeks.

Flucytosine. 5-flucytosine is deaminated in the fungal cell to 5-fluorouracil, which is incorporated into messenger RNA to produce garbled codons and faulty proteins. It has a narrow-spectrum of activity, which includes many *Candida* and most *C. neoformans*, but most filamentous fungi are resistant. Resistance develops readily during treatment. Therefore, flucytosine is often used only in combination with other drugs, usually amphotericin.

Imidazoles. Imidazoles interfere with the biosynthesis of ergosterol and bind fungal cell membrane phospholipids to cause leakage of cell contents. Fluconazole, itraconazole, ketoconazole, and miconazole are fungistatic against a wide range of yeasts, dimorphic fungi, and dermatophytes; they also have some antibacterial and antiprotozoal activity. Ketoconazole, itraconazole, and fluconazole are more active than miconazole and are the drugs favored for systemic administration because they can be given orally rather than intravenously. They produce few significant adverse effects in humans and animals, but liver damage has been reported in people given ketoconazole. They appear to be an effective treatment for many systemic fungal infections in dogs and cats, but there has been little experience with their use in other animal species. They have the disadvantage of fungistatic action; prolonged treatment may be necessary in serious infections to prevent the relapses that have occurred, and this is expensive.

Resistance to Antibacterial Drugs

The speed and scale with which resistance has emerged in many bacterial pathogens has caught many veterinarians and physicians by surprise. Resistance has increased markedly in the last two decades. In human medicine, the antibiotic resistance crisis has taken the approaches to treating some totally resistant bacterial infections back to the preantibiotic era, including surgery such as the amputation of infected limbs. The emergence and spread of highly resistant bacteria is a serious threat to modern medicine and surgery.

The potential for mutation and for genetic exchange between all types of bacteria, combined with the short bacterial generation time, is of major importance in limiting the use of antimicrobial drugs in controlling infection in animals and humans. The use of antimicrobial drugs does not induce resistance in bacteria but rather eliminates the susceptible bacteria and leaves the resistant bacteria already present in the population. The exposure of animals to antimicrobials is the basis of selection for the evolution and spread of resistance genes and resistant bacteria. The genetic processes involved in the development of resistance in bacteria are precisely those involved in the evolution of bacteria generally; it is natural, Darwinian, selection for "fitness."

Resistance to antimicrobial drugs can be classified as constitutive or acquired.

Constitutive Resistance

Microorganisms may be resistant to certain antibiotics because the cellular mechanisms required for antibiotic susceptibility are absent from the cell. Bacteria in the genus *Mycoplasma*, for example, are resistant to benzyl penicillin G because they lack a cell wall; similarly *E. coli* is resistant to penicillin G largely because the drug fails to penetrate into the cell.

Acquired Resistance

Acquired, genetically based, resistance can arise because of mutation or, more importantly, through horizontal gene transfer ("transferable drug resistance")—the acquisition of genetic material from other bacteria by different means (bacteriophages, plasmids, transformation, or transposons). Mutations, especially in the chromosome, tend to produce changes in bacterial cell structures, whereas horizontal gene transfer tends to encode synthesis of enzymes that modify antibiotics. Mutation-based resistance is often a gradual, stepwise process, whereas transferable resistance is often high-level, all-or-none, resistance.

Important mechanisms of acquired resistance include (1) enzymatic inactivation of antibiotics, (2) failure of bacterial permeability, (3) alteration in target receptors, (4) development of bypass mechanisms in metabolic pathways, (5) development of enzymes with low drug affinity, and (6) removing antimicrobial drugs from the cell through efflux pumps, or combinations of these mechanisms.

Mutation to Resistance. Mutation to resistance is a minor problem relative to horizontal gene transfer. Mutations to antibiotic resistance are spontaneous events involving changes in DNA sequences uninfluenced by the presence of antibiotics. Such mutations, especially in the chromosome, may lead to other changes that leave the cell at a disadvantage so that, in the absence of antibiotic selection, these mutants may gradually be lost. Mutation to antibiotic resistance can be dramatic, as in the case of single-step mutation to streptomycin resistance where MIC increases a thousandfold, or gradual, as in the case of chromosomal resistance to penicillin where a series of mutational events may gradually increase the MIC of the organisms. These differences occur because, when antibiotics affect one target site, chromosomal mutation is a single-step process, whereas when several targets are affected, mutation to resistance is a multistep process.

The rate of mutation differs for, and is characteristic of, each antibiotic. Sometimes, as discussed earlier, antibiotics are used in combination to overcome the possibility of mutation to resistance, since the chance of mutation to resistance to two antibiotics is the product of the chances of mutation for each antibiotic alone. In veterinary medicine, mutational resistance has limited the use of streptomycin, novobiocin, rifampin, and, to a lesser extent, erythromycin. It is increasingly limiting the use of fluoroquinolones. Interestingly, for fluoroquinolones, there are differences between species in the importance of single-step mutations in the development of resistance. For *C. jejuni* and *P. aeruginosa*, a single nucleotide change at a particular site in the *gyrA* DNA gyrase gene can lead to clinical resistance, whereas in *E. coli*, a single nucleotide change may lead to only a slight reduction in susceptibility.

A chromosomal mutation resulting in multiple antibiotic resistance has been described for clinically relevant bacteria. The region involved, the Mar (multiple antibiotic resistance) locus, controls efflux systems resulting in resistance to a variety of drugs without modification of the drugs.

Horizontal Drug Resistance Transfer. Horizontal gene transfer as a cause of antibiotic resistance is of major importance in veterinary and human medicine. Unlike chromosomal mutation to resistance, which occurs in individual bacteria, transfer of genetic material produces "infectious" resistance. The three ways in which bacteria can acquire foreign resistance genes are by transformation (uptake of naked DNA), by bacterial viruses (transduction), and by conjugation (mating by means of plasmids) (Figure 4.2). Depending on the type of horizontal gene transfer, this may result in transfer of resistance to several or even many antibiotics at one time, which can spread to and between bacteria from the original source. The extrachromosomal DNA molecules responsible for most infectious antibiotic resistance are usually plasmids, called R plasmids.

The development of resistance genes including those associated with horizontal gene transfer is often an enormously complex combination of different mobile genetic elements, but includes also mutation and recombination within these elements, all of which enable bacteria possessing these elements and genes to have selective advantage ("fitness") in surviving exposure to antibiotics (and sometimes concurrently to disinfectants and heavy metals) to which they may be exposed. To add further complexity, these same transferable elements may also acquire other determinants that enhance their fitness, such as the ability to form biofilms in the case of hospital-associated *Enterococcus* species.

Plasmids. Plasmids that carry DNA responsible for resistance can reproduce themselves within a cell and spread to other cells by conjugation. Plasmids themselves are commonly partly constructed from transposons and integrons (see the individual sections on "Transposons" and on "Integrons" immediately below).

Conjugation refers to plasmid-mediated transfer of resistance (Figure 4.2). In this common process of gene transfer,

FIGURE 4.2. *Mechanisms of horizontal gene transfer of resistance in bacteria.*

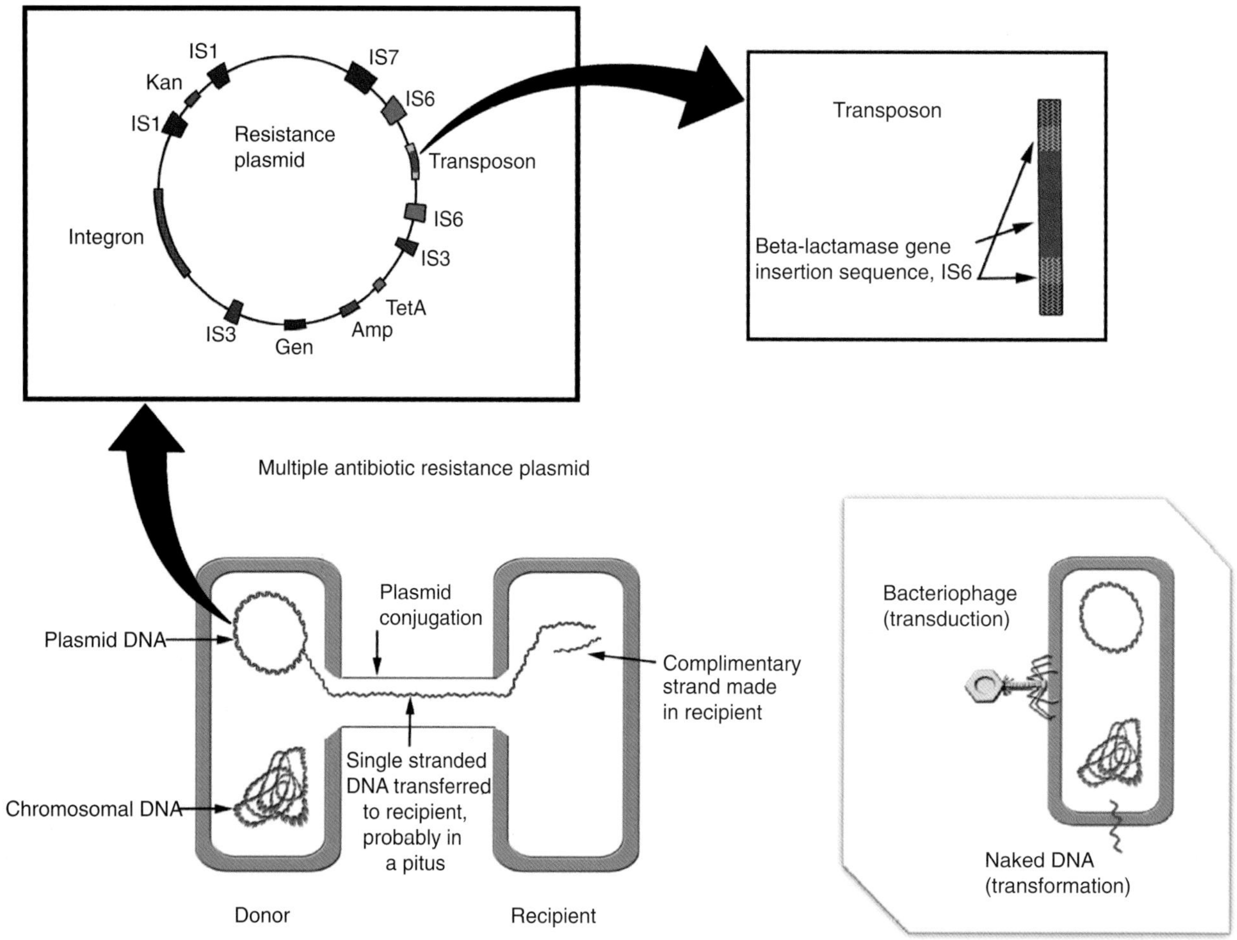

a donor bacterium synthesizes a sex pilus, which attaches to a recipient bacterium in a mating process, resulting in transfer of copies of plasmid genes to the recipients. The donor retains copies of the plasmid but the recipient has now become a potential donor. Conjugation can occur not only between species of the same genera but also across genera and families, so that similar plasmids can be found in a wide range of unrelated bacteria. The large intestine is a site where bacterial conjugation through resistance plasmids commonly occurs.

Much plasmid-mediated resistance, and indeed some chromosomally mediated resistance, is associated with transposons (Figure 4.2). The simplest form of transposon is a resistance gene flanked on either side by an insertion sequence, the smallest form of mobile genetic element. These short DNA sequences known as transposons ("jumping genes") can transpose from plasmid to plasmid, from plasmid to chromosome, or from chromosome to plasmid. A transposon copy usually remains at the original site. The frequency of transposition is characteristic of the particular transposon and bacterium. The importance of transposition as a key element in resistance transfer is that transposition is independent of the recombination process of the bacterial cell; homology with the interacting DNA is not required. Because of transposons, plasmids from diverse sources often possess identical antibiotic inactivating genes. Because of the widespread nature of insertion sequences in many bacteria, there is essentially no gene in bacterial genomes (including genes that encode resistance) that cannot be mobilized and moved to other bacterial genomes as a transposon. In addition, because of the DNA homology between insertion sequences, DNA recombination events frequently modify resistance plasmids that can combine to add DNA with additional resistance genes. Plasmids may also carry integrons encoding for resistance (as discussed later in this section on "horizontal gene transfer"). Conjugative transposons may cause bacteria to conjugate, in the way that conjugative plasmids will.

A well-known example of a resistance gene spread by plasmids is the *bla*$_{\text{CMY-2}}$ gene encoding resistance to third-generation cephalosporins. This gene, which likely originated from the chromosome of a *Citrobacter* spp., has spread among related plasmids within the Enterobacteriaceae, for example, to *Salmonella* serovars and to *E. coli*. The plasmids encoding *bla*$_{\text{CMY-2}}$ are relatively "promiscuous," so that the resistance gene has disseminated rapidly among commensal and pathogenic members of the Enterobacteriaceae. The emergence of this resistance has been encouraged by the use of third-generation cephalosporin antibiotics in animals in cattle and in chickens.

Bacteriophage. Bacterial viruses (bacteriophages) can transfer resistance genes originating in the chromosome or in plasmids between bacteria in a process known as transduction (Figure 4.2). An example is transfer of β-lactamase genes from penicillin-resistant to previously penicillin-susceptible staphylococci. The importance of transduction in spread of antimicrobial resistance may have been underestimated, although the narrow specificity of bacteriophages has likely limited their role.

Transformation. Transformation is a special type of horizontal gene transfer that occurs in some bacterial pathogens (Figure 4.2). Transformation describes a process by which DNA released by dying bacteria is taken up from the environment by other usually closely related bacteria and then recombines during DNA replication to produce novel forms of existing genes. The best-known example of this is the emergence of penicillin resistance in *Streptococcus pneumoniae*, an important human pathogen, through the development of novel PBPs.

Other Genetic Elements Associated with Resistance.

Integrons. Integrons are increasingly recognized as widespread genetic elements associated with multiple drug resistance in gram-negative enteric bacteria. An integron is a gene capture and dissemination system, consisting of an integrase gene and a site-specific integration site ("gene capture") into which the integrase can insert antimicrobial drug resistance "cassettes" ("gene dissemination"). Over nine types of integrons and over 60 different gene cassettes have been identified in gram-negative enteric bacteria, with some integrons containing as many as seven different resistance gene cassettes. In addition, some bacteria may carry cassettes in their genomes that have not incorporated into integrons but are capable of so doing. Integrons (with or without resistance-gene cassettes) may be found in the chromosome, in plasmids, or in transposons.

Genomic Resistance Islands. Genomic resistance islands are large chromosomal regions that contain multiple resistance genes, mostly associated with different integrons, and which can be moved between bacteria by plasmids. A well-known example is the *Salmonella* genomic island 1 associated with multidrug resistance in *S.* serovar Typhimurium DT104, but also found in strains of other multidrug resistant serovars, as well as in other Enterobacteriaceae.

Clinical Importance of Antimicrobial Drug Resistance

Acquired drug resistance has become a major problem in some pathogenic bacteria of veterinary importance and has been described as a crisis in human medicine. It is common in many bacterial species, although notably some bacteria, particularly gram-positive bacteria such as many streptococci and corynebacteria, have remained highly susceptible to commonly used drugs. As a result, diseases produced by these bacteria have in many cases declined considerably in importance, to be replaced by infections produced by bacteria that have the ability to evolve more readily.

Acquired resistance to penicillins is frequent in coagulase-positive staphylococci, and recently methicillin-resistant *S. aureus* and in dogs methicillin-resistant *S. pseudintermedius* infections have emerged in domestic animals on a global basis. Acquired multiple antibiotic resistance to many common antibiotics seriously limits their use in members of the family Enterobacteriaceae such as *Salmonella* and *E. coli*. In animals, acquired resistance is increasingly observed in nonenteric bacteria such as *Bordetella*, *Haemophilus*, and *Pasteurella*, and has been identified in virtually every pathogenic bacterial genus as well as in the normal flora.

There is to some extent a causal relationship between antimicrobial drug use and the development of resistance but its importance varies with different pathogens and essentially reflects their ability to adapt to changing circumstances, that is, to evolve, as well as to colonize different animal species.

The development of resistance is particularly notable among enteric bacteria in animals. The intestine is a major site of transfer of antibiotic resistance because of the vast numbers of bacteria present and their ability to transfer resistance genes horizontally, the use of oral antimicrobial drugs, and because of the opportunities for spread of these bacteria through focally contaminated environments. Within the intestine, "promiscuous" plasmids may transfer resistance between bacteria within families of bacteria, for example, between members of the Enterobacteriaceae such as from *E. coli* to *Salmonella* or *Proteus*, or even between bacteria belong to unrelated taxonomic families such as *E. coli* to *Bacteroides*. The emergence and spread of drug resistance in Enterobacteriaceae and other opportunist infections is increasingly well documented in individual companion animals such as dogs, and may reflect in some cases infections acquired from their owners through antibiotic use in human medicine.

Where multiple drug resistance genes are present on a plasmid or an integron, the use of any antimicrobial to which resistance is encoded by one of the genes present will help maintain the entire collection of resistance genes. Plasmids may gradually accumulate resistance genes through acquisition by their integrons of resistance cassettes or through acquisition of transposon-mediated resistance genes.

Intestinal *E. coli*. Extensive study of antimicrobial resistance in intestinal *E. coli* in food animals has provided considerable information on the mechanisms and ecology of antimicrobial resistance. These studies have shown the relationship between the extent of resistance and the degree of antimicrobial use. For example, resistance in *E. coli* from adult ruminants at pasture is slight, whereas it is pronounced in intensively reared young animals where antibiotic use is common and the intestinal flora is immature. As a result of plasmid-mediated resistance, these *E. coli* may be resistant to many clinically useful drugs. Among enterotoxigenic *E. coli* from farm animals, plasmid-mediated resistance to tetracyclines, sulfonamides, and streptomycin is now practically universal. Antibiotic-resistance encoding plasmids in enterotoxigenic *E. coli* in swine and calves may also include genes for virulence determinants such as toxin production or adhesins.

Within the intestine, R plasmids are found in *E. coli* and in the more dominant anaerobic flora of the large bowel. Within a short time of treating an animal with an antibiotic, the *E. coli* and much of the anaerobe population become resistant to that antibiotic, principally because of selection of resistant strains but also because of enhanced transfer of R plasmids. In the absence of antimicrobials, conditions in the large bowel seem generally to prevent the transfer of R factors. Short-term oral use of antimicrobials is followed by high levels of *E. coli* resistance, which fall once the antimicrobials are removed because the majority of R plasmid bearing *E. coli* are not good intestinal colonizers. However, the continuous presence of antimicrobials is associated with extensive resistance, which persists long after the antimicrobial is removed since resistant *E. coli* that are good intestinal colonizers have been selected.

Salmonella. Multiple antimicrobial resistance is a major problem in selected serovars and in individual strains within serovars of *Salmonella*, including serovar Typhimurium. It is often the result of a chromosomally incorporated genomic island containing integrons. Among *S.* Typhimurium strains, clones of certain phage types such as DT104 are characterized by the presence of a multiple-antimicrobial resistant genomic island, which has spread to other serovars. The extent of resistance can be marked among calf isolates because the extensive use of antimicrobials in some types of calf rearing and because the nature of salmonellosis in calves apparently provides an opportunity for the development and spread of resistant *Salmonella*. Multiply resistant and more virulent clones of *S.* Typhimurium have a history of emerging to spread within some cattle populations, and to spread from cattle into other species including humans, and then to decline in importance. For example, the multiply resistant clone DT 104 disseminated widely through cattle on a global basis before declining after a decade. This clone had a region containing florfenicol and tetracycline resistance encoding gene flanked by two integrons carrying a β-lactamase and streptomycin resistance gene cassette. This cluster of genes formed part of the larger, distinctive, *Salmonella* genomic island 1, which may have been a plasmid integrated into the chromosome. This island or its variants has also been identified in other *Salmonella* serovars, such as *S.* Agona and *S.* Newport. *Salmonella* carrying these multidrug resistance genes have caused serious infections in people.

As discussed earlier, use of third-generation cephalosporins in farm animals has been associated with selection of *Salmonella* strains carrying plasmids encoding the $bla_{\text{CMY-2}}$ gene encoding resistance to these antibiotics. For example, in Canada and the United States, use of ceftiofur injection of eggs to prevent navel infections has resulted in selection of ceftiofur-resistant *S.* Heidelberg as well as ceftiofur-resistant *E. coli*. These resistant *S.* Heidelberg have reached and caused serious illnesses in people. The significance of this is that third-generation cephalosporins are drugs of choice for serious *Salmonella* infections in infants and pregnant women.

Hospital-Acquired Resistant Infections. Acquired antimicrobial resistance in resident hospital bacteria is a major problem in human hospitals and is increasingly recognized in veterinary hospitals. In human medicine, hospital-associated infections with multiresistant bacteria belonging to the so-called ESKAPE group can become a major problem. The ESKAPE bacteria are *Enterococcus faecium*, *Staphylococcus aureus*, *Klebsiella* species, *Acinetobacter baumannii*, *P. aeruginosa*, and *Enterobacter* species. Resistance is by no means restricted to hospital-acquired infections but hospitals are inevitably a breeding ground for the development and selection of resistance in bacterial pathogens. There is a causal relationship between antimicrobial use in hospitals and the development of resistance in bacteria. Colonization of patients by resistant opportunist bacteria is hard to prevent because of shared air spaces and environment, utensils, and veterinary staff. In addition, patients with serious and sometimes immunosuppression-associated illnesses may be repeatedly treated with numerous broad-spectrum antimicrobial drugs, thus removing the normal colonization resistance of the body, including the large intestine, provided by the normal microbial flora. Under such circumstances these patients can readily be colonized by bacteria that are either intrinsically resistant to many antimicrobial drugs (ESKAPE group) or that have acquired resistance.

Public Health Aspects of Antimicrobial Resistance in Animal Pathogens

The use of antimicrobial agents in animals can result in antimicrobial-resistant bacteria and their resistance genes reaching the human population through a variety of routes Figure 4.3). The scale of the contribution via these routes has not been determined and indeed, because of the complexity of resistance in bacterial pathogens, is hard to determine.

Most antimicrobial resistance in human pathogens comes from antimicrobial use in human medicine. However, antimicrobial-resistant bacteria of animal origin, such as *Enterococcus* spp. *E. coli* and *Salmonella*, can colonize the intestines of people. Heavily exposed humans (e.g., farmers who use feed containing antimicrobials, slaughterhouse workers, cooks, and other food handlers) often have a higher incidence of resistant *E. coli* in their feces than the general population. Contamination of meat by intestinal bacteria at slaughter is extensive and an important route by which resistant bacteria reach people. Although many of these bacteria are nonpathogenic, many pathogenic bacterial species from the intestines of animals cause zoonotic infections in humans (e.g., *Salmonella* and *C. jejuni*) and these infections may be harder to treat because of acquired resistance. The nonpathogenic bacteria of animals acquired by humans are a potential source of resistance genes for human pathogenic bacteria other than the zoonotic bacteria. These bacteria may reach humans not only through the food chain but also through water contaminated by resistant bacteria of animal origin.

The topic of the contribution of antimicrobial use in food animals, particularly for growth promotion and disease prophylactic purposes, to resistance in human

FIGURE 4.3. *Summary of routes of spread of resistant bacteria and their genes between humans, animals, and the environment.*

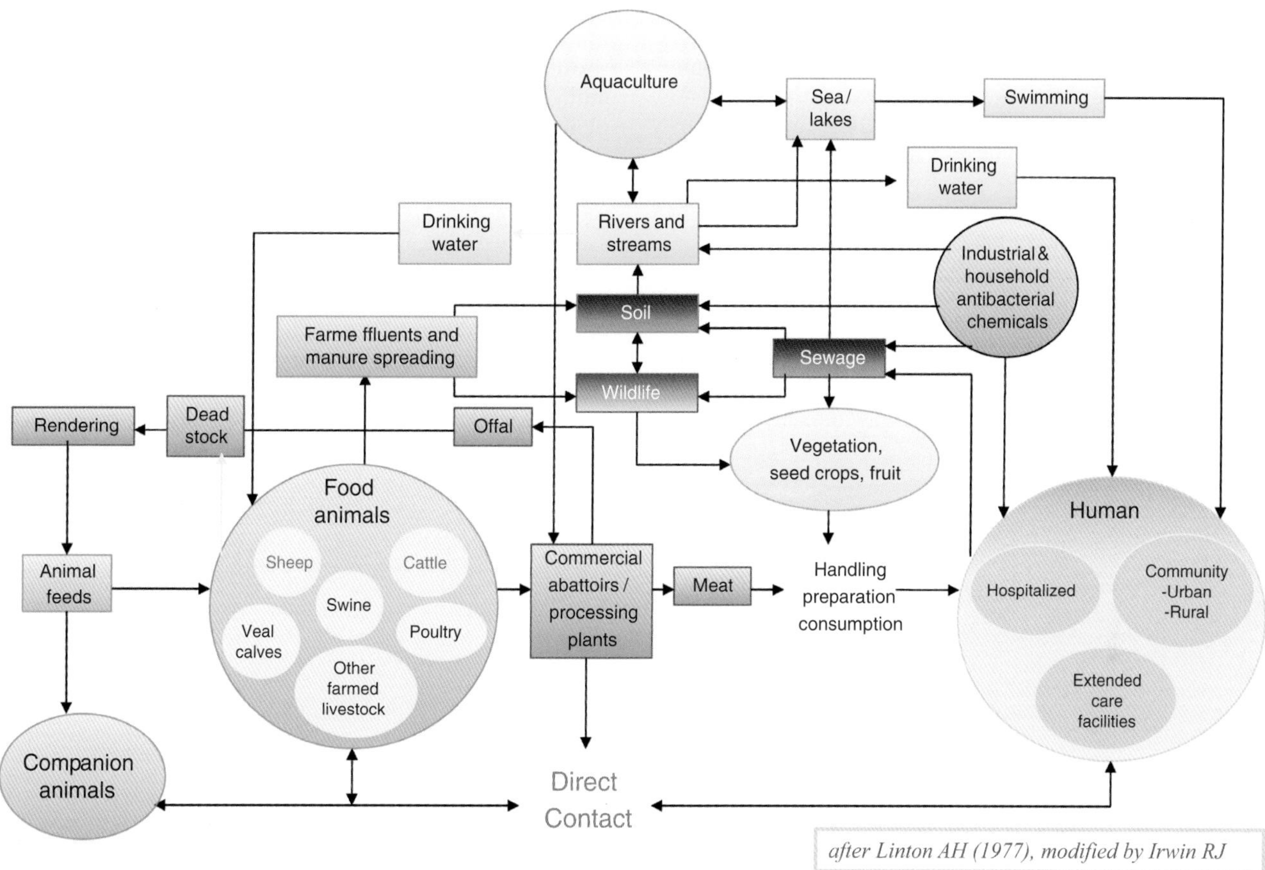

pathogens has been the subject of repeated review over many years, but the last 15 years has seen the issue subject to the most intense scrutiny. The major driving force for the renewed debate on the prudence of using antimicrobial drugs in food animals for growth promotion and disease prophylactic purposes has been the alarming increase in resistance in human pathogens, particularly those causing "community-acquired" (e.g., *S. pneumoniae*) infections rather than hospital-acquired infections. Resistance has left the hospital to enter the community. This has led to a total reappraisal of the use of all antimicrobial drugs in all circumstances. Another factor driving the change is evidence from Europe that vancomycin-resistant *E. faecium* (VRE), a serious and essentially untreatable hospital-acquired pathogen of immunocompromised human patients, was being selected in intensively reared farm animals by the use of avoparcin, a glycopeptide antimicrobial drug used as a growth promoter and disease prophylactic. These VREs were almost universal in the intestines of treated animals and were found in a small proportion of healthy humans in Europe. Paradoxically, they were not present in healthy humans in the United States, where the drug was not used. The European findings were a demonstration of the scale of the movement of resistant bacteria from animals to humans, which was clearly measurable. Another factor was the entry of Sweden into the European Union (EU) in 1999. Since Sweden had banned the use of all antimicrobial drugs as growth promoters and disease prophylactics for many years, in order to bring its practices into line with those of other EU countries either it had to change its regulations or it had to change to those of the EU. It used the VRE evidence to persuade the EU to change policies on the use of antimicrobial growth promoters, most of which (avoparcin, bacitracin, spiramycin, and tylosin) were banned in Europe in late 1999. A similar ban has occurred in Australia.

In the United States, there has also been extensive reexamination of the use of antimicrobials in animals. One notable decision in 2001 was to reverse the approval of fluoroquinolones for treatment of *E. coli* septicemia in chickens because of the rapid development of fluoroquinolone-resistance in *C. jejuni*. It was estimated that as many as 14 000 people annually treated for campylobacteriosis had their treatment affected because they were infected with resistant bacteria acquired from fluoroquinolone-treated chickens. In 2003, the Center for Veterinary Medicine of the US Food and Drug Administration developed a guidance document for the evaluation of the impact of resistance as part of the regulatory approval of new antimicrobial drugs. The document takes into account the relative importance of different antimicrobial drug classes in human medicine and analyzes the risks of production of resistance and its acquisition by humans, depending on the proposed usage of the drug. In 2010, the Center for Veterinary Medicine developed a "judicious use" guidance document that promoted two principles, the first that use of antibiotics in animals be limited to prevention, treatment, and control of disease (i.e., not for growth promotion) and that all use in feed be under veterinary oversight (i.e., not available over-the-counter).

It seems likely that antimicrobial drugs important in human medicine will be removed from use as growth promoters or long-term disease prophylactics throughout the world. This is in keeping with the important prudent-use principle that antimicrobial drugs should only be used when the benefits are clear and substantial.

Control of Antimicrobial Resistance

Avoiding the use of a drug is the best way to control antimicrobial resistance. Most major national veterinary medical associations have published prudent-use guidelines for the optimal use of antimicrobial agents that are readily available on their web sites. Prudent use is defined as optimizing the efficacy of antimicrobial drug use while minimizing the development and spread of resistance. Although these guidelines are general in scope, they are increasingly supplemented by species or veterinary practice type guidelines that are sometimes case specific. Further refinement of such guidelines will occur into the future and are part of a global movement of antibiotic stewardship in medicine and veterinary medicine. The topic of antibiotic stewardship is beyond the scope of this book, but includes appropriate choice of antibiotics and optimal dosage based on susceptibility and understanding of pharmacokinetic and pharmacodynamic principles, implementing effective infection control measures to limit spread of bacteria, and finding alternatives to antibiotics in controlling infection.

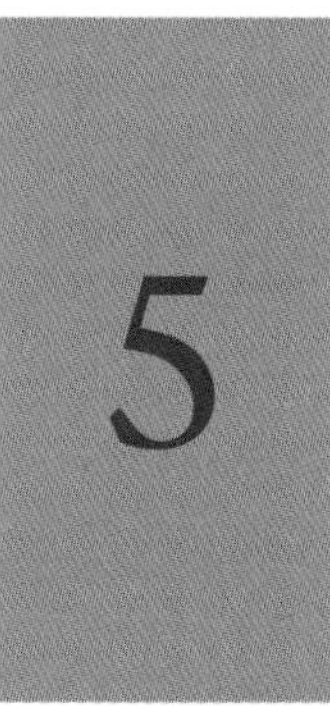

Vaccines

Ronald D. Schultz and D. Scott McVey

Introduction

Vaccines are substances that are used to elicit immune responses to prevent or minimize disease produced by infectious agents. Vaccines can be composed of the infectious agent itself (either live or killed), a portion of the agent that induces a protective immune response (toxoid or subunit vaccine), or a product of the agent. Products containing a killed bacterial agent are more properly called bacterins. Products that have toxic activities are called toxins, and toxins that have been inactivated are called toxoids.

To be effective, vaccines should stimulate an immune response that ideally prevents infection but, at the very least, should interfere with the development of severe disease.

Humoral Immunity

Antibodies function immunologically by binding to epitopes on the surface of the infectious agent and/or one of its products. By binding to the surface of an infectious agent, antibodies interfere with attachment to host target cells by stearic interference and/or by changing the charge or hydrophobicity of the surface of the agent (enhancing phagocytosis by multiple cell types), and trigger the complement cascade generating products that are opsonic (lie antibodies) and products that are damaging to agents that have surface membranes. Antibodies that bind to products of infectious agents can block the attachment of the product to receptors on cellular targets and/or change the configuration of the product resulting in a change in binding affinity.

Cell-Mediated Immunity

Cell-mediated immunity (CMI) is an immune response that results in the generation of "activated" macrophages and/or specific cytotoxic T lymphocytes. This aspect of the immune response concerns agents that live inside of cells, which are thus protected from interaction with the elements of the humoral components of the system.

Activated macrophages are mononuclear phagocytic cells that have come in contact with interleukin 1 (IL-1) and interferon gamma (INF-γ). Such cells have increased phagocytic and enzymatic activity, contain increased amounts of nitric oxide, and have increased production of cytokines, such as tumor necrosis factor (TNF) and IL-1, and increased expression of major histocompatibility complex class I (MHC-I). This increase in activity is thought to be responsible for the destruction of infectious agents that non-activated mononuclear cells cannot destroy following uptake. Some term this immune state (i.e., activation of macrophages) cellular hypersensitivity.

Cytotoxic T lymphocytes recognize affected and infected host cells (e.g., cells infected with viruses or bacteria). In so doing, these lymphocytes secrete substances that result in the death of the affected host cell. If the affected host cell contained an infectious agent, that agent would now be either destroyed or liberated from the cell and be in contact with other host immune effectors (e.g., antibodies, complements, and activated macrophages).

Generation of the Immune Response

Antigens that are processed by antigen-processing cells via the exogenous pathway elicit antibodies. Thus, extracellular bacteria (live or killed), inactivated viral particles, portions (subunits) of a virus, and products are processed by the exogenous pathway. Epitopes are presented to the immune system in context of MHC-II by an antigen-presenting cell that secretes IL-1 and little, if any, IL-12. T helper cells (T_{H2} subset of CD4 lymphocytes) respond to this stimulus by secreting cytokines that trigger an antibody response (IL-4, IL-5, and IL-13).

Some infectious agents replicate within cells. If the agent multiplies within a mononuclear phagocyte, then antigens are processed by way of the exogenous and/or endogenous pathways (see below). As outlined above with extracellular antigens, antigens of intracellular agents are presented in context of MHC-II, but the antigen-presenting cell secretes IL-1 and IL-12. IL-12 stimulates T helper cells (T_{H1} subset) while turning off cells of the T_{H2} subset. T_{H1} cells secrete INF-γ, resulting in the activation of mononuclear phagocytic cells. Some of these "intracellular" agents (some viruses, bacteria, and fungi) replicate in the cytoplasm of

Veterinary Microbiology, Third Edition. Edited by D. Scott McVey, Melissa Kennedy and M.M. Chengappa.

mononuclear phagocytic cells. Antigens from these agents are also processed by the endogenous pathway, as are antigens liberated within nonphagocytic cells, so that epitopes are presented to the immune system in context of MHC-I. Epitopes presented in this fashion are recognized by CD8 cytotoxic lymphocytes. These lymphocytes function by lysing infected targets, that is, cells expressing epitope–MHC-I complexes.

DNA Vaccines

DNA vaccines are those in which the gene encoding the antigen in question is inserted into a plasmid vector that has a strong promoter (e.g., cytomegalovirus immediate/early promoter and SV40 early promoter) that will result in expression of the target gene, a termination sequence (polyA tail), and a number of cytidine-phosphate–guanosine (CpG) motifs. The function of the CpG motif (a motif common in bacterial genomes) is to direct the antigen-processing cell to secrete lymphokines that favor T_{H1} lymphocytes. The construct is administered in any number of ways (intramuscular, intradermally, upon a mucosal surface), but intramuscularly is the most common. Myocytes that become transfected serve as antigen-presenting cells and express antigens in context of MHC-I (turn on CD8 T lymphocytes). It is unclear how an antigen is expressed in context of MHC-II (for CD4 T lymphocytes). Possibilities include MHC-II antigen-presenting cells (macrophages/dendritic cells/B lymphocytes) becoming transfected, or transfected myocytes transferring the plasmid construct to MHC-II antigen-presenting cells.

DNA vaccines have been experimentally successful in eliciting protective immune responses (both humoral and cellular) to a variety of bacterial, viral, and protozoal microorganisms. Commercial DNA vaccines are now available for vaccinating horses against the West Nile virus and as an oral therapeutic vaccine for dogs to treat malignant melanomas.

Adjuvants

Adjuvants are used to influence the types of immune response elicited by an antigen. The response is influenced at various stages, depending upon the adjuvant. Some adjuvants function as depots, so that the antigen is slowly released over an extended period of time to maximize the immune response. Examples include water/oil emulsions, minerals/salts (bentonite and aluminum), and inert particles (microspheres). Other adjuvants direct activity to the processing step in the initiation of the immune response. Examples include "immune-stimulating complexes" (ISCOMs) composed of cholesterol–phospholipid structures that contain the immunogen, and liposomes (lipid vesicles). "Targeting" various components by using various cytokines as adjuvants can influence immune responses. For example, IL-1 activates T lymphocytes, IL-12 and INF-γ influence the helper T lymphocyte subset selection, and granulocyte macrophage colony-stimulating factors activate macrophages and increase efficiency of antigen processing.

Viral Vaccines

Immunization of animals with viral vaccines is critical to the prevention of many viral diseases. The basis of an effective vaccine is its ability to induce an immune response or responses capable of eliciting protection to subsequent field exposure to pathogenic viruses. A multitude of vaccine preparations have been developed and used over the years, with variable success. The success of a potential vaccine is primarily dependent on safety and efficacy; however, economics also determine vaccine design, development, and ultimate production on a commercial basis.

Various approaches to vaccination have been employed over the years. These include (1) administering a live virulent virus in an anatomical site so that the target tissue or tissues are not infected, (2) administering a live virulent virus to animals at a time of relative resistance to disease expression, (3) concurrent administration of a live virulent virus and immune serum, which no longer is acceptable for obvious reasons, (4) use of live avirulent viral strains (e.g., attenuated or "modified live" viruses), and (5) use of inactivated viruses. In recent years, additional approaches to vaccine development have become available. These include subunit, synthetic peptide, and recombinant products. Regardless of the vaccine type, the desired result is to induce immune responses specific for viral antigens expressed on the virion surface or on the surface of infected cells, so that the immunized host is immune when exposed to the virulent virus. The rational development of an efficacious viral vaccine requires an understanding of viral pathogenesis, of protective immune responses induced following infection, and of their protein specificities. The latter point is of obvious importance for developing recombinant and synthetic peptide vaccines.

Concerning pathogenesis, the following three general types of viral infections occur:

1. Infections that are confined to the mucosal surfaces of the respiratory or gastrointestinal tracts. In such instances, local immunity in the form of a secretory antibody (e.g., IgA) is important. The role of CMI is less well characterized in such infections.
2. Infections that begin at mucosal surfaces but then cause a systemic infection with viremia, and subsequent infection of distant target tissues. In these infections, both immunity at the mucosal surface and systemic immunity are important.
3. Infections that gain direct entry into the host's circulation via insect bite (arthropod-borne viruses), inadvertent inoculation, or a traumatic break in an epithelial surface. In such infections, systemic immunity is the primary line of defense.

These mechanisms of viral infection and subsequent dissemination must be considered in vaccine development. Modified live (attenuated) and inactivated (killed)

Table 5.1. Types of Viral Vaccines

1. Live viral vaccines
   a. Attentuation for low virulence of viruses that produce natural diseases.
   b. Host-range mutants—use of different viral strains infecting different host species that are related antigenically to the virus strain that produces a natural disease in the original host.
   c. Recombinant heterologous viral vector vaccines—construction of an infectious viral recombinant that expresses protective antigen(s) of another virus that produces a natural disease. Construction of a recombinant virus with insertion of genes with known antiviral activities or with known immunoregulatory functions.
   d. Recombinant homologous viral strains attenuated by targeted mutations on deletions of genes coding for specific virulence factors that produce a natural disease.
   e. Nonreplicating recombinant viral vector vaccines capable of replicating to high titer *in vitro* but unable to grow efficiently *in vivo*.
2. Inactivated viral vaccines
   a. Inactivated viral vaccines by chemical methods.
   b. Inactivated viral vaccines by physical methods.
   c. Purified viral antigens using monoclonal antibody immunoaffinity chromatography.
   d. Cloned viral protein subunit vaccines produced in eukaryotic or prokaryotic cells by recombinant DNA technology.
   e. Synthetic viral polypeptide vaccines representing immunologically urpident domains of viral surface antigens.
   f. Direct injection of plasmid DNA encoding viral protective antigens into tissues *in vivo*.
   g. Use of anti-idiotypic antibodies as antigens to induce an antiviral antibody response.

virus vaccines dominate the veterinary vaccine market (Table 5.1).

Live Attenuated Viral Vaccines

The attenuated viral vaccines include artificially attenuated (modified live) strains of viruses or naturally occurring viruses with reduced virulence for the host. The origin of these naturally attenuated isolates may be the natural host, or a closely related virus isolated from a different host; for example, the cowpox virus was initially used to vaccinate humans against smallpox. The major requirements of such an approach are that it induces adequate immunity and that the attenuation (lack of virulence) of the vaccine strain be stable. The majority of vaccines currently used today in veterinary medicine are attenuated viruses. The most common approach to viral attenuation is the development of host-range mutants. Other approaches include development of temperature-sensitive and cold-adapted mutants (missense mutations), deletion mutants, and recombinant viruses.

Host-range mutants are developed by serial passage in a host system different from the natural host to be vaccinated, usually laboratory animals, embryonated chicken eggs, or, increasingly, cell cultures. Upon serial passage in these systems, viruses often lose their virulence for the natural host due to accumulation of mutations in the viral genome that result in changes in virus-specified proteins. The basis of attenuation of many modified live virus vaccines, however, is poorly characterized, and the possibility of reversion to virulence after growth in the natural host is always a concern.

Conditional lethal mutants have been generated with the intent that such viruses would exhibit limited replication in the host and so serve as vaccines. Temperature-sensitive mutants are typically created by mutagenesis and phenotypically selected on the basis of temperature. Cold-adapted mutants are generated by propagation at successively lower temperatures, the end product being incapable of replication at normal body temperatures. The cold-adapted mutants typically acquire multiple mutations in genes encoding virulence and are relatively more stable than temperature-sensitive mutants.

A unique approach to expression of cloned viral genes is the use of heterologous viral expression vectors. The vaccinia virus has widely been used for many years as an infectious vaccine expression vector because it is a virus that has widely been used as a human vaccine and the fact that at least 22 kilobases of the vaccinia genome can be deleted without loss of infectivity. The latter attribute provides ample space in which to insert foreign cloned genes and has the potential to permit insertion of multiple foreign viral genes for the purpose of designing multivalent and multiviral vaccines. A major potential advantage of such infectious vaccine vectors is the potential for induction of both humoral and cellular immunity by inserting expressed viral proteins into the host cell membrane in context with histocompatibility antigens.

Construction of deletion mutants is another potential mechanism of virus attenuation; thus, the selective deletion of genes that express factors for virulence, persistence, or immunosuppression can often be accomplished without compromising viral replication. This approach requires a thorough understanding of the virus and the pathogenesis of the respective disease. A deletant vaccine has been developed to prevent pseudorabies in swine. The thymidine kinase gene is deleted in the pseudorabies vaccine strain, which is able to induce an immune response without producing disease. Furthermore, the genes encoding virus glycoproteins gpI, gpIII, or gpx are deleted in the vaccine strain. The presence of an antibody to these specific virus antigens can be used to differentiate field-strain infected animals from vaccinated animals, an important advance in defining the epidemiology and control of this disease. These vaccines are referred to as DIVA (differentiation of infected from vaccinated animals) vaccines.

Nonreplicating recombinant viral vectors that are not capable of replication *in vivo* but that can express foreign proteins during abortive infections can induce humoral and CMI in immunized hosts. Experimental studies show that dogs or cats are resistant to wild-type rabies viral challenge when inoculated with avian pox-rabies glycoprotein recombinant viruses. There are effective commercial recombinant canarypox-vectored vaccines for canine distemper (hemagglutinin and fusion protein antigens), for and for the feline leukemia virus, and rabies (glycoprotein G) vaccine for cats. This type of viral vaccine has the distinct advantage of being safe even in the immunosuppressed host.

Table 5.2. Relative Advantages and Disadvantages of Live versus Inactivated Virus Vaccines

Criteria	Live	Inactivated
Immunity	Long	Short
Adjuvant	No	Yes
Safety	Variable	Usually very safe
Complications (potential)	Reversion to virulence, spread to susceptible animals	Sensitization
Potential contamination	Possible	Minimal
Interference	Possible	Minimal
Cost	Minimal	Significant
Immunomodulation	Not required	Required
Vaccine marker	Possibly genetic marker	Serologic marker
Stability	Poor	Good
CMI induction	Yes	No
Local secretory immunity	Yes	No
Reassortment/ recombination	Possible	No
Persistent	Yes	No

There are advantages and disadvantages to all vaccines including the attenuated viral vaccines. Table 5.2 lists the general characteristics of live attenuated as compared to killed viral vaccines. A major advantage of live viral vaccines is their ability to replicate within the host and thereby elicit both humoral and cellular immune responses. In the case of viral infections attacking primarily the mucosal surfaces of the respiratory and gastrointestinal tracts, administering attenuated viruses by nasal or oral routes stimulates local immunity. Therefore, local routes of administration are often more effective than systemic administration. Economic considerations also favor attenuated vaccines due to the lower cost of production and the typical absence of a requirement for adjuvants, immunopotentiating agents, and the need for multiple immunizations.

While attenuated viral vaccines continue to be the most commonly used veterinary vaccines, there are serious disadvantages to their use. With some vaccines, attenuation may result in complete or partial loss of immunogenicity. Thus, modified live vaccine strains of viruses may require a compromise between loss of virulence of the virus and loss of its immunogenicity because some viruses exhibit reduced immunogenicity as they become attenuated. Furthermore, accurate assessment of viral attenuation can often be difficult since experimental reproduction of clinical disease is difficult with certain viruses. In such instances, a vaccine virus considered to be attenuated may not provide complete protection or it may produce clinical disease under special circumstances, involving stress, physiologic imbalance, or concurrent infections with other organisms. If any of these circumstances occurred, the vaccine would be removed from the market and improved. Viruses that have a wide host range are also problematic. Virus attenuated for one animal species may retain virulence for more susceptible species. If the vaccinated animals shed the attenuated virus in the environment, transmission to susceptible species may occur.

A major concern in the use of attenuated viruses is reversion to virulence. This phenomenon has plagued vaccine development and licensing over the years. Reversion to virulence is a more serious possibility with those viruses that enjoy a wide host range or that are biologically transmitted by arthropod vectors. While the virus may appear stable in the host for which the vaccine was intended, reversion to virulence may occur in the vector or in other species. Vaccination of pregnant animals may also be of concern, since attenuated viruses may be pathogenic for the developing fetus. Vaccinating animals with reduced immunologic responsiveness can result in expression of clinical disease and death.

Additional negative features of attenuated virus vaccines include (1) the potential for reassortment (viruses with segmented genomes) or recombination between vaccine strains or with wild-type viruses to create new viruses, (2) lack of a vaccine marker for serologic differentiation of vaccine and wild-type virus exposure, (3) development of persistent infections, (4) poor stability of vaccine viruses, especially in hot tropical areas, and (5) replication interference between viruses in multivalent vaccines. Viruses that exhibit continued antigenic drift present another dilemma since new isolates must be continually attenuated and tested for safety and efficacy.

Inactivated Virus Vaccines

Many inactivated vaccines have been developed for use in veterinary medicine. Virus inactivation has most commonly employed formalin, β-propiolactone, acetyl ethyleneimine, or binary ethyleneimine. Additional methods include ultraviolet light, gamma irradiation, psoralen compounds, and ozone gas. The primary advantage of inactivated virus vaccines is safety—many potential disadvantages of live virus vaccines are eliminated since no virus replication occurs. Viruses for inactivation have been produced in laboratory animals, embryonated chicken eggs, and, most commonly today, in cell cultures. From an economic viewpoint, viruses that grow to high titer in cell cultures and exhibit first-order inactivation kinetics provide the best candidates for vaccine preparation. Adjuvants are typically required to induce good immunity with killed viral products, and multiple doses are usually required to provide an active immunity. Some highly effective adjuvants can lead to undesired consequences that include severe local tissue reactions, reduced weight gain in growing animals, systemic hypersensitivity, and even death. With the continued development of better adjuvants and ISCOMs, inactivated vaccines will become more effective. Inactivated vaccines are also relatively stable under adverse environmental conditions, and their potential for strain interference in multivalent preparations is reduced compared to attenuated vaccines.

There are, however, certain disadvantages associated with the use of inactivated virus vaccines. Some inactivating agents are toxic, and some are carcinogenic. Also, inactivating agents may be present at very low concentrations in the final product. Unlike a live virus, an inactivated vaccine virus is not quantitatively amplified, so it requires adjuvant and multiple inoculations. Furthermore, such preparations do not induce strong cellular immunity, since inducing such responses requires that the antigen be presented in association with histocompatibility antigens on cell surfaces (processed via the endogenous pathways, see the preceding text). Nor are such vaccines associated with development of local secretory immunity due to the usual parenteral route of vaccination.

The success of viral inactivation depends on the inactivant and viral characteristics. While most viruses can be successfully inactivated, the retention of critical antigenic integrity is variable. Antigens responsible for inducing protective immunity must be preserved. A possible complication of inactivated vaccine use is the potential for animal sensitization such that an exacerbated clinical disease is experienced upon exposure to a virulent field virus. This sensitization is not well understood, but it is often immunologically precipitated by atypical immune responses such as incomplete antibody responses that lack effective avidity, antibody responses to nonneutralizing epitopes, preferential stimulation of IgE (antibodies that mediate type I hypersensitivities), or other aberrant stimulation of immune-mediated inflammation.

Development of new subunit vaccines is currently an area of extensive research; it includes purification of viral subunits, recombinant technology, and peptide synthesis. The basis of a subunit vaccine is an immunogenic protein (or peptide sequences) capable of eliciting protective immunity. Such proteins would typically be found on the virion surface and contain epitopes capable of inducing neutralizing antibodies. Vaccines can be prepared by disruption of the virus followed by protein purification. The potential cost of such preparations has sometimes precluded their commercial development, but recent biotechnological advances have offered alternatives via recombinant DNA and peptide synthesis technologies.

The approach to developing recombinant vaccines involves insertion of DNA that contains the desired viral genomic coding sequences into an appropriate expression vector. The viral or complementary DNA (cDNA) is inserted into a plasmid or bacteriophage followed by infection of susceptible prokaryotic cells such as *Escherichia coli*, yeast cells, or mammalian cells. Multiple strategies have been used to construct vaccine expression vectors, and most include a strong promoter (constitutive or inducible). Following infection of the cell with the plasmid, the cloned cDNA can be expressed and the desired gene product purified for vaccine use. Over the last 15 years, attention has also been focused on the inoculation of plasmid DNA encoding viral antigens directly into animals. Such DNA vaccines offer the potential advantage of having viral proteins and glycoproteins expressed on the surface of transfected cells and inducing immunity without interference from passively acquired viral antibodies.

Synthetic peptide vaccines have also been developed. As with cloned viral vaccines, the successful development of synthetic peptide vaccines requires extensive knowledge of the viral proteins involved in inducing protective immunity. Two basic approaches are available for determining critical peptide sequences: (1) indirectly, from nucleotide sequences derived from cloned viral genes, and (2) directly, by sequencing purified peptides. Immunologically based peptide and epitope mapping to determine the regions involved in protective immunity facilitate the latter approach. An additional approach to determining critical peptide sequences is based upon the projected tertiary structure of the viral protein, with the areas that demonstrate hydrophilic characteristics serving as candidate sequences. One major drawback of synthesizing peptide vaccines is the potential for critical epitopes to be formed by the tertiary structure (an epitope formed by juxtaposition of two separated peptide sequences). Such epitopes confound attempts to deduce the peptide sequence and realize such complex configurations in the synthetic product.

The use of anti-idiotypic antibodies as immunogens to stimulate the production of viral neutralizing antibodies has also been explored. The advantage of this type of immunogen may overcome viral variability problems by inducing broadly neutralizing antibodies. However, this type of vaccine induces only antibody responses in most cases. Production and formulation technologies have not been developed for these vaccines.

Toxoids, Bacterins, and Bacterial Vaccines

As with viral vaccines, the basis of an effective toxoid, bacterin, or bacterial vaccine is the ability to induce an immune response or responses capable of eliciting protection from field exposure to the pathogenic microorganism. Most of the principles outlined above with respect to viral vaccines apply to products designed to induce protective immunity to bacterial agents. The development of an efficacious product depends on understanding the pathogenesis of the bacterial disease that is to be prevented. However, in general, it is more difficult to develop a vaccine to a bacteria or fungal pathogen than it is to a virus. Most pathogenic bacteria have multiple virulence factors, and neutralization of one such factor may only partially reduce the virulence of the infection. Vaccines to bacterial infections often do not prevent infection. In contrast, many attenuated viral vaccines will prevent infection.

In general terms, diseases produced by bacteria can be grouped into three categories: (1) those that result from association with a bacterial toxin, (2) those that result from the sequelae of extracellular multiplication of the bacterial agent, and (3) those that result from the sequelae of intracellular multiplication.

Toxoids

Bacterial toxins are of two kinds: exotoxins and endotoxins. Endotoxins are strictly defined as the lipopolysaccharide portion of the gram-negative cell wall (it is the lipid A portion that is specifically responsible for the "toxic" manifestations). Muramyl dipeptide, which is present in gram-positive cell walls and to a lesser extent in gram-negative, also has "toxic" properties. We have used quotation marks around "toxic" because both endotoxin and muramyl dipeptide elicit their "toxic" activities by inducing the production of a variety of cytokines by host cells. It is the degree of vigor of the host response that defines the toxicity. Exotoxins are proteins that interact with host cells (usually after binding to a specific receptor), resulting in deregulation of host cell function without undue harm to the cell, interference of the normal physiology of the host cell(s), or death of the host cell.

Antibodies elicited to various epitopes on toxins that result in neutralization are sometimes called antitoxins. As mentioned previously, an antibody may block interaction between a toxin and its cellular receptor or change the configuration of the toxin so that it no longer has an effect on the host cell. Antibodies to exotoxins have been shown to be efficacious in preventing disease. Antibodies to endotoxins have had mixed results as far as preventing disease.

Toxoids are toxins without toxic activity that can elicit an immune response, that is, antibodies (see above for explanation). Toxoids can be produced by chemical inactivation of the native toxin or by manipulations of the gene encoding the toxin so that the toxin is inactivated. For example, in the case of A–B toxins (see Chapter 8), where the A subunit is responsible for the toxic activity of the toxin and the B subunits are responsible for binding of the toxin to the host, the gene encoding the A subunit can be eliminated and a toxoid produced that is composed of B subunits. An antibody to lipopolysaccharide (endotoxin) is elicited by immunization with mutants (called "rough" mutants) that produce very little of the O-repeat unit of the lipopolysaccharide (see Chapter 8).

The main advantage of toxoids is that they are safer than the disease-associated toxin. Toxoids administered parenterally elicit antibodies (IgM and IgG) that interfere with toxin–host cell interactions that are not at a mucosal surface. On the other hand, the administration of toxoids on a mucosal surface elicits antibodies (sIgM and sIgA) that interfere with toxin–host cell interaction at the mucosal surface. The main disadvantage of toxoids used for immunization by way of a mucosal surface is their extremely short half-life, thus they are unable to stimulate an immune response that is sufficient for protection.

Bacterins

Bacterins are killed pathogenic bacteria. They are usually produced by chemical killing of the infectious agent, with the aim to preserve bacterial structures expressing epitopes important in eliciting a protective immune response. The immune response to bacterins is an antibody response similar to toxoids as described above in the toxoids section.

The advantage of bacterins is that they are safe. If administered parenterally, the antibody elicited will be effective if the bacterin is made from a pathogen that has an extracellular life style. If the bacterin is administered by way of a mucosal surface, the antibody elicited (sIgM and sIgA) will interfere with interactions of pathogens with host cells. The disadvantage is that the main immune response is an antibody so that only antibody-mediated protection will occur. Thus, bacterins and toxoids administered parenterally are not as effective against intracellular pathogens. Bacterins placed on a mucosal surface have extremely short half-lives, a serious disadvantage. Another disadvantage is that the pathogen is usually grown *in vitro*, and epitopes expressed *in vivo* may not be expressed. This can result in a product that elicits antibodies with inappropriate specificities.

Bacterial Vaccines

Bacterial vaccines are composed of attenuated versions of the pathogen; that is, they are live but reduced in virulence. Attenuation may be accomplished in a number of ways: selection of a naturally occurring attenuated strain, repeated passage on artificial media, or elimination of a virulence trait by mutation of the gene encoding the trait.

The major advantages of bacterial vaccines are directly related to their being alive. Live vaccines not only have longer half-lives than their dead counterparts (regardless of location) but they will also express epitopes that may only be expressed *in vivo*, thus eliciting antibodies to epitopes that the pathogen will also express following infection. Another advantage is that live vaccines will elicit antibody and cellular immunity. A major disadvantage is that live vaccines may produce disease, for example, through reversion to the virulent phenotype. Also, if the vaccinated host has reduced resistance or if used in alternative host species, then the vaccine may produce disease.

Further Reading

Bassett JD, Swift SL, and Bramson JL (2011) Optimizing vaccine-induced CD8(+) T-cell immunity: focus on recombinant adenovirus vectors. *Expert Rev Vaccines*, **10** (9), 1307–1319.

Gilbert SC (2012) T-cell-inducing vaccines—what's the future. *Immunology*, **135** (1), 19–26. doi:10.1111/j.1365-2567.2011.03517.x

Hillaire ML, Osterhaus AD, and Rimmelzwaan GF (2011) Induction of virus-specific cytotoxic T lymphocytes as a basis for the development of broadly protective influenza vaccines. *J Biomed Biotechnol*, 2011, 939860. Epub October 5, 2011.

Lousberg EL, Diener KR, Brown MP, and Hayball JD (2011) Innate immune recognition of poxviral vaccine vectors. *Expert Rev Vaccines*, **10** (10), 1435–1449.

Meeusen EN (2011) Exploiting mucosal surfaces for the development of mucosal vaccines. *Vaccine*, **29** (47), 8506–8511. Epub September 22, 2011.

Murtaugh MP and Genzow M (2011) Immunological solutions for treatment and prevention of porcine reproductive and respiratory syndrome (PRRS). *Vaccine*, **29** (46), 8192–8204. Epub September 17, 2011.

Pinheiro CS, Martins VP, Assis NR *et al.* (2011) Computational vaccinology: an important strategy to discover new potential S. mansoni vaccine candidates. *J Biomed Biotechnol*, 2011, 503068. Epub October 15, 2011.

PART II

Bacteria and Fungi

Family Enterobacteriaceae

RODNEY MOXLEY

The family Enterobacteriaceae currently includes 46 genera and 263 names species and subspecies (Table 6.1). Some species are significant causes of intestinal or extraintestinal disease in food and companion mammals, poultry, other avian species, reptiles, and humans. Extraintestinal infections often involve the urinary tract, respiratory tract, bloodstream, and wounds. The genera that contain significant pathogens of animals and humans include *Citrobacter, Cronobacter, Enterobacter, Escherichia, Klebsiella, Morganella, Plesiomonas, Proteus, Providencia, Salmonella, Serratia, Shigella,* and *Yersinia*. Some genera predominantly include pathogens of plants (*Brenneria, Dickeya, Erwinia, Pantoea,* and *Pectobacterium*) and insects or nematodes (*Arsenophonus, Buchnera, Photorhabdus, Shimwellia, Wigglesworthia,* and *Xenorhabdus*).

Descriptive Features

Morphology and Staining

These organisms are gram-negative straight rods (Figure 6.1), most ranging from 0.3 to 1.0 μm wide by 0.6–6.0 μm long (Figure 6.2). Members of the family Enterobacteriaceae are indistinguishable from one another based simply on morphology.

Cellular Structure and Composition

The cell wall is consistent with that of other gram-negative bacteria, containing both inner (cytoplasmic) and outer membranes (OM), a thin peptidoglycan layer, and periplasm (Figure 6.3). The OM is an asymmetric bilayer with phospholipids on its inner surface, and lipid A (endotoxin), the hydrophobic anchor of lipopolysaccharide (LPS) on the outside. The OM contains proteins, (Braun's) lipoproteins, and an acidic polysaccharide known as the enterobacterial common antigen (ECA). OM phospholipids are similar in composition to those in the cytoplasmic membrane. Outer membrane proteins (OMP) vary considerably, but OmpA and other porins are major components. Porin proteins are assembled as trimers, forming pore-like structures with hydrophilic lumens, allowing ions and aqueous solutions to pass through the otherwise hydrophobic lipid bilayer. ECA contains *N*-acetyl-D-glucosamine, *N*-acetyl-D-mannosaminuronic acid, and 4-acetamido-4,6-dideoxy-D-galactose.

The proximal portion of the LPS macromolecule consists of the hydrophobic lipid A region. This region is a polar lipid in which a backbone of glucosaminyl-β-(1→6)-glucosamine is substituted usually with six or seven saturated fatty acid residues. Distally, the lipid A backbone is connected to the inner core polysaccharide region, and both the inner core and the lipid A backbone contain many charged groups, most of which are anionic. The outermost region of the LPS consists of the hydrophilic, O-antigen polysaccharide region. Core polysaccharide is positioned between the lipid A region on the proximal side (inner core) and the O-antigen region on the distal side (outer core) (Figure 6.4). The lipid A component is a polar lipid in which a backbone of glucosaminyl-β-(1→6)-glucosamine is substituted usually with six or seven fatty acid residues, all of them saturated. In bacteria that produce smooth LPS, the core polysaccharides are divided into two regions: inner core (lipid A proximal) and outer core. The outer core region provides an attachment site for O-polysaccharide (O-antigen). Within family and genus, the structure of the inner core tends to be well conserved. The inner core typically contains residues of Kdo and L-glycero-D-mannoheptose (Figure 6.2).

The somatic antigens (O-antigens) are composed of repeat units that can differ in the monomer glycoses, the position and stereochemistry of the O-glycosidic linkages, and the presence or absence of noncarbohydrate substituents (Figure 6.2). O-repeat units from different structures may comprise varying numbers of monosaccharides, may be linear or branched, and may form homopolymers or more frequently, heteropolymers. Extensive heterogeneity in the sizes of molecules occurs due to variations in the chain length of the O-polysaccharides, giving rise to the classical "ladder" pattern in sodium dodecyl sulfate–polyacrylamide gel electrophoresis, where each "rung" in the ladder represents a lipid A-core molecule substituted with an increment of one additional O-unit.

Veterinary Microbiology, Third Edition. Edited by D. Scott McVey, Melissa Kennedy and M.M. Chengappa.

Table 6.1. Taxa of the Family Enterobacteriaceae[a]

Genus	Number of Species and Subspecies	Type Species
Arsenophonus	1	*nasoniae*
Brenneria	5	*salicis*
Buchnera	1	*aphidicola*
Budvicia	2	*aquatica*
Buttiauxella	7	*agrestis*
Cedecea	3	*davisae*
Citrobacter	11	*freundii*
Cosenzaea	1	*myxofaciens*
Cronobacter	9	*sakazakii*
Dickeya	6	*chrysanthemi*
Edwardsiella	4	*tarda*
Enterobacter	21	*cloacae*
Erwinia	17	*amylovora*
Escherichia	5	*coli*
Ewingella	1	*americana*
Hafnia	2	*alvei*
Klebsiella	7	*pneumoniae*
Kluyvera	4	*ascorbata*
Leclercia	1	*adecarboxylata*
Leminorella	2	*grimontii*
Lonsdalea	3	*quercina*
Moellerella	1	*wisconsensis*
Morganella	3	*morganii*
Obesumbacterium	1	*proteus*
Pantoea	20	*agglomerans*
Pectobacterium	9	*carotovorum*
Photorhabdus	16	*luminescens*
Plesiomonas	1	*shigelloides*
Pragia	1	*fontium*
Proteus	4	*vulgaris*
Providencia	8	*alcalifaciens*
Rahnella	1	*aquatilis*
Raoultella	3	*planticola*
Salmonella	8	*enterica*
Samsonia	1	*erythrinae*
Serratia	16	*marcescens*
Shigella	4	*dysenteriae*
Shimwellia	2	*pseudoproteus*
Sodalis	1	*glossinidius*
Tatumella	5	*ptyseos*
Thorsellia	1	*anopheles*
Trabulsiella	2	*guamensis*
Wigglesworthia	1	*glossinidia*
Xenorhabdus	22	*nematophila*
Yersinia	18	*pestis*
Yokenella	1	*regensburgei*

[a]Total: 46 genera, 263 species and subspecies (when subspecies are present, they replace the respective species in the total).
Adapted from the Leibniz-Institut DSMZ-Deutsche Sammlung von Mikroorganismen und Zellkulturen GmgH Bacterial Nomenclature Up-to-Date database, http://old.dsmz.de/microorganisms/bacterial_nomenclature.php (accessed March, 20, 2013), and the J.P. Euzéby: List of Prokaryotic Names with Standing in Nomenclature, http://www.bacterio.cict.fr (accessed January 10, 2013).

The O-antigen serological specificity of an organism is defined by the structure of the O-polysaccharide; however, there is great variability in the numbers of unique O-antigens within a species. The O-antigen portion of the LPS molecule provides protection against phagocytosis. Further, loss of the more proximal part of the LPS core ("deep

FIGURE 6.1. E. coli, *gram-negative rods, magnification 1000 ×. (Courtesy of Hans Newman, Bacteria in Photos, Copyright 2011, www.bacteriainphotos.com, accessed January 10, 2013.)*

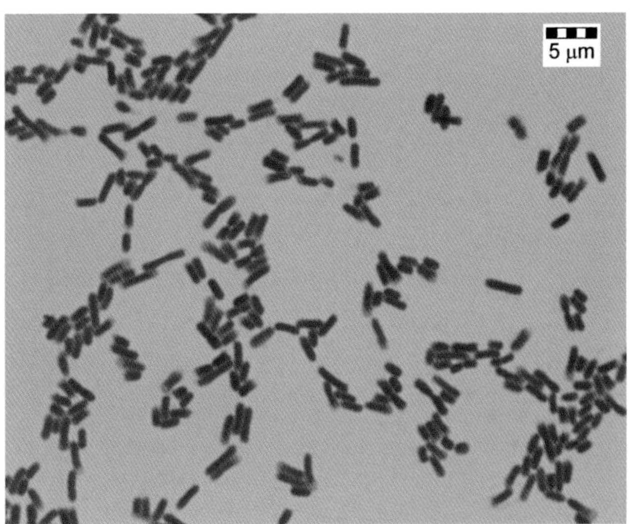

rough" mutants) makes the strains exceptionally sensitive to many different hydrophobic compounds. These include dyes, antibiotics, bile salts, other detergents, and mutagens; thus, this area is involved in maintaining the barrier property of the OM. The lipid A component is essential for the assembly of the OM.

Enterobacteriaceae often expresses a capsule that consists of an acidic polysaccharide. Two types of capsular polysaccharides may be produced. The first type, known as M (mucous) antigen, consists of colanic acid and is produced by most strains. M antigen is thought to provide protection against desiccation. The second type, known as K antigen, K for *kapsel* (capsule in German), is a component of the serotype and may provide antiphagocytic, serum resistance, and mucosal adherence properties depending on the chemical composition.

Many members of this group express adhesins that generally behave as lectins, recognizing oligosaccharide residues of glycoproteins and glycolipids. These adhesins consist of proteins embedded in the outer cell membrane that are composed of subunits and assembled into organelles, or consist of a single OMP. Those assembled into organelles include fimbria (pili) and afimbrial (nonfimbrial) adhesins.

Fimbriae are hair-like appendages that are arranged diffusely on the surface of the bacterial cells. Fimbriae are thinner and typically shorter and more numerous than flagella; they range from 2 to 8 nm in diameter, and usually number 100–1000 per cell. The fimbriae bind to receptors on the surfaces of host cells, and different types of fimbriae vary in their binding specificities. A single bacterial isolate can express multiple fimbrial types. The term "pili" (plural) is used interchangeably with fimbriae, although some authors reserve "pili" for those structures (F pili) that are involved in conjugation.

The fimbrial structure consists of a shaft and an adhesin tip, with the latter conferring binding specificity to the

FIGURE 6.2. *Colorized scanning electron photomicrograph (magnification 6836 ×) of gram-negative* E. coli *O157:H7. (Courtesy of US Health and Human Services, Centers for Disease Control and Prevention, Public Health Information Library, ID# 10068.)*

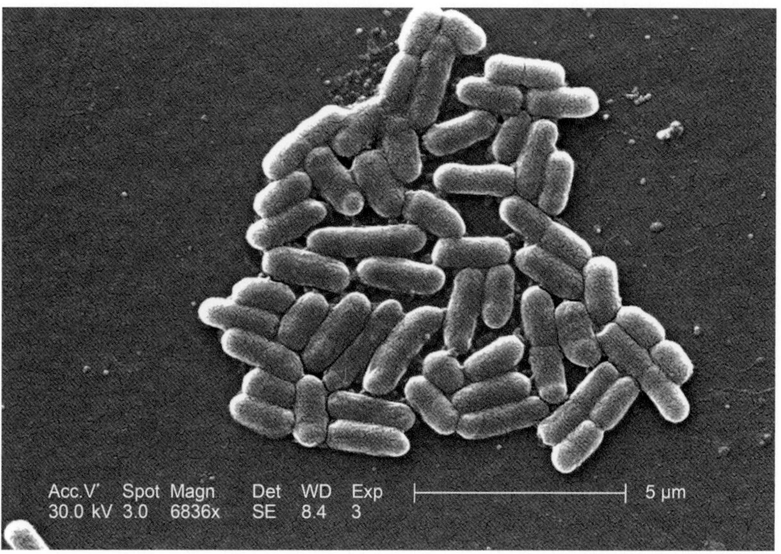

host cell. The construction of fimbriae requires the coordinated folding, secretion, and ordered assembly of multiple distinct protein subunits. Both shaft and adhesin tip are made up of repeating protein subunits called fimbrins. The fimbrin composition of the shaft and the adhesin tip may differ or be the same. The fimbrin proteins are antigenic, and these properties have been used to group them into F-types. The adhesive properties of fimbriae have also been used for their classification, for example, whether or not they bind to mannose-containing host cell receptors. The binding of fimbriae to a mannose-containing receptor can be inhibited by exposing the fimbriae to mannose prior to

FIGURE 6.3. *Molecular model of the inner and outer membranes of* E. coli *K-12. Ovals and rectangles represent sugar residues, as indicated, whereas circles represent polar head groups of various lipids. PPEtn, ethanolamine pyrophosphate; LPS, lipopolysaccharide; Kdo, 2-keto-3-deoxyoctulosonic acid; MDO, membrane-derived oligosaccharide. (Reproduced by permission of Raetz and Whitfield 2002; original publication in black and white, Raetz et al. 1991.)*

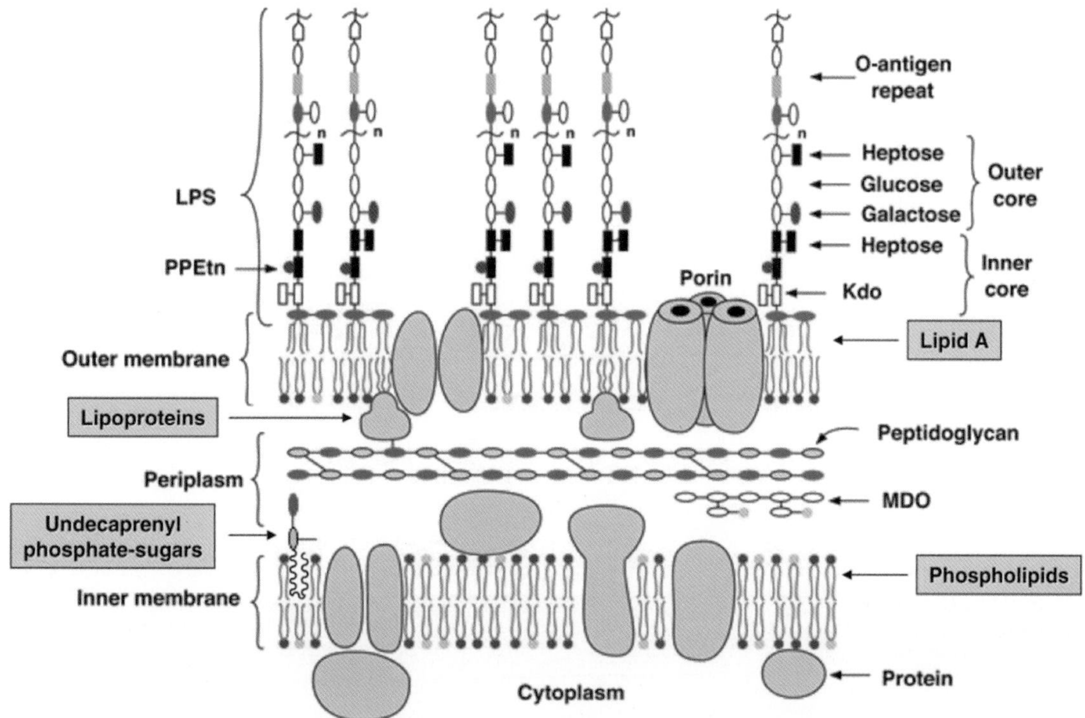

FIGURE 6.4. *Chemical structure of endotoxin from E. coli O111 : B4 according to Ohno and Morrison 1989. Hep, l-glycerol-d-manno-heptose; gal, galactose; Glc, glucose; Kdo, 2-keto-3-deoxyoctonic acid; NGa, N-acetyl-galactosamine; NGc, N-acetyl-glucosamine. (Reproduced by permission of Dr Fakhreddin Jamali, Editor,* J Pharm Pharmaceut Sci*; Magalhães et al. 2007.)*

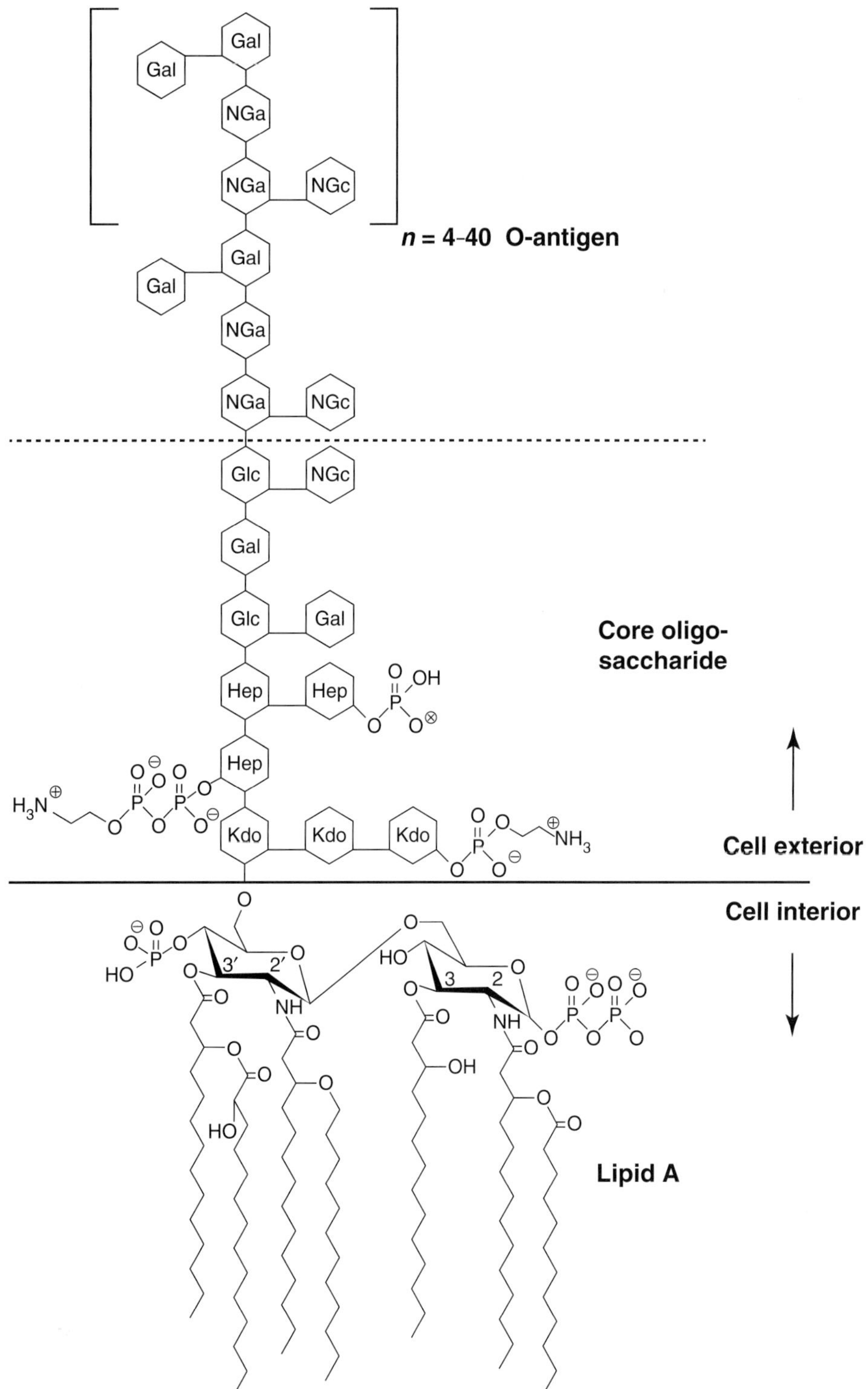

exposure to the receptor; those that are inhibited are called "mannose-sensitive" (MS) and those that are not are called "mannose-resistant" (MR). The type 1 fimbria of *Escherichia coli*, also known as F1, is an example of an MS adhesin. Mannose-containing receptors are found on the surfaces of red blood cells of different species; hence, hemagglutination reactions have been used to test for the presence of MS and MR fimbria. Molecular-based methods that are more practical and specific are now more commonly used for diagnostic purposes, for example, assays such as polymerase chain reaction, which may be used to detect the genes that encode fimbrin proteins.

Afimbrial adhesins are associated with an amorphous capsule-like, outer membrane-associated structure, and do not form visible fimbriae on the bacterial surface. The first afimbrial adhesin discovered was found on certain uropathogenic *E. coli* strains and named AFA (for afimbrial adhesin). Afimbrial adhesins were later found on the surfaces of some pathogenic *E. coli* in calves and lambs (see Chapter 7).

Most wild-type strains of the Enterobacteriaceae family are motile, a property imparted by flagella. The number of flagella expressed varies, but typically there are about 5–10 per cell, and they are arranged in a peritrichous pattern. Each flagellum is typically about 5–10 μm in length and 20 nm in diameter. The extracellular portion includes, from proximal to distal, the following structures made up of specific proteins (in parentheses): a curved hook region (FlgE) that extends from the surface of the outer cell membrane; a hook–filament junction (FlgK and FlgL); a long helical filament (FliC); and a filament cap (FliD). The filament consists of flagellin (FliC) subunits arranged in a cylindrical or tubular pattern, giving it a hollow lumen. Despite having a hollow structure, the filament is rigid, making it suitable for its function as a propeller. The flagellum is anchored in the cell envelope by its basal body. The basal body also has an approximately cylindrical symmetry, and consists of a rod and a set of five rings. The rings—L, P, M, S, and C—are named for the plane in which they are found—LPS, peptidoglycan, membrane (cytoplasmic), supramembrane, and cytoplasm, respectively.

The mol% guanine-plus-cytosine (G+C) content of the DNA is 38–60.

Cellular Products of Medical Interest

Cellular products of medical interest common to all or most of the members of the family are endotoxins and various siderophores. Products produced by many include serine protease transporters of Enterobacteriaceae and extended spectrum β-lactamases.

Endotoxin. Endotoxin (lipid A) elicits severe toxic reactions in animals due to its effects on the innate immune and coagulatory systems. Lipid A binds to LPS-binding protein (a serum protein), which converts oligomeric micelles of LPS into a monomer for delivery to CD14. CD14 concentrates lipid A for binding to the TLR4–MD2 complex, found on the surfaces of macrophages, dendritic cells, and endothelial cells. TLR4 is a transmembrane protein that complexes with MD2 and CD14. Binding of lipid A to CD14 triggers a signal transduction cascade that results in expression of proinflammatory cytokines. This binding results in the association of the cytosolic domain of TLR4 with myeloid differentiation factor 88 (MyD88) adaptor protein, which is necessary for the recruitment of the protein kinases interleukin-1 receptor-associated kinase 1 (IRAK1) and IRAK6 and TNF receptor-associated factor 6 (TRAF6) to the complex. Ultimately, the IκB kinase is phosphorylated, which phosphorylates IκB, which allows nuclear factor (NF)-κB to translocate to the nucleus and activate the transcription of TNF-α, IL-1β, and IL-6. In addition, expression of tissue factor by endothelial cells and B7 costimulatory molecules by macrophages and dendritic cells is activated. These proinflammatory and procoagulatory responses are responsible, in part, for the clinical signs associated with endotoxemia. However, the elicitation of this pathway is also necessary for host resistance to the bacteria. Diversity in lipid A molecules among bacterial species prevents the innate immune systems of some hosts from responding. This is especially true with some of the most virulent members of the Enterobacteriaceae, for example, *Yersinia pestis*, and host species that are susceptible to sepsis with the respective pathogen. In contrast to *E. coli*, whose lipid A is hexa-acylated with five 14-carbon and one 12-carbon fatty acids, *Y. pestis* is tetra-acylated with four 14-carbon fatty acids. Consequently, *Y. pestis* lipid A is poorly recognized by the TLR4s of some host species, thereby preventing, among other functions, costimulatory molecule expression, which is needed for activation of T helper cells and ultimately macrophages, which interferes with the host's ability to clear the infection.

Siderophores. Iron is an important inorganic cation micronutrient as it is present in almost all bacterial cells. Iron is a cofactor for many different metalloproteins needed for bacterial growth and survival, for example, heme-containing proteins such as cytochromes; iron–sulfur proteins, for example, some enzymes involved in amino acid and pyrimidine biosynthesis, the electron transport chain, and the tricarboxylic acid cycle; and non-iron–sulfur proteins, for example, some enzymes required for DNA synthesis, amino acid synthesis, and antioxidant activity. Although animal hosts contain abundant amounts of iron, it is not readily available to bacteria, since it is tightly bound to such carrier proteins as transferrin and lactoferrin. Also, in culture conditions, iron availability is affected by the pH of the media and aeration. In aerobic conditions, iron is present in the ferric (Fe^{3+}) state and forms insoluble oxyhydroxide polymers at neutral pH. In contrast, ferrous (Fe^{2+}) iron is relatively soluble and accessible to bacterial cells growing under anaerobic conditions. To obtain ferric iron that is tied up in insoluble complexes, bacteria synthesize and release small iron-chelating molecules into the environment called siderophores. Siderophores have a molecular mass generally less than 1 kDa, are synthesized only under iron-deficient conditions, and have an affinity and specificity for iron in the ferric state. More than 100 different siderophores have been described in bacteria; however, all are broadly categorized as either catecholates or hydroxamates. Enterobacterin (also known as enterochelin) is the prototype catecholate siderophore and is commonly found among members of the Enterobacteriaceae family. Some strains also produce the hydroxamate siderophore aerobactin. When in low iron conditions, the bacteria synthesize and release siderophores that bind to Fe^{3+} ions and in turn bind to a receptor on the outer cell membrane, which then transports the ferrisiderophore complex into the cell. A given bacterial cell may also utilize siderophores synthesized by other bacterial species and even fungi. When in relatively high environmental concentrations of ferric iron, bacteria utilize a low-affinity system that functions without a siderophore. Iron is taken across the outer cell membrane by several different transport systems. In *E. coli*, six Fe^{3+} transport systems can function in aerobic conditions, and another, for Fe^{2+} transport, functions under anaerobic conditions. Five of these transport systems utilize siderophores and include enterochelin, aerobactin, citrate–Fe^{3+}, ferrichrome, and ferrioxamine B hydroxamate. These five systems have separate outer membrane receptors but share a dependency on an inner membrane protein called TonB for functioning of the outer membrane receptor proteins. In addition, there is a low-affinity system that functions at high concentrations of Fe^{3+} without a siderophore transport cofactor. The genes governing aerobactin uptake may be on the chromosome in some organisms, or on a plasmid, such as the ColV class plasmids in enteric bacteria. Once accumulated within the cell, the iron cations are either incorporated into iron-specific proteins (both heme- and non-heme-containing) or stored in either of two *E. coli* iron storage proteins, namely ferritin and bacterioferritin.

Growth Characteristics

Members of this group of microorganisms are nonsporeforming, nonacid-fast, facultative anaerobes, which grow rapidly under aerobic or anaerobic conditions. Their ability to grow in the presence or absence of oxygen reflects both a respiratory and fermentative metabolism, although fermentation is the more common method of utilization of carbohydrates, and often with production of acid and gas. Almost all members of this group ferment glucose to pyruvic acid via the Embden–Meyerhof pathway. Some produce succinic acid, acetic acid, formic acid, and ethanol by way of the mixed acid fermentation pathway, whereas others produce butanediol from pyruvic acid. These microorganisms utilize a variety of simple substrates for growth, although most have simple growth requirements. Some are capable of utilizing D-glucose as the sole source of carbon. Under aerobic conditions, the range of suitable substrates includes organic acids, amino acids, and carbohydrates. Members of this family are usually motile with peritrichous flagella, catalase positive, and oxidase negative (due to a lack of cytochrome c), and reduce nitrate to nitrite. Most grow well on MacConkey medium, and on peptone or meat extract without supplements or sodium chloride; however, some require vitamins and/or amino acids. Most grow well at 22–35 °C.

Resistance

Members of this group are susceptible to killing by sunlight, drying, pasteurization, and common disinfectants, for example, chlorine-, phenol-, and quaternary ammonium-based compounds. They can survive for weeks to months in moist, shaded environments, such as pastures, manure, litter, and bedding. Although many are susceptible to broad-spectrum antimicrobial agents, their susceptibility is not accurately predictable and can change rapidly through acquisition of R plasmids, or resistance-encoding DNA cassettes (which may insert into numerous integrons located in the genome and in plasmids) (see Chapters 4 and 5). Persistent use of antibiotics to treat infections (e.g., swine herds with enzootic enteric colibacillosis) may potentially select for and result in an increased herd-level prevalence of pathogens resistant to the antibiotics being used.

Variability

Variability of one isolate of enteric organism as compared to another within the same species or genus depends upon the genetic basis for the trait under consideration. Differences in the capsular, somatic, or flagellar antigens account for variability among isolates of the same genus and species. Some variation among members of the same genus and species in the family, as well as among members of different genera and species, is accounted for by the presence of genes residing on plasmids encoding certain phenotypic traits. Such traits as resistance to antimicrobial agents, production of toxin, or secretion of hemolysin may be plasmid encoded and will vary depending on the presence or absence of a particular plasmid.

Transition from the smooth to the rough phenotype occurs with all members of the family, and is often the result of phase variation. Likewise, change in the O-antigens has been shown to occur following lysogeny by certain bacteriophages (lysogenic conversion).

Susceptibility to various bacteriophages (phage typing) is sometimes useful in demonstrating differences in isolates (strains) of the same genus and species. Phage typing is a useful epidemiological tool.

Laboratory Diagnosis

The family is composed of a large number of related, facultatively anaerobic, oxidase-negative, nitrate-reducing, gram-negative rods. Differentiation within the family is accomplished by some or all of the following: culture, biochemical tests, immunological tests (i.e., serotyping of O : K : H antigens and detection of virulence products), and PCR. 16S rRNA sequencing is beginning to be used in some clinical laboratories to identify organisms that cannot be cultured or phenotypically classified.

A number of manuals deal exclusively with this family, and because of the extreme clinical importance and prevalence of these organisms, an increasing number of programmed and/or computerized identification schemes are becoming commercially available.

Morphology and Staining

All are gram-negative rods have similar morphological features (Figures 6.1 and 6.2).

Cultural Characteristics

Methods used to isolate members of the Enterobacteriaceae family vary depending upon whether the sample normally contains intestinal or other background flora, or is normally sterile. When the source is normally sterile

FIGURE 6.5. *Colonies of* E. coli *growing on blood agar culture medium. (Courtesy of Hans Newman, Bacteria in Photos, Copyright 2011, www.bacteriainphotos.com, accessed January 10, 2013.)*

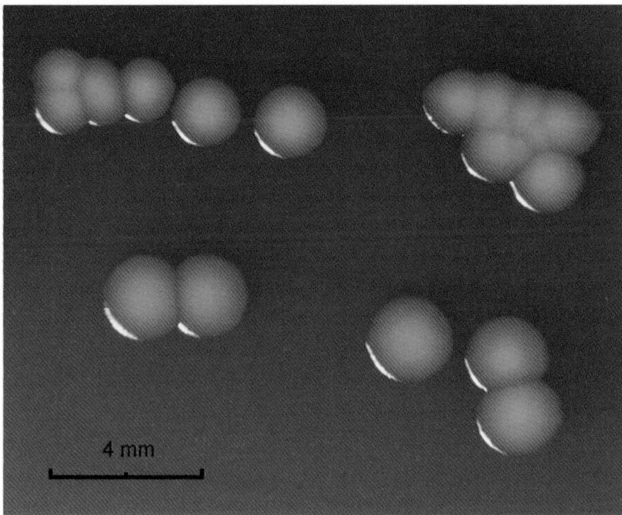

and proper aseptic procedures during sample collection (e.g., extraintestinal specimen) are used, isolation of any member of the Enterobacteriaceae family is significant. The medium for this purpose is sheep blood agar, and incubation is at 35–37 °C (Figure 6.5). In the case of intestinal samples, commensal strains of *E. coli* will be present and cannot be differentiated from pathogenic strains of *E. coli* simply by colony phenotype on such standard culture media as blood agar or MacConkey agar. In the case of some targeted serotypes (e.g., *E. coli* O157:H7), commercially available chromogenic media are available, and these media are designed to allow for presumptive differentiation of the pathogen from other flora on the plates.

Different enteric media have been devised to favor the identification of *Salmonella, Shigella, Yersinia,* or *E. coli* O157:H7 or other Shiga toxin-producing *E. coli*. The bases of the media are as follows:

1. An inhibitory substance, for example, bile salts, a dye, or antibiotics. These substances inhibit gram-positive or other competing enteric bacteria from growing.
2. A substrate whether utilized or not by the pathogen of interest.
3. A pH indicator to tell if the substrate has been changed, for example, utilization of a carbohydrate with production of fermentation products.

The following are useful selective media for isolating enteric pathogens.

Brilliant Green Agar

Inhibitor. Brilliant green dye (suppresses the growth of most members of the family except nontyphoidal *Salmonella*).

Substrate. Lactose and sucrose—*Salmonella* (and some strains of *Proteus*) does not ferment these sugars. Neither does *Shigella*, but *Shigella* grows poorly (if at all) on this medium.

Phenol Red. If sugars are not fermented (alkaline), colonies will be red; if sugars are fermented (acid), colonies will be yellow-green (due to the color of the background dye).

Usefulness. Excellent for isolating *Salmonella*.

Cefsulodin–Irgasan™–Novobiocin (*Yersinia* Selective Agar)

Inhibitor. Bile salts, crystal violet, cefsulodin, Irgasan, novobiocin.

Substrate. Mannitol.

Neutral Red. If mannitol is fermented (acid), colonies will be colorless with a red center ("bulls-eye" appearance); if mannitol is not fermented (alkaline), they will remain colorless, translucent.

Usefulness. Excellent for isolating *Yersinia enterocolitica*.

Eosin Methylene Blue (EMB). Agar, Levine.

Inhibitor. Eosin Y, methylene blue (these dyes inhibit gram-positive bacteria to a limited degree).

Substrate: Lactose

Eosin Y and Methylene Blue. These dyes play a role in differentiating between lactose-fermenters and nonfermenters. Bacteria that ferment lactose, especially the coliform bacterium *E. coli*, appear as colonies with a green metallic sheen or blue-black to brown color. Bacteria that do not ferment lactose appear as colorless or transparent, light purple colonies.

Usefulness. Isolation of gram-negative enteric bacteria with good differentiation between *Escherichia* and *Enterobacter* species.

Hektoen Enteric Agar

Inhibitor. Bile salts.

Substrate. Lactose and salicin—*Salmonella, Shigella,* and some species of *Proteus* and *Providencia* are lactose-negative and salicin-negative.

Ferric Salt. Organisms producing H_2S will form black-centered colonies.

Bromthymol Blue. Fermentors of salicin and/or lactose will form yellow to orange colonies; isolates not fermenting these sugars will form green or blue-green colonies.

Usefulness. Excellent for *Salmonella* and *Shigella*.

MacConkey Agar

Inhibitor. Bile salts and crystal violet (inhibit gram-positive bacteria).

Substrate. Lactose—*Salmonella*, *Shigella*, and *Proteus* do not ferment lactose.

Neutral Red. If lactose is fermented (acid), colonies will be pink; if lactose is not fermented (peptides digested—basic), colonies will be colorless.

Usefulness. Very permissive medium. *Salmonella* and *Shigella* readily grow on this medium (as do most other Enterobacteriaceae and *Pseudomonas*).

Sorbitol MacConkey Agar

Inhibitor. Bile salts and crystal violet (inhibit gram-positive bacteria).

Substrate. Sorbitol. More than 98% of *E. coli* ferment sorbitol within 24 h; *E. coli* O157:H7 is an exception.

Neutral Red. If sorbitol is fermented (acid), colonies will be pink; if sorbitol is not fermented (peptides digested—basic), colonies will be colorless.

Usefulness. Screening for *E. coli* O157:H7. The addition of 4-methylumbelliferyl-β-D-glucuronide (MUG) or 5-bromo-4-chloro-3-indolyl-β-D-glucuronide (BCIG) to the medium increases its specificity for *E. coli* O157 : H7 (see Sorbitol MacConkey Agar BCIG, cefixime, and potassium tellurite).

Sorbitol MacConkey Agar BCIG, cefixime, and potassium tellurite

Inhibitor. Bile salts and crystal violet inhibit gram-positive bacteria. Addition of cefixime and potassium tellurite inhibits sorbitol nonfermenters (e.g., *Proteus* and *Providencia*).

Substrate. Sorbitol. More than 98% of *E. coli* ferment sorbitol within 24 h; *E. coli* O157:H7 is an exception.

Neutral Red and BCIG. The nonsorbitol-fermenting and β-glucuronidase-negative *E. coli* O157:H7 will appear as straw-colored colonies. Organisms with β-glucuronidase activity will cleave the substrate, leading to a distinct blue-green coloration of the colonies.

Usefulness. Presumptive detection of *E. coli* O157:H7.

Xylose Lysine Deoxycholate Agar

Inhibitor. Bile salts.

Substrate. (1) Xylose—not fermented by *Shigella* (*Salmonella* ferments xylose). (2) Lysine—isolates that ferment xylose, but not lactose and sucrose, and are lysine decarboxylase-negative (*Proteus mirabilis*) produce colonies that will be amber-orange. *Salmonella* decarboxylates lysine. The ratio of xylose to lysine is such that an alkaline pH predominates (more decarboxylation). *Shigella* does not decarboxylate lysine. (3) Lactose and sucrose—*Salmonella* and *Shigella* do not ferment these sugars rapidly.

(4) Ferric salt—colonies of organisms producing H_2S (*Salmonella*; *Proteus*) will have black centers (iron sulfide).

Phenol Red. Acid colonies (non-*Salmonella* or non-*Shigella*) will be yellow. Alkaline colonies (possible *Salmonella* or *Shigella*) will be red.

Usefulness. An excellent all-purpose medium for both *Salmonella* and *Shigella*.

Enrichment Media. At times, the numbers of *Salmonella* or *Shigella* in fecal samples may be too low ($<10^4$/g) to be detected on the primary plating media discussed above. Therefore, in addition to being plated directly to a selective medium, the fecal sample is placed in an enrichment medium. To detect *Salmonella* by utilizing enrichment methods, at least 100 salmonellae/g are needed.

For *Salmonella*, enrichment may be achieved by incubating feces for 12–18 h in selenite F broth or tetrathionate broth. During this time, the growth of organisms other than *Salmonella* is suppressed, whereas the growth of *Salmonella* is not. After the 12–18 h has elapsed, an aliquot of the broth is streaked onto a plate of selective medium (e.g., brilliant green agar).

Enrichment for *Shigella* is not easy because it is rather sensitive to commonly used inhibitory substances found in selenite F and tetrathionate broths. An enrichment broth called gram-negative (or GN broth) is used in the same manner as selenite is used for *Salmonella*. GN broth and trypticase soy broth with novobiocin are both excellent for enrichment of fecal samples for *E. coli* O157:H7.

Members of the genus *Pseudomonas* (especially *P. aeruginosa*) may be found in feces, but this is probably an insignificant finding. *Pseudomonas* (not a member of the family Enterobacteriaceae) will grow on enteric media. This microorganism does very little to the substrates other than the peptides and peptones and thus mimics *Salmonella* and *Shigella* on selective media. *Pseudomonas* is oxidase-positive, a useful distinction.

References

Magalhães PO, Lopes AM, Mazzola PG *et al.* (2007) Methods of endotoxin removal from biological preparations: a review. *J Pharm Pharmaceut Sci*, **10** (3), 388–404.

Ohno N and Morrison DC (1989) Lipopolysaccharide interaction with lysozyme. Binding of lipopolysaccharide to lysozyme and inhibition of lysozyme enzymatic activity. *J Biol Chem*, **264**, 4434–4441.

Raetz CRH and Whitfield C (2002) Lipopolysaccharide endotoxins. *Ann Rev Biochem*, **71**, 635–700.

Raetz CR, Ulevitch RJ, Wright SD *et al.* (1991) Gram-negative endotoxin: an extraordinary lipid with profound effects on eukaryotic signal transduction. *FASEB J*, **5**, 2653.

Further Reading

Abbott, SL (2011) *Klebsiella, Enterobacter, Citrobacter, Serratia, Plesiomonas*, and other *Enterobacteriaceae*, in *Manual of Clinical Microbiology*, 10th edn (ed. J Versalovic), ASM Press, Washington, DC, pp. 639–657.

Atlas RM and Snyder JW (2011) Reagents, stains, and media: bacteriology, in *Manual of Clinical Microbiology*, 10th edn (ed. J Versalovic), ASM Press, Washington, DC, pp. 272–303.

Farmer, JJ III, Boatwright KD, and Janda JM (2007) *Enterobacteriaceae*: introduction and identification, in *Manual of Clinical Microbiology*, vol. 1, 9th edn (eds PR Murray, EJ Baron, JH Jorgensen, ML Landry, and MA Pfaller), ASM Press, Washington, DC, pp. 649–669.

7 Enterobacteriaceae: *Escherichia*

RODNEY MOXLEY

The genus *Escherichia* contains five species: *albertii, coli, fergusonii, hermannii,* and *vulneris;* the species *blattae* has recently been moved into the *Shimwellia* genus. *Escherichia* is the type genus of the Enterobacteriaceae family, with *coli* the type species of the genus. *Escherichia coli* is the only species that includes important pathogens of animals. Many *E. coli* are commensals of the intestinal tract, especially the large intestine; however, many are opportunistic or primary pathogens too. Pathogenic *E. coli* are broadly divided into diarrheagenic and extraintestinal strains. Diarrheagenic *E. coli* are economically important pathogens of neonatal piglets, calves, and lambs. Postweaning diarrheal infections are also important in swine. Extraintestinal infections commonly occur in the urinary tract, umbilicus, blood, lung, and wounds in any location, and these infections occur in most animal species. *E. coli* causes septicemia in neonates of most species, but especially calves, piglets, lambs, foals, puppies, and kittens, and causes opportunistic septicemia in older immunosuppressed animals. In avian species, *E. coli* is an important cause of air sacculitis, pneumonia, septicemia, and omphalitis. Zoonotic infections with Shiga toxin-producing *E. coli* (STEC) and host-specific diarrheagenic and extraintestinal infections are of major importance in human medicine.

Descriptive Features

Cellular Structure and Composition

Escherichia are straight, cylindrical, gram-negative rods with rounded ends that are approximately 0.5 μm in diameter and 1.0–3.0 μm in length (see Figures 7.1 and 7.2). The cell wall contains lipopolysaccharide (LPS), outer membrane proteins, lipoproteins, porins, and a thin peptidoglycan layer (see Figure 7.3). Cells with a complete LPS layer will typically express an O-antigen, although not all are typable. Cells may express a capsule (K-antigen), flagella (H-antigen), and adhesins.

Cellular Products of Medical Interest

Adhesins. Adhesins are composed of protein subunits assembled into organelles or consist of a single outer membrane protein, in either case forming a filamentous structure that projects out from the surface of the cell. Those assembled into organelles include fimbria (pili) and afimbrial (nonfimbrial) adhesins. The construction of fimbriae requires the coordinated folding, secretion, and ordered assembly of multiple distinct protein subunits. In *E. coli*, fimbriae are assembled by several pathways, but the chaperone-usher pathway is the most frequent in pathogenic strains. Most *E. coli* produce type 1 (F1) fimbriae, and these bind to mannose. Thus, F1 are called mannose-sensitive because their ability to bind can be blocked by pretreatment with mannose. Mannose-resistant fimbriae, which include many fimbrial types on pathogenic strains, are not inhibited by mannose. F1 plays a role in *E. coli* urinary tract infections in which it mediates adherence to uroepithelium by binding to uroplakin.

Fimbrial adhesins found on *E. coli* that cause disease (colibacillosis) in animals include F4 (with ab, ac, and ad subtypes), F5 (K99), F6 (987P), F11 (PapA), F17 (with a, b, c, and d subtypes), F18 (with ab and ac subtypes, formerly known as F107), F41, and F165 complex ($F165_1$ and $F165_2$). Several of the fimbriae on enterotoxigenic *E. coli* (ETEC) isolates from humans are called colonization factor antigens (CFA), for example, CFA/I (also known as F2), CFA/II (also known as F3), and others. Some fimbriae in ETEC isolates from humans are called coli-surface (CS) antigens, for example, CS1, CS2, CS3, and others. Finally, other ETEC fimbriae from human isolates are called putative colonization factors (PCF), also numbered sequentially. Approximately 75% of ETEC isolates from humans express CFA/I, CFA/II, or CFA/IV.

In animals, strains that express F4, F5, F6, F18ac, or F41 fimbria are ETEC and cause enteric colibacillosis manifested as diarrhea. Genes for expression of F4, F5, and F6 are usually carried on plasmids, whereas those for F41 are on the chromosome. F4, formerly known as K88, mediates adherence to brush border receptors on small intestinal enterocytes of piglets (Figure 7.1). In pigs, the resistant and susceptible phenotypes for F4ab and F4ac are inherited as a monogenetic trait, with the susceptibility allele being dominant over the resistance one. The F4ab/ac receptor is a mucin-like sialoglycoprotein that is encoded on a locus distal to the mucin-4 gene on chromosome 13. Piglets

Veterinary Microbiology, Third Edition. Edited by D. Scott McVey, Melissa Kennedy and M.M. Chengappa.

FIGURE 7.1. *The photomicrograph taken at an objective magnification of 60× shows mucosal epithelium in the jejunum of an 11-day-old gnotobiotic piglet infected with porcine-origin enterotoxigenic* E. coli *(ETEC) strain WAM2317 (O8:K87:H⁻:F4). Immunohistochemistry was used to demonstrate the bacteria that are adherent to the enterocytes. Rabbit anti-O8 was used as the primary antiserum. Alkaline phosphatase-labeled goat antirabbit serum and fast red were subsequently used in the staining procedures.*

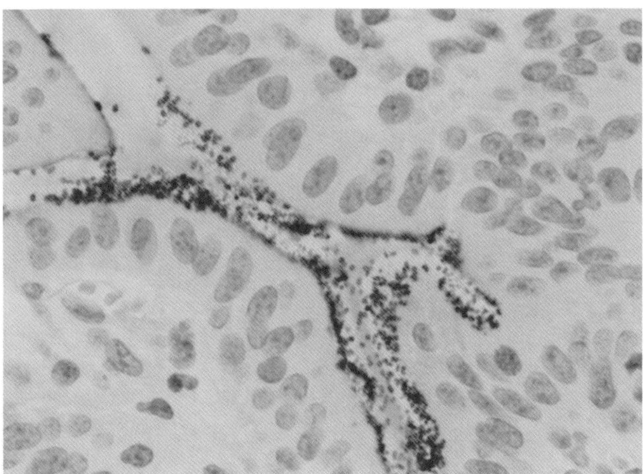

expressing the F4ab/ac receptor are susceptible to F4ab- or F4ac-mediated fimbrial adherence. Enterotoxigenic colibacillosis caused by F4-positive strains is often clinically severe, and may be seen in piglets only a few hours old to approximately 8 weeks of age. F4-positive bacteria adhere to the full length of the small intestine, a feature that greatly increases the severity of disease. F5-positive fimbria mediate adherence to receptors on the brush borders of enterocytes in the distal half of the small intestine.

FIGURE 7.2. *β-Hemolysis produced by α-hemolysin. Porcine-origin enterotoxigenic* E. coli *strain 3030-2 (O157:H⁻:F4) was streaked for isolation on tryptic soy agar containing 5% sheep red blood cells, and incubated at 37 °C for 24 h. (Xing 1996.)*

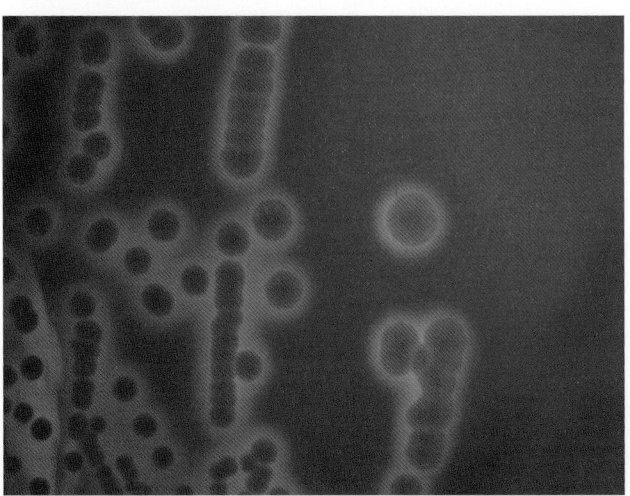

FIGURE 7.3. *Higher magnification scanning electron photomicrograph of colon of neonatal gnotobiotic calf. Shiga toxin-producing* E. coli *strain 84-5406 (serotype O5:K4:H⁻, arrow) cover the apical cell membranes of enterocytes. Cuplike or pedestal-like distortions of the apical cell membranes (arrowhead) are present at sites where bacteria were detached during tissue processing. Microvilli between attached bacterial cells are prominent and elongated. Enterocytes are swollen and are in the process of detachment from the mucosal surface (original negative magnification 5000×; bar = 1 μm). (Copyright © American Society for Microbiology. Moxley RA and Francis DH 1986; with permission.)*

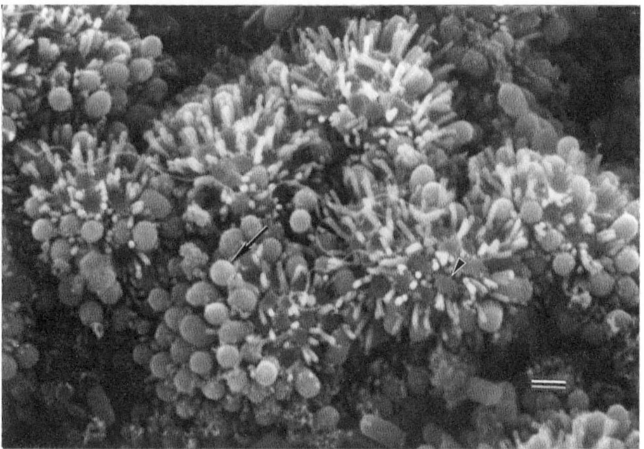

Strains expressing F5, formerly known as K99, cause diarrhea in piglets less than 1 week old and in calves and lambs during only the first few days of life. In pigs, resistance to F5-mediated fimbrial adherence results from a decrease in the number of receptors on the intestinal epithelium. Similar to F5, F6-positive fimbriae mediate colonization of only the distal small intestine. Strains expressing F6, formerly known as 987P, cause diarrhea only in piglets, and clinical disease is usually limited to piglets less than 1 week old. Age-mediated resistance to F6 results from shedding of fimbrial receptors into the intestinal lumen, facilitating bacterial clearance rather than colonization. F18ab- and F18ac-positive fimbriae mediate colonization of the small intestine in postweaned swine. Strains that express F18ab typically produce Shiga toxin-2e and cause edema disease. Strains that produce F18ac are typically enterotoxigenic. F18ab colonization may occur in either the proximal or distal part of the small intestine.

F17-positive *E. coli* are typically isolated from 4- to 21-day-old calves with diarrhea or septicemia. Approximately half of the F17-positive *E. coli* strains isolated from calves with diarrhea are resistant to complement and produce aerobactin, suggesting a role in septicemia. Approximately, one-fourth of the F17-positive *E. coli* strains isolated from calves produce cytotoxic necrotizing factor-2 (CNF-2) and afimbrial adhesin (Afa), findings also suggesting a role in extraintestinal infections. Most bovine strains expressing F17c subtype fimbriae also produce the afimbrial CS31A adhesin. Genes for expression of F17c fimbria are often found on a self-transmissible plasmid that also encodes for CS31A adhesin, aerobactin, and antibiotic resistance.

$F165_1$ and $F165_2$ fimbriae have also been found on *E. coli* isolates from piglets and calves with septicemia. F165-positive isolates from piglets are usually nonenterotoxigenic, serogroup O115, and express F11 (PapA) fimbriae, aerobactin, K "V165" O-antigen capsule, and additional virulence factors, many of which are found other in extraintestinal pathogenic *E. coli* strains. F165-positive strains colonize the distal small intestine of piglets, but cause septicemia and polyserositis instead of diarrhea. The bacteria are thought to enter extraintestinal tissues by translocation from the intestine and are known to resist phagocytic killing by porcine neutrophils. Both $F165_1$ fimbriae and the K"V165" capsule are required for complete resistance to killing by neutrophils.

Curli are thin, coiled, fibrillar fimbriae that promote adherence to extracellular matrix proteins, for example, fibronectin and laminin. Curli fimbriae play a role in biofilm formation, which assists bacterial survival in the environment. Curli fimbriae are produced by both pathogenic and nonpathogenic strains of *E. coli*, as well as by other members of the Enterobacteriaceae family.

Aggregative adherence fimbriae (AAF/I and AAF/II) mediate adherence of enteroaggregative *E. coli* (EAEC) to HEp-2 cells *in vitro*. Following growth, adherent bacteria form an autoaggregative, "stacked-brick" pattern on the surfaces of the host cells. EAEC are an important cause of persistent diarrhea in children and adults in developing and developed countries. In humans, EAEC are thought to primarily colonize the colon. EAEC with ability to cause disease usually contain a large set of virulence genes regulated by the AggR transcription activator. These include plasmid (pAA) genes encoding the AAF, a protein coat secretion system (Aat), secreted dispersin protein (Aap), plasmid-encoded toxin (Pet; a serine protease autotransporter that targets spectrin), Shf (a protein involved in intercellular adhesion), and Aai (a putative type VI secretion system). EAEC also express virulence factors that are encoded by genes on the chromosome. Protein Involved in Colonization (Pic) (which is a type of serine protease autotransporter of Enterobacteriaceae (SPATE)) that functions as a secreted mucinase and Irp2 (yersiniabactin, a siderophore) are two important virulence factors encoded on the chromosome. A newly emergent EAEC clone of serotype O104:H4 is highly virulent in humans. It produces most of the aforementioned EAEC virulence factors, plus Shiga toxin (Stx)-2, aerobactin (*iutA*), *iha* (IrgA homolog adhesin), extended spectrum β-lactamases, and two additional SPATEs rarely found in EAEC (SepA (unknown function) and SigA (which cleaves the cytoskeletal protein spectrin)). Based on detection of aggregative adherence, EAEC have been detected in piglets and calves, but these isolates contained almost none of the virulence factors found in human EAEC isolates, and consequently were not likely to be pathogens of animals or humans.

The bundle-forming pilus (Bfp) is a fimbrial adhesin produced by class I (typical) enteropathogenic *E. coli* (EPEC). These fimbriae form "bundles" and mediate localized adherence to HEp-2 cells in culture. *In vivo*, together with the type III secreted outer membrane protein known as EspA, they mediate the first stage of EPEC adherence to small intestinal epithelial cells. EPEC are one of the most important causes of infantile diarrhea in humans in the world. EPEC infections occur naturally in pigs, calves, dogs, and cats, but only a small fraction of the causative strains produce Bfp.

Afimbrial (nonfimbrial) adhesins in various pathogenic *E. coli* include CS31A, AfaE-VII, Afa-VIII, AIDA-I, LifA, Efa1, ToxB, Paa, Saa, OmpA, Iha, and TibA. CS31A is typically found on neonatal calf septicemia isolates that are also positive for F17c fimbria and aerobactin. CS31A is present as fine, wiry, fibrillae that collapse onto the surface of the bacterium, forming a capsule-like structure. CS31A mediates adherence to *N*-acetylneuraminic acid receptors on host cells. Afa-VII and Afa-VIII are afimbrial adhesins found on bovine isolates. Afa-VII has been found on isolates from diarrhea cases and Afa-VIII has been found on isolates from diarrhea and septicemia cases in calves. Isolates expressing Afa-VIII usually also produce CNF-1 or CNF-2. Afa-VIII is produced more often than Afa-VII by bovine isolates, as is CNF-2 than CNF1. AIDA-I (adhesin involved in diffuse adherence) is an autotransporter produced by diffusely adherent *E. coli* (DAEC) of humans, and mediates the diffusely adherent phenotype. AIDA-I has been found in isolates from pigs with edema disease and postweaning diarrhea. Many porcine isolates that are genotypically positive for AIDA-I are also positive for heat-stable enterotoxin-b (STb) alone or in combination with enteroaggregative *E. coli* heat-stable toxin-1 (EAST1). LifA (lymphostatin) in EPEC and its homolog Efa1 (enterohemorrhagic *E. coli* (EHEC) factor for adherence) in EHEC mediate enterocyte adherence. LifA also inhibits lymphocyte activation and production of certain cytokines. Efa1 is produced by non-O157 EHEC strains and it mediates adherence to epithelial cells *in vitro* and in the bovine intestine. ToxB is a homolog of LifA and Efa1 and is produced by EHEC O157:H7. Paa (porcine attaching-and effacing-associated) factor is found in porcine EPEC and EHEC isolates; its role in the pathogenesis is unknown. Saa (STEC-autoagglutinating adhesin) is found in non-O157 STEC strains that lack the locus of enterocyte effacement (LEE) and is much more highly prevalent in cattle than human isolates. OmpA (outer membrane protein A) is a putative adhesin used by EHEC in adherence to large intestinal enterocytes. OmpA is also produced by meningitis-associated *E. coli* in human isolates. Saa (STEC autoagglutinating adhesin) is produced by EHEC. Iha (IrgA homolog adhesin) is produced by EHEC O157:H7, EAEC O104:H4 and many STEC isolated from cattle. TibA is produced by a subset of ETEC isolates of humans.

E. coli cell surface antigens are subject to phase variation. Phase variation is the reversible change of one or more cell surface antigens of a bacterium at a high frequency, and involves the regulation of genes at the transcriptional level. Phase variation of uropathogenic *E. coli* (UPEC) fimbrial *pap* genes involves the switching "on" or "off" of transcription in response to environmental signals. Similarly, ETEC F4 fimbriae are expressed *in vitro* when cultured on blood agar at 37 °C, but suppressed at 18 °C. Hence, through phase variation, the bacteria sense environmental signals and expend energy and nutritional resources only to the extent necessary (e.g., shut off fimbrial expression when it is not needed).

FIGURE 7.4. *Transmission electron photomicrograph of rectum of neonatal gnotobiotic calf inoculated with Shiga toxin-producing* E. coli *strain 84-5406. The attachment of bacteria to this enterocyte results primarily in pedestal-like cell membrane evagination (P), with occasional cuplike invagination (Cp). Microvilli between sites of bacterial attachment are elongated (arrow). Some bacteria are in the process of binary fission (arrowhead). The cytoplasm lacks a discernible terminal web and contains numerous vacuoles (original negative magnification × 15 000; bar = 1 μm). (Copyright © American Society for Microbiology, Moxley RA and Francis DH 1986; with permission.)*

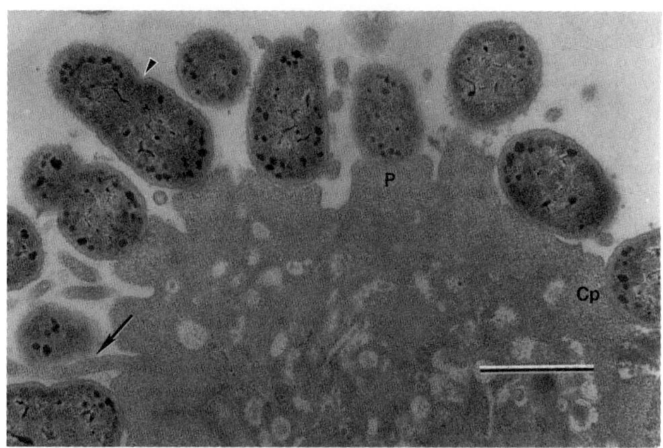

Capsule. The capsule consists of an acidic, high molecular weight polysaccharide that is anionic and hydrophilic. The negative charge of the capsule helps protect the bacteria against phagocytosis, since the phagocytes also have a negative charge on their cell surfaces. The capsule is usually antigenic, and if so, listed as a K-antigen type. Some capsular antigen types (e.g., K87) impart the bacteria with "serum resistance"; that is, it protects the outer cell membrane from the membrane attack complex of the complement cascade (C5b-C9). This property is especially important for survival of pathogenic strains causing extraintestinal infections.

Cell Wall. The cell wall is typical of the Enterobacteriaceae family (see Figure 7.3). The LPS layer in the outer membrane is an important virulence determinant by virtue of the biological effects of lipid A (endotoxin) and the O-antigen repeat unit (see Figure 7.4). The effects of lipid A are described in detail in Chapter 6. A thick O-antigen layer may provide effects similar to a K-antigen capsule. These effects may include protection against phagocytosis and the membrane attack complex of the complement system. Thick O-antigen layers that mediate these protective effects are sometimes referred to as an O-antigen capsule.

Enterotoxins

Some pathogenic strains, especially those belonging to the diarrheagenic class known as ETEC, may produce one or more enterotoxins. These enterotoxins are protein exotoxins encoded by genes usually carried on transmissible plasmids. *E. coli* produces four different enterotoxins: heat-labile enterotoxin (LT), heat-stable enterotoxin-a (STa), STb, and EAST1. LT is labile when heated to 70 °C for 10 min, whereas STa and STb are stable at 100 °C for 15 min.

Heat-Labile Enterotoxin. LT is very similar structurally, antigenically, and functionally to cholera toxin. The genes for LT expression, *eltAB*, are organized in an operon and typically carried on a large, transmissible plasmid. Expression of the *eltAB* operon is enhanced by exposure of the cells to free glucose. This is due to derepression as a result of inhibition of the cAMP receptor protein (CRP). Enhanced expression upon exposure to glucose is the opposite to the effects of glucose exposure on expression of the genes for STa and STb, both of which are subject to catabolite repression. Since an individual ETEC strain often carries both LT and STb or LT and STa, expression of one or the other toxin is enabled in either condition.

LT is a rather large macromolecule with a molecular weight of approximately 86 000 daltons. The LT holotoxin includes one 28-kDa A-subunit and five 11.5 kDa B-subunits. The A-subunit contains a serine-protease cleavage site that allows for separation into an A2- and an enzymatically active A1-chain. The A-subunit is linked noncovalently to the B-subunit via the A2-chain, and the A1- and A2-chains are bridged together by a disulfide bond. The B subunits are arranged in a homopentamer around the A subunit, and bind with greatest affinity to Galβ3GalNAcβ4(NeuAcα3)Glcβ1-ceramide, more commonly known as monosialoganglioside G_{M1}. The B-subunits also bind with lower affinity to the disialoganglioside GD1b, and to terminal galactose units on other molecules, for example, intestinal glycoproteins. Lipid rafts in the apical cell membranes of intestinal epithelium are enriched in G_{M1}, and this serves as a route by which LT enters the host cell. While either in the intestinal lumen or upon binding to the apical membrane of the cell, the A subunit is proteolytically cleaved ("nicked") into A1- and A2 chains. Trypsin is able to cleave the A subunit, but the identity of the protease(s) involved in this step is not actually known. Following this nicking event, the two chains remain attached by the disulfide bond.

Based on studies with cholera toxin, after being bound to G_{M1}, the holotoxin is taken up by a variety of endocytic mechanisms, including clathrin- and caveolin-dependent, as well as caveolin- and dynamin-independent ones. Following uptake, the holotoxin traffics through early and recycling endosomes, and then enters the trans-Golgi network. From there it bypasses the Golgi cisternae and travels to the endoplasmic reticulum (ER), utilizing v- and t-SNARES, and other transmembrane vesicle fusion proteins. From the initial endocytic step to entry into the ER, the B-subunit is bound to G_{M1}. While in the ER lumen, the A1-chain is unfolded by protein disulfide isomerase and dissociates from the A2-chain and the B-subunits. The unfolded A1-chain is then recognized by the ER Hsp70 chaperone BiP and solubilized by the ER-associated degradation lumenal pathway. At this point, the A1-chain retro-translocates into the cytosol by an as yet unidentified pathway; the Sec61 translocon and the Hrd-1 complex are hypothetically possible routes. Upon reentry into the cytosol, the A1-chain refolds into its native conformation, and catalyzes the ADP-ribosylation of arginine 201 of the α-subunit of the host G_s

protein that regulates adenylyl cyclase. This modification leads to inhibition of the GTPase activity of Gsα of the host G_s protein. Adenylyl cyclase, located at the basal surface of the cell, is constitutively activated.

Constitutive activation of adenylyl cyclase results in a marked intracellular increase in cAMP, which causes activation of protein kinase A. Protein kinase A causes phosphorylation of the cystic fibrosis transmembrane conductance regulator (CFTR), an anion channel in the apical cell membrane. Phosphorylation opens the channel, resulting in excessive secretion of Cl^- and bicarbonate ion (HCO_3^-) into the gut lumen. Secretion mainly occurs by cryptal enterocytes, making the electric potential of these cells negative and their serosal potential positive, both relative to the lumen. The transmural potential drives the diffusion of Na^+ through the tight junctions into the gut lumen. The increased Na^+ concentration in the gut lumen results in an increased osmotic pressure and corresponding diffusion of water into the gut lumen, which presents clinically as diarrhea.

A second mechanism by which LT may cause secretory diarrhea is through stimulated synthesis of prostaglandins of the E series (e.g., PGE_2) and platelet-activating factor (PAF). Binding of the B subunit to G_{M1} activates phospholipase A_2, resulting in release of arachidonic acid and generalized enhancement of cyclooxygenase activity, that is, production of PGE_2. Fibroblasts, mast cells, and leukocytes are major sources of prostaglandins and leukotrienes. Binding of the B subunit to these cells could potentially stimulate electolyte transport and motility in the intestine through induced synthesis of PGE_2. Prostaglandins, including PGE_2, have prosecretory and antiabsorptive effects on the intestine through induction of Ca^{2+} uptake, activation of protein kinase C, and increased intracellular cAMP in such target cells as neurons and epithelial cells. In addition, PGE_2 causes increased transcription of proinflammatory cytokines, for example, interleukin-6 (IL-6).

A third mechanism by which LT may cause secretory diarrhea is through stimulation of the enteric nervous system (ENS). The ENS has highly significant control over secretion and absorption in the intestine. Both cholera toxin and LT cause the release of vasoactive intestinal polypeptide (VIP), an ENS neurotransmitter that acts on epithelial cells and has prostimulatory and antiabsorptive effects. VIP binds to its receptor on secretory epithelial cells. The VIP receptor is a G protein-linked activator of adenylyl cyclase; hence, VIP binding to its receptor has the same result on these cells as does the direct binding by cholera toxin or LT. Cholera toxin also causes release of two other prosecretory and antiabsorptive neurotransmitters that LT does not, namely, serotonin and substance P. This effect has been proposed as an explanation for why cholera toxin tends to be a more potent toxin than LT.

In addition to its pathogenic effects, LT is antigenic and a mucosal adjuvant. Antibodies against the B subunit neutralize the toxin by preventing its binding to G_{M1}. Active and toxoided LT holotoxin have marked adjuvant activity, and both have been used to boost the immune responses to a large variety of antigens, especially those applied mucosally. The A subunit of the toxin provides the adjuvant effects.

Heat-Stable Enterotoxin-a. STa (STI, ST) is a small, nonimmunogenic polypeptide of approximately 2.0 kDa, and encoded by *estA* which is carried on transmissible plasmids. Expression of *estA* is subject to catabolite repression; hence, exposure of cells to free glucose results in gene repression. ETEC strains isolated from pigs express a form of STa referred to as STp (STIa), which is an 18-amino acid variant. Isolates from humans express either STp or a 19-amino acid variant called STh (STIb). The receptor for both forms of STa is the transmembrane protein, guanylyl cyclase-C (GC-C), located in the apical cell membrane of intestinal epithelial cells. STa is active on enterocytes of a variety of species (e.g., humans, mice, pigs, and cattle) and causes fluid accumulation in ligated intestinal loops of neonatal mice and pigs, and in the natural disease mainly causes diarrhea in the neonatal animal.

The mature 18- or 19-amino acid STa peptide is initially produced as a 72-amino acid pre-pro form. The latter is cleaved by a signal peptidase to a 53-amino acid pro-STa peptide. Another protease then cleaves this precursor to form the mature toxin. Upon binding to GC-C, this enzyme is activated to convert guanosine triphosphate (GTP) to cyclic 3′,5′-monophosphate (cGMP), causing an increased intracellular concentration of cGMP in the cell. This causes activation of a cGMP-dependent protein kinase (protein kinase G), which phosphorylates the CFTR, opens the channel, causing secretion of Cl^- and accumulation of Na^+ and water in the intestinal lumen. Guanylin, a hormone produced by goblet cells, is the natural ligand for GC-C, and bears significant amino acid homology to STa. The enterotoxic domain of STa is homologous to the active site of guanylin and the enterotoxic domains of EAST1 and *Yersinia enterocolitica* heat-stable toxin. In the case of guanylin, its natural function is thought to be the hydration of mucus secreted by goblet cells.

Heat-Stable Enterotoxin-b. STb is synthesized as a 71-amino acid precursor, and contains a 23-amino acid N-terminal signal sequence that is cleaved during export to the periplasm. The mature STb (STII) enterotoxin is secreted as a nonimmunogenic 48-amino acid peptide of approximately 5.2 kDa. The gene for Stb (*estB*) is carried on a transmissible plasmid and is often linked (i.e., in close proximity to the genes for LT). Similar to *estA*, *estB* is subject to catabolite repression; glucose represses gene expression.

STb is unrelated to STa in terms of its amino acid sequence and mode of action. STb does not cause an increase in intracellular cAMP or cGMP, in contrast to LT and STa. STb is thought to only be involved in disease in pigs, because with few exceptions it is active only on enterocytes of pigs (rat enterocytes are an exception). STb is inactivated in the gut lumen by trypsin. Diarrheic piglets less than 1 week old have a lower incidence of carriage of *estB*-positive ETEC strains. Studies with gnotobiotic piglets inoculated with isogenic and complemented *estB* mutants support the hypothesis that STb is less effective as a virulence factor in neonatal piglets. The high content of trypsin in the small intestines at this age may play a significant role in this regard. Studies with gut loop assays and carriage of *estB*-positive strains both provide evidence that STb is more important as virulence factor in weaned pigs, that is, postweaning colibacillosis. *E. coli* strains that produce AIDA as the adhesin and either STb alone or in conjunction with EAST1 have the potential to cause of diarrhea in pre- or postweaned swine.

The receptor for STb on enterocytes is a glycosphingolipid known as sulfatide. STb is internalized and stimulates a pertussis toxin-sensitive GTP-binding regulatory protein. This results in an influx of Ca^{2+} through a receptor-dependent ligand-gated calcium channel, which activates calmodulin-dependent protein kinase II. This activates the opening of an intestinal ion channel, and may also activate protein kinase C and consequently, the CFTR. The increased calcium level regulates phospholipases A_2 and C activities, and the release of arachidonic acid from membrane phospholipids leading to the formation of PGE_2 and serotonin. As noted earlier, PGE_2 and serotonin both have prosecretory and antiabsorptive effects on the intestine. STb causes HCO_3^- and Cl^- (but especially the former) secretion from the enterocytes, which results in diffusion of Na^+ and osmotic accumulation of water into the gut lumen.

Enteroaggregative *E. coli* Heat-Stable Toxin-1. EAST1 is a 38-amino acid peptide of approximately 4.1 kDa. EAST1 is encoded by the *astA* gene, which may be carried on plasmids or the chromosome, in one or more copies. EAST1 shares 50% identity with the enterotoxic domain of STa, binds to the same receptor as STa, guanylyl cyclase-C, and causes increased cGMP concentrations in target host cells. However, anti-STa antibodies do not neutralize EAST1, and EAST1 does not contain an N-terminal signal sequence region as does STa, hence the two toxins differ significantly outside of their enterotoxic domains. EAST1 has been demonstrated to be freely secreted from the bacterial cell.

EAST1 was first detected in an EAEC strain isolated from a child with diarrhea, hence the name. However, besides EAEC, EAST1 has since been found to be highly prevalent among EHEC, atypical EPEC, ETEC, DAEC, and other bacterial genera such as *Salmonella*. In *astA*-positive *E. coli* isolates from diarrheic swine, *astA* is found most often as the sole enterotoxin gene. The second most common presentation is carriage of *astA* in conjunction with the STa gene (*estA*). Detection of *astA* in combination with genes for STb, LT, Stx2e, and fimbrial F4, F5 F6, or F18 genes is also seen. The *astA* gene is highly prevalent among diarrheagenic *E. coli* isolated from preweaned piglets, but also has been associated with postweaning diarrhea and edema disease isolates. The *astA* gene has been found in *E. coli* bacteremia isolates from cattle. In these extraintestinal isolates, carriage of *astA* was significantly associated with carriage of the *clpG* gene encoding the major subunit of CS31A, and with *afa-8*. EAST1 has been detected in conjunction with STb in *E. coli* isolates from diarrheic pigs that express AIDA-I. Despite the *in vitro* evidence for activation guanylyl cyclase-C, no *in vivo* studies have shown that EAST1 by itself will cause diarrhea. In each study, diarrhea has been caused by *astA*-positive strains that produced at least one other enterotoxin. Hence, clarification is still needed on the role of EAST1 in diarrhea, in addition to other clinical manifestations of disease.

Other Toxins

Shiga Toxin. The Shiga toxin family includes the prototype Shiga toxin (Stx) produced by *Shigella dysenteriae* serotype 1, and the closely related Stx types produced by *E. coli* strains present in reservoir hosts, food, environment or other sources, known as STEC. Those STEC strains isolated from human patients with hemorrhagic colitis and/or hemolytic uremic syndrome (HUS) are known as enterohemorrhagic *E. coli*, and are discussed below.

Stx produced by *E. coli* strains were previously called Shiga-like toxins, and all members of the Stx family are also known as verotoxins or verocytotoxins. The Stx produced by *E. coli* strains fall into two major immunologically noncross-reactive groups, Stx1 and Stx2. The prototypical Stx1 and Stx2 toxins have 55% and 57% sequence identity in the A and B subunits, respectively. Stx1 exists as two variants; one (called Stx1) is identical to or varies by only one amino acid from Stx produced by *S. dysenteriae* serotype 1. The other, Stx1c, has only 97.1% and 96.6% amino acid sequence identity to Stx1. Stx2 variants include Stx2, Stx2c, Stx2d, Stx2e, and Stx2f; the last four are 84–99% homologous to Stx2. Stx2e is the toxin that causes edema disease in swine.

E. coli strains acquire the genes for all Stx except Stx2e through infection with lambdoid bacteriophages. These phage become integrated in the chromosome, but in response to stress may be induced to excise from the chromosome and assume a cytosolic replicating form (lytic cycle). Treatment of patients with some antibiotics (e.g., quinolones) is contraindicated because it may cause induction of prophage with cytosolic replication the phage; this results in increased expression of Stx and bacterial lysis, releasing much greater Stx products than before.

Stx family members have an AB_5 molecular configuration, in which the B subunits bind to receptors on the plasma membranes of target cells, and the A subunit mediates the toxic activity following endocytosis of the holotoxin. Functionally, the Stx belong to a larger family of ribosome-inactivating toxins that includes such other potent toxins such as ricin, produced by castor beans, although the activity of Stx is not limited to inhibition of protein synthesis. The host cell receptor for all Stx except Stx2e is the neutral glycosphingolipid globotriaosylceramide (Gb3, also known as CD77). The Stx2e B subunits bind to globotetraosylceramide (Gb4). The molecular mass of the A subunit is 32 kDa, whereas that of each B subunit is 7.7 kDa. Similar to LT, the holotoxin assembles in the periplasm and consists of a B-subunit homopentamer surrounding and becoming noncovalently bound to the A subunit. Although some EHEC contain genes for a type II secretion system, to date there is no evidence that Stx is actively secreted by the bacterium. Instead, Stx is released following death of the cell, and phage-mediated lysis is thought to play a major role in this process.

Trafficking of Stx in the target cell also bears many similarities with the mechanisms employed by LT, described earlier. Following contact with the receptor, the holotoxin molecule is endocytosed into the cell via clathrin-dependent and -independent mechanisms. During the early entry process, probably at the stage of the early endosomes, a protease-sensitive loop located in the C-terminal region of the A-subunit is cleaved by the membrane-associated endoprotease furin. This "nicking" process divides the A-subunit into the catalytic A1 fragment and a B-subunit-associated A2 fragment. The A1 fragment remains linked to the A2-B subunit complex via a disulfide bond. This disulfide bond is ultimately reduced in the ER lumen, releasing the enzymatic A1 fragment, which is thought to use the ER-associated protein degradation pathway to become subsequently retro-translocated to the cytosol. The N-terminal 27-kDa fragment of A1 acts as an *N*-glycosidase and removes an adenine from the 28S rRNA of the 60S ribosomal subunit. This causes an alteration of rRNA and prevents elongation factor (EF)-1-dependent binding of aminoacyl tRNA to the ribosome.

The result of Stx intoxication of a cell depends, at least in part, on the cell type. Endothelial cells respond to Stx intoxication by apoptosis, the initial stage of vascular damage. Some cell types may primarily undergo actin and microtubular rearrangement. Some cells, such as, circulating monocytes are not killed by Stx but respond by upregulation of proinflammatory cytokines, for example, GM-CSF and tumor necrosis factor (TNF). TNF in the circulation induces the expression of Gb3 by endothelial cells, thus exacerbating the exposure of the latter cells to Stx. In those cells that respond to Stx intoxication by intracellular signaling, a ribotoxic stress response is generated that may activate kinases such as JUN N-terminal kinase and mitogen-activated protein kinase p38.

The clinicopathologic effect of Stx-mediated tissue damage is mainly seen in the human host and is manifested as bloody diarrhea caused by hemorrhagic colitis and HUS. Most of these effects stem from the direct and indirect effects of Stx (apoptosis of endothelium and upregulated cytokine expression by monocytes, macrophages and other cells).

Cyclomodulins. Cyclomodulins are a family of bacterial toxins and effectors that interfere with the eukaryotic cell cycle. Pathogenic strains of *E. coli* are known to produce any of three different ones, including CNF, cytolethal distending toxin (CDT), and cycle inhibiting factor (Cif). The effects of these toxins have mainly been studied *in vitro*; other studies have tried to assess the relationships between carriage of a respective virulence gene and natural disease. In general, these toxins cause cell death or interference with cell function, both of which arguably increase the potential for colonization or invasion of an epithelial surface. A study of *E. coli* isolates from calves and dogs with diarrhea, cystitis, or no disease revealed that the *E. coli* isolates positive for cyclomodulin genes were almost always from cases of disease (diarrhea or cystitis). In another study involving bovine isolates, the *cnf2* and *cdt*-III genes were found to be colocalized on the Vir plasmid. It is thought that the different cyclomodulins may be synergistic in their effects.

Cytotoxic Necrotizing Factor. CNFs are large (110–115 kDa), monomeric proteins that cause permanent activation of the Rho, Rac, and Cdc42 GTPases of target cells by deamidation of a glutamine residue. There are two types of CNF, CNF1 and CNF2, which are immunologically related and similar in size. The activation of Rho GTPases causes reorganization of the actin cytoskeleton with formation of stress fibers, membrane ruffles, and filopodia. The cells become flattened and multinucleated and are increased in their phagocytic behavior. CNF also activates NF-κB, resulting in increased expression of proinflammatory cytokines, and protection of the cell against apoptotic stimuli. The gene encoding CNF1 is located on the chromosome on a pathogenicity island (PAI), whereas that encoding CNF-2 is located on a plasmid. CNF1 is produced by extraintestinal *E. coli* isolates from humans, especially UPEC and *E. coli* that cause meningitis in the human infant. The PAI carrying *cnf1* in these strains also contains genes that encode for α-hemolysin (*hlyA*) and fimbriae (*papC* and *sfa*). CNF-2 is produced by *E. coli* isolates from the intestines of calves with diarrhea, or the blood of calves or lambs with bacteria.

Cytolethal Distending Toxin. The CDTs are a family of related toxins that affect the mammalian cell cycle. They cause growth arrest at the GM2/M phase of the cell cycle, which ultimately leads to cell death. Three adjacent genes, *cdtA*, *cdtB*, and *cdtC*, are required for protein expression, and five CDT types (CDT-I to CDT-V) have been described. The CDTs have not been associated with any particular pathogenic type of *E. coli* except for a few isolates of EPEC, and a role in pathogenicity has not been determined. Strains that express CDT may produce a number of other virulence factors.

Cycle-Inhibiting Factor. Cif is mainly produced by EPEC and EHEC. *In vitro*, Cif causes irreversible cytopathic effects characterized by the progressive recruitment of focal adhesions, assembly of stress fibers, and arrest of the cell cycle at the GM2/M phase.

Serine Protease Autotransporters of Enterobacteriaceae. The SPATEs are a subfamily of serine protease autotransporters that are produced by diarrheagenic *E. coli*, UPEC, and *Shigella* spp.

Plasmid-Encoded Toxin. Pet is a 104-kDa SPATE that cleaves spectrin (also known as α-fodrin, a part of the cytoskeleton) and is produced by EAEC. Fodrin cleavage disrupts the actin cytoskeleton in intestinal epithelial cells, causing loss of stress fibers and release of focal contacts. These changes also stimulate an inflammatory response. Diarrhea is thought to result from prostaglandin synthesis by the recruited PMNs and affected epithelial cells, as well as activation of various inositol-signaling pathways within affected host cells. The net result is the secretion of chloride ions and water. Pet is encoded on a large virulence plasmid in close proximity to the gene encoding AAF.

Protein Involved in Colonization. Pic is a SPATE produced by UPEC, EAEC, EIEC, and *Shigella* spp. It is a mucinase and a protease. The *pic* gene is encoded on the chromosome, in the same locus but on the opposite DNA strand from the gene encoding *Shigella* enterotoxin 1 (ShET1). Pic is thought to be involved in the early stages of the pathogenesis of EAEC infection, and most likely promotes intestinal colonization. It does not damage epithelial cells, cleave fodrin, or degrade host defenses (e.g., secretory IgA, lactoferrin, or lysozyme) embedded in the mucus layer. Pic also induces intestinal mucus hypersecretion, which is thought to enhance biofilm formation.

Hemolysins. *E. coli* produce at least three hemolysins: α-hemolysin, enterohemolysin (Ehx for enterohemorrhagic *E. coli* toxin), and cytolysin A (Cly).

α-Hemolysin. α-Hemolysin (Hly) is the prototype of the RTX toxin family. RTX is an acronym for repeats-in-toxin, and named on behalf of the repeats in glycine-rich sequences within the protein. Hly is a pore-forming protein exotoxin that is secreted by a type I secretion system. Hly is commonly produced by extraintestinal *E. coli* isolates in humans and animals and is also ubiquitous in F4-positive ETEC isolates from swine. Hly is encoded by the operon, *hlyCABD*, and loss or gain of *hly* by genetic manipulation produces corresponding changes in virulence of extraintestinal *E. coli* strains. In human extraintestinal isolates, *hly* genes are carried on PAIs on the chromosome, in conjuction with *pap* and *prs* genes. In contrast, in porcine ETEC isolates *hly* genes are carried on transmissible plasmids. Hly causes hemolysis, and is detected by the presence of β-hemolytic zones surrounding isolated colonies on blood agar medium (Figure 7.2). Lysis of erythrocytes provides a source of iron, but perhaps even more important is its effects on granulocytes. Neutrophils exposed to sublytic concentrations of Hly have impaired capabilities of responding to chemotactic signals, phagocytosis, and bacterial killing. In addition, exposure of neutrophils to sublytic concentrations of Hly causes release of inflammatory mediators that can cause tissue damage and increase the ability of the bacteria to evade the epithelial barrier.

Enterohemolysin. Enterohemolysin (Ehx, for enterohemorragic *E. coli* toxin) also is an RTX toxin, and is produced by many STEC serotypes. Its virulence features are essentially the same as that of α-hemolysin. The genes for *ehx* are carried on large plasmids along with other virulence genes for a catalase-peroxidase (KatP) and an extracellular serine protease (EspP).

Cytolysin A. A gene encoding a cryptic hemolysin called *clyA* (cytolysin A), *sheA* (for silent hemolysin) or *hlyE*, is found on the chromosome of essentially all *E. coli* strains. The hemolytic protein is 34-kDA and a pore-former. Both activators and repressors regulate the transcription of the gene. Since the protein has hemolytic activity, it is presumed to have a potential *in vivo* role in iron release from erythrocytes.

Iron Acquisition. Iron is an absolute growth requirement for most, if not all, living things. Siderophores (e.g., aerobactin) that remove iron from host iron-binding proteins are necessary if a microbe is to have invasive capabilities (see Chapter 6).

Acid Tolerance. RNA polymerase containing RpoS (the sigma factor associated with stationary phase) preferentially transcribes genes responsible for acid tolerance (survival at pH, 5), allowing safe transit through the stomach.

Locus of Enterocyte Effacement. The LEE is a PAI on the chromosome in EPEC and EHEC strains that contains genes needed for proteins that cause attaching-and-effacing (A/E) lesions in the host cell (Figures 7.3 and 7.4).

Intimin and Translocated Intimin Receptor. Intimin is a transmembrane, outer membrane protein encoded by *eae* located in the LEE5 operon. The N-terminus of intimin is in the periplasm, and the C-terminus projects out above the surface of the bacterial cell. The N-terminus has a rather constant amino acid sequence, whereas the C-terminus is variable and forms the basis of intimin types and subtypes. At least 17 different intimin types and subtypes have been described, and these are differentiated by Greek letter and number designations (e.g., $\alpha1$, $\alpha2$, $\beta1$, and $\beta2$). The C-terminus of the intimin molecule binds to another secreted bacterial protein, translocated intimin receptor (Tir), encoded by *tir*, also located in the LEE5 operon. The Tir protein is inserted into the host cell membrane with the C- and N-termini located in the host cell cytoplasm and the mid-region of the polypeptide external to the cell forming a hairpin loop. It is this hairpin loop to which the C-terminus of the intimin molecule binds. Numerous adjacent intimin-Tir molecular complexes result in an intimate anchoring of the bacteria to host cell membrane, significantly enhancing colonization.

Type III Secretion System. The genes encoding a type III secretion system (an assemblage of proteins—more than 20—that form a hollow tube-like structure through which effector proteins are injected into host target cells) are also encoded on the LEE (see LEE).

***E. coli* Secreted Protein.** The genes encoding *E. coli* secreted protein (Esp) proteins are also located on the LEE. EspA forms the hollow, syringe-like structure through which Tir, EspB, EspD, and other effectors are injected into the host cell. EspB and EspD form the pore in the host cell. Several other effectors elicit cytoskeletal rearrangements leading to effacement of the microvilli. Other less-well defined effectors, such as Cif and Map, are thought to mediate toxic effects to the host cell, for example cell cycle arrest and mitochondrial damage. Diarrhea occurs secondary to increases in intracellular calcium ions and activation of protein kinase C. Protein kinase C is responsible for phosphorylation of proteins composing the chloride channels resulting in loss of chloride and water into the intestinal lumen, as well as the phosphorylation of the membrane associated ion transport proteins resulting in blockage of absorption of NaCl.

Variability

One measure of variability of *E. coli* resides in the antigenic makeup of the O-repeat units (type of sugar subunits, how the subunits are hooked together, and the length of the chain), the composition of the flagellar protein (flagellin), and the composition of the capsule. The O-, H-, and

K-antigens are used in serotyping a particular isolate. There are 174 O-antigens, at least 80 distinct K-antigens, and 53 H-antigens in the international serotyping scheme. The O-antigens are numbered 1–181, but several numbers have been deleted due to cross-reactivity with other antigens. For example, O8:K87:H19 describes an isolate with antigens of the O-antigen number 8, capsular-antigen number 87, and flagellar-antigen number 19.

Ecology

Reservoir and Transmission

Strains of *E. coli* capable of producing disease reside in the lower gastrointestinal tract and are abundant in environments inhabited by animals. Transmission is through the fecal-oral route. The lower intestinal tract has been termed the "primary habitat" and the environment outside the animal, the "secondary habitat" of *E. coli*. This reflects the importance of the lower intestine in providing the necessary nutrients and warm temperatures for *E. coli* (a mesophile) to be in a positive growth state, and also the need for it to exit one host in order to enter a new one to complete its "life cycle."

Pathogenesis

Mechanisms and Disease Patterns

In order for *E. coli* to produce disease, it must have the necessary genes encoding the virulence factors needed to do so. If the genes are acquired (by transduction, conjugation, or transformation), the nonpathogenic strain may be changed to one with pathogenic potential. This lateral form of gene acquisition, often through bacteriophages or plasmids, is of paramount importance in the emergence of new pathogenic types. Also, the type of disease produced depends upon the genes acquired.

Enterotoxigenic Diarrhea. This disease occurs in neonatal pigs, calves, and lambs, and in weanling pigs. It has been reported in dogs and horses.

Enterotoxigenic diarrhea is caused by strains of *E. coli* that produce adhesins that promote attachment to glycoproteins on the surface of epithelial cells of the jejunum and ileum, and an enterotoxin(s) that affects the epithelial cell (to which the enterotoxigenic strain of *E. coli* is adhered), resulting in fluid secretion and diarrhea. Both traits are necessary for disease to result, since unless the ingested strain adheres to these cells, peristalsis will move it into the large bowel. The cells of the jejunum and the ileum are susceptible to the action of enterotoxin; the cells of the large bowel are not.

As discussed above, at least four fimbrial adhesins may be found on ETEC, F4, F5, F6, and F41. They possess some host species specificity: F4 and F6 are almost always associated with isolates from swine; F5 with isolates from cattle, sheep, and swine; and F41 with those from cattle. The epithelial cell receptors for these adhesins regulate the age incidence of this disease as well. In calves and lambs, the receptors appear transiently during the first week or so of life. Analogous receptors are present in pigs throughout the first 6 weeks of life. There are many uncharacterized adhesins that probably play a role.

Also as discussed above, some enterotoxigenic strains of *E. coli* express fimbria known as curli. Curli fimbria mediate adherence to glycoproteins on the surface of epithelial cells and to extracellular matrix proteins, and are important in the formation of biofilms. The presence of curli may explain the increase in the window of age susceptibility to enterotoxigenic disease in animals concurrently infected with rotavirus or *Cryptosporidium parvum*, two agents that may cause enough tissue damage to lead to exposure of extracellular matrix proteins.

In addition to adherence to the target tissues of the small intestine, enterotoxigenic strains must have the genetic capability of synthesizing enterotoxins. As noted above, there are four different enterotoxins produced by ETEC strains, and although there are clones that have become highly prevalent throughout the world (e.g., porcine strains that produce the combination of F4, LT, and STb), with time and extensive testing (usually by PCR), just about every possible combination is detected.

Some of the adhesins and enterotoxins are encoded on plasmid DNA. As a consequence, it is difficult to predict which strain of *E. coli* possesses the genetic information necessary to produce disease. Some adhesins prefer to be associated with certain serotypes. In particular, the genes encoding the protein for the F41 adhesin are almost always found within strains of *E. coli* of the O9 and the O101 serogroups. As might be expected, the genes encoding the proteins for F41 adhesin are located on chromosomal DNA.

Following ingestion by the host, enterotoxigenic strains of *E. coli* adhere to target cells, multiply, and secrete enterotoxin (Figure 7.1). Fluid and electrolytes accumulate in the lumen of the intestine, resulting in diarrhea, dehydration, and electrolyte imbalances. In time, the infecting strain is moved distally away from the target cell, and the disease process stops, due probably in part to the cessation of expression of the adhesin along with a decrease in available substrate following the almost explosive multiplication of the strain in the small intestine. Unless steps are taken to correct the fluid and electrolyte imbalances, the disease has high mortality.

The diarrhea produced is watery and nonbloody. There are minimal inflammatory changes, if any, in the small intestine. Bacteria will be observed histologically coating the villi of the mid to distal portions of the small intestine.

Enteroaggregative *E. coli*. As noted above, strains of *E. coli* that express the AAF and therefore defined as EAEC have been isolated from weaned pigs and calves with diarrhea. However, these isolates contained almost none of the other virulence factors found in human EAEC isolates, and consequently were not likely to be pathogens of animals or humans. EAEC are noted pathogens of humans and have a number of other virulence factors that are described earlier.

Extraintestinal *E. coli*. Association of susceptible animals (usually a neonate that has received inadequate amounts of colostrum or colostrum of inadequate quality) with strains of *E. coli* that have some ability to invade the gut epithelium and are able to survive outside of the intestine may occur by way of the conjunctivae, an inadequately treated umbilicus, or ingestion. If these strains are acquired by ingestion, they first adhere to target cells in the distal small bowel. Adherence is probably related to expression of afimbrial adhesins, namely CS31A, AfaE-VII, and AfaE-VIII. Likewise, the fimbrial adhesin F17c and the siderophore aerobactin originally described on a plasmid termed Vir (so-called because of its association with virulent *E. coli*) are prevalent on these *E. coli* strains. Following adherence, these strains may induce their own uptake by expression of either CNF1 or CNF2, resulting in an endocytotic process that allows them to enter the intestinal epithelial cells. Entry into the lymphatics and subsequently the bloodstream follows. The mechanism by which these strains gain access to lymphatics after uptake by the epithelial cell is unknown. Likewise, the mechanism of entry into lymphatics after association with conjunctivae or the umbilicus is unknown. Once the epithelial surface is traversed, expression of adhesins is repressed (otherwise adhesin-expressing bacteria could adhere to host phagocytic cells with disastrous consequences for the bacterium).

The infecting strain multiplies in the lymphatics and bloodstream and endotoxemia develops. Death of the host occurs if antibacterial therapy, the immune system, or both do not remove the microorganism.

Extraintestinal *E. coli* have special qualities, for example, they must escape phagocytosis, complement-mediated lysis, and must have a mechanism to acquire iron. Capsule and various outer membrane proteins confer resistance to complement-mediated lysis (serum resistance). How capsules protect the outer membrane from insertion of the membrane attack complex is not known. Certain capsules (such as K1) are chemically similar to the surface of host cells in that they are composed mainly of sialic acid. Complement components associating with surfaces composed of sialic acid are shunted to degradative pathways rather than amplification and formation of membrane attack complexes.

Escape from phagocytosis is also related to capsule and certain outer membrane proteins. How outer membrane proteins function as antiphagocytic factors is not known.

The genes encoding the adhesin (e.g., CS31A and F17) and those responsible for siderophore production reside on plasmids. As mentioned above, the genes encoding F17 have been associated with the plasmid Vir, as has the gene encoding CNF2; those responsible for siderophore production have been associated with the plasmid pColV. In the latter instance, the siderophore genes are linked closely with the genes for the production of colicin V. The siderophore, aerobactin, has a high affinity for iron.

Many of the strains with invasive capability, except those from foals, produce α-hemolysin (Hly) and are β-hemolytic on blood agar.

Histopathologically there are inflammatory changes in liver, spleen, joints, and meninges. There may be hemorrhages on the pericardium, peritoneal surfaces, and adrenal cortices.

Enteropathogenic *E. coli*. Enteropathogenic strains of *E. coli* produce diarrhea in all animal species, including human beings. EPEC do not produce ST, LT, or other enterotoxins. Most notably, they cause A/E lesions in the small intestines in humans, which they colonize the small intestine. In animals, EPEC colonize and cause A/E lesions in both the distal small intestine and the large intestines. The characteristic lesion is named so because the microvilli are effaced and at these sites of effacement, the bacteria are intimately attached to the apical plasma membrane. Cytoskeletal rearrangements induced by effector proteins (discussed earlier) cause the formation of pedestals, to which the bacteria attach (Figures 7.3 and 7.4).

Shiga Toxin-Producing *E. coli*. As described above, STEC that produce intimin and other LEE gene products are called enterohemorrhagic *E. coli* (EHEC). These strains have a greater virulence since they most likely have the ability to produce A/E lesions and they produce Stx. *E. coli* O157:H7 is the prototype of the EHEC and is thought to have evolved from EPEC O55:H7, a human infantile diarrhea pathogen. *E. coli* acquire Stx genes via lysogeny with the bacteriophage(s) that encode Shiga toxin (Stx)-1 and/or -2. Cattle are reservoir hosts for STEC; for some reason, the bovine intestine has become a natural primary habitat for these organisms. Many different serotypes of *E. coli* are now known to be STEC; however, a much smaller subset of these contain the LEE PAI. As noted above, some non-O157 STEC that lack the LEE genes produce an alternative adhesin known as Saa. Human patients are highly susceptible to the effects of Stx, whereas cattle are not. Cattle lack the Gb3 receptor for Stx on their vascular endothelial cells; in addition Stx that enters into the enterocytes of cattle ends in the lysosomes instead of the trans-Golgi and ER, which prevents toxic effects. Human patients are susceptible to vascular necrosis, thrombosis and infarction of the large intestine, which is manifest as hemorrhagic colitis. Approximately 5–10% of these patients develop postdiarrheal sequelae, namely, HUS. Although the pathogenesis is complex, Stx plays a major role through the direct causation of endothelial apoptosis and induction of cytokine production by leukocytes, which in turn increase the expression of Gb3 on the endothelial cells. Clinically, HUS is characterized by microangiopathic hemolytic anemia, thrombocytopenia, and uremia.

All affected animals acquire EPEC and STEC by fecal-oral transmission. Both STEC and EPEC have zoonotic potential, but STEC strains are of greater concern due to the potentially life-threatening effects of Stx. Human beings primarily become infected following ingestion of contaminated food and water, or through direct contact with reservoir hosts (all ruminants). Petting zoos have become a source of infection. At slaughter, the surface of the carcass becomes contaminated with fecal microorganisms. The surfaces of cuts of meat derived from an infected carcass are usually adequately decontaminated by cooking. However, when meat is ground, the microorganisms on the surface become introduced throughout the product. Though proper cooking will readily kill surface microorganisms, including STEC O157:H7, those inside may not be killed. Currently in the

United States, non-O157 STEC cause more cases of illness than does O157:H7. In the United States, six serogroups, namely, O26, O45, O103, O111, O121, and O145, cause approximately 71% of the cases of non-O157 STEC-related illness in humans. Recently, the USDA-FSIS declared these serogroups, in addition to O157:H7 as adulterants in beef.

Edema Disease. Edema disease is an acute, often fatal enterotoxemia of weaned pigs. The disease is characterized by subcutaneous and subserosal edema, and neurological signs that reflect infarcts in the brain stem. These lesions are caused by absorption of Stx2e from the intestine. Causative strains are usually of certain serotypes, for example, O141:K85, O138:K81, and O139:K82, and usually express α-hemolysin and F18ab fimbria. F18ab fimbrial expression enhances bacterial colonization of the distal small intestine. Stx2e is absorbed from the intestine into the blood stream, and binds predominantly to the surfaces of erythrocytes, which are rich in Gb4. Erythrocytes are thought to then deliver the toxin to endothelial cells, which also express the Gb4 receptor. Stx2e enters the endothelial cells as described earlier and intoxicates the cells by inactivating the ribosomes, shutting down protein synthesis, and causing cell death. Vascular leakage and thromboses result in edema and infarcts, respectively, in different tissues and organs. Grossly, pigs typically exhibit subcutaneous edema of on the forehead, in the eyelids, and also in the wall of the stomach, mesocolon, and other areas.

Avian-Pathogenic *E. coli*. Avian-pathogenic *E. coli* (APEC) cause colibacillosis of fowl, which is economically important to the poultry industry. APEC are invasive, extraintestinal strains of *E. coli* that are usually of certain serotypes, and bear several virulence genes in common with UPEC of humans. One common serotype is O1:K1:H7. Notably, K1 is a capsular antigen that plays an important role in the pathogenesis of infection of human infants, causing meningitis in these cases. In addition, O1 is notably an invasive serogroup. Virulence factors in common with human UPEC strains include the siderophores enterobactin, aerobactin, salmochelin, and yersiniabactin, as well as a hemin uptake system. In addition, both APEC and human UPEC strains produce Pap and type 1 fimbriae.

The disease takes many forms in fowl, depending upon the age of the host and mode of infection. In the case of egg infections, the egg surface may be contaminated with potentially pathogenic strains at the time they are laid. The bacteria penetrate the shell and infect the yolk sac. If the bacteria grow, the embryo dies, usually late in incubation. Embryos that survive may die shortly after, with losses occurring as late as 3 weeks after hatching. A very important clinical manifestation in poultry is respiratory and septicemic disease. The course may be rapidly fatal or chronic, manifested by debilitation, diarrhea, and respiratory distress. Air sacculitis and pneumonia are common presentations. Other clinical syndromes caused by APEC include cellulitis, synovitis, pericarditis, salpingitis, and panophthalmitis.

Adherent-Invasive *E. coli*. Adherent-invasive *E. coli* (AIEC) were first described in human patients with Crohn's disease. They have been significantly associated with Crohn's disease, but a definite cause-and-effect relationship has yet to be determined. AIEC have also been found in dogs with histiocytic ulcerative colitis, and in this disease there is considerable scientific evidence for an etiological role. AIEC adhere to and invade intestinal epithelial cells. Entry into these cells is dependent upon induction of actin microfilament and microtubule recruitment. The bacteria then gain entrance into macrophages beneath the epithelial layer, within which they replicate in endocytic vacuoles without causing host cell death. Infection of the macrophages induces these cells to produce large amounts of TNF-α. This upregulation of cytokine production is thought to significantly exacerbate inflammation and tissue damage.

Immunologic Aspects

Immunologic defense against diseases produced by pathogenic *E. coli* occurs at two levels: at the site of attachment to the target cell and through destruction of the bacteria or neutralization of its products.

Enterotoxigenic Diarrhea. Specific anti-adhesin antibody (sIgA and sIgM) found in colostrum and milk prevents bacterial attachment to small intestinal enterocytes. Likewise, specific anti-LT neutralizes LT enterotoxin, although the importance of this effect is incompletely understood. LT has been shown to be delivered directly to the enterocyte by the bacteria, which may bypass the effect of luminal antibodies.

Extraintestinal Disease. The neonate acquires immunity from the dam, and depending upon the isotype of the immunoglobulin (IgA, IgG, or IgM), the type of protection differs. For the first 36 h or so of life, ingested IgG and IgM attach to receptors on the surface of epithelial cells of the small intestine. Transfer across the cell into the systemic circulation follows attachment. If the antibodies are specific for a virulence determinant, then disease may not result if the neonate encounters a pathogenic strain expressing that virulence determinant. For example, anticapsular antibodies acquired from the dam will protect the newborn from fatal invasive disease by strains of *E. coli* possessing that particular capsule.

EPEC and STEC Infections. Specific antibodies to intimin and type III secreted proteins that mediate A/E lesions may provide some degree of protection. Studies with a type III secreted vaccine for STEC O157:H7 have shown efficacy in cattle. In the case of the neonate, sIgA and sIgM found in colostrum and milk are thought to prevent attachment to enterocytes.

Edema Disease. Antibody specific for Stx2e prevent endothelial and vascular damage, further preventing ischemic lesions. It is imperative, therefore, that the dam be exposed either naturally or artificially to the microorganism and its virulence determinants before parturition. Such exposure allows for antibodies to be made for secretion into colostrum and milk.

Laboratory Diagnosis

Demonstration of Enterotoxigenic Strains of *E. coli*. The currently preferred diagnostic method for microbiological diagnosis of ETEC is detection of virulence genes, that is, fimbrial and enterotoxin, in isolated *E. coli* colonies on culture plates by polymerase chain reaction (PCR). A multiplex PCR format is commonly used in diagnostic laboratories that targets a variety of virulence genes besides those of concern with ETEC, for example, Stx, intimin, and others. Bacterial isolates chosen for PCR should first be subcultured onto a nutrient medium (e.g., blood agar), both to ensure purity and to remove the possibility of inhibitors of the DNA polymerase.

Histopathology on animals submitted for necropsy should be conducted, preferably on an acutely affected animal that has been euthanatized. Selection of an acutely affected animal that has not undergone postmortem autolysis and postmortem bacterial overgrowth will greatly enhance the chances of detecting the pathogen among a background of commensal flora. Detection of bacterial adherence to enterocytes in the small intestine is pathognomonic. Immunohistochemistry also could be conducted if the laboratory has antiserum that includes most of the common serogroups (Figure 7.1). However, culture is needed for detection of the specific pathogen involved from the standpoint of virulence factor production. Culture on blood and MacConkey agars are standard procedures for ETEC diagnosis, although detection of some fimbrial types may be enhanced by culture on additional media, namely, E medium for F4; Minca medium for F5 and F6; and E or Minca medium for F41. Detection of large numbers of *E. coli*, that is, 10^8 to 10^9 colony-forming units per milliliter of luminal contents, is supportive of a diagnosis of ETEC infection.

Immunological approaches may still be used, for example, slide agglutination tests run on each colony using antiserum specific for the various adhesins. An enzyme-linked immunosorbent assay may be used to measure directly the presence of F4 and F5 adhesin-expressing bacteria in feces. Fluorescent-labeled antibody techniques still provide an easy method of detection of fimbria. Bacterial colonies or smears of scrapings taken from the small intestine are flooded with antisera that are specific for the various adhesins. After treatment with fluorescent-labeled secondary antiserum, preparations are examined for labeled bacteria adhering to the epithelial cells. STa or LT enterotoxin production by isolated strains of *E. coli* can be detected with an ELISA test. This test is reputed to detect 140 pg/ml of STa (>100 times more sensitive than the suckling mouse assay) and 290 pg/ml of LT.

Demonstration of Extraintestinal Strains. The microbiological diagnosis of extraintestinal disease is based upon the demonstration of *E. coli* in normally sterile sites or locations (joint, bone marrow, spleen, or blood). In fowl, the same sites are cultured, plus those grossly affected (lung, air sac). Dead in-shell embryos are cultured. Culture of the liver is to be avoided even though the Kupffer cells remove bacteria from the blood, because retrograde movement of enteric bacteria during the agonal stages of the disease complicates the microbiologic findings.

Demonstration of EPEC and STEC Strains. Histopathology can allow for detection of A/E bacteria, but will not result in definitive identification of the pathogen. Specific protocols and special media for isolation of *E. coli* from fecal or intestinal samples are now available. Other media, for example, for non-O157 STEC are also available, but have not been validated for all serogroups of interest. Some of the selective media for this purpose, for example, sorbitol-MacConkey, are described in Chapter 6. Once *E. coli* isolates that are suspect to be STEC (e.g., showing the proper phenotype on chromogenic media) are obtained in cases of animal infection, detection of Stx genes by PCR is the preferred method for confirmation of these organisms as STEC. The most important virulence gene targets are *stx1*, *stx2*, and *eae*; *ehx* is also a useful target for diagnostic purposes. Fecal isolates also may be obtained from a more general-purpose selective medium for *E. coli* (e.g., MacConkey agar), and these can be tested by PCR.

Demonstration of Strains-Producing Edema Disease. The microbiological diagnosis of edema disease depends upon the isolation and demonstration of certain serotypes that have been shown to play a role in this disease. The characteristic gross and microscopic tissue changes make this disease relatively easier to diagnose pathologically than microbiologically.

Treatment, Control, and Prevention

Treatment of an animal that has diarrhea due to an infectious cause centers on correcting fluid and electrolyte imbalances. If the animal is in shock due to cardiovascular collapse, then the fluid and electrolytes (sodium bicarbonate, KCl) are given IV; if not, oral electrolyte solutions are given. Since the animals are acidotic, sodium bicarbonate is included. Adding glucose to oral electrolytes will enhance the absorption of the sodium ions being excreted. The use of antimicrobials is controversial. Because the concentration of antimicrobic achievable (and available) in the lumen of the bowel is not known, the results of *in vitro* susceptibility tests to guide therapy are of doubtful reliability. Administration of nonabsorbable antimicrobics (such as neomycin) will sufficiently reduce the numbers of *E. coli* in the upper small bowel to allow correction of fluid and electrolyte imbalances. Such reduction occurs even though *in vitro* tests show that strains of *E. coli* commonly test "resistant" to neomycin. The fact that *in vitro* tests measure susceptibility to microgram amounts, whereas milligram amounts may be available locally accounts for the discrepancy.

Antimicrobial agents, fluid, and electrolyte augmentation are necessary to successfully treat septicemic disease produced by invasive strains of *E. coli*. Invasive disease results in an endotoxemia progressing to a lactic acidosis because of decreased organ perfusion secondary to hypotension and disseminated intravascular coagulation. This should be taken into account when the electrolyte replacement is chosen. Antimicrobial agents should be chosen according to susceptibility trends in the practice area. Usually *E. coli* isolated from farm animals are susceptible to gentamicin or amikacin, trimethoprim-sulfonamides, and ceftiofur. They are usually resistant to tetracyclines, streptomycin, sulfonamides, ampicillin, and kanamycin. The severity of the signs of endotoxemia has been reduced experimentally by administering antibodies to the lipid A portion of the LPS.

Prevention and control of the enteric diseases produced by pathogenic strains of *E. coli* are one and the same. The key is sound husbandry practices. It is important that the dam be exposed to the antigenic determinants of the various virulence factors expressed on or by the infecting strains. Exposure can be provided naturally by placing the dam into the environment in which parturition will take place or artificially by vaccinating the dam with preparations containing the antigenic determinants perceived to be a threat to the newborn. Commercially produced preparations containing monoclonal antibodies to the adhesins (for ETEC) can be given orally to the neonatal animal. Although this practice will not significantly reduce the incidence of diarrhea, it will reduce the severity and mortality.

Other Coliforms

There are a few other medically important members of the family Enterobacteriaceae. Like *E. coli*, the bacteria usually ferment lactose, resulting in the traditional reddish-pink colonies on MacConkey agar. The genera *Klebsiella, Enterobacter, and Citrobacter* are also facultative anaerobes. These organisms are not hemolytic on blood agar and although they produce some toxins, these bacteria are generally opportunistic pathogens.

Klebsiella

The most common pathogens in veterinary medicine are *Klebsiella pneumoniae* and *K. oxytoca*. These bacteria, like most coliforms, are commensals of the intestinal tract of animals. Therefore, fecal-contaminated environments are often the source of perinatal infections of young ruminants. However, bovine mastitis attributed to *K. pneumoniae* spp. *pneumoniae* can be a very serious condition with case-fatality rates ranging from 10% to 80%. This form of coliform mastitis is associated with cool, wet weather and various forms of sawdust bedding. Many of the affected cattle develop severe mammary gland infections with septicemia and endotoxic shock.

Klebsiella spp. have been associated with many forms of opportunistic infections. Contaminated obstetric equipment, surgical equipment, cleaning devices, and clinic surfaces may contribute to the probability of infection. Once tissue infection is established, the organism may spread and eventually cause a fulminating septicemia. *Klebsiella* will also rapidly acquire extended spectrum β-lactamase resistance. Virulence factors associated with *Klebsiella* are similar to other Enterobacteriaceae. The capsule is essential for resistance to host defense mechanisms (phagocytosis, opsonization, and cytolysis). Endotoxins, adhesins, enterotoxins, siderophores, and cell wall components are also important.

Klebsiella are easily identified through routine diagnostic laboratory culture at 37 °C. The colonies on blood agar are nonhemolytic, large and very mucoid. *Klebsiella* ferment lactose and are generally indole-negative (see Table 7.1).

Table 7.1. Properties of *Klebsiella, Enterobacter*, and *Citrobacter*

Properties	*Klebsiella*	*Citrobacter*	*Enterobacter*
Lactose fermentation	+	−	+
Urea hydrolysis	(+)	V	V
Citrate utilization	(+)	(+)	(+)
Hydrogen sulfide	−	(+)	−
Voges–Proskauer	+	−	+
Motility	−	(+)/weak	+
Common species	*pneumoniae* *oxytoca*	*freundii* *rodentium*	*cloacae* *aerogenes*

+, positive; (+), most positive; −, negative; V, variable.

Enterobacter and Citrobacter

Like *Klebsiella*, bacteria of the genera *Enterobacter* and *Citrobacter* are opportunistic pathogens. These bacteria often cause infections in contaminated wounds or the urogenital tract. Both *Enterobacter* and *Citrobacter* are identified using traditional colony morphology and biochemical testing (Table 7.1). *Enterobacter* are usually motile. The *Citrobacter* produce hydrogen sulfide in triple sugar-iron slant agar tubes, thus sometimes these cultures may be confused with *Salmonella*. These bacteria are notably resistant to most penicillins and cephalosporins and rapidly acquire other forms of antibiotic resistance.

References

Moxley RA and Francis DH (1986) Natural and experimental infection with an attaching and effacing strain of Escherichia coli in calves. *Infect Immun*, **53**, 339–346.

Xing J (1996) Pathogenicity of an enterotoxigenic *Escherichia coli* Hemolysin (hlyA) mutant in gnotobiotic piglets. MS Thesis. University of Nebraska-Lincoln. R.A. Moxley, Advisor.

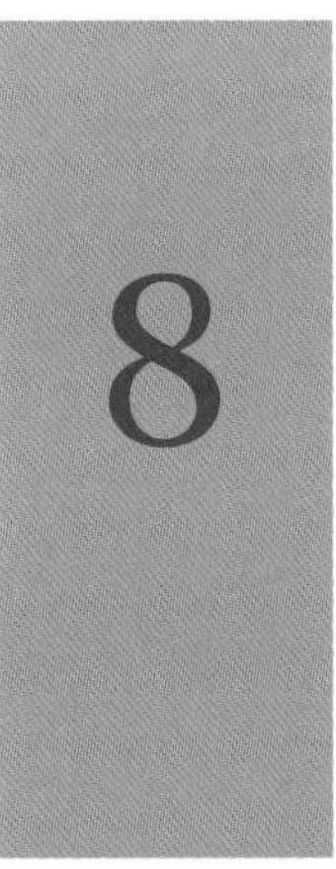

Enterobacteriaceae: *Salmonella*

Rodney Moxley

The genus *Salmonella* is a member of the family Enterobacteriaceae, and is composed of three species: *S. bongori*, *S. enterica*, and *S subterranea*. *S. enterica* contains six subspecies (Table 8.1); these include *enterica* (also known as subspecies I), *salamae* (subspecies II), *arizonae* (subspecies IIIa), *diarizonae* (subspecies IIIb), *houtenae* (subspecies IV), and *indica* (subspecies VI). Subspecies V was reclassified as *S. bongori*. The type species is *S. enterica* ssp. *enterica*. The type strain is *S. enterica* ssp. *enterica* serotype Typhimurium strain LT2 (Lilleengen strain type 2). Subspecies I strains are commonly isolated from humans and warm-blooded animals. *S. enterica* includes more than 2500 serotypes, also known as serovars (ser.) or varieties (var.), and approximately 60% of these fall within subspecies I. In the United States, approximately 99% of the reported *Salmonella* isolates from humans belong to subspecies I. *S. bongori* and *S. enterica* subspecies II, IIIa, IIIb, IV, and VI mainly infect cold-blooded vertebrates and live in the environment. *S. subterranea* is a recent addition to the genus and was isolated from low pH subsurface sediment contaminated with nitrate and hexavalent to tetravalent uranium.

The *Salmonella* nomenclature has been problematic for many years due to the use of several different taxonomic schemes and the listing of serotypes as species. In 2005, Judicial Opinion 80 was published in the *International Journal of Systematic and Evolutionary Microbiology* and clarified many of these issues. Serotypes of *S. enterica* ssp. *enterica* are written in Roman letters in which the first letter is upper case; others are denoted by antigenic formulae.

In this chapter, the subspecies designation will not be used unless important to the discussion. For example, *S. enterica* ssp. *enterica* serovar Typhimurium will first be denoted as *S. enterica* serovar Typhimurium, and then, simply *S.* Typhimurium.

Descriptive Features

Cellular Description and Composition

There is one capsular type, a polysaccharide antigen that has been named Vi (for virulence). Vi is produced by serovar Typhi and Paratyphi C strains, some *Citrobacter* strains, and occasionally by strains of serovar Dublin. The cell wall is typical of gram-negative bacteria, composed of lipopolysaccharide (LPS) and protein. As described in Chapter 6, the kind and the number of sugars together with the linkage between them in the outermost portion of the LPS macromolecule determine the O-antigen serogroup of the particular isolate. The O-antigens, together with the antigenic determinants on the surface of the flagella (H-antigens), which are possessed by most salmonellae, define the serotype. This classification is called the Kauffmann–White scheme.

Cellular Products of Medical Interest

Adhesins. Depending on the serotype, *S. enterica* contains gene clusters for more than 10 different fimbriae. *S.* Typhimurium potentially encodes at least 13 fimbrial operons: *agf* (*csg*), *fim*, *pef*, *lpf*, *bcf*, *saf*, *stb*, *stc*, *std*, *sth*, *sti*, and *stj*). Production of at least 11 of these fimbriae has been detected, with expression being dependent on growth conditions. The fimbria mediates adherence to mucosal epithelial in the gastrointestinal tract. Because of their relative hydrophobicity, fimbrial adhesins may also promote association with the membrane of phagocytic cells. Adhesins are important virulence factors only when the microbes are on mucosal surfaces.

Of the aforementioned fimbriae, there is evidence for Pef, Agf, and Lpf as being important adhesins for the intestinal tract. Pef (plasmid encoded fimbriae) mediate attachment to murine small intestinal epithelial cells. The genes for Pef are carried on the virulence plasmid of *S.* Typhimurium, pSLT. Mutations in *pef* increase the oral lethal dose 50 (LD_{50}) by about 2.5-fold. Agf (thin aggregative fimbriae, or curli) are analogous to curli fimbriae of *Escherichia coli* (see Chapter 7). Agf promote autoaggregation, biofilm formation, and virulence. Agf also mediate attachment to small intestinal epithelial cells. Lpf (long polar fimbriae) mediate attachment of *S.* Typhimurium to M cells, but not to the absorptive enterocytes. Mutations in *lpf* increase the oral LD_{50} by about fivefold, and delay death

Veterinary Microbiology, Third Edition. Edited by D. Scott McVey, Melissa Kennedy and M.M. Chengappa.

Table 8.1. Subspecies of *S. enterica*

Numeral Designation	Nomenclature
I	*enterica*
II	*salamae*
IIIa	*arizonae*
IIIb	*diarizonae*
IV	*houtenae*
VI	*indica*

by about 3 days compared to the wild-type parent strain. The Pef, Lpf, and Agf fimbriae are thought to be functionally redundant. Inactivation of all three genes results in an increase in the oral LD_{50} by about 30-fold.

Capsule. The Vi capsule is a linear homopolymer of α-1,4-2-deoxy-2-*N*-acetylgalactosamine uronic acid, which can be acetylated at the C-3 position. The role of the capsule (Vi) is unclear. Since salmonellae are primarily intracellular parasites, possession of a capsule does not seem to be a strategy that is consistent with the role this structure has in other microorganisms (i.e., antiphagocytic). However, Vi protects the outer membrane from effective interactions with membrane attack complexes generated by the complement system. This is useful in protecting salmonellae when extracellular.

Cell Wall. As described in detail in Chapter 6, the LPS in the outer membrane is an important virulence determinant. Not only is the lipid A component toxic (endotoxin), but the length of the side chain in the O-repeat unit hinders the attachment of the membrane attack complex of the complement system to the outer membrane. LPS binds to LPS-binding protein (a plasma protein), which in turn transfers it to the blood phase of CD14. The CD14–LPS complex binds to Toll-like receptor (TLR)-4 protein (see Chapter 6) on the surface of macrophages triggering cell-signaling pathways that ultimately cause release of proinflammatory cytokines. Recent studies have shown that TLR signaling is required for the virulence of *S.* Typhimurium. Recognition of *S.* Typhimurium is largely mediated by TLR2, TLR4, and TLR5. Mice deficient in both TLR2 and TLR4 are highly susceptible to *S.* Typhimurium, consistent with reduced innate immune function. TLR signaling enhances the rate of acidification of the *Salmonella*-containing phagosome, and inhibition of this acidification prevents induction of the *Salmonella* pathogenicity island 2 (SPI-2). Hence, *S.* Typhimurium fails to induce virulence genes when deprived of innate immune signals.

Flagella. All salmonellae except *S. enterica* serotype Pullorum and *S. enterica* serotype Gallinarum are motile. Motility is mediated by peritrichous flagella. The flagella are highly immunogenic. Subspecies I, II, IIIa, and VI are biphasic, capable of producing two and sometimes three types of functional and immunologically distinct flagella. Serological distinction among the H-antigens constitutes the second part of the Kauffmann–White scheme. Phase 1 H-antigens are designated by lower case letters, "a" through "z" and then "z1," "z2," "z3," and so on. Phase 2 antigens are designated by numerals, "1," "2," "3," and so on. As with O-antigens, the H-antigens are determined by agglutination testing using specific antiserum.

SPI, Type III Secretion Systems, and Effector Proteins. Many genes responsible for *Salmonella* virulence are located on pathogenicity islands (PAIs). PAIs are large contiguous blocks of DNA on the chromosome that contain insertion sequences and genes for virulence factors, integrases, and mobility factors. In *Salmonella*, the PAIs are known by name as *Salmonella* pathogenicity islands (SPIs); to date there are 22 reported SPIs, numbered SPI-1 through SPI-22. *S. bongori* contains a different collection of SPIs than different serotypes of *S. enterica*. No strain studied has contained all 22 PAIs, and there is variation in the SPIs among *S. enterica* serotypes. This variation in SPIs reflects the variation in host range and the degree of adaptation of the pathogen for the host. *S. bongori* contains SPI-1, SPI-3A, SPI-3B, SPI-4, SPI-9, and SPI-22. *S.* Typhimurium contains SPI-1 through -6, -9, -12 through 14, and -16. *S.* Enteritidis and *S.* Gallinarum contain SPI-1 through SPI-6, SPI-9, SPI-10, SPI-12 through SPI-14, SPI-16, SPI-17, and SPI-19. *S.* Typhi contains SPI-1 through SPI-10, SPI-12, and SPI-15 through SPI-18. SPI-1 through SPI-5 each contain genes encoding type III secretion systems (T3SS), and these are named according to the SPI in which they are located; for example, T3SS-1 is on SPI-1 and T3SS-2 is on SPI-2. Each T3SS consists of an assembly of more than 20 proteins that form a hollow tube-like structure through which effector proteins are injected into host target cells.

The major function of SPI-1 is to promote invasion of the intestinal epithelium. It does so by induction of actin cytoskeletal rearrangement (membrane ruffle formation), which results in bacterial entry into the enterocyte (Figure 8.1). The SPI-1 locus contains approximately 35 genes that encode components of a T3SS apparatus, several effector proteins, transcriptional regulators of genes encoded both within SPI-1 and elsewhere in the chromosome, and chaperones required for assembly of the apparatus or secretion of effectors. The effector proteins encoded on SPI-1 include SipA (SspA), AvrA, and SptP. SPI-1 also encodes translocon proteins SipB, SipC, and SipD. Effectors secreted by the SPI-1 T3SS that are encoded on other PAIs include SopA, SopB (SigD), SopD, SopE (SopE1), SopE2, SspH1, and SlrP. SopE, SopE2, and SopB promote actin rearrangement by acting as GDP/GTP exchange factors for Rac1, Cdc42, and RhoG. Rac1, Cdc42, and RhoG are Rho family GTPases, and their activation results in extensive actin rearrangement in the host cell. SopB is an inositol phosphatase and produces a molecule that acts as an indirect activator of Cdc42. SipA and SipC are actin-binding proteins that promotes bacterial-mediated endocytosis. Binding of SipA to actin decreases the critical concentration required for actin polymerization and binding of T-plastin. SipC is a two-domain protein that nucleates and bundles actin. SptP is a GTPase-activating protein for both Cdc42 and Rac1 that promote actin depolymerization, opposing the activating functions of SopE, SopE2, and SopB. These depolymerization events return the cell to a normal architecture. SipB, also a member of the translocon, interacts with caspase

FIGURE 8.1. *SPI-1 T3SS-induced changes in host cells. On contact with the epithelial cell, salmonellae assemble the SPI-1-encoded T3SS and translocate effectors (yellow spheres) into the eukaryotic cytoplasm. Effectors, such as SopE, SopE2, and SopB, then activate host Rho GTPases, which results in the rearrangement of the actin cytoskeleton into membrane ruffles, induction of MAPK pathways, and destabilization of tight junctions. Changes in the actin cytoskeleton, which are further modulated by the actin-binding proteins SipA and SipC, lead to bacterial uptake. MAPK signaling activates the transcription factors AP-1 and NF-κB, which turn on production of the proinflammatory PMN leukocyte chemokine IL-8. SipB induces caspase-1 activation in macrophages, with the release of IL-1β and IL-18, so augmenting the inflammatory response. In addition, SopB stimulates Cl^- secretion by its inositol phosphatase activity. The destabilization of tight junctions allows the transmigration of PMNs from the basolateral to the apical surface, paracellular fluid leakage, and access of bacteria to the basolateral surface. However, the transmigration of PMNs also occurs in the absence of tight-junction disruption and is further promoted by SopA. The actin cytoskeleton is restored and MAPK signaling is turned off by the enzymatic activities of SptP. This also results in the downmodulation of inflammatory responses, to which SspH1 and AvrA also contribute by inhibiting activation of NF-κB. (Reproduced from an original kindly provided by A. Haraga, University of Washington, USA; Haraga* et al. *2008.)*

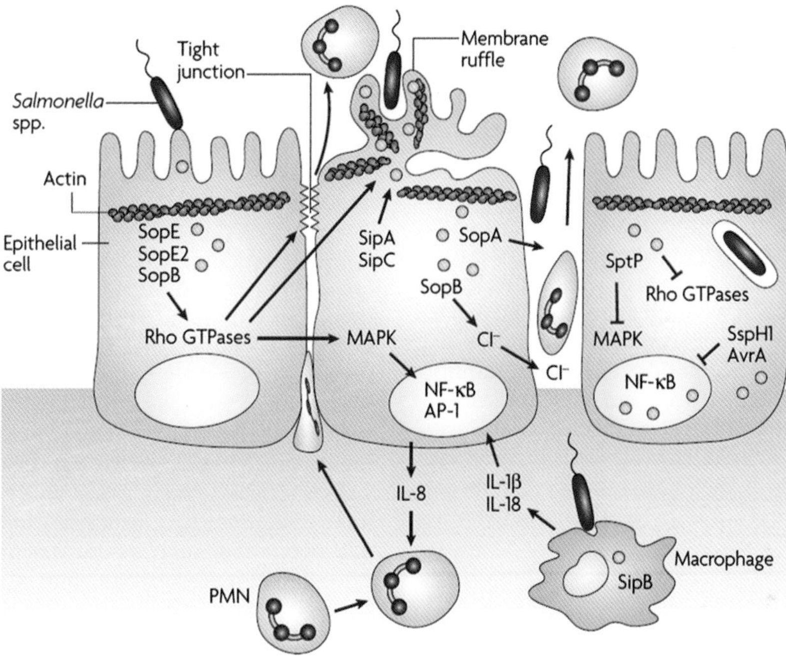

1 to cause apoptosis of macrophages. The expression of the SPI-1 T3SS is controlled in response to environmental signals; for example, it is activated in response to high osmolarity and low oxygen. Regulation is mediated primarily by control of the level of HilA, a transcriptional regulator that itself is encoded on SPI-1. HilA is regulated by other SPI-1-encoded proteins, namely, HilC and HilD, and by other gene products encoded outside the SPI-1. PhoPQ and PhoBR, both two-component regulatory systems, repress expression of the SPI-1 T3SS; PhoBR does so through repression of expression of *hilA*. SirA/BarA is another two-component regulatory system that is required for maximal expression of *hilA*.

The stimulation of Cdc42 by SopE, SopE2, and SopB also triggers several mitogen-activated protein kinase (MAPK) pathways, including the Erk, Jnk, and p38 pathways, which results in the activation of the transcription factors activator protein-1 (AP-1) and nuclear factor-κB (NF-κB) (Figure 8.1). These transcription factors then direct the production of proinflammatory cytokines, such as interleukin (IL)-8, which stimulate polymorphonuclear neutrophil (PMN) transmigration and the inflammatory response leading to diarrhea. Activation of Rho family GTPases by SopB, SopE, SopE2, and SipA also promotes intestinal disease by causing disruption of tight junctions. SipB (SspB) adds to the inflammatory response by increasing production of IL-1β and IL-18 through binding and activating caspase-1. SopA and SopD also contribute to enteritis in calves. Inflammation of the intestine in calves and many other species is typically fibrinosuppurative and often severe (Figures 8.2 and 8.3).

The major function of SPI-2 is to promote survival within macrophages. SPI-2 encodes a T3SS and effectors that play an important role in survival in macrophages; expression of the SPI-2 genes is induced once the bacterium is within the macrophage (Figure 8.4). There are at least 21 known SPI-effector proteins in addition to the translocon proteins SseB, SseC, and SseD. These include GogB, PipB, PipB2, SifA, SifB, SopD2, SpiC, SpvB, SseF, SseG, SseI (SrfH), SseJ, SseK1, SseK2, SseL, SspH2, SteA, SteB, and SteC. The functions of GogB, PipB, SifB, SseK1, SseK2, SteA, SteB, and SteC are unknown. PipB2 and SopD2 contribute to *Salmonella*-induced filament (Sif) formation. Sifs are long, filamentous membrane structures necessary for the proper positioning of the *Salmonella*-containing vacuole (SCV) in close proximity to the Golgi apparatus and near the perinuclear

FIGURE 8.2. *Jejunum of a 7-day-old calf naturally infected with* S. Typhimurium. *The mucosa is hyperemic and edematous, with erosions, and is overlaid by an adherent fibrinosuppurative exudate that extends into the lumen.*

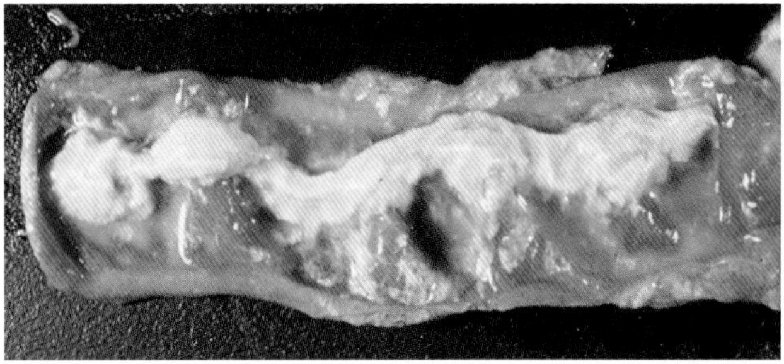

region of the host. Sif tubules extend from the surface of the SCV and appear to be derived from late endosomal compartments. They contain lysosomal associated membrane protein 1 (LAMP-1), vacuolar adenosine triphosphatase, lysobisphosphatidic acid, and cathepsin. SifA induces Sif formation, maintains the integrity of the SCV, and downregulates kinesin recruitment to the SCV. SpiC interferes with endosomal trafficking. SpvB is an actin-specific ADP-ribosyltransferase and downregulates Sif formation. SseF and SseG contribute to Sif formation and microtubule bundling. SseI (SrfH) contributes to host cell dissemination. SseJ maintains the integrity of the SCV and has deacylase activity. SseL is a deubiquitinase. SspH1, SspH2, and SrlP contribute to virulence in calves. SspH2 inhibits the rate of actin polymerization. SspH1 inhibits NF-κB signaling and IL-8 secretion and has E3 ubiquitin ligase activity. SrlP and SspH1 are also encoded on SPI-1.

FIGURE 8.3. *Photomicrograph of jejunum from a 2-week-old calf naturally infected with* S. Typhimurium. *There is severe diffuse villus atrophy with an attenuated, regenerative epithelial layer where intact. Neutrophils diffusely infiltrate the mucosa and submucosa, and are especially numerous at the mucosal surface which is necrotic and eroded. Capillaries and venules in the mucosa and submucosa are hyperemic. The lesions are compatible with severe acute diffuse necrosuppurative enteritis caused by salmonellosis.*

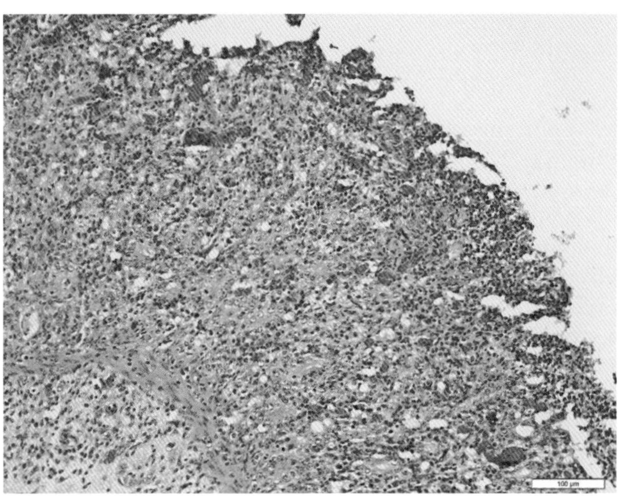

The functions of the genes located on the other SPIs are less well understood. The effector proteins associated with SPI-3 include Mgts (magnesium transport system, encoded by a number of *mgt* genes, located within SPI-3). These genes (e.g., *mgtC*) are induced by low concentration of magnesium ions (as occurs within macrophages), and the encoded proteins appear to be important for survival inside of macrophages. Different studies have concluded that SPI-4 genes are required for both the intestinal and systemic phases of disease. SPI-4 is a 27-kilobase (kb) region that carries six genes designated *siiABCDEF*. SiiC, SiiD, and SiiF form a type I secretion apparatus for the secretion of SiiE. SiiE is an adhesin that contributes to the colonization of bovine intestines, and is required for efficient translocation of SPI-1 effectors in *S.* Typhimurium. All six genes (*siiABCDEF*) are required for *S.* Typhimurium virulence in a mouse model. Like SPI-1, SPI-4 and SPI-5 are under the control of the SirA/HilA global regulatory cascade.

Enterotoxin. *Salmonella* has been reported to produce an enterotoxin called Stn (*Salmonella* enterotoxin). Original reports noted that Stn induced water and electrolyte secretion by host target cells. However, subsequent studies, one very recently conducted, have found no evidence that Stn is enterotoxigenic, nor has a role in virulence. The latter study suggests that Stn may play a role in maintenance of membrane integrity of the bacterium.

Siderophores. In response to iron limitation, all pathogenic *Salmonella* serovars produce the catecholate siderophore enterobactin, and all salmonellae with the exception *S. bongori* produce the glycosylated enterobactin derivative salmochelin. *Salmonella* mutants deficient in salmochelin but not enterochelin synthesis or secretion exhibit reduced virulence during systemic infection of mice.

Stress Proteins. Stress proteins are expressed when the bacterium is placed under stressful conditions (e.g., heat, cold, low pH, high pH, oxidative, hyperosmotic, and other environments). Different RNA polymerase (Rpo) sigma factors govern transcription initiation when the cell is under environmental stress; for example, RpoS is a general response factor, and RpoH responds to heat shock and RpoE to hyperosmotic states. In addition to Rpo sigma factors, other regulatory proteins are involved in response to these signals, and are needed for survival. Exposure to mild stress prior to more severe stress helps the bacteria adjust. *S.* Typhimurium can survive extremely low pH after growth in mildly acidic conditions (pH 4–5), a process termed the acid tolerance response (ATR). *S.* Typhimurium contains two different ATR systems, one in log and another in stationary phase. The log phase ATR induces the expression of more than 50 proteins, termed acid shock proteins. Several regulatory proteins are required for the log phase ATR, including RpoS, Fur, and PhoPQ. A second ATR system in *S.* Typhimurium is an RpoS-independent stationary phase ATR regulated by

FIGURE 8.4. *Formation of the SCV and induction of the SPI-2 T3SS within the host cell. Shortly after internalization by macropinocytosis, salmonellae are enclosed in a spacious phagosome that is formed by membrane ruffles. Later, the phagosome fuses with lysosomes, acidifies, and shrinks to become adherent around the bacterium. This is called the SCV, which contains the endocytic marker LAMP-1 (purple). The SPI-2 T3SS is induced within the SCV and translocates effector proteins (yellow spheres) across the phagosomal membrane several hours after phagocytosis. The SPI-2 T3SS effectors SifA and PipB2 contribute to Sif formation along microtubules (green) and regulate microtubule motor (yellow star shape) accumulation on the Sif and the SCV. SseJ is a deacylase that is active on the phagosome membrane. SseF and SseG cause microtubule bundling adjacent to the SCV and direct Golgi-derived vesicle traffic toward the SCV. Actin accumulates around the SCV in an SPI-2 T3SS-dependent manner, in which SspH2, SpvB, and SseI are thought to have a role. (Haraga* et al. *2008.)*

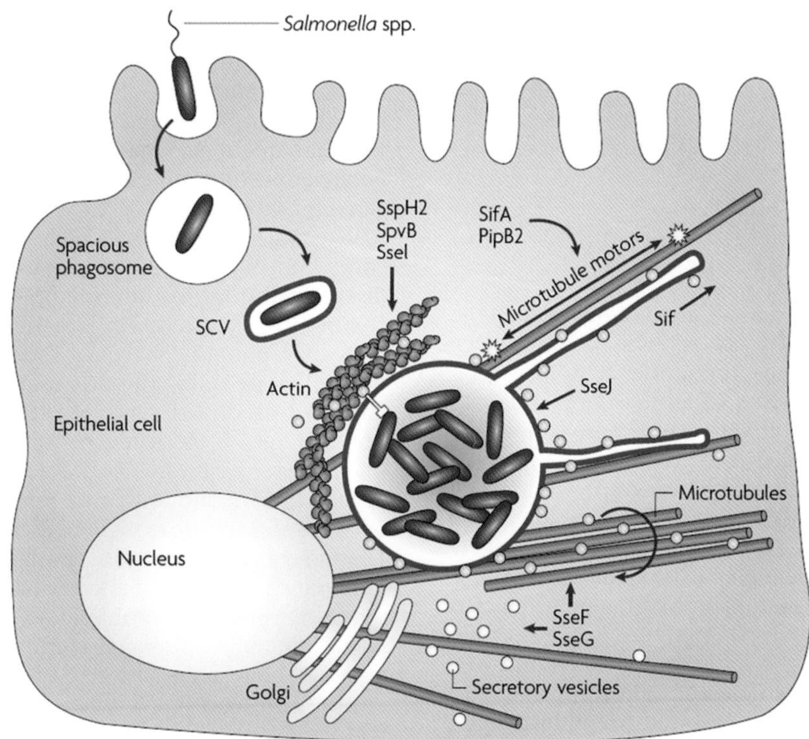

OmpR/EnvZ. RNA polymerase containing RpoS regulates genes found on *Salmonella* virulence plasmid (Spv) (see in the following text). Many other stressful environmental conditions require similar types of responses involving different regulatory proteins. Some of these are encoded on the Spv (see Section "Virulence Plasmids").

Virulence Plasmids. Salmonellae possess plasmids of various sizes, some of which have been associated with virulence. The most notable is a family of large (~50–100 kb) plasmids, termed Spv plasmids that are found within those serovars with potential to produce disseminated disease. Within subspecies I, nine serovars, namely, Abortusovis, Abortus-equi, Choleraesuis, Dublin, Enteritidis, Gallinarum, Pullorum, Sendai, and Typhimurium, are known to harbor a serovar-specific virulence plasmid that contains the *spv* operon. The *spv* operon consists of five genes, *spvRABCD*. The *spvR* gene product regulates *spvABCD*. In addition to the virulence plasmid, the *spv* operon can be found in the chromosome of subspecies I, II, IIIa, IV, and VII. The *spv* genes are essential for virulence of the different serovars in their specific hosts. Expression of *spv* genes is induced in the intracellular environment of the phagolysosome. Expression of these genes is regulated by the conditions the bacterium is exposed to, for example, those within the phagosome of the macrophage; carbon starvation; low pH and low iron environment in the presence of carbon; and stationary phase under the control of RpoS (see Section "Stress Proteins"). Other genes on these plasmids are responsible for serum resistance and may be involved in adherence and invasion of the cellular target. The virulence plasmids modulate the immune reaction, including complement activation (serum sensitivity), of the animal host in favor of the infecting salmonellae. There are a number of loci that influence the serum sensitivity of the organism. The *rck* gene is required for serum resistance; it encodes an outer membrane protein that prevents C9 insertion into the bacterial outer cell membrane.

Miscellaneous Products. The transcriptional regulator, SlyA (for salmolysin), is in part responsible for survival of salmonellae within macrophages, by activating the expression of proteins that afford protection from the toxic products generated by oxygen-dependent pathways. The products of the *phoP/phoQ* operon (PhoP and PhoQ) comprise a two-component system. PhoPQ regulates genes (e.g., *pagABC* for pho-activated genes) important for survival in macrophages, resistance to cationic proteins (defensins), acidic pH, and invasion of epithelial cells. The following conditions are sensed by PhoQ and activate PhoP: carbon starvation, nitrogen starvation, low pH, and high oxygen levels. PhoQ is a kinase that phosphorylates (activates) PhoP, which is a transcriptional regulator of other target genes, thereby transmitting the signal. *phoP* mutants are avirulent. The products of Pho-repressed genes (*prg*) are mainly located in the outer membrane, and assist in secretion of proteins through the outer membrane.

The product of the *shdA* (for shedding) gene governs fecal shedding of salmonellae by an infected host. This gene is restricted to serotypes of subspecies I. Arc (for aerobic regulation control) is a two-component global regulator system involved in intracellular survival.

Ecology

Reservoir

The reservoir for members of the genus *Salmonella* is the gastrointestinal tract of warm- and cold-blooded animals. Sources of infection include contaminated soil, vegetation, water, and components of animal feeds (such as bone, meat, and fish meal), particularly those containing milk-, meat-, or egg-derived constituents, and the feces of infected individuals. Lizards and snakes are commonly infected with several serotypes, although these infections are usually subclinical. Subspecies I is almost exclusively found in warm-blooded mammals and birds (evidence suggests that the possession of the *shdA* gene product is responsible).

Some salmonellae have become adapted to certain hosts; that is, they are not usually detected in host species other than the one to which they have adapted. Examples include Abortus-equi in horses, Abortus-ovis in sheep; Choleraesuis in swine (and occasionally humans); Dublin in cattle (and occasionally humans); Gallinarum (the cause of fowl typhoid) in poultry; Pullorum (the cause of pullorum disease) in poultry; Typhi (the cause of typhoid fever) in humans; and Paratyphi (also a cause of typhoid fever) in humans.

Some salmonellae are non-host-adapted, that is, capable of infecting many different host species. These include Anatum, Derby, Newport, Tennessee, and Typhimurium.

Transmission

Salmonellae are primarily transmitted by the fecal–oral route, often through ingestion of contaminated food and water. The outcome of the interaction between the host and *Salmonella* depends upon the state of the colonization resistance of the host, the infectious dose, and the particular species or serotype of *Salmonella*. Disease may or may not occur following ingestion. If it occurs, it may do so immediately, or at some later date. In the latter instance, the initial interaction may result in the colonization (without disease) of the host, but with a change in the intestinal environment, brought on, for example, by stress or antibiotics (activities that affect the normal flora), and disease may follow.

Pathogenesis

Mechanisms

The most common clinical manifestation of salmonellosis is diarrhea. In certain instances (defined by host factors, the strain of *Salmonella*, and dose) septicemia occurs. Host factors include age, immune status, concurrent disease, and composition of the normal flora (i.e., providing resistance to colonization).

Stationary phase salmonellae appear best suited to initiate disease, because under these conditions, RNA polymerase containing the alternative sigma factor, RpoS, initiates transcription of genes responsible for acid tolerance and subsequent survival through the stomach. Also, RNA polymerase containing RpoS is a positive regulator for the genes found on the Spv plasmids.

The target cells are the M cells in the follicle-associated epithelium overlying gut-associated lymphatic tissue in the distal small intestine and the upper large bowel. Lack of competitive flora caused by poor nutrition, stress, or antibiotics may potentially reduce the infectious dose. Adhesion to the M cell is the first step in the disease process, mediated by one or more of the adhesins, namely, Agf, Pef, and Lpf, or by others yet to be determined. Following adhesion, salmonellae are internalized following the induction of membrane ruffles in the target cells triggered by Ssps and Sops subsequent to their injection by the T3SS. The target cell is irreversibly damaged by this interaction, undergoing apoptosis. Salmonellae are now found within the target cells, the lymph nodule, and submucosal tissue. An inflammatory response is initiated by release of various chemokines from affected host cells, as well as release of proinflammatory cytokines following host interaction with cell wall LPS—activities that result in an influx of PMN leukocytes and macrophages. The influx of PMNs may be reflected in a transient peripheral neutropenia. PMNs are highly efficient in phagocytosing and killing salmonellae, whereas nonactivated macrophages are less so. If the immune status of the host and the characteristics of the salmonellae are such, the infectious process is arrested at this stage. Diarrhea is thought to result from prostaglandin synthesis by the recruited PMNs (and perhaps by the affected host cells), as well as activation of various inositol-signaling pathways within affected host cells. The net result is the secretion of chloride ions and water.

If the infecting strain of *Salmonella* has properties that allow dissemination (possession of SPI-2, SPI-3, SPI-4, and SPI-5—associated gene products that allow growth within macrophages; Spv plasmid encoding ability to grow intracellularly and serum resistance; PhoQ/PhoP system allowing resistance to defensins; SlyA allowing resistance to oxygen-dependent by-products; *arcA*), septicemia may result. The likelihood of this occurring is increased if the immune status of the host is diminished. Salmonellae disseminate and multiply within phagocytic cells (macrophages mainly) within phagosomes. Following systemic dissemination of the salmonellae, septicemia and endotoxic shock may develop. Strains producing this form of disease escape destruction by the host and multiply within macrophages of the liver and spleen, as well as intravascularly. During the dissemination process, salmonellae are occasionally outside of the intracellular environment and therefore at risk from the formation of complement membrane attack complexes on their surfaces. This occurrence is discouraged by at least two mechanisms: a product of the Spv plasmid and the length of the O-repeat unit of the LPS (there is a direct correlation between O-repeat length and virulence). Invasive salmonellae are capable of secreting a siderophore, salmochelin that removes iron from the iron-binding proteins of the host. Uncontrolled multiplication of the organism results in endotoxemia, severe vascular damage, and death.

Pathology

If the infectious process is limited to the intestinal tract, the lesions will consist of a fibrinosuppurative, necrotizing and hemorrhagic inflammation of the distal small intestine and large bowel. Necrosis of the intestine is at first erosive and frequently becomes ulcerative, resulting in the formation of a diphtheritic membrane. This lesion is especially common in cattle (Figures 8.2 and 8.3) and swine. The liver is frequently affected with random, multifocal necrotizing inflammation that reflects bacterial spread via the portal vein and phagocytosis by Kupffer cells without effective bacterial killing. In the septicemic form of the disease, there may be fibrinoid change in blood vessels in many different organs as well as vasculitis, thromboembolism, hemorrhages, and infarcts. In swine with septicemic *S.* Choleraesuis infection, the spleen is usually markedly enlarged due to hyperemia, and the ears of white-skinned pigs may be dark blue from thrombosis and venous congestion.

Disease Patterns

Ruminants. Salmonellosis is a significant disease of ruminants, mainly cattle. The disease affects young (usually 4–6 weeks of age) as well as adult animals, although neonatal calves may also be affected, especially in dairies. Animals in feedlots and dairies are commonly affected. The disease may be a septicemia or be limited to an enteritis or enterocolitis (Figures 8.2 and 8.3). Pneumonia, hematogenously acquired, is a common presenting sign in calves with septicemia due to *S.* Dublin. Abortion may follow septicemia. *S.* Typhimurium, *S.* Dublin, and *S.* Newport are the serotypes commonly isolated from cattle, and *S.* Typhimurium the main serotype affecting sheep.

Swine. Salmonellosis in swine can present as an acute, fulminating septicemia or as a chronic debilitating intestinal disease. The form depends upon the strain of *Salmonella*, the dose, and the colonization resistance of the infected animal. The disease is seen most often in pigs that have been stressed. Such conditions occur often in feeder pigs, an age group in which salmonellosis commonly occurs. *S.* Typhimurium and *S.* Choleraesuis are the predominant serotypes.

Horses. Adult horses are commonly affected with *Salmonella*. The pattern is diarrhea, though septicemia is seen occasionally. Colic, gastrointestinal surgery and antimicrobial agents predispose the horse to the development of clinical signs. The agent is either carried normally (as in ~3% of clinically normal horses) or acquired from other sources (e.g., a veterinary hospital). *S.* Typhimurium and *S.* Anatum are most commonly isolated.

Dogs and Cats. Salmonellosis is uncommon in dogs and cats, although carriage is reportedly high in clinically normal pound dogs (upward of 35%). When outbreaks occur they are usually associated with a common source, such as contaminated dog food or "treats" (e.g., dried pig's ears). *Salmonella* should be high on the microbiological differential list for cats with signs of septicemia.

Poultry. See Section "Salmonellosis of Poultry."

Epidemiology

Salmonella spp. are ubiquitous geographically and zoologically. Some serotypes are relatively host-specific (*S.* Dublin—cattle; *S.* Typhisuis—swine; *S.* Pullorum—fowl), while others, notably *S.* Typhimurium, *S.* Anatum, and *S.* Newport, affect a wide host range among which feral birds and rodents play important roles in interspecific dissemination of infection. Long periods of subclinical and convalescent shedding ensure widespread, unchecked distribution of the organisms.

Clinical outbreaks are correlated with depressed immune states, as in newborn animals (e.g., calves and foals) and stressed adults, parturient cows, equine surgical patients, and swine with systemic viral diseases. All animals are at increased risk of developing disease if their normal flora is disrupted (e.g., stress and antibiotics). These circumstances render animals susceptible to exogenous exposure or activation of silent infections.

Humans appear to be susceptible to all *Salmonella* serotypes, with typhoid fever caused by *S.* Typhi, a disease restricted to humans, and infections with other serotypes being food-borne zoonoses. Poultry and poultry products (eggs) are a major source of salmonellosis in humans. *S.* Enteritidis (e.g., phage type 4) is especially adapted for egg transmission. Whether a person develops disease following ingestion of salmonellae from the environment depends upon the dose of organisms, the serotype of *Salmonella*, and the colonization resistance of the infected individual. *S.* Typhimurium is most common, usually producing gastroenteritis. Some serotypes have greater invasion potential and greater potential for causing septicemia, for example, *S.* Choleraesuis (from swine) and *S.* Dublin (contaminated milk).

S. Typhimurium DT104 is a more virulent strain in both animals and humans than most other strains of this serotype. The case-fatality rate with DT104 is 3%, compared to 0.1% with other nontyphoid salmonellae. DT is the definitive type designation, which specifies a particular phage type. In addition to increased virulence, DT104 isolates are multidrug resistant, by definition, resistant to ampicillin, chloramphenicol, streptomycin, sulfonamides, and tetracycline. DT104 infection in humans is usually acquired by eating contaminated beef, pork, or poultry, or by direct contact with animals, particularly those with diarrhea (e.g., cattle and cats). In the United States, the prevalence of *S.* Typhimurium isolates with the five-drug pattern of resistance increased from less than 1% in 1979–1980 to 34% in 1996, most of which were DT104 with one pulsed-field electrophoresis pattern predominating among the DT104 types. Reptiles have also become an important source of *Salmonella* in humans, with pets (e.g., turtles) in classrooms a common means of exposure.

Immunological Aspects

Protection depends upon both innate and adaptive immunity. Competitive floras help reduce the numbers of pathogens by competing for nutrients, masking receptors, and producing toxic compounds. Direct-fed microbials, for example, certain strains of *Lactobacillus acidophilus* or other bacteria, may help prevent infections through providing competitive exclusion. However, complete protection can only be afforded by an adaptive immune response in the form of specific antibodies and T cells. Antibodies specific for surface structures of *Salmonella*, possibly adhesins, prevent adherence to target cells. The neonate is protected passively by ingesting specific sIgA or IgG_1 (bovine). The immunologically mature animal is protected by the active secretion of specific immunoglobulins (IgM, IgG, or IgA) into the intestinal lumen by plasma cells in the lamina propria, which prevent bacteria from adhering and invading gut epithelial cells.

Antibodies in the circulation act as opsonins and promote the phagocytosis of the organism. Destruction of the salmonellae that have been phagocytosed follows the immunological activation of the macrophages by specifically stimulated lymphocytes (T_H1 cells) though activated macrophages are damaged or killed by Ssps. NK cells lyse *Salmonella*-infected cells.

Acquired immunity revolves around activation of macrophages, which takes place as follows. After initial interaction between salmonellae and macrophage, IL-12 is released by the affected macrophage. IL-12 activates the T_H1 subset of T helper cells. This subset secretes, among other cytokines, interferon-γ, which activates macrophages. Activated macrophages are efficient killers of intracellular salmonellae.

Artificial immunization against salmonellae is difficult. Bacterins have had limited success. Apparently, they do not stimulate strong cellular immunity, even though abundant antibody is produced. Antibodies that are produced locally or passed in colostrum or milk interfere with adsorption to the target cell and protect against disease in this location. Macrophages can be activated and antibody production stimulated in response to modified live vaccines. If given orally, these vaccines stimulate local secretory immunity and cell-mediated activation of phagocytic cells. Aromatic-dependent mutants of *Salmonella* show promise as effective modified live vaccines, especially for calves. *aroA* mutants of *Salmonella* cannot multiply within the host since vertebrate tissue does not contain the needed precursors for aromatic acid synthesis.

FIGURE 8.5. *Colonies of* S. enterica *ssp. enterica serotype Enteritidis on blood agar. Bacteria were cultivated for 24 h in an aerobic atmosphere at 37 °C. (www.bacteriainphotos.com, accessed January 3, 2013.)*

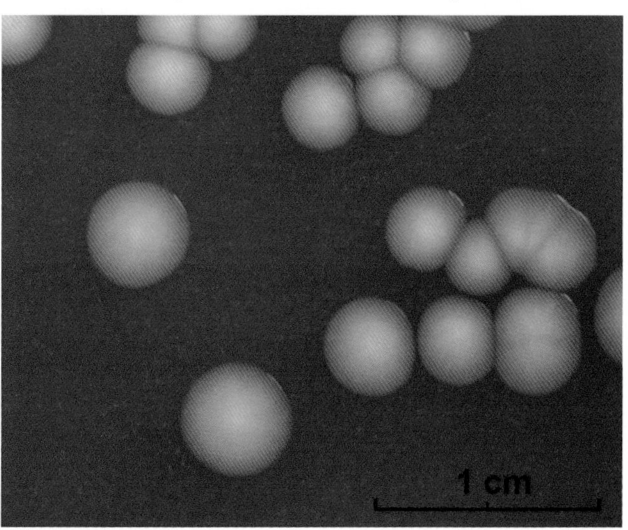

Laboratory Diagnosis

In cases of intestinal infection, fecal samples are collected; in systemic disease, a blood sample is collected for standard blood culture. Spleen and bone marrow are cultured for the salmonellae when postmortem diagnosis of systemic salmonellosis is required.

Fresh fecal samples are placed onto nutrient, for example, blood agar (Figure 8.5), and one or more selective media, including MacConkey agar (Figure 8.6), xylose lysine deoxycholate (XLD) agar (Figure 8.7), Hektoen

FIGURE 8.6. *Colonies of* S. enterica *ssp. enterica serotype Enteritidis on MacConkey agar. Bacteria were cultivated for 24 h in an aerobic atmosphere at 37 °C. (www.bacteriainphotos.com, accessed January 3, 2013.)*

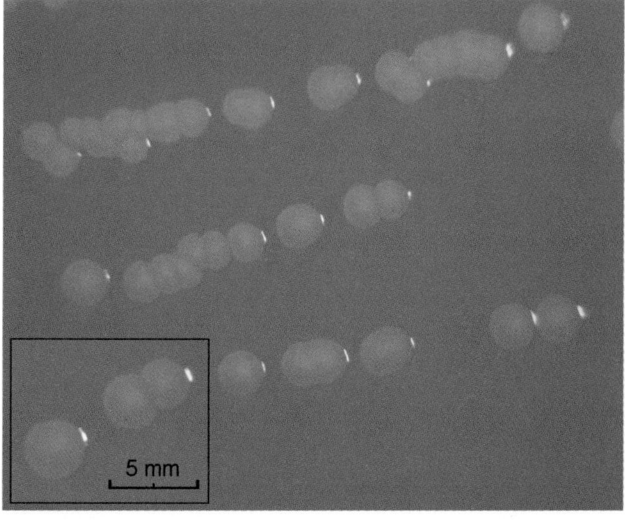

FIGURE 8.7. *Salmonella colonies, XLD agar. When xylose lysine (XL) agar is supplemented with sodium thiosulfate, ferric ammonium citrate, and sodium deoxycholate, it is then termed XLD agar. The presence of any black-colored area indicates the deposition of hydrogen sulfide (H_2S), under alkaline conditions, and is highly suggestive of Salmonella. (US Health and Human Services, Centers for Disease Control and Prevention, Public Health Information Library, ID# 6619.)*

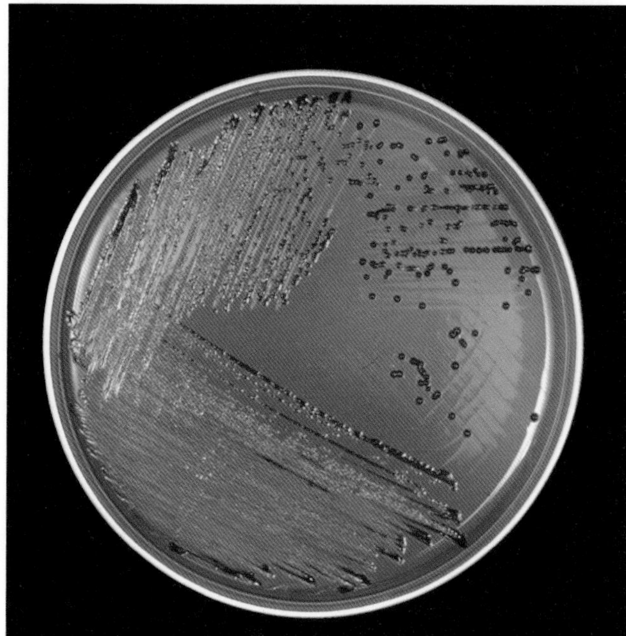

enteric medium, and brilliant green agar. For enrichment, selenite F, tetrathionate, or gram-negative broth is recommended.

Salmonellae appear as lactose-non-fermenting colonies on lactose-containing media (Figure 8.6). Since most serotypes of salmonellae produce H_2S, colonies on iron-containing media (e.g., XLD agar), they will have a black center (Figure 8.7). Suspicious colonies can be tested directly with polyvalent anti-*Salmonella* antiserum or inoculated into differential media and then tested with antisera.

To cultivate salmonellae from tissue, blood agar (Figure 8.5) can be used.

Definitive identification involves determination of somatic and flagellar antigens and possibly bacteriophage type.

Various *Salmonella*-specific DNA probes and primers for the polymerase chain reaction have been developed for identification as well as detection in samples (food, feces, and water) containing other microorganisms.

A multiplex polymerase chain reaction assay using primers designed to detect the common diarrhea-associated microorganisms of swine (*Brachyspira hyodysenteriae, Lawsonia intracellularis,* and *Salmonella*) has been described.

Treatment, Control, and Prevention

Nursing care is the principal treatment for the enteric form of salmonellosis. The use of antimicrobial agents is controversial. Some studies show that antibiotics do not alter the course of the disease. In addition, there is evidence that antibiotics promote the carrier state and select for resistant strains. Treatment of the systemic form of salmonellosis includes nursing care and appropriate antimicrobial therapy as determined by retrospectively acquired susceptibility data. Since salmonellae survive in the phagocytic cell, the antimicrobial drug should be one that penetrates the cell. Examples of those that distribute in this manner include ampicillin, enrofloxacin, trimethoprim–sulfonamides, and chloramphenicol/florfenicol. Treatment options may be compromised due to acquisition of R plasmids or integrons encoding resistance to multiple antibiotics. A serious global epidemic of *S.* Typhimurium DT104, a type of salmonella that affects humans and other animals worldwide, contains a cluster of antibiotic resistance-encoding genes within its chromosome. This cluster, called *Salmonella* genomic island 1 (SGI1), contains the genes for resistance to ampicillin, chloramphenicol/florfenicol, streptomycin/spectinomycin, sulfonamides, and tetracyclines bounded by two integrons. SGI1 has moved into *S. enterica* serotype Albany (fish in Southeast Asia) and *S. enterica* serotype Paratyphi B (tropical fish in Singapore).

Salmonellosis is controlled through strict attention to protocols designed to curtail the spread to susceptible animals of any contagious agent found in feces. Artificial immunization with modified live products has shown promise (e.g., *aroA* mutants). Attempts have been made to treat and prevent the endotoxemia produced by the systemic form of the disease by administering serum containing antibodies to the core LPS. Likewise, the administration of J5, a rough variant of *E. coli*, has been shown to stimulate the production of antibody to the core LPS. Both methods appear to prevent and control the signs of disease produced by systemic salmonellosis.

Salmonellosis of Poultry

Paratyphoid. "Paratyphoid" of poultry (in quotation marks because true paratyphoid is a disease of humans caused by paratyphoid serotypes of *Salmonella*) is salmonellosis produced by any of the motile strains of *Salmonella*. All salmonellae except *S. enterica* serotype Pullorum and *S. enterica* serotype Gallinarum are motile. The disease produces its highest losses in the first 2 weeks of life as a septicemic disease. Survivors become asymptomatic excretors. Infection is through ingestion. The source is usually feces or fecally contaminated materials (e.g., litter, fluff, and water).

Diagnosis is made by culturing the organism from affected tissue (e.g., spleen and joints) from birds that had been showing clinical signs of disease. It is more difficult to detect a subclinical carrier because such carriers only periodically shed the organism in feces. Some have suggested that culture of fluff and litter could be used to detect carrier flocks.

Treatment does not eliminate carriers, although it does control mortality. Treatment regimens have included avoparcin, lincomycin, furazolidone, streptomycin, and gentamicin. Exclusion of salmonellae by feeding "cocktails" of normal flora has been used with some success to reduce the number of salmonellae shed by carrier birds (competitive exclusion).

Pullorum Disease. Pullorum disease, caused by *S.* Pullorum, is rare in North America but not in the rest of the world. The disease has almost been eliminated in the United States due to a breeding flock testing program.

S. Pullorum infects the ova of turkeys and chickens. Thus, the embryo is already infected when the egg is hatched. The hatchery environment is contaminated following hatching of an infected egg, leading to infection of other chicks and poults. Mortality is due to septicemia and is greatest in the second to third weeks of life. Surviving birds carry the bacterium and may pass it to their offspring. It is difficult to detect infected breeding hens by bacteriologic means. Agglutination titers, produced 3–10 days after infection, are used to detect carrier birds.

Eliminating infected breeding birds detected serologically controls this disease. Treatment with antimicrobial agents (mainly sulfonamides) reduces mortality in infected flocks.

Fowl Typhoid. Fowl typhoid, caused by *S.* Gallinarum, is an acute septicemic or chronic disease of domesticated adult birds, mainly chickens. Fowl typhoid is rare now in the United States due to control programs.

The disease is diagnosed by culturing the organism from liver or spleen. It is treated with antimicrobial agents, mainly sulfonamides (sulfaquinoxaline) and nitrofurans. Fowl typhoid is controlled by management and eliminating infected birds. A bacterin made from a rough variant of *S.* Gallinarum, 9R, has been shown to decrease mortality.

Avian Arizonosis. *S. enterica* ssp. *arizonae* and *S. enterica* ssp. *diarizonae* are most often isolated from reptiles and fowl, although these species can be isolated from any animal. Turkeys are most commonly affected. There are 55 serologic types affecting fowl, with type 7: 1, 7, and 8 most commonly isolated in the United States.

S. enterica ssp. *arizonae* and *S. enterica* ssp. *diarizonae* are maintained in turkey flocks via hatching eggs, which become infected following ingestion by the hen. Feces also spread it.

Diagnosis is made by culturing salmonellae from the liver, spleen, blood, lungs, or kidneys of affected birds, or from dead poults and hatch debris.

Most serotypes of *S. enterica* ssp. *arizonae* and *S. enterica* subsp. *diarizonae* possess R plasmids, which sometimes makes it difficult to prevent and treat this disease. Various antimicrobial agents such as furazolidone and sulfamerazine added to feed have shown some success in lowering mortality. Injection of day-old poults with gentamicin or spectinomycin decreases mortality, but survivors still harbor (and shed) the organism.

Control measures should be aimed at prevention rather than treatment. Because of the multiplicity of serotypes, no effective vaccine is available.

Reference

Haraga A, Ohlson MB, and Miller SI (2008) Salmonellae interplay with host cells. *Nat Rev Microbiol*, **6**, 53–66.

Further Reading

Ellermeier CD and Slauch JM (2006) The genus *Salmonella*. *Prokaryotes*, **6**, 123–158.

Euzéby JP (2012) List of prokaryotic names with standing in nomenclature—genus *Salmonella*, http://www.bacterio.cict.fr/s/salmonella.html (accessed January 3, 2013).

Nataro JP, Bopp CA, Fields PI *et al.* (2011) *Escherichia, Shigella,* and *Salmonella*, in *Manual of Clinical Microbiology*, 10th edn (ed. J Versalovic), ASM Press, Washington, DC, pp. 603–626.

Enterobacteriaceae: *Yersinia*

RODNEY MOXLEY

The genus Yersinia is included in the family Enterobacteriaceae. Yersinia includes 17 species: *aldovae, aleksiciae, bercovieri, enterocolitica, entomophaga, frederiksenii, intermedia, kristensenii, massiliensis, mollaretii, nurmii, pekkanenii, pestis, pseudotuberculosis, rohdei, ruckeri,* and *similis*. *Yersinia enterocolitica* includes two subspecies, *enterocolitica* and *palearctica*. The type species is Y. pestis.

Disease caused by *Yersinia* infection is called yersiniosis. Yersinioses are zoonotic infections that predominantly affect rodents, pigs, and birds. Humans and nonhuman primates are affected only by *Y. pestis*, *Y. pseudotuberculosis*, and *Y. enterocolitica*. *Y. pestis* is the cause of plague, a septicemic disease of major importance in humans, rodents, and occasionally domestic animals that is primarily acquired through bite wounds of rodent fleas. *Y. enterocolitica* mainly causes disease in domestic animals and primates, and is the most prevalent species in humans. *Y. pseudotuberculosis* mainly affects birds and rodents, and only occasionally domestic animals and primates. *Y. enterocolitica* and *Y. pseudotuberculosis* infections are food- and water-borne illnesses that result in mesenteric lymphadenitis, terminal ileitis, acute gastroenteritis, and septicemia.

The three main pathogenic species have several features in common, including tropism for lymphoid tissues; capacity to resist nonspecific immune responses; behavior as facultative intracellular pathogens; ability to resist phagocytosis by macrophages; cause formation of extracellular colonies in tissues; carriage of a plasmid of 70–75 kb that contains virulence genes, pCD1 in *Y. pestis*, pYV (also known as pCad and pIB1) in *Y. pseudotuberculosis*, and pYV in *Y. enterocolitica*; carriage of a pathogenicity island known as a high-pathogenicity island (HPI) on the chromosome; production of *Yersinia* outer proteins (Yops); and having animals as a reservoir, with transmission to humans occurring directly or indirectly.

Yersinia ruckeri affects only fish and causes red mouth, a septicemic disease of salmon and trout. The zoonotic aspects of *Y. intermedia*, *Y. frederiksenii*, and *Y. kristensenii* are uncertain. *Yersinia aldovae*, *Y. rohdei*, *Y. mollaretii*, and *Y. bercovieri* are without known pathogenic potential.

Descriptive Features

Morphology and Staining

Members of the genus *Yersinia* are gram-negative coccobacilli (Figure 9.1) that exhibit bipolar ("closed safety pin") staining, especially when seen in smears from tissue specimens and stained with Giemsa (Figure 9.2). Most species are flagellated at ambient temperatures.

Growth Characteristics

Yersinia grow on blood, chocolate, MacConkey, and other ordinary laboratory media incubated at 35 °C in ambient air, although their rate of growth is relatively slow compared to most other members of the family Enterobacteriaceae. Hence, they may be outcompeted by other bacteria in cultures of clinical and environmental samples. Yersiniae grow well at a temperature range of 4–43 °C, with optimum temperatures ranging from 25 °C to 28 °C, and form 1–2 mm diameter colonies after 48 h of incubation (Figure 9.3). The ability of yersiniae to grow at 4 °C is a concern for blood banks because some donors may carry species such as *Y. enterocolitica* asymptomatically.

Yersiniae in culture yield colonies that range from <1 to 1.5 mm in diameter, with those at the low end of the spectrum being more typical of *Y. pestis*. Yersiniae are not hemolytic on blood agar (Figure 9.3). They are catalase-positive, oxidase-negative, and ferment glucose with the production of acid but no gas. Yersiniae do not typically grow well nor form turbid suspensions in liquid media. All *Yersinia* spp. except *Y. pestis* are motile at 25 °C.

Y. pestis (Plague Bacillus)

Y. pestis is the cause of the disease called plague. As are all yersinioses, plague is a zoonotic disease with rodents, the reservoir for the pathogen. In human patients and susceptible domestic animal species (mainly cats), plague is manifested as a local lymphadenitis called a bubo (bubonic

Veterinary Microbiology, Third Edition. Edited by D. Scott McVey, Melissa Kennedy and M.M. Chengappa.

FIGURE 9.1. *Y. pestis, gram stain, showing gram-negative bacilli. (Courtesy of Larry Stauffer, Oregon State Public Health Laboratory, and US Health and Human Services, Centers for Disease Control and Prevention, Public Health Image Library, ID#1914.)*

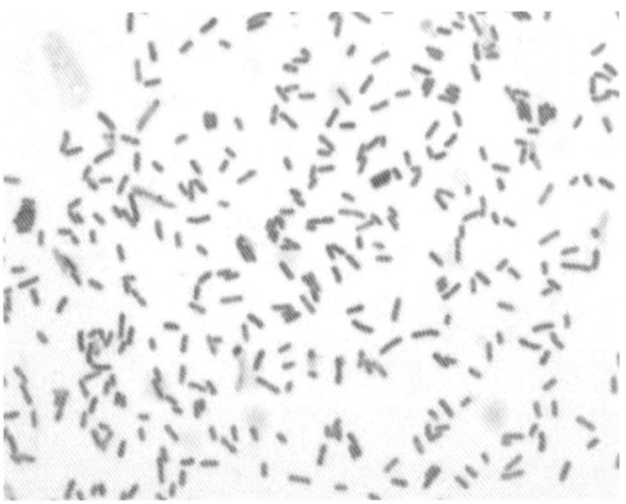

plague, Figures 9.4 and 9.5), pneumonia (pneumonic plague, Figure 9.6), or septicemia (septicemic plague, Figures 9.7 and 9.8). Analysis of DNA sequences of the genes encoding the 16S ribosomal RNA indicates that *Y. pestis* is a subspecies of *Y. pseudotuberculosis* that has lost a number of the enteropathogenic *Yersinia* virulence genes.

Historically, there have been three pandemics: AD 541–544 (Justinian plague), AD 1330–1346 to 1600s, and AD 1855 to present. The second pandemic was called "the Black Death." It was called "black" because this was the appearance of acral necrosis caused by infarcts as a component of septicemia affecting the digits of the hands and feet (Figures 9.7 and 9.8). The Black Death pandemic was characterized by extremely high mortality, especially from about 1347 to 1351. An estimated 17–28 million people in Europe died from the Black Death during this time, representing 30–40% of the European population. Epidemics during modern times are often seen in war-torn countries (e.g., an epidemic occurred in Vietnam in the 1960s and 1970s). From 1990 to 1995, about 12 000 cases and 1000 deaths occurred worldwide; these were mainly seen in Africa, Vietnam, China, South America, and India.

FIGURE 9.2. *Y. pestis, Wright's stained blood smear from a plague victim showing dark stained bipolar ends of bacteria. (Courtesy of US Health and Human Services, Centers for Disease Control and Prevention, Public Health Image Library, ID#2050.)*

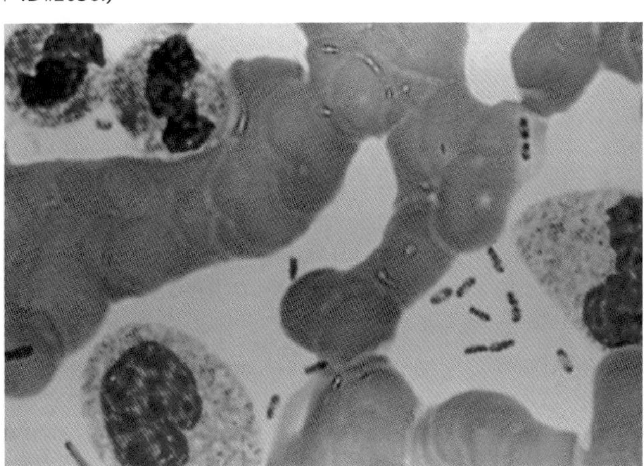

FIGURE 9.3. *Y. pestis colonies on sheep blood agar after 72 h of culture. Y. pestis grows well on most standard laboratory media. After 48–72 h of incubation, colonies are grey-white to slightly yellow opaque and raised, and have an irregular "fried egg" appearance. Alternatively, colonies may have a "hammered copper" shiny surface. (Courtesy of US Health and Human Services, Centers for Disease Control and Prevention, Public Health Image Library, ID#1921.)*

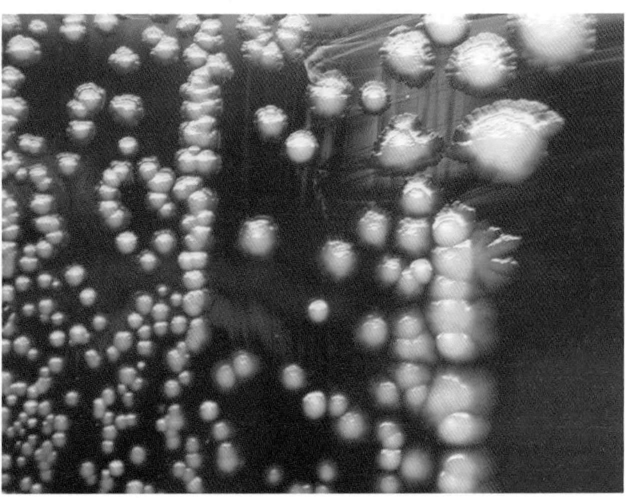

FIGURE 9.4. *An axillary bubo and edema exhibited by a patient with bubonic plague. After the incubation period of 2–6 days, symptoms of the plague appear including severe malaise, headache, shaking chills, fever, and pain and swelling, or adenopathy, in the affected regional lymph nodes, also known as buboes. (Courtesy of US Health and Human Services, Centers for Disease Control and Prevention, Public Health Image Library, ID#2061.)*

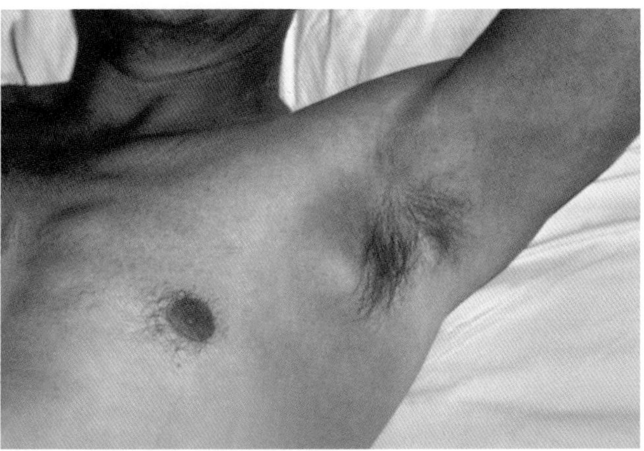

FIGURE 9.5. *Histopathology of lymph nodes in fatal human plague. Medullary necrosis with fluid and Y. pestis. (Courtesy of US Health and Human Services, Centers for Disease Control and Prevention, Public Health Image Library, ID#731.)*

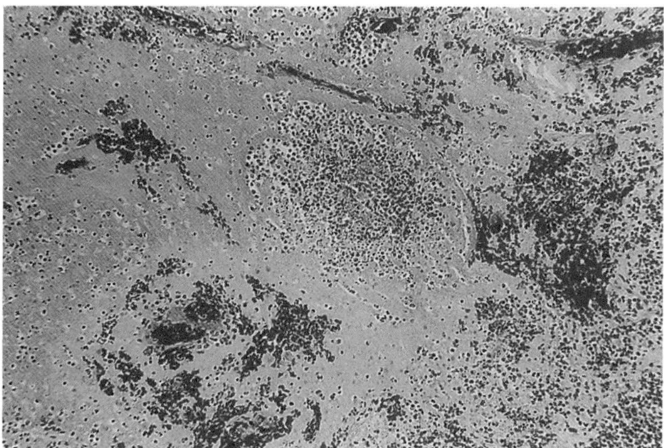

Initial signs and symptoms in human plague victims appear 2–6 days after contact with the organism. They have fever, headache, chills, and swollen tender lymph nodes (buboes). Buboes usually involve the inguinal and femoral lymph nodes, which is reflective of lymphatic drainage of organisms originating from fleabites on the lower legs. If untreated, plague often progresses to septicemia, which is characterized clinically by prostration, lethargy, high fever, and seizures.

In humans, presepticemic plague if untreated has a 40–60% case-fatality rate, and if treated has a 14% case-fatality rate. Septicemic plague, if untreated, has a 100% case-fatality rate; with treatment, it has a 30–50% case-fatality rate. Pneumonic plague can be a rare secondary complication of bubonic or septicemic plague or can be the primary infection following direct inhalation of aerosolized organisms from other pneumonic cases (human or animal), infected tissues, or cultured organisms. The case-fatality rate in untreated pneumonic cases is essentially 100%, and often exceeds 50% in treated cases.

Necropsy of animals infected with plague is a distinct risk factor for veterinarians. In 2007, a fatal case of

FIGURE 9.6. *Radiograph of the thorax of a patient with pneumonic plague. There is bilateral involvement, with greater consolidation of the left side of the lung. (Courtesy of US Health and Human Services, Centers for Disease Control and Prevention, Public Health Image Library, ID#4068.)*

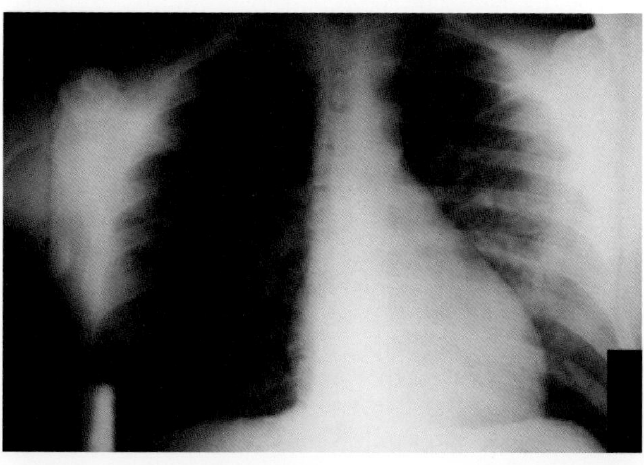

FIGURE 9.7. *Acral gangrene of the digits of the right foot of a patient with septicemic plague. Systemic infection with Y. pestis resulted in thrombosis and infarction of the terminal segments of the digits. It was because of this type of lesion that the disease became known as the "Black Death." (Courtesy of US Health and Human Services, Centers for Disease Control and Prevention, Public Health Image Library, ID#4139.)*

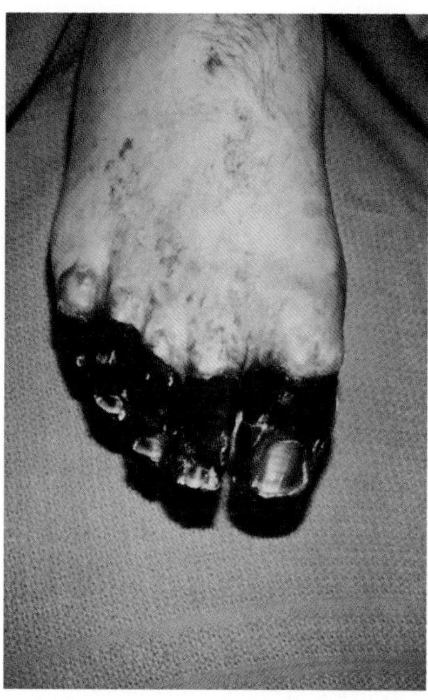

FIGURE 9.8. *A shaved anterior thoracoabdominal region of a rock squirrel, Spermophilus variegatus, afflicted with the plague. This squirrel is displaying a petechial rash, which is similar in appearance to those found on humans also afflicted with Y. pestis. (Courtesy of US Health and Human Services, Centers for Disease Control and Prevention, Public Health Image Library, ID#6720.)*

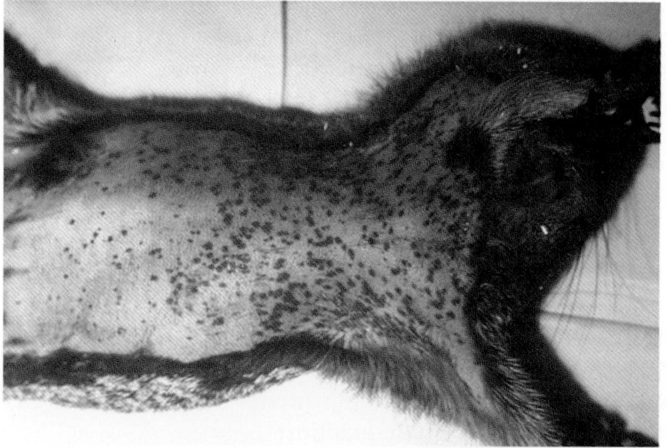

pneumonic plague occurred in a Grand Canyon National Park wildlife biologist who had necropsied an infected mountain lion carcass 7 days earlier. Face-to-face contact with infected pets and laboratory exposure are two other examples of hazards associated with veterinary practice (see Sections "Ecology," and "Pathogenesis").

Descriptive Features

Cellular Composition and Products of Medical Importance. The majority of *Y. pestis* strains regardless of biotype or origin contain three virulence plasmids: pCD1 (70–75 kb encoding the type III secretion system, Yops, and low calcium response genes); pMT1 (100–110 kb encoding the Caf1 (F1) capsule and *Yersinia* murine toxin (Ymt); and pPCP1 (9.5 kb encoding pesticin, coagulase, and plasminogen activator (Pla). The *ybt* genes encoding the siderophore, yersiniabactin, are found on the 35 kb HPI, which in turn is within the 102 kb *pgm* (pigmentation) locus on the chromosome. An additional operon within the *pgm* region and unique to *Y. pestis* is the 6 kb *hms* locus. The *hms* genes encode hemin storage proteins, which enable biofilm formation and proventricular blockage in fleas. Also located on the chromosome are the genes encoding the protein Gsr (global stress requirement).

Capsule (Fra1, Caf1, or F1). The capsule plays many roles, the most important of which are interference with phagocytosis, and the protection of the outer membrane from the deposition of membrane attack complexes generated by activation of the complement system. The capsule of *Y. pestis* is called Fra1 for fraction 1 or Caf1 (for capsular antigen fraction 1) or F1 (fraction 1 antigen), and is encoded by genes that reside on the 110 kb plasmid pMT1 (which also carries the genes encoding the toxin Ymt, see Section "Toxins"). In contrast to Ymt, F1 is expressed at temperatures >30 °C and during mammalian infection. Upon flea inoculation of *Y. pestis*, some of the bacteria are engulfed and transported to regional lymph nodes by macrophages. Here, during intracellular growth, F1 is expressed and forms a capsule on the bacterial surface. Subsequent to release of *Y. pestis* from its intracellular location, the antiphagocytic properties of the new F1 surface enable widespread dissemination and replication and result in host sepsis.

Cell Wall. *Y. pestis* has lost the genetic capacity to express a complete lipopolysaccharide (LPS) layer; hence, it lacks an O-antigen. This organism does, however, elicit clinical effects typical of those due to endotoxemia. This is the result of LPS binding to the LPS-binding protein and then to Toll-like receptor (TLR)-4. The mechanism of endotoxin-mediated effects is described further in Chapter 6.

High-Pathogenicity Island. The HPI is so-called because its presence is related to increased virulence as compared to strains that do not contain it. It is a pathogenicity island that contains genes encoding the siderophore, yersiniabactin, and hemin storage proteins (see Sections "Hms Phenotype" and "Iron Acquisition").

Hms Phenotype. The Hms (for hemin storage) phenotype is associated with iron acquisition and colonization of fleas (see Section "Iron Acquisition"). In addition to playing a role in iron acquisition, the hms locus encodes proteins that serve to block the proventriculus of the flea with aggregated bacteria. This causes regurgitation and repeated attempts at feeding. Although this enhances the possibility of transmission of the bacteria to new rodent hosts, it also eventually causes death of the flea. Hemin is Fe^{2+} heme and contains chloride. The Hms^{+} phenotype is dark greenish-brown colonies on hemin agar.

Iron Acquisition. Iron is an absolute growth requirement and must be removed from iron-binding proteins of the host. The genes encoding products involved with iron acquisition reside on the HPI, an integrase protein, a specific insertion site, and mobility. The HPI of *Y. pestis* encodes the genes for the iron-acquiring siderophore yersiniabactin, and the Hms (for hemin storage) phenotype. Colonies growing on the surface of blood agar plates that display the Hms phenotype appear pigmented (they are not) due to the binding of hemoglobin (dark greenish-brown) or Congo red if present. It is probable that bound hemoglobin is used as a source of iron. The genes responsible are encoded by the *pgm* (for pigment) locus.

Type III Secretion System. The type III secretion system consists of an assemblage of proteins (more than 20) encoded by *ysc* (Yop secretion apparatus) genes that form a hollow tube-like structure through which effector proteins (Yops and LcrV) are injected into host target cells. The *ysc* genes encoding the proteins needed by the type III secretion system reside on plasmid pYV (along with the genes encoding Yops and LcrV, see Section "Toxins"). Most of the proteins of the type III secretion system make up the membrane-spanning channel that will eventually fuse with the eukaryotic cell to form the injection pore. Genes for the core of the membrane-spanning complex are expressed at 37 °C. Contact with the eukaryotic cell is not needed for this core to form, only exposure to body temperature (37 °C).

Toxins. *Y. pestis* produces a number of toxins and other effector proteins:

1. *Yops*: Following their injection into macrophages, Yops (for *Yersinia* outer protein) interfere with the actin cytoskeleton, thereby blocking phagocytosis, and downregulating the inflammatory responses by the inhibition of nuclear factor-κB. Injection of Yops into neutrophils results in a decrease in the expression of endothelial cell adhesion proteins, thereby reducing effective inflammatory responses. The genes encoding Yops reside on the pCD1 or pYV plasmid. The genes residing on this plasmid encode Yops, LcrV, and the type III secretion system. They are downregulated at 26 °C, and upregulated at 37 °C and low calcium ion concentrations.

   The six Yops that are injected into the target cell, namely, YopB, YopD, YopE, YopH, YopM, and YopT, are not secreted unless contact with the cell is made.

YopB and YopD are translocated early; they form the portion of the pore that transits the membrane of the eukaryotic cell. However, the low Ca^{2+} response keeps the channel closed in the absence of contact. The cytoplasm of the eukaryotic cell is low in free Ca^{2+} due to its content of calcium-binding proteins, for example, calmodulin. Exposure of the tip of the secretion apparatus to the low calcium environment of the eukaryotic cytoplasm is thought to be the signal that causes the pore to open. If Ca^{2+} concentrations are high, the protein gate remains closed and no effector proteins are translocated. YopB and YopD form the part of the pore that transits the eukaryotic cell membrane. YopH blocks phagocytosis and inhibits the oxidative burst. It also elicits tyrosine phosphatase activity, which blocks signal transduction pathways in the phagocyte. YopE depolymerizes actin filaments in phagocytes, providing an antiphagocytic effect. YopM prevents thrombin-platelet aggregation, and this reduces inflammatory response and clot formation. YopT disrupts actin filaments by inactivation of Rho GTPases.

2. *LcrV*: LcrV (for low calcium response virulence, also known as factor V) is a protein located on the surface of *Y. pestis*. LcrV has several roles: it aids in the injection of effector proteins (e.g., Yops) into target cells; after injection into phagocytic cells, it reduces the excretion of proinflammatory cytokines and inhibits neutrophil chemotaxis. The genes encoding LcrV reside on the plasmid pYV (also known as pCD1). As noted earlier, the genes residing on this plasmid encode Yops, LcrV, and the type III secretion system, and they are downregulated at 26 °C, and upregulated at 37 °C and low calcium ion concentrations.
3. *Ymt*: The genes encoding Ymt (for *Yersinia* murine toxin) reside on the plasmid pMT (which also contains the genes for the F1 capsule, see Section Capsule (Fra1, Caf1 or F1)). Ymt is a phospholipase D, and previous studies have indicated that this protein is toxic to mice and rats, causing circulatory collapse of the animal. However, it is poorly expressed at 37 °C. More recent studies have shown that it is expressed at lower temperatures (e.g., 25 °C), more typical of the flea vector. Its main function is to enhance bacterial colonization within the midgut of the flea, by helping to protect it from digestive enzymes.
4. *Pesticin*: Pesticin is a bacteriocin produced by *Y. pestis* with an uncertain role in the production of disease. Genes on plasmid pPCP1 encode pesticin (along with Pla). Pesticin inhibits growth of *Y. pseudotuberculosis* serotype IA and IB, highly invasive serovar O:8 isolates of *Y. enterocolitica*, and certain clinical strains of *Escherichia coli*. Pesticin utilizes siderophore receptors to enter into sensitive bacteria, and their antibacterial activity can be inhibited by exogenous Fe^{3+} that downregulates these receptors. Yersiniae that produce pesticin are protected by a periplasmic immunity protein encoded on pPCP1.
5. *Pla and coagulase*: Pla is an outer membrane protein of *Y. pestis* that provides prothrombin activation (coagulase), plasminogen activation (fibrinolysis), and complement C3 proteolytic activity. Genes on plasmid pPCP1 encode Pla (along with pesticin and the periplasmic protein that confers immunity to pesticin). Pla is closely related to OmpT of *E. coli*, an outer membrane protein found in many enteric bacteria. Pla enhances the ability of *Y. pestis* to colonize the viscera and thus cause lethal infection. Adherence to host basement membranes and extracellular matrix is dependent upon Pla expression, where plasminogen activation facilitates bacterial metastasis. The fibrinolytic and coagulase activities of Pla are temperature dependent. The fibrinolytic and proteolytic activities are higher at 37 °C than at 28 °C, whereas the coagulase activity is higher at 28 °C than at 37 °C. When Pla protease is activated, it lyses the blood clot in the proventriculus of the flea. This liquefies the blood and lets the bacteria pass through the flea's midgut and hindgut (providing it with nourishment). Bacterial replication and production of coagulase (e.g., at 28 °C) results in blockage of the proventriculus; consequently, the flea regurgitates blood and bacteria out of its mouthparts, transmits the bacteria to the mammalian host, and starves.
6. *Gsr*: Gsr is expressed at 37 °C while *Y. pestis* is within the macrophage phagolysosome. The Gsr protein is responsible for the survival of *Y. pestis* within this environment.
7. *Ypk*: Ypk (for *Yersinia* protein kinase) is a serine/threonine kinase that interferes with signal transduction events in the phagocyte.
8. *PsaA*: PsaA (for pH 6 antigen) is a fibrillar protein that provides entry into macrophages and mediates delivery of certain Yop proteins (e.g., YopE) into the phagocyte. It is named for the observation that it is expressed at acidic pH (5–7). It is also expressed at low calcium concentrations and at 37 °C. Acidic conditions in the phagolysosome induce its expression. It is expressed when bacteria infect the spleen and liver.

Variability. *Y. pestis* is serologically uniform. There are four biotypes (also known as biovars) based on carbohydrate fermentation and ability to reduce nitrate: Antiqua, Medievalis, Orientalis, and Microtus. Genetic analyses suggest that the biotype Microtus is the closest ancestral relative of *Y. pseudotuberculosis*.

Ecology

Reservoir. Tolerant rodents in endemic areas (see Section "Epidemiology") constitute the plague reservoir. They rarely develop fatal disease and are called maintenance or enzootic hosts. In North America along the coastal regions of California, the meadow mouse *Microtus californicus* is such a host. In the urban cycle, the rat is the main intermediate host and the oriental rat flea is the main vector.

Transmission. Transmission is by fleas (Figure 9.9). They may carry *Y. pestis* to more susceptible, epizootic, or

FIGURE 9.9. *Xenopsylla cheopis, oriental rat flea, with a proventricular plague mass. During feeding, the flea draws viable Y. pestis organisms into its esophagus, which multiply and block the proventriculus just in front of the stomach, later forcing the flea to regurgitate infected blood unto the host when it tries to swallow. (Courtesy of US Health and Human Services, Centers for Disease Control and Prevention, Public Health Image Library, ID#2025.)*

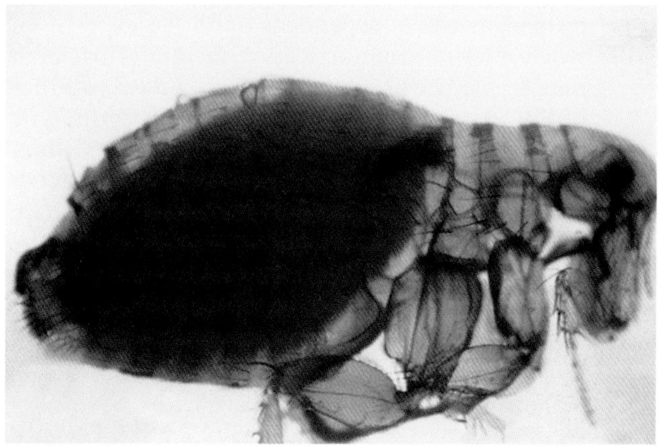

amplification hosts, such as ground squirrels or rats. In sylvatic (rural) environments, squirrels, prairie dogs, deer mice, gerbils, voles, rats, and rabbits—are all intermediate hosts. Some species are more resistant than others to full-blown disease and septicemia. However, like humans, prairie dogs, ground squirrels, and many other species develop bubonic or septicemic plague (Figure 9.8). When these die, still other hosts, such as humans, are attacked. Infected mammals may spread plague by the airborne route. Oral acquisition is by predation, cannibalism, and scavenging.

Pathogenesis

Fleas feed on an infected host. *Y. pestis* in the midgut of the fleas proliferate until they block (obstruct) the flea's proventriculus (function of Ymt and Hms), a process that takes about 2 weeks. Blocked fleas infest a new host and contaminate the feeding site with *Y. pestis* when attempting to feed. At flea temperature, the type III secretion system, Yops, LcrV, Caf1, and Gsr are not produced. The bacteria, thus introduced into a vertebrate host, lack defense against the host's innate immune system, and are killed when ingested by neutrophils (an inflammatory response is generated due to products of the flea bite along with the gram-negative cell wall components of *Y. pestis*). In mononuclear phagocytes, at mammalian temperatures, and low calcium ion concentrations, and while protected by Gsr, *Y. pestis* activates the type III secretion system; produces Yops, LcrV, and F1; and is released from the phagocytic cell following initiation of apoptosis. Yersiniae acquire resistance to further phagocytosis and intracellular killing by neutrophil and mononuclear phagocytes (LcrV reduces the excretion of proinflammatory cytokines and inhibits neutrophil chemotaxis; injected Yops prevent phagocytosis; Caf1 prevents phagocytosis and promotes serum resistance). Thus, early in the disease process, *Y. pestis* is an intracellular parasite, and later, an extracellular one.

Extracellular multiplication made possible by iron acquisition systems and capsule production elicits a hemorrhagic inflammatory lesion, followed by local lymph node involvement (bubo). This form is called bubonic plague.

The infection commonly becomes septicemic and, if untreated, terminates fatally (an endotoxemia aided by the function of Pla, which accelerates initiation of disseminated intravascular coagulation). Some individuals develop plague pneumonia and shed *Y. pestis* in sputum and droplet nuclei. Others contract primary pneumonic plague from this source and transmit it by the same route. Under epidemic conditions this form is nearly always fatal.

Among domestic animals, cats acquire natural clinical infection, often by ingestion of infected prey. Signs include regional (particularly mandibular) lymphadenitis, fever, depression, anorexia, sneezing, coughing, and occasionally central nervous system disturbances. Most cases end fatally. Lesions, mainly in the respiratory and alimentary tracts, include lymphadenitis, tonsillitis, cranial and cervical edema, and pneumonia. Cattle, horses, sheep, and pigs are apparently not susceptible to clinical plague. However, goats and camels are susceptible.

Human plague can be acquired directly from infected cats, ingestion of meat from infected animals (e.g., goats or camels), and necropsy of infected animals (e.g., rodents and mountain lions). In the case of domestic cats, suspected inoculation routes are via cuts, bites, scratches, and airborne and flea-borne pathways, although the latter is unlikely since the cat flea (*Ctenocephalides felis*) does not become blocked.

Epidemiology. Plague is concentrated in certain endemic areas in southern and southeastern Asia, southern and west central Africa, western North America, and north central South America. Endemicity largely parallels presence of enzootic and epizootic rodent hosts. Human plague epidemics have historically been precipitated by importation of infected rats on board ships coming from endemic regions. Today, most human cases result from infection following contact with rural wild animals (sylvatic plague).

Plague is a disease of rodents. The organism is maintained in endemic hosts (certain species of *Microtus* and *Peromyscus*, i.e., voles and meadow mice). Endemic hosts are infected following the bite of infected fleas. Although endemic hosts are fairly resistant to development of serious disease, when their populations rapidly increase and spread of *Y. pestis* is rapid, dying-off of endemic hosts occurs. Infected fleas, having a shortage of preferred hosts, feed on epidemic, highly susceptible species such as prairie dogs, rats, mice, and ground squirrels. What constitutes an endemic host and an epidemic host is somewhat clouded since there is considerable overlap between the two.

In endemic areas, infections are clustered during the warm months. "Off-season" plague mostly affects persons handling infected rabbits, bobcats, and occasionally house cats. Carnivores such as canids (wild and domestic), bears, raccoons, and skunks, as well as raptors, seroconvert following infection (ingestion and flea bite), but rarely develop clinical disease. Cat fleas and dog fleas, *C. felis*, and *C. canis* do not transmit *Y. pestis* efficiently because neither flea becomes blocked. Thus, infection of humans from an infected cat (rarely dogs) occurs from infections of scratches or bites with infected saliva or from inhalation of infected droplets.

Immunologic Aspects

Specific resistance to plague probably requires antibody and cell-mediated responses. Capsular antigens (F1 antigen) evoke opsonin formation. Antibody to the LcrV antigen is protective. Disposal of intracellular organisms depends on activated macrophages. Immunity following recovery is good, but temporary.

Detection of antibodies to *Y. pestis* in resistant species (e.g., canids) is a way of determining the presence of the organism in a particular environment.

Laboratory Diagnosis

Diagnostic attempts should be supervised by qualified public health personnel (see Section "Treatment and Control"). Samples from affected sites (i.e., edematous tissues, lymph nodes, and nasopharynx), transtracheal aspirates, cerebrospinal fluid, and blood (for culture and serology) are collected.

Direct smears are examined following immunofluorescent, Wayson's staining, or gram staining. Culture is done on blood or infusion agar. Identification is confirmed by immunofluorescence or bacteriophage susceptibility. Mice or guinea pigs injected subcutaneously with *Y. pestis* die within 3–8 days. DNA techniques utilizing molecular probes or the amplification of specific DNA sequences by the polymerase chain reaction are available.

Serologic tests (hemagglutination, hemagglutination-inhibition, and enzyme-linked immunosorbent assay) are useful for retrospective studies.

Treatment and Control

If plague is suspected in domestic cats, the following recommendations from the Centers for Disease Control apply:

1. Arrange immediately with local and state public health officials for laboratory diagnostic assistance and steps to prevent spread and contamination.
2. Place all suspect cats in strict isolation.
3. When handling such cats, wear gown, mask, and gloves.
4. Treat every suspect for fleas (5% carbaryl dust for residual effect).

Flea elimination should precede rodent control.

Aminoglycosides, chloramphenicol, fluoroquinolones, and tetracycline are effective antimicrobics. No vaccines for animals are available. Protection of humans by bacterins is transient.

Y. pseudotuberculosis

Y. pseudotuberculosis is associated with mesenteric lymphadenitis, terminal ileitis, acute gastroenteritis, and septicemia, affecting mainly birds and rodents, and only occasionally domestic animals and primates. *Y. pseudotuberculosis* is closely related to *Y. pestis*, and many consider *Y. pestis* to be a subspecies.

Descriptive Features

Cellular Composition and Products of Medical Importance. *Y. pseudotuberculosis* contains the plasmid pYV (encodes the type III secretion system, Yops, and LcrV). A chromosomal locus called the HPI contains the genes for iron uptake. Also located on the chromosome are the genes encoding the proteins Ail, Inv, YadA, and Gsr.

Adhesins. *Y. pseudotuberculosis* produces three adhesins that are responsible for adherence to β-integrins on the luminal surface of M cells and the basolateral surface of ileal epithelial cells—Ail, Inv, and Yad:

1. Ail (for attachment invasion locus) adheres to receptors on the surface of M cells. Ail also protects the outer membrane from insertion of the membrane attack complexes generated by activation of the complement system.
2. Inv (for invasin) adheres to receptors on the surface of M cells and the basolateral surface of ileal epithelial cells.
3. Yad (for *Yersinia* adhesin) adheres to receptors on the surface of M cells and the basolateral surface of ileal epithelial cells. Yad also protects the outer membrane from insertion of the membrane attack complexes generated by activation of the complement system.

Cell Wall. The cell wall of *Y. pseudotuberculosis* has O-antigens (smooth phenotype). The cell wall of the members of this genus is one typical of gram-negatives. The LPS in the outer membrane is an important virulence determinant. Not only is the lipid A component toxic (endotoxin), but the length of the side chain in the O-repeat unit hinders the attachment of the membrane attack complex of the complement system to the outer membrane. LPS binds to LPS-binding protein (a plasma protein), which in turn transfers it to the blood phase of CD14. The CD14–LPS complex binds to TLR proteins (see Chapter 6) on the surface of macrophage cells, triggering the release of proinflammatory cytokines.

High-Pathogenicity Island. See Section "Cellular Composition and Products of Medical Importance," under "*Y. pestis* (Plague Bacillus)."

Iron Acquisition. Iron is an absolute growth requirement and must be removed from iron-binding proteins of the host. The genes encoding products involved with iron acquisition reside on a chromosomal pathogenicity island.

The HPI of *Y. pseudotuberculosis* encodes the genes for the iron-acquiring siderophore yersiniabactin.

Type III Secretion System. See Section "Cellular Composition and Products of Medical Importance," under "*Y. pestis* (Plague Bacillus)."

Gsr. See Section "Cellular Composition and Products of Medical Importance," under "*Y. pestis* (Plague Bacillus)."

Toxins. *Y. pseudotuberculosis* produces toxins that are involved with pathogenicity:

1. *Yops*: See Section "Cellular Composition and Products of Medical Importance," under "*Y. pestis* (Plague Bacillus)."
2. *LcrV*: See Section "Cellular Composition and Products of Medical Importance," under "*Y. pestis* (Plague Bacillus)."

Variability

There are 21 serotypes based on variability of the somatic (O) antigens.

Ecology

Reservoir. *Y. pseudotuberculosis* is a parasite of wild rodents, lagomorphs, and birds, but it infects other mammals and reptiles and persists in the environment. The cat is the most commonly infected domestic mammal. Minor epidemics occur among sheep, pigs, nonhuman primates, fowl, and pet birds.

Transmission. Transmission is fecal–oral, with exposure primarily through ingestion of contaminated food and water.

Pathogenesis

Y. pseudotuberculosis attaches to M cells of lymphoid nodules of the distal small intestine following expression of the cell surface proteins Inv, Ail, and YadA. Attachment triggers actin cytoskeletal changes resulting in a "zippering" phenomenon that leads to the enclosure of the cell membrane around the attached yersiniae, resulting in their internalization. Internalized microorganisms pass through to the lymphoid nodule where they are phagocytosed by macrophages within the nodule. Expression of Gsr permits intracellular survival. Within macrophages (37 °C, low calcium), the type III secretion apparatus is activated, and Yops and LcrV are produced. Ingested yersinae are released after initiation of apoptosis of the macrophage. Now extracellular, yersiniae interfere with further phagocytosis. Invasion of the basolateral surface of ileal epithelial cells occurs following attachment of YadA and Inv, and internalization follows. Inflammation induced by extracellular yersiniae (lps), together with interferon secretion by natural killer cells and $\gamma\delta$ T cell recognition of infected epithelial cells (as well as LPS), results in an influx of polymorphonuclear neutrophil (PMN) leukocytes. Extracellular yersiniae avoid phagocytosis (Yops), and destruction by complement-mediated mechanisms by expression of Ail and YadA, both of which impart complement resistance. *Y. pseudotuberculosis* acquires iron from iron-binding proteins of the host following secretion of yersiniabactin (encoded within the HPI). Diarrhea is thought to result from prostaglandin synthesis by the recruited PMNs (and perhaps by the affected host cells), as well as activation of various inositol-signaling pathways within affected host cells. The net result is the secretion of chloride ions and water. Septicemia results from the host's inability to "clear" yersiniae from infected sites (serum resistance, antiphagocytic traits, and iron scavenging). The result is enteritis and septicemia.

Y. pseudotuberculosis causes intestinal infections with formation of necrotic foci in the intestinal wall, abdominal lymph nodes, and viscera, particularly liver (Figure 9.10) and spleen. There may be vomiting, diarrhea, or constipation, and weight loss, pale to subicteric mucous membranes, and depression. Fever is inconsistent. Few cases are diagnosed clinically antemortem. Mastitis is seen in cattle and abortion in ruminants and monkeys. In immunocompetent humans, the disease is generally an enteritis and abdominal lymphadenitis that is self-limiting or responsive to treatment.

Epidemiology. Pseudotuberculosis occurs worldwide. Cases tend to cluster in the cold months. In cats, prevalence is biased toward adult, rural, outdoor cats.

Immunologic Aspects

Natural infection leaves surviving individuals immune. Avirulent live vaccine protects against homologous challenge. It is not available commercially.

Laboratory Diagnosis

Diagnosis involves isolation of the agent antemortem from feces or lymph node aspirates. Isolation, particularly from mixed sources, is enhanced by cold enrichment, that is, incubation of a 10% mixture of inoculum in a minimal medium for several weeks at 4 °C. DNA techniques utilizing molecular probes or the amplification of specific DNA sequences by the polymerase chain reaction are available.

Treatment and Control

Pseudotuberculosis responds to the same antimicrobics as plague.

Y. enterocolitica

Y. enterocolitica is associated with mesenteric lymphadenitis, terminal ileitis, acute gastroenteritis, and septicemia in domestic animals and primates.

Descriptive Features

Cellular Composition and Products of Medical Importance. *Y. enterocolitica* contains the plasmid pYV (encodes

FIGURE 9.10. *Histopathologic tissue sections from the liver of a captive Perodicticus potto (a "prosimian" primate belonging to the Lorisidae family) that died from yersiniosis. The animal was found dead, and at necropsy had multiple 1–2 mm white foci in all liver lobes. Histopathologic sections of liver, as shown in this figure, revealed severe multifocal coalescing massive necrosis associated with bacterial colonies. Y. pseudotuberculosis was isolated. Sections of lung were affected with diffuse pulmonary hyperemia and edema with intravascular bacterial colonies consistent with those seen in the liver. (A) Hematoxylin and eosin stain, and (B) Brown-and-Brenn gram stain.*

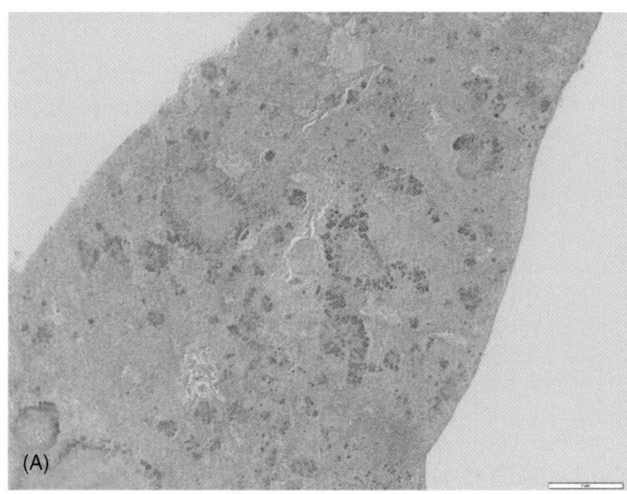

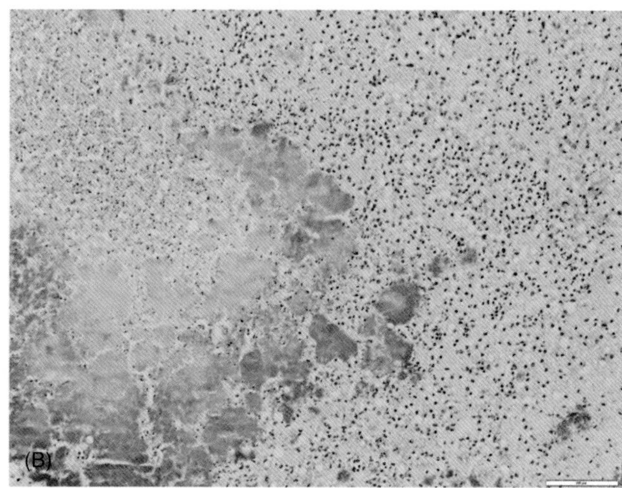

the type III secretion system, Yops, and LcrV). A chromosomal locus called the HPI contains the genes for iron uptake. Also located on the chromosome are the genes encoding the proteins Ail, Inv, YadA, Gsr, and Yst.

Adhesins. See Section "Cellular Composition and Products of Medical Importance," under "*Y. pseudotuberculosis*."

Cell Wall. See Section "Cellular Composition and Products of Medical Importance," under "*Y. pseudotuberculosis*."

Gsr. See Section "Cellular Composition and Products of Medical Importance," under "*Y. pestis* (Plague Bacillus)."

High-Pathogenicity Island. See Section "Cellular Composition and Products of Medical Importance," under "*Y. pestis* (Plague Bacillus)."

Iron Acquisition. See Section "Cellular Composition and Products of Medical Importance," under "*Y. pseudotuberculosis*."

Type III Secretion System. See Section "Cellular Composition and Products of Medical Importance," under "*Y. pestis* (Plague Bacillus)."

Toxins. *Y. enterocolitica* produces a number of toxins that are involved with pathogenicity:

1. *Yops*: See Section "Cellular Composition and Products of Medical Importance," under "*Y. pestis* (Plague Bacillus)."
2. *LcrV*: See Section "Cellular Composition and Products of Medical Importance," under "*Y. pestis* (Plague Bacillus)."
3. *Yst*: Yst (for *Yersinia* stable toxin) is a chromosomally encoded enterotoxin unique to *Y. enterocolitica*. Yst affects the guanylyl cyclase system by deregulating cGMP synthesis (increase in intracellular cGMP leads to the opening of chloride channels with the resultant flow of chloride and water into the intestinal lumen), resulting in fluid and electrolyte accumulation in the bowel lumen subsequent to blockage of sodium and chloride ion (and thus water) absorption (tip cells) and loss of chloride ions (crypt cells) (see also, STa enterotoxin of *E. coli*, Chapter 7).

Variability

Y. enterocolitica includes two subspecies, *enterocolitica* and *palearctica*. The *enterocolitica* subspecies was proposed for strains with the 16S rRNA type of American origin, whereas *palearctica* was proposed for strains of European origin. *Y. enterocolitica* strains are differentiated by bio- and serotyping. Serotyping is based on reactivity to O-antigen polysaccharides. There are more than 70 serotypes, although only a small number are pathogenic. O groups 3, 5, 8, 9, and 27 are associated with classical disease of the gastrointestinal tract in human patients. There are six biogroups (biotypes), namely, BT1A, BT1B, BT2, BT3, BT4, and BT5. BT1A strains are mostly nonpathogenic; the rest (BT1B through BT5) are pathogenic. BT1B predominates in the United States. BT1A and BT2 through BT5 are found in Europe. The biogroups (or biotypes) are differentiated on the basis of reactivity to esculin, indole, D-xylose, trehalose, pyrazinamidase, β-D-glucosidase, and lipase. Strains are also referred to by a combination of the serotype and biotype; for example, a strain that is serotype O:3 and BT4 is referred to as serobiotype O:3/4.

Ecology

Reservoir and Transmission. *Y. enterocolitica* has been isolated from a wide range of sources, for example, soil, water, food (fruits, vegetables, milk, retail meat products, cheese, and eggs), and animals. The number of species of animals from which it has been isolated is also numerous and includes pets (cats and dogs), stock (chinchilla, mink, pig, rabbit, cow, goose, horse, sheep, and buffalo), zoo animals (monkeys), wild animals (raccoon, fox, snail, frog, beaver, deer, ocelot, crab, flies, fleas, birds, oysters, and many species of small rodents). Pathogenic BT2 through BT5 are mainly isolated from animals (sheep, cattle, goat, and poultry) or food. Serobiotype O:3/4 strains are frequently isolated from pigs; O:9/2 strains are often isolated from cows and goats; and O:2,3/5 strains are isolated from sheep, rabbits, and goats. Expression of certain virulence determinants at 22–25 °C suggests that mammals acquire *Y. enterocolitica* from a "cold" source (e.g., water and food) rather than a warm-blooded animal. Infection follows ingestion of organisms expressing the adhesin. One of the major sources of human infection with serobiotype O:3/4 is through the handling of swine and consumption of pork. Pigs are known to carry the organism in their oropharynx, nasopharynx, and their intestine. Human-to-human transmission may also occur, although it is rarely documented.

Transmission. Transmission is by the fecal–oral route. Infection is mainly acquired through ingestion of food and water that has been contaminated with animal feces or by direct contact with animal feces (e.g., abattoir worker). Children younger than 5 years are much more prone to *Y. enterocolitica* infections.

Pathogenesis

The pathogenesis of disease produced by *Y. enterocolitica* is the same as *Y. pseudotuberculosis* (see Section, "Pathogenesis", under "*Y. pseudotuberculosis*"). In addition to diarrhea associated with invasion of epithelial cells and inflammation (as with *Y. pseudotuberculosis*), *Y. enterocolitica* produces Yst.

Epidemiology. As noted earlier, certain subspecies, serotypes, and biotypes are geographically restricted. Subspecies *enterocolitica* is found in the United States and subspecies *palearctica* is found in Europe. BT1B predominates in the United States. BT1A and BT2 through BT5 are found in Europe. Serotype O:8 is indigenous to the United States but not the rest of the world. Until recently, serotype O:3 was rarely isolated in the United States but is common in the rest of the world, and is becoming more so in the United States. Serotype O:9 has not been reported outside of Europe.

Immunologic Aspects

Y. enterocolitica is an extracellular microorganism. Phagocytic cells readily destroy it, even though the microorganism excretes proteins (Yops) that interfere with this process. Most often, *Y. enterocolitica* disease is self-limiting due to the innate immune response: phagocytosis, lysis of infected epithelial cells, iron sequestration, and complement proteins.

A serologic relationship between O:9 serotype, common in swine, and *Brucella* spp. has complicated swine brucellosis eradication programs.

Laboratory Diagnosis

Samples of feces, lymph node biopsy, and biopsy from affected tissues are examined microbiologically. Selective media containing bile salts are somewhat inhibitory to *Y. enterocolitica*, especially at 37 °C. MacConkey agar is least inhibitory. There are special media designed for the isolation of *Y. enterocolitica* (e.g., cefsulodin–Irgasan–novobiocin medium; see Chapter 6). Cold enrichment of the sample at 4 °C aids in attempts to isolate small numbers of *Y. enterocolitica* from a contaminated environment. Isolation from tissue necessitates the use of blood agar plates incubated at 37 °C. DNA techniques utilizing molecular probes or the amplification of specific DNA sequences by the polymerase chain reaction are available.

Treatment and Control

Antimicrobial agents useful for treating disease produced by *Y. enterocolitica* are the fluoroquinolones, tetracycline, trimethoprim–sulfonamides, and chloramphenicol. R plasmids are common in *Y. enterocolitica*, and genes encoding resistance to tetracycline and streptomycin are most commonly found.

Y. ruckeri

"Enteric redmouth" is a hemorrhagic inflammation of the perioral subcutis of freshwater fish, particularly rainbow trout. Infection is systemic and causes significant mortality in hatcheries of North America, Australia, and Europe. The agent is disseminated by asymptomatic carrier fish and possibly riparian mammals (muskrats). Outbreaks appear to be related to massive exposure.

The pathogenesis of this disease has not been described. A protease, Yrp (*Y. ruckeri* protease) appears to play an important role since inactivation of the encoding gene significantly reduces virulence.

Outbreaks are brought under control with antimicrobics (e.g., sulfonamides, tetracycline, trimethoprim–sulfonamide), and bacterins have been successful in lowering mortality.

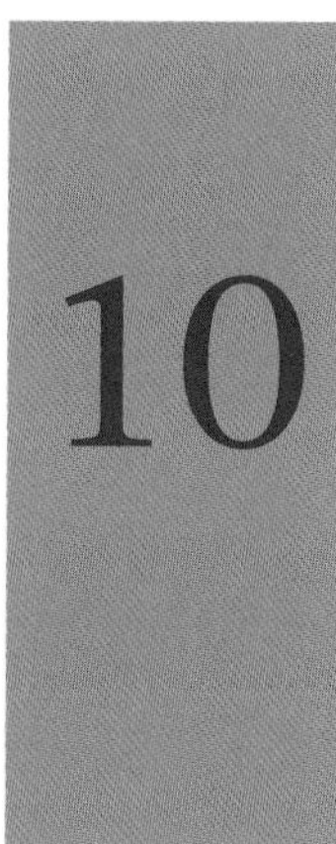

Enterobacteriaceae: *Shigella*

Rodney Moxley

Members of the genus *Shigella* belong to the family Enterobacteriaceae and cause bacillary dysentery (shigellosis) in human and nonhuman primates. The genus includes four species: (1) *Shigella dysenteriae*, (2) *Shigella flexneri*, (3) *Shigella boydii*, and (4) *Shigella sonnei* (Table 10.1). These species are also known as serogroups (or subgroups) A, B, C, and D, respectively. The type species for the genus is *S. dysenteriae*. The chromosomal DNAs of the four members of the *Shigella* genus are nearly identical to *Escherichia coli*, for example, the sequence divergence between *S. flexneri* and *E. coli* K-12 is 98.5%. The exception is *S. boydii* serotype 13, which has been reclassified as *Escherichia albertii*. Based on the extensive DNA sequence homology between *Shigella* and *E. coli*, some taxonomists have proposed that the four species of *Shigella* be reclassified as serological biotypes of *E. coli*. However, this reclassification has not occurred. The main reason is that the medical community prefers to continue to associate the distinctive clinical disease with the name shigellosis. Enteroinvasive *E. coli* (EIEC) share biochemical characteristics, essential virulence factors, and clinical features with *Shigella* spp. The EIEC organism is even more closely related to *Shigella* spp. than to commensal *E. coli* strains. Comparative genomics studies indicate that *Shigella* spp. and EIEC evolved from multiple *E. coli* strains by convergent evolution.

In nonhuman primates, shigellosis occurs almost exclusively in captive animals and appears to be related to stressful situations (e.g., transportation, crowding) or immunological dysfunctions (e.g., simian acquired immunodeficiency syndrome). Cases in nonhuman primates are due to infection with *S. flexneri*, *S. boydii*, or *S. sonnei*, whereas cases in humans may be due to any of these or *S. dysenteriae*. In both humans and nonhuman primates, lesions of shigellosis are limited to the colon, and may be focal or diffuse (Figure 10.1).

Descriptive Features

Cellular Structure and Composition

The structure of each of the *Shigella* spp. is typical for the family Enterobacteriaceae. Though closely related genetically, *Shigella* spp. lack many of the traits characteristic of *E. coli*. They express neither capsules (K antigens) nor flagella (H antigens). The latter trait is the result of mutations in or complete loss of the master operon of flagellar synthesis, *flhDC*. While *E. coli* are usually prototrophic, *Shigella* spp. are auxotrophic. *Shigella* isolates do not grow on synthetic media with Simmon's citrate, and are negative for the deaminases for phenylalanine and tryptophan. They are also negative for arginine and lysine decarboxylase, growth in KCN medium, liquefaction of gelatin, oxidation of gluconate, production of H_2S (on triple-sugar-iron agar), urease, and utilization of Christensen's citrate or malonate. Like *E. coli*, shigellae yield both a positive methyl red and a negative Voges-Proskauer reaction. As do all Enterobacteriaceae, they ferment glucose, but, with the exception of *S. flexneri* type 6, *S. boydii* types 13 and 14, and *S. dysenteriae* type 3, they do not produce gas. *S. dysenteriae*, *S. flexneri*, and *S. boydii* do not ferment lactose, but after several days of culture, *S. sonnei* and *S. boydii* serotype 9 do yield lactose-positive results. Similarly, *S. sonnei* slowly ferments saccharose. *Shigella* spp. do not ferment adonitol, inositol, or salicin.

Shigella spp. have a typical gram-negative (GN) cell wall that includes lipopolysaccharide and, like other Enterobacteriaceae, express an O-antigen that is useful for serogrouping and serotyping. Serogroup determination is required for the identification of the species of *Shigella*. Slide agglutination assays with commercially available specific antisera are used to determine the serogroup (subgroup) and serotype. *S. dysenteriae* has 15 serotypes; *S. flexneri* has 6 serotypes and 2 variants, with serotypes 1–5 subdivided into 11 subserotypes; *S. boydii* has 19 serotypes, and *S. sonnei* has only 1 serotype (Table 10.1). *S. boydii* serotypes are numbered from 1 to 20, but serotype 13 was removed as it has been reclassified as *E. albertii*. *S. sonnei* undergoes phase variation from a smooth, virulent phase I to a rough, avirulent phase II, which has lost the capacity to synthesize its O-side chains. Conversion of one serotype to another within a species is under the regulation of the genes contained within the Shi-O pathogenicity island (PAI), as described below.

Veterinary Microbiology, Third Edition. Edited by D. Scott McVey, Melissa Kennedy and M.M. Chengappa.

Table 10.1. *Shigella* Serogroups, Species, and Serotypes

Serogroup	Species	Number of Serotypes
A	*dysenteriae*	15
B	*flexneri*	6
C	*boydii*	19
D	*sonnei*	1

Cellular Products of Medical Interest

Cell Wall. The cell wall of the members of this genus is one typical of GNs, and also participates in the pathogenesis by typical means, that is, through the effects of lipid A (endotoxin) and resistance to complement-mediated lysis (both described in detail for Enterobacteriaceae in Chapter 6).

Type III Secretion System (T3SS) and Invasion Proteins. A requisite step in the pathogenesis of shigellosis is invasion of the large intestinal epithelium, which occurs through M cells (Figure 10.2). The initial contact between the bacterium and the host cell is at lipid raft domains and is mediated by the receptors CD44 and $\alpha_5\beta_1$ integrin. This binding induces early actin cytoskeletal rearrangements, but efficient and complete bacterial uptake requires T3SS effector proteins that are encoded on a large virulence (220-kb) plasmid. The virulence plasmid contains a mosaic of approximately 100 genes.

Invasion Plasmid Antigen (Ipa) and Ipg Proteins. Ipa effector proteins, viz., IpaA, IpaB, IpaC, and IpaD are encoded by one group of genes that are carried on the large virulence plasmid. The Ipa proteins are secreted by the T3SS and mediate invasion of M cells and escape from the phagosome (Figure 10.3). IpaB and IpaC mediate the formation of a translocon (pore) in the host cell plasma membrane, the insertion of which is guided by IpaD. IpaA is injected through the translocon into the host cell, and targets β1 integrins, vinculin, and the GTPase, Rho. This induces entry of the bacteria into the host cell into a phagosome by triggering actin cytoskeletal rearrangement and formation of membrane ruffles (pseudopodia) that engulf the bacteria. IpaC targets actin and β-catenin, causing effects on actin polymerization that assist in membrane ruffle formation. In addition, IpaC is thought to disrupt the integrity of the phospholipid bilayer, causing rupture of the phagosome and escape of the bacteria into the cytoplasm. IpgB1 is secreted by the T3SS and plays a significant role in bacterial invasion by mimicking the GTPase RhoG, and thereby activating Rac1 through the ELMO-Dock180 pathway. IpgB1 also activates Cdc42, but to a lesser extent. Activation of Rac1 and Cdc42 induce membrane ruffling through their effects on actin cytoskeletal rearrangement. The gene encoding IpgB1 (*ipgB1*) is located upstream of the *ipaBCDA* operon on the large virulence plasmid.

IpaBa and IpaC also cause release from the phagosome in macrophages. Release of IpaB into the cytoplasm of the macrophage results in it being integrated into organellar membranes in a cholesterol-dependent manner. This causes the proteolytic activation of procaspase-1 to caspase-1, and resultant causation of apoptosis of the macrophage. This process also results in the cleavage and activation of proinflammatory cytokines IL-1β and IL-18, which results in release of these cytokines and elicitation of the marked inflammatory response that characterizes shigellosis.

FIGURE 10.1. *Diffuse hemorrhagic inflammation of the colon in a Rhesus monkey affected with shigellosis. (US Department of Health and Human Services, Centers for Disease Control and Prevention, Public Health Information Library, PHIL_5166.)*

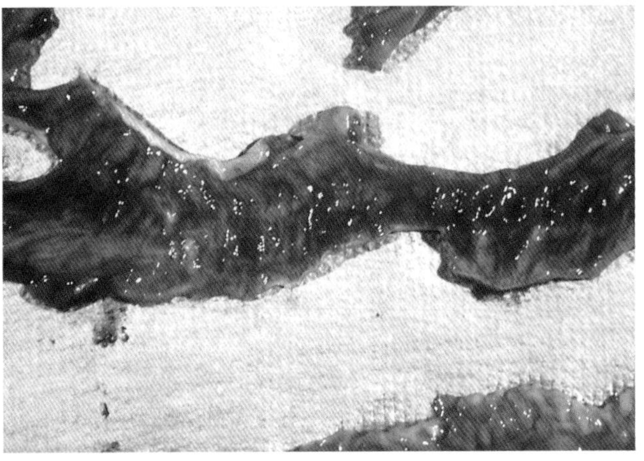

Mxi-Spa T3SS. A second group of genes on the large virulence plasmid encode for the more than 25 proteins needed for the molecular structure, assembly, and function of the T3SS apparatus (Figure 10.3). These include the membrane expression of *ipa* (*mxi*) and surface presentation of *ipa* antigen (*spa*) genes. The Mxi-Spa T3SS consists of four main parts: (1) a basal body that spans the bacterial envelope; (2) a hollow needle structure that is anchored in the basal body and protrudes extracellularly; (3) a translocon at the needle tip; and (4) a cytoplasmic ring that energizes and mediates the transport of proteins from the bacterial cytoplasm into the needle structure.

A third group of genes on the large virulence plasmid encodes for two transcriptional activators, VirB and MxiE, which regulate T3SS-associated genes. A fourth group of genes encodes chaperones (*ipgA*, *ipgC*, *ipgE*, and *spa15*) needed to unfold and insert proteins into the needle complex. Approximately 25 proteins are secreted by the T3SS.

Intercellular Spread (Ics) Proteins. Another group of genes on the large virulence plasmid encodes the Ics proteins. Once in the host cell, the bacterium uses the Ics proteins to move within the cytoplasm and spread to adjacent epithelial cells (ECs). The IcsA (VirG) protein moves to one pole of the bacterium and targets N-WASP (neural Wiskott–Aldrich syndrome protein). Binding of N-WASP allows for nucleation of actin at that site. Once actin polymerization at one pole of the bacterium has begun and progresses, it propels the organism through the host cell cytoplasm (Figure 10.4). Positioning of IcsA to one pole of the organism is mediated by PhoN2, an apyrase (adenosine diphosphatase). IcsB

FIGURE 10.2. *Cellular pathogenesis of* Shigella spp. *Shigella flexneri passes the epithelial cell (EC) barrier by transcytosis through M cells and encounters resident macrophages. The bacteria evade degradation in macrophages by inducing an apoptosis-like cell death, which is accompanied by proinflammatory signaling. Free bacteria invade the EC from the basolateral side, move into the cytoplasm by vectorial actin polymerization, and spread to adjacent cells. Proinflammatory signaling by macrophages and EC further activates the innate immune response involving NK cells and attracts polymorphonuclear (PMN) cells. The influx of PMNs disintegrates the EC lining, which initially exacerbates the infection and tissue destruction by facilitating the invasion of more bacteria. Ultimately, PMN phagocytose and kill* Shigella, *thus contributing to the resolution of the infection. (Reproduced by permission of Schroeder and Hilbi 2008.)*

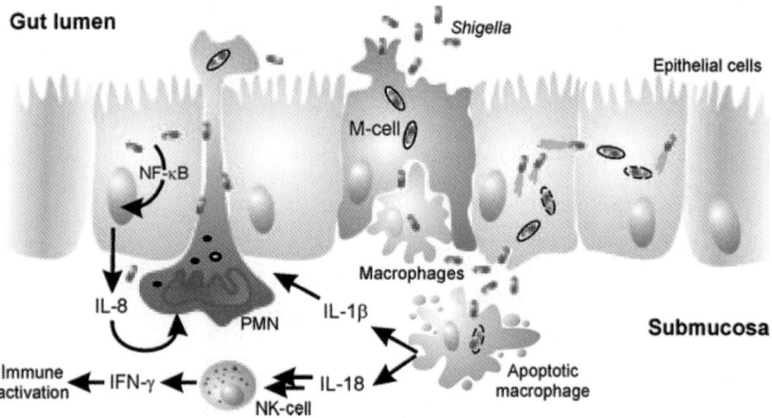

camouflages IcsA to prevent it from autophagic recognition and destruction. IcsA does not utilize the T3SS; it enters the host cell by its properties as an autotransporter protein. IcsP (SopA) is a serine protease that cleaves IcsA and modulates the actin-based motility.

Virulence A (VirA) Protein. VirA, also encoded by a gene on the large virulence plasmid, is secreted by the T3SS. VirA is a cysteine protease that targets α-tubulin and assists in the mediation of intracellular motility by causing disassembly of microtubules (Figure 10.4).

***Shigella* Enterotoxin 2 (ShET-2).** ShET-2 is encoded by genes (*sen*, for Shigella enterotoxin) on the large virulence plasmid. ShET-2 is produced by *S. dysenteriae*, *S. sonnei*, and *S. flexneri*. In contrast, ShET-1, is encoded by *set1A* and *set1B* genes on the chromosome (described below), and produced only by *S. flexneri*. ShET-1 and ShET-2 are thought to cause the watery diarrhea that precedes dysentery. Watery diarrhea occurs in all patients, but dysentery does not; hence, the enterotoxins should be considered as important virulence factors.

Proteins Encoded by Genes on Pathogenicity Islands (PAIs). *Shigella* spp. isolates may contain as many as five PAIs on their chromosomes, four of which are referred to as *Shigella* pathogenicity islands (SHI), and one of which is called SRL (for *Shigella* resistance locus). SHI-1 contains *sigA*, *pic*, and *set* genes, which encode, respectively, an immunoglobulin A-like cytopathic protease (SigA), a serine protease/mucinase (Pic), and *Shigella* enterotoxin 1 (ShET-1). SigA is a cytopathic toxin, Pic causes mucus permeabilization, and ShET-1 induces intestinal fluid accumulation. SHI-2 and SHI-3 contain copies of the genes (*iucA* to *iucD*) for production of aerobactin, although SHI-3 is only found in *S. boydii*. SHI-O contains genes for modification of the O antigens and serotype conversion. SRL contains genes encoding for iron acquisition (*fecA* to *fecE*, *fecI*, and *fecR*), and resistance to antibiotics. SRL genes encode resistance to tetracycline (*tetA* to *tetD*, and *tetR*), chloramphenicol (*cat*), ampicillin (*oxa-1*), and streptomycin (*aadA1*).

Shiga Toxin (Stx). With rare exceptions, *S. dysenteriae* serotype 1 is the only member of the genus that contains the genes for Stx production. As in essentially all Shiga toxin-producing *E. coli* (STEC), except edema disease strains, the Stx genes in *S. dysenteriae* are carried on the chromosome. However, unlike STEC, *S. dysenteriae* serotype 1 does not carry intact Stx-converting phages. This is thought to be the result of loss of essential phage genes caused by transposition and recombination events. A human isolate of *S. sonnei* with an integrated bacteriophage carrying Stx genes has been detected. Experimentally, other *S. sonnei* strains could be lysogenized with the phage and thereby produce Stx. The *stx* DNA sequence in this phage was more closely related to stx_2 than stx_1. These findings suggest that Stx-positive *S. sonnei* and other Stx-positive species of *Shigella* may possibly emerge as important pathogens in the future.

The production of Stx is iron-regulated (by way of Fur (ferric uptake regulator), see Section "Regulatory Genes"), with more toxin being produced in conditions of low iron concentration. Although the other virulence factors described above are important in the pathogenesis, the virulence of a particular *S. dysenteriae* strain is also directly related to the amount of Stx produced. As described for STEC, Stx causes severe vascular lesions in the colonic mucosa, renal glomeruli, and other organs that result in hemorrhagic colitis and, in some cases, hemolytic uremic syndrome (HUS). The molecular, cellular, and pathophysiologic mechanisms of Stx toxicity and the corresponding clinical effects are described in detail in Chapter 7.

FIGURE 10.3. *Architecture of the* Shigella flexneri *Mxi-Spa type III secretion system (T3SS). The S. flexneri Mxi-Spa T3SS consists of four main parts. The seven-ringed basal body spans the bacterial inner membrane (IM), the periplasm, and the outer membrane (OM). The hollow needle is attached to a socket and protrudes from the basal body to the bacterial surface. Contact with host membranes (HM) triggers the IpaD-guided membrane insertion of the IpaB-IpaC translocon at the needle tip. The T3SS is completed by the cytoplasmic C ring, which is comprised of proteins that energize the transport process and mediate the recognition of substrates, chaperone release, and substrate unfolding. (Reproduced by permission of Schroeder and Hilbi 2008.)*

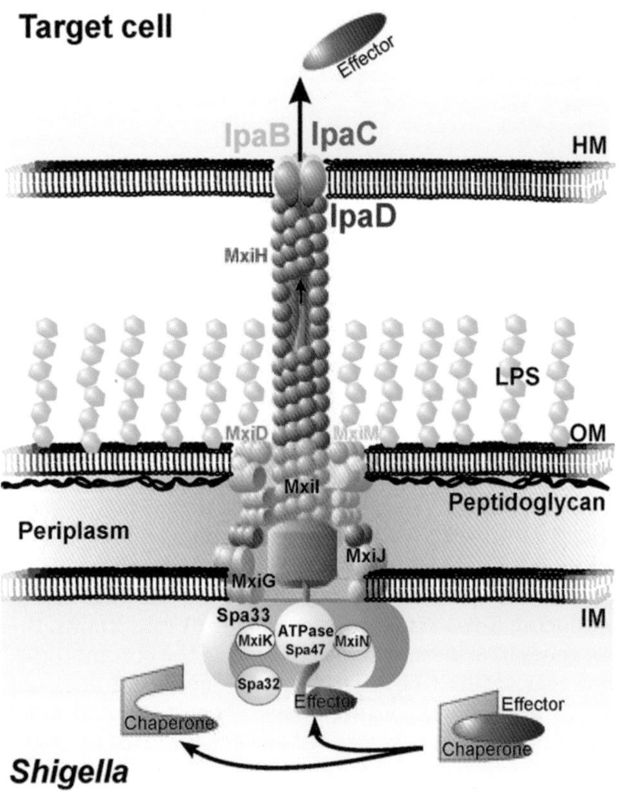

Regulatory Genes. Shigellae possess a number of genes whose activation results from specific environmental cues. The primary elements of the regulatory cascade that sense and respond to environmental changes are encoded on the chromosome. A change in pH, temperature (increase to 37 °C), or change in osmolarity would be sensed by chromosomally encoded sensor proteins (e.g., VirR), which would activate expression of *virF* on the virulence plasmid. VirF then activates transcription of *icsA* and *virB*, also located on the virulence plasmid. VirB activates T3SS assembly genes (*ipa*, *mxi*, *spa*), and "first-set" effectors. The "first-set" effectors lead to increased transcription of "second-set" T3SS effectors. In this manner, an environmental change indicating presence of the bacterium in the host would initiate a cascade of sequential gene activation steps culminating in bacterial invasion of the colonic epithelium. Some genes that are activated in this process serve as negative regulators, preventing wasted energy usage by the bacteria as they invade the host.

FIGURE 10.4. *Intracellular movement of* Shigella flexneri *by directed actin polymerization. Due to the activity of the serine protease SopA/IcsP,* S. flexneri *IcsA localizes to one pole of the bacterium, where it interacts with the host cell N-WASP (neural Wiskott–Aldrich syndrome protein). The IcsA/N-WASP complex recruits and activates the Arp2/3 complex, thereby mediating actin nucleation. Elongation of the actin tail pushes* S. flexneri *through the cytoplasm. The movement is facilitated by VirA, which opens a path by degradation of the microtubule network. To avoid sequestration by the autophagy defense system, an autophagy recognition site on IcsA is masked by the protein IcsB. (Reproduced by permission of Schroeder and Hilbi 2008.)*

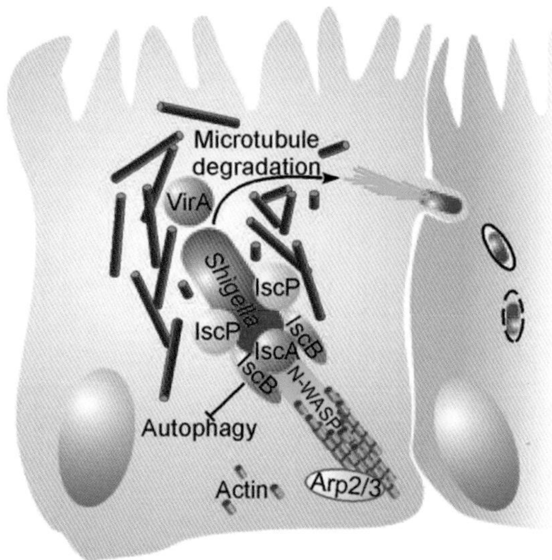

Fur and an RNA polymerase containing RpoS are additional regulatory genes. The Fur protein "senses" available iron concentration, and when low (as would be inside the host, since most iron is bound to host iron-binding proteins) it activates the synthesis and secretion of aerobactin, ShET-1, and Stx (see Sections "Proteins Encoded by Genes on pathogenicity islands (PAIs)" and "Shiga Toxin (Stx)"). RNA polymerase containing RpoS preferentially transcribes genes effecting acid tolerance (survival at pH 5), providing protection against the acidic pH of the gastric lumen.

Variability

Shigellae are serogrouped and serotyped solely on the basis of the O-antigen, since no H or K antigens are expressed. Serogroup determination is essential for the identification of the species of *Shigella*, and within three of the four species, there are a multiple serotypes (see Table 10.1).

Ecology

Reservoir

The distribution of *Shigella* is essentially limited to the intestinal tracts of humans and large, captive primates in which shigellosis naturally occurs, and sewage. Humans are the reservoir host; there is no evidence that the disease occurs naturally in nonhuman primates in the wild without prior contact with humans. Shigellae are consistently present in sewage, and accidental contamination of water supplies by sewage effluents often causes outbreaks of shigellosis in humans. In humans, *Shigella* is endemic throughout the world, although 99% of the cases occur in the developing world.

Transmission

The disease is transmitted by the fecal-oral route, but the infective dose is so small (only 10–100 cells) and the organisms survive long enough that fomites also play a role. *S. flexneri* serotype 4 is associated with periodontal disease of nonhuman primates; the mode of transmission is unknown, but it is assumed to be feces. Antimicrobial drugs, stress, or dietary changes promote risk by reducing colonization resistance (by decreasing the numbers of the competing normal flora), which may lead to disease in subclinically infected nonhuman primates or humans, or by lowering the oral dose needed for infection and subsequent disease. Studies have demonstrated that an important vehicle for transmission of shigellosis is the hand, which points out the importance of thorough hand washing in disease prevention. *S. dysenteriae* serotype 1 survives for up to 1 h in culturable form on human skin.

Clinical Disease

The classical disease begins as watery diarrhea, then after 3–4 days the feces becomes scant and contains blood and mucus. There is fever, abdominal pain, cramping, and straining. There may be malaise, myalgia, and anorexia.

The severity of the clinical course usually varies with the species. *S. sonnei* mainly causes a watery diarrhea, whereas *S. flexneri* and *S. dysenteriae* produce more severe signs (e.g., more pronounced blood in the stool with either *S. flexneri* or *S. dysenteriae* and systemic complications such as HUS or brain damage in the case of *S. dysenteriae*). In all forms of shigellosis, microscopic examination of the stool will reveal large numbers of leukocytes.

Shigellosis is characterized pathologically by a mucopurulent and hemorrhagic colitis. Microscopic abscesses may be seen in the colonic mucosa, involving the crypts or intercryptal regions. Crypt abscesses often slough, producing ulcers.

HUS may be seen in human patients infected with *S. dysenteriae* 1, mainly the result of the effects of Stx production. Reiter's syndrome, characterized by arthritis, sometimes appears after the intestinal infection has passed. This syndrome also may be seen with the other bacterial infections, viz., *Yersinia enterocolitica*, *Salmonella enterica* var. Typhimurium, *Klebsiella pneumoniae*, and *Campylobacter jejuni*.

Pathogenesis

Within 12 h after ingestion, the bacteria multiply in the small intestine to concentrations of 10^7–10^8 viable cells per ml of luminal contents. Abdominal pain, cramping, and fever occur while the bacteria are localized in the small intestine.

The bacteria pass to the colon and invade the colonic mucosa by a series of steps (Figure 10.2). The events at the molecular level are described above. Shigellae adhere to the surfaces of M cells, and are taken up into phagosomes. The bacteria escape from phagosomes, multiply in the cytoplasm, and move to adjacent enterocytes by causing the induction of actin cytoskeletal rearrangement at one pole of the organism. This propels the bacteria through the cytoplasm and allows contact to be made with adjacent ECs. Spread to adjacent absorptive ECs occurs by induction of endocytosis through the cell membranes of both cells. The bacteria continue to spread through the epithelial layer in this manner and the cycle continues to be repeated. Phagocytosis of bacteria by neutrophils and macrophages occurs, but the bacteria cause apoptotic cell death of macrophages, thereby reducing the effectiveness of the host defense and causing the release of IL-1β and IL-18, which exacerbate the inflammatory response. Neutrophils effect bacterial killing, but also cause tissue damage that enhances bacterial spread. Infiltration and death of neutrophils generates the lesion, purulent colitis. Bacteria are released by dead or dying ECs and macrophages, and drain via the lymphatics into gut-associated lymphoid tissue, where they are ultimately killed.

In addition to the effects of inflammation and necrosis of the colonic mucosa, diarrhea is brought about by the activation of phospholipase C leading to increase in intracellular calcium ions, activation of protein kinase C, and subsequent phosphorylation of proteins of the chloride ion channels and those of the membrane-associated ion transport proteins involved in NaCl absorption.

Based on mutagenesis and animal model studies, ShET-1 and ShET-2 are thought to play a significant role in the causation of watery diarrhea; however, the mechanism for these effects is poorly understood.

Stx produced by *S. dysenteriae* serotype 1 causes apoptosis of vascular endothelial cells and activation of leukocytes with upregulation and expression of tumor necrosis factor-α (TNF-α). TNF-α induces increased expression of the Gb3 receptor for Stx, which increases the extent of endothelial toxicity and vascular damage. The vasculature in the mucosa of the colon is affected by Stx toxicity, causing thrombosis and infarction of the colonic mucosa. These effects exacerbate those of colonic inflammation and cause hemorrhagic colitis. Stx may also affect the vasculature in extraintestinal locations, for example, the kidneys and brain, resulting in the development of the HUS. The effects of Stx are described in more detail in Chapter 7.

Epidemiology

As noted above, among animals, the disease is seen almost exclusively in large, captive primates. Humans are the reservoir host. In developed countries, shigellosis is a disease of the disadvantaged and those having close contact in group settings. In the United States, shigellosis is also mainly a disease of children 1–4 years old, and is caused by *S. sonnei*. Outbreaks are often seen in preschool children and toddlers in day care centers. Outbreaks are also seen in mental institutions. Large urban outbreaks have been seen following accidental contamination of a city water supply by sewage effluents. Worldwide in humans, *S. flexneri* and *S. sonnei* are typically responsible for endemic shigellosis, whereas *S. dysenteriae* 1 is responsible for the epidemic form of the disease.

Immunologic Aspects

Protection from bacillary dysentery is by specific secretory immunoglobulin in the intestinal lumen. These antibodies prevent adherence and subsequent uptake. Shigellae are serum-sensitive (i.e., they are susceptible to complement-mediated lysis), and they are susceptible to killing by neutrophils. As a result, shigellae do not typically cause septicemia.

Whether nonhuman primates are resistant to reinfection following recovery from shigellosis is not known. Reinfection or exacerbation does occur in humans in stressful situations such as in prisoner-of-war camps. Bacterins given orally or parenterally have been ineffective. Some protection has been demonstrated following vaccination with avirulent, live oral vaccines, but these are not universally available.

Laboratory Diagnosis

Fecal samples from the live animal, or in the case of necropsy, colonic samples, should be plated onto a selective medium that is less inhibitory than media for isolation of salmonellae. There is no reliable enrichment medium for all shigellae; however, GN broth is preferred for general use. Selenite broth and tetrathionate broth, both primarily intended for enrichment of *Salmonella*, are usually too inhibitory. For the optimal isolation of *Shigella*, both a medium of low selectivity, viz., MacConkey agar, and a more selective agar medium, such as xylose-lysine-deoxycholate (XLD) agar should be used. Hektoen enteric (HE) medium is a suitable alternative to XLD (Figure 10.5), whereas *Salmonella-Shigella* (SS) agar is often too inhibitory for some strains of shigellae, for example, *S. dysenteriae* 1. *Shigella* will not grow on more inhibitory media primarily intended for isolation of *Salmonella*, for example, brilliant green agar.

Shigellae appear as lactose-nonfermenting colonies on lactose-containing media, although some species (*S. sonnei* and *S. boydii* serotype 9) ferment this sugar after several days of incubation. Suspicious colonies are tested directly with shigellae-specific antisera or inoculated into differential media and then tested with antisera.

Primers have been designed to amplify (by the polymerase chain reaction) DNA targets specific for shigellae. This assay has been used to detect and identify members of this genus. However, there are no FDA-approved nucleic acid detection methods for the clinical diagnosis of *Shigella* infections.

FIGURE 10.5. *Shigella boydii, isolated colonies on Hektoen enteric (HE) agar. This photograph depicts the colonial morphology displayed by S. boydii bacteria cultivated on a HE agar surface; colonies of S. boydii bacteria grown on HE agar display a raised, green, and moist appearance. (US Department of Health and Human Services, Centers for Disease Control and Prevention, Public Health Information Library, PHIL_6688.)*

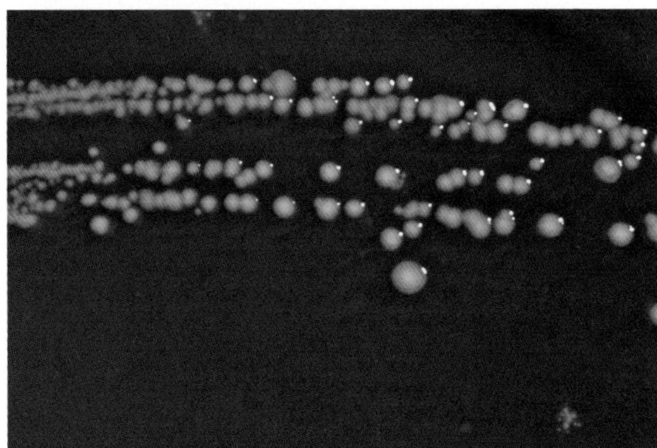

Treatment, Control, and Prevention

Treatment of shigellosis involves nursing and supporting care. Antimicrobial agents are indicated in serious cases but not routinely since their use in an animal facility selects for resistant strains. The first choices are ampicillin or trimethoprim-sulfonamide, and if the causative organism is resistant to these, a fluoroquinolone; these are effective against most strains and these drugs do not disrupt the normal flora (colonization resistance) as much as other antimicrobials.

Further Reading

Germani Y and Sansonetti PJ (2006) Chapter 3.3.6. The genus *Shigella*. *Prokaryotes*, vol. **6**, Springer, pp. 99–122.

Nataro JP, Bopp CA, Fields PI *et al.* (2011) Chapter 35. *Escherichia*, *Shigella*, and *Salmonella*, in *Manual of Clinical Microbiology*, 10th edn (ed. J Versalovic), ASM Press, Washington, DC, pp. 603–626.

Schroeder GN and Hilbi H (2008) Molecular pathogenesis of *Shigella* spp.: controlling host cell signaling, invasion, and death by type III secretion. *Clin Microbiol Rev*, **21**, 134–156.

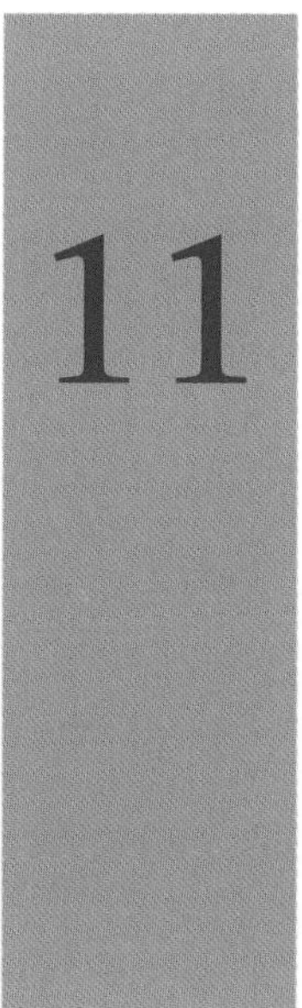

11 Pasteurellaceae: *Avibacterium, Bibersteinia, Mannheimia,* and *Pasteurella*

Amelia R. Woolums

The family Pasteurellaceae contains many organisms that contribute to animal disease. Many are normal inhabitants of the upper respiratory and gastrointestinal tracts and cause disease opportunistically when other factors enhance their ability to advance to deeper levels of these systems. Others are infrequently isolated from normal individuals and cause severe disease when animals are exposed to these agents.

There have been many changes in the taxonomy of the family Pasteurellaceae since the second edition of this textbook was written, and more changes will likely occur in the future. At the time of this writing, there are 16 genera included in the family: *Actinobacillus, Aggregatibacter, Avibacterium, Basfia, Bibersteinia, Chelonobacter, Gallibacterium, Haemophilus, Histophilus, Lonepinella, Mannheimia, Necropsobacter, Nicoletella, Pasteurella, Phocoenobacter,* and *Volucribacter*. Bacteria from genera that contribute to important diseases of animals are described here and in Chapters 13 and 14. At this time bacteria in the genus *Aggregatibacter* do not appear to be importantly associated with animals. The sources of agents in the genera *Basfia, Chelonobacter, Lonepinella, Necropsobacter, Nicoletella,* and *Necropsobacter* are listed in Table 11.1, but these agents are not discussed further here.

All the members of the family Pasteurellaceae are gram-negative coccobacilli. They are facultative anaerobes, and typically oxidase-positive (which sets them apart from members of the family Enterobacteriaceae).

Discussed in this chapter are the genera *Avibacterium, Bibersteinia, Mannheimia,* and *Pasteurella*, whose members play an important role in diseases of several animal species (Table 11.1). Briefly discussed is also *Ornithobacterium rhinotracheale*, a bacterium that is not a member of the family Pasteurellaceae, but phenotypically (and clinically) resembles some strains of *Avibacterium paragallinarum*.

Also discussed in the chapter are *Actinobacillus* (*A.*) *equuli* ssp. *equuli, A. equuli* ssp. *haemolytica, A. lignieresii, A. suis, A. pleuropneumoniae,* and members of the genus *Gallibacterium*. Additional information is provided in Chapter 12 on *Actinobacillus*. As with other members of the family Pasteurellaceae, all of these agents are gram-negative coccobacilli. They are facultative anaerobes, and are typically oxidase-positive (which sets them apart from members of the family Enterobacteriaceae).

Original chapter written by Drs. Dwight C. Hirsh and Ernst L. Biberstein.

Descriptive Features

Morphology and Staining

Members of the genera *Avibacterium, Bibersteinia, Pasteurella,* and *Mannheimia* are gram-negative coccobacilli measuring 0.2 μm by up to 2.0 μm. Bipolarity, that is, the staining of only the tips of cells, may be demonstrable with polychrome stains (e.g., Wright's stain).

Structure and Composition

Capsules contain acidic polysaccharides. The capsule of *Pasteurella multocida* type A is made of hyaluronic acid, the capsule of type D is made of heparin, and the capsule of type F is made of chondroitin (see Section "Variability" for discussion of *P. multocida* capsule nomenclature). Some *P. multocida* and *Mannheimia haemolytica* strains express adhesins.

Cell walls are typical of gram-negative microorganisms consisting mainly of lipopolysaccharides and proteins. Some of the latter are iron-regulated (i.e., they are expressed under iron-poor conditions).

Veterinary Microbiology, Third Edition. Edited by D. Scott McVey, Melissa Kennedy and M.M. Chengappa.

Table 11.1. Some Members of the Family Pasteurellaceae of Importance in Animal Disease

Genus and Species	Associated Disorder or Site
Avibacterium avium (formerly *Pasteurella avium*)	Normal respiratory flora of chickens
Avibacterium endocarditidis	Endocarditis in chickens
Avibacterium gallinarum[a] (formerly *Pasteurella gallinarum*)	Respiratory disease in poultry
Avibacterium paragallinarum[a] (formerly *Haemophilus paragallinarum*)	Infectious coryza in chickens
Avibacterium volantium (formerly *Pasteurella volantium*)	Normal respiratory flora of chickens
Basfia succiniciproducens	Normal rumen flora
Bibersteinia trehalosi[a]	Respiratory disease in ruminants, bacteremia in lambs
Chelonobacter oris	Various infections in tortoises
Lonepinella koalarum	Tannin-degrading bacterium in normal koala feces
Mannheimia glucosida	Mastitis in sheep, respiratory disease in ruminants
Mannheimia granulomatis	Respiratory and other infections in deer, ruminants, and hares; skin disease (lechiguana) in cattle; mastitis in sheep
Mannheimia haemolytica[a]	Respiratory disease in ruminants, mastitis in sheep
Mannheimia ruminalis	Normal rumen flora, mastitis in sheep
Mannheimia varigena	Respiratory infections and bacteremia in ruminants and swine, mastitis in cattle
Necropsobacter rosorum	Isolated from birds, significance uncertain
Nicoletella semolina	Respiratory disease in horses
Pasteurella aerogenes	Gastroenteritis in swine, abortion in swine
Pasteurella caballi	Respiratory disease in horses
Pasteurella canis[a]	Respiratory and oral infections in dogs, canine bite wound infections
Pasteurella dagmatis	Normal respiratory flora of birds, respiratory and oral cavity infections in dogs and cats, canine or feline bite wounds
Pasteurella langaaensis (formerly *Pasteurella langaa*)	Normal respiratory flora of birds
Pasteurella lymphangitidis	Bovine lymphangitis
Pasteurella mairii	Abortion in swine, bacteremia in piglets
Pasteurella multocida ssp. *gallicida*[a]	Fowl cholera-like disease in birds
Pasteurella multocida ssp. *multocida*[a]	Fowl cholera, respiratory disease in ruminants and swine, bacteremia/septicemia in ruminants, mastitis in ruminants, respiratory disease and other infections in rabbits, respiratory and oral cavity infections in dogs and cats, canine and feline bite wound infections
Pasteurella multocida ssp. *septica*[a]	Fowl cholera-like disease in birds, respiratory and oral cavity infections in dogs and cats, canine and feline bite wound infections, respiratory and other infections in bats
Pasteurella pneumotropica[a]	Respiratory disease in rodents
Pasteurella skyensis	Bacteremia/septicemia in farmed Atlantic salmon
Pasteurella stomatis[a]	Respiratory and oral cavity infections in dogs and cats, canine and feline bite wound infections
Pasteurella testudinis	Infections in tortoises and turtles
Phocoenobacter uteri	Isolated from uterus of harbor porpoise, significance uncertain

[a]Organisms that cause disease of particular importance, as defined by relatively frequent identification of infection and relative severity of disease associated with infection.

Cellular Products of Medical Interest

Adhesins. Some and probably all members of the family Pasteurellaceae produce adhesins (and possibly more than one kind). A type 4 fimbria (adhesin) has been described for avian strains of *P. multocida*, and an adhesin (termed Adh1) is expressed by *M. haemolytica*. As with other microorganisms, the expression of adhesins probably depends upon environmental cues. That is, adhesins are expressed while the microorganism inhabits an epithelial surface, but repressed when the microorganism is inside the host where adherence to a phagocytic cell could be disastrous. *M. haemolytica* and *Bibersteinia trehalosi* produce fibrinogen-binding proteins. The role of these proteins is unclear at present, but in the streptococci (see Chapter 28) fibrinogen-binding proteins impart an antiphagocytic property to the streptococcal particle by "coating" the bacterial cell, thereby "covering" sites for complement activation (and thus decrease opsonization, and the generation of functional membrane attack complexes) as well as those recognized by serum proteins (collectins/ficolins) that opsonize foreign particles. The hyaluronic acid capsule of type A strains *P. multocida* serves as an adhesin probably similar to hyaluronic acid encapsulated *Streptococcus pyogenes* (Chapter 28), which binds to human epithelial cells via CD44, a hyaluronic acid-binding glycoprotein

Capsule. Several species within these genera produce capsules. The capsule plays many roles, the most important of which are interference with phagocytosis (antiphagocytic) and the protection of the outer membrane from the deposition of membrane attack complexes generated by activation of the complement system. The amount of capsule produced is inversely proportional to the amount of available iron. *In vivo,* where the amount of available iron is low, the amount of capsule formed is less (but sufficient to protect the microorganism from phagocytosis and complement-mediated lysis). *P. multocida* type A capsules are made of hyaluronic acid, type D capsules are made of heparin, and type F capsules are made of chondroitin. These substances are similar (if not identical) to host tissue components, and are thus poorly antigenic; they also bind complement components poorly (and are therefore antiphagocytic). The hyaluronic acid capsule also serves as an adhesin for respiratory tract epithelial cells as in the case of capsule type A strains of *P. multocida* (see above "Adhesins").

Cell Wall. Lipopolysaccharide (LPS) elicits an inflammatory response following binding to LPS-binding protein (a serum protein), which in turn transfers it to CD14 on the surface of leukocytes. The CD14–LPS complex then binds to Toll-like receptor 4 on the surface of macrophages and other leukocytes, triggering the release of proinflammatory cytokines and inducing local or systemic inflammatory responses. LPS also acts synergistically with the *M. haemolytica* leukotoxin by increasing expression of the leukotoxin receptor, CD18, on the surface of macrophages and other leukocytes (see below, "RTX toxin").

Toxins. *Bibersteinia, Mannheimia,* and *Pasteurella* produce a number of proteins with toxic activity. At least two of these are important in the pathogenesis of disease: an RTX, and a Rho-activating toxin:

1. *RTX toxin*: The RTX (repeats in toxin, so-called because of the common feature of repeats in glycine-rich sequences within the protein) type of toxin is a leukotoxin produced by all species of *Mannheimia* (with the exception of some isolates of *Mannheimia ruminalis*) and *B. trehalosi*. Though similar in amino acid sequence to other members of the RTX family, leukotoxin specifically affects bovine leukocytes and erythrocytes; cells of nonruminant species are resistant to the effects of leukotoxin. The effect on erythrocytes probably has little importance *in vivo*, but is responsible for the hemolysis observed when most *Mannheimia* and *B. trehalosi* isolates are grown on blood agar plates. Leukotoxin binds to CD18 (a β_2 integrin), which is expressed on the surface of bovine leukocytes (neutrophils, macrophages, platelets, and lymphocytes). At low concentrations, leukotoxin causes target cell activation, at higher concentrations, apoptosis is initiated, and at very high concentrations, necrosis is produced (due to production of transmembrane pores). Upon contact with leukotoxin, neutrophils degranulate releasing potent enzymes that induce as well as aggravate inflammation, macrophages release proinflammatory cytokines (magnified in the presence of LPS), lymphocytes undergo apoptosis and necrosis, and platelets respond by increased adhesion. In addition, tissue mast cells degranulate releasing vasoactive amines. In summary, leukotoxin drives a tissue-destroying inflammatory response. The importance of leukotoxin in the pathogenesis of ruminant pneumonia due to *M. haemolytica* is evidenced by the fact that strains of *M. haemolytica* with the gene for leukotoxin disrupted produce much less severe disease than strains that can express leukotoxin normally.
2. *Rho-activating toxin*: The Rho-activating toxin is produced by *P. multocida* capsule type D, associated with atrophic rhinitis of swine. The toxin, Pmt (*P. multocida* toxin), stimulates two different signaling proteins: the small GTPase Rho and heterodimeric G proteins. Unlike similar toxins (cytotoxic necrotizing factor produced by *Escherichia coli*, see Chapter 8; and dermonecrotic toxin produced by *Bordetella bronchiseptica*, see Chapter 15), Pmt does not enzymatically affect either of these regulatory proteins. However, the interaction of Pmt with either results in toxicity mediated by increases in intracellular calcium. In addition, Pmt binds to vimentin, an intracellular intermediate filament responsible for providing mechanical strength to the cell.
3. *Miscellaneous toxins*: Some strains of *P. multocida* produce hyaluronidase and neuraminidase. The role played by these enzymes in the pathogenesis of disease is unclear. It is tempting to speculate that hyaluronidase is active *in vivo* and may be responsible for the microorganism's ability to "spread" through tissue. Neuraminidase has been postulated to play a role in the colonization of epithelial surfaces by removing terminal sialic acid residues from mucin, thereby modifying normal host innate immunity.

Iron Acquisition. Because iron is an absolute growth requirement, microorganisms must acquire this substance if they are to exist within the host. Some avian strains of *P. multocida* produce a siderophore, multicidin, which is neither a phenolate nor hydroxamate-type siderophore. Siderophores have not been demonstrated in *Pasteurella* or *Mannheimia* from other sources or species. However, *Pasteurella* and *Mannheimia* bind transferrin–iron complexes by virtue of iron-regulated outer membrane proteins expressed under iron-poor conditions (so-called transferrin-binding proteins, or Tbps). Iron is acquired from the transferrin–iron complexes that bind to the surface of the microorganism. Iron-regulated outer membrane proteins are also upregulated in conditions of low iron availability. *P. multocida* also binds heme and hemoglobin, which are other possible sources of iron.

Miscellaneous Products. Some avian strains of *P. multocida* express an outer membrane protein that is toxic to phagocytic cells. It is unclear what role this protein might play in the pathogenesis of disease. If capsule formation is downregulated *in vivo* due to low available iron concentrations, then the toxic outer membrane protein might serve to protect the microorganism from phagocytosis.

Growth Characteristics

Avibacterium, Bibersteinia, Mannheimia, and *Pasteurella* grow best in the presence of serum or blood. After overnight incubation (35–37 °C), colonies are up to 2 mm in diameter, clear to grayish, and smooth or mucoid. *Mannheimia haemolytica*, *M. glucosida*, and some isolates of *B. trehalosi* produce hemolysis on ruminant blood agar. All are gram-negative, nonmotile coccobacilli. They are facultative anaerobes, typically oxidase-positive, reduce nitrates, and attack carbohydrates fermentatively. The pattern of carbohydrates fermented can be used to differentiate individual species.

Members of these genera vary in their requirement for β-nicotinamide adenine dinucleotide (β-NAD, also known as V factor), with *Avibacterium avium*, *A. volantium*, and some isolates of *A. paragallinarum* requiring β-NAD and the remaining members of these genera characterized to date not requiring β-NAD. *A. paragallinarum* isolates not requiring β-NAD are designated as biovar 2 isolates, while isolates requiring β-NAD are designated as biovar 1. Phenotypically, *A. gallinarum*, *A. endocarditidis*, and biovar 2 isolates of *A. paragallinarum* can be difficult to differentiate from *Gallibacterium anatis* (see Chapter 12), but differentiation is possible based on differences in the ortho-nitrophenyl-β-D-galactopyranoside (ONPG) reaction and fermentation of glycerol, D-mannitol, D-galactose, and maltose. Biovar 2 isolates of *A. paragallinarum* can also be difficult to differentiate phenotypically from *O. rhinotracheale*, another bacterial pathogen also associated with respiratory disease in poultry (see Section "*O. rhinotracheale*"). Differentiation of these agents is best accomplished by use of polymerase chain reaction (PCR) testing.

Pasteurella aerogenes and *Actinobacillus rossii* (Chapter 13), both of which can be associated with reproductive tract infections in sows, can be difficult to differentiate based on phenotypic and even genotypic testing. *B. trehalosi* and *P. multocida* can both overgrow *M. haemolytica* in culture (and possibly *in vivo*), a fact that may be relevant to accurate diagnosis of cases of ruminant respiratory disease.

Resistance

Cultures die within 1 or 2 weeks. Disinfectants, heat (50 °C for 30 min), and ultraviolet light are promptly lethal. *P. multocida* survives for months in bird carcasses.

Pasteurella and *Mannheimia* have become increasingly resistant to penicillins, tetracyclines, and sulfonamides, to which they were originally susceptible. The gene encoding tetracycline resistance is unique to *Pasteurella* and *Mannheimia*. Resistance encoding genes are frequently associated with R plasmids.

Variability

P. multocida consists of 5 capsular serogroups (A, B, D, E, and F) and 16 somatic serotypes (1–16). Serotypes are often related to host specificity and pathogenicity. The serotype is designated with a letter designating the capsule type and a number designating the somatic type (e.g., A : 1).

M. haemolytica consists of 12 capsular types (1, 2, 5–9, 12–14, 16, and 17), while *B. trehalosi* consists of four (3, 4, 10, and 15). Capsular typing alone cannot be used to identify *M. haemolytica* as some other species within the genus *Mannheimia* also react with typing sera used to classify *M. haemolytica*. *A. paragallinarum* is also encapsulated, with evidence suggesting that there may be differentiation in capsule composition similar to that seen among different capsular types of *P. multocida*. There are three serotypes of *A. paragallinarum* (Page serotypes A, B, and C).

Ecology

Reservoirs

Bacteria in the genera *Avibacterium*, *Bibersteinia*, *Mannheimia*, and *Pasteurella* are carried on mucous membranes (most commonly in the oropharyngeal region) of susceptible host species. Carriage may be widespread, as with *P. multocida* in carnivores, or exceptional, as with avian cholera-producing strains in birds or hemorrhagic septicemia-producing strains in ruminants. One host species may serve as reservoir for another, as has been recognized for avian cholera and for respiratory disease due to *M. haemolytica* in bighorn sheep.

Transmission

Infection is by inhalation, ingestion, or bites and scratch wounds. Many infections are probably endogenous. In bovine hemorrhagic septicemia and avian cholera, environmental contamination contributes to indirect transmission.

Pathogenesis

Mechanisms

In general, there are three manifestations of disease induced by bacteria in the genera *Avibacterium*, *Bibersteinia*, *Mannheimia*, or *Pasteurella*: respiratory tract disease, septicemia, and trauma-associated conditions:

1. Respiratory tract involvement is either pneumonia or pleuropneumonia or upper respiratory tract disease (e.g., atrophic rhinitis in swine and infectious coryza in chickens). Pneumonia is seen most frequently in ruminants and is usually associated with *M. haemolytica*, *P. multocida*, or *B. trehalosi*. Environmental stress (e.g., recent shipment or weaning), virus infection, or other bacterial infections (e.g., mycoplasma) usually precede pneumonia, and are thought to decrease host defenses of the tract, allowing commensal bacteria living in the upper respiratory tract (*M. haemolytica*, *P. multocida*, or *B. trehalosi*) to infect the lung. *M. Haemolytica* or *B. trehalosi* from the upper respiratory tract is deposited in the lung, and secrete Lkt and, along with LPS from their cell walls, initiate an intense inflammatory response with fibrin deposition and thrombosis. Although *P. multocida* has not been shown to produce Lkt, its deposition in the lung initiates an inflammatory response by virtue of having LPS. Capsule, iron-scavenging abilities, and perhaps binding of fibrinogen enhance survival of the bacteria within the lesion.

   A. paragallinarum causes outbreaks of primarily upper respiratory tract disease in chickens (infectious coryza). Likewise, *P. multocida* in combination with *B. bronchiseptica* (Chapter 15) causes the serious upper respiratory tract disorder known as progressive atrophic rhinitis in swine. In this disease, *B. bronchiseptica* first adheres to the nasal mucosa and secretes a toxin called dermonecrotic toxin, which mildly damages the epithelium. Capsule type D strains of *P. multocida* adhere to this mildly damaged epithelium (these strains do not readily adhere to normal epithelium) and secrete *P. multocida* toxin (Pmt). It is Pmt that is responsible for the destruction of the nasal turbinates. The action of *B. bronchiseptica* toxin alone, without the participation of *P. multocida*, results in a mild, nonprogressive turbinate hypoplasia.

2. Bacteremic and septicemic disease is produced by *P. multocida* in ruminants and avian species. *P. multocida* ssp. *multocida* causes hemorrhagic septicemia in cattle (currently a disease exotic to the United States). *P. multocida* ssp. *multocida* and *B. trehalosi* cause septicemia in sheep, and *P. multocida* ssp. *multocida* causes avian cholera in avian species. Why these strains and not others in the family Pasteurellaceae are able to cause bacteremia and septicemia is not understood. However, characteristics of their capsules and iron scavenging mechanism may be relevant. Outer membrane proteins on avian strains of *P. multocida* appear to play some role by decreasing phagocytosis. Signs and outcomes of these diseases are attributable to severe systemic inflammatory response and multiorgan infection.
3. Trauma-related conditions are those in which "mouth" microorganisms (*Pasteurella* is the most common) are inoculated into the site of infection. Examples include canine or feline bite wounds and infections caused by dogs and cats licking compromised sites (e.g., surgical wounds).

Pathology

Lesions vary with site of infection, virulence of strains, and host resistance. In septicemias, vascular damage results in hemorrhage and fluid loss but little cellular inflammatory response. Focal necrosis in parenchymatous organs or ulcerations of mucous membranes may occur. Mammals develop generalized hemorrhagic lymphadenopathy. In chronic fowl cholera, caseopurulent inflammation occurs in joints, middle ear, ovaries, or wattles.

In ruminant pneumonias, due to *Mannheimia, Bibersteinia,* and *Pasteurella*, gross lesions are those of bronchopneumonia or pleuropneumonia. *M. haemolytica* infection of cattle can induce a severe fibrinous necrotizing pleuropneumonia, with much fibrin deposition and exudation of proteinaceous fluid in the pleural space. Gross lesions due to *B. trehalosi* or *P. multocida* are more commonly limited to bronchopneumonia without pleural reaction. Microscopically, the inflammatory response mirrors the gross lesions, with massive neutrophil infiltration and necrosis, hemorrhage, fibrin deposition, and thrombosis seen in acute *M. haemolytica* infection. In contrast, infiltration of neutrophils in airways and alveoli (purulent bronchopneumonia) without tissue necrosis and fibrin deposition is more commonly seen in pneumonia associated with *B. trehalosi* or *P. multocida*.

Atrophic rhinitis of pigs (see also under *B. bronchiseptica*, Chapter 15) is a chronic rhinitis accompanying disturbed osteogenesis adjacent to the inflamed areas. Increased osteoclastic and diminished osteoblastic activity destroys the turbinates and bones of the snout, resulting in distortions of facial structures. Histologically, fibrous tissue replaces osseous tissue. Bone atrophy is accompanied by inflammation of varying acuteness.

The pathology of lesions that are "mouth" related is unremarkable with neutrophils predominating.

Disease Patterns

Cattle

Pneumonia. The most common form of bovine "pasteurellosis," which most commonly involves *M. haemolytica* or *P. multocida* ssp. *multocida*, is "shipping fever," a bronchopneumonia or fibrinous pleuropneumonia seen when cattle, especially recently weaned calves, are transported, assembled, and handled under stressful conditions. The onset, 1–2 weeks after shipment, is marked by fever, inappetence, and listlessness. Respiratory signs (nasal discharge and cough) are few and variable. At more advanced stages, the fever may drop but respiratory distress will be obvious. Abnormal lung sounds can be detected, especially over the apical lobes, which are first and most severely affected.

P. multocida ssp. *multocida* is commonly isolated from young dairy calves with pneumonia, which can occur either in an endemic pattern (enzootic calf pneumonia) or in epidemics (epizootics). It is likely that other insults, such as primary viral respiratory infection, environmental factors such as poor air quality and crowding, and inadequate host immunity all enhance the ability of *P. multocida* to advance into the lung and cause disease. Serogroup A isolates of *P. multocida* are most commonly associated with ruminant respiratory disease in North America and Europe.

Hemorrhagic Septicemia. Hemorrhagic septicemia is an acute systemic infection with *P. multocida* ssp. *multocida*, serotype B (southern and Southeast Asia) or E (Africa), occurring in tropical areas as seasonal epidemics with high morbidity and mortality. Signs include high fever, depression, subcutaneous edema, hypersalivation and diarrhea, or sudden death. All excretions and secretions are highly infectious.

Sheep and Goats

Septicemia. Septicemic pasteurellosis, usually due to *B. trehalosi* in feeder lambs and *M. haemolytica* in nursing lambs, resembles bovine hemorrhagic septicemia, although intestinal involvement is often absent and the morbidity rate is much lower.

Pneumonia. As is the case in cattle, pneumonia in sheep and goats can occur following shipment, or in groups of animals in either enzootic or epizootic patterns. *M.*

haemolytica, *B. trehalosi*, and *P. multocida* are most commonly involved. As described earlier for calves, other factors including coinfection with viral pathogens, environmental stressors, and inadequate host immunity enhance the ability of *P. multocida* to cause bronchopneumonia in small ruminants.

Mastitis. Mastitis in small ruminants can be caused by various *Mannheimia* species or *P. trehalosi*. Disease often occurs late in lactation, when large lambs bruise the udder and provide the inoculum from their oropharyngeal flora. Acute systemic reactions accompany disease of the udder, parts of which undergo necrosis ("blue bag") and may slough.

Swine

Atrophic Rhinitis. Atrophic rhinitis of young pigs (3 weeks to 7 months) leading to turbinate destruction and secondary complications results from synergistic nasal infection by *P. multocida* (usually serogroup D or A) and *B. bronchiseptica*. In addition, ammonia (in concentrations sometimes found in swine-rearing houses) acts synergistically with Pmt.

Signs include sneezing, epistaxis, and staining of the face due to tear duct obstruction. Skeletal abnormalities produce lateral deviation of the snout or wrinkling due to rostrocaudal compression. Secondary pneumonia is due in part to the elimination of the turbinates as defenses of the respiratory tract.

Pneumonia. As is the case for ruminants, bronchopneumonia can occur in swine following shipment, or in groups of swine in enzootic or epizootic patterns. *P. multocida* ssp. *multocida* is commonly isolated from such cases. As for ruminants, it is likely that other insults such as primary viral respiratory infection, environmental factors such as crowding and poor air quality, and inadequate host immunity enhance the ability of *P. multocida* to cause bronchopneumonia.

Rabbits

Respiratory Tract Conditions. "Snuffles," a mucopurulent rhinosinusitis of rabbits due to *P. multocida* ssp. *multocida*, develops when bacteria normally residing in the nasopharynx cause disease following stress of pregnancy, lactation, or mismanagement. Coinfection with other pathogens, particularly *B. bronchiseptica*, may exacerbate disease. Complications include bronchopneumonia, middle and inner ear infection, conjunctivitis, and septicemia.

Genital Tract Disease. In the genital tract, *P. multocida* may cause orchitis, balanoposthitis, and pyometra.

Avian Species

Infectious Coryza. Infectious coryza (caused by *A. paragallinarum*) is an acute contagious infection of chickens, which is usually confined to the upper respiratory tract. It affects birds of practically all ages. Signs include nasal discharge, swelling of sinuses, facial edema, and conjunctivitis. Air sac and lung involvement may occur in severe cases. When disease is uncomplicated, mortality is low, and loss of production is the most important consequence. Superimposed infections with mycoplasmas and helminth parasites exacerbate and prolong outbreaks. Of other species, only Japanese quail are highly susceptible.

Avian Cholera. Avian cholera, a systemic infection due to *P. multocida* ssp. *multocida* (most commonly serogroup A), is acquired by ingestion or inhalation and mainly affects turkeys, waterfowl, and chickens. The peracute form kills about 60% of infected birds without preceding signs of illness. The acute type, marked by listlessness, anorexia, diarrhea, and nasal and ocular discharges, may last several days and be about 30% lethal. The subacute form is mostly respiratory and is manifested by rales and mucopurulent nasal discharges. In chronic fowl cholera, there is localization of caseous lesions. Inapparently infected carrier birds appear to be important in the epidemiology of fowl cholera. *Avibacterium gallinarum* is sometimes isolated from chronic cases.

Dogs and Cats

Mouth-Related Conditions. *P. multocida* (cats) and *P. canis* (dogs) are found alongside predominantly anaerobic flora in oral cavity infections, bite wound infections, serositides (e.g., feline pyothorax), and oral cavity-related foreign body lesions.

Equine

Respiratory Tract Conditions. *Pasteurella caballi* occurs in equine respiratory disease, usually in association with *Streptococcus equi* ssp. *zooepidemicus*.

Laboratory Rodents. *P. pneumotropica*, a common commensal, may contribute to opportunistic infections such as pneumonia. Phenotypically similar organisms in other hosts probably belong to different species (e.g., *P. dagmatis*).

Immunity

Basis of Immunity

Circulating antibody is significant in protection against hemorrhagic septicemia and fowl cholera. The type-specific capsular antigens are essential immunogens in hemorrhagic septicemia. In birds recovering from infection with *A. paragallinarum*, immunity provides heterologous protection across various capsular types. With other forms of disease associated with *Pasteurella* and *Mannheimia*, the picture is less clear. Both antitoxic and antibacterial antibodies are important in protection; for example, antileukotoxin antibodies are an important requirement for immunity to severe disease induced by *M. haemolytica* challenge.

Vaccination

Vaccines against *A. paragallinarum* are commercially available and can protect chickens from disease following experimental exposure to the bacteria, but vaccines must contain the challenge serotype to be most effective.

Vaccines to prevent bronchopneumonia associated with *P. multocida* in swine and cattle, and bronchopneumonia or pleuropneumonia associated with *M. haemolytica* in cattle, are commercially available. These vaccines can prevent disease associated with experimental challenge, but their efficacy in the field is less consistent. Vaccines manufactured for use in cattle are sometimes administered to sheep and goats, but in general these are unlikely to provide much benefit because different serotypes of *Mannheimia* and *Pasteurella* not included in bovine vaccines are most commonly associated with disease in small ruminants.

In countries where bovine hemorrhagic septicemia occurs, vaccines are used to prevent disease and can be effective for up to 2 years. Antiserum is useful for short-term protection.

The essential attributes of an effective avian cholera vaccine are not known. Field performance of bacterins has been inconsistent. Most promising have been live vaccines containing attenuated organisms. Attenuation appears inversely related to immunogenicity.

P. multocida and *B. bronchiseptica* bacterins with toxoid are commercially available and are useful in the control of atrophic rhinitis.

Laboratory Diagnosis

Isolation and Identification

Bacteria in the genera *Avibacterium, Bibersteinia, Mannheimia,* and *Pasteurella* overnight (35–37 °C) on media containing blood or serum and are identified using differential tests. Capsule and somatic typing can be done, but these tests are more often used in research applications and may not be available at regional veterinary diagnostic laboratories. DNA probes and primers designed to amplify specific regions of the bacterial chromosome by PCR can be used to identify specific species. Definitive identification of members of the family Pasteurellaceae is typically completed through sequencing 16S ribosomal RNA gene sequences and, if necessary, the rpoB (β-subunit of the RNA polymerase) gene sequence, but this is beyond the scope of most diagnostic laboratories.

Treatment and Control

Bacteria in the genera *Avibacterium, Bibersteinia, Mannheimia,* and *Pasteurella* are susceptible to a variety of antimicrobials effective against gram-negative bacteria. Strains from carnivores are generally susceptible to almost all antimicrobials; strains from ruminants and swine can be more variable in susceptibility. Metaphylactic administration of the antimicrobials oxytetracycline, tilmicosin, or florfenicol is used to prevent shipping fever associated with *M. haemolytica* infection in cattle.

Vaccination is used to control disease associated with infection by *M. haemolytica* in cattle, *P. multocida* in swine, cattle, and avian species, and *A. paragallinarum* in chickens. While vaccines against these agents are effective in preventing disease following experimental infection, efficacy in the field is more variable and likely depends on a variety of factors related to relative severity of challenge, ability of vaccinated animals to respond appropriately to vaccination, and the severity of environmental stressors that exacerbate host susceptibility to disease.

O. rhinotracheale

O. rhinotracheale is a gram-negative rod that resembles some members of the family Pasteurellaceae. It is a facultative anaerobe whose growth is enhanced by carbon dioxide; it is oxidase-positive and attacks carbohydrates fermentatively. It requires neither hemin (factor X) nor β-NAD (factor V). It is important to note, however, that it is not a member of the family Pasteurellaceae, and in fact is not a member of any recognized group of microorganisms. Based upon the sequence of the DNA encoding, the 16S ribosomal RNA, it is more closely related to *Riemerella* and *Capnocytophaga*. There are 12 serotypes (A–L), with A being the most common.

O. rhinotracheale causes (by unknown mechanisms) respiratory tract disease (sinusitis, airsacculitis, and pneumonia) in birds (domestic and wild). In turkeys and chickens, respiratory tract disease may be relatively mild, resulting in poor performance, or severe with increased mortality. Transmission is horizontal (aerosols and contaminated fomites) or vertical; it is unclear whether vertical transmission is transovarian or through cecal contamination of eggs.

With the appearance of NAD-independent strains of *A. paragallinarum* (see Section "Growth Characteristics"), differentiation of *A. paragallinarum* from *O. rhinotracheale* can be difficult by classical culture techniques. A PCR-based test quickly and easily differentiates the two organisms.

Most isolates of *O. rhinotracheale* are susceptible to ampicillin, erythromycin, penicillin, tetracycline, and tylosin. Vaccination with autogenous bacterins may reduce morbidity.

Further Reading

Dabo SM, Taylor JD, and Confer AW (2007) *Pasteurella multocida* and bovine respiratory disease. *Anim Health Res Rev*, **8**, 129–150.

Dousse F, Thomann A, Brodard I *et al.* (2008) Routine phenotypic identification of bacterial species of the family Pasteurellaceae isolated from animals. *J Vet Diagn Invest*, **20**, 716–724.

Harper M, Boyce JD, and Adler B (2006) *Pasteurella multocida* pathogenesis: 125 years after Pasteur. *FEMS Microbiol Lett*, **265**, 1–10.

Rice JA, Carrasco-Medina L, Hodgins DC, and Shewen PE (2007) *Mannheimia haemolytica* and bovine respiratory disease. *Anim Health Res Rev*, **8**, 117–128.

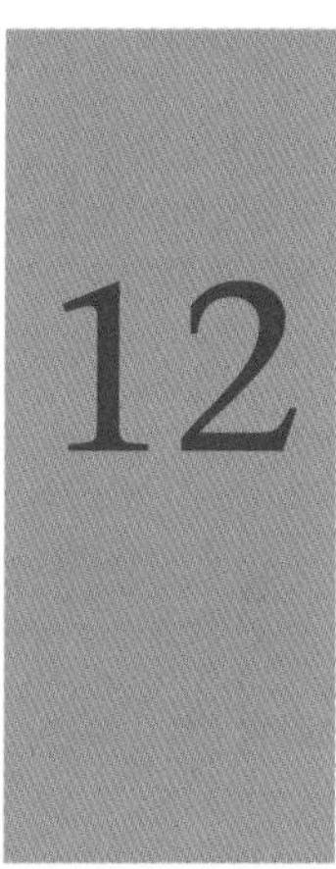

12 Pasteurellaceae: *Actinobacillus*

BRADLEY W. FENWICK AND AMELIA R. WOOLUMS

The family Pasteurellaceae contains the genera *Actinobacillus, Gallibacterium, Haemophilus, Histophilus, Lonepinella, Mannheimia, Pasteurella,* and *Phocoenobacter*. Most if not all of these genera contain species of medical importance as opportunistic pathogens generally characterized by septicemia and associated sequelae.

Although they are genetically distinct, the genera *Actinobacillus, Gallibacterium,* and *Pasteurella* overlap phenotypically. As is the case with the genus *Pasteurella*, the genus *Actinobacillus* is undergoing considerable taxonomic change. As of this writing, there are 17 species and 2 subspecies in the genus *Actinobacillus*, many of which are associated with disease in animals (Table 12.1). The relatively newly defined genus *Gallibacterium* includes avian isolates previously classified as *Pasteurella haemolytica*-like, "*Actinobacillus salpingitidis*," or *Pasteurella anatis*. These bacteria can be isolated from a variety of birds with salpingitis, peritonitis, bacteremia/septicemia, and other infections. The recently characterized genus *Volucribacter* includes bacteria isolated mainly from psittacines and chickens with signs of respiratory disease or bacteremia/septicemia.

While phenotype-based and molecular methods have been developed to identify and differentiate some of the most common taxa, the restricted host range and characteristic disease conditions associated with each species allow for a reliable presumptive etiological diagnosis. Like may others, the genus *Actinobacillus* has and likely will continue to undergo taxonomic reclassification. Depending on the level of evaluation, the genus *Actinobacillus* contains 21 species or species-like taxa, many of which are associated with disease in several animal species (Table 13.1). A case can be made that about half of these are sufficiently unrelated to *Actinobacillus sensu stricto* and should be regrouped into different genera. *Actinobacillus actinomycetemcomitans* is now classified as *Aggregatibacter actinomycetemcomitans*.

Discussed in this chapter are *Actinobacillus equuli* ssp. *equuli* (previously *A. equuli*, the case of neonatal septicemia of foals), *A. equuli* ssp. *haemolytica* (previously *A. suis*-like, which is an equine pathogen and occurs mainly in respiratory tract disease of horses), *A. lignieresii* (the agent of pyogranulomatous inflammatory processes, primarily of ruminants), *A. suis* (associated with respiratory, septicemia, and localized infectious in swine), and *A. pleuropneumoniae* (the agent of porcine pleuropneumonia).

Original chapter written by Drs. Dwight C. Hirsh and Ernst L. Biberstein.

All the members of the family Pasteurellaceae are gram-negative coccobacilli. They are facultative anaerobes, and typically oxidase-positive (setting them apart from members of the family Enterobacteriaceae). Most are commensal parasites of the respiratory tract and oral cavity of animals that sporadically cause disease in individuals. The most notable exception being *A. pleuropneumoniae*, which like other actinobacilli can be asymptomatically carried, is viewed as a primary pathogen because of its ability in a dose-dependent fashion to cause significant disease outbreaks in healthy pigs characterized by high morbidity and mortality.

Descriptive Features

Morphology and Staining

Members of the genus *Actinobacillus* are nonmotile, gram-negative pleomorphic coccobacilli, approximately 0.5 μm wide and variable in length, that produce a "Morse code"-like series of dots and dashes. In older cultures the degree of pleomorphism increases.

Structure and Composition

Capsules and Polysaccharide. The cell wall is typical of gram-negative microorganisms consisting mainly of lipopolysaccharides (LSP) and proteins. Considerable effort has been applied to the detailed chemical–structural characterization of the LPS and capsule of various actinobacilli, particularly between different serotypes of *A. pleuropneumoniae*. The genetic basis behind these structural differences has been determined. Variations in the structures of the LPS and capsule to a greater degree are responsible for serotype differentiation, to some degree virulence differences between serotypes, and are the basis of serotype-specific serological tests and vaccine-induced

Veterinary Microbiology, Third Edition. Edited by D. Scott McVey, Melissa Kennedy and M.M. Chengappa.

Table 12.1. Some Members of the Genera *Actinobacillus*, *Gallibacterium*, and *Volucribacter* that are of Importance in Animal Disease

Genus and Species	Associated Disorder or Site
Actinobacillus arthritidis	Bacteremia and septicemia in foals
Actinobacillus capsulatus	Arthritis in rabbits
Actinobacillus delphinicola	Bacteremia and septicemia in sea mammals
Actinobacillus equuli ssp. *equuli*[a]	Bacteremia/septicemia in foals, respiratory disease in horses, pericarditis in horses, abortions in mares (mare reproductive loss syndrome), bacteremia/septicemia in swine
Actinobacillus equuli ssp. *haemolyticus* (formerly *A. suis*-like) [a]	Respiratory disease in horses, pericarditis in horses, abortions in mares (mare reproductive loss syndrome)
Actinobacillus indolicus	Respiratory disease in swine
Actinobacillus lignieresii[a]	Chronic pyogranulomatous glossitis in cattle ("wooden tongue"), pyogranulomas of the proximal gastrointestinal tract in cattle
Actinobacillus minor	Respiratory disease in swine
Actinobacillus muris	Respiratory disease in rodents
Actinobacillus pleuropneumoniae[a]	Respiratory disease in swine
Actinobacillus porcinus	Respiratory disease in swine
Actinobacillus rossii	Reproductive tract infections in sows
Actinobacillus scotiae	Bacteremia and septicemia in harbor porpoises
Actinobacillus seminis	Epididymitis in rams
Actinobacillus succinogenes	Normal rumen flora
Actinobacillus suis	Respiratory disease and bacteremia/septicemia in swine
Gallibacterium anatis	Salpingitis, peritonitis, bacteremia/septicemia, and other infections in birds
Gallibacterium melopsittaci	Salpingitis, bacteremia/septicemia in psittacines
Gallibacterium salpingitidis	Salpingitis in ducks
Gallibacterium trehalosifermentans	Bacteremia/septicemia in budgerigars
Volucribacter psittacicida	
Volucribacter amazonae	

[a]Organisms that cause disease of particular importance, as defined by relatively frequent identification of infection and relative severity of disease associated with infection.

immunity. Sequence similarities and antigenic cross-reactions between the LPS of different actinobacilli species have been demonstrated. Growth condition-dependent expression (particularly iron availability) of proteins and the amount of surface polysaccharide have been described *in vitro* with indirect evidence of their expression *in vivo*.

Actinobacillus has a polysaccharide capsule; whether members of the genus *Gallibacterium* express a capsule has not been defined. The cell wall of members of these genera is typical of gram-negative microorganisms consisting mainly of LSP and proteins. Some of the latter are iron regulated (i.e., they are expressed under iron-poor conditions).

Cell Products of Medical Interest

Adhesins. Colonization is often the first step toward the occurrence of disease. The role of adhesins, as in other microorganisms, is to allow the bacterium expressing them to adhere to cells lining a particular niche, as well as to the surface of the so-called target cells prior to the initiation of disease (in some cases, niche and target cells may be the same). The expression of adhesins depends upon various environmental cues and dictates both the location of colonization (carrier vs. disease) and the transmission potential. Probably all members of the family Pasteurellaceae that colonize animals express a number of adhesins. This is likely to be particularly true for the actinobacilli given the natural habitat of most is the oral cavity and respiratory tract (particularly the tonsils).

Except of *A. pleuropneumoniae*, little is known about the adhesins of the other actinobacilli associated with diseases of animals. *A. pleuropneumoniae* adheres to different cell types, the epithelium of the nasal cavity and tonsillar crypts (as in the case with carrier animals), and to a greater degree the cells of the terminal bronchiole and alveoli (antecedent to disease). Whether colonization of the upper respiratory tract is required for lower respiratory tract disease is not known, but the 48 h delay in the development of acute clinical disease following experimental nasal or aerosol challenge suggests that it is.

A. pleuropneumoniae produces at least two structures that function as adhesins. The first is an adhesion in the classic sense, that is, a structure composed of protein subunits whose main function is to bind to the surface of host cells. These adhesins are type 4 fimbriae that in the case of *A. pleuropneumoniae* adhere to cultured primary lung epithelial cells but are only expressed under nicotinamide adenine dinucleotide (NAD)-restricted growth conditions in some but not all strains. A 55 kDa and a 60 kDa outer membrane protein as well as an autotransporter protease has also been described to be associated with culture condition-dependent adhesion. In addition, *A. pleuropneumoniae* is reported to bind to or interact with respiratory tract mucus, collagen, fibronectin, and double-stranded DNA. The other, cell wall LSP, is not usually considered an adhesion. Nevertheless, the LSP (in particular the core portion) of *A. pleuropneumoniae* is likely involved in the adherence of this microorganism to cells of the lower respiratory tract of swine by interacting with specific surface glycoproteins. Gene expression following contact with porcine lung cells and involving the *tad* locus-specific genes suggest the mechanism for the occurrence of rough phenotypes (waxy) that are common on primary culture but lost after laboratory passage (mucoid).

Capsules. The capsule plays many roles, the most important of which are interference with phagocytosis (antiphagocytic) and protection of the outer membrane from the deposition of membrane attack complexes generated by activation of the complement system (serum resistance). In addition, capsules (perhaps in association with LPS) provide sufficient space between surface-activated membrane attack complexes induced by antipolysaccharide antibodies and the cell wall such that the microorganism survives. In the case of *A. pleuropneumoniae*, the capsule is the primary basis of resistant to the complement-mediated killing of normal and immune serum as well as opsonophagocytosis. The amount of capsules produced is regulated by growth conditions and inversely proportional to the amount of available iron. *In vivo*, where the amount of available iron is low, the amount of capsules formed is less (but sufficient to protect the microorganism from phagocytosis and complement-mediated lysis).

Biofilm. Biofilms are structured bacterial communities surrounded by a polymer matrix that they produce to support attachment and provide protection from hostile environments, including host immune responses and antibiotics. Odds are good that most, if not all, actinobacilli can under the right conditions form biofilms. The conditions necessary to induce the expression of biofilms is not well understood, and the phenotype can be easily repressed under standard laboratory growth conditions. In the case of *A. pleuropneumoniae* and likely other species, biofilm production is enhanced under anaerobic conditions. The biofilm produced by *A. pleuropneumoniae* when grown on polystyrene is highly hydrated polyglucosamine.

Cell Wall. LSP elicits an inflammatory response following associated with LSP-binding protein (serum protein), which in turn transfers it to the blood phase of CD14. The CD14–LPS complex binds to Toll-like receptor proteins (see Chapter 2) on the surface of macrophage cells, triggering the release of proinflammatory cytokines. The outer LPS core can interact with RTX-type toxins in a Ca^{2+}-dependent fashion that enhances hemolytic and cytotoxic potential. In addition, the LPS plays a role in antiphagocytosis, serum resistance, and serotyping.

Toxins. Members of the genus *Actinobacillus* produce a least two products that have toxic activity. The most important is an RTX-type toxin, and the other is the enzyme urease:

1. *RTX-type toxin*: The RTX-type toxin (repeats in toxin, so called because of the common feature of repeats in glycine-rich sequences within the protein; see also *Escherichia coli* hemolysin in Chapter 7, Pasteurella/Mannheimia leukotoxin in Chapter 12, adenylyl cyclase toxin of *Bordetella* in Chapter 15, and *Moraxella* cytotoxin in Chapter 18) is produced by *A. pleuropneumoniae*, *A. suis*, and *A. rossii*. The toxin is termed Apx (for *A. pleuropneumoniae* toxin). *A. equuli* ssp. *haemolytica* produces a similar toxin, Aqx (for *A. equuli* toxin). Even though *A. lignieresii* contains the genes encoding Apx, it does not express them (lacks a functioning promoter). The central importance of Apx toxins in the development of clinical disease is well established in that they are necessary for full virulence but are not in themselves fully sufficient. As with other RTX-type toxins, there is a dose effect. At low concentrations these toxins interfere with macrophage and neutrophil function by triggering degranulation, and at higher concentrations they are cytolytic for macrophages, neutrophils, and alveolar epithelial cells. In addition, the RTX-type toxins lyse erythrocytes (explaining the hemolytic phenotype of actinobacilli expressing them when grown on blood agar), and they are responsible for CAMP reaction when cross-streaked with a β-toxin-producing strain of *Staphylococcus* (see Chapter 26). The effect on erythrocytes probably plays little if any role in disease production, except perhaps increasing the availability of iron. There are four types of Apx toxins (ApxI, ApxII, ApxIII, and ApxIV), each with a different degree of cytotoxicity (ApxI is the most potent of the four, followed by ApxIII, and then ApxII—the potency of ApxIV is unknown because it is not produced *in vitro* under standard laboratory conditions). Actinobacilli may contain the genes encoding any combination of the four toxins. In the case of *A. pleuropneumoniae* (see Section "Variability"), serotypes 1, 5, 9, 10, 11, and 14 produce Apx1, and all the serotypes (except serotypes 10 and 14) produce ApxII; serotypes 2, 3, 4, 6, 8, and 15 produce ApxIII, and all the serotypes produce ApxIV *in vitro*. *Actinobacillus rossi* produces ApxII and ApxIII, whereas *A. suis* produces ApxI and ApxII.
2. *Urease*: However, urease produced by *A. pleuropneumoniae* has been shown to be a virulence factor (it is unknown whether this enzyme plays a role in the diseases produced by the other urease-positive species of actinobacilli). Urease is responsible for the liberation of ammonia from urea (the association constant of *A. pleuropneumoniae* urease is extremely high, allowing effective association with the very low concentration of urea found in blood and tissue fluids). In addition to attracting and activating neutrophils and macrophages, ammonia inhibits phagolysosome fusion and increases the pH within phagolysosomes, thereby reducing the effectiveness of various acid hydrolase. These effects not only result in a decrease in the host's ability to clear the microorganisms from the lung but also support colonization of the upper respiratory tract, thereby promoting the carrier state (mutants unable to produce urease are cleared more rapidly from the respiratory tract).

Iron Acquisition. Because iron is an absolute growth requirement, microorganisms have developed multiple high-affinity systems to obtain it from their environment or hosts. For several reasons free iron is maintained at extremely low concentrations (10^{-18} M) by the host via a number of iron-binding proteins. Actinobacilli acquire iron via a number of mechanisms including from transferrin–iron complexes by virtue of iron-regulated outer membrane proteins expressed under iron-poor conditions (so-called transferrin-binding proteins or Tbps). Iron is acquired from the transferrin–iron complexes that bind to the surface of the microorganism via a 60 kDa lipoprotein. Interestingly, in the case of *A. pleuropneumoniae* only porcine transferrin binds, which could contribute to the basis for only pigs being susceptible. In addition to acquiring iron by way of Tbps, *A. pleuropneumoniae* binds to hemin and hemoglobin and utilizes siderophores (hydroxamates, catechols, and possibly others) produced by other species of bacteria even though it does not produce them itself.

Miscellaneous Products. Other products produced by actinobacilli (specifically *A. pleuropneumoniae*) that may play a role in disease production include IgA and IgG proteases (prevent adherence and opsonization, respectively) and periplasmic superoxide dismutase (suggested as a strategy to prevent digestion within the phagolysosome by inactivating superoxide molecules). In addition, high-molecular-weight surface carbohydrates associated with the capsule and LPS may play a role in scavenging free toxic oxygen radicals. Like iron, nickel is held as low concentrations by the host but is required for urease activation. To account for this, *A. pleuropneumoniae* has a high-affinity nickel uptake system. Finally, while the most common locations of the actinobacilli are oxygen rich, within lesions oxygen concentrations can be low. In the case of *A. pleuropneumoniae*, alternate terminal electron acceptors have been identified and it appears that oxygen-poor environments induce the expression of some virulence factors.

Growth Characteristics

Actinobacillus grows on blood and serum-containing media at 20–42 °C as facultative anaerobes. Colony sizes at 24 h reach 1–2 mm and may be very sticky, particularly primary cultures. Some actinobacilli (*A. indolicus*, *A. minor*, *A. pleuropneumoniae* biotype 1, and *A. porcinus*) require NAD for growth, while *A. pleuropneumoniae* biotype 2 does not. They are variably hemolytic on blood agar, depending upon expression of ApxI, ApxII, or Apx (toxins with hemolytic activity). Expression of hemolytic toxins may change following *in vitro* passage, and erythrocytes from some species are more sensitive than others.

Carbohydrates are fermented without gas production. Urease, orthonitrophenyl-β-D-galactopyranosides (ONPGase, "β-galactosidase"), and nitratase are typically present; no indole is produced and some strains grow on MacConkey agar (but poorly as very small colonies). Cultures die within a week and may be difficult to recover after as few as 3 days. They are typically oxidase-positive.

Resistance

A. pleuropneumoniae contains R plasmids encoding resistance to sulfonamides, tetracycline, and penicillin G.

Variability

A. lignieresii and *A. equuli* are antigenically diverse. The six somatic types of *A. lignieresii* have some relation to geographic and host species predilection, but autoagglutinating strains are common. There are 15 somatic serotypes of *A. pleuropneumoniae* (1–15), and two biotypes (biotype 1 requires NAD for growth, but biotype 2 does not). *A. suis* has at least two somatic serotypes (1 and 2).

Ecology

Reservoir

Actinobacilli (except possibly *Actinobacillus capsulatus*) are commensal parasites on mucous membranes, perhaps added by the formation of biofilms, and toxins and proteases that interfere with host defenses. *Actinobacillus pleuropneumoniae* colonizes the tonsils of healthy pigs but is more closely associated with the respiratory tracts of sick or recovered animals and is viewed as an obligate parasite of pigs as no other host has been identified and is environmentally fragile. *A. equuli* ssp. *hemolyticus* is a pathogen restricted to horses.

Transmission

Except in neonates where infections likely originate from their mothers or the environment, most actinobacilloses are probably endogenous infections. Neonatal foals acquire *A. equuli* ssp. *equuli* before, at, or short after birth from their dams, commonly via the umbilicus. For *A. pleuropneumoniae*, transmission is both via direct contact and aerosol exposure with clinical disease as opposed to colonization being dependent on immunity and exposure dosage.

Pathogenesis

Mechanisms

Most diseases produced by members of the genus *Actinobacillus* result from "contamination" (infection) of a normally sterile, compromised site by microorganisms living on a contiguous site (niche). Common compromises are viral infections, trauma, or stress. At times it is difficult to determine the nature of the antecedent event. In neonates with septicemia, failure of passive transfer is suspected and maternal immunity is often protective. Deposition of actinobacilli into a normal sterile site results in initiation of an inflammatory response due to the LSP of the cell wall, and urease if the infecting strain produces this enzyme. The capsule interferes with phagocytosis (antiphagocytic) and protects the outer membrane from the deposition of membrane attack complexes generated by activation of the complement system. Transferrin-binding proteins participate in iron acquisition. The RTX-type toxins (Apx and Aqx) intensify the inflammatory response by activating and damaging neutrophils and macrophages. If the infectious process involves the lungs, alveolar epithelial cells are also damaged. Urease-producing actinobacilli that are phagocytosed resist destruction by generating ammonia, and perhaps superoxide dismutase. Opsonization is reduced by the production of IgG protease.

In the case of neonatal septicemia (*A. equuli* spp. *equuli*, in particular), actinobacilli gain access to the systemic circulation. Capsules and Tbps permit multiplication within the bloodstream resulting in an endotoxemia (see Figure 8.1).

Pathology

Lung lesions (usually produced by *A. equuli* ssp. *haemolytica*, *A. pleuropneumoniae*, and *A. suis*) are suppurative. Inflammatory cells are prominent, with erythrocytes, neutrophils, and mononuclear cells appearing and predominating successively. The tissue appearance changes accordingly from reddish-black to red, pink, and gray. Localized to more generalized pleuritis is common, especially in pigs. The lung lesions may nearly fully resolve over several months so that, depending on the age of the pig, prior disease may not be apparent at the time of slaughter. Making slaughter checks an unreliable means of determining the health status of a herd.

A soft tissue process, mainly produced by *A. lignieresii*, is a chronic granuloma in the ruminant tongue and occasionally other tissues. At its center is a colony of *A. lignieresii*, ringed by eosinophilic, club-like processes forming a "rosette." The complex is surrounded by neutrophils and granulation tissue containing macrophages, plasma cells, lymphocytes, giant cells, and fibroblasts. Plant fibers are often present. Through coalescence, larger granulomas (1 cm or more in diameter) may be found. Infection spreads to lymph nodes, producing granulomas along the way. The proliferative tissue reaction causes the tongue to protrude from the mouth. Other tissues in the vicinity, and occasionally among the gastrointestinal tract, may be involved, along with adjacent lymph nodes. Superficial lesions often ulcerate. In sheep, suppurative infectious occur around the head and neck and in the skin and mammary gland. Tongue involvement is not typical.

Disease Patterns

Ruminants. Actinobacillosis or "wooden tongue" involving *A. lignieresii* occurs in ruminants and, rarely, dogs, horses, and rats. In ruminants, the agent (normally inhabitant of the nasopharynx and can be recovered from the rumen) is probably inoculated by trauma (plant fibers), initiating the process described. As such, course poor-quality hay has been implicated as the basis for increased disease frequency in some herds. The course is protracted and healing is slow. Interference with feed intake causes weight loss and dehydration. On occasion it may cause mastitis.

Swine

Pneumonia. *A. pleuropneumoniae* occurs worldwide (serotypes 1 and 5 are more common in North America; serotype 2 is more common in Europe) and causes a primary pneumonia of swine (Figure 12.1). Clinical disease in its most aggressive form is remarkable among bacterial diseases in its speed, severity, and host specificity. Disease can occur at any age in susceptible animals, but significant "outbreaks" are particularly common in 2- to 6-month-old pigs. Transmission is favored by crowding and poor ventilation that under the right conditions may result in exposure levels sufficient to cause clinical disease. Early signs include lameness, fever, and reduced appetite, followed within a day or less by acute respiratory distress. In the paracute form of the disease, animals may die within 24 h or sooner. Morbidity may reach 40%, with mortality up to 24%. Survivors show intermittent nonproductive cough and unsatisfactory weight gains, regardless of antimicrobial treatment. Chronic infections, often without preceding acute episodes, are the source of persistent herd problems. Lesions consist of fibrinous pneumonia and pleuritis. Arthritis, meningitis, and abortion occur as complications. Pneumonia in older animals may be caused by *A. suis* that is difficult to differentiate from acute *A. pleuropneumoniae* infection.

FIGURE 12.1. *Consolidated lung lesion of a 3-month-old pig infected with* A. pleuropneumoniae.

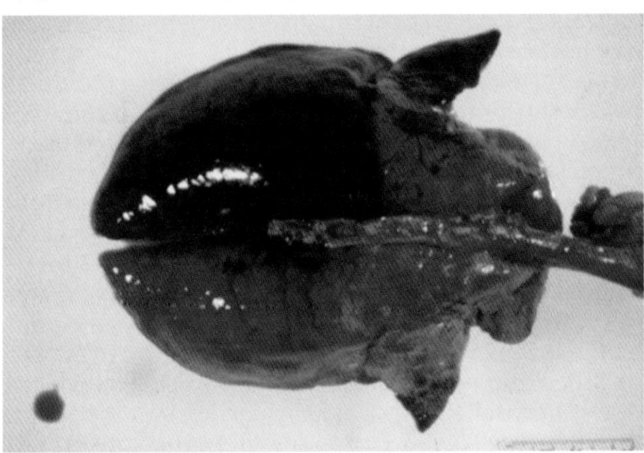

Septicemia. Septicemia of young pigs, as well as arthritis, petechial hemorrhage, and endocarditis, is sometimes associated with *A. suis* and *A. pleuropneumoniae*. Clinically this can be confused with erysipelas.

Horses

Pneumonia. Bacterial pneumonia in horses (of any age) is usually associated with a mixture of beta hemolytic streptococci (usually *S. equi* ssp. *zooepidemicus*) and gram-negative microorganisms (commonly *A. equuli* spp. *haemolytica*).

Septicemia. Foal septicemia due to *A. equuli* ssp. *equuli* ("sleepy foal disease") occurs within a few days of birth and is marked by fever, inappetence, prostration, and diarrhea (see Figure 74.1). Animals surviving the first day typically develop lameness due to (poly)arthritis. Some foals develop umbilical infections with this microorganism ("navel ill").

It can also be isolated from verminous aneurysms associated with *Strongylus vulgaris*. Sporadically, *A. equuli* ssp. *haemolyticus* is associated with metritis, abortion, endocarditis, meningitis, and other sequelae of septicemia.

Other Species. Rare actinobacilli infections (except *A. pleuropneumoniae*, which is restricted to pigs) occur in other species, including humans, and are often associated with contact with horses and pigs.

Avian Species. Members of the genus *Gallibacterium* have been isolated from birds with salpingitis, peritonitis, and bacteremia/septicemia. *Gallibacterium anatis* has been associated with these infections in a variety of avian species, while to date *Gallibacterium melopsittaci* has been isolated mostly from psittacines, and *Gallibacterium* salpingitidis has been isolated from a duck with salpingitis. The pathogenesis of these conditions has not yet been characterized.

Epidemiology

Actinobacilli are opportunistic pathogens producing disease when their host's integrity is compromised, as by trauma, immaturity, or other stress. Trauma to mucous membranes of ruminants by rough feed may cause herd outbreaks of *A. ligieresii* suggestions of transmissible disease.

In the case of porcine pleuropneumonia, chronic asymptomatic carriers are the reservoir and the basis for unexpected disease "outbreaks" and transmission between herds. Disease occurs when nonimmune animals are exposed to subclinically infected individuals that sporadically shed at sufficient levels to cause infection and at higher levels clinically apparent disease. That prevalence highest in the colder months is due probably more to management (i.e., the mixing of individuals with different exposure histories) than climate factors.

Immunologic Aspects

The pathology of "wooden tongue" suggests cell-mediated hypersensitivity. Antibodies of no known protective function appear during infection. The benefits of bacterins have not been established. Antibody to *A. pleuropneumoniae* is opsonizing and colostrum protects piglets. Antibody to RTX-type toxin and a host of other antigens are protective from clinical disease, but do not reliably prevent colonization or transmission.

Laboratory Diagnosis

The generally restricted host range and characteristic disease conditions caused by the various *Actinobacillus* species are of considerable aid in arriving at reliable presumptive etiological diagnosis. Actinobacilli can often be demonstrated in gram-stained exudates. They grow best on blood agar under increased amounts of carbon dioxide (35–37 °C). Colonies are often sticky. In most cases, speciation is accomplished by cultural and biochemical tests, which are continually being refined. A positive CAMP reaction is particularly valuable in the identification of *A. pleuropneumonia*. Because of a high degree of variability, biochemical methods alone may not be adequate to reliably determine the species. Increasingly, 16S rDNA sequence is used to confirm species identity, particularly when isolated from unusual tissues and hosts. While 16S rDNA is viewed as a reliable means to determine species, there are recognized differences in virulence between strains of the same 16S rDNA-determined species.

Serological testing has become the primary tool in control of disease and in preventing transmission of *A. pleuropneumoniae* within and between herds. Enzyme immunoassay-based methods focused on a number of species and serotype-specific antigens are more reliable than complement fixation tests. Apx toxins are good antigens, and toxin neutralization tests provide a means to differentiate vaccinated and infected pigs because vaccines generally fail to produce strong toxin-neutralizing titers.

Treatment and Control

Good management and environmental practices are the key to controlling the transmission and disease caused by actinobacilli. Porcine pleuropneumonia is controlled and treated by a combination of management practices, immunoprophylaxis, and antimicrobial therapy. Management practices including minimizing contact of piglets with mature (carrier) animals (e.g., "all in, all out," "age segregation," and "early weaning" rearing practices; and the identification and elimination of carriers by serological testing, culture, and/or by polymerase chain reaction using primers) are the most useful. Vaccination strategies include bacterins (do not prevent carrier states) and modified live vaccines (*A. pleuropneumoniae* with Apx and urease deletion mutants). Apx toxins are not stable, and the ability to induce neutralizing antibodies in the absence of a vaccine reaction has been challenging. While vaccines help to reduce the occurrence and severity of clinically apparent disease, they do not prevent colonization and shedding. Interestingly, while infection with one serotype confers strong immunity from disease caused by the other serotype, vaccine-provided protection is serotype specific. Potentially useful antimicrobial agents include penicillin G, tetracycline, gentamicin, kanamycin, cephalosporins, tilmicosin, tiamulin, florphenicol, ceftiofur, enrofloxacin, and trimethoprim–sulfas.

Autogenous bacterins are used but have not been critically evaluated for the prevention or control of *A. suis*-related disease in neonatal pigs.

In "wooden tongue" iodides given orally or intravenously promptly reduce the inflammatory swelling, which is the main clinical problem. Avoidance of harsh, dry feed reduces the likelihood of developing this condition.

Good foaling hygiene, including naval disinfection, reduces the likelihood of foal septicemia. Prophylactic use of antimicrobials is occasionally warranted. Potentially effective antimicrobial treatment of septicemia produced by *A. equuli* ssp. *equuli* include penicillin G, ceftiofur, and gentamicin.

Actinobacillus equuli spp. *haemolytica* responds to most antibiotics.

Further Reading

Chiers K, De Waele T, Pasmans F *et al.* (2010) Virulence factors of *Actinobacillus pleuropneumoniae* involved in colonization, persistence and induction of lesions in its porcine host. *Vet Res*, **41**, 65–81.

Christensen H and Bisgaard M (2004) Revised definition of *Actinobacillus sensu strict* isolated from animals. A review with special emphasis on diagnosis. *Vet Microbiol*, **99**, 13–30.

Dousse F, Thomann A, Brodard I *et al.* (2008) Routine phenotypic identification of bacterial species of the family Pasteurellaceae isolated from animals. *J Vet Diagn Invest*, **20**, 716–724.

Ramjeete M, Deslandes V, Gouré J, and Jacques M (2008) *Actinobacillus pleuropneumoniae* vaccines: from bacterins to new insights into vaccination strategies. *Anim Health Res Rev*, **9**, 25–45.

Rycroft AN and Garside LH (2000) *Actinobacillus* species and their role in animal disease. *Vet J*, **159**, 18–36.

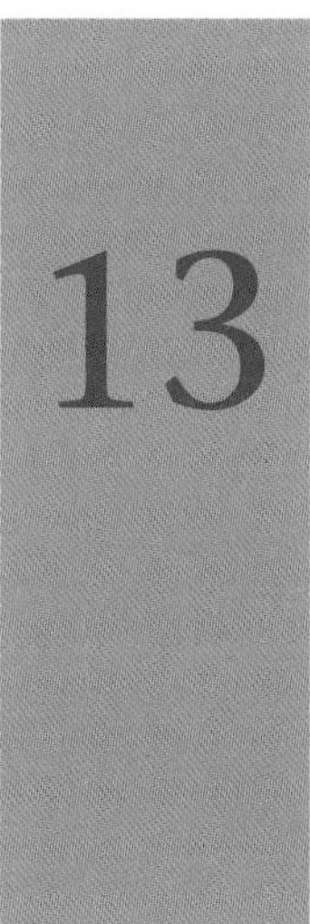

Pasteurellaceae: *Haemophilus* and *Histophilus*

Amelia R. Woolums

The family Pasteurellaceae contains many organisms that contribute to animal disease. Many are normal inhabitants of the upper respiratory and gastrointestinal tracts and cause disease opportunistically when other factors enhance their ability to advance to deeper levels of these systems. Others are infrequently isolated from normal individuals and cause severe disease when animals are exposed to these agents.

There have been many changes in the taxonomy of the family Pasteurellaceae since the second edition of this textbook was written, and more changes will likely occur in the future. At the time of this writing, there are 16 genera included in the family: *Actinobacillus*, *Aggregatibacter*, *Avibacterium*, *Basfia*, *Bibersteinia*, *Chelonobacter*, *Gallibacterium*, *Haemophilus*, *Histophilus*, *Lonepinella*, *Mannheimia*, *Necropsobacter*, *Nicoletella*, *Pasteurella*, *Phocoenobacter*, and *Volucribacter*. Bacteria from genera that contribute to important diseases of animals are described here and in Chapters 12 and 13. Discussed in this chapter are the genera *Haemophilus* and *Histophilus*, whose members play an important role in diseases of several animal species (Table 13.1).

All the members of the family Pasteurellaceae are gram-negative coccobacilli. They are facultative anaerobes, and typically oxidase-positive (which sets them apart from members of the family Enterobacteriaceae). Members of the genus *Haemophilus*, beyond sharing the traits of the family Pasteurellaceae, require for propagation one or both of two growth factors: porphyrins (hemin) or β-nicotinamide adenine dinucleotide (β-NAD), originally called X (heat-stable) and V (heat-labile) factors, respectively. Some other members of the family Pasteurellaceae also show these needs even though they are genetically unrelated to bacteria in the genus *Haemophilus*.

Original chapter written by Drs. Dwight C. Hirsh and Ernst L. Biberstein.

Discussed in this chapter are *Haemophilus parasuis*, the cause of a septicemic disease of swine characterized by polyserositis, polyarthritis, and sometimes meningitis (also known as Glässer's disease), and *Histophilus somni*, the cause of septicemic, respiratory, and genital tract disease in cattle and sheep. *H. somni* is the name now given to those microorganisms formerly named "*Haemophilus somnus*," "*Haemophilus agni*," and "*Histophilus ovis*."

Descriptive Features

Morphology and Staining

Members of the genera *Haemophilus* and *Histophilus* are gram-negative rods, <1 μm wide and usually 1–3 μm long, but sometimes forming longer filaments.

Structure and Composition

Some members of the genus *Haemophilus*, including some isolates of *H. parasuis*, can produce capsules. *H. somni* has not been shown to produce a capsule. The cell wall of bacteria in the genera *Haemophilus* and *Histophilus* is similar to other gram-negative microorganisms in that it contains lipopolysaccharide (LPS) or, in *Histophilus*, lipooligosaccharide (LOS). Other proteins are also contained in the cell wall, some of which are iron-regulated (i.e., they are expressed under iron-poor conditions).

Cellular Products of Medical Interest

Adhesins. The role of adhesins, as in other microorganisms, is to allow the bacterium expressing them to adhere to cells lining a particular niche, as well as to the surface of the so-called target cells prior to the initiation of disease (in some cases, niche and target cells may be the same). The expression of adhesins depends upon various environmental cues. Some and probably all members of the family Pasteurellaceae express adhesins (and possibly more than one kind).

Veterinary Microbiology, Third Edition. Edited by D. Scott McVey, Melissa Kennedy and M.M. Chengappa.

Table 13.1. Some Members of the Genera *Haemophilus* and *Histophilus* of Importance in Animal Disease

Genus and Species	Associated Disorder or Site
Haemophilus aegyptius	Meningoencephalitis in sheep
Haemophilus felis	Respiratory disease and conjunctivitis in cats
Haemophilus haemoglobinophilus	Cystitis and (possibly) vaginitis and balanoposthitis in dogs, neonatal infection of puppies
Haemophilus paracuniculus	Mucoid enteritis in rabbits
Haemophilus parahaemolyticus	Respiratory disease in swine
Haemophilus parainfluenzae	Respiratory disease in rabbits and guinea pigs
Haemophilus parasuis[a]	Fibrinous polyserositis, polyarthritis, and meningitis (Glässer's disease) in swine, respiratory disease in swine
Histophilus somni[a]	Respiratory disease in ruminants, bacteremia/septicemia in cattle, septic polyarthritis in cattle, thromboembolic meningoencephalitis in cattle, reproductive infection and abortion in ruminants, myocardial abscesses or pericarditis in cattle

[a]Organisms that cause disease of particular importance, as defined by relatively frequent identification of infection and relative severity of disease associated with infection.

H. somni produces a particular surface protein, which appears as fibrils when the agent is viewed with an electron microscope. These structures are responsible for the binding of the microorganism to endothelial cells, in which apoptosis is triggered with subsequent vascular leakage, fibrin deposition, and thrombosis (see Section "Mechanisms"). The protein comprising this fibrillar network is one of two immunoglobulin-binding proteins (IgBPs) produced by *H. somni*—in particular, the so-called high-molecular-weight IgBP (see Section "Immunoglobulin-Binding Proteins"). Little else is known about specific adhesins expressed by *Haemophilus suis* or *H. somni*.

Cell Wall. The cell wall of *H. parasuis* contains LPS, which can elicit a host inflammatory response following its binding to LPS-binding protein (a serum protein), which in turn transfers it to CD14 on the surface of leukocytes. The CD14–LPS complex then binds to Toll-like receptor 4 on the surface of macrophages and other leukocytes, triggering the release of proinflammatory cytokines and inducing local or systemic inflammatory responses. In *Histophilus*, the cell wall LPS is termed LOS. LOS, under the direction of the gene *lob* (for LOS biosynthesis), undergoes phase variation resulting in periodic changes in epitope expression due to periodic changes in the carbohydrate portions of the LOS. This phase variation of LOS helps *H. somni* evade the adaptive arm of the host immune response; it also renders the bacteria resistant to complement-mediated lysis (a major component of the innate immune response). As a result, isolates that undergo phase variation are more virulent. Clinical isolates from animals with disease have been shown to undergo phase variation, while isolates from the normal flora of the upper respiratory tract or distal urogenital tract do not undergo phase variation.

Immunoglobulin-Binding Proteins. There are two different IgBPs expressed on the surface of *H. somni*, a 41 kDa protein and a high-molecular-weight protein of 100–350 kDa. Both IgBPs bind immunoglobulin, but the high-molecular-weight protein preferentially binds IgG_2. Immunoglobulin molecules bind to IgBPs by way of the Fc portion, rendering the antibody ineffective for opsonization or triggering complement activation; this helps *H. somni* evade the host immune response. In addition, the high-molecular-weight IgBP serves as an adhesin (see above "Adhesins").

Capsule. Some strains of *H. parasuis* can produce capsules; *H. somni* has not been shown to produce a capsule. Bacterial capsules play many roles, the most important of which are interference with phagocytosis and the protection of the bacterial outer membrane from the deposition of membrane attack complexes generated by activation of the complement system.

Iron Acquisition. Because iron is an absolute growth requirement, microorganisms must acquire this substance if they are to exist within the host. Members of the genera *Haemophilus* and *Histophilus* bind transferrin–iron complexes by virtue of iron-regulated outer membrane proteins expressed under iron-poor conditions (so-called transferrin-binding proteins, or Tbps). Iron is acquired from the transferrin–iron complexes that bind to the surface of the microorganism.

Growth Characteristics

Members of the genera *Haemophilus* and *Histophilus* are facultative anaerobes, typically oxidase-positive, and attack carbohydrates fermentatively. *H. somni* may produce a yellowish pigment. Carbon dioxide at 5–10% enhances growth of some species of *Haemophilus* and is essential for isolation of *Histophilus*. Within 24–48 h at 35–37 °C and on adequate media, members of these genera produce turbidity in broth media or colonies on solid medium that are 1 mm in diameter. While members of the genus *Haemophilus* generally require hemin (X factor) or β-NAD (V factor), *H. somni* requires neither. *H. parasuis* requires β-NAD but not hemin. A medium, which provides both hemin and β-NAD, is "chocolate agar," a blood agar prepared by addition of blood when the melted agar is at 75–80 °C (rather than 50 °C as is the case when making regular blood agar). This procedure liberates β-NAD from cells and inactivates enzymes destructive to β-NAD.

An alternate way of providing hemin and β-NAD when attempting to identify bacteria that require these factors is to inoculate a "feeder" bacterium (e.g., *Staphylococcus*) across plates where *Haemophilus* has been streaked. The feeder bacterium will produce through metabolism the hemin and β-NAD required by the *Haemophilus*. On otherwise inadequate media, growth of small *Haemophilus* colonies can be seen only near the feeder streak, a phenomenon called "satellitism" or "satellite growth." It may be duplicated by commercially prepared X and V factor-impregnated filter papers placed on the inoculated area.

Resistance

Haemophilus and *Histophilus* are readily killed by heat and die rapidly in culture and storage unless freeze-dried or stored at −70 °C.

Variability

There are at least 15 serovars of *H. parasuis*, with different serovars demonstrating different levels of virulence. Although isolates of *H. somni* have been shown to be variable based on assessment of genetic or antigenic characteristics, serotypes of *H. somni* have not been defined at the time of this writing.

Ecology

Reservoirs

Like many members of the family Pasteurellaceae, members of the genera *Haemophilus* and *Histophilus* are normal inhabitants of the upper respiratory tract; in addition, they may be found among the normal flora of the distal urogenital tract. From these sites they may extend inward to the normally sterile regions of these organ systems and cause disease, Alternately, they may cross the epithelium of these sites and move through the host via the vascular system. *H. parasuis* lives in the nasopharynx of normal swine, while *H. somni* is found in normal cattle and sheep both in the lower genital tract (prepuce and vagina) as well as in the upper respiratory tract.

Transmission

Mechanisms of transmission of *H. parasuis* and *H. somni* have not been well characterized. It may be that infection occurs when endogenous bacteria on the upper respiratory or distal urogenital mucosa convert by some mechanism to an invasive phenotype, cross the epithelium of the mucosal surface of these sites, and move through the bloodstream to other sites in the body. Alternately, these agents may extend on the mucosal surface to the deeper and normally sterile sites in these organ systems when other insults disrupt the physical and functional barriers provided by the normal mucosa. Transmission may also occur through close contact or short distance aerosol from other infected animals. Indirect transmission (through fomites) may be important during outbreaks of *H. parasuis* infection in swine.

Pathogenesis

Mechanisms

Disease is induced when *H. parasuis* or *H. somni* invades normally sterile sites. Whether an invasive phenotype is triggered by some as yet undefined event, or whether it is happenstance "contamination" of a previously sterile site due to some primary insult such as trauma, primary viral infection, or immunocompromise associated with the stress of transport or other environmental factor, is currently not known.

In septicemic disease produced by *H. somni*, the microorganism is resistant to complement-mediated lysis and the adaptive immune response due to LOS phase variation. Both *H. parasuis* and *H. somni* can resist killing inside phagocytic cells, although the mechanisms by which they do so are not defined. Iron is acquired by removal of iron from transferrins in host plasma. In addition, antibody (especially belonging to the IgG_2 isotype) binds to IgBPs on *H. somni* by the Fc region of the antibody molecule. Antibody bound in such fashion does not trigger complement activation, nor does it serve as an opsonin. By all of these mechanisms, these bacteria are able to proliferate within the bloodstream and spread throughout the body, particularly affecting joints and the central nervous system. *H. somni* also adheres to endothelial cells by way of the high-molecular-weight IgBPs, and triggers apoptosis of these cells. Endothelial cell death through apoptosis induces thrombosis, which likely contributes to tissue necrosis and inflammation through local hypoxia due to interrupted blood flow through small blood vessels. Intravascular multiplication of bacteria and cellular injury induces a local or systemic inflammatory response.

Extension of *H. somni* or *H. parasuis* into the lower respiratory tract likely stimulates an inflammatory response by virtue of their cell wall LOS or LPS. Iron is acquired from transferrin, aiding bacterial survival. In *H. somni*, immune evasion occurs because of LOS phase variation, as well as IgBPs sidetracking antibody-mediated opsonization and complement activation. Both bacteria can survive intracellularly within phagocytic cells. While the pathogenesis of reproductive infection due to *H. somni* is not well characterized, the mechanisms described earlier are likely operative.

Disease caused by members of the genera *Haemophilus* and *Histophilus* are generally species specific.

Pathology

All infections have suppurative components brought about by the gram-negative cell wall, which triggers the release of proinflammatory cytokines from macrophages with resultant influx of neutrophils. Infection of lungs, body cavities, and joints tends to be serofibrinous to fibrinopurulent. Because of the ability of *H. somni* to induce apoptotic death of endothelial cells, which leads to platelet aggregation and thrombus formation, thrombosis is a characteristic microscopic finding in lesions caused by *H. somni*. For example, colonization of *H. somni* in the microvasculature of the central nervous system produces thrombotic vasculitis leading to encephalitis and meningitis. Thrombosis also leads to vascular leakage and decreased blood flow to tissues downstream of the thrombus; thus, hemorrhagic, necrotizing lesions are often a feature of pathology caused by *H. somni*.

Disease Patterns

Ruminants

Bovine Thrombotic Meningoencephalitis. Thrombotic meningoencephalitis (also known as "infectious thromboembolic meningoencephalitis"—an inaccurate designation as embolus formation does not appear to be a component of the pathogenesis of the disease) is a consequence of septicemia produced by *H. somni* leading to endothelial cell injury and then thrombosis in the microvasculature of the cerebrum and cerebellum. Thrombus formation leads to infarcts, interrupted blood flow, and necrosis, which leads to inflammation and thus meningoencephalitis. Affected animals show clinical abnormalities referable to the inflammatory process in the affected regions of the central nervous system, with depression and stupor being common. The pre-encephalitic stage is marked by high fever.

Pneumonia and Pleuropneumonia. *H. somni* can cause suppurative bronchopneumonia or fibrinous pleuropneumonia in ruminants, most commonly in cattle. The agent commonly contributes to the development of "shipping fever" in recently transported cattle, along with viral agents, mycoplasmas, and *Mannheimia haemolytica* and *Pasteurella multocida* ssp. *multocida*. Cattle with pneumonia due to *H. somni* may have concurrent septic arthritis in one or more joints, which is also due *H. somni*.

Bacteremia/Septicemia. *H. somni* can cause bacteremia and septicemia in ruminants, resulting in signs of a systemic inflammatory response and sometimes leading to arthritis, myocarditis, or abortion.

Myocarditis and Pericarditis. *H. somni* can cause myocarditis, myocardial abscesses, and/or pericarditis in cattle; these conditions can be common in feedlot cattle, particularly in the Northwestern United States and Western Canada. Affected cattle often die acutely with no previous signs of disease.

Abortion, Reproductive Infections, and Mastitis. Abortion due to *H. somni* sometimes occurs in ruminants. Whether this is most often secondary to bacteremia or to ascending infection from the urogenital tract has not been determined. Reproductive infections (such as metritis or epididymitis) or mastitis in ruminants can also be caused by *H. somni*.

Swine

Bacteremia/Septicemia. In young weaned pigs, *H. parasuis* causes polyserositis, polyarthritis, and sometimes meningitis (also known as Glässer's disease). Infection leads to an acute inflammatory response with fibrinous polyserositis, which can affect the pleura, peritoneum, mediastinum, pericardium, joints, and meninges. Weaning, transport, and management stress are predisposing causes. The disease strikes sporadically within days of the predisposing event. Morbidity and mortality are often low because of widespread acquired resistance, but they may be high in previously unexposed herds (e.g., specific pathogen-free herds). Disease manifestations include fever and general malaise, respiratory distress and abdominal discomfort, lameness, and paralytic or convulsive signs. Disease can be fatal, or recovery can follow, typically in 1–2 weeks. Similar syndromes can be caused by *Mycoplasma hyorhinis*.

Respiratory Disease. *H. parasuis* can cause bronchopneumonia in swine; this may be secondary to virus infections (e.g., due to swine influenza). Other bacteria (e.g., *Pasteurella* spp. and *Mycoplasma* spp.) may also participate.

Dogs. *Haemophilus haemoglobinophilus*, a commensal of the canine lower genital tract, sometimes causes cystitis and neonatal infections. Its role in canine balano-posthitis and vaginitis, where it is frequently found, is uncertain.

Cats. *Haemophilus felis* can be associated with conjunctivitis and respiratory disease in cats.

Immunity

Basis of Immunity

Circulating antibody develops in infected individuals and has a protective function. Immunity to *H. parasuis* occurs after experimental or natural infection; however, immunity to the infecting serotype is more consistent than is cross-protective immunity to other serotypes.

Infection or vaccination of cattle with *H. somni* can induce production of IgE directed against the agent, which has been associated with disease of increased severity. This is probably due to IgE-mediated degranulation of mast cells and eosinophils and resultant release of inflammatory mediators. In cattle, coinfection with bovine respiratory syncytial virus (a common respiratory virus of cattle) and *H. somni* has been shown to increase production of *H. somni*-specific IgE more than that which occurs in cattle infected with *H. somni* alone.

Vaccination

Vaccines are commercially available for use to prevent and control respiratory disease due to *H. somni* in cattle. While vaccination can decrease the incidence of respiratory disease in at-risk animals (such as feedlot cattle), protection is not inevitable. The efficacy of these vaccines in preventing meningoencephalitis, polyarthritis, reproductive, or cardiac disease in cattle is not well characterized.

In the United States, a modified live vaccine is commercially available for control of disease due to *H. parasuis* in swine. Autogenous vaccines have also been used to prevent disease due to *H. parasuis*. It is important for isolates used in autogenous vaccines to represent the virulent serotype causing disease; nonvirulent serotypes of *H. parasuis*, which may not induce protective immunity, can be concurrently isolated from diseased animals.

Laboratory Diagnosis

Recovery of members of the genera *Haemophilus* and *Histophilus* from infected tissues or fluids is usually required to establish a diagnosis. However, these agents can be fastidious relative to other commensal or contaminating organisms that may also be present in samples; thus, it is important for veterinarians submitting samples to diagnostic laboratories to specifically request that the laboratory attempt to isolate *Haemophilus* or *Histophilus* if disease due to these agents is suspected. Identification of genus and species-specific DNA by polymerase chain reaction (PCR) may be easier than culture of these agents if the laboratory offers this test; however, diagnosis made in this manner will not result in an isolate that can be used to identify serotype (in the case of *H. parasuis*) or antimicrobial susceptibility profile. Also, some studies have shown PCR to be less sensitive than culture for isolation of *H. parasuis*.

Organisms requiring X factor cannot convert delta-aminolevulinic acid to urobilinogen and porphyrin. The porphyrin test determines this ability and X factor requirement most reliably. Definitive assignment to a species usually requires additional tests.

Treatment and Control

Bacteria in the genera *Haemophilus* and *Histophilus* are generally susceptible to antimicrobials effective against gram-negative organisms; they may also be susceptible to antimicrobials not usually chosen for treatment of gram-negative organisms, such as penicillin. Resistance to antimicrobials does not appear to be an important problem at this time. Effective treatment of infection by these organisms is thus possible, and some antibiotics are specifically labeled for treatment of respiratory disease due to *H. somni* in cattle. However, effective treatment of some conditions caused by *Haemophilus* or *Histophilus somni* may be difficult if the nature of the pathologic lesion is such that a long course of therapy is required (e.g., septic arthritis in a feedlot steer). In such cases, it may not be practically feasible to treat the animal effectively due to management or financial constraints.

Control of disease due to these agents can be aided in some cases by vaccination (see Section "Vaccination"). Management to prevent or limit primary insults that may increase susceptibility to infection, such as primary viral respiratory infection, may also help to limit disease due to these agents.

Further Reading

Dousse F, Thomann A, Brodard I *et al.* (2008) Routine phenotypic identification of bacterial species of the family Pasteurellaceae isolated from animals. *J Vet Diagn Invest*, **20**, 716–724.

Nedbalcova K, Satran P, Jaglic Z *et al.* (2006) *Haemophilus parasuis* and Glässer's disease in pigs: a review. *Vet Med (Praha)*, **51**, 168–179.

Oliveira S and Pijoan C (2004) *Haemophilus parasuis*: new trends on diagnosis, epidemiology, and control. *Vet Microbiol*, **99**, 1–12.

Siddaramppa S and Inzana TJ (2004) *Haemophilus somnus* virulence factors and resistance to host immunity. *Anim Health Res Rev*, **5**, 79–93.

14 Bordetella

BRADLEY W. FENWICK

Members of the genus *Bordetella* are gram-negative coccobacilli belonging to the family Alcaligenaceae and related to *Alcaligenes* and *Achromobacter*. Currently there are nine species described, most of which are important pathogens of humans and other animals (Table 14.1), and numerous isolates with uncertain phylogeny that are most closely related to the *Bordetella*. *Bordetella pertussis* is the type strain, which with *B. parapertussis*, *B. bronchiseptica*, and *B. avium* are referred to as the "classic" *Bordetella* species. *B. pertussis and B. parapertussis* are genetically closely related to and evolved from a historical lineage of *B. bronchiseptica*. *B. avium* is genetically distinct. Associated with the adaption to being a human-specific pathogen, *B. pertussis* has a genome that is reduced in size while maintaining the virulence factors of associated with the other *Bordetella* species. Based on 16S rDNA sequence, *B. pertussis* and *B. holmesii* are closed related. Interestingly, while the genes may be present the expression of key virulence factors varies between the classic *Bordetella* species. For example, only *B. pertussis* expresses pertussis toxin but is transcriptionally silenced in *B. parapertussis* and *B. bronchiseptica*.

All but one (*Bordetella petrii*) are aerobic bacteria that are highly adapted to be parasites of ciliated respiratory epithelium. *B. petrii* is a facultative anaerobe that lives in the environment and is occasionally associated with human infection and disease in compromised individuals. *B. pertussis* (and, rarely, *B. parapertussis and B. hinzii*) causes whooping cough or whooping cough like disease in humans. On rare occasions *B. hinzii*, *B. ansorpii*, and *B. avium* cause opportunistic infections in humans. Of veterinary importance, and the main topic of discussion in this chapter are *B. bronchiseptica*, which has been implicated in porcine atrophic rhinitis, canine and feline kennel cough, and bronchopneumonia in other species and *B. avium*, the cause of rhinotracheitis of birds (mainly turkeys). To be complete, *B. parapertussis* infection in sheep and *B. hinzii* infection of poultry are briefly reviewed.

Original chapter written by Drs. Dwight C. Hirsh and Ernst L. Biberstein.

Descriptive Features

Morphology and Staining

Bordetellae are pleomorphic gram-negative coccobacilli, about 0.5 μm × up to 2 μm in size.

Structure and Composition

The cell wall is typical of gram-negative bacteria being composed of lipopolysaccharide (LPS) and protein. *B. bronchiseptica* produces a capsule. All members of the genus that have been evaluated produce fimbrial adhesins (pili) and biofilms. *B. bronchiseptica* and *B. avium* are motile by peritrichous flagella.

Cellular Products of Medical Interest

With few exceptions, *B. pertussis*, *B. parapertussis*, *B. bronchiseptica*, and *B. avium* produce (or at least have the genes to produce) many of the same products important in the pathogenesis of disease (Table 14.2).

Adhesins. The role of adhesins, as in other microorganisms, is to allow the bacterium expressing them to adhere to cells lining a particular niche, as well as to the surface of so-called target cells prior to the initiation of disease (in some cases, niche and target cells may be the same). The expression of adhesins depends upon various environmental cues. Binding followed by adherence appears to be at least a two-step process involving sequential involvement of different adhesins.

Bordetellae produce a number of structures that are responsible for adherence to host cells. These adhesins include fimbriae (or pili), filamentous hemagglutinin (FHA), pertactin, cell wall LPS, tracheal colonization factor (Tcf), and pertussis toxin. All are positively regulated by the BvgAS regulon (see Section "Regulation of the Cellular Products of Medical Interest").

1. *Fimbriae*: Fimbriae are protein structures composed, in part, of subunits (pilins) responsible for adherence to receptors on host cells. While not required for colonization, *Bordetella* fimbriae adhere to ciliated epithelial cells and mucus of the respiratory

Veterinary Microbiology, Third Edition. Edited by D. Scott McVey, Melissa Kennedy and M.M. Chengappa.

Table 14.1. Members of the Genus *Bordetella* and There Usual Source or Associated Condition

Species	Usual Source or Associated Condition
Bordetella pertussis	Whooping cough in humans, chimpanzees
B. parapertussis	Whooping cough-like disease in humans; chronic nonprogressive pneumonia in sheep (human and sheep strains are different)
B. bronchiseptica	Atrophic rhinitis in swine, respiratory tract disease in many animals
B. avium	Rhinotracheitis in poultry (especially turkeys, coryza) and wild birds
B. hinzii	Commensal in poultry, rare respiratory disease in turkeys, septicemia in humans
B. holmesii	Whooping cough-like disease and septicemia in humans
B. trematum	Opportunistic infections in humans
B. petrii	Opportunistic infections in humans
B. ansorpii	Opportunistic infections in humans

tract and are necessary for persistence. They are in the same family as the type 1 fimbriae produced by enterobacteria and are encoded by four structural genes fim2, fim3, fimX, and fimA that are distributed in the genome. Fimbrial proteins are strongly antigenic, responsible for agglutination by immune sera, and are the basis of different serotypes (see Section "Variability"). Expression of fimbrial proteins is regulated by the BvgAS system as well as can undergo phase variation caused by slipped-strand mispairing during replication. The independent location of fimbrial genes allows of protein-specific phase variants, serotype switching, and perhaps enhanced survive in the face of a host immune response. Binding is via sulfated glycoconjugates on epithelial cells that can increase the expression of CR3 integrin to which FHA binds.

2. *Filamentous hemagglutinin*: FHA is a generally highly conserved very large complex protein adhesin that has a number of activities associated with various domains within the protein. The FHA of *B. holmesii* is distinct. FHA undergoes significant posttranslational modification that results in a 220 kDa mature protein from a 370 kDa precursor forming a 50-nm long filamentous molecule that includes a hairpin fold. It crosses the outer membrane via a two-partner secretion system. The N-proximal region is similar to various other adhesins and toxins produced by other gram-negative pathogens. Minor variations in critical binding domains may, in part, explain species- and strain-dependent differences in host specificity, virulence, and persistence. There is clear evidence that FHA is required but not sufficient for adherence to ciliated epithelial cells of the respiratory tract and for binding to macrophages. This is accomplished by way of heparin-binding, carbohydrate-binding, and/or a "Arg-Gly-Asp" (RGD) sequence that targets CR3 integrin. The heparin-binding domain is responsible for hemagglutinin, except in *B. avium*. FHA is also involved in biofilm formation. It induces a strong protective antibody response.
3. *Pertactin*: Prn (for pertactin, so names because of being a protective antigen) is an outer membrane protein that functions as an adhesion and is a member of a family of proteins know as "autotransporter" which are virulence factors in many gram-negative bacteria (e.g., *Neisseria* IgA protease). Numerous other autotransport proteins have been

Table 14.2. Cellular Products of Medical Interest within Members of the Genus *Bordetella*

Product	*B. pertussis*	*B. parapertussis*	*B. bronchiseptica*	*B. avium*
Adhesins and others				
Fimbria	+	+	+	+
Filamentous hemagglutinin	+	+	+	+
Pertactin	+ (69 kDa)	+ (70 kDa)	+ (68 kDa)	−
Tracheal colonization factor	+	−	−	ND
Pertussis toxin	+	−[a]	−[a]	−
Biofilm	+	+	+	ND
Toxins				
Tracheal cytotoxin	+	+	+	+
Dermonecrotic toxin	+	+	+	+
Adenylate cyclase toxin	+	+	+	−
Pertussis toxin	+	−[a]	−[a]	−
Osteotoxin	+	−[a]	+	+
Other				
Capsule	−	−	+	−
Iron Scavenging	+	+	+	+
Type III secretion system	+	+	+	−
Brk	+	+	+	−
BatB	−	+	+	−

[a]Genes encoded but protein is not produced.
ND, not determined.

identified among the bordetellae (including BatB), but their role in the ecology of *Bordetella* infection and pathogenesis of disease is not known. Like FHA, pertactin contains an "Arg-Gly-Asp" or RGD sequence involved in the binding to host cell integrins. Though a particular host target cell has not been identified for Prn, it is likely that ciliated epithelial cells of the respiratory tract, as well as phagocytic cells are the targets. It also has two areas of repetitive amino acids (GGXXP and PQP) that vary in number and responsible for the difference in size of the mature protein (68–70 kDa) between different species and strains, and are protective epitopes.

4. *Tracheal colonization factor*: Tcf is a protein adhesin this is similar to pertactin (e.g., autotransporter, contains Arg-Gly-Asp sequences, and proline-rich regions) that binds to ciliated epithelial cells of the respiratory tract. It appears to target the trachea and produced by *B. pertussis* and not by either *B. parapertussis* or *B. bronchiseptica*.
5. *Pertussis toxin*: Ptx (for pertussis toxin) is composed of five unique subunits and functions as both an ADP-ribosylating toxin (see Section "Exotoxins") and as an adhesin. Synthesized only by *B. pertussis*, a portion of Ptx is excreted from the bacterial cell, and a portion remains attached to its surface. It is the surface-associated portion that serves as the adhesin. The host cell types to which Ptx adheres are ciliated epithelial cells of the respiratory tract, and phagocytic cells. While the genes for Ptx are present in both *B. parapertussis* and *B. bronchiseptica*, they are not expressed because of a number of point mutations, particularly in the promoter.
6. *Biofilm*: Biofilms are produced by a majority of pathogenic bacteria, providing a degree of protection against environmental and host factors, as well as provide resistance to a number of antimicrobial agents. While poly-glucosamine (PGA) is not required for the formation of biofilms by *Bordetella*, it contributes to biofilm stability. A xylose polymer is also produced as part of the biofilm. As with other virulence factors, biofilm production is regulated by BvgAS system, and there is evidence that fimbria, FHA, and pertactin could be involved in the formation and/or stabilization of biofilms. *In vivo* evaluation demonstrates that biofilm contributing to the attachment of *B. bronchiseptica* to nasal epithelium.

Capsule. The capsule plays many roles, the most important of which are interference with phagocytosis (antiphagocytic) and protection of the outer membrane from the deposition of membrane attack complexes generated by activation of the complement system.

Cell Wall. The cell wall of the members of this genus is one typical of gram-negative bacteria being composed of carbohydrates, lipids, and protein. Bordetellae possess LPS and outer membrane proteins that are important virulence determinants:

1. *Lipopolysaccharide*: Cell wall LPS of *B. avium*, and by inference *B. pertussis*, *B. parapertussis*, and *B. bronchiseptica*, serves as an adhesin by binding to ciliated epithelium of the respiratory tract, and as a "shield" to cover the outer membrane protecting it from the action of membrane attack complexes generated by the complement system. The LPS in the outer membrane is an important virulence determinant, interacting with the innate and adaptive immune responses, and likely acting in association with other toxins. Not only is the lipid A component toxic (endotoxin), but the length of the side chain in the O-repeat unit hinders the attachment of the membrane attack complex of the complement system to the outer membrane and imparts resistance to antimicrobial proteins (defensins) found in respiratory tract secretions and within phagocytic cell granules. LPS binds to LPS-binding protein, which transfers it to the blood-phase of CD14. The CD14-LPS complex binds to Toll-like receptor proteins (see Chapter 2) on the surface of macrophage cells triggering the release of proinflammatory cytokines including tumor necrosis factor. The composition of the LPS (presence or absence of the O-repeat portion, its length, charge, and fatty acid substitutions) influences the extent of protection against the complement system and antimicrobial peptides and may be involved in differences in virulence between strains. *B. pertussis* has two types of LPS, LPSI and LPSII. LPS composition is regulated by the BvgAS regulon (see Section "Regulation of the Cellular Products of Medical Interest").
2. *Outer membrane protein*: Brk (for *Bordetella* resistance to killing) is an outer membrane protein and provides resistance against serum-mediated killing. Brk imparts resistance to damage by the complement system and may also function as an adhesion (contains two Arg-Gly-Asp regions as well as binding locations for sulfated glycoconjugates). Brk is regulated by the BvgAS regulon (see Section "Regulation of the Cellular Products of Medical Interest").

Exotoxins. There are five described exotoxins produced by the bordetellae that play important roles in diseases associated with members of this genus: tracheal cytotoxin, dermonecrotic toxin (DNT), adenylyl cyclase toxin, pertussis toxin, and osteotoxin. All, except and osteotoxin and tracheal cytotoxin (a portion of the cell wall, are regulated by the BvgAS regulon (see Section "Regulation of the Cellular Products of Medical Interest").

1. *Tracheal cytotoxin*: Produced by the "Classic" *Bordetella* species plus *B. avium*, tracheal cytotoxin is a fragment of the *Bordetella* peptidoglycan cell wall that is identical to *Neisseria gonorrhoeae* ciliostatic anhydropeptidoglycan that in other gram-negative bacteria is recycled is released instead released. Acting in association with LPS, tracheal cytotoxin damages ciliated epithelial cells by interfering with DNA synthesis (LPS). Tracheal cytotoxin also induces the

production of interleukin-1 (IL-1) and excessive amounts of nitric oxide from macrophages.

2. *Dermonecrotic toxin*: DNT is a member of a family of toxins with similar structures and biological activity. The other "dermonecrotic" toxins include Pmt produced by *Pasteurella multocida* (see Chapter 11), and CNF1 and CNF2 produced by *E. coli* (see Chapter 7). These toxins are so named because dermonecrosis follows their injection into the skin, an occurrence that does not occur naturally (DNT is not secreted). DNT deaminates and transglutamates (preferred) the small GTP-binding protein Rho blocking its GTPase activity (i.e., GTPase activating proteins are unable to correctly bind to modified Rho). These modifications result in changes in the actin cytoskeleton of affected cells (actin stress fibers) and inhibition of differentiation of osteoblasts in bone tissue. DNT expression is required for *B. bronchiseptica* to cause turbinate atrophy in pigs and pneumonia in mice, and for *B. avium* to be pathogenic.
3. *Adenylyl cyclase toxin*: Adenylyl cyclase toxin is a bifunctional protein with independent adenylyl cyclase as well as hemolytic activity that is produced by classic *Bordetella* species but not *B. avium.* Adenylyl cyclase toxin is the only known *Bordetella* exotoxin that is secreted without proteolytic cleavage. It enters the host cell and following "activation" by calmodulin, increases the intracellular concentration of cAMP. Affected cells lose control of intracellular levels of cAMP, resulting in an inability to regulate ion and fluid flow into and out of the "target" cell (respiratory tract epithelium). Loss of control of cAMP levels in phagocytic cells results in reduction of this cell's ability to phagocytose and kill. The hemolytic activity is associated with an RTX motif (repeats in toxin, so-called because of the common feature of repeats in glycine-rich sequences within the protein, see also *E. coli* hemolysin in Chapter 7, *Pasteurella/Mannheimia* leukotoxin in Chapter 11, *Actinobacillus* hemolysin in Chapter 12, *Moraxella* cytotoxin in Chapter 18). By virtue of the RTX-type toxin activity, adenylyl cyclase toxin is also a pore-forming protein that targets neutrophils, macrophages, and lymphocytes. Taken together, adenylyl cyclase production is necessary for infection and plays a central role in virulence.
4. *Pertussis toxin*: Pertussis toxin (Ptx) is an ADP-ribosylating toxin that ribosylates "activated" heterotrimeric G proteins (GTP-bound), rendering them incapable of returning to the inactive state (GDP-bound). "Activated" G proteins stimulate adenylyl cyclase leading to increased levels of intracellular cAMP. Abnormally high concentration of cAMP results in loss of fluid and ion flow into and out of the cell, and if the cell has phagocytic function, interference with uptake and intracellular killing. While Ptx causes considerable dysfunction in a number of metabolic pathways, the host cell typically is not killed. The role of Ptx as an adhesin is discussed earlier. Ptx induces a significant and fully protective immune response.
5. *Osteotoxin*: Osteotoxin is produced by *B. avium, B. pertussis,* and *B. bronchiseptica* but not by *B. parapertussis.* It is lethal to tracheal and bone cells via the reactive products of cleaved extracellular cysteine.

Iron Acquisition. Because iron is an absolute growth requirement, microorganisms must acquire this substance if they are to exist within the host. Bordetellae acquire iron by secreting a siderophore and utilizing siderophores made by other species of microorganism. In addition, they utilize the iron found in heme and hemoproteins.

Under conditions of iron starvation (as would occur in the host), bordetellae secrete a hydroxamate-type siderophore called alcaligin. Bordetellae also have the ability to utilize enterobactin, a siderophore produced by members of the family *Enterobacteriaceae,* as well as xenosiderophores. These siderophores (alcaligin and enterobactin) remove iron from the iron-binding proteins of the host (transferrin and lactoferrin), making it available to the bacterium.

Heme and hemoproteins (albumin and hemopexin) are additional sources of iron. The outer membrane protein that binds these substances, BhuR (for Bordetella heme uptake receptor), is regulated by levels of available iron by means of the extracytoplasmic sigma factor Rhu (for regulation of heme uptake) and the Fur regulon (see *E. coli,* Chapter 7).

Type III Secretion System. A type III secretion system has been identified in the *B. bronchiseptica* and *B. parapertussis* (under the control of the BvgAS regulon, see Section "Regulation of the Cellular Products of Medical Interest"). While the genes are present in *B. pertussis* and human strains of *B. parapertussis,* evidence of production is lacking, *B. avium* appears to lack the required genes. The type III secretion system consists of an assemblage of proteins (more than 20) that form a hollow tube-like structure through which effector proteins are "injected" into host "target" cells. As yet, *Bordetella* effector proteins have not been identified, but host "target" cells (tracheal epithelial cells, phagocytic cells) undergo apoptosis as a result of effector protein "injection," resulting in loss of epithelial integrity, and evasion of the immune system of the host (decreased phagocytosis, and decreased antigen processing which leads to reduced immune responses).

Regulation of the Cellular Products of Medical Interest. Bordetellae transcriptionally regulated by a two-component system, the genes encoding products involved in the production of disease. These include the genes encoding all of the adhesins (fimbriae, FHA, pertactin, the character of the cell wall LPS, Tcf, and pertussis toxin), pertactin, Brk, toxins (adenylyl cyclase, DNT, pertussis toxin), alcaligin, biofilm, and the type III secretion system. All are regulated by the products of the genes encoded in bvgA and bvgS (for *Bordetella* virulence genes) and are referred to as the BvgAS regulon. BvgS is a histidine kinase that acts as a "sensor" of environmental cues, resulting in autophosphorylation of one of its histidine residues. This phosphate is then serially transferred to an aspartate residue, then to another histidine before being used to phosphorylate BvgA. Phosphorylated BvgA is a transcriptional activator of the genes encoding the products mentioned above and is responsible for phenotype modulation and phase variation. Not all virulence factor expression is regulated to the same degree under different environmental conditions, thus producing a continuum of phenotypes. It is unclear exactly what the environmental cues are that are "sensed" by *Bordetella*. Growth at 37 °C in low concentrations of $MgSO_4$ and nicotinic acid activates the regulon. Though growth at 37 °C is compatible with a parasitic state, it is unclear what role $MgSO_4$ and nicotinic acid concentrations play *in vivo*.

Growth Characteristics

All but one of the species of Bordetella is strict aerobes, deriving energy from oxidation of amino acids. *B. petrii* (the exception) is a facultative anaerobe. They are fastidious and can be difficult to culture, particularly on primary isolation, forming mature colonies in 1–3 days. Growth can be inhibited by fatty acids, particularly in the case of *B. pertussis*, which requires the use of specialized media. *B. bronchiseptica* and *B. avium* grow on ordinary laboratory media (35–37 °C), including MacConkey agar, under atmospheric conditions; the former is inconsistently hemolytic on blood agar. *B. bronchiseptica*, *B. avium*, and *B. hinzii* are motile.

Biochemical Activities

B. avium and *B. bronchiseptica* are catalase and oxidase-positive, ferment no carbohydrates, and utilize citrate as an organic carbon source. *B. bronchiseptica*, *B. avium*, and *B. hinzii* are oxidase-positive. Only *B. bronchiseptica* reduces nitrate and produces urease, *B. parapertussis* is weakly urease-positive.

Resistance

Bordetella spp. are killed by heat or disinfectants. They are susceptible to broad-spectrum antibiotics and polymyxin, but not to penicillin. Their environmental survival is epidemiologically significant.

Variability

An assortment of typing schemes has been developed, mainly for epidemiological purposes. At least four serotypes have been described for bordetellae based upon the Fim protein (see Section "Adhesins"). Except for *fimA*, the fimbrial genes of *B. avium* are not shared with the *Bordetella*. Related to differences in the number of proline-rich repeats, pertactin varies both in size and in antigenic character between *Bordetella* species and also within strains of the same species.

B. bronchiseptica dissociates into four phases varying in colonial characteristics, hemolytic activity, suspension stability in saline, ease of colonization, and toxicity. Some strains appear to be host specific. Some 20 heat-labile (K) and heat-stable (O; 120 °C/60 min) antigens exist. Many are common to several species. Others are species and type specific. *B. bronchiseptica* from pigs appear different from the strains from dogs and horses (which are also different from each other). Other strain-specific disease, phenotype, and molecular differences have been identified and hypothesized to be the basis for vaccine failures.

Three serotypes, based on surface agglutinins, are recognized in *B. avium*.

B. parapertussis strains that infect and cause disease in humans are distinct from those strains that cause chronic nonprogressive pneumonia in sheep.

Ecology

Reservoir

Bordetella spp. are mainly parasites of ciliated respiratory tract tissue. Bordetellae are found in the nasopharynx of healthy animals. *B. bronchiseptica* associated disease (either as a primary or secondary infection) occurs in wild and domestic carnivores, wild and laboratory rodents, swine, rabbits, and occasionally horses, koalas, seals, other herbivores, primates, and turkeys.

B. avium inhabits the respiratory tract of infected wild and domestic fowl, resulting in disease principally in turkeys (coryza).

Transmission

Mammalian infections are primarily airborne, but environmental contamination is a significant factor in some cases, while in turkeys (*B. avium*) indirect spread via contaminated water and litter is common. Experimentally, as few as 10 organisms can establish an infection. Transmission can occur rapidly resulting in significant acute disease outbreaks. Environmental conditions (temperature, humidity) and host density influence the frequency and severity of clinical disease. The hypothesis is that phenotype shifts (loss of adhesins) associated with the BvgAS system promote transmission and that once deposited in a new host the appropriate environmental are recognized thus reactivating the BvgAS system resulting in adhesion and toxin expression.

Pathogenesis

Mechanisms

Bordetellae "sense" various environmental cues, leading to activation of the BvgAS regulon and upregulation of the various genes encoding the products discussed earlier (see Section "Cellular Products of Medical Interest"). Attachment of bordetellae to ciliated epithelial cells follows expression of adhesins (fimbriae, FHA, pertactin, cell wall LPS, Tcf, and biofilms—see Table 14.2 for listing of which adhesins are produced by which bordetellae). Multiplication occurs (iron is scavenged from host iron-binding proteins—lactoferrin and transferrin—and from heme and hemoproteins; bordetellae outer membrane is protected from complement-generated membrane attack complexes by capsule, LPS, Brk) and inflammation is initiated (LPS; death of epithelial cells due to "injection" of effector proteins; tracheal cytotoxin). Inflammation and loss of the ability to control fluid and ion flow into and out of tracheal epithelial cells (increased production of cAMP from effects of increased activity of adenylyl cyclase) leads to increased mucus and fluid accumulation in the upper respiratory tract. Ciliated epithelial cells become ineffectual in clearing secretions (cilial paralysis due to increased levels of cAMP and cytoskeletal changes brought about by the action of DNT; death of ciliated cell due to tracheal cytotoxin, and the unidentified effector protein "injected" by way of the type III secretion system). Unencapsulated bordetellae adhere to inflammatory cells (by way of FHA, pertactin, and pertussis toxin), and release adenylyl cyclase (interferes with phagocytosis and killing), pertussis toxin (interferes with phagocytosis and killing), and "injection" of an effector protein (interferes with phagocytosis). If phagocytosis occurs, bordetellae survive within phagolysosomes (nature of their LPS) and also escape into endocytic compartments that do not lead to lysosomal fusion.

The consequences of Bordetella-induced changes in the ciliated portions of the respiratory tract are varied: depression of respiratory clearance mechanisms, facilitating secondary complications (e.g., pneumonia); in pigs, *B. bronchiseptica* provides nasal irritation, rendering the turbinates susceptible to the action of the DNT (Pmt) of *P. multocida*, which has emerged as the primary agent of atrophic rhinitis ("progressive atrophic rhinitis," see Chapter 11). If *P. multocida* does not become involved, DNT as well as all of the products described above, produces a mild, reversible turbinate hypoplasia ("nonprogressive atrophic rhinitis"). Pneumonia, if this occurs, is due to inflammatory responses and the inability of host phagocytic cells and complement system to easily clear bordetellae.

Pathology

The attachment and destruction of ciliated respiratory epithelium is the hallmark of Bordetella-initiated disease. The process is a suppurative one affecting various portions of the tract (rhinitis, sinusitis, tracheitis). Compromise of the clearance mechanisms of the upper respiratory tract may lead to a suppurative pneumonia and airsacculitis with *Bordetella* itself and often secondary superinfections with other bacteria that can significantly enhance disease severity.

Disease Patterns

Swine

Atrophic rhinitis. The progressive form of atrophic rhinitis is due to combined infection with *P. multocida* and *B. bronchiseptica*, and was discussed in Chapter 11. The nonprogressive form of this disease follows infection with *B. bronchiseptica* alone and is transient and self-limiting, most frequently causing disease (sneezing and nasal discharge) in pigs 3–4 weeks old.

Pneumonia. Compromise of the host defenses of the upper respiratory tract sometimes leads to secondary pneumonia associated with *B. bronchiseptica* or some other microorganism. Primary pneumonia caused by *B. bronchiseptica* occurs in neonatal pigs (3–4 days old) and is characterized by coughing, dyspnea, and at times high morbidity and mortality. Disease outbreaks are likely associated with failure of passive transfer or low material immunity.

Dogs and Cats

Canine Infectious Tracheobronchitis (Kennel Cough). Kennel cough is associated with *B. bronchiseptica*; with clinical disease being most common in young dogs, mature vaccinated dogs are susceptible under the right circumstances. The natural disease may be accompanied by canine parainfluenza virus, canine adenoviruses 1 and 2, and canine herpesvirus. Rapidly progressing disease outbreaks occur in kennels and animal hospitals. The incubation period is around a week followed by acute coughing, in the most severe cases gagging and retching. While most dogs recover within a few weeks without treatment, the bacterium can persist for months and relapses are possible. Transfer of the same strain to susceptible cats has been demonstrated.

Pneumonia. *B. bronchiseptica* is sometimes isolated from samples collected from pneumonic lungs, often from dogs with canine distemper.

Cats. *B. bronchiseptica* produces a mild upper respiratory tract infection in cats (tracheobronchitis, conjunctivitis) that spontaneously resolves in less than 10 days. Clinical disease is most notably in cat colonies (upper respiratory tract infections in cats are also associated with herpesvirus, calicivirus, *Mycoplasma*, *Chlamydophila*). Coughing is not common. Cats, like dogs, carry the organism asymptomatically (up to 19 weeks) following recovery. Secondary bronchiopneumonia in kittens and immunocompromised cats has been reported. Transfer of the same strain to susceptible dogs has been demonstrated.

Poultry

Turkey Coryza. Turkey poults infected with *B. avium* develop tracheobronchitis, sinusitis, and airsacculitis. Signs include nasal exudate, conjunctivitis, sneezing, tracheal rales, and dyspnea. Morbidity can be very high, but mortality, except by secondary infection, is generally low (<5%). Recovery may begin after 2 weeks, although some illnesses may last 6 weeks and is associated with stunted growth and tracheal collapse. Chickens and other birds may be infected with *B. avium* and opportunistically causes disease. *B. hinzii* is generally viewed as a commensal but under the right environmental conditions is capable of causing mild respiratory disease in turkeys. There have been a number of cases of *B. hinzii* in humans whooping cough-like disease and septicemia in human, particularly when asplenic.

Laboratory and Wild Animals

Rabbit bordetellosis. *B. bronchiseptica* infections in rabbits are usually asymptomatic but may cause mild upper respiratory disease (snuffles). However, in association with other infectious agents (e.g., *P. multocida*) can be involved with bronchopneumonia. In guinea pigs, *B. bronchiseptica* outbreaks can be clinically significant, resulting in acute development of respiratory disease associated with high mortality. Wild birds commonly asymptomatically carry *B. avium* and *B. henzii*.

Epidemiology

Atrophic rhinitis affects pigs under 6 weeks old, when osteogenesis and bone remodeling are most active. Affected pigs spread *B. bronchiseptica*. The ultimate sources are carrier sows, in which carrier rates decline with age.

Canine kennel cough usually affects young, nonimmune dogs or adults following introduction of new strains from recovered healthy carriers. Environmental contamination can be a significant factor.

B. avium causes disease mainly in young turkey poults and causes opportunistic disease in chickens and perhaps other birds. A contaminated environment is important in perpetuating and transferring infection between flocks.

Immunologic Aspects

Pathogenic Factors

Many of the virulence factors produced by the *Bordetella* function to either directly or indirectly overcome the host's innate immune response resulting in persistent infection, disease, and transmission. Depressed cell-mediated responses have been observed in experimental *B. avium* infections. *B. bronchiseptica* can alter the response of dendritic cells, which results in a decrease production of IL-10 and interferon.

Protective Role

Local antibody is believed to prevent *B. bronchiseptica* colonization in dogs, but evidence is lacking and questioned because of the protection provided via injected vaccines. The significant degree of common antigens as well as *Bordetella* species and strain-specific differences make it difficult to assess the degree of immunity to infection or disease.

B. avium antiserum is ineffective in protecting turkeys, but maternal immunization reduces losses in challenged progeny. Antibody to adhesins prevents adherence to tracheal epithelia.

Immunization Procedures

Vaccines appear to afford some protection against disease but often to not prevent colonization. Bacterins used on pregnant sows provide some colostral immunity to piglets, especially when including toxigenic *P. multocida* strains. Bacterin-toxoid preparations protect piglets.

Parenteral administered killed and antigen extracts as well as intratracheal live attenuated vaccine have been beneficial but provide unreliable protection against kennel cough in dogs and cats. As in the case with vaccine failures against *B. pertussis* in humans, this is likely related to critical antigenic differences, particularly with pertactin, between vaccine and wild-type strains of *B. bronchiseptica*. Localized reactions, typical of a type III hypersensitivity occasionally occur with parenteral vaccines. Of *B. avium* vaccines, those using attenuated live organisms intratracheally have been most effective.

Laboratory Diagnosis

Nasal swabs (atrophic rhinitis and kennel cough), sediment of transtracheal washes (canine tracheobronchitis), and tracheal swabs (coryza of turkeys) are cultured on blood and MacConkey agars. Selective media are helpful in limiting overgrowth by faster growing bacteria. As in the case with the primary isolation of *B. pertussis*, the use of Bordet-Gengou and charcoal blood agar can be helpful in the initial recovery of *B. bronchiseptica*. Colonies of *B. bronchiseptica* and *B. avium* can easily be overlooked on primary isolation, as they are often less than 1 mm in size after 48-h incubation and variably hemolytic. Routine laboratory tests are used for identification with differential agglutination of sheep and guinea pig red blood cells being helpful for differentiating *B. avium* and *B. bronchiseptica*. A polymerase chain reaction-based assay utilizing primers designed to amplify various species-specific segments of DNA is available for determining the presence of bordetellae as well as for identification purposes.

B. avium reacts like *Alcaligenes faecalis* in routine laboratory tests and can be differentiated by cellular fatty acid analysis. In addition, *B. avium* must be differentiated from *B. hinzii*. A microagglutination test is used for serodiagnosis.

Treatment and Control

The basis of *Bordetella* disease control is basic infectious disease control focused on preventing transmission between healthy carriers and fully susceptible new hosts, either directly by aerosol or indirectly by mechanical transfer. Significant disease outbreaks, in contrast to subclinical infection, are often associated with less than optimal environmental conditions. Vaccination reduces the likelihood of clinical disease but appear to have marginal impact on the potential of infection.

The progressive form of atrophic rhinitis is not treatable. Preventive measures include maintenance of an aged sow herd with a low carrier rate; preventing transmission from sow to piglet via mediated and/or segregated early weaning methods; thorough disinfection and cleanup of farrowing houses and nurseries after each use (all-in/all-out production); vaccination (see Section "Immunization Procedures"); prophylactic use of sulfonamides in feed or water; and elimination of carrier sows based on nasal swabs.

Canine tracheobronchitis responds inconsistently to antibiotics. Vaccination (see Section "Immunization Procedures"), fumigation of kennels, adequate ventilation, and isolation of affected dogs are useful preventive practices. Prior infection, with or without clinical disease, does not provide durable protection against reinfection. Tetracycline remains the drug of choice and there is widespread resistance to cephalosporins.

B. avium is susceptible to tetracycline, erythromycin, and nitrofurantoin, but resistant to penicillin G, strep to mycin, and sulfonamides. Medication during the early stages of a disease outbreak can be economically beneficial. Mass medication and vaccination may prevent outbreaks without eliminating the infection.

15 Brucella

Steven Olsen and Brian Bellaire

The genus *Brucella* encompasses a group of gram-negative bacteria that survive almost exclusively in infected hosts with preference for localization in intracellular compartments of phagocytic, reticuloendothelial, and specialized epithelial cells. The genus has traditionally been divided into species based on microbial characteristics and host preference, but most *Brucella* species are capable of infecting many hosts. Clinical disease caused by infection with bacteria in this genus, brucellosis, is generally associated with chronic infections and pathologic effects in reproductive tissues.

One of the most important characteristics of brucellae is the number of species in the genus that are capable of causing zoonotic infections. Human brucellosis is a significant, resurging, worldwide zoonosis with particularly high prevalence in Middle East, central Asia, and Mediterranean countries. Because clinical symptoms are not pathognomonic, human brucellosis is frequently misdiagnosed. Addressing the disease in animal reservoirs is the most economic approach for preventing human brucellosis.

Descriptive Features

The *Brucella* genus has traditionally been characterized as having six species: *B. abortus, B. melitensis, B. suis, B. canis, B. ovis,* and *B. neotomae.* The high degree of homology at the genomic level has led to it being proposed that the genus is actually composed of only one species, *B. melitensis,* with the other classical species proposed as strains of *B. melitensis.* Recent isolations of new *Brucella* species from sea mammals, voles, a prosthetic breast implant, and Austrian foxes may expand the number of species included in the *Brucella* genus. Some of the classical species (*B. melitensis, B. abortus,* and *B. suis*) are divided into biovars based on biochemical, phenotype, and antigenic properties. Although division into biovars has been used for epidemiologic purposes, biotyping can be somewhat subjective because it is based on subtle differences such as requirements for higher CO_2 tensions for growth, production of hydrogensulfide, growth on media containing dyes (thionin or basic fuchsin), and agglutination with monospecific A and M antisera.

Morphology and Staining

Brucellae are gram-negative coccobacilli that are usually single but can be in pairs or small groups. Coccobacilli are usually 0.6–1.5 μm in length and 0.5–0.7 μm I width. Pleomorphic forms are rare except in old cultures. Brucellae are nonmotile and do not have capsules or form spores. True bipolar staining is not observed. Although not truly acid-fast, they are resistant to decolorization with weak acids and therefore stain red with a modified Zehl–Nielsen stain.

B. abortus, B. suis, B. melitensis, and *B. neotomae* are considered to have a smooth colony morphology; a characteristic associated with expression of the lipopolysaccharide (LPS) O-side-chain. In comparison, *B. ovis* and *B. canis* have rough colony morphologies and do not express the LPS O-side-chain. Smooth colonies appear round, glistening, and blue-green in color and do not take up crystal violet stain. In comparison, rough colonies have a dry, granular appearance, yellowish-white color and stain with crystal violet.

Cellular Structure and Composition

The cell wall of *Brucella* is typical for gram-negative bacteria. The outer membrane, approximately 4–5 nm in thickness, is composed of asymmetric layers of LPS and phospholipids and is supported by an underlying 3–5 nm layer of peptidoglycan. Some proteins, such as OmpA, are covalently bound to the peptidoglycan layer and stabilize the outer membrane. The hydrophobic region of the membrane provides an anchor for proteins and forms a functional and structural barrier between the periplasm and the exterior of the cell. The periplasmic space varies from 3 to 30 nm. Porins in the outer membrane function as channels to the interior of the cell. Other proteins, such as lipoproteins, are also embedded in the outer membrane.

The LPS of *Brucella* is composed of lipid A, core oligosaccharides, and O-poly-saccharides. The structure of LPS in *Brucella* differs from gram-negative enteric bacteria in that the backbone sugar of the lipid A is different and the LPS has a low phosphate content. The LPS protects the bacteria from cationic peptides, oxygen metabolites, and complement-mediated lysis. The O-polysaccharide on the LPS, expressed by smooth strains, is very immunogenic

Veterinary Microbiology, Third Edition. Edited by D. Scott McVey, Melissa Kennedy and M.M. Chengappa.

and can express A and/or M antigens dependent upon the species of *Brucella*. The *Brucella* cell envelope, LPS, lipoproteins, and flagellin display a reduced pathogen-associated molecular pattern (PAMP) for recognition by innate immunity, most likely due to hydrophobic moieties of the outer membrane including ornithine lipids. The altered PAMP of *Brucella* fails to induce a robust innate immune response that contributes to the pathogen's *in vivo* stealth.

Cellular Products of Medical Interest

The lipid A of *B. abortus* LPS has been demonstrated to haveimmunostimulatory properties with reduced toxicity as compared to LPS from other gram-negative bacteria. A 14-kDA protein present in all traditional *Brucella* species can function as a lectin by binding IgGs from several animal species and also has hemagglutination properties. *Brucella* bacteria and LPS are also very poor activators of complement. The potent ability of heat-killed *B. abortus*, its LPS, and/or lipoproteins to elicit β-chemokines, Th-1 cytokines and stimulate expression of stimulatory and adhesion molecules on antigen-presenting cells has led to its proposed use as an adjuvant for human HIV vaccines

In phagocytic cells, virulent *Brucella* spp. inhibit phagolysosome fusion and may express proteins that bind to human Rab GTPase molecules and influence intracellular trafficking, and/or maturation of phagosome-derived vacuoles into replicative vacuoles. *Brucella* can also produce guanosine monophosphate, adenine and other compounds that interact with neutrophils to reduce myeloperoxidase activity, prevent primary granule release, and inhibit production of reactive oxygen compounds.

Growth Characteristics

Brucellae are aerobic and many strains require carbon dioxide for growth. Thiamine, nicotinamide, and biotin are also required for growth. Addition of 5–10% serum to media may stimulate growth, but bile salts, tellurite, and selenite inhibit growth. Growth in liquid media is usually slow unless vigorous aeration is provided. Colonies generally become visible on solid media in 3–5 days but samples should be incubated for at least 7–10 days before considered negative. Typical colonies of virulent strains are round with smooth margins, convex, translucent and appear pearly white in color.

Resistance

Although brucellae can survive freezing and thawing, freeze/thaw cycles are associated with reductions in viability. Long-term survival under environmental conditions is highest under cool, moist conditions with minimal exposure to ultraviolet light. *Brucella* is susceptible to most disinfectants for gram-negative bacteria. Lysis by bacteriophages is frequently used under laboratory conditions to type *Brucella*. Pasteurization of milk is effective for killing *Brucella*.

Diversity

Most brucellae have two circular chromosomes encoding approximately 2.1 and 1.2 Mbp. The genome of *B. suis* biovar 3 is the exception in that it has a single chromosome of 3.1 Mbp. The origin of replication of the large chromosome is typical of bacterial chromosomes while that of the small chromosome is plasmid like. The G+C content of the two chromosomes is nearly identical with an average GC content of approximately 58–59%. The genus is highly homogeneous with DNA–DNA pairing studies demonstrating greater than 90% homology across all species. Only 7000 single nucleotide polymorphisms were identified in the 3.1 Mb of genomic sequences shared across *Brucella* spp. Differences in genomic structure were primarily due to occurrence of genomic islands and deletions related to these genomic islands were found in *B. abortus* and *B. ovis*. Though many bacterial genetic islands encode pathogenicity factors, most of the *Brucella* genomic islands encode hypothetical proteins and enzymes commonly found associated with horizontally acquired DNA such transposases and integrases. The genomes of the *Brucella* species display an average of >94% identity at the nucleotide levels with *B. abortus* and *B. melitensis* being the most closely related. A close relationship has also been detected between *B. canis* and *B. suis*, while *B. neotomae* and *B. ovis* demonstrate greater divergence levels from other *Brucella* species. With the exception of biovar 5, *B. suis* isolates cluster together.

Brucellae have multiple mechanisms to protect against DNA mutations and the genome is very stable. This trait prevents the use of restriction fragment length polymorphism techniques to characterize strain lineages within biovars. No mechanisms of genetic exchange have been found in the genus.

Ecology

Zoologic and Geographic Reservoirs

Members of the genus *Brucella* exist as intracellular pathogens in mammalian hosts. Most species of *Brucella* are obligate pathogens in that they do not exist as commensals nor are they found free living in the environment. However, more recently identified species, that is, *Brucella microti*, may have genetic differences that support a free-living as compared to a host-associated life style. Although traditional species of *Brucella* may temporarily be recovered from environmental samples associated with infected animals, environmental persistence is generally not believed to be of epidemiologic importance. Because direct or close contact is generally believed to be required for transmission, maintenance of brucellosis in an animal or human population generally requires continual infection of susceptible hosts.

The preferred host of *B. abortus* is cattle, but it can also naturally infect numerous other species including bison (*Bison bison*), elk (*Cervus elaphus*), camels (*Camelus dromedaries* and *Camelus bactrianus*), yaks (*Bos grunniens*), African buffalo (*Syncerus caffer*), and swine. Biovars 1 and 2 have widespread worldwide distribution although biovar 3 is predominantly found in India, Egypt, and Africa. Several countries in Northern and Central Europe, Canada, Australia, Japan, and New Zealand are considered to be free of this pathogen.

Sheep and goats are the preferred hosts of *B. melitensis*, but this species of *Brucella* is also known to infect cattle, camels, and other species. *B. melitensis* is considered to be endemic in parts of Central and South America, Africa, Asia, the Middle East, and countries in the Mediterranean region. Areas considered to be free of *B. melitensis* include Canada, the United States, Southeast Asia, northern and central Europe, Australia, and New Zealand.

Domestic and feral swine are the preferred hosts for biovars 1, 2, and 3 of *B. suis*. Biovars 1 and 3 of *B. suis* can also infect cattle and horses. Biovar 2 can establish infection in hares (*Lepus capensis*) and has a geographical distribution in a broad range between Scandinavia and the Balkans. Biovar 4 is predominantly associated with infection in caribou (*Rangifer tarandus*) but has also been found in moose, arctic foxes, and wolves in subarctic areas. Biovar 5 has been exclusively isolated from wild rodents in the former USSR. Porcine brucellosis (biovars 1, 2, and 3) has widespread distribution in domestic and feral swine globally, but prevalence is higher in some areas such as Southeast Asia and South America. It should be noted that unlike biovars 1, 3, and 4, biovar 2 of *B. suis* is not considered to be important for causing human brucellosis.

Dogs and sheep are the preferred hosts of *B. canis* and *B. ovis*, respectively, and both species of *Brucella* have widespread geographic distribution. *B. neotomae* was isolated from desert wood rats in the Great Salt Lake Desert of Utah and appears to have a restricted host range and limited geographic distribution.

Marine strains of *Brucella* have been identified in both Atlantic and Pacific oceans although current knowledge is not sufficient to characterize geographic and host population distributions. Information on other new species of *Brucella* (i.e., *B. microti* and *B. inopinata*) is insufficient to determine distribution.

Transmission

Transmission of brucellae in preferred hosts primarily occurs through aerosol, oral, and/or venereal mechanisms across mucosal surfaces. Transmission can be best described by dividing the species into highly virulent (*B. abortus* and *B. melitensis*) and low virulence (*B. ovis* and *B. canis*) groups, with *B. suis* differing by sharing characteristics of both groups. For *B. abortus* and *B. melitensis,* transmission primarily occurs laterally through fluids or tissues associated with the birth or abortion of infected feti, or vertically to offspring through the milk. Abortion events are the most important route for transmission of *B. abortus* and *B. melitensis* with fetal fluids and placenta tissues having colonization as high as 10^9 to 10^{10} CFU/gm. Venereal transmission is not considered to be of importance for *B. abortus* or *B. melitensis*.

Venereal transmission is an important route for infection by *B. suis*, *B. ovis*, and *B. canis* in preferred hosts. *B. suis and B. canis* can also be shed by excretion in urine, milk, or from mucosal surfaces, and *B. canis* has also been recovered from feces. Bitches can shed *B. canis* for 4–6 weeks after abortions and vaginal discharges may contain bacterial numbers as high as 10^{10} CFU/ml. In general, animals infected with *B. suis* and *B. canis* effectively transmit *Brucella* for longer periods of time than animals infected with *B. abortus* or *B. melitensis* through shedding from mucosal surfaces or within urine.

The mechanisms for transmission of *Brucella* in marine mammals are unknown but may differ from other brucellae. The demonstration that marine *Brucella* are almost exclusively localized within gut and uterine tissues of lungworms (*Parafilaroides* and *Phocoena*) in an infected Pacific harbor seal and harbor porpoise suggests an intriguing possibility that parasites may play a role in transmission.

Pathogenesis

Brucellae generally enter across mucosal membranes, and initially localize in lymphatic tissues draining the site of entry. If bacteria do not become localized and are not killed in regional lymph nodes draining the site of infection, bacteria may replicate and spread to other lymphoreticular tissues and organs via lymph and blood. Distribution to reproductive and mammary tissues occurs during the bacteremic phase. Once localized in the immunoprivileged environment of the pregnancy uterus, or lumens of ducts within the mammary gland, immunologic mechanisms to eliminate brucellae are severely impaired.

The internalization of *Brucella* into phagocytic cells differs between rough and smooth organisms. The LPS O-side-chain of nonopsonized smooth *Brucella* interact with lipid rafts, which contain glycosphingolipids, cholesterol, and glycosyl-phosphatidylinositol anchored proteins, on the surface of phagocytes. Internalized *Brucella* initially localize within phagocytes in an acidified membrane-bound compartment (phagosome) where they are exposed to free oxygen radicals generated by the respiratory burst. Cyclic β-1,2-glucans may help target *Brucella* to their replicative niche in the endoplasmic reticulum. Exposure to an acidified environment induces a type IV secretion system that interferes with phagosomal maturation and interacts with the endoplasmic reticulum to neutralize the pH of the phagosome. The modified phagosome ("brucellosome") resists phagosome maturation and fusion with lysosomes. Although most brucellae (approximately 70–85%) are eliminated by phagolysosome fusion, creation of the brucellasome allows intracellular survival of some. Brucellae use stationary-phase physiology and siderophores to scavenge iron as a mechanism for long-term survival within the nutrient-poor environment of the modified phagosome. Brucellae have multiple molecular mechanisms to detoxify free radicals since oxidative killing is the primary mechanism employed by host phagocytes to control replication of intracellular pathogens. The O-side-chain on the LPS appears to be a key molecular for invasion, protection from oxidative killing, cationic peptides, and complemented mediated lysis. The capacity of *Brucella* to maintain long-term residence within macrophages serves as the basis for their ability to establish and maintain chronic infection.

In contrast to entry via lipid rafts, opsonization of *Brucella* strains increases entry 10-fold with entry targeted to phagosomes that mature and fuse with lysosomes to form phagolysosomes. Localization within phagolysosome compartments increases intracellular killing of brucellae by phagocytic cells.

During persistent infection some brucellae reside in a dormant, nonreplicative state in phagocytic cells. Calves infected with *B. abortus* at young ages often do not demonstrate seroconversion until after reaching puberty. Recrudescence of clinical brucellosis is a significant problem in human patients. Molecular mechanisms controlling recrudescence, or host physiology influencing *in vivo* replication of brucellae have not been identified at this time.

The erythritol genes are highly conserved in *B. abortus*, *B. suis*, and *B. melitensis*, and erythritol is preferentially metabolized and can promote the growth of some *Brucella* strains. Although it has been hypothesized that the preferential localization of *B. abortus* within the reproductive tract is related to the high concentration of erythritol in fetal placenta, data suggest that erythritol is not an essential carbon source for *B. suis* in intracellular environments.

Epidemiology

Human brucellosis, caused by *B. melitensis*, *B. suis*, and *B. abortus* infection, occurs worldwide, but prevalence tends to be higher in parts of the Mediterranean basin, Central and South America, the Middle East, sub-Saharan Africa, and central Asia. Human brucellosis caused by *B. canis* or marine *Brucella* strains have also been reported in South America and New Zealand. Brucellosis is estimated to infect more than 500 000 people yearly in nonindustrialized countries of the world with estimates of disease prevalence ranging from <1 per 100 000 people in the United Kingdom, United States, and Australia to >70 per 100 000 people in some countries in the Middle East and central Asia. Of particular concern is the observation that children appear to represent a high proportion of human brucellosis cases. Economic instability, socioeconomic factors, and insufficient regulatory programs in domestic livestock over the last 10–15 years are likely contributing factors to the re-emergence of brucellosis in both livestock and humans in a number of countries.

Brucellosis in humans is most frequently a disease of farm workers, veterinarians, and laboratory or abattoir workers but can also occur through consumption of non pasteurized dairy products. Direct contact with infected animals, or materials associated with abortion, can lead to human infection through aerosolization into respiratory tissues, oral consumption, or opportunistic penetration through breaks in the skin. Veterinarians can also develop brucellosis from infection with vaccine strains of *B. abortus* or *B. melitensis* with inadvertent needle sticks being a frequent cause of infection. As prevention of human brucellosis is primarily related to the control of the disease in animals, human brucellosis has a low incidence in countries in which livestock brucellosis has been controlled.

It should be noted that *B. suis* has unique zoonotic features due to the long bacteremia and prolonged shedding from infected swine. Processing of infected swine in an abattoirsetting has frequently resulted in large numbers of workers becoming infected with brucellosis. In addition to the prolonged bacteremia in pigs, the observed infections in abattoirs may also be related to the fact that *B. suis* can be readily isolated from urine within the bladder of infected swine. Processing of infected swine may be associated with aerosolization of *B. suis* from urine or other body fluids.

The incubation period associated with human infection is variable and can range from less than a week to several months. The pathophysiology of brucellosis in humans differs from the characteristics of brucellosis in animal models. Clinical symptoms in humans are not pathognomonic and can include recurrent pyrexia (undulant fever), cephalalgia, malaise, joint and muscle pain, night sweats, and even neurologic manifestations. *Brucella* can distribute to almost any tissue or *in vivo* site with clinical symptoms related to inflammatory lesions associated with bacterial localization. Osteoarticular disease is the most common complication and can include peripheral arthritis, sacroiliitis, and spondylitis. Although human brucellosis is generally associated with low mortality, endocarditis associated primarily with *B. melitensis* infection is the principal cause of human mortality. Although reports are rare, human-to-human transmission of brucellosis through venereal transmission or through breast milk have been reported.

Characterization of Infection in Animal Populations

As mentioned previously, most *Brucella* spp. have widespread worldwide distribution in domestic livestock populations. Susceptibility to infection, clinical effects, and disease prevalence are influenced by vaccination status, sexual maturity, and pregnancy status. Localization in the reproductive tract or mammary gland is associated with the most severe pathology and capability to transmit infection. In general, preferred hosts are more susceptible to infection with brucellae during pregnancy although host mechanisms responsible for the increased susceptibility are not characterized at this time. In the absence of vaccination, infected herds frequently demonstrate seroprevalence rates of 40–60%. Vertical transmission of brucellosis to offspring can occur through infected milk. With *B. abortus* it has been shown that infection in young animals may remain latent until the initiation of puberty.

The most common clinical manifestation of *B. melitensis*, *B. suis*, and *B. abortus* in natural hosts is reproductive losses. With the exception of third trimester abortions, birth of weak offspring, and infertility in males and females, clinical symptoms of brucellosis in natural hosts are relatively rare. In uniparous species, abortions are generally fresh with minimal autolysis. In multiparous animals, abortion may not be as common due to physiologic mechanisms that maintain pregnancy while viable fetuses remain in utero. Brucellae also frequently infect mammary glands causing mastitis and reduced milk production. Occasionally, *Brucella* can localize in joints, bones, or other aberrant locations in natural hosts leading to inflammation and associated pathology. Osteomyelitis/spinal meningitis in swine infected with *B. suis* can lead to hind limb paralysis.

Transmission of *B. ovis* infection in sheep generally occurs during the breeding seasons. The ewe acts as a mechanical vector for transmitting infection between infected and noninfected rams. Homosexual activity of rams may be another mechanism for transmitting infection. The most common clinical manifestation of *B. ovis* infection is infertility in rams with scrotal palpation being a mechanism for identification of infected rams.

Because of the capability to be transmitted venereally, husbandry practices and management practices can contribute to the introduction of *B. suis* and *B. canis* into noninfected herds or kennels. Entry of infection can occur by the purchase of infected animals, male or female, or by the communal use of a male, who may transmit the disease mechanically or who may be excreting *Brucella* in semen. Use of *B. suis* infected semen for artificial insemination is also a potential route for introduction of infection into swine herds.

Immunologic Aspects

Immune Mechanisms in Pathogenesis

Cellular immune responses are generally felt to play the critical role in protection against intracellular pathogens such as *Brucella*. Development of adaptive immunity, involving presentation of epitopes by antigen presenting cells, production of TH-1 type cytokines (interferon-γ, tumor necrosis factor, interleukins 2, 12, and 18), and clonal expansion of antigen-specific CD4+ and CD8+ T cells are key to development of protective immunity. In generally, it is felt that antigens derived from outside and which enter the antigen-processing cell through phagocytosis for degradation in the phagolysosome are presented through the Class II MHC (major histocompatibility complex) or exogenous pathway. In comparison, antigens synthesized within the antigen-presenting cell cytoplasm and transported to the endoplasmic reticulum are presented with class I MHC and processed through endogenous pathways. The intracellular location or entry of antigen into the cell is important as processing via the endogenous pathway tend to evoke a Th1 response associated with cell-mediated immune responses. However, antigens processed via the exogenous pathway are typically associated with a nonprotective Th2 response. This may explain why efficacious brucellosis vaccines are composed of live bacteria, whereas vaccination with killed bacteria generally fails to induce adequate protection.

In general, antibodies are considered to play a minor role in long-term protection against brucellosis, although they may opsonize bacteria and facilitate phagocytosis and may lead to processing/presentation of *Brucella* epitopes on antigen-presenting cells. Cytotoxic T lymphocytes may play an important role in *in vivo* protection by killing infected cells, and releasing intracellular bacteria within the cells for uptake and destruction by activated macrophages. As some smooth *Brucella* strains downregulate genes associated with apoptosis, prevention of host cell apoptosis may also be a mechanism used by *Brucella* to facilitate intracellular survival and persistence.

The roles of Toll-like receptors that facilitate interactions between bacteria and phagocytic cells have been of interest for their role in induction of innate and adaptive immunity. Dendritic cells are of particular interest as they express receptors that function *in vivo* as immunologic sensors for detection of pathogens. When pathogen-recognition receptors are triggered, the dendritic cells integrate the signals and migrate to the T cell areas of secondary lymphoid organs to stimulate naive T cells. The observation that *Brucella* display reduced PAMP signals to dendritic cells may be a mechanism the bacteria use to elude innate immune responses.

Mechanisms of Resistance and Recovery

Long-term protection against brucellosis is associated with stimulation of cellular immunity, whereas antibodies are considered to play a minor role in protection. Although specific correlates of protective immunity are currently not know, it is believed that protection is mediated by the Th1 subset of CD4+ lymphocytes and is associated with production of IFN-γ and other cytokines associated with cellular immunity. The ability of preferred hosts to clear infection, with or without treatment, remains controversial because of the intracellular location of the pathogen, and observations of recrudescence of infection under field conditions.

Vaccination

Vaccination is a critical tool for control or eradication of brucellosis that primarily prevents clinical effects of disease (i.e., abortions or infected offspring) that lead to transmission. Approved vaccines are available to prevent *B. abortus* in cattle and *B. melitensis* in sheep and goats. Approved vaccines are not available for other hosts or brucellae, although the *B. melitensis* Rev1 vaccine has been recommended for use in preventing *B. ovis* infections. In regards to *B. melitensis* and *B. abortus* preferred hosts, vaccination programs have not included males, as males are not considered to have a significant role in disease transmission. The most efficacious vaccines are live attenuated strains that are frequently administered to prepubescent animals. Rough vaccine strains of *B. abortus* (i.e., RB51 or killed 45/20) that do not express the O-side-chain on the LPS that function as differential (differentiation of infected from vaccinated animals) vaccines for diagnostic purposes have been utilized. Conjunctival administration of vaccine strains has also been used, particularly in adult animals, in an effort to reduce positive responses on brucellosis serologic tests. Brucellosis vaccine strains have disadvantages in that they may induce abortions in pregnant animals, be shed in milk of lactating animals, and are themselves potential zoonoses.

Laboratory Diagnosis

Specimens

As brucellosis is one of the most common laboratory-acquired infections, manipulations of live cultures of zoonotic *Brucella* spp. should be handled under Biosafety level 3 conditions using appropriate safety procedures. All work should be conducted in biologic safety cabinets and avoid procedures that produce aerosols. Biosafety level 2 conditions are recommended for processing of routine clinical specimens of human or animal origin. In the United States, *B. abortus*, *B. melitensis*, and *B. suis* (vaccine strains are exempt) are classified as potential bioweapons and must be handled in accordance with Select Agent regulations.

Optimal microbiologic samples for diagnosis would include milk or vaginal swabs from live animals; lung and/or gastric contents from aborted fetuses; or tissues such as uterus, mammary gland, male reproductive tissues, lymphatic tissues associated with the mammary gland or reproductive tract obtained at necropsy, or bursitis/hygroma fluid. Although blood collected in anticoagulant may be beneficial for isolation of *B. canis* or *B. suis*, it is generally a poor sample for bacteriologic evaluation for other brucellae due to the fact that bacteremias associated with infection are generally of very short duration.

Direct Examination

Gross lesions caused by *Brucella* spp. are not pathognomonic, but can include variable necrosis of cotyledons across the placenta, thickening of intercotyledonary areas, and retained placenta. Common histologic lesions of maternal tissues include necrotic placentitis and lymphosuppurative or lymphohistiocytic interstitial mastitis. In males, orchitis with multiple abscess, epididymitis, vesicular adenitis, and testicular degeneration have been reported. The most frequent fetal lesion is a multifocal, histiocytic bronchopneumonia with, or without, suppurative infiltrates. Fetal lesions may also include variable foci of necrotizing arteritis, necrosis, and granulomas in the lung and other tissues.

Additional lesions caused by *B. suis* infection in pigs include fibrinopurulent arthritis in compound or large joints, osteomyelitis in lumbar vertebral epiphysis, and military uterine nodules *B. abortus* is known to cause bursitis and hygromas in cattle. Horses are an aberrant host of *B. abortus* and can have suppurative and granulomatous bursitis lesions at the supraspinous (fistulous withers) or atlantal (poll evil) bursae.

Isolation

Because brucellae are slow growing in relation to other bacteria, contaminants may overgrow and severely impair the ability to isolate *Brucella* spp. For that reason samples obtained for culture should preferentially be obtained aseptically. Alternatively, selective media (i.e., Farrell's media or Kuzdas and Morse media) have been developed to inhibit the growth of contaminants and facilitate the isolate of *Brucella* spp. Regardless, *Brucella* spp. will at minimum take 72 h for colonies to be visible on media, and samples should be incubated a minimum of 7–10 days before determined to be negative.

Identification

Traditionally, after isolation of gram-negative coccobacilli with culture and biochemical characteristics consistent with identification as *Brucella*, species differentiation has been based on phage and dye sensitivity, CO_2 dependence for growth, production of H_2S, and serum agglutination tests. However, as microbial isolation can be slow and tedious, other more rapid methods have been developed for identification. Classifying *Brucella* isolates into biovars has been used for epidemiologic purposes, but is somewhat subjective because it is based on subtle differences including requirements for higher CO_2 tensions for growth, production of hydrogen sulfide, growth on media containing dyes (thionin or basic fuchsin), and agglutination with monospecific A and M antisera.

Serologic Tests

For serologic detection of *B. suis*, *B. abortus*, and *B. melitensis* in preferred hosts, the immunodominant antigen involved in the serologic responses is the O-side-chain of the LPS. Most standard brucellosis serologic tests (agglutination, complement fixation, fluorescence polarization assay, and enzyme-linked immunosorbent assays (ELISAs)) use the polysaccharide O-side-chain from *B. abortus* as antigen and were initially developed for detection of *B. abortus* infections in cattle. Although considered adequate for use in detection of *B. melitensis* infection in small ruminants and cattle, they are generally felt to have reduced sensitivity and specificity in detection of *B. suis* infections in swine. Sensitivity and specificity of standard brucellosis serologic tests may differ by host species and the *Brucella* spp. causing infection. The structural component of the O-side-chain (repeated residues of 4-formamindo-4, 6-dideoxymanose linked in α-1,2 or α-1,3 conformation) is also similar to epitopes on the LPS of other bacteria such as *Yersinia enterocolitica* O:9, *Escherichia coli* O:157, and others, and can lead to reductions in specificity under some conditions.

For detection of *B. ovis* in sheep, complement fixation, ELISA, and agar gel immunodiffusion (AGID) tests have been utilized. For detection of *B. canis* infection in kennels, tube agglutination, AGID, ELISA, indirect fluorescence, and rapid slide agglutination (*B. ovis* as antigen) tests have been recommended.

The delayed-type hypersensitivity reaction (allergic skin test) based on the use of S-LPS free *Brucella* cytoplasmic proteins (widely known as brucellin) extracted from rough *B. melitensis* strain B115 has been used as a diagnostic in many countries. The brucellin test has been proposed to be beneficial in differentiating seropositive responses caused by infection with *Y. enterocolitica* O:9.

Molecular-Based Tests

Multiple polymerase chain reaction (PCR) techniques are currently available for differentiating *Brucella* species. However, current PCR techniques have not been able to fully differentiate all biovars within all *Brucella* spp.

Because of the stability of *Brucella* genomes, molecular assays designed to assess genetic relationships between isolates (i.e., restriction fragment length polymorphism) are ineffective for epidemiologic investigations or strain comparisons. A new molecular technique, variable nuclear tandem repeats, which evaluates strings of nucleotide repeats in noncoding areas of the chromosome, has been used to compare genetic and epidemiological relationships between strains. However, molecular biotyping is more complicated than that of standard PCR methods and requires special equipment that may limit their use by diagnostic laboratories.

Treatment

In general, no treatment strategies are recommended for preferred hosts for *B. abortus*, *B. suis*, and *B. melitensis* due to the requirement for long-term treatment and the inability to adequately insure total clearance of *Brucella* from its intracellular niche, and prevent re-emgergence in regulatory programs. In some countries, antibiotic treatment (oxytetracycline), alone or in combination with test-and-slaughter, has been used to minimize clinical and economic impact of disease in infected swine or sheep farms.

Treatment of humans usually involves a prolonged course of antibiotic therapy and relapse of infection of treatment is not uncommon. Relapses are usually not associated with the emergency of antibiotic resistant strains.

Control and Prevention

Control Methods for *B. abortus, B. melitensis,* and *B. suis*

Many countries have programs to control or eradicate zoonotic brucellae (*B. abortus, B. melitensis,* and *B. suis*) from domestic livestock. Although brucellosis can cause severe economic losses to livestock producers, most regulatory programs for brucellosis were developed to reduce brucellosis in animal reservoirs as a mechanism to prevent human infections. Multiple studies have demonstrated that the most cost-efficient mechanism for controlling human brucellosis is to control brucellosis in animal reservoirs.

As brucellae are intracellular pathogens, most test and removal programs are based on removal of animals which are positive on serologic tests that detect antibodies against the immunodominant O-side-chain of the *Brucella* LPS. Although antibodies indicate that the individual's immune response has responded to infection with brucellae, it should be emphasized that seropositive responses do not necessarily indicate the animal is currently infected or capable of transmitting brucellosis.

The full depopulation of all animals on infected premises is the strategy of choice for controlling brucellosis. However, because this strategy may be too expensive or not acceptable to the owner, other approaches may need to be utilized.

Regulatory programs for cattle and small ruminants can include sanitation programs to prevent disease transmission, vaccination programs to reduce herd susceptibility, and test and removal programs to eliminate animals infected with brucellosis. Efficacious vaccines are effective tools in both control and eradication programs. Although vaccination is highly effective in reducing production losses (i.e., abortions or weak offspring) caused by brucellosis, it is less effective at preventing infection after exposure to field strains or seroconversion after exposure. Although vaccination is an effective tool in controlling brucellosis, vaccination alone has never been effective in eradicating brucellosis. With the exception of depopulation, the most effective brucellosis programs incorporate combinations of sanitation, vaccination, and test and removal procedures.

For control of *B. suis* in swine, regulatory efforts, including serologic surveillance, to control or eradicate *B. suis* in swine should be directed toward herds, rather than individual animals. Owing to the present lack of effective tools to manage brucellosis in swine, whole-herd depopulation appears to be the only viable option to eradicate *B. suis* from domestic swine herds. If feral swine or other wildlife reservoirs were the source of infection, management practices may need to be modified to prevent reintroduction of brucellosis.

Control Methods for *B. ovis*

Use of a test and slaughter approach based on scrotal palpation and/or serologic testing (complement fixation, ELISA, or gel diffusion test) has been successfully used to eradicate *B. ovis*. As shedding in semen can be intermittent, a single negative sample is not accurate. Antibody responses are also unreliable as only 35% of infected rams develop detectable lesions. Vaccination is considered the most viable method of control with the *B. melitensis* Rev-1 strain the current recommended vaccine. As mentioned previously, antibiotic therapy for 7–21 days resulted in cessation of shedding and improvement in sperm motility in 80–100% of rams. In some instances, culling of the entire ram flock may be the most economical approach for eradication of *B. ovis*.

Control Methods for *B. canis*

Best control in infected kennels is removal of seropositive dogs and desexing of infected animals. Disinfection of the kennel after removal of infected dogs is recommended. Treatment of infected dogs is not encouraging due to frequent failure of antibiotic regimens or relapse of infection. Best results have occurred using long-term treatment (90 days) with a combination of antibiotics combined with monitoring for reversion to negative status on serologic tests (AGID). Repeat testing 3–6 months after negative tests is required to check for relapse of infection. Relapse of infection is possible. Owners should be warned of possible zoonotic infections with *B. canis*. Prevention of reentry of brucellosis into kennels is prevented by isolation of new additions and serologic testing.

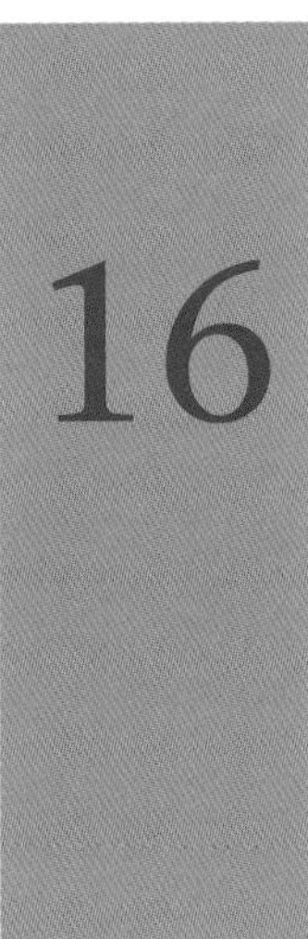

16 *Burkholderia mallei* and *Burkholderia pseudomallei*

Sanjeev Narayanan

Members of the genus *Burkholderia* are gram-negative, aerobic rods belonging to phylum Proteobacteria, class Betaproteobacteria, order Burkholderiales, and family Burkholderiaceae. As of this writing, there are more than 60 species belonging to this genus, most of which live in soil and/or produce disease in plants. Members of the *Burkholderia cepacia* and *B. gladioli* species groups produce disease in compromised human patients (e.g., those with cystic fibrosis, chronic granulomatous disease, immunosuppression, and nosocomial infections). Two members of *Burkholderia pseudomallei* species group, *B. mallei* (the cause of "glanders" primarily in equids) and *B. pseudomallei* (the cause of "melioidosis" in a variety of species) are important in veterinary medicine, and are the topics of discussion in this chapter. Both produce pyogranulomatous disease and have gained notoriety as category B bioterrorism agents by Centers for Disease Control and Prevention, USA, and are considered emerging and reemerging infectious agents of humans by National Institutes of Health, USA.

B. mallei

B. mallei is a facultative intracellular bacterium that causes a systemic pyogranulomatous disease called "glanders," once a worldwide disease of Equidae, and remains endemic in parts of Asia, Africa, and South America. Focal outbreaks were also reported in the former USSR in 2007. No naturally occurring cases of glanders have been reported in North America since the 1940s. Natural infections have been reported in dogs, camels, horses, goats, and sheep, but felids are particularly susceptible. Guinea pigs and hamsters are highly susceptible to glanders and are, therefore, used in diagnostic testing or experimental studies. Glanders varies in severity and can be an acute, chronic, or latent disease.

At one time or other, this bacterium was called *Pseudomonas mallei, Bacillus mallei, Actinobacillus mallei, Acinetobacter mallei, Malleomyces mallei, Pfeiferella mallei*, and *Loefferella mallei*.

Descriptive Features

Morphology and Staining. *B. mallei* organisms are gram-negative rods 0.5 μm wide and variable in length. The bacilli may be arranged singly, in pairs end to end, in parallel bundles, or palisades.

Structure and Composition. *B. mallei* produces a carbohydrate capsule. The cell wall is typical of gram-negative bacteria composed of lipopolysaccharide (LPS) and protein. Being nonmotile, flagella are not produced (differentiating it from *B. pseudomallei*, which is motile).

Cellular Products of Medical Interest

Capsule. The only demonstrable function the capsule plays in disease produced by *B. mallei* is to protect the outer membrane from membrane attack complexes generated following activation of the complement system (which is manifest as a serum-resistant phenotype). Capsule-negative mutants show significant reduction in virulence.

Cell Wall. The cell wall of *B. mallei* is typical of gram-negative bacteria. The LPS in the outer membrane is an important virulence determinant. LPS consists of lipid A, a core region, and cell wall (O) antigens. Not only is the lipid A component toxic (endotoxin), but the length of the side chain in the O-repeat unit hinders the attachment of the membrane attack complex of the complement system to the outer membrane. LPS binds to LPS-binding protein in serum, which transfers it to the blood phase of CD14. The CD14–LPS complex binds to Toll-like receptor protein-4 (see Chapter 2) on the surface of antigen-presenting cells, triggering the release of proinflammatory cytokines and chemokines.

Miscellaneous Products. *B. mallei* possesses type IV pili, type III (animal and plant types), and type VI secretion systems. Although many effector proteins injected into the

Veterinary Microbiology, Third Edition. Edited by D. Scott McVey, Melissa Kennedy and M.M. Chengappa.

host cells by the type III secretion apparatus have been identified, their exact function is not known. Many effectors have been hypothesized to play an integral role in bacterial survival in intracellular (including cytosolic) environments in the host cells (predominantly macrophages).

Proteases, lipases, and a phospholipase C have been demonstrated in the culture fluids of *B. mallei*. None of these products have been shown to play a significant role in disease.

Growth Characteristics. The organism grows in routine bacteriological media, but media containing glycerol or blood are the best. Nonhemolytic colonies develop in ≥48 h at 20–41 °C (optimal 37 °C). They range from mucoid to rough forms. Confluent growth is common. *B. mallei* does not grow on MacConkey agar or at 42 °C. *B. mallei* grows on MacConkey agar.

Biochemical Characteristics. *B. mallei* is aerobic, nonmotile and oxidase variable, catalase-positive, indole-negative, and resistant to colistin and polymyxin B; it reduces nitrates (without gas) and hydrolyzes urea. Glucose is catabolized oxidatively.

Resistance. Resistance is unremarkable, although in dark, damp, and cool environments the agent can survive for months. Aminoglycosides, chloramphenicol, fluoroquinolones, macrolides, sulfonamides, trimethoprim, imipenem, ceftazidime, piperacillin, and tetracyclines inhibit *B. mallei in vitro*.

Ecology

Reservoir. Infected Equidae are the reservoir.

Transmission. Exposure occurs via contaminated feed, water, and fomites, and sometimes through inhalation and wounds. Skin exudates and respiratory secretions are the most common source of infection in equids, especially in crowded and unsanitary conditions. Carnivores can be infected by ingesting meat from infected animals.

Pathogenesis

Pathology. *B. mallei* produces typical pyogranulomas characterized by a central core of necrotic debris admixed with fibrin and intact and degenerate neutrophils (Figure 16.1). This core is surrounded by a layer of histiocytes, epithelioid macrophages, and multinucleated giant cells. The entire nodule is surrounded by an outer rim of collagenous capsule embedded with small to large infiltrates of lymphocytes and few plasma cells. A multifocal and coalescing distribution is common in systemic infections, and in lesions near epithelial surfaces, ulceration is common. Strain variations determine the suppurative versus granulomatous predominance in lesions.

Mechanisms. Although toxins are suspected in pathogenesis, the mechanisms are uncertain. Primary lesions form at the point of entry—the pharynx, for example. Infection spreads along lymphatics, producing nodular lesions on the way to lymph nodes and the bloodstream, which disseminates the agent. Monocytes and macrophages are suspected to carry the bacterium to draining lymph nodes because *B. mallei* is facultative intracellular bacterium capable of surviving and replicating in the cytosol of macrophages. Metastatic lesions form in the lungs or other organs, such as spleen, liver, and skin, producing cutaneous glanders ("farcy"). Lesions in the nasal septum may be primary, hematogenous, or secondary to a pulmonary focus.

FIGURE 16.1. *Section from the nasal cavity of a horse with B. mallei infection (H&E). There is leukocytoclastic vasculitis in many vessels and their lumens contain thrombi.*

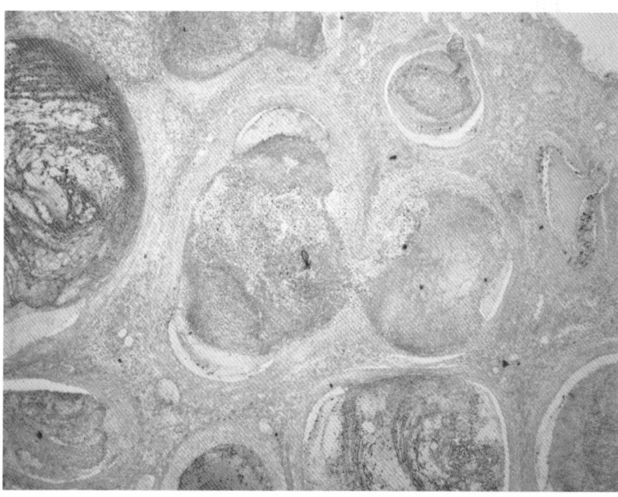

Disease Patterns

Glanders. The disease predominates in the upper and lower respiratory tracts and in the skin. Multiple nodules and ulcers develop in the upper airways and nasal cavity, which rupture to release thick mucopurulent nasal discharge. Lung lesions are multifocal coalescing pyogranulomas with caseous or calcified centers. Cutaneous glanders (farcy) is characterized by subcutaneous abscesses. Local, regional, or generalized lymphadenopathy is typical in all types of glanders.

Acute infections are characterized by fever, nasal discharge, and lymphadenitis of head and neck, with swelling along the upper respiratory tract. They tend to end fatally in about 2 weeks and predominate in donkeys and felids, less so in mules.

In horses, protracted chronic and subclinical infections are typical; signs, if present, include occasional fever, persistent respiratory problems, skin abscesses ("farcy buds"), and nodular induration of cranial lymph nodes.

Natural infections in humans are traced to acutely ill horses and may lead to acute or chronic infections.

Epidemiology

The persistence of glanders depends on an infected horse population. Movement of animals contributes to the spread of disease in facilities and in geographic regions.

Susceptible nonequids acquire glanders from infected horses or horsemeat, and appear to be dead-end hosts.

Immunologic Aspects

Humoral and cell-mediated responses occur.

Apparent recovery from glanders, including loss of dermal hypersensitivity, has been observed under natural conditions, but without increased resistance to reinfection.

Killed whole-cell preparations, polysaccharide-based preparations, and live-attenuated bacteria have all been tested as vaccine candidates and have shown to provide some protection. However, no vaccines are commercially available.

Laboratory Diagnosis

Nodular contents are cultured on blood or glycerol agar. They may be examined for gram-negative rods and by immunofluorescence.

Guinea pigs and hamsters are highly susceptible to fatal infection with virulent strains.

Any suspect isolates should be submitted to a qualified reference laboratory. Differentiation from *B. pseudomallei* is important.

Serologically, glanders is diagnosed by complement fixation tests employing aqueous bacterial extracts as antigens. Enzyme-linked immunosorbent assays (ELISAs), indirect hemagglutination, counterimmunoelectrophoresis, immunoblotting, and indirect fluorescent testing are used for diagnostic purposes in some areas. However, complement fixation tests and ELISAs are approved for international trade. The intradermo-palpebral mallein test detects cell-mediated hypersensitivity, which indicates infection and has served as a basis for glanders eradication. Mallein is a heat extract of old *B. mallei* broth cultures.

Polymerase chain reaction–based assays have high sensitivities of detection; however, due to high genetic variability of *B. pseudomallei*, differentiation between *B. mallei* and *B. pseudomallei* using DNA-based techniques is complicated.

Differential diagnoses for equine glanders include strangles (*Streptococcus equi*), epizootic lymphangitis (*Histoplasma farciminosum*), sporotrichosis(*Sporothrix schenckii*), ulcerative lymphangitis (*Corynebacterium pseudotuberculosis*), and melioidosis (*B. pseudomallei*).

Treatment and Control

Although glanders is treatable by many antimicrobials (see the section on resistance above), treatment is inappropriate in countries committed to glanders eradication. Equine imports from endemic areas are mallein-tested, and reactors are destroyed.

B. pseudomallei

B. pseudomallei organisms are aerobic gram-negative, facultative intracellular rods that cause a pyogranulomatous disease called "melioidosis," a disease superficially resembling glanders. Important distinctions are that (1) melioidosis affects a wide host range and (2) the agent is a saprophyte (an endosymbiont of amoebae living in the environment), whose prevalence is unaffected by elimination of infected animals.

Previous synonyms for this bacterium include *Pseudomonas pseudomallei*, *Bacillus pseudomallei*, *Bacterium whitmori*, *Malleomyces pseudomallei*, and *L. mallei*.

Descriptive Features

Morphology and Staining. *B. pseudomallei* organisms are gram-negative rods 0.5 μm wide and variable in length. They frequently appear as long bundles of densely packed organisms. The bacterium in clinical samples may occasionally appear bipolar (safety-pin shaped).

Structure and Composition. *B. pseudomallei* produces a carbohydrate capsule. The cell wall is typical of gram-negative bacteria composed of LPS and protein. Being motile, flagella are produced (differentiating it from *B. mallei*, which is nonmotile).

Cellular Products of Medical Interest

Adhesin. *B. pseudomallei* adheres to amoebic trophozoites of *Acanthamoeba* species prior to uptake (and by inference adherence to phagocytic cells). Adherence is by means of the flagellar protein Fli (for flagellin). Surface proteins of *B. pseudomallei* (BoaA and BoaB) that affect its adherence to respiratory epithelium have been characterized.

Capsule. The only demonstrable function the capsule has been shown to play in *B. pseudomallei* is to protect the outer membrane from membrane attack complexes generated following activation of the complement system (which is manifest as a serum-resistant phenotype). Capsules may play an integral role in intracellular survival of this bacterium, and mutants that lack functional genes encoding the capsule are avirulent.

Cell Wall. The cell wall of *B. pseudomallei* is typical of gram-negative bacteria. The LPS in the outer membrane is an important virulence determinant. Not only is the lipid A component toxic (endotoxin), but the length of the side chain in the O-repeat unit hinders the attachment of the membrane attack complex of the complement system to the outer membrane. LPS binds to LPS-binding protein (a serum protein), which transfers it to the blood phase of CD14. The CD14–LPS complex binds to Toll-like receptor proteins on the surface of macrophage cells, triggering the release of proinflammatory cytokines.

Miscellaneous Products. The chromosome of *B. pseudomallei* possesses at least one pathogenicity island (a cluster of genes encoding virulence determinant(s), an integrase protein, a specific insertion site, and mobility) encoding a type III secretion system. Studies have shown that the type III secretory system of *B. pseudomallei* is extensive and the genome contains at least three separate gene clusters. A Bsa type III secretion system has been shown to be vital for the escape of this bacterium from the primary endosomes into the cytoplasm of host cells, thereby playing a critical role in replication and persistence in the host cell. A type VI secretory system is also present.

Proteases, lipases, and a phospholipase C have been demonstrated in the culture fluids of *M. pseudomallei* grown *in vitro*. None of these products have been shown to play a significant role in disease production.

Growth Characteristics. *B. pseudomallei* can grow in routine bacteriological media, especially those containing blood. In sheep blood agar, the organism reveals small, smooth colonies, which after a few days will appear dry and wrinkled. Unlike *B. mallei*, *B. pseudomallei* grows on MacConkey agar, in the presence of 2% sodium chloride, and at 42 °C.

Biochemical Characteristics. *B. pseudomallei* is aerobic, motile and oxidase-positive, catalase-positive, indole-negative, and resistant to colistin and polymyxin B; it reduces nitrate to nitrogen gas (often produces only one small bubble of gas) and hydrolyzes urea.

Resistance. *B. pseudomallei* is killed by disinfectants and does not survive chilling and freezing in biologic specimens. It is generally susceptible to imipenem, doxycycline, and minocycline. Most clinical strains have been shown to be resistant to amoxicillin, ticarcillin, cefoxitin, cefoperazone, cefsulodin, and aztreonam. Resistance to ceftazidime (drug of choice) is on a rise. Majority of the clinical isolates are also resistant to fluoroquinolones, aminoglycosides, and macrolides.

Ecology

Reservoir. *B. pseudomallei* is considered a soil and water dweller (most likely an endosymbiont of amoebae). Although most prevalent between 20° northern and southern latitude, extratropical foci do exist, for example, in France, Iran, China, and North America.

Transmission. Direct contact with contaminated soil and surface waters is the most likely source of initial infection. Inhalation, ingestion, wound infection, transplacental (in goats), and possibly arthropod bites introduce infection. Animal to animal and sexual transmission are rare. In humans, inhalation and consumption of infected animal products may be significant.

Pathogenesis

Pathology. The lesions are primarily pyogranulomatous. Single to multiple suppurative or caseous nodules may be a predominant feature in affected organs. Lungs, spleen, liver, and associated lymph nodes are commonly affected. Small abscesses tend to coalesce, developing into larger suppurative foci or granulomas.

Mechanisms. Being an endosymbiont of amoebae, *B. pseudomallei* is adapted to survive within phagocytic cells of the host. Microorganisms are taken up by a process of "coiling" phagocytosis and survive within the cell by being resistant to lysosomal contents (e.g., defensins), and by escaping phagosomes and phagolysosomes. Actin-based motility has been observed within phagocytic cells (see Chapters 11 and 33), and actin-associated "budding" occurs from affected to unaffected cells. Host cells infected with *B. pseudomallei* release proinflammatory cytokines and undergo apoptosis.

Disease Patterns

Melioidosis. Also called Whitmore's disease is typically systemic, although it can be localized to specific systems (as in pulmonary melioidosis). They can be acute, chronic, subclinical, latent, or fulminant disease. Manifestations depend on the extent and distribution of lesions. Strain differences and overall innate and adaptive immune status of the host have been demonstrated to play a role in disease presentation and manifestation. The equine disease may mimic glanders. In cattle, acute and chronic infections can localize in lung, joints, and uterus. Arthritis and lymphadenitis occur in sheep. Goats suffer loss of condition, respiratory and central nervous system disturbances, arthritis, and mastitis. Similar signs are seen in swine, along with abortions and diarrhea. Dogs develop a febrile disease with localizing suppurative foci.

Epidemiology

Clinical disease is usually sporadic. The host range is virtually unlimited. Melioidosis has been reported in sheep, goats, pigs, cattle, horses, deer, camels, alpaca, dogs, cats, dolphins, wallabies, kangaroo, koala, and primates. Nonmammal cases have been documented in birds, tropical fish, and reptiles. Human infections range from the rapidly fatal to the subclinical. A wet environment, such as a swampy terrain or rice paddies, is related to exposure. Many recent studies have shown that persons with uncontrolled diabetes are highly prone for melioidosis.

Immunologic Aspects

Complement-fixing and indirect hemagglutinating antibodies are produced during infections. Cell-mediated hypersensitivity has been demonstrated in infected goats. Successful vaccination of horses and zoo animals is reported.

Laboratory Diagnosis

The methods for isolating and identifying *B. mallei* apply to *B. pseudomallei*. Chilling and freezing of specimens should be avoided. Motility, growth on citrate, growth at 42 °C, and reduction of nitrates to gaseous nitrogen distinguish *B. pseudomallei* from *B. mallei*. Polymerase chain reaction-based assays are available for detection and identification. They are however not as effective in differentiating *B. pseudomallei* from *B. mallei*.

Treatment and Control

Treatment in animals is expensive, prolonged, and often unsuccessful. Companion and zoo animals may be treated after antimicrobial susceptibilities are verified by laboratory tests. Vaccines are not commercially available.

Further Reading

Maxie GM (ed.) (2007) *Pathology of Domestic Animals*, vol. 2, 5th edn, Saunders-Elsevier, pp. 623–624, 633–634.

NCBI. *Bacterial Taxonomy*, http://www.ncbi.nlm.nih.gov/Taxonomy/ (accessed January 8, 2013).

Quinn PJ, Carter ME, Markey B, and Carter GR (1999) *Clinical Veterinary Microbiology*, Mosby, pp. 237–242.

Snyder JW (2008) *Sentinel Laboratory Guidelines for Suspected Agents of Bioterrorism—Burkholderia mallei and B. pseudomallei*, American Society for Microbiology.

17 *Francisella tularensis*

Peter C. Iwen

Introduction

Francisella tularensis is a facultative intracellular bacterium that causes an acute zoonosis known as tularemia (rabbit fever, deerfly fever, or lemming fever). The disease is generally characterized by systemic symptoms frequently with the formation of a localized cutaneous ulcer. Although the disease has been reported throughout the United States, most cases occur in the southern and south-central states including Missouri, Kansas, Arkansas, Oklahoma, and Texas with an average of 123 human cases reported annually since 2000 in the United States (CDC 2012). Tularemia is a nationally notifiable disease through the National Public Health Surveillance System. A case definition for reporting is considered a clinically compatible case with confirmatory laboratory results.

Classification

F. tularensis is a species that belongs to a large group of intracellular bacteria that includes the mycobacteria, *Listeria, Legionella, Brucella, Coxiella*, and *Rickettsia*. The genus *Francisella*, named after Edward Francis, an American bacteriologist who extensively studied the etiological agent and pathogenesis of tularemia, is comprised of seven valid species and eight subspecies (http://www.bacterio.cict.fr/f/francisella.html, accessed February 19, 2013). Of these species, only *F. tularensis* is considered a true pathogen to humans and animals. The species epithet *tularensis* pertains to Tulare County, California, where the disease was first described in rodents. *F. tularensis* has three widely accepted subspecies known to cause infections. These include *F. tularensis* ssp. *tularensis* (also referred to as type A), *F. tularensis* ssp. *holarctica* (also referred to as type B), and *F. tularensis* ssp. *mediasiatica*. A fourth ssp. *F. tularensis* ssp. *novicida* has also been proposed but has not been widely acknowledged and currently has been elevated to valid species status (*F. novicida*) (Johansson *et al.* 2010). Most cases of tularemia are caused by the type A and type B strains. These strains have been typed using pulsed-field gel electrophoresis, with the type A strain identified as containing two distinct type A genotypes, type A.I and type A.II (Kugeler *et al.* 2009). These strains and subtypes appear to have distinct pathological characteristics and geographical distributions. The type strains for each subspecies are described in Table 17.1

Epidemiology

F. tularensis is endemic in Europe, Asia, and in North America. The type A strains are found mostly in North America, while the type B strains are found more widespread in Europe and Asia as well as in North America. *F. tularensis* spp. *mediasiatica* on the other hand has been isolated only in Kazakhstan and Turkmenistan. For the type A subtypes, the A.I strains appear to be more common in the eastern part of the United States while the A.II strains are more commonly observed in the western United States (Farlow *et al.* 2005). Both the type A and type B strains are associated with sporadic outbreaks of tularensis in the United States. *F. tularensis* has been seen in a variety of environments to include more than 100 species of wild mammals, domestic animals, blood-sucking arthropods, water, and soil. Animals associated with acute disease after exposure include rodents such as the muskrat, water vole, domestic mouse, prairie dog, rat, and beaver; lagomorphs such as the cotton tail rabbit, hare, and jackrabbit; and insectivores such as red-toothed shrew. Domestic animals include the sheep and cat. Outbreaks of disease in humans frequently follow an increase of tularemia in animals.

Due to this widespread association with animals and the environment, there are numerous diverse modes of transmission for *F. tularensis*. These include direct contact with infected mammals (e.g., skinning of rabbits), bites of infectious arthropods (e.g., deer flies and ticks), ingestion of contaminated water or food (e.g., raw milk and undercooked meat), inhalation of contaminated aerosols or dusts, and bites from infected animals (e.g., cats) (WHO 2007). There is, however, no evidence for person-to-person transmission. Transmission from infected animals to humans can occur in a variety of ways. Arthropods are frequent vectors for disease transmission with ticks considered a common means of transmission east of the Rocky Mountains and flies common vectors in Utah, Nevada, and California

Veterinary Microbiology, Third Edition. Edited by D. Scott McVey, Melissa Kennedy and M.M. Chengappa.

Table 17.1. Description of *F. tularensis* Subspecies

Subspecies	PFGE Type	Strain Designation	Type Strains[a]	Isolate Information
tularensis	A.I	SCHU S4	FSC 237	Human ulcer, 1941, Ohio
tularensis	A.II	B-38	ATCC 6223 FSC 230	Human lymph node, 1920, Utah
holarctica	B	LVS	ATCC 29684 FSC 155	Live vaccine strain, Russia, 1936
mediasiatica	NA		FSC 147 GIEM 543	Miday gerbil, 1965, Kazakhstan

PFGE, pulse-field gel electrophoresis; FSC, *Francisella* strain collection, Swedish Defense Research Agency, Umea, Sweden; ATCC, American Type Culture Collection, Manassas, Virginia, USA; GIEM, Gamaleya Scientific Research Institute of Epidemiology and Microbiology, Moscow, Russia; NA, not applicable.
[a]Prepared from the List of Procaryotic Names With Standing in Nomenclature, J.P. Euzeby curator, Societe de Bacteriologie Systamatique et Veterinaire, France, http://www.bacterio.cict.fr/ (accessed October 19, 2012).

(Petersen *et al.* 2009). Cases of tularemia from occupational and recreational exposure to an *F. tularensis*-contaminated tick tend to be seasonal and occur in late spring and summer. Overall, tularemia is considered one of the major tick-borne illnesses in the United States (Graham *et al.* 2011). The tick vectors most commonly associated with transmission are *Amblyomma americanum* (lone star tick, South Central and Eastern United States), *Dermacentor andersoni* (Rocky Mountain wood tick, Western North America), and *Dermacentor variabilis* (American dog tick, Eastern, Central, and Southern North America). A differential diagnosis of tularemia from other tick-borne diseases is necessary following initial presentation of a patient. Tularemia is characterized by a high fever, headache, normal WBC count, and elevated liver transaminases without a rash (the rash is typical of Lyme disease and Rocky Mountain spotted fever) or anemia (this sign is typical of ehrlichiosis and babesiosis).

Clinical Manifestations

F. tularensis ssp. *tularensis* is one of the most infectious pathogens to humans. An infectious dose of as little as 10 organisms are known to cause an acute infection. Type A-caused tularemia is generally associated with the more severe disease, with the type A.I subtype causing more serious disease than the type A.II serotype. Type B-caused tularemia is generally associated with milder symptoms and frequently occurs after exposure to an *F. tularensis*-contaminated stream, pond, lake, or river, or to an infected semiaquatic animal such as a muskrat or beaver. Therefore, this disease is sometimes considered to be a water-borne disease. *F. tularensis* ssp. *mediasiatica* has rarely been reported as a cause of human disease, and *F. novicida* is considered of low virulence and only occasionally causes disease in immunocompromised patients. The incubation period following exposure to the type A and B strains is usually 3–5 days, range 1–21 days. Tularemia is a potential lethal infectious disease characterized by seven different clinical syndromes (WHO 2007). **Ulceroglandular** is the most common condition recognized, which occurs after exposure to infected animal tissue (direct contact) or by the bite of an insect vector, which has fed on an infected animal. This condition is characterized by the formation of a primary ulcer (painful, maculopapular lesion) that develops at the site of bacterial exposure with the presence of acutely inflamed regional lymph nodes. **Glandular** disease is characterized by a regional lymphadenopathy with no ulcer present. This disease may have originated with a primary ulcer, but at presentation, the ulcer may not be detected. The **oropharyngeal** form occurs in individuals who ingest *F. tularensis*-contaminated water or food. The patient with this form presents with an ulcerative–exudative stomatitis and pharyngitis with or without tonsillar involvement. The disease is also associated with an excessive regional neck lymphadenitis (cervical lymphadenopathy), which may mimic streptococcal disease. This condition may also occur in patients who may have been exposed to an infected insect or tick bite to the head and neck region without the detection of an ulceroglandular lesion. The **pneumonic** or respiratory form of tularemia is contacted by inhalation of aerosolized *F. tularensis*. This form occurs after exposure to the carcasses of rodents or lagomorphs found in the environment after death from tularemia (Matyas *et al.* 2007). Respiratory tularemia may present with symptoms of pneumonia, including cough, chest pain, and an increased respiratory rate. An intentional aerosol release of *F. tularensis* type A would be expected to result in clinical manifestations similar to those recognized in natural respiratory tularemia (fever, dry cough, chest pain, and hilar adenopathy). Other rare forms of tularemia include **oculoglandular** disease characterized by severe conjunctivitis and preauricular lymphadenopathy, **typhoidal** tularemia characterized by high fever, hepatomegaly, and splenomegaly, and **intestinal** disease characterized by intestinal pain, vomiting, and diarrhea.

Pathogenesis

F. tularensis is an intracellular pathogen, and the pathogenesis of this organism is the ability of the organism to replicate and survive within macrophage cells (Foley and Nieto 2010). Although the course of infection involves the spread of the organism to multiple systems to include the lungs, liver, spleen, and lymphatic system, the ultimate course of disease differs depending on the route of infection. The cell surface of *F. tularensis* contains a carbohydrate that is a unique version of lipopolysaccharide (LPS), which leads to phagocytosis via the formation of asymmetrical pseudopod loops. Once inside the cell, *F. tularensis* avoids phagolysosomal fusion, exits the phagosome, and is able to replicate within the cytosol of the cells (Cowley and Elkins 2011). Following a period of replication, the bacteria are released from the cell and quickly infect another phagocytic cell. The ability to cause disease is related to a large set of virulence genes, including *mgl*A and *mgl*B (macrophage growth locus) and the *Francisella* pathogenicity island (FPI)

(Backer and Klose 2007). The FPI contains 19 genes that encode for essential qualities of intracellular growth and virulence (Foley and Nieto 2010). Both the type A and type B strains are noted for causing disease; however, differences in virulence have been noted among the subtypes of type A and between type A and type B strains. The type A.I tends to produce a severe form of tularemia with a higher mortality rate, while type A.II and type B strains produce less severe and rarely fatal infections in humans. Evidence suggests that this difference in virulence is related to genomic properties of the strains, potentially leading to a broader range of immunosuppression that likely contributes to increased virulence.

Immunology

The bulk of data on immune responses to *F. tularensis* infection has been generated using mammalian animal models of infection and by studying responses in humans following vaccination (Elkins *et al.* 2003; Cowley and Elkins 2011). Additional information has been compiled following studies on individuals who have had natural infection. Studies following the administration of the attenuated vaccine strain derived from type B *F. tularensis*, designated LVS for "live vaccine strain," have been a model for intracellular pathogens although this information should not be assumed to apply directly to fully virulent *Francisella*. This vaccine has not been licensed by the US Food and Drug Administration (FDA) because of a lack of understanding of the basis of attenuation and the mechanism of pathogenesis. This attenuated vaccine was derived by repeated passage of a Russian vaccine strain on peptone cysteine agar and subsequent manipulations including lyophilization and serial passage through mice. The LVS strain is administered by the dermal route using a scarification method to produce an ulceroglandular lesion at the site of inoculation. Following immunization, a robust specific anti-*Francisella* antibody response occurs; however, the contribution of B cells toward protective immunity has been found to offer little advantage in intracellular infections (Elkins *et al.* 2003). On the other hand, activation of the specific T cells response involving memory cells is known to have a protective response following both vaccination and natural disease. Similar to other intracellular pathogens, long-term protective immunity to *Francisella* infection relies primarily upon T cells. T cells use a variety of both soluble and contact-dependent mechanisms to ultimately control and eliminate *Francisella* infection. Multiple research groups are studying the essential role for the various T cells subsets to characterize the mechanisms for providing protection against tularemia.

Vaccination

Numerous approaches have been employed to develop a tularemia vaccine ranging from crude culture extracts to subunit vaccines (Oyston 2009; Conlan 2011). So far, these approaches have failed to achieve good levels of protection against virulent strains. LPS appears to be a key component that is recognized by the human immune system with a search for other protective antigens continuing. Part of the hope in the development of a subunit vaccine is in the availability of new adjuvants, such as immune-stimulating complexes. However, use of this adjuvant system has not been evaluated in humans. Thus, the attenuated strain of *F. tularensis* type B (LVS) continues to be the only vaccine available for protection in humans. Although this vaccine has been utilized successfully for decades to immunize large groups of people, the vaccine has not been licensed by the regulatory agencies. There are many reasons for this; however, the lack of understanding of the basis of attenuation and the inability to do clinical studies due to the infectious nature of the organism are some key reasons why a universal vaccine is not available. Recently, the FDA issued a new regulation in 2002 as an alternative licensing pathway for pharmaceutical products that target highly lethal pathogens (Crawford 2002). This regulation called by some the "animal rule" has been used in the development of biodefense vaccines. This allows for approval based on animal efficacy data conducted under Good Laboratory Practice controls and human safety and immunogenicity data conducted under Good Clinical Practice controls, which support the correlation of protection defined in the animal model (Sullivan *et al.* 2009). The animal rule is intended to be used as a pathway for regulatory review only when there are no other ways to license a vaccine. However, utilization of this regulation still requires an understanding of the mechanism of pathogenesis, which is not available. Additionally, the immunological responses in animals differ significantly from those in humans. This makes it unlikely animal studies will totally predict what happens in humans. Currently, the LVS strain continues to be the lead candidate to protect individuals in the event of a deliberate release, based on its long history of use in humans.

Laboratory Diagnosis

The laboratory diagnosis of tularemia is based on recovery of the causative agent or detection of specific antigen or DNA in a clinical specimen or recognition of a serological response to *F. tularensis* in serum. The Council of State and Territorial Epidemiologists has described, based on laboratory criteria, a presumptive case of tularemia as an elevated serum antibody titer to *F. tularensis* antigen (without documented fourfold or greater change) in a patient with no history of tularemia vaccination or detection of *F. tularensis* in a clinical specimen by a fluorescent assay. A confirmatory case of tularemia is isolation of *F. tularensis* in a clinical specimen or a fourfold or greater change in serum antibody titer to *F. tularensis*-specific antigen (when testing acute and convalescent sera).

Laboratory Response Network

Special precautions are necessary when working with cultures or specimens suspected to contain *F. tularensis* since this organism is considered a risk group 3 agent by the US National Institutes of Health and a select agent by the federal government (CDC 2005; DHHS 2009). As a part of the bioterrorism preparedness program in the United States for the evaluation of specimens and isolates potentially containing *F. tularensis*, the CDC has developed a network of sentinel level clinical microbiology laboratories, which comprise part of the US Laboratory Response Network (LRN). The CDC and the Association of Public Health Laboratories in coordination with the American Society for Microbiology have developed protocols designed to assist these sentinel laboratories with information and techniques to rule out microorganisms that might be suspected as agents of bioterrorism (such as *F. tularensis*), or to refer suspect isolates to LRN reference laboratories (e.g., public health laboratories) for confirmation testing.

Serological Methods

Serology is the most common method used for the confirmation of tularemia. Antibody responses against *F. tularemia* are detected in patients about 10–20 days after infection. Agglutination protocols using antigens such as *Francisella*-specific LPS, an outer membrane carbohydrate–protein fraction, or whole killed cells are used as antigens to measure the immune response. Testing of both acute and convalescent sera is necessary to demonstrate a fourfold rise in specific antibody titer for confirmatory diagnosis of tularemia.

Morphology and Staining

F. tularensis is a tiny, pleomorphic, nonmotile, gram-negative, facultative intracellular coccobacillus (0.2–0.5 μm by 0.7–1.0 μm) (see Figure 17.1). From culture, the organism stains poorly and may be difficult to interpret because of this small size and poor staining (Figure 17.1).

FIGURE 17.1. *Gram stain of* F. tularensis *showing poor staining tiny gram-negative coccobacillus mostly seen as single cells, original magnification × 1000. (Courtesy of Larry Stauffer, CDC Public Health Image Library.)*

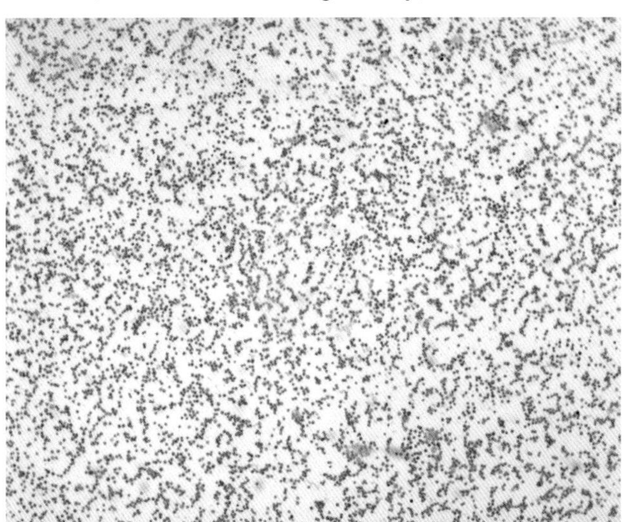

FIGURE 17.2. *Culture of* F. tularensis *on cysteine heart agar after 72 h incubation showing colonies that are 2–4 mm, smooth, entire, greenish-white with an opalescent sheen. (Courtesy of Larry Stauffer, CDC Public Health Image Library.)*

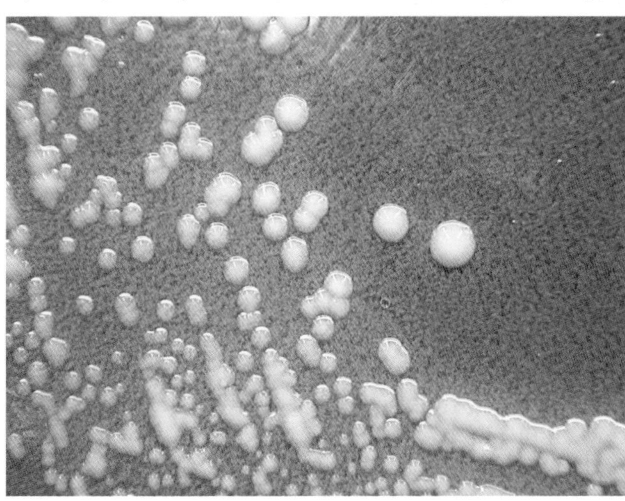

Culture Isolation

F. tularensis can be isolated from specimens of blood, skin, ulcers, lymph node drainage, gastric washings, or respiratory tract in cases of tularemia. Isolation of *F. tularensis* in culture provides a confirmed diagnosis of tularemia and also provides an isolate for molecular, epidemiological, and susceptibility testing (Splettstoesser *et al.* 2005). As a fastidious aerobe, this organism has preference to grow on medium supplemented with cysteine (e.g., cysteine hemoglobin agar), but this organism will also grow on other enriched media such as chocolate agar and modified Thayer-Martin agar. However, growth on sheep blood agar is generally poor. Adequate growth generally takes ≥48 h at 35–37 °C in 5% CO_2 after which time the colonies are about 2–4 mm in diameter, white to grey opaque, flat with an entire edge, smooth, and have a shiny surface (see Figure 17.2). *F. tularensis* will not grow on gram-negative selective/differential media such as MacConkey or eosin methylene blue agars, but will grow in commercial blood culture media (Figure 17.2).

Preliminary Biochemical Reactions

F. tularensis is oxidase-negative, weakly catalase-positive (3% hydrogen peroxide), β-lactamase-positive (e.g., Cefinase test reagent), urease-negative (e.g., Christensen agar), negative for satelliting, and shows no requirement for factor X (hemin) and factor V (nicotinamide adenine dinucleotide) for growth. Sentinel laboratories, which cannot rule out a potential *F. tularensis* at this point, are requested to consult with their LRN reference laboratory to determine the next step for submission of confirmation testing.

Limitations of Culture

Commercial identification systems should not be used to identify *F. tularensis* since they have a high probability of misidentification with the potential for generating aerosols during set up. The most common misidentification of *F. tularensis* is *Haemophilus influenzae* (which generally satellite or have a growth requirement for X and V factors) and *Actinobacillus actinomycetemcomitans* (which generally are β-lactamase-negative).

Antigen Detection Methods

Antigen detection methods are most useful for the direct detection of *F. tularensis* in clinical specimens. Direct fluorescent antibody staining, using a fluorescein isothiocyanate (FITC)-labeled rabbit antibody directed toward whole-cell killed *F. tularensis*, is commonly used. Additionally, immunohistochemical staining, using a monoclonal antibody directed against the LPS, can be used to visualize *F. tularensis* in formalin-fixed tissues.

Molecular Methods

Numerous polymerase chain reaction (PCR) methods have been described for the molecular detection of *F. tularensis* from clinical specimens and for confirmation identification from culture isolates (Larson *et al.* 2011). The majority of PCR tests have been either conventional or real-time PCR methods targeted at the genes *fopA* or *tul4* encoding the outer membrane proteins (Backer and Klose 2007). The increased sensitivity and specificity along with the rapidity over other diagnostic methods makes molecular testing attractive for future diagnostics. However, the lack of standardization of assays and validation testing protocols limits the use of molecular methods for confirmation testing at the present time. Genomic methods using sequence analysis comparison have also been used for the accurate identification of isolates recovered in culture. Targets within the rDNA complex (e.g., 16S rDNA) have been shown to be useful for identification purposes. Additional targets are being evaluated now that complete genomes for the *F. tularensis* ssp. are publically available (ssp. *holarctica*, GenBank Accession no. CP000803 and no. CP000437; ssp. *mediasiatica*, no. CP000915; and ssp. *tularensis*, no. CP001633 and no. NC006570).

Treatment

Parenteral administration of an aminoglycoside is the first choice for treatment of tularemia in adults and children (WHO 2007). The drug of choice is gentamicin at 5 mg/kg divided into two or three doses and monitored by assay of serum concentrations of the drug. This drug, when available, is a viable alternative, which can be given by intramuscular injection for a daily dose of 2 g for up to 10 days. However, streptomycin is not widely used because of its potential to cause vestibular toxicity and a frequent appearance of hypersensitivity reactions among personnel involved in its administration. For postexposure prophylaxis where an accidental exposure has been known to occur to laboratory personnel, a recommended therapy is either ciprofloxacin (1000 mg daily, divided in two doses) or doxycycline (200 mg daily, divided in two doses) for up to 14 days. In cases where exposure may have occurred without verification, the potentially exposed person should be instructed to be alert to the development of fever within 14 days of exposure and a readiness to treat is warranted. Antimicrobial susceptibility testing is not routinely done for *F. tularensis* since no natural resistance to antibiotics used for clinical therapy has been documented. However, the potential for *F. tularensis* to be used for bioterrorism makes resistance an area of concern. Thus, standardized methods for antimicrobial susceptibility testing are available to test *F. tularensis* to various antibiotics to include aminoglycosides (gentamicin and streptomycin), tetracyclines (doxycycline and tetracycline), quinolones (ciprofloxacin or levofloxacin), and chloramphenicol (CLSI 2010).

Safety Measures

Both the general public and laboratorians are at high risk of infection when exposed to infected arthropods, infected animals, or when handling cultures in the laboratory. To prevent exposure in the environment, individuals should be protected against arthropod bites by wearing protective clothing and by using insect repellents with frequent inspection for and removal of ticks from the skin and scalp. Children should be instructed not to handle dead or sick animals. Landscape workers should be aware of the potential for inhalation infection when creating aerosols (e.g., lawn mowing) where infected carcasses might be present (Matyas *et al.* 2007). Hunters, trappers, and food preparers should be instructed to wear rubber gloves or other protection when handling the carcasses of wild rabbits and other potentially infected animals. Game meats should also be cooked thoroughly. For laboratorians and researchers handling specimens and cultures in the laboratory, special precautions must be considered. Tularemia has been reported as the fourth most commonly reported laboratory-associated infection worldwide caused by bacteria behind brucellosis, Q fever, and typhoid fever (Singh 2009). The US Department of Health and Human Services provides a document for guidance in the laboratory when handling *F. tularensis* (DHHS 2007). Additionally, the CDC has published a guideline for managing potential laboratory exposures to *F. tularensis* (http://www.cdc.gov/tularemia/, accessed October 26, 2011). This guideline provides guidance on how to determine if the exposed individual should be managed by fever watch and who would benefit from immediate prophylaxis.

F. tularensis as a Biological Weapon

The high virulence of the pathogen in humans, the low infectious dose (10–50 organisms), and the ease of dissemination by aerosol have led to the concerns of *F. tularensis* for utilization as a bioweapon. Therefore, the US government has classified *F. tularensis* as a select agent that requires the handling and possession of this agent to be highly regulated (CDC 2005). Any laboratory (human or veterinary) where diagnostic testing is performed must document destruction of confirmed cultures of *F. tularensis* or be registered by the national Select Agent Program to have viable cultures in their possession.

References

Backer J and Klose K (2007) Molecular and genetic basis of pathogenesis in *Francisella tularensis*. *Ann NY Acad Sci*, **1105**, 138–159.

Centers for Disease Control and Prevention (2005) Possession, use, and transfer of select agents and toxins, final rule. *Fed Regist*, **70**, 13293–13325.

Centers for Disease Control and Prevention (2012) Summary of notifiable diseases—United States, 2010. *Morbidity and Mortality Weekly Reports*, **59**, 97–99.

Clinical and Laboratory Standards Institute (2010) *Methods for Antimicrobial Dilution and Disk Susceptibility Testing of Infrequently Isolated or Fastidious Bacteria; Approved Guideline, M45-A2*, Clinical and Laboratory Standards Institute, Wayne, PA.

Conlan JW (2011) Tularemia vaccines: recent developments and remaining hurdles. *Future Microbiol*, **6**, 391–405.

Cowley SC and Elkins KL (2011) Immunity to *Francisella*. *Front Microbiol*, **2**, 1–21.

Crawford LM (2002) New drug and biological drug products: evidence needed to demonstrate effectiveness of new drugs when human efficacy studies are not ethical or feasible. *Fed Regist*, **67**, 37988–37998.

Department of Health and Human Services (2007) *Biosafety in Microbiology and Biomedical Laboratories*, 5th edn, US Government Printing Office, Washington, DC.

Department of Health and Human Services (2009) *NIH Guidelines for Research Involving Recombinant DNA Molecules, September 2009*, US Government Printing Office, Washington, DC.

Elkins KL, Cowley SC, and Bosio CM (2003) Innate and adaptive immune responses to an intracellular bacterium, *Francisella tularensis* live vaccine strain. *Microbes Infect*, **5**, 135–142.

Farlow J, Wagner DM, Dukerich M *et al.* (2005) *Francisella tularensis* in the United States. *Emerg Infect Dis*, **11**, 1835–1841.

Foley JE and Nieto NC (2010) Tularemia. *Vet Microbiol*, **140**, 332–338.

Graham J, Stockley K, and Goldman RD (2011) Tick-borne illnesses, a CME update. *Pediatr Emerg Care*, **27**, 141–150.

Johansson A, Celli J, Conlan W *et al.* (2010) Objections to the transfer of *Francisella novicida* to the subspecies rank of *Francisella tularensis*. *Int J Syst Evol Microbiol*, **60**, 1717–1718.

Kugeler KJ, Mead PS, Janusz AM *et al.* (2009) Molecular epidemiology of *Francisella tularensis* in the United States. *Clin Infect Dis*, **48**, 863–870.

Larson MA, Fey PD, Bartling AM *et al.* (2011) *Francisella tularensis* molecular typing using differential insertion sequence amplification. *J Clin Microbiol*, **48**, 2786–2797.

Matyas BT, Nieder HS, and Telford SR, III (2007) Pneumonic tularemia on Martha's Vineyard: clinical, epidemiologic, and ecological characteristics. *Ann NY Acad Sci*, **1105**, 351–377.

Oyston PCF (2009) *Francisella tularensis* vaccines. *Vaccine*, **27**, D48–D51.

Petersen JM, Mead PS, and Schriefer ME (2009) *Francisella tularensis*: an arthropod-borne pathogen. *Vet Res*, **40**, 1–9.

Singh K (2009) Laboratory-acquired infections. *Clin Infect Dis*, **49**, 142–147.

Splettstoesser WD, Tomaso H, Al Dahouk S *et al.* (2005) Diagnostic procedures in tularemia with special focus on molecular and immunological techniques. *J Vet Med*, **52**, 249–261.

Sullivan JJ, Martin JE, Graham BS, and Nabel GJ (2009) Correlates of protective immunity for Ebola vaccines: implications for regulatory approval by the animal rule. *Nat Rev Microbiol*, **7**, 393–401.

World Health Organization (2007) *WHO Guidelines on Tularemia*, WHO Press, World Health Organization, Geneva, Switzerland.

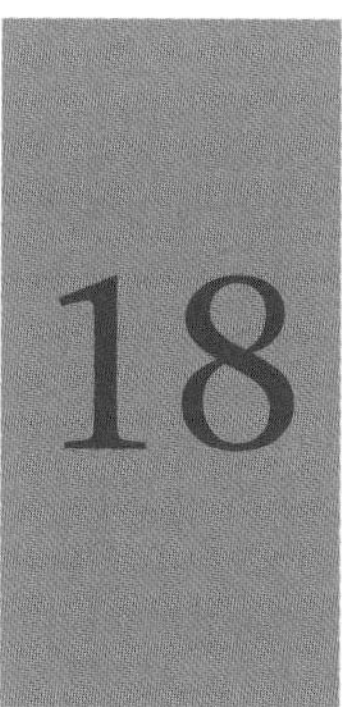

18 Moraxella

HUCHAPPA JAYAPPA AND D. SCOTT MCVEY

Members of the genus *Moraxella* are gram-negative rods and cocci belonging to the family Moraxellaceae (or Gammaproteobacteria). The genus *Moraxella* had been previously subdivided into two subgenera, *Moraxella* (containing the rod-shaped members of the genus) and subgenus *Branhamella* (the coccoid members). Some of the coccoid species were also formerly classified as *Neisseria*. There are several members of this genus (see Table 18.1), some of which are associated with diseases of human patients. From a veterinary perspective, *Moraxella bovis* is the most important member of the group. *M. bovis* is the cause of infectious bovine keratoconjunctivitis (IBK), the most common ocular disease of cattle.

Descriptive Features

Morphology and Staining

Moraxellae are short, plump gram-negative rods, 11.5 μm × 1.5–2.5 μm, and are often arranged in pairs ("diplo bacilli") or short chains (Figure 18.1).

Structure and Composition

The cell wall is typical of gram-negative bacteria being composed of lipopolysaccharide (LPS) and protein. The LPS of moraxellae does not contain O-repeat units, in contrast to many other gram-negative microorganisms (e.g., members of the family Enterobacteriaceae).

The fimbrial adhesins (pili) of *M. bovis* are virulence determinants and can be lost in subculture (see Section "Variability"). Capsules may be present on fresh isolates.

Cellular Products of Medical Interest

Adhesins. The role of adhesins, as in other microorganisms, is to allow the bacterium expressing them to adhere to cells lining a particular niche, as well as to the surface of the so-called target cells prior to the initiation of disease (in some cases, niche and target cells may be the same). *M. bovis* produces a type 4 pilus (fimbria) that adheres to conjunctival and corneal epithelial cells. This pilus is similar to those of *Pseudomonas aeruginosa, Neisseria gonorrhoeae, Dichelobacter nodosus, Pasteurella multocida*, and *Vibrio cholerae*. Mutants unable to produce this adhesin are avirulent.

Capsule. The capsule plays many roles, the most important of which are interference with phagocytosis (antiphagocytic), and protection of the outer membrane from the deposition of membrane attack complexes generated by activation of the complement system.

Cell Wall. The cell wall of the members of this genus is one typical of gram-negative bacteria (except for the absence of the O-repeat unit). The LPS in the outer membrane is an important virulence determinant. LPS binds to LPS-binding protein (a serum protein), which transfers it to the blood phase of CD14. The CD14–LPS complex binds to Toll-like receptor proteins (see Chapter 2) on the surface of macrophage cells, triggering the release of proinflammatory cytokines.

Exotoxins. The most noteworthy toxin produced by *M. bovis* is an RTX (repeats in toxin, so called because of the structural repeats of glycine-rich sequences within the protein) type of cytotoxin (see also *Escherichia coli* hemolysin, Chapter 7; *Pasteurella/Mannheimia* leukotoxin, Chapter 11; *Actinobacillus* hemolysin, Chapter 12; and adenylyl cyclase toxin of *Bordetella*, Chapter 14). This cytotoxin, sometimes referred to as "hemolysin" due to its behavior on blood agar plates, has been termed Mbx (for *M. bovis* toxin). Mbx is a pore-forming toxin with specificity for conjunctival and corneal epithelial cells, and neutrophils. Mutants unable to produce Mbx are avirulent.

Iron Acquisition. Because iron is an absolute growth requirement, microorganisms must acquire this substance if they are to exist within the host. Moraxellae acquire iron from the iron-binding proteins of the host (transferrin and lactoferrin) by expressing Tbp and Lbp (for transferrin- and lactoferrin-binding proteins, respectively) on their surface. Tbp and Lbp bind their respective proteins giving moraxellae access to iron.

Miscellaneous Products. A number of proteins with toxic activities are produced *in vitro* by *M. bovis*. These include

Veterinary Microbiology, Third Edition. Edited by D. Scott McVey, Melissa Kennedy and M.M. Chengappa.

Table 18.1. Members of the Genus *Moraxella* and Their Usual Source or Associated Condition

Species	Usual Source or Associated Condition
Moraxella atlantae (CDC group M-3)	Septicemia in human patients
M. boevrei	Respiratory tract of normal goats
M. bovis	IBK in cattle
M. bovoculi	Respiratory tract and ocular surfaces of cattle
M. cuniculi	Respiratory tract of rabbits
M. canis	Respiratory tracts of normal dogs and cats
M. caprae	Respiratory tracts of normal goats and sheep
M. catarrhalis	Middle ear infections in children; upper respiratory tract infections in human patients
M. caviae	Respiratory tract of guinea pigs
M. lacunata	Conjunctivitis and keratitis in human patients
M. lincolnii	Respiratory tract of human patients
M. nonliquefaciens	Respiratory trace of normal human patients; blood, cerebral spinal fluid, and lungs of compromised patients
M. ovis and *M. oblonga*	Keratoconjunctivitis in sheep
M. osloensis	Nematodes; various conditions in human patients
M. phenylpyruvica	Respiratory tract of normal human patients; bloodstream of compromised human patients

FIGURE 18.1. M. bovis *in the cornea of an experimentally infected calf. There is evidence of digestion of corneal substance around the bacterial cells. Scanning electron micrograph, 22 000×. (Courtesy of Dr Doug Rogers, University of Nebraska Veterinary Diagnostic Center.)*

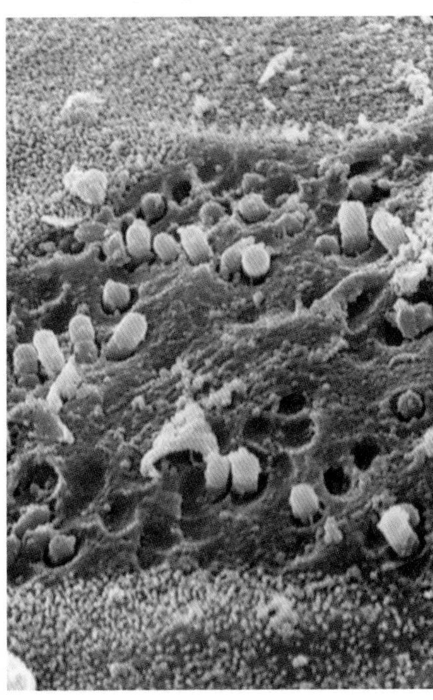

complement-degrading proteases, lipases, phosphoamidases, peptidases, and proteases. There is little evidence showing that any of these play a role *in vivo*.

Growth Characteristics

M. bovis grows best at 35 °C in the presence of serum and blood. No growth occurs on MacConkey agar or anaerobically. In 48 h, fresh isolates produce flat, hemolytic, friable colonies, about 1 mm in size, that corrode the agar and autoagglutinate when suspended in saline.

Biochemical Activities

M. bovis is oxidase-positive, asaccharolytic, nonfermenting, and catalase-variable. Nitrates and urea are not digested, but proteins are digested. Most other species of *Moraxella* do reduce nitrate and nitrite.

Resistance

Resistance to physical and chemical agents is not remarkable. It is usually susceptible to commonly used antibiotics including penicillin. Some isolates of *M. bovis* are resistant to tetracyclines and tylosin. *Moraxella catarrhalis* is the only species that commonly produces a β-lactamase.

Variability

In culture, *M. bovis* undergoes colonial dissociation (phase variation) producing smooth butyrous colonies composed of cells, which lack pili (due to inversion of the pilin-encoding gene) and infectivity, and are less autoagglutinable. Pili are immunogenically diverse, and this trait is responsible for a classification scheme based on serological similarities. Nonhemolytic variants are nonpathogenic.

Ecology

The Moraxellaceae are generally normal flora of the upper respiratory mucosal surface and ocular surface. Most of these bacteria are not pathogens.

Reservoir

M. bovis occurs worldwide on the bovine conjunctiva and upper respiratory mucosa, often without clinical manifestations.

Transmission

Dissemination is by direct and indirect contact, including flying insects and possibly other airborne transmission.

Pathogenesis

Mechanisms

Disease produced by *M. bovis* is closely linked to cytotoxin (Mbx) and pili. Attachment (pili) to conjunctival

FIGURE 18.2. *(A and B) Calves with infectious IBK.*

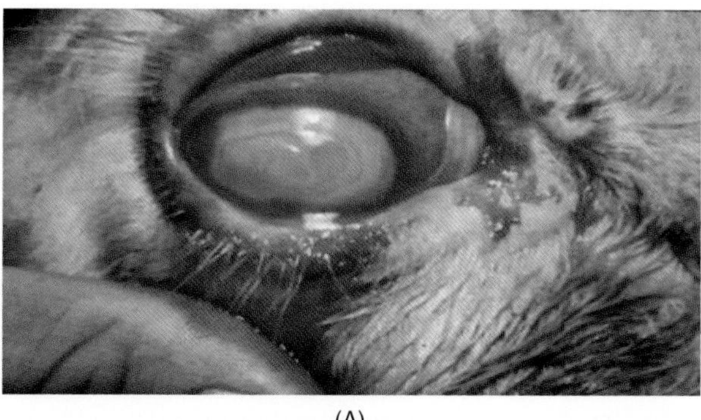

(A)

(B)

epithelium is followed by destruction (Mbx) of conjunctival and corneal cells. Growth of *M. bovis* in the conjunctival and corneal lesions leads to inflammation (gram-negative cell wall). Mbx-mediated lysis of neutrophils amplifies inflammation and tissue destruction.

Environmental factors implicated include ultraviolet irradiation, flies, dust, and woody pasture plants, all of which contribute to irritation of the target tissues. Concurrent infections with viruses, such as bovine herpesvirus 1 (infectious bovine rhinotracheitis virus) and adenovirus, mycoplasma (*Mycoplasma bovoculi*), bacteria (*Listeria monocytogenes*), and nematodes (Thelazia), may complicate the disease.

Disease Pattern and Pathology

Infectious Bovine Keratoconjunctivitis. IBK begins with invasion of conjunctiva and cornea by *M. bovis*, resulting in edema and a predominantly neutrophilic inflammatory response. It may progress from mild epiphora and corneal clouding to production of severe edema, corneal opacities, vascularization, ulceration, and rupture, leading to uveal prolapse and panophthalmitis (Figure 18.2 and Chapter 74). Healing of the ulcers proceeds from the periphery and requires several weeks. Central scarring may persist for months. Although it is a self-limiting disease, losses occur because vision-impaired animals do not forage and lose condition.

Epidemiology

IBK is a highly infectious disease, mostly of beef cattle. Young animals are preferentially affected, probably due to lack of acquired immunity. Lack of eyelid pigmentation and prominent placement of eyes are apparent predisposing factors, as is vitamin A deficiency.

Prevalence is greatest during summer and early fall, when environmental stresses are maximal.

Immunologic Aspects

Antibodies of all isotypes are produced during infection, with secretory IgA predominating locally. Temporary resistance to reinfection follows recovery. The relative roles in immunity and recovery of general versus local responses and humoral versus cell-mediated responses are unsettled.

Experimental bacterins and fimbrial antigens stimulate resistance, optimally to homologous challenge. Apparently, fimbrial proteins, Mbx, and proteolytic enzymes have protection-inducing activity. Fimbrial vaccines are commercially available.

Laboratory Diagnosis

The agent may be demonstrated in smears of exudate, most convincingly by immunofluorescence (by using the antibody specific to *M. bovis* antigens). Exudate is cultured on blood agar, and *Moraxella* is identified by colonial characteristics, oxidase activity, hemolysis, proteolysis, and failure to ferment carbohydrates. Specific fluorescent antibody conjugates can be applied directly to suspect colonies on plates for identification even of dissociant colonies (epifluorescence). Polymerase chain reaction-based assays utilizing *M. bovis*-specific primers are available for detection and identification.

Treatment and Control

Affected animals should be placed in a dark stall, free from dust and flies. Topical corticosteroids may relieve the inflammation, while antimicrobial drugs, given topically or systemically, may be beneficial. Long-acting tetracycline or florfenicol is considered the drug of choice.

Fimbrial vaccines are the most promising specific prophylactics. However, immunity is serotype specific and broad-spectrum antigenic coverage is generally not available.

Further Reading

Alexander D (2010) Infectious bovine keratoconjunctivitis: a review of cases in clinical practice. *Vet Clin North Am Food Anim Pract*, **26** (3), 487–503.

Pseudomonas

SANJEEV NARAYANAN

Members of the genus *Pseudomonas* are gram-negative aerobic rods. Although there are more than 200 characterized and uncharacterized species and subspecies of *Pseudomonas*, most veterinary diseases are caused by *Pseudomonas aeruginosa*. Previously named pseudomonads of veterinary importance, *Pseudomonas mallei* and *Pseudomonas pseudomallei*, have been moved to the genus *Burkholderia* (see Chapter 16).

P. aeruginosa is very rarely involved with primary disease, although it is extremely important in clinical medicine. Most strains are resistant to the commonly used antimicrobial agents and are, therefore, sometimes difficult to eliminate when they contaminate a compromised site.

Descriptive Features

Morphology and Staining

The organisms are gram-negative rods, 1.5–5.0 μm by 0.5–1.0 μm.

Cellular Anatomy and Composition

Pseudomonads produce a typical gram-negative cell wall, surrounded by a carbohydrate-containing capsule. All members of the genus are motile by means of polar flagella. Pili (fimbrial adhesins) are produced.

Cellular Products of Medical Interest

Adhesins. *P. aeruginosa* produces several products that serve as adhesins. These include a fimbrial adhesin that has affinity for certain glycoproteins on epithelial cells. In addition, there are nonfimbrial adhesins, an outer membrane protein with affinity for mucin, and another, the lipopolysaccharide (LPS) of the cell wall that has affinity for chloride channel proteins. Fimbrial adhesins induce proinflammatory cytokines via the Toll-like receptors (see Chapter 2) on the surface of macrophages.

Capsule. The capsule protects the outer membrane from the membrane attack complex of the complement cascade. The capsule also inhibits attachment to, and ingestion by, phagocytic host cells.

Cell Wall. The cell wall of the members of this genus is one typical of gram-negative bacteria. The LPS in the outer membrane is an important virulence determinant. Not only is the lipid A component toxic (endotoxin), but the length of the side chain in the O-repeat unit hinders the attachment of the membrane attack complex of the complement system to the outer membrane. LPS binds to LPS-binding protein, which transfers it to the blood phase of CD14. The CD14–LPS complex binds to Toll-like receptor proteins, triggering the release of proinflammatory cytokines.

Iron-Acquiring Systems. Iron is an absolute growth requirement for all living things. *P. aeruginosa* produces the iron-acquiring siderophores pyochelin and pyoverdin, as well as using the siderophores produced by other bacteria living in its environment (e.g., enterobactin and aerobactin). These products are used to remove iron from host iron-binding proteins.

Exotoxins. *P. aeruginosa* produces a number of protein exotoxins: exotoxins A, S, T, U, and Y, elastase, and a number of other proteins with biological activity (proteases and phospholipases). Exotoxins S, T, U, and Y are "injected" into host cells by way of a type III secretion apparatus (an assemblage of proteins—more than 20—that form a hollow tube-like structure through which effector proteins are "injected" into host "target" cells):

1. *Exotoxin A*: Exotoxin A inhibits protein synthesis by ribosylation of elongation factor-2 following receptor-mediated endocytosis.
2. *Exotoxins S and T*: Exotoxins S and T ribosylate host cell GTP-binding proteins, interrupting cell functions relying on the actin cytoskeleton (e.g., phagocytosis).
3. *Exotoxin U*: Exotoxin U is cytotoxic, but the mechanism is undefined.
4. *Exotoxin Y*: Exotoxin Y is an adenylate cyclase that raises the amount of intracellular cAMP (cyclic AMP) to damaging levels.

Miscellaneous Products. *P. aeruginosa* produces bacteriocins (pyocins) and pigments (pyocyanins). Pyocins are

Veterinary Microbiology, Third Edition. Edited by D. Scott McVey, Melissa Kennedy and M.M. Chengappa.

useful for tracing epidemics within the hospital environment. Pyocyanin has toxic activity and is used as an aid in the laboratory identification of *P. aeruginosa*. Pyocyanin reacts with oxygen to form reactive oxygen radicals that are toxic to eukaryotic and prokaryotic organisms. Pyocyanin has been shown to inhibit lymphocyte proliferation in the host. *P. aeruginosa* protects itself from the toxic effects of pyocyanin by increasing synthesis of catalase and superoxide dismutase.

Product Regulation. Regulation of the expression and excretion of cellular products involved in the pathogenesis of disease produced by *P. aeruginosa* is complex. Secretion of products that are secreted by way of the type III secretion apparatus (exotoxins S, T, U, and Y) is initiated following bacteria–host cell interaction. The remaining bacterial cell products are under the control of the "quorum-sensing" system of *P. aeruginosa*. The genes that encode these products are expressed when concentrations of bacterially produced homoserine lactones reach a threshold level (a "quorum"). All *P. aeruginosa* cells excrete homoserine lactones, but the concentration is too low to trigger virulence gene expression until a critical number of bacterial cells is reached. Finally, exotoxin A and an endoprotease are also regulated by levels of pyoverdin. When free iron concentrations are low (as would be the case *in vivo*), these two proteins are expressed and excreted.

Growth Characteristics

P. aeruginosa is an obligate aerobe, deriving energy from the oxidation of organic materials and using oxygen as a terminal electron acceptor. It grows on all common media over a wide range of temperatures, 4–41 °C.

Ecology

Reservoir

Most members of the genus *Pseudomonas* live in soil and water. *P. aeruginosa* may also be found in the feces of normal animals, but not as a member of the normal flora (i.e., they are transients).

Transmission

Environmental or endogenous exposure is constant, and most infections are secondary to compromised host defenses.

Pathogenesis

Mechanisms

P. aeruginosa can cause infection of almost any location in the host, although it does not cause clinical illness in a healthy host. *P. aeruginosa* contaminates areas of the body that possess reduced numbers of normal flora. Disruption of the normal flora is almost always due to antimicrobial agents. Since *P. aeruginosa* is resistant to most commonly used antimicrobial agents, it will replace the normal flora. If the site colonized is compromised or contiguous to a compromised site, there is risk of infection of the site. Tissue destruction is due to liberation of exotoxins and pyocyanin from the bacterium and release of proinflammatory cytokines and reactive oxygen intermediates from the host.

P. aeruginosa is also isolated from certain sites of animals that have no history of antimicrobial therapy.

Disease Patterns

Dogs and Cats

P. aeruginosa infection is associated with otitis externa, lower urinary tract infection, pyoderma, and occasional ocular infections.

Horse

P. aeruginosa is associated with metritis (vaginitis) secondary to prolonged treatment with antimicrobial agents, keratitis, and conjunctivitis following treatment of corneal ulcers with topical steroid–antibiotic mixtures.

Bovine

P. aeruginosa is associated with mastitis (uncommon).

Miscellaneous

P. aeruginosa is an uncommon cause of septicemia in immunocompromised animals, but a frequent cause of bacteremia in human beings with burns, leukemia, or cystic fibrosis.

Epidemiology

The organism is ubiquitous in the environment, and therefore, it is impossible to prevent exposure. Disease determinants, therefore, lie largely with the hosts and their immediate environment. The organism is nonfastidious, and in a veterinary hospital a number of situations favor selection of this organism. *P. aeruginosa* thrives in wet, poorly aerated environments within the hospital, especially in surgery areas within support bags that have not been properly dried, in hoses on anesthetic machines that have not been cleaned and dried properly, or in disinfectant solutions that have not been changed frequently. These situations result in an increase in the number of pseudomonads in the environment of the compromised animal (site), thereby increasing the risk of infection (contamination).

Immunologic Aspects

Specific immune responses do not seem to play much of a role in pathogenesis or resistance, though artificial protection has been shown to occur in animals vaccinated with extracts of the organism or exotoxin A. The most important consideration is to decrease the risk of infection by reducing the concentration of the organism in the environment of the patient, in addition to reducing the extent of compromise, for example, by cleaning and drying an infected ear.

Laboratory Diagnosis

P. aeruginosa grows well on blood agar medium. The colonies are somewhat large, >1 mm in diameter, gray (gunmetal), rough, usually with a zone of hemolysis. A plate containing *P. aeruginosa* has a characteristic odor, reminiscent of corn tortillas. Besides being oxidase-positive, a trait that sets it apart from members of the family Enterobacteriaceae, it turns triple sugar iron agar slightly alkaline (without gas), utilizes glucose oxidatively, grows at 42 °C, and forms a blue-green, chloroform-soluble pigment, pyocyanin. Resistance to some antimicrobials is due to permeability barrier of the *Pseudomonas* cell wall, and to others because of inactivation due to products encoded by plasmid-based genes (R plasmids).

Treatment and Control

Treatment involves correction of compromise and, if necessary, the use of an antimicrobial agent. *P. aeruginosa* is usually susceptible to gentamicin, tobramycin, amikacin, carbenicillin, ciprofloxacin, and ticarcillin–clavulanic acid, and these agents are used for the treatment of soft tissue infections. In the canine urinary tract, tetracycline achieves concentrations sufficient to kill most isolates. Most pseudomonads are susceptible to levels achieved by antimicrobial agents in otic preparations: enrofloxacin, neomycin, polymyxin, chloramphenicol, and gentamicin. It should be noted that there are no *in vitro* tests that predict susceptibility/resistance of an isolate from infectious processes that will be treated topically (e.g., the ear).

Further Reading

Greene CE (ed.) (2006) *Infectious Diseases of Dog and Cat*, Saunders-Elsevier, pp. 320–321, 815–817, and 884–885.

NCBI. *Bacterial Taxonomy*, http://www.ncbi.nlm.nih.gov/Taxonomy/ (accessed January 8, 2013).

Quinn PJ, Carter ME, Markey B, and Carter GR (1999) *Clinical Veterinary Microbiology*, Mosby, pp. 237–242.

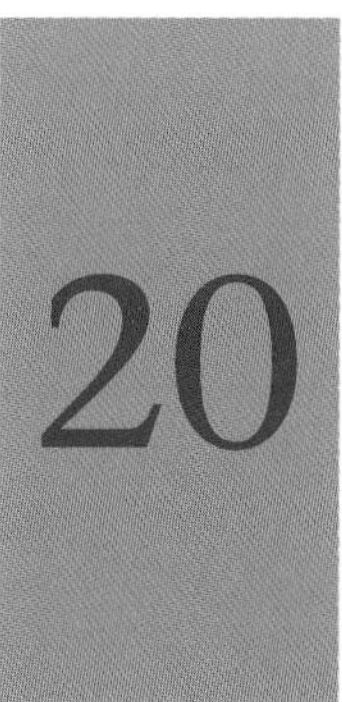

Taylorella

Megan E. Jacob

Members of the genus *Taylorella* are gram-negative, nonmotile, rods or coccobacilli. Equid species appear to be the natural host of *Taylorella* organisms. The genus contains two known species: *Taylorella equigenitalis*, the causative agent of contagious equine metritis (CEM), and *Taylorella asinigenitalis*, which has been associated with the genital tract of stallions or jacks. While *T. equigenitalis* has significant clinical and economic importance, *T. asinigenitalis* has rarely been associated with natural infection.

T. equigenitalis

T. equigenitalis is the causative agent of an acute, suppurative, self-limiting disease of the uterus of mares called CEM. The disease was first described in Europe in 1977; in 1978, CEM was classified as a reportable disease in the United States. CEM can result in temporary infertility or rarely early abortion in mares. The organism is highly contagious, and long-term asymptomatic carriage of *T. equigenitalis* can follow initial infection. Stallions develop no clinical signs of disease, but are important long-term carriers. Because of the costs associated with outbreak investigations, testing, and loss of reproductive efficiency, CEM has significant economic implications for the equine industry.

Descriptive Features

Morphology and Staining. *T. equigenitalis* is a gram-negative short rod or coccobacillus approximately 0.8 μm by 5–6 μm in size (Figure 20.1). The organism may exhibit bipolar staining and is nonmotile.

Structure and Composition. The cell wall structure of *T. equigenitalis* is typical of gram-negative bacteria, composed of lipopolysaccharide and protein. It is inconsistently fimbriated (typically in culture), and the outer membrane is covered by a capsule. The immunodominant outer membrane protein appears to resemble porin proteins from *Bordetella pertussis* and several *Neisseria* species.

Original chapter written by Drs. Ernst L. Biberstein and Dwight C. Hirsh and illustrations by Dr. Peter Timoney.

Growth Characteristics. *T. equigenitalis* is a fastidious organism that grows optimally between 35 °C and 37 °C under microaerophilic conditions. The organism generally grows well on a rich base medium with 5% chocolate sheep blood, and antimicrobials can be added to the medium to improve the selectivity of the assay. Visible colonies can be seen after 48–72 h of incubation, although growth may take up to 14 days. Current protocols recommend an incubation period of 7 days before confirming samples are negative. Overgrowth of other urogenital tract organisms may interfere with the culture and identification of *T. equigenitalis*; however, supplemental antimicrobials may improve recovery. Colonies of *T. equigenitalis* are variable in size (2–3 mm in diameter) and are shiny, smooth, and grayish-yellow. The organism is oxidase, catalase, and phosphatase-positive and otherwise biochemically unreactive, producing no acid from carbohydrates.

Resistance. Although there are two biotypes of *T. equigenitalis*—one is susceptible to streptomycin and another is resistant—*T. equigenitalis* isolates are generally susceptible to a broad range of antimicrobials with no obvious resistance patterns and are susceptible to various disinfectants.

Variability. Molecular methods such as random amplification of polymorphic DNA and pulse-field gel electrophoresis of restriction endonuclease-digested DNA have identified different strains of *T. equigenitalis*. Some reports have suggested that differing strains vary in their ability to cause clinical disease in exposed mares; however, this association is not fully understood. In addition, strains can differ in their susceptibility to streptomycin; the clinical significance of this observation is unknown.

Ecology

Reservoir. The equine genital tract is the only known natural host of *T. equigenitalis*. Mares and stallions that carry the organism asymptomatically are the most important reservoirs. The foci of carriage in mares are the clitoral fossa and sinuses; in stallions, the organism is typically a surface contaminant of the external genitalia or urogenital

Veterinary Microbiology, Third Edition. Edited by D. Scott McVey, Melissa Kennedy and M.M. Chengappa.

FIGURE 20.1. *A Gram stain of* T. equigenitalis. *(Courtesy of Peter Timoney and Mike Donahue.)*

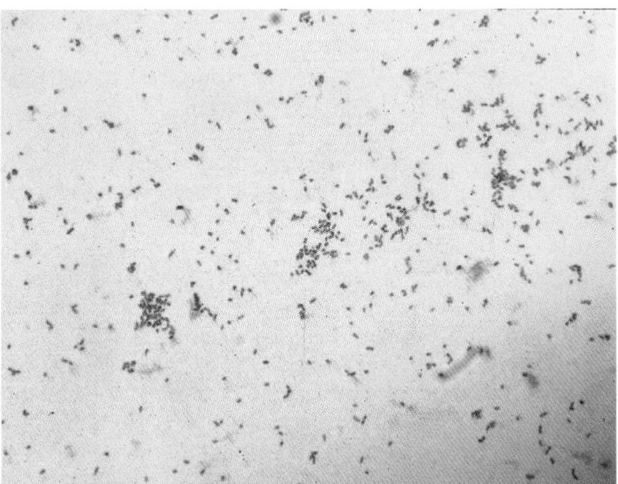

FIGURE 20.2. *A mare with vaginal discharge associated with* T. equigenitalis *infection. (Courtesy of Peter Timoney and Donald Simpson.)*

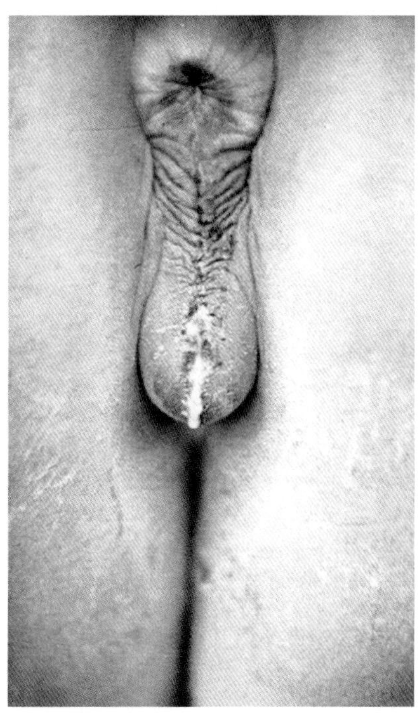

membranes including the urethra, urethral fossa, urethral sinus, and penile sheath. Stallions in particular can carry *T. equigenitalis* for an extended length of time, up to several years. Although antibodies to the agent have been found in species other than horses, no natural infections have been reported.

Transmission. *T. equigenitalis* is communicable, with an extremely high transmission rate. The organism is most commonly transmitted sexually, often through an asymptomatic carrier stallion. Foals born to infected mares can also be infected and become chronic carriers of *T. equigenitalis*. Indirect transmission can occur by contaminated fomites and hands, or through artificial insemination. There is no evidence to suggest that the organism can persist in the environment for an extended time and be transmitted independent of the horse.

Pathogenesis

Infection of mares with *T. equigenitalis* can result in variable clinical disease, ranging from asymptomatic to acute and overt. The incubation period for infection is generally 2–14 days. In acute clinical cases, a mucopurulent endometritis develops with variable amounts of discharge within days (2–12) of infection (Figure 20.2). The main damage is to uterine epithelium (exclusive of glands), which becomes covered by neutrophilic exudate. The cellular infiltrate in the endometrial stroma is predominantly mononuclear. The epithelium can be eroded or undergo severe degenerative changes. The uterine infection usually subsides spontaneously within several weeks. Endometrial repair is complete and there is no lasting impairment of breeding performance. Infection has been demonstrated in placentas and newborn foals, but abortions are rare. There is no fever or other sign of illness. The only apparent effect may be failure of conception. In chronic cases, there is often less obvious discharge and a more mild inflammation of the uterus. Carrier mares and stallions remain asymptomatic, but are still highly infectious.

Epidemiology. The carrier state of stallions and mares has been described as the single most important factor in the dissemination and persistence of *T. equigenitalis* in horse populations. Dissemination of infection is most commonly tied to breeding operations and the movement and use of infected animals. CEM has been reported in horse populations throughout the world including Europe, Africa, Japan, Australia, and North and South America. Some countries have successfully eradicated the organism. As recently as 2011, the United States Department of Agriculture's (USDA) National Veterinary Services Laboratories confirmed a positive stallion in the United States. Prior cases were identified in 2008 and 2010, with the 2008 source stallion being linked to 27 other *T. equigenitalis*-positive horses.

Immunologic Aspects

Immunity to *T. equigenitalis* is weak and animals may become reinfected; however, recovered animals show increased resistance for several months, manifested by milder signs and a lower concentration of bacteria. The mechanism of resistance is not fully understood.

Serum antibodies can persist in mares for 3–7 weeks postacute infection; however, they may not be detectable until 15–21 days after recovery. Titers are unrelated to the carrier status. Antibody is present in vaginal mucus, but its relation to infection is unknown. Stallions will not mount an antibody response to colonization with *T. equigenitalis*.

Diagnosis

Several diagnostic tests are available for *T. equigenitalis*; however, federal regulations require approved laboratories provide the testing service for routine import and export purposes. Confirmative diagnosis of CEM and *T. equigenitalis* carriers requires demonstration of the organism in the genital tract. In clinical cases, the agent can be demonstrated in the uterine exudate by Gram stain; however, this is only suggestive and not confirmatory for CEM disease. Most commonly, *T. equigenitalis* is diagnosed based on a positive bacterial culture on a selective medium. In mares, the most appropriate culture sites include the uterus, cervix, clitoral sinuses and fossa, or vaginal exudate, if present. Appropriate samples from stallions include urethral fossa and sinus, distal urethra, and the external surface of the penis. Samples sent for *T. equigenitalis* testing should be transported in appropriate medium (i.e., Amies transport media with charcoal). Isolates exhibiting *Taylorella* characteristics (slow-growing, gram-negative coccobacilli that are oxidase-positive) should be evaluated for reactivity with antiserum.

Other available testing strategies include serology (e.g., complement fixation test). These tests are often of limited value because they may only detect acutely infected mares; carrier mares and stallions will not demonstrate an antibody response. Serologic testing has not been reliable as a stand-alone test for diagnosis and control of *T. equigenitalis*.

Test breeding is a strategy to evaluate stallions for carriage of *T. equigenitalis*. Test breeding involves breeding a stallion to two pretested *T. equigenitalis*-negative mares. The mares would be sampled and evaluated for *T. equigenitalis* for up to 35 days postbreeding to declare the stallion negative.

Finally, several molecular tests have been reported that can identify and differentiate *T. equigenitalis* from other *Taylorella* species (*T. asinigenitalis*). A polymerase chain reaction (PCR)-based assay has been developed and found to be more sensitive than traditional culture techniques used to identify *T. equigenitalis*-affected animals and isolates; however, it is not routinely used by CEM-approved laboratories. More recently, a real-time PCR assay was developed in Europe. These are promising new tests that should improve diagnosis of *T. equigenitalis*; however, further validation is required before their routine use.

Treatment and Control

Treatment with antibiotics and disinfectants has been successful in eliminating *T. equigenitalis*. Topical treatment of affected carrier mares consists of a cleansing of the clitoral fossa with 4% chlorhexidine followed by liberal application of nitrofurazone ointment (0.2%) for 5 days. In stallions, a thorough cleansing of the urethral fossa and sinus, prepuce, and penis with a 2% chlorhexidine solution and 0.2% nitrofurazone ointment for 5 continuous days has been proposed. Surgery or ablation of the clitoral sinuses has been suggested in female carrier animals. Uterine infusions of disinfectants or antimicrobials and systemic antibiotic treatment have been used in attempts to reduce the severity and duration of illness and perhaps abort the carrier state. Currently, there is no effective vaccine available for controlling this organism; control is achieved through preventing transmission from infected animals.

In CEM-endemic countries, attempts to control CEM have included mandatory veterinary examinations, negative cultures of all animals intended for breeding, and supervision of the movement of horses. Because of subclinical infection or asymptomatic carriage by stallions, detection of the disease can be challenging. Biosecurity measures are very important in preventing the introduction and transmission of *T. equigenitalis*. The USDA has established import and export regulations for the United States, which include CEM treatment and testing requirements on mares and stallions imported from CEM-affected countries.

T. asinigenitalis

T. asinigenitalis is a gram-negative rod that is phenotypically similar to *T. equigenitalis*. The two organisms can be distinguished by PCR and differ after sequence analysis of 16S rRNA. *T. asinigenitalis* can cross-react with some of the identification tests for *T. equigenitalis*; however, it tends to grow more slowly in culture and may exhibit a slightly different colony appearance.

T. asinigenitalis has been reported in the genital tract of donkey jacks and a naturally infected stallion. It can be transmitted to mares by natural service. Depending upon the strain of *T. asinigenitalis* that is used, some affected mares develop clinical disease that is similar to CEM. However, mares do test positive when the complement fixation test is used to identify animals infected with *T. equigenitalis*. This, coupled with the fact that isolates of *T. asinigenitalis* and *T. equigenitalis* are similar phenotypically, makes identification of horses with *T. equigenitalis* (an economically devastating disease) difficult. At this time, the significance (other than making control of CEM more difficult) of *T. asinigenitalis* is not known.

Further Reading

Bleumink-Pluym NMC and Van Der Zeijst BAM (2005) Genus IX. *Taylorella*, in *The Proteobacteria, Parts A–C, Bergey's Manual of Systematic Bacteriology*, Vol. **2** (eds GM Garrity, DJ Brenner, NR Krieg, and JT Staley), Springer, Verlag.

Heath P and Timoney P (2008) Contagious equine metritis, in *OIE Terrestrial Manual, World Animal Health Information Database*, pp. 838–844.

Kristula M (2007) Contagious equine metritis, in *Equine Infectious Diseases* (eds DC Sellon and MT Long), Saunders-Elsevier, St. Louis, MO, pp. 351–353.

Timoney PJ (1996) Contagious equine metritis. *Comp Immun Microbiol Infect Dis*, **19**, 199–204.

Timoney PJ (2011) Contagious equine metritis: an insidious threat to the horse breeding industry in the United States. *J Anim Sci*, **89**, 1552–1560.

United States Department of Agriculture Animal and Plant Health Inspection Service (2009) *Veterinary Services Factsheet. Questions and Answers: Contagious Equine Metritis*, http://www.aphis.usda.gov/publications/animal_health/content/printable_version/faq_CEM09.pdf (accessed January 9, 2013).

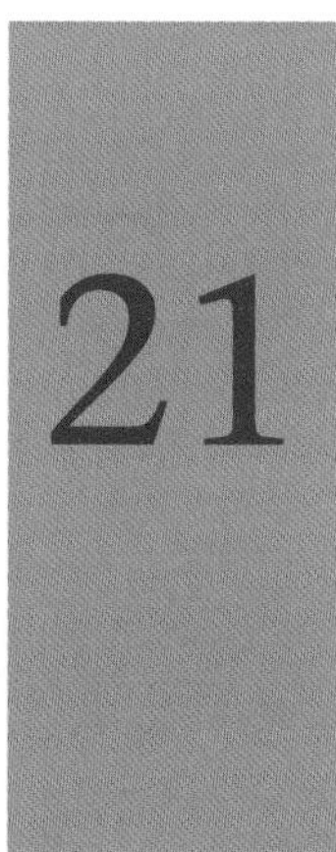

21 Spiral-Curved Organisms I: *Borrelia*

Rance B. LeFebvre

Borreliae are spirochetes transmitted and maintained primarily by ticks. The infections they cause have blood-borne phases accompanied or followed by general and localizing manifestations.

Animal pathogens include *Borrelia anserina*, the fowl spirochetosis agent; *Borrelia theileri*, a mild pathogen mainly of cattle; and *Borrelia burgdorferi* sensu lato, comprised of three genospecies, the cause of Lyme disease in dogs, humans, horses, and possibly other mammals. Tick-borne relapsing fever borreliae of humans occurs asymptomatically in feral mammals, birds, and reptiles.

Descriptive Features

Morphology and Staining

Borreliae measure 0.2–0.5 μm by 8–30 μm and are gram-negative. For demonstration by light microscopy, polychrome strains (Giemsa and Wright's) are best. Dark-field examination reveals spirals and motility.

Cellular Anatomy and Composition

Borreliae have a structure like other spirochetes consisting of an outer sheath encasing the axial fibrils consisting of 15–20 endoflagella (depending on species).

Borrelia spp. are unique among prokaryotes in that they have a linear double-stranded chromosome of approximately 900 kbp and a multiplicity of linear and circular plasmids, which may in fact constitute components of the genome. Genes expressing major outer surface proteins may be found on any of the genetic elements.

Growth Characteristics

Of the *Borrelia* spp. pathogenic for animals, *B. anserina* is propagated in embryonated hen's eggs, and *B. burgdorferi* sensu lato is cultivated at 33 °C on modified Barbour–Stoenner–Kelly (BSK) medium, an enriched serum broth made selective by inclusion of kanamycin and 5-fluorouracil.

The organisms are slow-growing microaerophiles (doubling times: 12–18 h). They ferment glucose and possibly other carbohydrates.

Survival of borreliae is about a week at room temperature in blood clots, several months at 4 °C, and indefinite at <20 °C.

Variability

A number of genes encoding outer surface proteins have been identified in several *Borrelia* species. The spirochetes control the expression of these genes at the transcriptional level. The antigenic variability available to the spirochetes is utilized for immune evasion in the relapsing fever borreliae. Lyme disease spirochetes are also equipped to express a wide range of outer surface proteins both at the intragenic and intergenic levels. Although not utilized like the relapsing fever borreliae, an immune evasion function may still be involved in their maintenance and expression in these spirochetes.

Ecology

Reservoir and Transmission

Pathogenic borreliae of animals are vectored by ticks. Ticks become infected at some stage in their life cycle by feeding on infected animals. Other arthropods may serve as short-term vectors. Infection occurs by wound contamination, usually during feeding by infected ticks. Passage via placenta, milk, and urine has been documented. During an outbreak in birds, infection may occur by coprophagia and cannibalism.

Animal Borrelioses

B. anserina

B. anserina causes fowl spirochetosis in chickens, turkeys, geese, ducks, pheasants, pigeons, canaries, and some species of wild birds. Onset of disease is marked by fever,

Veterinary Microbiology, Third Edition. Edited by D. Scott McVey, Melissa Kennedy and M.M. Chengappa.

depression, and anorexia. Affected birds are cyanotic and develop a greenish diarrhea. Later signs may include paralysis and anemia. Mortality ranges from 10% to almost 100%. Necropsy reveals splenomegaly and widespread hemorrhages. The enlarged liver may contain necrotic foci. Peripheral blood is often sterile.

Avian spirochetosis occurs on all continents and in all ages of birds. The young suffer high mortality rates and die at earlier septicemic stages of infection. Following an outbreak the agent generally disappears from the flock within 30 days.

The leading vector, *Argas persicus*, can remain infected for over a year and can pass the agent transovarially.

Temporary immunity, apparently antibody mediated, follows recovery. Antisera confer protection for several weeks. Inactivated vaccines made from infected blood or egg-propagated *B. anserina* are beneficial.

Spirochetes are demonstrable in blood by dark-field microscopy, stained smear, or immunofluorescence. Suspect material (i.e., blood, spleen, or liver suspension) may be inoculated into the yolk sac of 5- to 6-day embryonated eggs. Spirochetes will appear within 2 or 3 days. Antigen or antibody may be demonstrated in agar gel diffusion tests.

B. anserina is susceptible to penicillin, tetracycline, chloramphenicol, streptomycin, kanamycin, and tylosin. Immune serum has protective potential, and bacterins produce long-lasting immunity.

Control of ectoparasites is essential.

B. theileri

B. theileri causes a mild febrile anemia, most often in African and Australian cattle, and occasionally in sheep and horses. The disease is associated with several species of ixodid ticks. The pathogenic mechanism is not understood. Most information comes from field cases, which may be complicated by other tick-borne infections. Although not routinely treated, animals respond to tetracycline. Tick control is advisable.

Lyme Borreliosis

Lyme disease is caused by *B. burgdorferi* sensu lato, a pathogenic spirochete. Genetic analysis now defines three genospecies: *B. burgdorferi* sensu stricto, *B. garinii*, and *B. afzelii*. *B. burgdorferi* sensu stricto is the predominant pathogen of North America.

Distribution and Transmission

Endemic areas include the Atlantic states, Minnesota and Wisconsin, parts of the American South and far West, most of continental Europe and Britain, Russia, Asia, Japan, and parts of New South Wales in Australia. May through October is the time of peak prevalence. Increasing spread of the disease is attributed to increased deer populations, increasing human movement into rural areas, and the dissemination of infected ticks by migratory birds. The agent is harbored by several ixodid ticks (primarily *Ixodes scapularis* and *Ixodes pacificus* in North America). The tick has a 2-year life cycle comprised of a larval, nymph, and adult stage, requiring a blood meal at each molt. Deer and white-footed mice, and other small rodents serve as reservoirs for the spirochete. *B. burgdorferi* has been isolated from the urine of dogs and cows as well as milk from infected cows, potentially serving as alternate routes for exposure and infection.

Human Lyme borreliosis, caused by *B. burgdorferi*, typically begins with a skin lesion (erythema migrans), often followed weeks or months later by neural, cardiac, and arthritic complications. Endotoxin, hemolysin, immune complexes, and immunosuppression may be involved in pathogenesis.

In animals, dogs are most often affected, with manifestations of polyarthritis, fever, and anorexia the most common ailment. Malaise, lymphadenopathy, carditis, and renal disease have also been noted in dogs.

Borreliosis in horses and cattle has also been reported. In horses, polyarthritis, ocular and neural involvement, and foal mortality have been reported.

Diagnosis

Diagnosis involves demonstration of the agent in tissues and fluids (dark-field immunofluorescence microscopy), antibody in serum or other fluids (indirect immunofluorescent test and enzyme-linked immunosorbent assays), or DNA amplification of tissue or fluid samples using genus-specific DNA primers and the polymerase chain reaction.

Culture is laborious and often unrewarding. However, culturing ear punch biopsies from infected dogs and mice has proven to be reliable. Culture of synovial fluid from affected joints is also possible. BSKII is a good isolation medium. The spirochetes grow best at 33 °C.

Treatment and Control

Tetracycline, doxycycline, enrofloxacin, erythromycin, and penicillin are generally effective, though not invariably so. Tick control is vital. Evidence of antibiotic resistance may be due to biofilm formation and could explain chronic, persistent infections.

Immunologic Factors

A humoral immune response appears essential for protection against *B. burgdorferi* as in all spirochetal infections. Most animals appear to self-immunize with little or no apparent clinical manifestations subsequent to exposure to the spirochete.

Prevention

Antibodies produced in response to vaccination with *B. burgdorferi* have proven effective in preventing infection of laboratory animals. These observations have led to the development of a commercially available whole-cell bacterin for use in canines. However, protective immunity appears to be of short duration and limited in range. Moreover, the potential for the induction of an autoimmune response has shifted the focus from a whole-cell vaccine to a subunit vaccine approach. Subunit vaccines are commercially available.

Further Reading

Barbour A and Hayes SF (1986) Biology of *Borrelia species*. *Microbiol Rev*, **50**, 381.

Burgess E, Gendron-Fitzpatrick A, and Wright WQ (1987) Arthritis and systemic disease caused by *Borrelia burgdorferi* in a cow. *J Am Vet Med Assoc*, **191**, 1468.

Cohen ND (1996) Borreliosis (Lyme disease) in horses. *Eq Vet Educ*, **4**, 213–215.

Gross WB (1984) Spirochetosis, in *Diseases of Poultry*, 8th edn (eds MS Hofstad *et al.*), Ames, Iowa.

Johnson RC, Hyde FW, Schmid GP, and Brenner DJ (1984) *Borrelia burgdorferi* sp. nov.: etiologic agent of Lyme disease. *Int J Syst Bacteriol*, **34**, 496.

Johnson SE, Klein GC, Schmid GP *et al.* (1984) Lyme disease: a selective medium for isolation of the suspected etiological agent, a spirochete. *J Clin Microbiol*, **19**, 81.

Kiptoon JC, Maribel JM, Kamau LJ *et al.* (1979) Bovine borreliosis in Kenya. *Kenya Vet*, **3**, 11.

Levy SA (1992) Lyme borreliosis in dogs. *Canine Pract*, **17**, 5–14.

Madigan JE and Teitler J (1988) *Borrelia burgdorferi* borreliosis. *J Am Vet Med Assoc*, **192**, 892.

Magnarelli LA, Anderson JF, Schreier AB, and Ficke CM (1987) Clinical and serologic studies of canine borreliosis. *J Am Vet Med Assoc*, **191**, 1089.

Schmid GR (1985) The global distribution of Lyme disease. *Rev Inf Dis*, **7**, 41.

Schwann TG (1996) Ticks and *Borrelia:* model systems of investigating pathogen-arthropod interactions. *Infect Agents Dis*, **5**, 167–181.

Smibert RM (1975) Spirochetosis, in *Isolation and Identification of Avian Pathogens* (eds SB Hitchner, CH Domermuth, HG Purchase, and JE Williams.), American Association of Avian Pathologists, College Station, Texas, pp. 66–69.

Smith RD, Miranpuri GS, Adams JH, Ahrens EH (1985) *Borrelia theileri:* isolation from ticks (*Boophilus microplus*) and tick-borne transmission between splenectimized calves. *Am J Vet Res*, **46**, 1396.

Tunev SS, Hastey CJ, Hodzic E *et al.* (2011) Lymphadenopathy during Lyme borreliosis is caused by spirochete migration-induced specific B cell activation. *PLoS Pathog*, **7** (5), e1002066. doi:10.1371/journal.ppat.1002066.

Von Stedingk LV, Olsson I, Hanson HS *et al.* (1995) Polymerase chain reaction for detection of *Borrelia burgdorferi* DNA in skin lesions of early and late Lyme borreliosis. *Eur J Clin Microbiol*, **14**, 1–5.

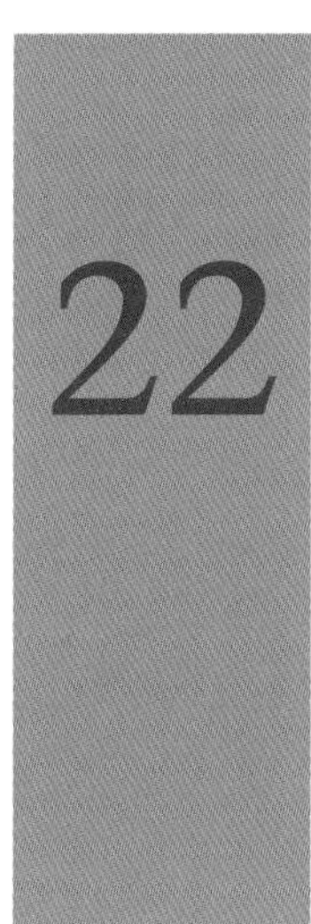

22 Spiral-Curved Organisms II: *Brachyspira* (*Serpulina*) and *Lawsonia*

Jerome C. Nietfeld

Members of the genera *Brachyspira* and *Lawsonia* are gram-negative, curved, or spiral-shaped bacilli associated with enteritis in multiple species. *Brachyspira* are oxygen-tolerant, obligate anaerobic bacteria belonging to the family Spirochaetaceae. *Lawsonia intracellularis*, the only member of the genus, is an obligate intracellular bacterium in the family Desulfovibrionaceae and does not appear to be phylogenetically related to any other species of pathogenic bacteria.

Brachyspira

All members of the genus colonize the large intestine and are able to move through fluid media by rotation of their flagella, which is a characteristic of all spirochetes. Seven species are recognized and three are proposed (see Table 22.1). Of the 10 *Brachyspira* species, only *B. aalborgi* and "*B. canis*" have not been found in birds, and only *B. aalborgi*, "*B. canis*," and "*B. pulli*" have not been identified in pigs. *B. aalborgi* has been found only in humans and nonhuman primates, whereas *B. pilosicoli* has been identified in many mammalian and avian species.

The most important and by far the best-characterized species is *Brachyspira hyodysenteriae* (previously named *Treponema hyodysenteriae*, *Serpula hyodysenteriae*, and *Serpulina hyodysenteriae*), which causes swine dysentery, a worldwide, mucohemorrhagic colitis of weaned, growing pigs. *B. hyodysenteriae* is also recognized as a cause of necrotizing typhlocolitis of the common rhea.

Brachyspira pilosicoli (*Anguillina coli*) is the cause of porcine intestinal spirochetosis and avian intestinal spirochetosis, which are characterized by mild, chronic diarrhea in pigs, and diarrhea, decreased egg production, and increased mortality in mature laying hens and occasionally in turkeys and game birds. *Brachyspira intermedia* and *Brachyspira alvinipulli* also cause avian intestinal spirochetosis. *B. pilosicoli* has been isolated from nonhuman primates, dogs, horses, mice, and opossums, with and without diarrhea. In humans the bacterium is recognized as a cause of mild, watery, or mucoid diarrhea referred to as intestinal spirochetosis or human intestinal spirochetosis. *B. pilosicoli* bacteremia is rarely reported in people, and affected individuals are usually immunocompromised. The organism is also commonly isolated from healthy people, especially those in economically underdeveloped and rural areas. *B. aalborgi* is another cause of human intestinal spirochetosis, but *B. pilosicoli* is more common. Animals are considered potential reservoirs of *B. pilosicoli* for human infection.

In addition to being associated with avian spirochetosis, *B. pilosicoli*, *B. intermedia*, and *B. alvinipulli* are all commonly isolated from healthy chickens. *Brachyspira innocens*, *B. murdochii*, and "*B. pulli*" are considered part of the normal large intestinal flora of chickens. Reports suggest that *B. intermedia* and *B. murdochii* might rarely cause mild typhlocolitis in swine, but neither species is considered pathogenic for pigs, nor is *B. innocens*.

"*B. canis*" is the most common *Brachyspira* species identified in stools of dogs with and without diarrhea. Most surveys do not find a significant association between it and diarrhea. Diarrhea and isolation of *B. pilosicoli* from canine feces are associated in some surveys.

"*Brachyspira suanatina*" has been isolated from pigs with swine dysentery-like disease and from healthy mallard ducks in Sweden and Denmark. Based on growth and biochemical characteristics, "*B. suanatina*" cannot be differentiated from *B. hyodysenteriae*, but the two organisms are genetically distinct. Experimentally, the organism causes diarrhea in weaned pigs, but not in mallards.

Researchers in several countries, including the United States, have isolated *Brachyspira* species from pigs with swine dysentery-like disease that have phenotypic features

Original chapter written by Dr. Dwight C. Hirsh. Contribution no. 12-193-B from the Kansas Agricultural Experiment Station.

Veterinary Microbiology, Third Edition. Edited by D. Scott McVey, Melissa Kennedy and M.M. Chengappa.

Table 22.1. Species of *Brachyspira*, Their Primary Hosts, and the Major Diseases with which They Are Associated

Species	Primary Host(s)	Major Disease
B. hyodysenteriae	Swine	Swine dysentery
B. pilosicoli	Swine, birds, humans	Porcine, avian, and human spirochetosis
B. intermedia	Swine, birds	Avian spirochetosis
B. innocens	Swine, birds	None recognized
B. murdochii	Swine, birds	None recognized
B. alvinipulli	Birds	Avian spirochetosis
B. aalborgi	Humans	Human spirochetosis
"*B. canis*"	Dogs	None recognized
"*B. suanatina*"	Swine, mallards	Diarrhea in pigs
"*B. pulli*"	Birds	None recognized

Proposed species names are in quotation marks.

of *B. hyodysenteriae* but are genetically different from *B. hyodysenteriae* and "*B. suantina*." Some of these isolates likely represent new species.

Descriptive Features

Morphology and Staining. Brachyspiras are helical spirochetes that range from 3 to 19 μm in length and 0.25 to 0.6 μm in width. They stain weakly gram-negative, but this characteristic is not used to identify or detect them. Romanovsky's stains (e.g., Wright's and Giemsa), Victoria blue 4R, silver impregnation stains, or crystal violet are more useful in demonstrating these organisms (see Figure 22.1).

Cellular Anatomy and Composition. Cells are typical of spirochetes. They consist of a protoplasmic cylinder bounded by an inner cell membrane loosely attached to an outer cell membrane. The two membranes are separated by a periplasmic space that contains periplasmic flagella that vary in number with the species. The axial filament of *B. hyodysenteriae* is made up of 8–12 flagella inserted at either end that overlap in the center of the bacterial cell. *B. innocens* has 10–13 flagella, and *B. pilosicoli* has 4–6 flagella.

FIGURE 22.1. B. hyodysenteriae *in colonic crypts of a pig with swine dysentery. Warthin–Starry silver stain.*

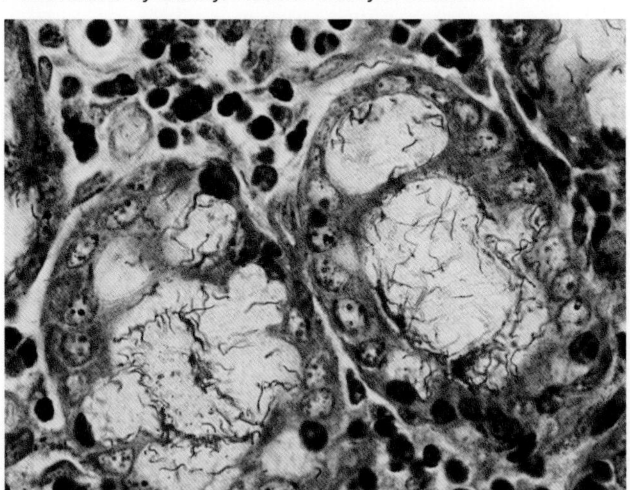

Cellular Products of Medical Interest

Cell Wall. The brachyspiras possess a gram-negative cell wall that differs somewhat from many gram-negative bacteria. The lipopolysaccharide (LPS) does not possess an outer layer of repeating polysaccharide side chains (O-antigens), or it only has an irregularly spaced, partial layer of polysaccharide side chains. The LPS is often referred to as lipooligosaccharide (LOS) and is a rough or semirough form of LPS. The LOS of different species varies in that LOS of *B. pilosicoli* has more complete O-antigen side chains and is thus smoother than LOS from *B. hyodysenteriae*. LOS has many of the same biological activities as LPS and is likely a virulence determinant. The lipid A component (endotoxin) is toxic and binds to the plasma protein LPS-binding protein (LBP), which then binds to CD14. The CD14–LPS complex binds to Toll-like receptors on the surface of macrophages and dendritic cells, triggering the release of proinflammatory cytokines. The length of O-antigen side chains is important in hindering the attachment of the attack complex of the complement system to the outer membrane. LOS of *Brachyspira* species is strongly immunogenic and is the basis for serotyping.

Hemolysin/Cytotoxin. An important virulence factor of *B. hyodysenteriae* is its hemolytic and cytotoxic activity. *B. hyodysenteriae* is strongly β-hemolytic, whereas other members of the genus are weakly β-hemolytic, except the newly proposed "*B. suanatina*," which is also strongly β-hemolytic. *B. hyodysenteriae* produces a β-hemolysin encoded by the *hlyA* gene that is cytotoxic for multiple continuous cell lines, primary cultures of porcine cells, and epithelial cells in ligated porcine intestinal loops. The bacterium also has three hemolysin regulatory genes: *tlyA*, *tlyB*, and *tlyC*. Isolates with mutations in either the *hlyA* or *tly* genes are not hemolytic and are significantly less virulent for pigs.

Flagella. Flagella are necessary for virulence. Motility is necessary to penetrate the intestinal mucus to gain access to target cells in the large intestine. Induced mutations to the flagella genes (*flaA* and *flaB*) of *B. hyodysenteriae* significantly reduce motility and virulence. Virulent, but not avirulent, strains of *B. hyodysenteriae* are attracted by pig intestinal mucin, and both motility and chemotaxis for mucin are necessary for full virulence. Strains of *B. pilosicoli* isolated from pigs, dogs, chickens, and humans possess varying attraction for pig intestinal mucin, but the effect of chemotaxis on virulence has not been studied.

Nicotinamide adenine dinucleotide phosphate (NADH) Oxidase. Although *Brachyspira* species are obligate anaerobes, they tolerate short exposure to oxygen, and when cultivated in broth, growth is enhanced by addition of 1% oxygen to the otherwise anaerobic environment. This resistance to oxygen toxicity is largely due to NADH oxidase and is an important *in vivo* virulence factor. NADH defective mutants are significantly less virulent in pigs than their parents. Oxygen tolerance likely assists colonization of the oxygenated mucosal surface of the large intestine and survival in the environment after being shed in feces.

Gene Transfer Agent of *B. hyodysenteriae, VSH-1*. The genome of *B. hyodysenteriae* codes for a mitomycin C induced bacteriophage-like gene transfer agent named VSH-1. Induced VSH-1 particles transfer random 7.5 kb genomic fragments between *B. hyodysenteriae* cells. Carbadox, an antimicrobial agent commonly used to treat and prevent enteric diseases in pigs, and metronidazole, a compound commonly used to treat anaerobic infections in humans and small animals, recently have been shown to induce VSH-1. The induced VSH-1 particles transmitted tylosin and chloramphenicol resistance to susceptible strains of *B. hyodysenteriae*. VSH-1 is likely important in the continuing development of antibiotic resistance of *B. hyodysenteriae*. The gene for VSH-1 has also been identified in several other *Brachyspira* species.

Plasmid of *B. hyodysenteriae*. Virulent strains of *B. hyodysenteriae* possess a 36 kb plasmid. Strains that lack the plasmid are significantly less virulent in pigs, suggesting that the plasmid carries genes important in disease expression.

Growth Characteristics. *Brachyspira* species are slow-growing obligate anaerobes. After 2–5 days of incubation on blood agar at 37–42 °C, they can be seen as a flat haze on the agar's surface surrounded by a zone of hemolysis (see Figure 22.2). *B. hyodysenteriae* is strongly β-hemolytic, a trait that is used to differentiate it from other *Brachyspira* species isolated from pigs (*B. innocens*, *B. intermedia*, *B. murdochii*, and *B. pilosicoli*), which are weakly β-hemolytic. However, "*B. suanatina*" and unclassified strains of *Brachyspira* occasionally isolated from pigs with swine dysentery-like disease are also strongly β-hemolytic.

Brachyspira species are resistant to high concentrations of several antibiotics, a characteristic used in isolating them from feces. *B. hyodysenteriae* and *B. pilosicoli* remain infective for long periods if enclosed within organic material, especially feces, at temperatures of 5–25 °C. They do not withstand drying or direct sunlight and are sensitive to most disinfectants.

FIGURE 22.2. *Strong β-hemolysis by* B. hyodysenteriae *and weak β-hemolysis by* B. murdochii *after 4 days of incubation. Note the ring of enhanced hemolysis (ring phenomenon) surrounding the cut in the agar with the* B. hyodysenteriae *isolate (arrow). (Curtesy of Joann M. Kinyon and Dr Kent Schwartz, Iowa State University, Ames, IA.)*

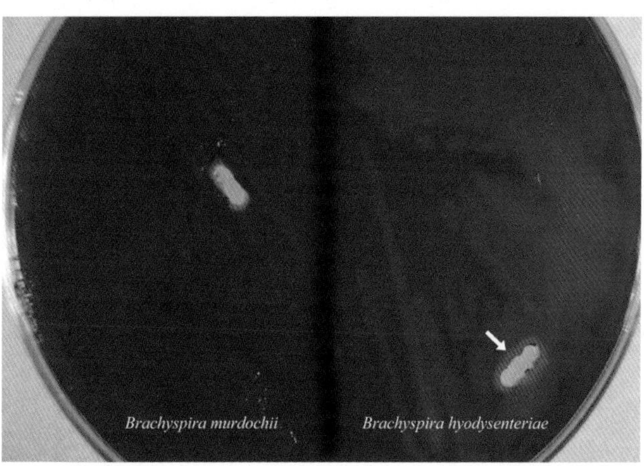

Variability. At least 12 LOS serotypes of *B. hyodysenteriae* exist. However, strains of the same serotype often vary greatly in virulence, and two strains of the same serotype can be quite different genetically. Consequently, serotyping is seldom used. Fingerprinting isolates by means of restriction length polymorphisms of whole-cell DNA, comparison of DNA sequences of ribosomal RNA genes, multilocus enzyme electrophoresis, multilocus sequence typing, and multiple-locus variable-number tandem-repeat analysis has demonstrated marked heterogeneity of *B. hyodysenteriae* and other members of this genus. For example, 111 isolates of *B. hyodysenteriae* were divided into 67 sequence types and 46 amino acid types by multilocus sequence typing. Using the same technique, 77 isolates of *B. intermedia* were divided into 71 sequence types and 64 amino acid types. Multiple-locus variable-number tandem-repeat analysis divided 172 isolates of *B. hyodysenteriae* into 44 types. In addition to demonstrating a high degree of genetic variability, fingerprinting allows isolates of a particular *Brachyspira* species to be aligned into clonal complexes with each complex containing multiple sequence types. Over time isolates of *B. hyodysenteriae* from individual pig farms tend to remain confined to a single clonal complex, but isolates of *B. pilosicoli* from chickens on a single farm often fall into multiple complexes.

Ecology

Reservoir and Transmission. The reservoir for *B. hyodysenteriae* is the gastrointestinal tract of pigs, especially asymptomatic carriers that have recovered from swine dysentery. The organism can survive in soil, lagoons, and pig feces for weeks to months depending on the temperature and environmental conditions. Transfer of the organism between pens and buildings on the footwear of workers and farm equipment is an important means of spread. *B. hyodysenteriae* has been isolated from the feces of dogs, rats, and mice living on farms where the disease exists. Mice probably constitute a real concern because experimentally they have been shown to shed *B. hyodysenteriae* for up to 6 months, whereas rats shed for only 2 days. *B. hyodysenteriae* has also been isolated from wild mallard ducks, rheas, and chickens, but any role played by birds in transmission is unknown. Asymptomatic carrier pigs are by far the most important reservoir. Many farms have eliminated swine dysentery, and as long as they do not reintroduce infected pigs into the herd, reacquiring the disease is rare.

B. pilosicoli has been isolated from many species, including dogs, birds, pigs, horses, mice, opossums, nonhuman primates, and humans. The concern is that humans can acquire *B. pilosicoli* from infected animals or animal products. Species normally associated with chickens, such as *B. alvinipulli*, *B. intermedia*, and "*B. pulli*," are occasionally isolated from dogs, and dogs are possibly infected by ingestion of uncooked or undercooked poultry products. *Brachyspira* species that have been isolated from wild mallard ducks include *B. hyodysenteriae*, "*B. suanatina*," *B. pilosicoli*, *B. intermedia*, *B. alvinipulli*, and "*B. pulli*." Whether infection is associated with diarrhea or whether mallards serve as a reservoir of *Brachyspira* species for domestic animals is unknown. Transmission of all *Brachyspira* species is by the fecal–oral route.

Pathogenesis and Clinical Signs

Swine dysentery can be reproduced by orally inoculating conventional pigs with pure cultures of *B. hyodysenteriae*, but germ-free pigs do not develop disease. Anaerobic bacteria that are part of the normal large intestinal flora, especially *Fusobacterium* and *Bacteroides* species, are necessary along with *B. hyodysenteriae* for development of clinical disease. Diet plays a role in development of swine dysentery because diets low in fiber and high in highly fermentable carbohydrates increase the severity of disease. *B. hyodysenteriae* multiplies and produces disease only in the large intestine. Flagella and chemotaxis to mucin allow the bacteria to penetrate the mucus layer that coats the mucosa and to closely associate with epithelial cells that cover the luminal surface and line colonic crypts. This results in superficial coagulative necrosis and loss (likely due to hemolysin/cytotoxin) of epithelial cells, edema, hyperemia, hemorrhage, and influx of neutrophils into the mucosa and submucosa. Hyperplasia of goblet cells occurs, followed by increased mucus production. Spirochetes are present in large numbers in the lumen of crypts (see Figure 22.1) and can be found in the lamina propria and within epithelial cells, especially goblet cells. Cellular attachment and invasion are not required for disease production. The diarrhea is due to decreased colonic absorption. Evidence of increased fluid secretion due to an enterotoxin or secondary to the inflammation has not been found.

Swine dysentery is most common in weaned pigs 2–4 months old, but can occur in pigs as young as 2–3 weeks. It is rare in nursing piglets and adults. The incubation period is usually about 10–14 days. Although pigs can die acutely without evidence of diarrhea, the most consistent sign is chronic diarrhea. Pigs are febrile and partially anorexic and initially pass semisolid, yellow-to-gray feces that do not contain blood. After a few days feces become more liquid and contain large amounts of mucus and increasing amounts of blood. Affected pigs become dehydrated and lose weight. Morbidity rates in susceptible pigs can be close to 90%, and mortality in untreated herds can be 20–40%. Duration of illness ranges from a few days to several weeks. Except for emaciation and dehydration, postmortem lesions are confined to the large intestine. The wall of the large intestine is thickened, eroded, and covered by fibrin and mucus containing flecks of blood. Survivors may be permanently stunted and remain asymptomatic shedders.

Intestinal spirochetosis of weaned pigs, chickens, nonhuman primates, and dogs associated with *B. pilosicoli* is characterized by mild, persistent diarrhea, decreased weight gain or weight loss, and low mortality. Clinical disease has not been reported in broiler chickens, but broilers hatched from flocks with clinical intestinal spirochetosis often grow slower than normal. Biopsies of the affected colon often contain a layer of spirochetes adhered by one end to the apical surface of the luminal epithelium forming a false brush border (see Figure 22.3). This "end-on" attachment is known to occur only with *B. pilosicoli* and *B. aalborgi*. Diarrhea is believed to result from malabsorption due to disruption of the microvilli of the apical surface of colonic epithelium. In cases of avian spirochetosis due to *B. intermedia* and *B. alvinipulli*, the bacteria do not attach to epithelium but are free in the lumen and the colonic crypts. Very little is known about the pathogenesis of disease caused by the latter two organisms.

FIGURE 22.3. B. pilosicoli *forming a false brush border (arrows) on the apical border of the colonic epithelium of a monkey. Hematoxylin and eosin stain.*

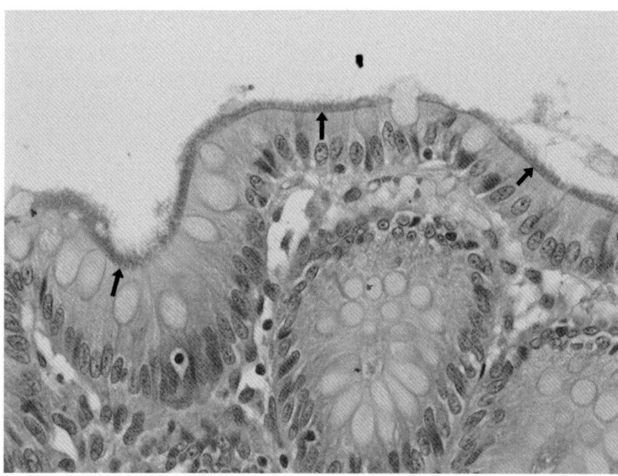

Immunologic Aspects

The immunologic aspects of these diseases are poorly understood. Some pigs that have recovered from swine dysentery are resistant to reinfection for up to approximately 4 months, but many pigs remain susceptible. Infection induces *B. hyodysenteriae* specific serum IgG and colonic IgA, but neither is highly protective. Bacterins have limited efficacy, and the immunity that does develop is serotype specific, so the vaccine must contain the serotype to which the pigs are exposed. Cell-mediated immune responses and changes in populations of CD4+ and CD8+ lymphocytes occur, but their role in immunity and/or disease production is unknown. Poultry and mammals with intestinal spirochetosis remain persistently infected, and if infection is eliminated by antimicrobial treatment, they are susceptible to reinfection.

Laboratory Diagnosis

Sample Collection. Lengths of colon or colon contents from several freshly necropsied animals are optimal, but fecal samples from clinically affected animals are

FIGURE 22.4. Brachyspira *spp. (arrows) in a smear prepared by scraping the large intestinal mucosa of a pig without diarrhea. Crystal violet stain.*

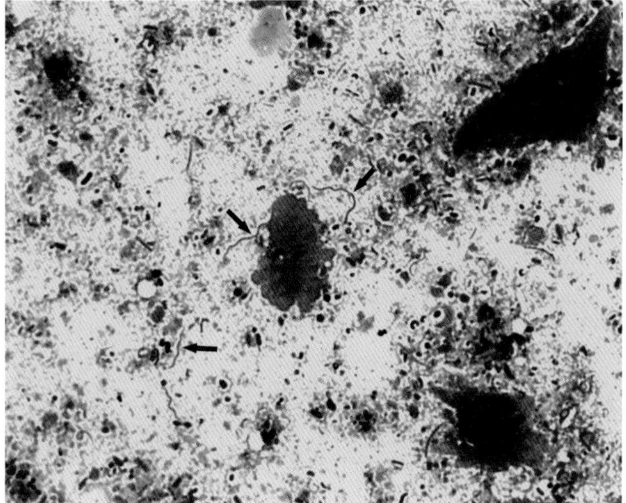

satisfactory. Samples should be chilled, but not frozen, and transported to the laboratory as soon as possible. Preventing samples from drying out en route is important.

Direct Examination. Smears of fecal material or scrapings of colonic mucosa can be examined by phase-contrast or dark-field microscopy or stained with a Romanovsky's stain (e.g., Wright's and Giemsa), carbol fuchsin, Victoria blue 4R, or crystal violet and examined by conventional light microscopy (see Figure 22.4). Observation of loosely coiled spirochetes is presumptive evidence of infection with *Brachyspira* species, but additional tests are necessary to differentiate pathogenic from nonpathogenic species.

Isolation. Isolation of *Brachyspira* species from fecal samples is accomplished by inoculation onto blood agar plates containing antibiotics to prevent overgrowth by faster-growing enteric bacteria. Agar plates for isolation of *B. hyodysenteriae* typically contain 400 μg/ml spectinomycin or some combination of spectinomycin, rifampin, spiramycin, vancomycin, polymixin, or colistin. Because *Brachyspira* species differ in antibiotic sensitivity, blood agar with 400 μg/ml spectinomycin and 25 μg/ml each of colistin and vancomycin are recommended as an all-around medium for *Brachyspira* species. The plates are incubated in an anaerobic environment containing 10% carbon dioxide. After 2–5 days of incubation, *B. hyodysenteriae* can be seen as a zone of strong β-hemolysis containing a surface film in which colonies are very small and difficult to identify. Other species will be surrounded by a zone of weak hemolysis. Making cuts in the agar helps with identification of *B. hyodysenteriae* because a zone of enhanced hemolysis (referred to as ring phenomenon) develops along the cuts on plates with strongly hemolytic isolates, but not with weakly hemolytic ones (see Figure 22.2). Plates without growth should be reincubated and reexamined every 2 days for 10 days. For phenotypic identification, obtaining a pure culture by cloning the isolate is important. This is difficult, especially with heavily contaminated plates, requires considerable experience, and can take 2 weeks or longer. For antigen detection and nucleic acid-based methods such as polymerase chain reaction (PCR), cloning the isolate is not as critical.

PCR assays for most *Brachyspira* species and multiplex PCR assays that simultaneously identify different combinations of *B. hyodysenteriae*, *B. pilosicoli*, *L. intracellularis*, and *Salmonella* species have been developed. In some instances, the PCR assays are performed directly on feces and test results are obtained within 1–2 days. In other instances, the PCR assays are used to identify organisms isolated on blood agar, which still greatly reduces the time required for identification of *Brachyspira* species. The best results are obtained when culture and PCR are used together. Unclassified *Brachyspira* isolates from pigs and poultry are not rare, and if only PCR tests are used for diagnosis, unclassified strains are not detected.

Identification. After isolation, *Brachyspira* species must be identified to differentiate pathogenic and nonpathogenic species. This is often done by observation of the strength of β-hemolysis and biochemical reactions. The tests commonly used are indole production, hippurate hydrolysis, α-galactosidase, α-glucosidase, and β-glucosidase tests (see Table 22.2), but there is some variability in biochemical results between strains of a given species and misidentification using phenotypic criteria is possible. For instance, strongly β-hemolytic, indole-positive isolates from pigs are identified as *B. hyodysenteriae* and weakly β-hemolytic, indole-positive isolates as *B. intermedia*. However, a few strains of *B. hyodysenteriae* are indole-negative. In addition, "*B. suanatina*" is indole-positive and strongly β-hemolytic. Similarly, weakly hemolytic, hippurate-positive isolates from pigs are identified as *B. pilosicoli*, but occasional strains of *B. pilosicoli* are hippurate-negative. Therefore,

Table 22.2. Phenotypic Characteristics of *Brachyspira* Species

Species	Hemolysis	Ind[a]	Hip[b]	α-Gal[c]	α-Gluc[d]	β-Gluc[e]
B. hyodysenteriae	Strong	+[f]	−	−	+	+
B. intermedia	Weak	+	−	−	+	+
B. innocens	Weak	−	−	+	±	+
B. murdochii	Weak		−	−	−	+
B. pilosicoli	Weak	−[f]	+[g]	±	±	−
B. alvinipulli	Weak	−	+	−	−	+
B. aalborgi	Weak	−	+	−	−	−
"*B. canis*"	Weak	−	−	−	+	+
"*B. suanatina*"	Strong	+	−	−	+	+
"*B. pulli*"	Weak	−	−	+		+

[a]Indole production.
[b]Hippurate hydrolysis.
[c]α-Galactosidase activity.
[d]α-Glucosidase activity.
[e]β-Glucosidase activity.
[f]Indole-negative strains of *B. hyodysenteriae* and indole-positive strains of *B. pilosicoli* have been identified.
[g]Hippurate-negative strains of *B. pilosicoli* have been identified.

laboratories increasingly identify *Brachyspira* isolates by species-specific PCR, sequencing the 16S rRNA gene, or molecular fingerprinting. The most common targets for species-specific PCR are the 23S rDNA and NADH oxidase genes.

Treatment, Control, and Prevention

Through the years many drugs have been used to treat swine dysentery, but several have been withdrawn from the market and others have limited effectiveness because of development of antimicrobial resistance. The most commonly used drugs are tiamulin, valnemulin, tylosin, and lincomycin. Because of resistance to tylosin and lincomycin, the pleuromutilins (tiamulin and valnemulin) are currently the most effective antimicrobials, but resistance to tiamulin and valnemulin is being reported from a few countries. Carbadox is used in the United States and it is usually effective, but it is approved for use only in pigs less than 34 kg (75 lb) and is not approved in Canada or Europe. Severely affected pigs sometimes require initial treatment with injectable antibiotics, but the preferred route of administration is usually through the drinking water. Presumably the same medications can be used to treat pigs with *B. pilosicoli* infection. Metronidazole is the recommended treatment for dogs with intestinal spirochetosis. No drugs are approved for treatment of avian intestinal spirochetosis. Recently, 30 of 30 *Brachyspira* isolates from chickens were reported to be sensitive to tylosin, valnemulin, tiamulin, and doxycycline. Two isolates showed decreased sensitivity to lincomycin. A problem in treating chickens is that the disease occurs in mature laying hens and long withdrawal times would be required before the eggs could be used for human consumption. In addition, chickens are likely to be reinfected when drug treatment is stopped.

The best prevention for swine dysentery is strict biosecurity so that only pigs from dysentery-free herds are brought onto the farm. To date, vaccines have met with limited success and are not commonly used. Vaccines for *B. pilosicoli* have so far proven ineffective.

Lawsonia

L. intracellularis is the only member of the genus *Lawsonia* and causes proliferative enteropathy, a diarrheal disease characterized by thickening of the intestinal mucosa because of hyperplasia of enterocytes. The bacterium is an obligate intracellular microorganism that grows in the apical cytoplasm of enterocytes (see Figure 22.5). Porcine proliferative enteropathy is a worldwide disease of pigs first recognized in the 1930s. Proliferative ileitis or proliferative bowel disease is a common disease of Syrian hamsters, and equine proliferative enteropathy is an important emerging disease of weaned foals. Sporadic cases of proliferative enteropathy due to *Lawsonia* infection have been reported in ferrets, foxes, dogs, rats, rabbits, sheep, deer, emus, ostriches, guinea pigs, and nonhuman primates, but not in humans. In the 1970s, *Campylobacter*-like bacteria were first observed in the apical cytoplasm of enterocytes, and a variety of *Campylobacter* species were proposed as possible causes. In 1991, *L. intracellularis* was isolated in cell culture and used to reproduce the disease.

FIGURE 22.5. L. intracellularis *(arrow) in the apical cytoplasm of enterocytes in the ileum of a weaned foal with equine proliferative enteropathy. Warthin–Starry silver stain.*

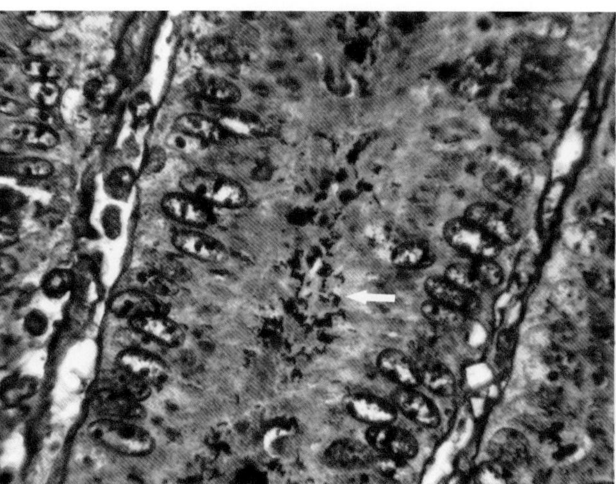

Descriptive Features

Morphology and Cellular Anatomy. *L. intracellularis* cells are straight to curved bacilli 1.25–1.75 μm long by 0.25–0.45 μm wide. They have a single polar flagellum, do not possess fimbriae, or form spores. Extracellular bacteria grown in cell culture have darting motility.

Cellular Products of Medical Interest

Cell Wall. The cell wall of *L. intracellularis* is typical of gram-negative bacteria. Little is known specifically about the biological effects of LPS from *L. intracellularis*, but typically LPS is an important virulence determinant. The lipid A component is toxic, and the length of the repeating polysaccharide side chains (O-antigens) hinders bacterial killing by complement. LPS also binds LPS-binding protein, which initiates a series of events that trigger the release of proinflammatory cytokines.

Type III Secretion System. Type III secretion systems are responsible for translocation of bacterial proteins into host cells. Protein components of a type III secretion system (IscN, IscO, and IscQ for *L. intracellularis* secretion component) were recently identified in multiple strains of *L. intracellularis*. The role of the Isc proteins is unknown, but they are expressed during natural infection and pigs react immunologically to the proteins.

Lawsonia *Surface Antigen A.* *Lawsonia* surface antigen A (LsaA) is a protein expressed *in vitro* and *in vivo*. The exact role of the protein is unknown, but it is involved in adherence to and invasion of epithelial cells. Pigs respond immunologically, and LsaA has been used as antigen to develop enzyme-linked immunoassays to identify infected pigs and rabbits.

Growth Characteristics. *L. intracellularis* has only been isolated in actively dividing eukaryotic cells maintained in a microaerobic atmosphere of 82.2% nitrogen, 8.8% carbon dioxide, and 8% oxygen.

Ecology

Reservoir. The reservoirs of *L. intracellularis* are the intestinal tracts and the environment of infected animals where it remains viable in feces for several weeks at 5–15 °C. Rodents trapped on pig and horse farms are commonly infected and are possible reservoirs.

Transmission. Infection occurs following ingestion of material contaminated with infected feces.

Pathogenesis

Proliferative enteropathy has been reproduced in conventional pigs, hamsters, and horses by oral inoculation with pure cultures of *L. intracellularis*. However, disease does not develop following oral inoculation of germ-free pigs. Interaction between *L. intracellularis* and unidentified normal intestinal flora is necessary for development of proliferative enteropathy.

Following oral inoculation of pigs and hamsters and *in vitro* inoculation of cultured epithelial cells, *L. intracellularis* cells attach to the apical border of target epithelial cells and are internalized into phagocytic vacuoles. Specific adhesions or attachment factors have not been identified. The bacteria do not have to be viable to invade cells, but treatments that inhibit cellular metabolism inhibit bacterial invasion. After internalization, the microorganisms escape from the vacuole into the cytoplasm where they multiply and inhibit cell maturation by an unknown mechanism. Cellular division continues and postmitotic daughter cells contain bacteria, which contributes to spread of bacteria throughout the length of the crypts. *L. intracellularis* also invades and spreads within the intestinal lamina propria, which likely contributes to infection of enterocytes throughout the length of the crypts. Immature secretory enterocytes, normally present in the crypts, replace goblet cells and absorptive villous enterocytes. This results in elongation of crypts, shortening of villi, increased fluid loss, decreased absorption, and loss of protein into the feces. Inflammation is variable and can be absent or consist of neutrophils, macrophages, and lymphocytes.

Following experimental infection, most bacterial invasion and multiplication initially occurs in the distal jejunum and ileum. Lesions in the large intestine are believed to be secondary infections caused by bacteria escaping from infected enterocytes in the small intestine.

Clinical Features and Lesions. Swine proliferative enteropathy (often referred to as proliferative enteritis or proliferative ileitis) is a disease complex that can occur in four forms: (1) intestinal adenomatosis, a chronic form characterized by thickening of the mucosa due to hyperplasia of the crypt epithelium (see Figure 22.6); (2) necrotic enteritis, a chronic form in which there is extensive necrosis and replacement of the mucosa by a necrotic membrane (see Figure 22.6); (3) regional ileitis, a chronic form with thickening of the smooth muscle wall resulting in a contracted, smooth segment of distal small intestine (sometimes referred to as "garden-hose gut"); and (4) proliferative hemorrhagic enteropathy, an acute form characterized by thickening of the small intestinal mucosa and acute hemorrhage into the intestinal lumen. The most consistent location of gross lesions is the distal jejunum and ileum, followed by the cecum, and spiral colon. Gross lesions in horses and hamsters also consist of mucosal hyperplasia and thickening of the distal small intestine (see Figure 22.7).

Proliferative hemorrhagic enteropathy usually affects pigs 4–12 months old, while the other forms usually affect younger pigs between 6 weeks and 5 months of age. Equine proliferative enteropathy primarily affects weaned foals. Hamsters are usually affected soon after weaning and are

FIGURE 22.6. *Small intestine from a pig with proliferative enteropathy. Note the diffuse rugose appearance of the serosa and the thickened and rugose appearance of the mucosa, which are characteristic of intestinal adenomatosis (single arrow). Also, note the replacement of the mucosa with a necrotic membrane, which is characteristic of necrotic enteritis (double arrows).*

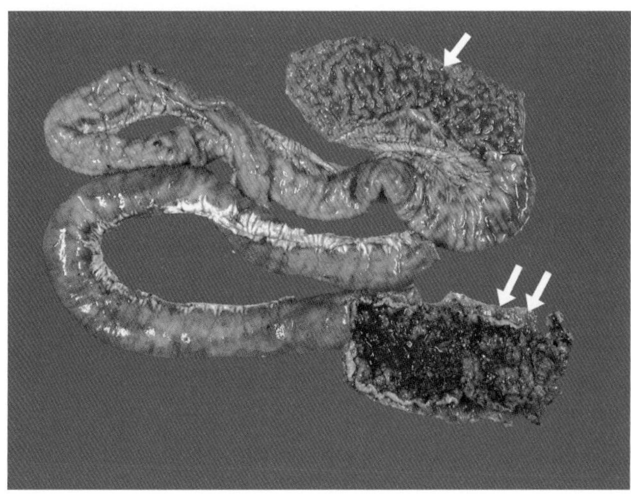

FIGURE 22.7. *Small intestine from a foal with equine proliferative enteropathy.*

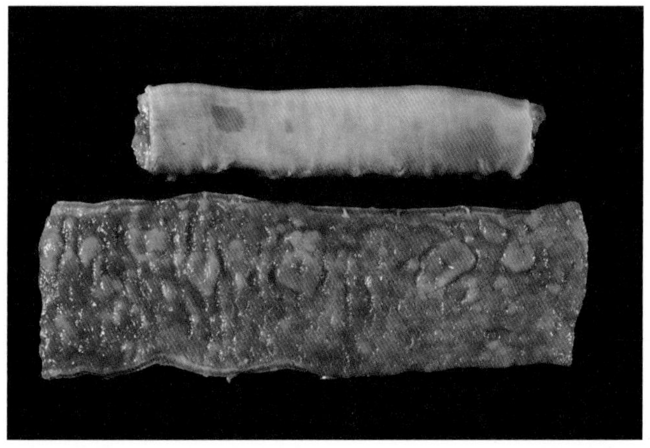

experimentally resistant by 10–12 weeks of age. Clinically affected pigs, horses, and hamsters develop diarrhea, become dehydrated, and lose weight. Hypoproteinemia and edema of the ventral neck, trunk, and/or limbs are common in foals. Poor weight gain is often the only manifestation of subclinical infection in pigs and possibly in other species.

Epidemiology. *L. intracellularis* occurs worldwide in pigs and probably in horses. Clinical disease in horses has been reported from the United States, Canada, Europe, South Africa, and Australia. Serologic surveys indicate that infection is widespread in horses in the United States, Canada, and Europe. The majority of pig herds in swine-raising areas are infected. Isolates from pigs, horses, hamsters, and deer have greater than 98% DNA homology, but there is no evidence that transmission between species is important. Experimentally, pig isolates were infective for hamsters and horses, and a horse isolate was infective for hamsters. However, the target species had to be immunosuppressed and infection was mild or subclinical.

Immunologic Aspects

Systemic humoral and cell-mediated immune responses are generated following infection of pigs and horses. Pigs, and most likely other species, develop specific IgA and cell-mediated responses in the intestinal mucosa. Pigs recovered from proliferative enteropathy are resistant to reinfection. An attenuated live *L. intracellularis* vaccine is available for pigs, and it is effective and widely used. Preliminary experiments with vaccines for foals show promising results.

Laboratory Diagnosis

Sample Collection. Fresh and formalin-fixed intestines, intestinal scrapings, and/or feces from affected animals are used for diagnosis.

Direct Examination. Modified acid-fast and Giminez stains of intestinal mucosal smears will demonstrate small curved bacilli in enterocytes of animals with proliferative enteropathy. The histologic intestinal changes are characteristic and can be used for a presumptive diagnosis. Silver and immunohistochemical stains are used to detect the bacteria in fixed tissue (see Figures 22.5 and 22.8).

Isolation. *L. intracellularis* can only be grown in living cells and has been isolated by only a few researchers. Isolation is not feasible for diagnosis.

Identification. The combination of macroscopic and microscopic lesions and identification of intracellular bacteria in enterocytes are considered diagnostic of *L. intracellularis* infection. Specific identification can be made by fluorescent antibody or immunochistochemical (see Figure 22.8). PCR assays that detect *L. intracellularis* alone or in combination with one or more common bacterial causes of diarrhea in pigs (*B. hyodysenteriae*, *B. pilosicoli*, and *Salmonella* species) are used by many veterinary laboratories.

FIGURE 22.8. *L. intracellularis* in the apical cytoplasm of small intestinal enterocytes (arrows) of a pig with proliferative enteropathy. Immunohistochemical stain with a hematoxylin counter stain.

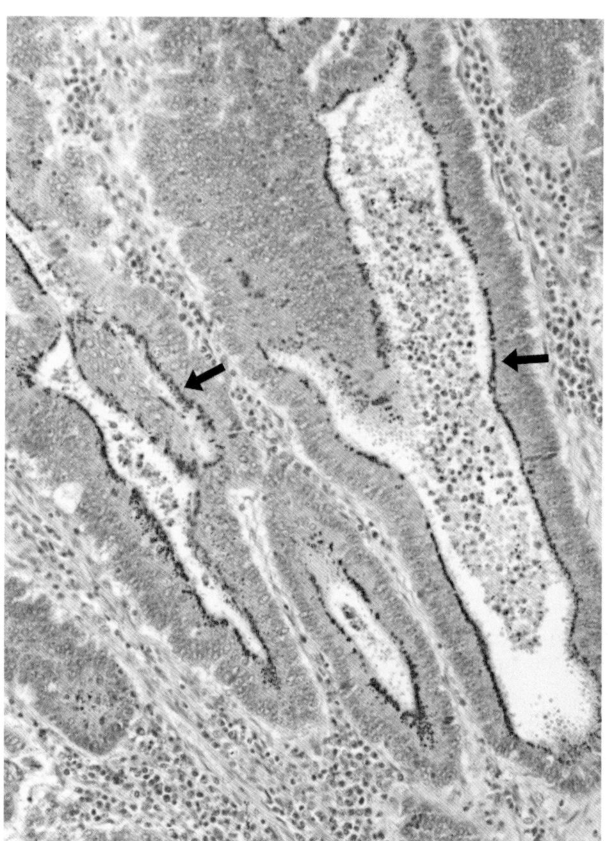

Treatment

Antimicrobials most commonly used to treat porcine proliferative enteropathy are tetracyclines, tylosin, tiamulin, lincomycin, and, where available, carbadox. There is little evidence of development of antibiotic resistance. Treatment in horses is by use of macrolide antibiotics alone or in combination with chloramphenicol, tetracyclines, or rifampin.

Excluding the organism from swine herds is very difficult as the disease occurs in many isolated "high health" herds. The most common method of control is oral vaccination with an attenuated, live vaccine. If vaccination is not possible, prevention is often by feeding antibiotics for 2–3 weeks beginning just before the expected onset of clinical disease. Experimental trials in horses with inactivated and attenuated vaccines have shown promise but require further evaluation.

Further Reading

Bellgard MI, Wanchanthuek P, La T *et al.* (2009) Genome sequence of the pathogenic intestinal spirochete *Brachyspira hyodysenteriae* reveals adaptations to its lifestyle in the porcine large intestine. *PLoS One*, **4** (3), e4641.

Boutrup TS, Boesen HT, Boye M *et al.* (2010) Early pathogenesis in porcine proliferative enteropathy caused by *Lawsonia intracellularis*. *J Comp Pathol*, **143**, 101–109.

Hampson DJ and Swayne DE (2008) Avian intestinal spirochetosis, in *Diseases of Poultry*, 12th edn (eds YM Saif et al.), Blackwell Publishing Ltd, Ames, Iowa, pp. 922–940.

Hidalgo Á, Rubio P, Osorio J, and Carvajal A (2010) Prevalence of *Brachyspira pilosicoli* and "*Brachyspira canis*" in dogs and their association with diarrhea. *Vet Microbiol*, **146**, 356–360.

Jacobson M, Fellström C, and Jensen-Waern M (2010) Porcine proliferative enteropathy: an important disease with questions remaining to be solved. *Vet J*, **184**, 264–268.

Jansson DS, Fellström C, Råsbäck T *et al.* (2008) Phenotypic and molecular characterization of *Brachyspira* spp. isolated from laying hens in different housing systems. *Vet Microbiol*, **130**, 348–362.

Kroll, JJ, Roof MB, Hoffman LJ *et al.* (2005) Proliferative enteropathy: a global enteric disease of pigs caused by *Lawsonia intracellularis*. *Anim Health Res Rev*, **6** (2), 173–197.

Primus A, Oliveira S, and Gebhart C (2011) Identification of a new potentially virulent *Brachyspira* species affecting swine. American Association of Swine Veterinarians 42nd Annual Meeting Proceedings, March 5–8, 2011, Phoenix, Arizona, pp. 109–110.

Pusteria N and Gebhart C (2009) Equine proliferative enteropathy caused by *Lawsonia intracellularis*. *Equine Vet Educ*, **21** (8), 415–419.

Råsbäck T, Jansson DS, Johansson K-E, and Fellström C (2007) A novel enteropathogenic, strongly haemolytic spirochaete isolated from pig and mallard, provisionally designated "*Brachyspira suanatina*" sp. nov. *Environm Microbiol*, **9** (4), 983–991.

Stanton TB, Humphrey SB, Sharma VK, and Zuerner RL (2008) Collateral effects of antibiotics: carbadox and metronidazole induce VSH-1 and facilitate gene transfer among *Brachyspira hyodysenteriae* strains. *Appl Environ Microb*, **74** (10), 2950–2956.

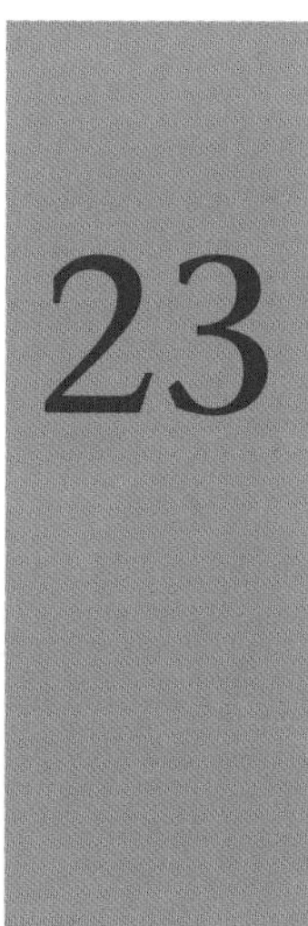

Spiral-Curved Organisms III: *Campylobacter* and *Arcobacter*

JEROME C. NIETFELD

Members of the genera *Campylobacter* and *Arcobacter* (previously classified within the genus *Campylobacter*) are small, gram-negative, curved rods associated with diseases of the reproductive and intestinal tracts. Both genera are members of the family Campylobacteraceae.

Descriptive Features

Morphology and Staining

Members of the genera *Campylobacter* and *Arcobacter* are gram-negative, nonspore-forming, curved rods that are 0.2–0.9 μm wide by 0.5–5 μm long. They have capsules and are motile by means of a polar flagellum at one or both ends. When two or more bacterial cells are placed together, they can form S or gull-winged shapes that can appear as "spirals" (see Figure 23.1).

Campylobacter

The genus contains 23 recognized species, several of which cause reproductive and gastrointestinal disease in animals and humans. Other species are commensal bacteria of the gastrointestinal tract of humans, domestic and wild mammals, birds, and shellfish. The species of veterinary importance are *Campylobacter fetus*, *C. jejuni* ssp. *jejuni*, *C. coli*, *C. lari*, *C. hyointestinalis*, *C. sputorum*, *C. helveticus*, *C. mucosalis*, and *C. upsaliensis* (see Table 23.1). *C. fetus* and *C. jejuni* are important causes of reproductive failure in ruminants. Several species, especially *C. jejuni* and *C. coli*, are important causes of gastroenteritis in humans and minor causes in animals.

C. fetus has two subspecies: *venerealis* and *fetus*. Disease caused by the two organisms is often referred to as vibriosis because *C. fetus* was originally classified in the genus *Vibrio*. *C. fetus* ssp. *venerealis* is host adapted to cattle and causes bovine venereal or genital campylobacteriosis, which is a venereal disease characterized by early embryonic death and infertility. The organism is of major importance because there are regulations to prevent transmission by international trade. *C. fetus* ssp. *venerealis* also causes sporadic bovine abortions. *C. fetus* ssp. *fetus* and *C. jejuni* ssp. *jejuni* are worldwide causes of abortion outbreaks in sheep and sporadic abortions in goats and cattle. *C. fetus* ssp. *fetus* has been isolated from aborted alpaca fetuses. *C. coli* also causes abortions in sheep, but much less commonly than either *C. fetus* or *C. jejuni*. Gastrointestinal colonization by *C. jejuni* occurs in many animal species. Infection is often accompanied by self-limiting diarrhea in young ruminants, puppies, and kittens, but in older animals infection is usually asymptomatic. The incidence of persistent, asymptomatic infection in poultry is especially high, but *C. jejuni* is not known to cause clinical disease in poultry. *C. coli* is most commonly isolated from the intestines of healthy pigs and poultry.

Campylobacters are a leading cause of food-borne, bacterial gastroenteritis of humans. More than 90% of human cases are caused by *C. jejuni* and *C. coli*, with *C. jejuni* being by far the more important cause. Other less common causes of gastroenteritis in people include *C. fetus* ssp. *fetus*, *C. upsaliensis*, *C. lari*, *C. hyointestinalis*, and *C. sputorum* (see Table 23.1). Most human infections result from ingestion of contaminated uncooked or undercooked food, unpasteurized milk, or contaminated water. Ingestion of poultry and poultry products is the most important risk factor for campylobacter enteritis in humans. Although human infection is uncommon, *C. fetus* ssp. *fetus* is the *Campylobacter* most likely to cause bacteremia and extraintestinal infection in people.

C. helveticus is most commonly isolated from feces of normal dogs and cats, but in some studies isolation is more frequent from pets with diarrhea. The bacterium is not known to cause disease in humans.

Original chapter written by Dr. Dwight C. Hirsh.

Veterinary Microbiology, Third Edition. Edited by D. Scott McVey, Melissa Kennedy and M.M. Chengappa.

FIGURE 23.1. C. jejuni *from a blood agar plate. Gram stain.*

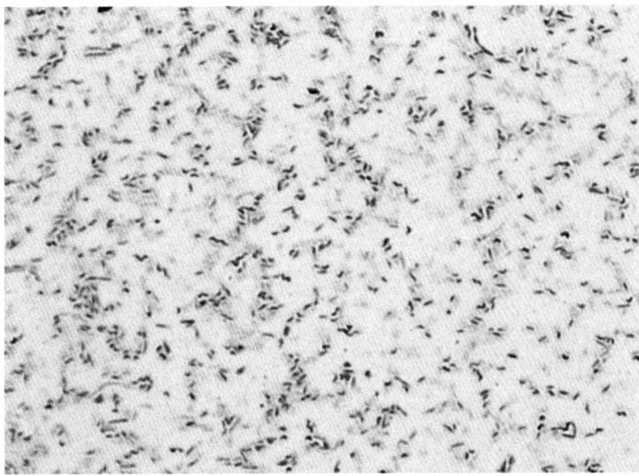

C. hyointestinalis and *C. mucosalis* were proposed as causes of porcine proliferative enteropathy, which was later proven to be caused by *Lawsonia intracellularis*. *C. hyointestinalis* is a rare cause of gastroenteritis in people, but *C. mucosalis* is not known to cause disease in animals or humans.

C. lari was originally isolated from feces of asymptomatic gulls (from which it gets its name). Since then the organism has been isolated from the feces of dogs, wild birds, and horses. *C. lari* is considered to be a sporadic cause of diarrhea and a rare cause of bacteremia in humans, but is not known to cause disease in animals.

C. sputorum has three biovars *sputorum, faecalis*, and *paraureolyticus* that are commensals of the oral cavity of humans, the gastrointestinal tract of ruminants, and the reproductive tract of cattle. The biovars are not specific as to location. It is important to differentiate *C. sputorum* from *C. fetus*. Strains from the reproductive tract of cattle that were previously classified as *C. sputorum* biovar *bubulus* have been reclassified as biovar *sputorum*. *C. sputorum* is associated with gastroenteritis in people.

C. upsaliensis is the most common *Campylobacter* isolated from dog feces. Cats are also commonly infected and the organism has been isolated from poultry. The bacterium is associated with diarrhea in puppies, but adult dogs and cats are usually asymptomatic. This microorganism has been reported to cause enteric disease, bacteremia, and abortion in humans.

Descriptive Features

Cellular Products of Medical Interest

Cell Wall. Campylobacters have a gram-negative cell wall. Although the lipid A component of lipopolysaccharide (LPS) is capable of binding LPS-binding protein in serum and triggering the host's immune system, the LPS of *C. fetus* has very low biological activity when compared to members of the Enterobacteriaceae. This is likely important in allowing the organism to establish persistent infection. The length of the repeating polysaccharide side chains (O-antigens) of LPS is important in resistance to killing in serum by complement, and serum resistant strains of *C. fetus* have long O-antigens. The LPS of *C. jejuni* lacks repeating polysaccharide side chains and is a rough form of LPS referred to as lipooligosaccharide (LOS). Most isolates of *C. jejuni* are from the intestines and are serum sensitive. Isolates from blood or other extraintestinal sites are often serum resistant, but that is because of their capsule and not the LOS. The LOS of *C. jejuni* is important in resistance to killing by cationic antimicrobial peptides (CAPs) or defensins, which are produced by host cells as part of the innate immune response. Intestinal isolates of *C. jejuni* have truncated LOS and are more sensitive to killing by CAPs in comparison to isolates from the meninges and blood. Mutations in the LOS genes also decrease adherence to and invasion of epithelial cells. Different forms of LOS are expressed by *C. jejuni* at 37 °C than at 42 °C, which likely helps it adapt to the different temperatures of mammalian and avian intestines.

Capsule. Peripheral to the outer membrane is a highly variable polysaccharide capsule. Mutations in the capsule genes of serum resistant strains of *C. jejuni* increase susceptibility to the bactericidal effects of serum. The capsule helps shield the LOS from host cell receptors, such as Toll-like

Table 23.1. *Campylobacter* Species of Veterinary Importance

Species	Animal Host(s)	Disease in Animals[a]	Disease in Humans[a]
C. fetus ssp. *fetus*	Sheep, goats, cattle	Abortion	Bacteremia, diarrhea
C. fetus ssp. *venerealis*	Cattle	Infertility, Abortion	None reported
C. jejuni ssp. *jejuni*	Poultry, ruminants, dogs, cats, humans	Abortion, diarrhea, asymp[b]	Diarrhea, bacteremia
C. coli	Pigs, poultry, sheep	Asymp, abortion	Diarrhea, bacteremia
C. upsaliensis	Dogs, cats, poultry	Asymp, diarrhea	Diarrhea, bacteremia
C. lari	Wild birds, dogs	None reported	Diarrhea, bacteremia
C. hyointestinalis	Cattle, pigs, sheep, poultry, pets, birds	None reported	Diarrhea
C. helveticus	Cats, dogs	Asymp, diarrhea	None reported
C. sputorum	Cattle, sheep	None reported	Diarrhea
C. mucosalis	Pigs	None reported	None reported

[a]The first entry is the most common.
[b]Asymp, asymptomatic.

receptors, which helps prevent stimulation of the innate immune response. The capsule plays a role in adherence of *C. jejuni* to epithelial cells, and isolates without a capsule do not efficiently colonize chick intestines. There is variation in expression of capsular antigens because of phase variation in expression of the responsible genes, which helps the organism to temporarily avoid the immune system. The capsular antigens are also used for serotyping.

Microcapsule or S-Layer of C. fetus ssp. fetus. A protein microcapsule called the S-layer (for surface layer) surrounds *C. fetus* ssp. *fetus* and is an important virulence factor. The S-layer resists phagocytosis and the bactericidal effects of serum by inhibiting binding by complement factor C3b. In sheep, the S-layer is necessary to cause systemic infection and abortion. Protective antibodies are produced to S-layer antigens, but phase variation in expression of S-layer proteins helps the organism temporarily avoid the immune system.

Adhesins. CadF is an outer membrane protein highly conserved in *C. jejuni* and *C. coli* that binds the cell matrix protein fibronectin and mediates adherence to host cells. Mutations in the CadF gene reduce bacterial adhesion and virulence in animal models. Peb 1 (also known as CBF1) is an adhesin of *C. jejuni* located in the periplasmic space that binds to aspartate and glutamate. Peb 1 deficient mutants do not efficiently colonize mice intestines. CapA is a lipoprotein that contributes to adherence of *C. jejuni* to epithelial cells and is important in colonization and establishment of persistent infection in chick intestines.

Flagella. The flagella of *C. jejuni* are essential for motility and for chemotaxis to mucin and to amino acids present in high levels in chicken intestines, which are important in intestinal colonization. *C. jejuni* has a flagellar export apparatus that functions similar to a type III secretion system (an assemblage of proteins that form a hollow tube-like structure through which proteins are "injected" into host "target" cells). Mutations in the flagellin (*fla*) genes, which code for the major proteins that comprise the flagella, abolish motility and secretion of Cia (*Campylobacter* invasion antigens) proteins, which are necessary for cell invasion.

Cytolethal Distending Toxin. Cytolethal distending toxin (CDT) is produced by *C. jejuni*, *C. coli*, *C. lari*, *C. fetus*, and *C. upsaliensis* and is the only toxin proven to be produced by *Campylobacter* species. The toxin causes apoptosis by arresting cells at the transition between the G_2/M phases of the cell cycle. Its role in disease production is uncertain. In humans, CDT stimulates production of interleukin-8 that recruits dendritic cells, macrophages, and neutrophils, thus increasing inflammation. However, clinical disease in humans caused by non-CDT-producing strains of *C. jejuni* was indistinguishable from disease caused by CDT producing strains.

Type II secretion system. *C. jejuni* possesses a type II secretion system that binds free DNA from the environment and transports it into the cytoplasm. Once in the cytoplasm, the DNA is incorporated into the genome or, in the case of a plasmid, it can replicate freely. The ability to acquire DNA from the environment is known as natural competence.

Type IV Secretion System (T4SS). The genome of *C. fetus* ssp. *venerealis* contains a unique segment of DNA (known as a genomic island) that contains genes believed to be responsible for adaption of *C. fetus* ssp. *venerealis* to the bovine reproductive tract. Within the genomic island are genes for a T4SS, which is an apparatus that mediates transfer of DNA and/or proteins between bacteria and/or eukaryotic host cells. Mutations to the T4SS genes reduce virulence of *C. fetus* ssp. *venerealis*.

Growth Characteristics. *Campylobacter* species are microaerobic, requiring an atmosphere containing 3–10% oxygen and 3–15% carbon dioxide. All species grow at 37 °C, but some, such as *C. jejuni*, *C. coli*, and *C. lari*, are thermotolerant and grow well at 42 °C, a characteristic often used in isolation from feces. Most species do not multiply below 30 °C and their numbers are greatly reduced by freezing and thawing. However, they can remain viable for days to weeks in organic material such as feces, meat, or milk, especially if chilled. Unlike members of the family Enterobacteriaceae, campylobacters are oxidase-positive. They do not ferment or oxidize carbohydrates, but generate energy from oxidation of amino acids or tricarboxylic acid intermediates through the respiratory pathway.

Variability. Campylobacters were originally classified on the basis of heat-stable LPS antigens A, B, and C. *C. fetus* ssp. *fetus* has serovars A-2 and B, and *C. fetus* ssp. *venerealis* has serovars A-1 and A-sub 1. Strains that express antigen C grow at 42 °C and are classified as *C. jejuni* and *C. coli*. The Penner serotyping system is based on extractable, heat-stable capsular antigens, and *C. jejuni* has 42 serotypes and *C. coli* has 18. More than 100 serotypes of *C. jejuni*, *C. coli*, and *C. lari* are identified by a system proposed by Lior based on heat-labile surface and flagellar antigens. Serologic typing is performed by only a few reference laboratories, because of the large number of typing sera required. Most typing is done by molecular methods such as ribotyping, restriction endonuclease analysis, pulse-field gel electrophoresis, amplified fragment length polymorphism, and PCR with genomic sequence analysis. Genetic analysis also indicates that there is marked genetic variability in individual enteric *Campylobacter* species, such as *C. jejuni*. However, a 2008 study of *C. jejuni* isolates from sheep abortions from different parts of the Unites States found that 66 of 71 isolates were derived from a single clone.

Ecology

Reservoir

C. fetus ssp. venerealis. The primary reservoir is the preputial crypts of persistently infected, carrier bulls. Approximately 1–2% of cows become persistent vaginal carriers and are also reservoirs.

C. fetus ssp. fetus. The reservoir is the intestinal tract and gall bladder of infected ruminants.

C. jejuni and Enteric Campylobacters. The reservoir of *C. jejuni* for sheep is primarily the intestinal tract and gall bladder of carrier sheep. Poultry, various birds, cattle, sheep, dogs, cats, and swine are also carriers of *C. jejuni*, and pigs and poultry are the primary reservoir for *C. coli*. The reservoir for other campylobacters is presumed to be the intestinal tract of infected animals (see Table 23.1).

Transmission

Reproductive Disease. Infection by *C. fetus* ssp. *venerealis* is predominately by coitus, but transmission by artificial insemination with contaminated semen and/or equipment is possible. Infection by *C. fetus* ssp. *fetus* and *C. jejuni* is by ingestion of organisms in food or water contaminated by feces of carrier ruminants or by fetal fluids and membranes from aborted fetuses.

Enteric Disease. Infection by campylobacters associated with enteric disease (*C. jejuni*, *C. coli*, etc.) occurs by the oral route by ingestion of contaminated food and water. For humans, consumption of poultry products is the single most important risk factor for gastroenteritis caused by *C. jejuni*, and ingestion of other meats, unpasteurized milk, and contaminated water are also important. Human-to-human transmission rarely occurs.

Pathogenesis and Clinical Signs

Reproductive Disease (Cattle). *C. fetus* ssp. *venerealis* is introduced into a susceptible female by an infected bull at coitus. The organisms multiply in the vagina but do not enter the uterus until the end of estrus, possibly because of increased numbers of neutrophils in the uterus during estrus. In the uterus, there is further multiplication and possibly active invasion that results in endometritis. Infection does not affect fertilization, but it creates an environment unsuitable for survival of the embryo. The female returns to estrus, usually at an interval of more than 25 days (21 days is normal). The process repeats itself until the female mounts an immune response sufficient to eliminate the agent from the uterus. Subsequently, the endometritis subsides and the animal conceives and pregnancy goes to term. On average, infected cattle go through about five estrus cycles before carrying a fetus to term.

Clinically, the signs are repeat breeding, irregular estrus cycles, increased calving intervals, and increased nonpregnant cows. If the herd remains closed, it develops immunity and fertility and calving intervals gradually return toward normal, but do not become normal without intervention.

Reproductive Disease (Sheep). Following ingestion, *C. fetus* ssp. *fetus* and *C. jejuni* invade the bloodstream and in pregnant sheep localize in the placenta. This results in placentitis, fetal infection, and abortion, usually 3–4 weeks after infection, but it can be as long as 2 months. The placenta, uterine fluids, and fetus contain large numbers of organisms. Abortions are usually in the second half of pregnancy and often occur in "storms" affecting up to 50% of pregnant animals, although approximately 25% is more typical. In the majority of cases, the macroscopic pathology consists only of placentitis, which is not specific for *Campylobacter* infection but is suggestive of bacterial infection (see Figure 23.2). Occasionally, the fetal liver contains tan-to-red foci of necrosis that often have a target- or donut-like appearance (see Figure 23.3). Abortions in cattle and goats infected with *C. fetus* ssp. *fetus* and *C. jejuni* typically occur as single, sporadic cases.

FIGURE 23.2. *Placentitis in the placenta of a sheep fetus infected by* Campylobacter fetus *ssp.* fetus.

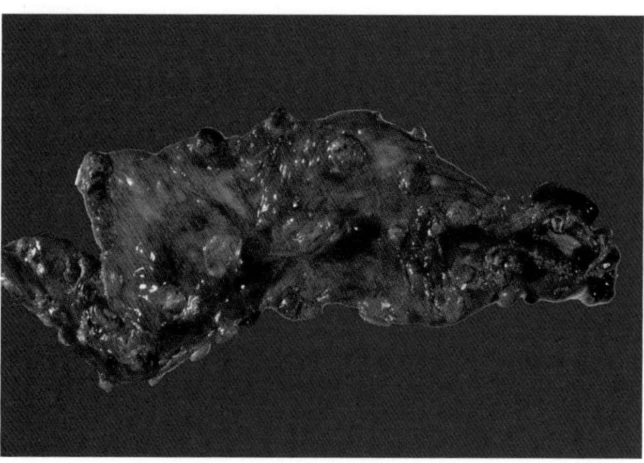

Enteric Disease. *C. jejuni* adheres to and invades epithelial cells of the distal small intestine and colon. Bacteria are translocated across the epithelium into the lamina propria. Invasive *C. jejuni* damage the epithelium and induce hemorrhage and inflammation with recruitment of neutrophils and production of interleukins and prostaglandins. Clinical signs include fever, abdominal cramps, and watery to bloody diarrhea that usually resolve on their own in a few days to a week in both animals and humans. The bactericidal effects of serum inactivate most campylobacters that reach the lymphatics and the systemic circulation. Only a small number of strains are serum resistant and cause systemic infection with extraintestinal localization. The

FIGURE 23.3. *Necrotic target- or donut-like lesions in the liver of an ovine fetus infected by* C. jejuni. Campylobacter fetus *ssp.* fetus *causes identical lesions.*

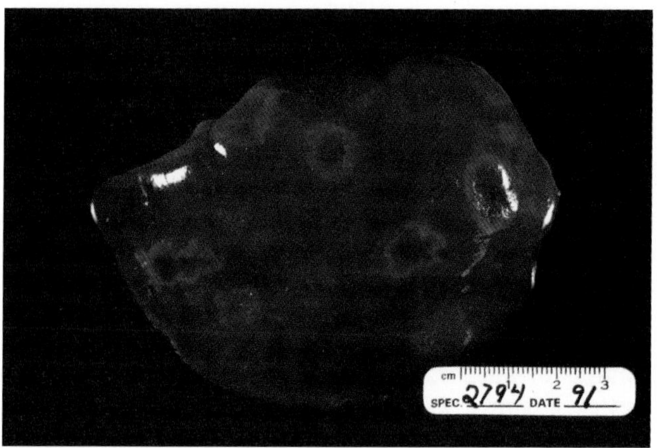

exception is *C. fetus* ssp. *fetus* in which almost all strains are resistant to killing in serum and to phagocytosis. Consequently, *C. fetus* is more important as a cause of systemic disease.

Epidemiology

Reproductive Disease (Cattle). Venereal campylobacteriosis occurs worldwide, but primarily occurs in beef cattle bred by a bull. The use of artificial insemination has almost eliminated the agent from dairy cattle, because it is easily inactivated in semen and on insemination equipment.

Reproductive Disease (Sheep). Abortions caused by *Campylobacter* species occur wherever sheep are raised. Historically, *C. fetus* ssp. *fetus* was the more important cause, but since the late 1980s, *C. jejuni* abortions have become more common and in some parts of the world outnumber those caused by *C. fetus*. *C. coli* causes sporadic abortions in sheep, but is not common in most parts of the world. However, in a few areas *C. coli* is isolated from up to 20% of *Campylobacter* abortions.

Enteric Disease. Feces from infected animals are a source of infection for other animals. Uncooked, undercooked and improperly handled contaminated poultry and other meats, raw milk and contaminated water are sources for human infection. The ceca of approximately 50% of chickens contain *C. jejuni*. At slaughter, the organism contaminates the environment, and as a consequence, almost all chicken carcasses in stores are contaminated. Infected pets and farm animals are potential sources of infection. Campylobacters are found in feces from healthy pets, but at lower prevalence and numbers than those with diarrhea. Dogs and cats from shelters and dogs fed homemade diets are more likely to carry *C. jejuni*. *C. jejuni* is commonly isolated from bovine feces and occasionally from cases of mastitis, which may help explain human outbreaks following ingestion of unpasteurized milk.

Immunologic Aspects

Reproductive Disease (Cattle). Protective immunity to *C. fetus* ssp. *venerealis* develops in the uterus and, although IgM is first produced, is primarily IgG based. Antibodies coat the bacteria and initiate the complement cascade resulting in bacterial lysis. IgG antibodies also act as opsonizing agents and bind capsular antigens that result in phagocytosis and destruction of the agent. Secretory IgA, IgG, and IgM bind surface antigens and prevent adherence of the organisms to epithelial cells. All isotypes of antibodies specific for flagellar antigens prevent movement of bacteria from the vagina to the uterus. The response in the vagina is primarily nonopsonizing IgA and it is less effective in clearing the organisms than the IgG response in the uterus. Most cattle clear *C. fetus* ssp. *venerealis* from the uterus in 2–3 months, but often require 6 months or more to clear the vagina. Vaginal clearance rarely takes more than 10 months, but 1–2% of cattle become persistent vaginal carriers. Reexposure to *C. fetus* ssp. *venerealis* results in vaginal infection that does not spread to the uterus in 30–70% of animals that eliminated the organism.

Bulls less than 4 years old rarely remain infected for longer than a few days, but older bulls can be infected for life, unless treated. The most commonly held explanation is that preputial crypts of older bulls are deeper and more hospitable than crypts of younger bulls. The immune response elicited by natural infection is ineffective in eliminating the bacteria from bulls. However, vaccination elicits specific IgG antibodies in serum and mucosal secretions that can prevent or eliminate infection from males and females.

Reproductive Disease (Sheep). Sheep are immune following abortion or vaccination, primarily because of IgM and IgG antibodies in the bloodstream and tissues. This results in removal by phagocytic cells and initiation of the complement cascade leading to bacterial lysis.

Enteric Disease. Circulating and mucosal antibodies develop following adherence to and invasion of the intestinal mucosa. This results in clearance of campylobacters from the intestinal mucosa but not from the intestinal lumen. The immune response does not prevent recolonization of the intestine, but it does help prevent clinical signs.

Laboratory Diagnosis

Sample Collection

Reproductive Disease (Cattle). Samples from males are much more likely to be positive than samples from females. Smegma or preputial scrapings are collected by aspiration into the tip of an insemination pipette. Samples from females are collected using a tampon placed in the anterior vagina. Samples should be chilled, but not frozen, and if they cannot be delivered to the laboratory within 6–8 h they should be placed into transport medium, such as Clark's or Lander's media, or thioglycollate broth. All bulls or 20 females or 10% of the herd, whichever is greater, should be sampled.

Reproductive Disease (Sheep). Abomasal fluid, lung and, liver from aborted fetuses are the best samples. Contamination makes it much more difficult to isolate the organisms from the placenta.

Enteric Disease. Fecal samples are used for the diagnosis of *Campylobacter* infections.

Direct Examination

Reproductive Disease (Cattle). Direct visualization of *C. fetus* ssp. *venerealis* in stained smears from infected bulls and/or cows is very unlikely, because of the low numbers of bacteria. Fluorescent antibody-stained preparations are useful and sometimes used in combination with culture to increase test sensitivity.

Reproductive Disease (Sheep). Gram or Romanovsky-stained preparations of stomach contents from aborted fetuses often contain small curved rods. Campylobacters have a characteristic rapid "corkscrew or tumbling" motility that can be seen in wet-mount preparations of abomasal contents viewed with phase-contrast or dark-field microscopy. Finding round or target-shaped necrotic foci on the liver (see Figure 23.3) also supports a presumptive diagnosis of *Campylobacter* infection.

Enteric Disease. Numerous slender, curved, gram-negative rods, blood, mucus, neutrophils, and cell debris are seen in stained fecal smears.

Isolation

Reproductive Disease (Cattle). Smegma, preputial scrapings, vaginal fluid, or stomach contents are plated onto selective media that contain antimicrobial agents to decrease the growth of contaminants. Vancomycin, polymyxin B or C, and trimethoprim are commonly used to decrease the growth of bacteria, and amphotericin B is sometimes included to inhibit fungal growth. It is important not to use selective media designed for isolation of *C. jejuni* and *C. coli* that contain cephalothin, such as Butzler's and Campy-BAP media, because both subspecies of *C. fetus* are sensitive to cephalothin. The plates are incubated at 37 °C in an atmosphere containing 6% oxygen and 5–10% carbon dioxide and examined in 48 h.

Reproductive Disease (Sheep). Abomasal contents, lung, and/or liver from fetuses are plated onto blood agar plates (with or without antimicrobials, depending upon the degree of contamination) and incubated at 37 °C in an atmosphere containing 6% oxygen and 5–10% carbon dioxide. Plates are examined in 48 h.

Enteric Disease. Enteric campylobacters are best isolated from intestinal samples on selective media containing antimicrobial agents (e.g., Campy-CVA medium containing cefoperazone, vancomycin, and amphotericin B or Skirrow medium). Media that contain cephalothin (such as Butzler's and Campy-BAP media) are suitable for isolation of *C. jejuni*, *C. coli*, and *C. lari*, but not *C. fetus* or *C. upsaliensis*. Because of the small size of *Campylobacter* species, an alternate method is to filter samples with 0.45 μm or 0.65 μm pore-size filters to reduce contamination and plate onto blood agar without antibiotics. The plates are incubated at 37 °C or 42 °C or both, in an atmosphere of 6% oxygen and 5–10% carbon dioxide.

Identification. Small, gram-negative, oxidase-positive, curved rods that grow at 37 °C or 42 °C in a microaerobic environment can be presumptively identified as *Campylobacter* or *Arcobacter* species. The two genera are difficult to differentiate based on phenotypic differences, but isolates that grow in an aerobic atmosphere at less than 30 °C can be presumptively identified as *Arcobacter*. The ability to grow microaerobically on MacConkey agar at 37 °C is further evidence that an isolate is an *Arcobacter* species, but failure to grow on MacConkey agar does rule out the possibility that it is an *Arcobacter*. *Campylobacter* isolates that grow at 42 °C and are hippurate-positive are identified as *C. jejuni*; however, hippurate-negative strains have been reported. Isolates can be identified as to species based on phenotypic characteristics (see Table 23.2), but there is variability between isolates of the same species and mistakes can be made. Because of the difficulty in differentiating *Campylobacter* species, molecular methods such as species-specific PCR, genomic fingerprinting, and sequencing of the ribosomal RNA genes are also used.

Table 23.2. Phenotypic Properties of Important *Campylobacter* and *Arcobacter* Species

	Growth 25 °C	Growth 37 °C	Growth 42 °C	Aerobic Growth	Catalase	Urease	Growth in 1% Glycine	Hippurate Hydrolysis	Indoxyl Acetate Hydrolysis	H_2S in TSI	Selenite Reduction	Growth in 4% NaCl	Cephalothin Sensitivity
C. fetus ssp. *fetus*	+	+	(−)[a]	-–	+	−	+	−	−	−	V		S
C. fetus ssp. *venerealis*	+	+	(−)[a]	−	+	−	−	−	−	−	V		S
C. jejuni ssp. *jejuni*	−	+	+	−	+	−	+	+[b]	+	−	V		R
C. coli	−	+	+	−	+	−	+	−	+	V	+		R
C. upsaliensis	−	+	(+)	−	−	−	+	−	+	−	+		S
C. hyointestinalis ssp. hyointestinalis	−	+	+	−	+	−	+	−	−	+	+		S
C. hyointestinalis ssp. *lawsonii*	−	+	+	−	+	+	V	−	−	+	+		S
C. sputorum biovar *sputorum*	−	+	+	−	−	−	+	−	−	+	V		S
C. sputorum biovar *faecalis*	−	+	+	−	+	−	+	−	−	+	V		S
C. sputorum biovar *paraureolyticus*	−	+	+	−	−	+	+	−	−	+	V		S
C. lari	−	+	+	−	+	V	+	−	−	−	V		R
C. helveticus	−	+	+	−	−	−	V	−	+	−	−		S
C. mucosalis	−	+	+	−	−	−	V	−	−	+	V		S
A. butzleri	+	+	(−)[a]	+	V	−	+	−	+	−	−	−	R
A. cryaerophilus	+	+	−	+	V	−	V	−	+	−	−	−	R
A. skirrowii	+	+	−	+	+	−	V	−	+	−	NT	+	S
A. thereius	+	+	−	+	+	−	+	−	+	−	−	−	NT

[a](−), most strains do not grow at this temperature.
[b]Approximately 5–10% of *C. jejuni* isolates are hippurate-negative.
V, variable results; NT, not tested; R, resistant; S, susceptible; TSI, triple sugar iron.

Serodiagnosis. *C. fetus* ssp. *venerealis* does not induce detectable serum antibodies, but antibodies in vaginal fluids are used for diagnosis. The vaginal mucus agglutination test identifies approximately 50% of infected cows, which is useful for herd but not individual cow diagnosis. Agglutinating titers are highest on 30–70 days after infection and persist for approximately 7 months. Samples should be collected 1–2 days before or 4–5 days after estrus to prevent excessive dilution of antibodies by the increased secretions during estrus. The presence of blood invalidates test results and the test cannot differentiate between infected and vaccinated animals. Antibodies in vaginal mucus can also be detected by an enzyme-linked immunosorbent assay (ELISA) that has better sensitivity and specificity. The ELISA test can be designed to detect IgA and differentiate between infected and vaccinated cattle.

Treatment

Reproductive Disease (Cattle). Two vaccinations, 3 weeks apart with a double dose of vaccine, will clear persistently infected bulls of *C. fetus* ssp. *venerealis*. Systemic streptomycin, topical streptomycin, and topical neomycin and erythromycin can effectively treat bulls, but if not vaccinated, they are susceptible to reinfection. Yearly vaccination is effective in treatment and prevention of disease in females.

Bovine venereal campylobacteriosis is best controlled by prevention. Use of virgin bulls from known negative herds, avoiding replacement females from herds with unknown histories, and not sharing pastures are good preventative methods. Artificial insemination is a very effective method to control and eliminate the disease.

Reproductive Disease (Sheep and Goats). Traditionally, treatment of *Campylobacter* abortion storms has consisted of parenteral tetracycline followed by tetracycline in the feed. However, resistance of *C. jejuni* to tetracycline has become increasingly common. The 2008 study in which a large majority of ovine abortion isolates of *C. jejuni* were from a single clone found that 100% were resistant to tetracycline. Potential alternatives include tilmicosin, erythromycin, tylosin, and florfenicol. Vaccination with *C. fetus* ssp. *fetus* and *C. jejuni* bacterins in the face of an abortion storm helps reduce the number of abortions. Vaccination prior to breeding helps prevent the disease.

Enteric Disease. Enteritis caused by *C. jejuni* and other campylobacters is usually self-limiting, but occasionally requires treatment. Macrolide antibiotics are the drugs of choice. Tetracyclines are often effective when macrolides cannot be used, but tetracycline resistance is becoming more common. Most campylobacters from animals are susceptible to fluoroquinolone antibiotics. However, because of the high rate of mutational resistance, fluoroquinolones are not the drugs of choice.

Control in the veterinary hospital and kennel requires meticulous adherence to hygienic measures, such as hand washing, cleaning, and disinfection protocols.

There are no vaccines effective in preventing enteritis or colonization by *C. jejuni*.

Arcobacter

Members of the genus *Arcobacter* are associated with diarrhea in livestock, mastitis in cattle, abortions in livestock, especially swine, and gastroenteritis in humans. The genus was created in 1991 to accommodate two species of *Campylobacter* that grew in air and it now contains 12 species. The six species that have been isolated from animals are *Arcobacter butzleri*, *A. cryaerophilus*, *A. skirrowii*, *A. thereius*, *A. cibarius*, and *A. trophiarium*. The remaining species are from shellfish, saltwater, plants, and sewage.

A. butzleri, *A. cryaerophilus*, and *A. skirrowii* are the only species isolated from both livestock feces and feces from humans with diarrhea, and are the species most likely to be animal pathogens. These species have been isolated from feces of pigs, cattle, sheep, and horses with and without diarrhea, and from dogs without diarrhea. In humans, *A. butzleri* is an emerging cause of food- and water-borne gastroenteritis and has been isolated from the blood. *A. cryaerophilus* and *A. butzleri* have been isolated from cases of bovine mastitis, and experimentally an *Arcobacter* isolate from milk caused clinical mastitis. Both species have also been isolated from milk from cows without mastitis. All three species are isolated from aborted calves, lambs, and piglets, with isolation of *A. cryaerophilus* from aborted piglets especially common. However, the organisms are not associated with pathologic changes, and the bacteria are also isolated from healthy piglets infected in utero and from amniotic fluid from normal litters.

A. thereius has been isolated from aborted piglets and cloacae of healthy ducks. Its role as a cause of pig abortions is unproven. *A. cibarius* was isolated from the carcasses of broilers at slaughter and *A. tropharium* from feces of healthy pigs. Neither organism has been associated with disease. Arcobacters are commonly isolated from feces of healthy poultry and are not associated with disease. The role of all *Arcobacter* species as a cause of animal disease is uncertain.

Descriptive Features

Cellular Products of Medical Interest. Arcobacters have a gram-negative cell wall and polar flagella. The LPS, LOS, and flagella of many gram-negative bacteria, such as *Campylobacter* species, play an important role in bacterial pathogenesis. However, the role of LPS, LOS, and flagella of *Arcobacter* are unstudied and unknown. Positive evidence of toxin production has not been found and virtually nothing is known about which genes are involved in virulence.

Growth Characteristics. *Arcobacter* species grow under both aerobic and microaerobic conditions and at temperatures as low as 15 °C. Except for a few strains of *A. butzleri*, they do not grow at 42 °C.

Ecology

Reservoir. The reservoirs of *Arcobacter* are presumably the intestinal tracts and the environment of infected animals. Asymptomatic swine, cattle, poultry, and possibly other animals may serve as an important reservoir for humans.

Transmission. Most animals are likely infected by ingestion or entry through other mucosal surfaces. Some are infected in utero.

Pathogenesis

Very little is known regarding the interactions of *Arcobacter* with the host.

Epidemiology. Asymptomatic infection of the intestinal tract of domestic livestock and poultry is common. Asymptomatic infection of dogs and horses also occurs, probably at lower prevalences. The bacteria are also isolated from the animals' environment, raw milk, and water, all of which serve as a reservoir for other animals and humans.

Immunologic Aspects

*Arcobacte*r specific antibodies were present in colostrum of naturally infected sows that farrowed piglets congenitally infected by *A. cryaerophilus*. Two weeks after birth, most congenitally infected piglets were no longer shedding *A. cryaerophilus* in their feces, but the role of colostral antibodies is unknown.

Laboratory Diagnosis

Sample Collection. Arcobacters have been isolated from stomach contents, kidney, liver, and placenta of aborted fetuses and milk from cattle. Fecal samples are used for diagnosis of *Arcobacter*-associated diarrhea and identification of carrier animals.

Direct Examination. In studies of swine abortion where fetal samples were directly examined for *Arcobacter* species, bacteria were not seen. It is impossible to differentiate *Arcobacter* from *Campylobacter* without some type of specific test, such as fluorescent antibody staining.

Isolation. The same media used to isolate campylobacters will support growth of *Arcobacter* species. Isolation from feces is enhanced by the use of commercial *Arcobacter* enrichment broth and agar supplemented with antimicrobial agents to reduce growth by other bacteria and fungi. One combination contains cefoperazone, amphotericin B, and teicoplanin and another procedure includes 5-fluorouracil, amphotericin B, cefoperazone, novobiocin, and trimethoprim. Culture plates are incubated at 25–30 °C and at 37 °C and examined daily for 3–5 days. Whether it is better to incubate aerobically or microaerobically is unproven. Common practices are to incubate all plates microaerobically or to incubate aerobically at 25–30 °C and microaerobically at 37 °C.

Identification. Small gram-negative, curved rods that are positive for oxidase, catalase, and indoxyl acetate hydrolysis and that grow aerobically and microaerobically and at 25–30 °C are presumptively identified as *Arcobacter* species. Growth on MacConkey agar at 37 °C is further evidence that an isolate is an *Arcobacter* species. Fermentation reactions are used to speciate *Arcobacter* isolates, but the results are often not definitive (see Table 23.2). Molecular methods such as PCR and sequencing of the 16SrRNA gene are more reliable.

Treatment

Most *Arcobacter* infections in humans are self-limiting, but in cases of prolonged or severe disease, fluoroquinolones and tetracyclines are most commonly used for treatment. However, resistance to nalidixic acid and ciprofloxacin has been reported. Treatment of *Arcobacter*-associated conditions in animals is poorly documented.

Further Reading

Blaser MJ, Newell DG, Thompson SA, and Zechner EL (2008) Chapter 23: Pathogenesis of *Campylobacter fetus*, in *Campylobacter*, 3rd edn (eds Nachamkin I, Szymanski CM, and Blaser MJ), American Society for Microbiology Press, Washington, DC, pp. 401–428.

Chaban B, Ngeleka M, and Hill JE (2010) Detection and quantification of 14 *Campylobacter* species in pet dogs reveals an increase in species richness in feces of diarrheic animals. *BMC Microbiol*, **10**, 73.

Collado L and Figueras MJ (2011) Taxonomy, epidemiology, and clinical relevance of the genus *Arcobacter*. *Clin Microbiol Rev*, **24**(1), 174–192.

Dasti JI, Tareen AM, Lugert R *et al.* (2010) *Campylobacter jejuni*: A brief overview on pathogenicity-associated factors and disease-mediating mechanisms. *Int J Med Microbiol*, **300**, 205–211.

Gorkiewicz G, Kienesberger S, Schober C *et al.* (2010) A genomic island defines subspecies-specific virulence features of the host-adapted pathogen *Campylobacter fetus* subsp. *venerealis*. *J Bacteriol*, **192**(2), 502–517.

Ho TKH, Lipman LJA, van der Graaf-van Bloois L *et al.* (2006) Potential routes of acquisition of *Arcobacter* species by piglets. *Vet Microbiol*, **114**, 123–133.

Merga JY, Leatherbarrow AJH, Winstanley C *et al.* (2011) Comparison of *Arcobacter* isolation methods, and diversity of *Arcobacter* spp. in Cheshire, United Kingdom. *Appl Environ Microbiol*, **77**(5), 1646–1650.

Mshelia GD, Amin JD, Woldehiwet Z *et al.* (2010) Epidemiology of bovine venereal campylobacteriosis: Geographic distribution and recent advances in molecular diagnostic techniques. *Reprod Domes Anim*, **45**, e221–e230.

Oporto B and Hutado A (2011) Emerging thermotolerant *Campylobacter* species in healthy ruminants and swine. *Foodborne Pathog Dis*, **8**(7), 807–813.

Sahin O, Plummer PJ, Jordan DM *et al.* (2008) Emergence of a tetracycline-resistant *Campylobacter jejuni* clone associated with outbreaks of ovine abortion in the United States. *J Clin Microbiol*, **46**(5), 1663–1671.

Young KT, Davis LM, and DiRita VJ (2007) *Campylobacter jejuni*: molecular biology and pathogenesis. *Nat Rev Microbiol*, **5**(9), 665–679.

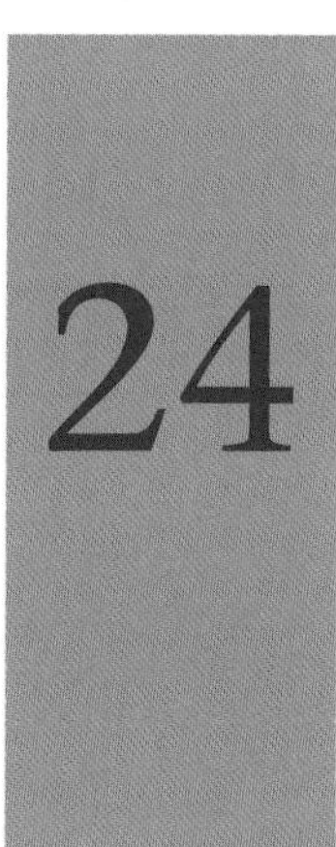

Spiral-Curved Organisms IV: *Helicobacter*

MEGAN E. JACOB

Spiral-shaped microorganisms have been noted throughout the gastrointestinal tract of animals for more than a century. After *Helicobacter pylori* was isolated from human gastric tissue in the 1980s, *Helicobacter* species were identified in animals including ferrets, birds, nonhuman primates, dogs, cats, and pigs (Table 24.1). These organisms have generated a great deal of interest because of their causal role in gastric disease. In humans, *H. pylori* can cause persistent gastritis and peptic ulcer disease, and also has been linked to the development of gastric adenocarcinoma and gastric mucosal-associated lymphoma. Other *Helicobacter* species, identified throughout the oral and gastrointestinal tract and/or liver of most animals, are associated with clinical signs ranging from cancer to gastritis to asymptomatic carriage.

The taxonomy of *Helicobacter* species is complicated, at least partially because of the rapidly expanding list of members and improved identification methods. Members of the genus are taxonomically distinct from the genus *Campylobacter*, where they were originally classified and which they resemble morphologically. There appear to be two broad groups of *Helicobacter*, those that are associated with gastric tissue and those associated with the lower intestine and hepatic regions. *Helicobacter* species from both groups are generally considered direct or opportunistic pathogens, and there is increasing recognition of the group as important zoonotic pathogens.

Descriptive Features

Morphology and Staining

Helicobacter species are gram-negative bacteria with morphologies ranging from tightly coiled spirals (e.g., *H. pylori*, *H. felis*, and *H. suis*) to slightly bent rods (e.g., *H. Mustelae* and *H. baculiformis*). Species vary in size with a length between 1.5 and 10 μm and a width between 0.3 and 1.2 μm. All known *Helicobacter* species express flagella, making them motile; the number (range between 4 and 23) and the location (biopolar, monopolar, etc.) of flagella differ between species.

Original chapter written by Dr. James G. Fox.

Virulence Factors

Helicobacter species possess several cellular products of importance; however, not all species produce all products. Some of the virulence factors represented by the genus include the following.

Flagella. Motility via multiple flagella is characteristic of *Helicobacter* species and vital for the organisms' ability to penetrate mucus and adhere to gastric epithelial cells. The number and location differ by species; however, all species possess flagella and most are sheathed.

Periplamic Fibrils. These fibers (present singly or in groups) wrap helically around the body of some *Helicobacter* species (e.g., *H. felis* and *H. bilis*), but are not present on all members. Although associated with motility of the organisms, periplasmic fibrils are distinct from flagella and are located under the outer membrane.

Urease. Urease hydrolyzes urea to ammonium and carbon. Ammonium ions neutralize stomach acid, thereby allowing the bacterium to live in the gastric environment. Urease is also associated with inflammation. Most *Helicobacter* strains produce urease; however, it seems to be variably produced by some enterohepatic species.

Adhesins. Adhesins are proteins that mediate adherence to target cells in the gastrointestinal tract comprising the niche for the strain. *H. pylori* express at least two adhesins with specificity for gastric epithelia, sialic acid-binding adhesin (SabA) and blood group antigen-binding adhesin (BabA). Similar adhesins have not been identified in all *Helicobacter* species.

Lipopolysaccharide. The lipopolysaccharide (LPS) in the outer membrane is an important virulence determinant.

Veterinary Microbiology, Third Edition. Edited by D. Scott McVey, Melissa Kennedy and M.M. Chengappa.

Table 24.1. Examples of Selected *Helicobacter* Species Reported from Animal Hosts

	Animal Species						
	Canine	Feline	Swine	Ovine	Bovine	Human	Other
H. pylori		+		+		+	Nonhuman primates
H. felis	+	+				+	Rabbit
Candidatus H. suis			+				Nonhuman primates
H. canis	+	+				+	
H. salomonis	+	+					Rabbit
"Flexispira rappini" or *H. rappini*	+	+		+		+	
H. bizzozeronii	+	+	+			+	Nonhuman primates
H. mustelae							Ferret
H. bilis	+		+				Mice
H. hepaticus							Mice
Candidatus H. bovis					+		
H. pullorum						+	Birds, Mice
H. cetorum							Dolphins, Whales

Not only is the lipid A component toxic (endotoxin) but the length of the side chain in the O-repeat unit also hinders the attachment of the membrane attack complex of the complement system to the outer membrane. *Helicobacter* LPS is important in the immune response as it is ultimately responsible for a release of proinflammatory cytokines and also has been associated with the adhesion process in gastric tissues.

cag Pathogenicity Island and CagA. The cag (for cytotoxin-associated gene) pathogenicity island (PAI) is associated with the pathogenesis of *H. pylori* strains. Specifically, the cag PAI encodes a type IV secretion system that mediates translocation of the CagA protein into host cells. Once inside the cell, CagA is phosphorylated, resulting in actin rearrangement. The PAI is heterogeneous between *H. pylori* strains, differing on the number of insertion sequences and related virulence. Various pieces of the cag PAI and type IV secretion systems have been found in other members of the genus.

Vacuolating Cytotoxin (Vac). The vacuolating cytotoxin, well described in *H. pylori*, has been associated with the colonization and persistence of the organism in the gastric epithelial cell barrier and stimulating an inflammatory response. Previous studies have shown the association between VacA activity *in vitro* and disease status. The vacA gene encodes the cytotoxin that ensures urea availability among other functions. VacA has been the subject of vaccine intervention research.

Cytolethal Distending Toxin. The cytolethal distending toxin (CDT) observed in *H. hepaticus* and *H. pullorum* is highly homologous to the CDT toxin produced by *Campylobacter jejuni*, which is associated with cell cycle arrest in eukaryotic cells.

Other miscellaneous cellular products including superoxide dismutase and catalase have also been described in *Helicobacter* species.

Growth Characteristics

Helicobacter organisms grow under microaerophilic conditions at 37 °C and typically appear as flat, nonpigmented, grayish white and nonhemolytic colonies, approximately 1–2 mm in size; however, some species do not form distinct colonies, but rather appear as a fine spreading film. Long incubation periods (up to one week) may be required for visible growth of *Helicobacter* colonies. Growth will not be observed under aerobic conditions; however, the growth of some species may be enhanced with atmospheric hydrogen, varying pH, or an enrichment step. The ability for *Helicobacter* species to grow at 42 °C is also variable, and may aide in identification.

Variability

A large degree of variability exists between and within *Helicobacter* species. Related to a high genomic heterogenicity, variability in phenotypic and growth characteristics, as well as virulence factors and sensitivity to antimicrobials is common. Urease production, nitrate reduction, and indoxyl acetate hydrolysis all can vary between and within *Helicobacter* species; this variability is often but not always differentiated between species common to the gastrointestinal tract verse enterohepatic species. In addition, some *Helicobacter* species can grow at 42 °C, and some require the presence of hydrogen for growth. The most recognizable difference between *Helicobacter* species is the number and placement of flagella, and the presence of periplasmic fibrils. Genomically, the G+C moles percent content can vary between 30% and 48% in different *Helicobacter* species.

Ecology

Reservoirs

Helicobacter species have been identified from numerous sites within animals including the stomach, liver, bile duct, and small and large intestine. The degree to which

Helicobacter species exclusively occupy specific niches within animals has not been well described with the possible exception of enterohepatic species of mice. In general, gastric *Helicobacter* species occupy the mucus layer or adhere to the gastric epithelium tissue. While some *Helicobacter* species can infect a number of different animal species, others are more specific, infecting only one known host. Multiple *Helicobacter* species have been shown to infect an individual animal.

It is estimated that a large proportion (>50%) of the human population carries *H. pylori* and potentially additional species within their gastrointestinal tract. *Helicobacter* organisms also appear to be highly prevalent in dogs and cats with studies finding 80–100% of subjects infected with at least one species. A number of non-*H. pylori* species have been identified in dogs including *Helicobacter bizzozeronii, felis, heilmannii,* and *bilis* among others. Studies evaluating *Helicobacter suis* prevalence in slaughter pigs found at least 60% of the population colonized. The enterohepatic *Helicobacter* species (*H. hepaticus* and *H. bilis*) are particularly prevalent and important in the mice population (including laboratory animals), and reports of >60% prevalence of *H. pullorum* have been reported in poultry populations. *Helicobacter* species have been found in virtually every animal examined including sheep, monkeys, ferrets, whales, dolphins, geese, and numerous others, although the prevalence of *Helicobacter* and the distribution of specific species in these populations is less well established.

Transmission

Both oral–oral and fecal–oral are hypothesized transmission routes for *Helicobacter* species. There is some evidence to support spread by both routes. The ability of organisms to survive outside of the gastrointestinal environment and be spread through other means is controversial and has not been resolved. Although additional vehicles may exist, they are not considered the primary mode of transmission.

Zoonotic Potential

There are strong indications that *Helicobacter* species can be zoonotically transferred between humans and animals. Humans have been infected by numerous different *Helicobacter* species, and contact with different animal species has been associated with infection. There is some evidence that similar strains are present in humans and their pets. *Helicobacter* species also have been isolated from milk products on several occasions. Zoonotic transmission is most commonly considered in non-*H. pylori* species, where human prevalence (estimated at 6%) is typically lower than *H. pylori* prevalence (estimated at 50%); however, cats harboring *H. pylori* have been reported as a zoonotic risk.

Pathogenesis

Numerous studies have shown that gastric *Helicobacter* species alter the gastric physiology. There also appear to be multiple mechanisms by which this can occur. Although the degree of pathology, the site of infection and the *Helicobacter* species differ by animal species, one common theme to clinical infection is the induction of a chronic inflammatory response. Previous work with experimentally *H. felis*-infected dogs reported no correlation between the number of organisms colonizing and the degree of gastric inflammation. Gastric *Helicobacter*-like organisms in cats have demonstrated good correlation between the degree of colonization and the lymphoid follicles; however, the correlation was not obvious in dogs. The lack of standard criteria for evaluating histological changes makes interpretation of these results difficult; however, it seems likely that individual host factors are large contributors to the degree and type of pathogenesis, with some individuals may remaining asymptomatic. Genes related to motility, acid neutralization/acclimation, chemotaxis, and adherence have been identified in numerous *Helicobacter* species. These, in addition to virulence factors like LPS, VacA, urease, and the cag PAI all likely contribute to the immune response, and subsequently, clinical manifestation.

Immunologic Aspects

The immune system is an important mediator for *Helicobacter*-induced pathogenesis. A chronic inflammatory response is typically associated with infection; however, the regulation of the immune response can also breakdown. The immune response mechanism leading to pathology has been most commonly studied in mice; however, likely differs between *Helicobacter* species and host animals. As an example, work with *H. felis* in mice revealed that cellular infiltrate was composed of neutrophils, B cells, and CD4 T cells. Of these, T cells were shown to be the most critical in pathology. *H. hepaticus*, which can induce hepatitis in mice, was shown to be related to a Th1-mediated immune response. The precise response from infection with different species of *Helicobacter* in different animal species is not fully understood.

Animals infected with *Helicobacter* generally produce a significant IgG response against the organisms, and specific serum IgG antibodies to gastric *Helicobacters* in animals have been used to diagnose both naturally and experimentally infected animals. Analyses of serum and mucosal secretions by enzyme-linked immunosorbent assay in *H. pylori* naturally infected cats reveal an *H. pylori*-specific IgG response, and elevated IgA anti-*H. pylori* antibody levels in salivary and local gastric secretions. Like humans, though helpful in diagnosis, neither secretory nor serum antibody responses appear protective from infection.

Laboratory Diagnosis

Direct Examination

Diagnosis of *Helicobacter*-associated chronic gastritis cannot be made with gross visual endoscopic examination. Other means of diagnosis vary in their degree of sensitivity. Spiral bacteria can be observed with cytologic examination of impression smears or with a Gram stain on homogenized gastric tissue. Gastric brushing cytology can be performed during routine endoscopy. Cells and mucus that adhere to the brush are applied to a glass slide, air-dried and stained with a Giemsa stain. For visualization of gastric *Helicobacter* organisms, oil immersion magnification (100×) is used. The urease activity of these gastric bacteria is frequently utilized as a diagnostic test, particularly for *H. pylori*. The urease test is commercially available, detecting urease activity in gastric tissue within 15 min to 3 h. Additionally, a gastric biopsy can be minced and placed directly into urea broth and a positive reaction obtained in 1 h gives a presumptive diagnosis.

Isolation and Identification

Samples from gastric or intestinal biopsies are ideal submissions for *Helicobacter* detection by culture or molecular methods (see Section "Molecular Methods"). Gastric or intestinal contents or feces can be submitted, although recovery is less predictable. Liver biopsies may also be submitted for detection in appropriate suspect patients. *Helicobacter* species are fastidious, microaerophilic, and biochemically unreactive. Higher hydrogen levels generally enhance recovery of the enterohepatic *Helicobacters* in culture; however, they can be isolated on the same medium as gastric *Helicobacters*. The organisms are typically isolated using a rich medium like brucella blood agar with antibiotics including trimethoprim, vancomycin, and polymyxin B. Some species remain difficult to isolate requiring specific pH or enrichment techniques and some may even be uncultivable. Because *Helicobacter* species may have different antibiotic susceptibilities, selection of antibiotics in culture media may aide in successful isolation. Finally, the use of 0.45 or 0.65 micron filters to selectively filter feces has been recommended to help minimize contamination from other enteric organisms during primary culture on selective agar.

Molecular Methods

DNA primers for genes encoding specific *Helicobacter* virulence proteins, as well as primers specific for segments of DNA encoding the 16S rRNA, have been described in the literature. Specialized polymerase chain reaction protocols are increasingly used for detection of "*Helicobacter* DNA" from gut contents in various animal species. In addition, the complete genome of several *Helicobacter* species including *H. pylori, H. suis* and *H. felis* have been sequenced and annotated, aiding in the rapid expansion of molecular identification techniques. New methods including FISH (fluorescence *in situ* hybridization) and Western blot analysis have recently been described as diagnostic techniques for human samples.

Treatment and Control

Treatment for *Helicobacter* infection is controversial and most commonly infection is thought to be subclinical. In addition, these organisms have been shown to quickly develop resistance to antimicrobials; therefore, treating *Helicobacter* infections should be based on lesions causing clinical illness. A combination of amoxicillin and metronidzole or clarithromycin with omeprazole or famotidine have been most commonly reported for treatment of dogs and cats with gastric *Helicobacter* infections; however, triple therapy may not result in long-term eradication of the organism from the host.

Further Reading

Mobley HLT, Mendz GL, and Hazell SL (eds) (2001) *Helicobacter pylori: Physiology and Genetics*, ASM Press, Washington, DC.

Haesebrouck F, Pasmans F, Flahou B *et al.* (2009) Gastric *Helicobacters* in domestic animals and nonhuman primates and their significance for human health. *Clin Microbiol Rev*, **22**, 202–223.

Harbour S and Sutton P (2008) Immunogenicity and pathogenicity of *Helicobacter* infections of veterinary animals. *Vet Immunol Immunopathol*, **122**, 191–203.

Neiger R and Simpson KW (2000) *Helicobacter* infection in dogs and cats: facts and fiction. *J Vet Intern Med*, **14**, 125–133.

Smet A, Flahou B, Mukhopadhya I *et al.* (2011) The other *Helicobacters*. *Helicobacter*, **16** (Suppl. 1), 70–75.

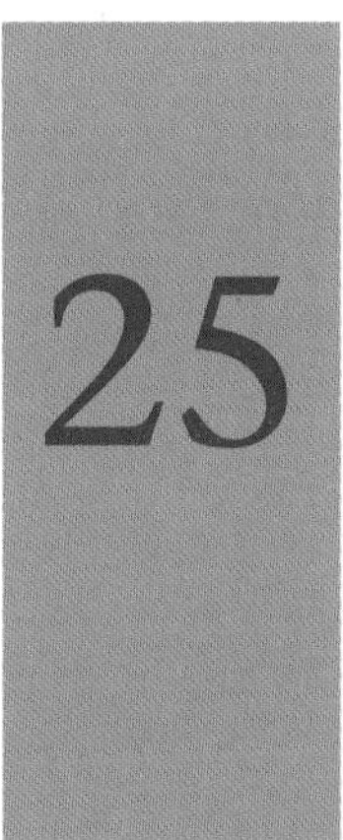

25 Spiral-Curved Organisms V: *Leptospira*

RANCE B. LEFEBVRE

Leptospirae are spirochetes, morphologically and physiologically uniform, but serologically and epidemiologically diverse. Domestic animals most commonly affected are dogs, cattle, swine, and horses. Late-term abortion is the hallmark manifestation in any pregnant animal, including humans, exposed to leptospirosis for the first time. The most common manifestations in canine leptospirosis are septicemic, hepatic, and renal. In cattle and swine, septic illness is largely confined to the young, while abortion is the principal manifestation in adults. Abortion and equine recurrent uveitis, or moon blindness, are the most common manifestations in horses. California sea lions are susceptible to acute, septicemic leptospiral infections. Other host species, though susceptible to infection, develop clinical signs less frequently. Leptospirosis in humans is typically an acute febrile disease.

Taxonomy studies, based on DNA analyses, have led to the description of eight pathogenic species: *Leptospira borgpetersenii*, *L. inadai*, *L. interrogans* sensu stricto, *L. kirschneri*, *L. meyeri*, *L. noguchii*, *L. santarosai*, and *L. weilii*. Leptospires have historically been classified by antigenic composition, which are divided into 23 serogroups and greater than 200 serovars. Reference to serovars is more common in clinical settings. Serovars important in North America and their principal hosts and clinical hosts (in parentheses) are as follows:

- *Leptospira icterohaemorrhagiae*: rodents (dogs, horses, cattle, and swine)
- *Leptospira grippotyphosa*: rodents (dogs, cattle, and swine)
- *Leptospira canicola*: dogs (swine and cattle)
- *Leptospira pomona*: cattle and swine (horses, sheep, and sea lions)
- Leptospira hardjo: cattle
- *Leptospira bratislava*: swine (horses and sea lions).

Descriptive Features

Morphology and Staining

Leptospirae are thin (Greek *leptos* = thin) spiral organisms 0.1 μm by 6–20 μm. Poorly staining, they require dark-field or phase-contrast microscopy for visualization. The spirals are best demonstrated by electron microscopy. Typical cells have a hook at each end making them S- or C-shaped. Wet mounts reveal them to be highly motile.

Leptospirae are gram-negative, but unrecognizable in routinely fixed stained smears. They can be demonstrated by fluorescent antibody or silver impregnation (Figure 32.1).

Cellular Anatomy and Composition

Leptospiral cells consist of an outer sheath, axial fibrils ("endoflagella"), and a cytoplasmic cylinder. The outer sheath combines features of a capsule and outer membrane. The cytoplasmic cylinder is covered by a cell membrane and the peptidoglycan layer of the cell wall.

A relatively feeble endotoxin is present in the cell wall. A hemolysin, sphingomyelinase C, is associated with some serovars, and cytotoxicity has been demonstrated *in vivo*.

Growth Characteristics

Leptospirae are obligate aerobes, which grow optimally at 29–30 °C. Generation time averages about 12 h. No growth occurs on blood agar or other routine media. Traditional media are essentially rabbit serum (<10%) in solutions ranging from normal saline to mixtures of peptones, vitamins, electrolytes, and buffers. Some newer media have substituted polysorbates and bovine albumin for rabbit serum. Protein is not required. Unlike most prokaryotes,

Veterinary Microbiology, Third Edition. Edited by D. Scott McVey, Melissa Kennedy and M.M. Chengappa.

leptospirae are not able to synthesize their own pyrimidines; thus, 5-fluorouracil is added to the media to inhibit other bacterial growth.

Most media are fluid or semisolid (0.1% agar). In fluid media, little turbidity develops. In semisolid media, growth is concentrated in a disk about 0.5 cm below the surface referred to as a dinger zone.

Biochemical Reactions

Leptospirae are oxidase- and catalase-positive; many have lipase activity. Some produce urease. Identification beyond genus is based on serology. However, the development of species-specific DNA primers in conjunction with the polymerase chain reaction (PCR) is a promising new development for a more accurate characterization of pathogenic leptospirae.

Resistance

Leptospirae are fragile bacteria and are killed by drying, freezing, heat (50 °C/10 min), soap, bile salts, detergents, acidic environments, and putrefaction. They persist in a moist, temperate environment at neutral to slightly alkaline pH (see Section "Epidemiology").

Variability

Greater than 200 serovars of pathogenic leptospirae exist. They vary in host, geographic distribution, and in virulence factors and thus, pathogenicity.

Ecology

Reservoir

Leptospira spp. inhabit the tubules of mammalian kidneys. Although leptospirae have been isolated from birds, reptiles, amphibians, and invertebrates, the epidemiologic significance of such associations is not established.

Rodents are the most frequent leptospiral carriers, with wild carnivores ranking second. No mammal can be excluded as a possible host. Typically reservoir hosts show minimal, if any, signs of disease. Abortion is always a problem in pregnant animals exposed for the first time. Leptospirae and serovars *L. icterohaemorrhagiae*, *L. canicola*, *L. pomona*, *L. hardjo*, and *L. grippotyphosa* occur on all continents.

Transmission

Exposure is through contact of mucous membranes or skin with urine-contaminated water, fomites, or feed. Other sources are milk from acutely infected cows and genital excretions from cattle and swine of either sex.

Pathogenesis

Clinical and pathological manifestations suggest toxic mechanisms. Filtrates of tissue fluids from experimentally infected animals contain cytotoxic factors producing vascular lesions.

The spirochetes enter the bloodstream subsequent to mucous membrane or reproductive inoculation, colonizing particularly liver and kidney, where they produce degenerative changes. Other affected organs may be muscles, eyes, and meninges, where a nonsuppurative meningitis may develop. Leptospirae damage vascular endothelium, resulting in hemorrhages. All serovars produce these changes to varying degrees. *L. pomona* in cattle causes intravascular hemolysis due to a hemolytic exotoxin. Autoimmune phenomena may also contribute to this condition. Secondary changes include icterus due to liver damage and blood destruction, and acute, subacute, or subchronic nephritis due to renal tubular injury. The cellular exudates predominantly contain lymphocytes and plasma cells. In surviving animals, leptospirae disappear from circulation with the appearance of serum antibody but persist in the kidneys for many weeks (Figure 32.1).

Disease Patterns

Most leptospiral infections run an inapparent course probably due to infection of the animal by a host-adapted serovar. Clinical infections manifesting overt symptoms are primarily due to non-host-adapted serovar infections. These occur mainly in dogs, cattle, and swine; increasingly in sea lions; occasionally in horses, goats, and sheep; exceptionally in cats.

Dogs. Leading serovars involved are *L. icterohaemorrhagiae* and *L. canicola*, with the latter the more common. Increasing numbers of acute renal failure due to *grippotyphosa* infections are being reported.

The most acute form affects young pups preferentially, produces fever without localizing signs, and is commonly fatal within days. Hemorrhages are often apparent antemortem on mucous membranes and skin, or manifested by epistaxis or by blood-stained feces and vomitus. Jaundice is absent.

The icteric type runs a slower course, and hemorrhages are less conspicuous. Icterus is prominent. Renal localization causes nitrogen retention, while renal casts and leukocytes appear in the urine.

The uremic type, centered in the kidneys, results subsequent to either of the type of infections described earlier or may develop in their absence. It may be acute and rapidly fatal with signs of gastrointestinal upsets, uremic breath, and ulcerations in the anterior alimentary tract; or it may run a slow course with delayed onset.

Cattle. The predominant manifestation of bovine leptospirosis is abortion, usually late term, but may occur at any time following infection. Abortion is due to primary fetal death rather than placental infection. Fetal retention with progressive autolysis is common. Abortion due to *L. hardjo*, the host adapted serogroup for cattle, is primarily a problem of heifers in dairies due to management practices that differ between beef cattle and dairy operations. *L. hardjo* infections affect calves in utero leading to either abortion or "weak-calf syndrome." These infections are often subclinical or may be marked by "milk-drop syndrome," reproductive failure, and infertility. Chronic infection of the kidneys and the shedding of leptospirae in urine are common.

Acute leptospirosis due to *L. pomona* mostly affects calves and sometimes adult cattle. It is marked by fever, hemoglobinuria, icterus, anemia, and a fatality rate of 5–15%.

In some parts of the world, *Leptospira grippotyphosa*, *L. icterohaemorrhagiae*, and *L. canicola* cause bovine leptospirosis.

Swine. The serovars implicated in porcine leptospirosis include *L. pomona*, *L. icterohaemorrhagiae*, *L. canicola*, *L. tarassovi*, *L. bratislava*, and *L. muenchen*. As in bovine leptospirosis, septicemia with icterus and hemorrhages occurs, especially in piglets, while abortion and infertility are the manifestations in sows.

Horses. Equine leptospirosis is due most often to serovars *L. pomona*, *L. grippotyphosa*, and *L. icterohaemorrhagiae*. Signs in natural infections have been fever, mild icterus, and abortion. Leptospirosis is probably involved in equine recurrent iridocyclitis (periodic ophthalmia).

Other Animals. In small ruminants, leptospirosis, usually due to *L. pomona*, resembles that seen in cattle. Infections with *L. hardjo* and *L. grippotyphosa* also occur. Epidemics due to *L. pomona* have caused high mortality among California sea lions periodically since the 1940s.

Humans. Humans are susceptible to all serovars with no host-adapted strains identified. Infections cause fever, icterus, muscular pains, rashes, and nonsuppurative meningitis, manifestations varying somewhat with the serovars involved. A malignant form, most often associated with *L. icterohaemorrhagiae*, can cause fatal liver or renal disease.

Epidemiology

Leptospirosis is perpetuated by the many tolerant hosts and the protracted shedder state. Indirect exposure depends on mild and wet conditions, which favor environmental survival of leptospirae. More direct transfer occurs by urine aerosols in milking barns, cattle sheds, or canine courting habits, which may explain the male bias of canine leptospirosis.

Contaminated bodies of water are important sources of infection to livestock, aquatic mammals, and humans. Animal handlers, sewer workers, field hands, miners, and veterinarians are at increased risk of exposure.

Immunologic Factors

Immune Mechanisms of Disease

Immunologic mechanisms may relate to some features of leptospiral disease:

1. The hemolytic anemia characteristic of septicemic leptospirosis due to *L. pomona* in ruminants is associated with the presence of cold hemagglutinins, suggesting an autoimmune process. The relative roles of this and the bacterial hemolysin are uncertain.
2. Canine chronic interstitial nephritis is common and may be a postleptospiral lesion. Evidence of biofilm formation could explain chronic degradation of kidney tissue and the intermittent shedding of leptospirae in otherwise healthy animals. A leptospiral etiology is suggested by a frequent history of leptospirosis and the presence of leptospiral antibody, particularly in urine.
3. Strong evidence of a leptospiral basis for equine recurrent iridocyclitis (uveitis, periodic ophthalmia, and moon blindness) rests in part on the actual culture of leptospirae from the eyes of affected horses, PCR-positive results of aqueous humor samples, and leptospiral titers in the serum of affected horses.

Mechanisms of Resistance and Recovery

Recovery from acute leptospirosis coincides with the cessation of septicemia and the appearance of circulating antibody, usually during the second week of infection. Protective antibody is of IgM and IgG isotype and is directed mainly at the outer sheath antigens.

Agglutinating antibody (mostly IgM), which may persist for years after recovery, is no indication of immunity, nor of the shedder state, which may exist in the absence of antibody or have terminated before its disappearance. Evidence of leptospiral biofilm formation may explain the cause of refractile, protracted infections.

Immunity following recovery is generally solid and serovar specific, but repeated abortions due to *L. hardjo* have been seen in cows.

Artificial Immunization

Vaccination by bacterins is used on dogs (bivalent containing *icterohaemorrhagiae* and *canicola*, or multivalent containing *pomona* and *grippotyphosa* added to the bivalent). Cattle swine use at least a pentavalent bacterin containing *hardjo*, *pomona*, *canicola*, *icterohaemorrhagiae*, and *grippotyphosa* with the addition of serovar *bratislava* and a second *hardjo* component in some vaccines. Humans may be vaccinated depending on their occupation, for example, sewer workers and slaughterhouse workers. Protection is serovar specific and temporary, requiring at least annual boosters. Vaccination prevents overt disease but not necessarily infection.

Laboratory Diagnosis

Diagnosis of leptospirosis must be established by laboratory confirmation.

Sample Collection

From living subjects, blood, urine, cerebrospinal fluid, uterine fluids, and placental cotyledons are examined. Blood is usually negative after the first febrile phase. Milk is destructive to leptospirae and not a promising source of cultures. Urine should always be tested.

From cadavers, including aborted fetuses, kidneys are most likely to harbor leptospirae. In septic fatalities (including abortions), many organs, especially the liver, spleen, lung, brain, and eye, may contain the agent.

Culturing is done promptly after sample collection, although leptospirae can survive in oxalated human blood for 11 days.

Direct Examination

Methods of direct visual demonstration are wet mounts, examined by dark-field (or phase) microscopy; immunofluorescent stains, and silver impregnation of fixed tissue.

Routine dark-field microscopy should be limited to urine. Other body fluids contain artifacts similar to leptospirae. Brief, low-speed centrifugation clears the specimen of interfering particles, but will not sediment leptospirae. Methods using formalinized urine have been described, but they destroy motility, and motility aids in the identification of leptospira. Negative results of direct examinations do not rule out leptospirosis.

Fluorescent antibody has been used on fluids, tissue sections, homogenates, organ impressions, and, most effectively, on aborted bovine fetuses, where examination of kidney was most rewarding. Silver-impregnated sections must be interpreted with caution, since argyrophilic tissue fibrils can mimic leptospirae.

DNA amplification using PCR and specific DNA primers has become an excellent diagnostic tool for detecting the presence of leptospirae in animal tissues and fluids.

Isolation and Identification

Ellinghausen-McCullough-Johnson-Harris medium (EMJH) is a good isolation medium, especially for *L. hardjo*, the slowest growing of the common serovars. Replicate inoculations are made into liquid media with and without selective inhibitors (5-fluorouracil, neomycin, and cycloheximide). Media are examined microscopically at intervals during incubation for up to several months.

Animal inoculation (hamsters or guinea pigs) eliminates minor contaminants from the primary inoculum, which is injected intraperitoneally. Blood is drawn periodically for culture starting a few days after inoculation. After 3–4 weeks, the animals are killed and their kidneys are examined and cultured for leptospirae. If infected with leptospirae, they will have developed antibody. Any isolate recovered by these methods can be identified morphologically as *Leptospira* sp. Definitive identification is carried out by reference laboratories (Center for Disease Control, Atlanta, GA, National Animal Disease Center, Ames, IA).

Serology. Since direct examination is often unreliable and culture laborious, expensive, and slow, serology is the most common diagnostic method. The microscopic agglutination test employing live antigen is most widely used. Others include macroscopic plate and tube agglutination tests, complement fixation tests, and enzyme-linked antibody assays. Paired samples are preferred: one collected at first presentation and the other 2 weeks later. If leptospirosis was the problem, a fourfold or greater rise in titer should have occurred in the interval. In bovine abortion, these relations may not hold. This is because *hardjo* infections of cattle elicit a very poor immune response, which is probably due to their adaptation to this animal species.

Antibody persists for extended periods postinfection. Postvaccination titers are lower and decline well before the vaccination immunity. Agglutination titers are type specific. Diagnostic laboratories generally maintain all common serovars for serologic testing.

Treatment and Control

Leptospirae are susceptible to penicillin, tetracycline, chloramphenicol, streptomycin, and erythromycin. Treatment, to be of benefit, has to be instituted early, possibly even prophylactically in cases of known exposure. Doxycycline is used to treat humans prophylactically. Streptomycin or dihydrostreptomycin is routinely used to eliminate the carrier state in animals. However, sustained leptospiral infection in the kidneys and reproductive tracts of cattle subsequent to antibiotic treatment is not uncommon, again suggesting the presence of leptospiral biofilm formation.

Vaccination generally prevents disease. It prevents neither infection nor shedding.

For More Information

CFSPH Technical Fact Sheets. Leptospirosis at http://www.cfsph.iastate.edu/DiseaseInfo/CDC website. Leptospirosis at http://www.cdc.gov/ncidod/dbmd/diseaseinfo/leptospirosis_g_pet.htm.

Further Reading

Acierno MJ (2011) Continuous renal replacement therapy in dogs and cats. *Vet Clin North Am Small Anim Pract.* **41**, 135–146.

Adler B and de la Peña Moctezuma A (2010) Leptospira and leptospirosis. *Vet Microbiol*, **140**, 287–296.

Burke RL, Kronmann KC and Daniels CC (2012) A review of zoonotic disease surveillance supported by the Armed Forces Health Surveillance Center. *Zoonoses Public Health*, **59**, 164–175.

Ellis WA (2010) Control of canine leptospirosis in Europe: time for a change? *Vet Rec*, **167**, 602–605.

Ellis WA and Little TWA (eds) (1986) *The present state of leptospirosis diagnosis and control*. Proceedings of the Seminar of the EEC Programme of Coordination of Research on Animal Pathology, 10–11 October 1984, Belfast, Northern Ireland. Martinus Nijhoff Publishers, Dordrecht/Boston/Lancaster, for the Commission of the European Communities, pp. 247.

Goldstein RE (2010) Canine leptospirosis. *Vet Clin North Am Small Anim Pract*, **40**, 1091–1101.

Hartskeerl RA, Collares-Pereira M and Ellis WA (2011) Emergence, control and re-emerging leptospirosis: dynamics of infection in the changing world. *Clin Microbiol Infect*, **17**, 494–501.

Koizumi N and Yasutomi I (2012) Prevalence of leptospirosis in farm animals. *Jpn J Vet Res*, **60** (Suppl), S55–S58.

Leshem E, Meltzer E and Schwartz E (2011) Travel-associated zoonotic bacterial diseases. *Curr Opin Infect Dis*, **24**, 457–463.

Marr JS and Cathey JT (2010) New hypothesis for cause of epidemic among native Americans, New England, 1616–1619. *Emerg Infect Dis*, **16**, 281–286.

Revich B, Tokarevich N and Parkinson AJ (2012) Climate change and zoonotic infections in the Russian Arctic. *Int J Circumpolar Health*, **23**, 18792.

Tulsiani SM, Graham GC, Moore PR et al. (2011) Emerging tropical diseases in Australia. Part 5. Hendra virus. *Ann Trop Med Parasitol*, **105**, 1–11.

Staphylococcus

MARK S. SMELTZER AND KAREN E. BEENKEN

The staphylococci are spherical gram-positive bacteria that divide in multiple planes to form irregular clusters. Other defining characteristics include the production of catalase, a unique peptidoglycan composition, and a G+C content below 40%. The staphylococci are present on the skin and epithelial surfaces of all warm-blooded animals. Based on modern era molecular typing schemes, the number of staphylococcal species continues to grow, but a primary distinction remains the production of coagulase. Coagulase is an enzyme capable of activating prothrombin, thereby promoting the coagulation of plasma. This distinction is important in that *Staphylococcus aureus* is without question the most prominent cause of disease in both man and animals, and unlike most other staphylococcal species, it is coagulase positive. In fact, given the predominance of *S. aureus*, it is often underappreciated that there are other important coagulase-positive species, and some of these are of particular importance in veterinary medicine. One example is species of the *Staphylococcus intermedius* group (SIG), which are a prominent if not predominant cause of canine pyodermas. It is also important to recognize that essentially all coagulase-negative species (CNS) are capable of causing infection in man and animals, one important example in veterinary medicine being bovine mastitis. Molecular characterization has also led to identification of clonal lineages within each species, and in some cases, these also appear to have general associations with infections in animals. For example, *S. aureus* isolates of the ST398 clonal lineage are a prominent cause of infections in pigs, and there is some evidence to suggest that this may reflect adaptations that favor colonization of the porcine host. Thus, it is important to consider the staphylococci in the specific context of veterinary medicine at the level of both species and clonal distinctions. Our goal here is not to be comprehensive in this regard but rather to provide the reader with a sufficient understanding of such differences to provide both the background necessary for practicing veterinarians to effectively diagnose and treat staphylococcal infections and the impetus for further research to explore and clinically exploit such differences.

Staphylococcal Species

The number of staphylococcal species continues to grow, largely owing to the development of detailed molecular typing techniques. A 1999 paper listed 39 species and subspecies and proposed guidelines for the identification of new staphylococcal species based on both phenotypic and genotypic criteria. Since that time, new species have been identified, one prominent example of particular importance in veterinary medicine being the SIG species *Staphylococcus pseudintermedius*. While species distinctions include consideration of phenotypic characteristics, the hallmark has become DNA sequence divergence as reflected either in DNA–DNA hybridization studies or more targeted comparisons between highly conserved genes, the most notable of these being those encoding ribosomal RNA. There is mounting evidence to suggest that these species distinctions also play an important role in defining host range, specific examples being *Staphylococcus caprae* (goats), *S. delphini* (dolphins), *S. equorum* (horses), *S. felis* (cats), *S. gallinarum* (chicken), *S. lentus* (goats), *S. hyicus* (pigs), *S. intermedius* and *S. pseudintermedius* (dogs), and *S. simiae* (monkeys). However, none of these host associations are absolute. Indeed, even a cursory search of the literature will reveal reports describing the isolation of each of these species from other hosts including humans, often in association with disease. As an example, *S. hyicus* is most commonly associated with exudative dermatitis in pigs, but it is also a prominent cause of bovine mastitis, and was recently described as a cause of bacteremia in a farmer that arose as a zoonotic infection.

Recent years have also seen the recognition of potentially important clonal lineages within a single staphylococcal species. As might be expected, this is particularly true with respect to *S. aureus*. Methods commonly used to make such distinctions include pulsed-field gel electrophoresis (PFGE), sequence typing of the genes encoding protein A (*spa* typing), and multilocus sequence typing (MLST), a method based on sequence divergence among seven highly conserved housekeeping genes. Related MLST (ST) types are sometimes included within the same clonal complex (CC).

Veterinary Microbiology, Third Edition. Edited by D. Scott McVey, Melissa Kennedy and M.M. Chengappa.

Among methicillin-resistant strains, particularly those of *S. aureus*, the SIG species, and the CNS *Staphylococcus epidermidis*, typing methods have also been developed on the basis of sequence variation in the staphylococcal chromosome cassette that contains the *mecA* gene (SCC*mec*), which encodes the alternative penicillin-binding protein that is the primary determinant of methicillin resistance in all staphylococcal species. Just as there is evidence to suggest that certain staphylococcal species exhibit distinct patterns of host colonization and consequently infection, there is also evidence that this is true of clonal lineages, particularly those of *S. aureus*. However, as with the species themselves, none of these are absolute, perhaps owing to widespread horizontal transfer of critical virulence factor genes between staphylococcal species. For example, *S. aureus* isolates of the ST398 lineage were first recognized as an important cause of infections in pigs, but it has since been demonstrated that livestock veterinarians are also at increased risk of infection with methicillin-resistant isolates of the ST398 clonal lineage.

FIGURE 26.1. *Hemolytic colonies of* Staphylococcus aureus *on blood agar.*

Descriptive Features

Morphology and Staining

Staphylococci are 0.5–1.5 μm in diameter and stain strongly gram-positive. In exudates, they form clusters, pairs, or short chains. They do not form spores but are extremely resilient and can survive in harsh environments and on inanimate objects for long periods. While often underappreciated, this resiliency is no doubt a major contributing factor to the pathogenesis of all staphylococcal infections because it allows the bacteria to persist in the immediate environment of their hosts, thus providing the opportunity for infection should conditions in the host allow. The staphylococci do not produce flagella and are not motile. On blood agar, colonies are round and relatively large (3–5 mm). A primary species distinction is that *S. aureus* produces carotenoid pigments that confer a golden color, particularly on certain types of media, while colonies of other species are generally white. This is not a trivial difference in that the production of these pigments has been directly associated with the increased virulence of *S. aureus*.

Unlike CNS, most strains of *S. aureus*, and to a somewhat lesser extent, other coagulase-positive species, are toxigenic. One manifestation of this is that they are hemolytic on blood agar (Figure 26.1). Toxins detectable on blood agar include α-, β-, and δ-toxin, each of which exhibits unique properties. α-Toxin is a pore-forming toxin that causes the complete lysis of appropriate erythrocytes, most notably those of rabbits. In contrast, β-toxin is an sphingomyelinase with increased activity against sheep erythrocytes. β-Toxin also generates a form of incomplete lysis that is enhanced by incubation at 4 °C, thus accounting for references to β-toxin as a "hot-cold" hemolysin. δ-Toxin is a phenol-soluble modulin closely associated with the *agr* (accessory gene regulator) regulatory system (see Section "Regulation of Pathogenesis"). The activity of α- and β-toxin is antagonistic, while that of β- and δ-toxin is synergistic. Because the staphylococci and streptococci are the cause of similar types of infection in both man and animals, it is important to distinguish these hemolytic reactions from those of the streptococci. Specifically, among streptococcal species, "β-hemolysis" refers to complete lysis of erythrocytes, which among the staphylococci is characteristic of α-toxin. The incomplete lysis that is characteristic of staphylococcal β-toxin has also been used to diagnostic advantage. For example, *Streptococcus agalactiae*, which is a Lancefield Group B species that, like *S. aureus*, is a common cause of bovine mastitis, produces an extracellular factor that is also synergistic with staphylococcal β-toxin, thus yielding a characteristic CAMP pattern of increased hemolytic activity when the two species are grown on blood agar in close proximity to each other (Figure 26.2). Interestingly, most *S. aureus* isolates associated with infections in cattle produce β-toxin, while most human isolates do not owing to the presence of a lysogenic prophage within the corresponding *hlb* gene.

When considering colony morphology and hemolytic reactions, it is important to recognize that many primary isolates from both animals and humans grow as small-colony variants (SCVs). These are metabolically inactive variants that yield much smaller colonies (<1 mm), are typically nonhemolytic irrespective of species, and, perhaps most importantly, exhibit reduced antibiotic susceptibility even in the absence of issues of acquired antibiotic resistance. The latter attribute greatly complicates treatment of staphylococcal infections in both man and animals, and is almost certainly why SCVs are responsible for persistent infections including bovine mastitis. In the diagnostic laboratory, this is a reversible phenotype in that subculture of SCVs on rich medium will result in the more typical colony morphologies and patterns of hemolytic activity,

FIGURE 26.2. *Hemolytic CAMP test reaction on blood agar, demonstrating zone of enhanced hemolysis at the intersection of group A* Staphylococcus aureus *and β-hemolytic streptococci.*

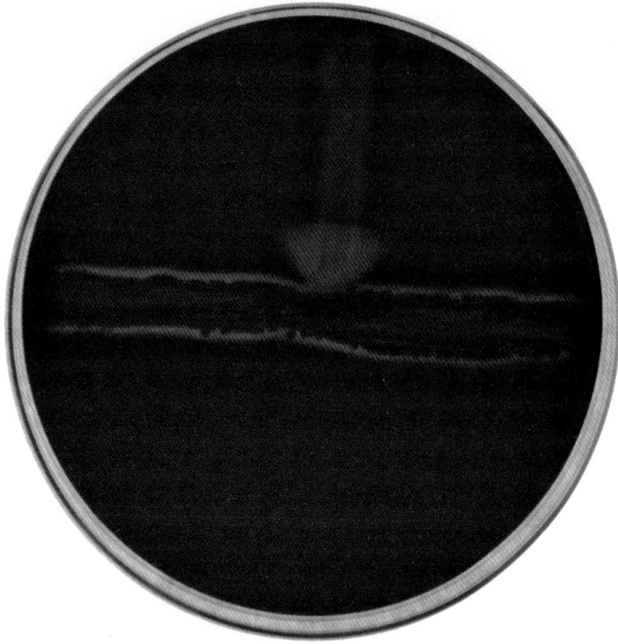

but it remains an important consideration that can impact critical issues including the failure to diagnose infection in a timely manner.

Most strains of *S. aureus* are encapsulated, with some reports suggesting the existence of as many as 11 capsular serotypes. However, four of these (serotypes 1, 2, 5, and 8) are by far the serotypes of primary medical interest. Isolates of serotypes 1 and 2 are heavily encapsulated to the point of appearing mucoid an agar medium, but they are rarely isolated by comparison to microencapsulated isolates of serotypes 5 and 8 irrespective of host species. Capsular polysaccharides contribute to pathogenesis by limiting neutrophil-mediated phagocytosis, which is a primary defense against all forms of staphylococcal infection. Coagulase-negative staphylococcal species are also encapsulated, but the capsules produced by these species have not been well characterized. In contrast, strains of both *S. aureus* and several CNS, most notably *S. epidermidis*, may produce a second exopolysaccharide that plays an important role in biofilm formation. This is referred to as either the polysaccharide intercellular adhesin (PIA), a designation that directly reflects its role in biofilm formation, or PNAG, a designation that reflects its structural identity as a β-1,6 poly-*N*-acetylglucosamine. Congo red agar (CRA) has been used as an indicator of PIA production and the relative capacity to form a biofilm, with biofilm-positive strains appearing black on this medium. There is also a report suggesting that both *S. epidermidis* and *S. aureus* produce a β-1,6 poly-*N*-succinylglucosamine (PNSG), particularly under *in vivo* conditions.

Biochemical Characterization

Most staphylococcal species are facultative anaerobes, but at least two species and/or subspecies (*S. aureus* ssp. *anaerobius* and *S. saccharolyticus*) include strains that cannot grow aerobically. These are also the only staphylococcal species that do not produce catalase, an enzyme that converts hydrogen peroxide to water and oxygen. The production of catalase by all other staphylococcal species allows for their easy discrimination from other medically relevant gram-positive cocci including streptococcal and enterococcal species, all of which are catalase-negative. All staphylococcal species are able to grow in high concentrations of salt and over a relatively wide temperature range.

At the species level, distinguishing characteristics include carbohydrate fermentation/oxidation patterns and other biochemical tests including those for nitrate reductase, alkaline phosphatase, arginine dihydrolase, ornithine decarboxylase, urease, and cytochrome oxidase. However, species classification based on such methods has largely been supplanted by the use of molecular techniques. Exceptions to this include the aforementioned production of coagulase and hemolytic activity, both of which remain mainstay diagnostic tests. Once again, while catalase-positive, coagulase-positive, hemolytic staphylococcal isolates are often identified as *S. aureus*, other species also exhibit all of these characteristics and are capable of causing infections in both man and animals. The most prominent example is the SIG species, primary members of which include *S. intermedius*, *S. pseudintermedius*, and *S. delphini*. These species have been isolated from dogs, cats, horses and birds, and they are difficult to distinguish from each other and from *S. aureus* without the use of molecular techniques because, in addition to being coagulase-positive, all produce similar extracellular proteins including hemolysins and a thermostable nuclease. However, SIG species typically do not produce clumping factor and consequently are generally negative in commercially available rapid identification kits for *S. aureus*. Other coagulase-positive or at least "coagulase-variable" species that are also sometimes confused with *S. aureus* include *S. schleiferi* ssp. *coagulans*, *S. lutrae*, *S. agnetis*, and *S. hyicus*. As an example of both this confusion and the possibility of zoonotic infection, a recent report described a clinical case of *S. hyicus* bacteremia in a farmer that was likely to have arisen from his close contact with pigs and was originally diagnosed as an *S. aureus* infection owing primarily to positive tests for catalase and coagulase.

Structure and Composition

The cell envelope of the staphylococci is highly complex. At its core, it consists of a thick, highly cross-linked peptidoglycan layer, with the cross-links themselves consisting of a unique pentaglycine bridge. These cross-links render staphylococcal species resistant to lysozyme but sensitive to lysostaphin, an enzyme currently being explored for therapeutic purposes. Other integral components include teichoic acids, which may be covalently linked to peptidoglycan (wall teichoic acids) or embedded in the cell membrane (lipoteichoic acids). Both of these forms contribute to the resistance of *S. aureus* and perhaps other staphylococcal species to cationic antimicrobial peptides, and in *S. aureus* at least they serve as adhesins to promote colonization. These components also act synergistically to cause septic shock, thus qualifying them within the strict definition of endotoxins.

Exposed on the surface of the peptidoglycan layer is a remarkable array of proteins capable of binding an equally diverse array of host proteins. As with the teichoic acids, some of these are covalently linked to peptidoglycan, while others are embedded in the cell membrane and/or excreted into the extracellular environment. Covalent anchoring occurs via an LPXTG motif and is mediated by the enzyme sortase A. Surface proteins anchored to peptidoglycan via this mechanism have been designated "microbial surface components recognizing adhesive matrix molecules" (MSCRAMM). The prototype example in *S. aureus* is protein A, but this species produces at least 19 such proteins, several of which have been shown to be highly immunogenic and are being pursued as vaccine candidates. The membrane anchored and secreted proteins, the latter being collectively referred to as "secretable expanded repertoire adhesive molecules" (SERAM), are far fewer in number but nevertheless potentially important.

When taken together, these surface proteins play defining roles in the colonization of host tissues. Most are highly conserved among different strains of *S. aureus*, but some are not, and this may play an important role in defining host specificity. For example, the *cna* gene, which encodes a collagen-binding MSCRAMM, is relatively rare among *S. aureus* isolates, but a recent report found that all ST398 isolates from poultry were *cna*-positive. Another potentially important MSCRAMM is *bbp*, which was first described based on the ability of the corresponding adhesin (Bbp) to bind bone sialoprotein. However, a recent report demonstrated that Bbp also binds human fibrinogen and, more importantly, that it does not bind the fibrinogen of cats, dogs, cattle, sheep, pigs, or mice. At the same time, another report examined "high-virulence" and "low-virulence" *S. aureus* isolates obtained from rabbits and found that *bbp* was conserved among the high-virulence strains. Similarly, *bap* (biofilm-associated protein) is present in a subset of *S. aureus* strains and several CNS, but to date it has been observed almost exclusively in animal isolates, most notably those associated with bovine mastitis. Finally, coagulase production is typically assessed using rabbit plasma, but a recent report described *S. aureus* variants that preferentially coagulate plasma from other host species. This was attributed to novel variants of a von Willebrand factor-binding protein, with the genes encoding these variants being located on a mobile pathogenicity island (SaPI) that exhibits sufficient host-range specificity to warrant species-dependent designations (e.g., SaPIbov4 vs. SaPIeq1). Whether any of these are cause-and-effect relationships that contribute to host range and/or the propensity to cause infection in different host species remains to be determined, but such reports nevertheless suggest that divergence among strains of *S. aureus*, as well as across different staphylococcal species, may play an important role in defining the host specificity of staphylococcal infection.

Although best characterized in *S. aureus*, functionally similar surface-exposed adhesins are present in the SIG group and CNS. In fact, an immunoglobulin-binding protein similar to *S. aureus* protein A has been identified in the SIG species *S. pseudintermedius* and in *S. hyicus*. Primary host proteins bound by these adhesins include fibronectin and fibrinogen, although as noted above there are potentially important differences across host species with respect to this binding specificity. There are also reports that capsular polysaccharides can mask these adhesins at least in *S. aureus*, but only when present in copious amounts. Although unproven, this could account for the prominence of serotype 5 and 8 strains by comparison to heavily encapsulated serotypes 1 and 2.

Toxins

The production of toxins is generally limited to coagulase-positive staphylococcal species, and this no doubt contributes to their predominance as a cause of serious infections. Strains of all of these species also typically produce multiple extracellular enzymes including proteases, lipases, and a thermostable nuclease. The list of toxins is extensive, particularly in *S. aureus*, but generally speaking they fall into one of five functional but overlapping categories: hemolysins/cytotoxins, phenol-soluble modulins (PSMs), enterotoxins, exfoliative toxins, and superantigens. The prototype example of a superantigen is toxic shock syndrome toxin-1, but several of the enterotoxins are also superantigenic. Like the number of staphylococcal species, the number of toxins continues to grow due to the availability of more precise methods of distinguishing between variants. However, perhaps the more important point is that essentially all strains of *S. aureus*, as well as most SIG species, produce some combination of these exotoxins, presumably to a point that makes a primary contribution to their increased virulence.

There is also evidence to suggest that the production of specific toxins may influence both host range and the relative capacity to cause disease. For example, the *S. aureus* exfoliative toxins are serine proteases that exhibit exquisite specificity for the desmosomal glycoprotein desmogein-1, thus accounting for the characteristic dermal lesions associated with staphylococcal scalded skin syndrome in humans. *S. hyicus* is a prominent cause of skin infections in pigs, and this species produces a form of exfoliative toxin that, by comparison to human desmoglein, selectively degrades porcine desmoglein-1. Similarly, examined 178 SIG isolates and found that only one harbored the human enterotoxin C gene (*sec*) while essentially all carried a canine variant. These isolates also had the gene for a unique exfoliative toxin designated the *S. intermedius* exfoliative toxin, and it is likely that this toxin contributes to the prominent role of SIG species as a cause of canine pyodermas. The SIG species also characteristically produce a hemolysin similar *S. aureus* β-toxin. This is potentially significant in that almost all *S. aureus* isolates associated with human infection are lysogenized with an *hlb*-converting

FIGURE 26.3. *Porcine dermatitis caused by* Staphylococcus hyicus. *(A) Generalized dermatitis referred to as greasy pig disease. (B) Histopathology of skin demonstrating inflammation and presences of many bacteria (Giemsa stain, 400×). (Courtesy of Dr Alan Doster, University of Nebraska Lincoln, Veterinary Diagnostic Center.)*

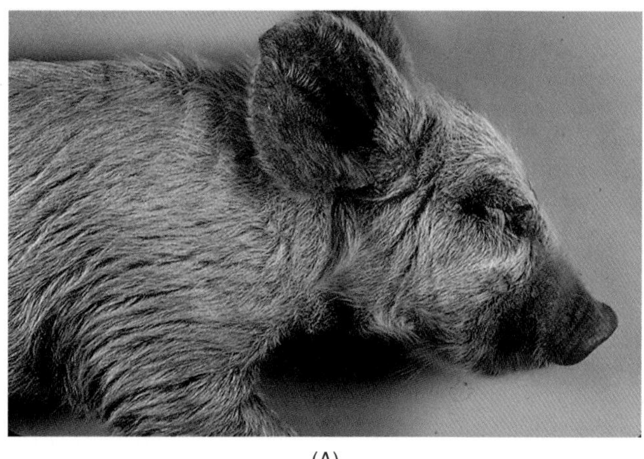

(A)

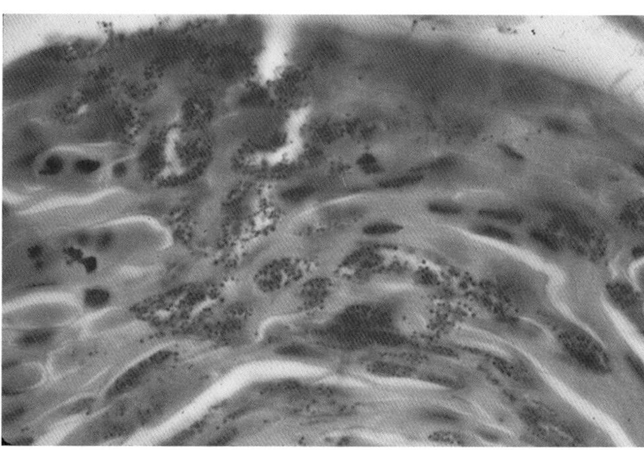

(B)

phage and consequently do not produce β-toxin, while this is rarely true of *S. aureus* isolates associated with several forms of animal infection including canine pyodermas and bovine mastitis (Figure 26.3). Based on this, it seems reasonable to suggest that the production of β-toxin may somehow contribute to host range in staphylococcal infection. Having said that, these phage also positively convert other virulence factors, several of which are known to modulate the host immune response, thus raising the possibility that this potentially important distinction is not directly related to the production of β-toxin itself.

Until recently, the important role of PSMs in the pathogenesis of staphylococcal infection was almost completely overlooked. This was due in part to the fact that these are very small molecules, the genes for which were not recognized in early genome annotation attempts. However, recent studies have confirmed that PSMs play a critical role in many forms of human infection owing to their capacity to lyse neutrophils. In fact, the production of PSMs in large quantities, together with the high-level production of α-hemolysin, appears to play a defining role in the hypervirulence of certain clonal lineages of *S. aureus*, most notably those of the PFGE-defined USA300 clonal lineage. Although the specific role of PSMs in animal infection has not been investigated, a recent report demonstrated that many *S. aureus* isolates associated with bovine mastitis, including the sequenced strain RF122, produce very high levels of α-toxin. This was associated with a single-nucleotide polymorphism (SNP) in the promoter region of the corresponding gene (*hla*), so it remains unclear if this extends to include the high-level production of PSMs. However, these same bovine mastitis isolates exhibited higher transcription levels of specific positive regulators of *hla* transcription including AgrA (see Section "Regulation of Pathogenesis"), which also positively regulates PSM production. Thus, it seems likely that PSMs may also play a critical role in at least some forms of animal infection. *S. pseudintermedius* also produces a biocomponent leukotoxin (LukI) similar to the Panton-Valentine leukocidin. This toxin is encoded by the cotranscribed genes *lukS* and *lukF*, and while such toxins also occur in a strain-dependent manner, found that these genes were present in all canine isolates of *S. pseudintermedius*.

Regulation of Pathogenesis

To adapt to changing conditions in the host, whatever that host may be, it is also important for a bacterial pathogen to control the production of critical virulence factors. These regulatory circuits involved in mediating this control are remarkably complex, at least as defined for *S. aureus*. For example, in their analysis of genome sequence data from the *S. aureus* human isolates N315 and Mu50, identified 124 genes encoding what they considered "transcription regulators." This included 17 two-component signal transduction systems and 63 regulators presumed to be DNA-binding proteins based on the presence of helix-turn-helix motifs. Most of these are conserved among different *S. aureus* strains, including those associated with infections in animals, but some are not. Many also have homologs in CNS species, although in most cases this remains an understudied area. Expression levels also vary dramatically between strains, and recent data strongly suggest that this is clinically relevant in both man and animals. Such variation, together with the use of different animal models of disease, also contributes to the many contrasting reports in the literature, and this makes it difficult to make definitive statements about the contribution of these regulatory elements to different forms of human and animal infection. However, it is becoming clear that, as with the virulence factors themselves, the regulatory circuits that modulate these processes exhibit important similarities and differences among the staphylococcal species that cause animal and human disease.

Mutations have been generated in just over 30 of *S. aureus* regulatory elements, and a complete discussion even of this subset is beyond the scope of this chapter. For this, we would refer the reader to previously published review, the caveat being the almost exclusive focus of this review on *S. aureus* and human infections. What we have chosen to do here is focus on the two regulatory systems that we consider the most central and the most highly conserved among diverse staphylococcal species. These are the *agr* and the staphylococcal accessory regulator (*sarA*), both of which have been shown to have a significant impact on both toxin production and other clinically relevant phenotypes including the ability to form a biofilm. The *agr* regulatory system has been studied in multiple staphylococcal species including *S. aureus*, the SIG group, and the CNS *S. epidermidis* and *S. lugdunensis*. Induction of *agr* results in the increased production of extracellular proteins, including toxins, and decreased production of surface-associated virulence factors. The *agr* regulatory system includes two divergent promoters (P2 and P3) that drive the production of transcripts designated RNAII and RNAIII, respectively. RNAII spans an operon (*agrACDB*) that encodes the elements of a two-component quorum-sensing system. Specifically, *agrC* encodes a membrane-bound sensor that is responsive to the accumulation of an *agrD*-encoded autoinducing peptide (AIP), production of which requires processing and export by the membrane-embedded AgrB. AIP binding to the AgrC sensor initiates a phosphorylation cascade that results in activation of the AgrA response regulator and increased transcription from both the P2 and P3 promoters. The functional result of *agr* activation is increased expression from the P3 promoter resulting in increased production of RNAIII. The RNAIII transcript spans the *hld* gene, which encodes δ-toxin, but it has been conclusively demonstrated that the regulatory effects of *agr* are mediated by RNAIII irrespective of the production of δ-toxin. Interestingly, δ-toxin is a PSM, and phosphorylated AgrA was recently shown to also bind to *cis* elements upstream of the *psm* gene clusters and induce the production ofPSMs. It has been suggested on this basis that the evolutionary basis of *agr*-mediated regulation revolved around AgrA-mediated control of PSM production, with the regulatory effects of RNAIII evolving later as a means of achieving more global regulatory control.

The phenotype of an RNAIII mutant is characterized by major changes at the transcriptional level. However, RNAIII itself functions primarily at a posttranscriptional level, with transcriptional changes associated with its production being the result of its impact on the production of accessory transcription factors. For instance, transcription of the gene encoding staphylococcal protein A (*spa*) is increased in the absence of RNAIII, but this is due to the fact that RNAIII normally represses production of other transcription factors (e.g., SarT, Rot, and ultimately SarS) that would otherwise promote *spa* transcription. Thus, in the absence of RNAIII, this repression does not occur, which results in the continued high-level expression of *spa*. Additionally, RNAIII binds *spa* mRNA in a manner that both limits translation and promotes RNase III-mediated degradation. This mechanism also plays a primary role in the RNAIII-mediated induction of toxin production via both direct and indirect pathways. For instance, the *hla* transcript forms a stem-loop structure that sequesters the Shine-Delgarno sequence, thus limiting translation and the production of α-toxin. RNAIII overcomes this by binding the *hla* transcript and relieving this stem-loop structure. The translation of *hla* is thus upregulated in the presence of RNAIII via a direct interaction between RNAIII and *hla* mRNA. In other cases, the regulatory functions are mediated indirectly via the interaction between RNAIII and the *rot* transcript. Specifically, the regulatory functions of *rot* (repressor of toxins) and *agr* are antagonistic, with RNAIII limiting the production of Rot by binding to the Shine-Dalgarno sequence of the *rot* transcript and, as with the *spa* transcript, both inhibiting translation and targeting the existing transcript for degradation by RNase III.

The *agr* regulatory system is also defined by the existence of subtypes even within a single species. For instance, in *S. aureus*, the *agr* system has four subtypes (I–IV), and these define *agr* interference groups. Specifically, variations in the AgrC sensor and the AgrD pheromone define groups that activate *agr* when matched with each other but inhibit *agr* expression when mismatched. A recent report examined mixed populations of *S. aureus* in an insect model and found that this interference occurs *in vivo*. At present, it is unclear whether this has an impact on host range, but cross-species interference does occur. For example, Lina *et al.* (2003) demonstrated that, in humans, colonization with *S. epidermidis* generally precluded concomitant colonization with *S. aureus*, and it seems reasonable to suggest that such cross-species interference could impact the host range of different staphylococcal species. One intriguing possibility in this regard is the SIG species, which produce a novel AIP by comparison to *S. aureus* that has been shown to be inhibitory to all four of the *S. aureus agr* subtypes.

Many reports have demonstrated that mutation of *agr* attenuates virulence in animal models of staphylococcal infection. Moreover, it is increasingly clear that the increased virulence of certain *S. aureus* isolates, most notably those of the USA300 clonal lineage, is a function of their high-level expression of *agr* and increased production of critical extracellular virulence factors including α-toxin and PSMs. As noted above, some *S. aureus* isolates from cases of bovine mastitis also exhibit *agr* expression levels that exceed even those of USA300 isolates, thus suggesting that this is a critical determinant of virulence in animal as well as human infections. However, this does not mean that *agr* expression plays a defining role in all forms of staphylococcal infection. Indeed, biofilm formation is a critical component of many forms of infection, and expression of *agr* at high levels has been associated with a reduced capacity to form a biofilm in both *S. aureus* and *S. epidermidis*. There is even evidence to suggest that activation of *agr* may constitute a specific means of dispersal from a biofilm. In fact, Yarwood *et al.* (2004) demonstrated that *agr*-negative variants arise spontaneously in *S. aureus* biofilms and that, over time, these variants become the dominant subpopulation. In humans, there are also multiple reports of the isolation of *agr* mutants from infected patients. Thus, while high-level expression of *agr* is clearly associated with virulence in both man and animals, it may also come at some cost to the pathogen with respect to both the metabolic burden placed on the bacterial cell and the ability to pursue alternative forms of avoiding host defenses, one potentially important example being the ability to form a biofilm on host tissues and/or implanted medical devices.

A second regulatory locus that plays an important role in the specific context of such biofilm-associated infections is the *sarA*. Like *agr*, *sarA* has a global impact on *S. aureus* virulence phenotypes and is conserved in both diverse staphylococcal species. The *sarA* locus encodes three overlapping transcripts, all of which share a common terminus and include the *sarA* gene. This gene encodes a DNA-binding protein that impacts gene transcription, at least in *S. aureus*, via both *agr*-dependent and *agr*-independent pathways. More directly, SarA has been shown to bind *cis* elements associated with *agr* in a manner that increases *agr* expression, an observation that suggests *agr* and *sarA* mutants would exhibit similar phenotypes. To some extent this is true, one example being that both *agr* and *sarA* mutants characteristically produce reduced amounts of critical extracellular toxins including α-toxin and PSMs. However, a recent report demonstrates that the mechanistic basis for these toxin-deficient phenotypes differs. Specifically, *agr* impacts the production of these exotoxins at the transcriptional and/or translational levels as described earlier, while the impact of *sarA* appears to be related to its impact on the production of extracellular proteases, with the increased production of proteases observed in *sarA* mutants resulting in reduced accumulation, rather than reduced production, of these exotoxins. In fact, this is a direct example of the importance of the *agr*-independent pathway in that mutation of *agr* characteristically results in reduced production of these proteases, while mutation of *sarA* has the opposite effect.

The impact of this is even more apparent in the clinically and therapeutically relevant context of biofilm formation in that mutation of *agr* enhances biofilm formation, while mutation of *sarA* has the opposite effect, an observation that in both cases as been correlated with the impact of these mutations on the production of extracellular proteases. Given the important role of biofilms in limiting the therapeutic efficacy of conventional antibiotics, either of these observations could potentially be exploited to therapeutic advantage. For instance, introduction of the *agr* AIP would result in increased expression of *agr*, the increased production of extracellular proteases, and a decreased capacity to form a biofilm, and when administered with an antibiotic this could significantly enhance the therapeutic outcome in infections in both man and animals. However, this would have the potentially adverse consequence of enhancing toxin production. In contrast, inhibitors of *sarA* expression and/or function could be used to enhance protease production and thereby limit both biofilm formation and toxin production. Given the importance of staphylococci as a cause of infection in both man and animals, and the persistent emergence of antibiotic resistance in essentially all staphylococcal species (see Section "Resistance and Antibiotic Treatment"), these are important observations that should be considered by investigators who focus on staphylococcal infections irrespective of the host species involved. In this respect, it should be noted that, while there are reports describing the role of *agr* in the context of veterinary medicine, there are essentially none we are aware of that have extended this consideration to other staphylococcal regulatory elements including *sarA*.

Iron Acquisition

The wealth of data regarding the staphylococci and their role in human and animal disease is almost overwhelming. We have attempted to focus in this chapter on the most critical issues that distinguish between staphylococcal species and may in fact contribute to host range and the development of infection in species other than humans. Based on this focus, we have also chosen to give specific consideration to mechanisms of iron acquisition. One reason for this is a recent report demonstrating that the surface-associated hemoglobin receptor IsdA of *S. aureus* preferentially binds human hemoglobin by comparison to the murine form, an observation that is likely to account for the need to employ a high infective dose in murine models of infection. This suggests that similar differences may also contribute to the relative propensity of different staphylococcal species to cause infection in different hosts, but once again this is an understudied area in the specific context of veterinary medicine. *S. aureus* has also at least two systems capable of acquiring iron from heme proteins. One of these was designated Isd (for *i*ron-responsive *s*urface *d*eterminants) and includes five transcriptional units (*isdA*, *isdB*, *isdCDEF-srtBisdG*, *isdH*, and *isdI*). The second (HtsABC for *h*eme *t*ransport *s*ystem) was identified in a genome search for proteins similar to ABC-type iron transporters (see below). The genes of the Isd system were first identified in an attempt to find sortase A (*srtA*) homologs in the *S. aureus* genome. This led to identification of the gene (*srtB*) encoding sortase B, which is part of a six gene operon designated *isdCDEF-srtBisdG*. One of these genes (*isdC*) encodes a protein with a unique NPQTN anchoring motif that is the only recognized substrate of sortase B, It has been demonstrated in a murine renal abscess model that mutation of *srtB* had little effect on virulence during the early stages of infection but did significantly attenuate virulence as the infection progressed, and based on this it was suggested that IsdC makes an important contribution to maintaining infection in the face of ongoing changes in the host. Two additional genes (*isdA* and *isdB*) are located upstream of the *isdCDEFsrtBisdG* operon and are divergently transcribed as monocistronic messages. Each of these genes, as well as the *isdCDEFsrtBisdG* operon itself, was subsequently shown to contain a Fur box and to be tightly regulated by the availability of iron. IsdA binds hemoglobin, transferrin, and the extracellular matrix proteins fibronectin and fibrinogen. This suggests that IsdA may function both in iron acquisition and as an adhesin. However, Torres *et al.* (2007) found that mutation of *isdA* has little impact on the ability to acquire iron from heme-containing proteins by comparison to IsdB.Kuklin *et al.* (2006) also demonstrated that immunization with IsdB protects against staphylococcal sepsis in both a murine model and in rhesus macaques. IsdB and IsdH are immunologically similar in that antibodies raised against IsdB are cross-reactive with IsdH, and immunization with purified IsdH also resulted in reduced nasal colonization in the cotton rat model. Other Isd proteins are responsible for transporting heme iron across the cytoplasmic membrane or for removing iron from heme once inside the cell.

Reniere *et al.* (2007) proposed three possible fates of heme iron once it is inside staphylococcal cells. First, intracellular heme is degraded by the monooxygenases IsdG and IsdI, thus releasing free iron which would likely be bound by staphylococcal ferritin (FtnA), a protein that stores iron in a nontoxic form for use when iron becomes restricted. Second, intact heme can be complexed with a membrane-associated heme-binding factor and used as a cofactor for specific *S. aureus* enzymes involved in energy production and/or protection against reactive oxygen species, one specific example of the latter being catalase. Third, given the toxicity of heme at high concentration, excess intracellular heme can be transported out of the cell via the ABC-type efflux pump HrtAB (*h*eme-*r*egulated *t*ransporter). Mutants defective in this transport system have a reduced capacity to grow in media with heme as the sole iron source but somewhat paradoxically exhibit increased virulence in a murine model of infection. This effect has been correlated with a reduction in the number of phagocytes recruited to the site of infection. Additionally, *hrtA* mutants produce elevated amounts of extracellular immunomodulatory proteins that inhibit phagocyte recruitment/activation and opsonophagocytosis. Based on this, it has been hypothesized that, once *S. aureus* encounters a heme-rich environment, the likelihood of which is increased by high levels of hemolytic activity; it avoids heme toxicity by activating the HrtAB system to promote efflux of heme iron while simultaneously reducing the production of specific virulence factors that would otherwise promote host tissue damage and further release of heme. Other components of this system include *hssRS*, which encode the response regulator (HssR) and sensor components (HssS) of bacterial two-component signal transduction system that modulates expression of *hrtAB*. This appears to be a highly specific regulatory system in that expression *hrtAB* is not affected by other environmental cues including the global regulators *agr* and *sarA*.

S. aureus also has at its disposal siderophore-based iron acquisition systems. Four siderophores have been identified to date including staphyloferrin A, staphyloferrin B, aureochelin, and staphylobactin. The enzymes required for production of staphylobactin are encoded within the nine-gene *sbnABCDEFGHI* operon, and mutation of one of these genes (*sbnE*) was shown to result in reduced growth in iron-limited media and reduced virulence in a murine kidney abscess model. Once siderophores bind extracellular iron, they are moved back into the cell by a number of iron-regulated ABC transporter systems that include iron-binding lipoproteins, an ATPase, and integral membrane proteins. Park *et al.* (2005) concluded that siderophore-mediated uptake plays a "dominant and essential role" in acquiring iron from transferrin, although as noted above certain of the Isd proteins also promote iron uptake from transferrin. Modun *et al.* (1999) has also identified a 42 kDa, cell wall-associated protein (Tpn) that binds human transferrin and is produced by both *S. aureus* and *S. epidermidis*. Further characterization confirmed that this protein is actually the glycolytic enzyme glyceraldehyde-3-phosphate dehydrogenase (GAPDH) and that it can bind transferrin without compromising its enzymatic activity. This is similar to the GAPDH of group A streptococci (subsequently renamed the streptococcal surface dehydrogenase), which is also capable of binding the extracellular matrix protein fibronectin while maintaining its enzymatic activity. Taylor and Heinrichs generated a GAPDH (*gap*) mutant in *S. aureus* and demonstrated that cell wall fractions from the mutant were indeed devoid of GAPDH enzymatic activity. However, the same cell wall fractions retained the capacity to bind transferrin. This led to identification of an additional transferrin-binding protein (SbtA) that is produced only when *S. aureus* is grown under iron-limited conditions. Mutation of the corresponding gene (*stbA*, *s*taphylococcal *t*ransferrin-*b*inding protein *A*) suggested that SbtA rather than Tpn (GAPDH) is responsible for transferrin binding in *S. aureus*.

Because *S. aureus* can acquire iron from different host proteins, Skaar *et al.* (2004) carried out directed studies to determine whether one iron source was preferred over another. Results from this analysis indicated that heme was the preferred source, although the ratio of heme to transferrin uptake decreased with samples taken later in growth. This led to the suggestion that *S. aureus* preferentially utilizes heme uptake via the HtsABC transport system during the early stages of infection and at sites rich in heme proteins but then shifts to siderophore-mediated iron uptake once the availability of heme proteins becomes limited. As with other aspects of this review, there are a number of other components to these iron acquisition systems, and it remains unknown whether the relative impact of these components differs among staphylococcal species in a manner that impacts their ability to cause infections in different mammalian hosts. Having said this, given the universal need for iron, the likely role of hemolysins in promoting heme-mediated iron uptake, and differences in hemolytic activity among staphylococcal species, it seems likely that important differences exist that remain to be explored.

Resistance and Antibiotic Treatment

As gram-positive cocci, the primary types of antimicrobial agents used to combat staphylococcal infection are inhibitors of cell wall biosynthesis. Primary examples include the β-lactams, most notably methicillin derivatives and early generation cephalosporins, and vancomycin. However, many classes of antibiotic have activity against staphylococci, the problem being that it is extremely difficult to predict which of these may be useful in the treatment of an infection caused by any given isolate. This reflects the widespread occurrence of antibiotic resistance among the staphylococci, and it emphasizes the need for rapid diagnostic methods that can be used not only to identify the offending pathogen but also to obtain information that can be used as a guide for determinative antimicrobial therapy. The polymerase chain reaction has been widely used to tremendous advantage in this regard, although once again this has been exploited primarily in the context of *S. aureus* and primarily in the specific context of methicillin resistance.

Absent issues of acquired resistance, penicillin remains the antibiotic of choice, but it has largely been rendered ineffective in all its forms owing to the widespread production of β-lactamases among all staphylococcal species. The semisynthetic penicillins represented by methicillin are the preferred alternative, but their use has also been increasingly compromised by the persistent emergence of resistance. This is true in all staphylococcal species including *S. aureus* and the SIG species, with the incidence of methicillin-resistant strains increasingly steadily in recent years is isolates causing both human and animal infections. Methicillin resistance is impacted by multiple factors, but the primary determinant is the *mecA* gene, which encodes an alternative penicillin-binding protein designated PBP2A or PBP2. The *mecA* gene is associated with some variant of a larger chromosomal insertion designated the SCC*mec* element. The SCC*mec* element occurs in various forms, and at least in humans these can be generally divided into larger elements typically associated with isolates causing healthcare-associated infections and somewhat smaller elements found in isolates causing community-associated infection. Not surprisingly given the economy of prokaryotic genomes, these size differences reflect the presence of absence of other genes, and in many cases, these include other antibiotic resistance genes. Thus, isolates carrying the larger SCC*mec* elements are more likely to be resistant to other classes of antibiotic, thus further limiting alternative therapeutic options.

At present, vancomycin is still considered the "last resort" antibiotic for the treatment of infections caused by methicillin-resistant staphylococci, but even this is being threatened by the appearance of both vancomycin-resistant *S. aureus* (VRSA) and vancomycin-intermediate *S. aureus* (VISA). Fortunately, VRSA remains remarkably rare among human isolates, and it has not been reported in any animal isolates we are aware of. VISA is much more common, particularly in patients undergoing long-term therapy, but at present, this too appears to be a significant problem primarily in humans. Nevertheless, the increasing prevalence of methicillin resistance among all staphylococcal species, including SIG, makes it imperative that veterinarians recognize the existence of VISA and the need to consider other alternatives when possible. There are also a number of newer alternatives including daptomycin, telavancin, linezolid, tigecycline, and the newest generation of cephalosporins (e.g., ceftobiprole), all of which are active even against methicillin-resistant strains.

Summary

Despite decades of intensive research, the staphylococci remain among the most important of all bacterial pathogens in both man and animals. Given the remarkable number of staphylococcal species, the diversity of virulence factors produced by these different species, and the fact that essentially all species are capable of causing disease in multiple mammalian hosts, it is impossible to be comprehensive in any discussion of their importance. It is also very important to recognize that spread between host species, and genetic exchange between staphylococcal species, creates a very dynamic environment that impacts all aspects of staphylococcal pathogenesis not only now but also predictably into the foreseeable future. This makes it imperative to remain diligent, and part of that diligence is recognizing that issues impacting humans will inevitably impact infections in animals and vice versa. Indeed, this is arguably the most important issue of all in that it emphasizes the fact that the control of staphylococcal infections will take an integrated and concerted effort among all practicing clinicians irrespective of whether they focus on human health, the world's food supply, or the remarkable role of companion animals in improving both our lives and theirs. This chapter was written in the hope of both making that point and providing information that can be used to further this indispensable objective.

References

Lina G, Boutite F, Tristan A *et al.* (2003) Bacterial competition for human nasal cavity colonization: role of Staphylococcal *agr* alleles. *Appl Environ Microbiol*, **69**, 18–23.

Modun B and Williams P (1999) The staphylococcal transferrin-binding protein is a cell wall glyceraldehyde-3-phosphate dehydrogenase. *Infect Immun*, **67**, 1086–1092.

Further Reading

Atalla H, Gyles C, and Mallard B (2011) *Staphylococcus aureus* small colony variants (SCVs) and their role in disease. *Anim Health Res Rev*, **12**, 33–45.

Atalla H, Wilkie B, Gyles C *et al.* (2010) Antibody and cell-mediated immune responses to *Staphylococcus aureus* small colony variants and their parental strains associated with bovine mastitis. *Dev Comp Immunol*, **34**, 1283–1290.

Beenken KE, Mrak LN, Griffin LM *et al.* (2010) Epistatic relationships between *sarA* and *agr* in *Staphylococcus aureus* biofilm formation. *PLoS One*, **5**, e10790.

Boerlin P, Kuhnert P, Hüssy D, and Schaellibaum M (2003) Methods for identification of *Staphylococcus aureus* isolates in cases of bovine mastitis. *J Clin Microbiol*, **41**, 767–771.

Casanova C, Iselin L, von Steiger N *et al.* (2011) *Staphylococcus hyicus* bacteremia in a farmer. *J Clin Microbiol*, **49**, 4377–4378.

Deurenberg RH, Vink C, Kalenic S *et al.* (2007) The molecular evolution of methicillin-resistant *Staphylococcus aureus*. *Clin Microbiol Infect*, **13**, 222–235.

Devriese LA, Vancanneyt M, Baele M *et al.* (2005) *Staphylococcus pseudintermedius* sp. Nov., a coagulase-positive species from animals. *Int J Syst Evol Microbiol*, **55**, 1569–1573.

Futagawa-Saito K, Sugiyama T, Karube S *et al.* (2004) Prevalence and characterization of leukotoxin-producing *Staphylococcus intermedius* in isolates from dogs and pigeons. *J Clin Micorbiol*, **42**, 5324–5326.

Kelesidis T and Tsiodras S (2010) *Staphylococcus intermedius* is not only a zoonotic pathogen, but may also cause skin abscesses in humans after exposure to saliva. *Int J Infect Dis*, **14**, e838–e841.

Kuklin NA, Clark DJ, Secore S *et al.* (2006) A novel Staphylococcus aureus vaccine: iron surface determinant B induces rapid antibody responses in rhesus macaques and specific increased survival in a murine S. aureus sepsis model. *Infect Immun*, **74**, 2215–2223.

Park RY, Sun HY, Choi MH, Bai YH, and Shin SH (2005) Staphylococcus aureus siderophore-mediated iron-acquisition system plays a dominant and essential role in the utilization of transferrin-bound iron. *J Microbiol*, **43**, 183–190.

Nickerson SC (2009) Control of heifer mastitis: antimicrobial treatment-an overview. *Vet Microbiol*, **134**, 128–135.

Reniere ML, Torres VJ, Skaar EP (2007) Intracellular metalloporphyrin metabolism in Staphylococcus aureus. *Biometals*, **20**, 333–345.

Skaar EP, Humayun M, Bae T, DeBord KL, and Schneewind O (2004) Iron-source preference of Staphylococcus aureus infections. *Science*, **305**, 1626–1628.

Smeltzer MS, Lee CY, Harik N, and Hart ME (2009) Molecular basis of pathology, in *Staphylococci in Human Disease*, 2nd edn (eds KB Crossley, KK Jefferson, GL Archer, and VG Fowler), West Sussex, UK, pp. 65–108.

Smetlzer MS, Gillaspy AF, Pratt FL *et al.* (1997) Prevalence and chromosomal map location of *Staphylococcus aureus* adhesion genes. *Gene*, **196**, 249–259.

Stranger-Jones YK, Bae T, and Schneewind O (2006) Vaccine assembly from surface proteins of *Staphylococcus aureus*. *Proc Natl Acad Sci USA*, **103**, 16942–16947.

Torres VJ, Stauff DL, Pishchany G *et al.* (2007) A Staphylococcus aureus regulatory system that responds to host heme and modulates virulence. *Cell Host Microbe*, **1**, 109–119.

Vuong C, Kocianova S, Yao Y *et al.* (2004) Increased colonization of indwelling medical devices by quorum-sensing mutants of *Staphylococcus epidermidis in vivo*. *J Infect Dis*, **190**, 133–139.

Werckenthin C, Cardoso M, Martel JL, and Schwarz S (2001) Antimicrobial resistance in staphylococci from animals with particular reference to bovine *Staphylococcus aureus*, porcine *Staphylococcus hyicus*, and canine *Staphylococcus intermedius*. *Vet Res*, **32**, 341–362.

Yarwood JM, Bartels DJ, Volper EM, and Greenberg EP (2004) Quorum sensing in Staphylococcus aureus biofilms. *J Bacteriol*, **186**, 1838–1850.

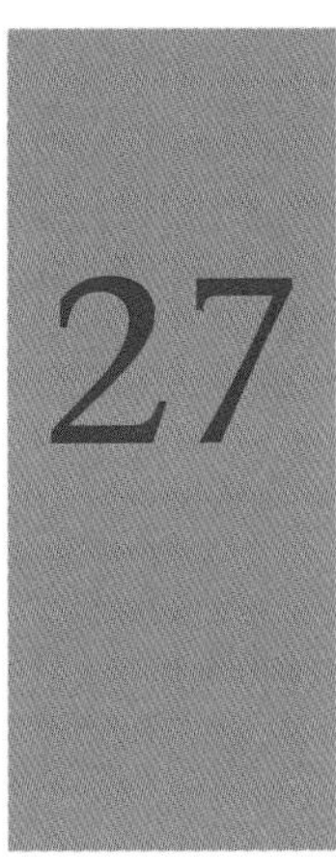

Streptococcus and *Enterococcus*

George C. Stewart

Streptococcus

Streptococci are gram-positive and catalase-negative cocci occurring in pairs and chains; they show considerable ecologic, physiologic, serologic, and genetic diversity. Currently there are 98 recognized species within the genus, but only a few are significant pathogens. These are listed in Table 27.1

On blood agar, the species exhibit various degrees of hemolysis, which can be used as an early step in identifying clinical isolates. Hemolysis produced by colonies on blood agar and Lancefield serological grouping are important factors in presumptive identification.

α-Hemolytic streptococci do not lyse erythrocytes but produce a zone of green discoloration around the colonies (hydrogen peroxide oxidation of the hemoglobin to methemoglobin). Most commensal streptococci of animals are α-hemolytic. Streptococci that do this are sometimes referred to as "viridans streptococci."

β-Hemolytic streptococci lyse erythrocytes and produce a complete zone of hemolysis around the colonies. Pathogenic streptococci tend to be β-hemolytic.

γ-Streptococci are nonhemolytic. Most are nonpathogenic.

Older classification schemes grouped the streptococcal species based on biological properties. These included the following:

Pyogenic group: The streptococci causing pyogenic infections in humans and animals; usually β-hemolytic.

Oral group: Primarily commensals on skin and mucous membranes; α- or nonhemolytic.

Lactic group: Associated with milk and dairy products. Now placed in the genus *Lactococcus*.

Enterococci group: Normal flora intestinal streptococci, opportunistically pathogenic. Most now belong to the genus *Enterococcus*.

Anaerobic group: Include anaerobic species of *Streptococcus* not related to the anaerobic general *Peptococcus* and *Peptostreptococcus*. Most of these species have been moved to other genera.

Lancefield Grouping Scheme

Streptococci are divided into 20 groups (designated A through V, but with no I or J) using a precipitin test based on extractable group-specific carbohydrate antigens. The Lancefield groups are further subdivided into types based on protein antigens. The type-specific antigens are the M, R, and T proteins. Whereas antibodies to the Lancefield group antigens are not protective, the M, R, and T proteins are protective, albeit type-specific, antigens. *Streptococcus pyogenes* has over 100 serotypes, based on M and other proteins, while *Streptococcus pneumoniae* has over 90 capsular polysaccharide types.

Descriptive Features

Morphology and Staining. Streptococci vary from spherical to ovoid cells, about 1 μm in diameter. Division occurs in one plane, producing pairs and chains, which is evident in liquid media or clinical samples. Some species, such as *S. pneumoniae*, are predominantly in pairs.

Young cultures stain gram-positive. In exudates and older cultures (>18 h), organisms often stain gram-negative, likely from effects of autolysins weakening the cell wall.

Structure and Composition. Streptococci have a typical gram-positive cell wall structure. Capsules are produced by some species. Cell wall-deficient forms (L forms) also occur.

Growth Characteristics. Streptococci have fairly exacting growth needs best satisfied by media containing blood or serum. After overnight incubation at 37 °C, streptococci produce clear colonies, usually <1 mm in diameter. Encapsulated forms, such as *Streptococcus equi* ssp. *equi*, produce larger mucoid colonies. Pathogenic species grow best at 37 °C in the presence of elevated CO_2 levels, such as with a candle jar or CO_2 incubator.

Veterinary Microbiology, Third Edition. Edited by D. Scott McVey, Melissa Kennedy and M.M. Chengappa.

Table 27.1. Clinically Important *Streptococcus* Species

Lancefield Group	Species Name	Type of Hemolysis	Most Important Hosts	Diseases
A	*S. pyogenes*	β	Humans	Respiratory infections, rheumatic fever, glomerulonephritis
B	*S. agalactiae*	α, β, γ	Humans, cattle	Neonatal sepsis, mastitis
None	*S. pneumonia*	α	Humans, horses, NH primates, laboratory animals	Pneumonia
C	*S. equi* ssp. *equi*	β	horses	Strangles
C	*S. equi* ssp. *zooepidemicus*	β	horses, swine, cattle, and humans	Pyogenic infections
C	*S. dysgalactiae* ssp. *equisimilis*	β	horses, swine, cattle, and humans	Pyogenic infections
C	*S. dysgalactiae* ssp. *dysgalactiae*	α, β, γ	horses, swine, cattle, and humans	Pyogenic infections, mastitis
E	*Streptococcus porcinus*	β	Swine	Cervical lymphadenitis
G	*S. canis*	β	Dogs	Metritis, mastitis, neonatal infections
L	Group L *Streptococcus*	β	Dogs	Urogenital infections
D, R, S, T	*S. suis*	α	Swine	Meningitis, pneumonia, septicemia
?	*S. uberis*	α, γ	Cattle	Mastitis
?	*S. parauberis*	α, γ	Cattle	Mastitis

?, unknown Lancefield group; NH, nonhuman.

Biochemical Activities. Streptococci are catalase-negative and obligately fermentative (can grow in the presence of oxygen but do not respire, deriving energy solely from fermentation).

Cellular Products and Activities of Medical Interest. The relation of specific streptococcal products to pathogenesis is largely speculative, with the following exceptions. The capsule of *S. pneumoniae* is a proven virulence factor. M protein is an important virulence determinant, and antibody to it is protective.

Adhesins. Streptococci produce a number of surface proteins that bind to a variety of extracellular matrix proteins of the host (fibronectin, fibrinogen, collagen, vitronectin, laminin, decorin, and heparin sulfate-containing proteoglycans). These adhesins have been termed MSCRAMMs (microbial surface components recognizing adhesive matrix molecules). Some MSCRAMMs, specifically the fibrinogen-binding M protein, impart an antiphagocytic property to the streptococcal cell. Coating of streptococcal cells with host proteins is thought to result in the masking of sites for complement activation (and thus decrease opsonization) as well as those recognized by serum proteins (collectins/ficollins) that opsonize foreign particles. The SeM protein of *S. equi* ssp. *equi* is a fibrinogen- and immunoglobulin-binding cell surface protein that is a major virulence factor of this bacterium.

M protein is an important virulence factor of *S. pyogenes* and *S. equi* ssp. *equi*. It binds fibrinogen, confers antiphagocytic properties, enhances adherence to epithelia cells of the nasal mucosa, and may be associated with the postinfection immune disease in the horse (purpura hemorrhagica). The FbsA protein is the fibrinogen-binding protein of *Streptococcus agalactiae*. The FOG protein is the analogous protein in the group G *Streptococcus dysgalactiae* ssp. *equisimilis*, and the Szp protein is the M protein equivalent of *S. equi* ssp. *zooepidemicus*.

The hyaluronic acid capsule of *S. pyogenes* is an adhesin (as well as imparting antiphagocytic effects, see Section "Capsule"), with affinity for human epithelial cells via CD44, a hyaluronic acid-binding glycoprotein. Whether the hyaluronic acid capsules of streptococci of veterinary importance also act as adhesins is unclear.

The BibA protein of *S. agalactiae* specifically binds to human C4-binding protein, a regulator of the classic complement pathway, and its deletion severely reduces the capacity of group B streptococci to resist opsonophagocytic killing by neutrophils.

Other adhesins are responsible for binding of streptococci to host cells. F protein and other proteins, such as Fnb and SFS, bind fibronectin and have been associated with bacterial adherence and internalization. PsaA (for pneumococcal surface adhesin) is a lipoprotein found on *S. pneumoniae*, *S. equi* ssp. *equi*, and *S. equi* ssp. *zooepidemicus* and is responsible for adherence to cells lining the upper and lower airways. E-cadherin, the cell junction protein in respiratory epithelial cells, has been shown to be a receptor for PsaA.

Capsule. Some species of streptococci produce a capsule. Group A and C streptococcal capsules are composed of hyaluronic acid. Hyaluronic acid, also a constituent of mammalian connective tissue, is poorly antigenic and does not readily bind complement components (and is, therefore, antiphagocytic). The capsules described for group B, E, and G organisms are polysaccharide in nature, but not hyaluronic acid.

Cell Wall. The gram-positive cell wall contains proteins and polysaccharides that are of medical interest. The lipoteichoic acids and peptidoglycan of the gram-positive cell wall interact with macrophage cells, resulting in the release of proinflammatory cytokines.

Streptococcal Pyrogenic Toxin Superantigens. Superantigens simultaneously bind to major histocompatibility complex class II molecules and T cell receptor molecules bearing a particular V-β region. This binding results in the activation of a large proportion of antigen-presenting cells and T cells, with subsequent release of high systemic levels of cytokines. Part of the systemic symptoms seen with streptococcal infections may be related to the cytokine storm that results from the large-scale T cell stimulation effected by these toxins. The streptococcal pyrogenic toxin superantigens (SPEs) produced by *S. pyogenes* (the group A streptococci) are the best studied. *S. pyogenes* produces several SPEs: SPEA, SPEC, SPEG, SPEH, SPEI, SPEJ, SPEK, SPEL, SPEM, SSA, and SMEZ (streptococcal mitogenic exotoxin Z). All known SPEs (with the exception of SMEZ, SPEG, and SPEJ) are localized on mobile DNA elements. As a consequence, each *S. pyogenes* isolate usually carries the genes for SMEZ, SPEG, and SPEJ, plus a variable combination of other SPE genes. *S. equi* ssp. *equi* has been shown to produce SPEs including SeeI, SeeL, and SeeM. These have been shown to stimulate proliferation of equine peripheral blood mononucleated cells. These SPEs are prophage encoded. Three SPEs have been identified in *S. equi* ssp. *zooepidemicus*. These are SzeF, SzeN, and SzeP and have been shown to stimulate the proliferation of equine peripheral blood mononuclear cells, and tumor necrosis factor α (TNF-α) and γ interferon (IFN-γ) production.

Miscellaneous Toxins and Enzymes. The streptococci produce a number of proteins that potentially act as virulence factors:

Streptolysins O and S: Oxygen-labile (O) and stable (S) hemolysins are additionally cytolysins that cause lysis of neutrophils, macrophages, and platelets. Streptolysin S is responsible for the large zone of β-hemolysis observed on sheep blood agar plates. The cytolytic spectrum of streptolysin S is broad, including the membranes of erythrocytes, leukocytes, platelets, tissue culture cells, and subcellular organelles such as lysosomes and mitochondria. The oxygen-labile and thiol-activated hemolysins, streptolysin O and the *S. suis* suilysin O, bind cholesterol in membranes. The toxin oligomerizes at or in the target membrane to form a hydrophobic protein complex integrated in the membrane with a hydrophilic channel forming center. The resulting pores are relatively large (up to 30 nm).

Streptokinase: It is encoded on a prophage and acts to activate plasminogen to plasmin. Plasmin is a protease that acts on host proteins, including fibrin, and thus degrades clots.

The streptococcal C5a peptidase ScpB of *S. agalactiae* is a multifunctional protein found in all group B *Streptococcus* clinical isolates and is required for mucosal colonization. ScpB is reported to inhibit neutrophil chemotaxis by enzymatically cleaving the complement component C5a.

Enzymes with potential roles in virulence produced by streptococci include hyaluronidase, DNases (e.g., SPEF), NADases, and proteases.

Regulation of the Cellular Products of Medical Interest. Expression of virulence-related genes in *S. pyogenes* is regulated by at least three global systems (whether these systems occur in other streptococci is unknown). The first is a "growth phase-related signal" that is undefined, but certain genes (including those encoding streptolysin S and DNases) are upregulated during stationary phase, while others (including those encoding capsule, streptokinase, streptolysin O, and a protein called multigene regulator in group A streptococci or Mga) are upregulated during late exponential phase of growth.

Regulation occurs by both activation and repression of gene expression by transcriptional regulator proteins and by two-component regulatory systems. Major regulator proteins include Mga, responsible for the activation of expression during exponential growth of genes involved in adhesion, internalization, and immune evasion, the RofA-like proteins including RofA and Nra, which regulate genes involved in persistence, FasA, which is involved in growth phase regulation of virulence gene expression, and Rgg (RopB), which activates expression of extracellular proteins such as the SpeB cysteine protease. Mga itself is regulated by growth phase as well as other undefined environmental cues.

The CovRS (control of virulence) two-component regulatory system regulates directly or indirectly 15% of the genome. Expression of several important virulence genes is directly regulated by the CovR response regulator protein, including those encoding the hyaluronic acid capsule operon, streptolysin S, streptokinase, *speB*, and *sda* (encoding the streptodornase DNase).

Resistance. β-Hemolytic streptococci can survive in dried pus for weeks. They are killed at 55–60 °C in 30 min, and inhibited by 6.5% sodium chloride and 40% bile (except *S. agalactiae*), 0.1% methylene blue, and low (10 °C) and high (45 °C) temperatures. Members of the genus *Enterococcus* tolerate these conditions. Viridans streptococci vary with respect to heat and bile resistance. Only *S. pneumoniae* is bile soluble. Streptococci tolerate 0.02% sodium azide, which is used in streptococcal isolation media.

Pathogenic streptococci are usually susceptible to penicillins, cephalosporins, macrolides, chloramphenicol, and trimethoprim–sulfonamides; they are often resistant to aminoglycosides, fluoroquinolones, and tetracycline.

Ecology

Reservoir. Most streptococci of veterinary interest live commensally in the upper respiratory, alimentary, and lower genital tracts.

Transmission. Streptococci are transmitted by inhalation and ingestion, sexually, congenitally, or indirectly via hands and fomites.

Pathogenesis

Streptococci cause pyogenic infections primarily of the skin, respiratory tract, reproductive tract, umbilical stump, and mammary gland. Septicemia may result from hematogenous spread of the primary infection. Clinically, the streptococcal diseases are usually characterized at some stage by febrile symptoms, alone or associated with symptoms of septicemia. The local areas exhibit pus formation that can be observed draining from the lesion. Abscesses form where this drainage is prevented. Toxemia and immune-mediated lesions are common sequela of the disease.

Pathology. The basic pathologic process resembles that of staphylococcal infection; that is, the typical lesion is an abscess, an inflammatory focus in which participating cells have been destroyed by the combined effects of bacterial and inflammatory cell activity. This confrontation between leukocytes and microorganisms produces pus, a mixture of host cell debris and bacteria, living and dead. In an abscess, pus is surrounded by intact leukocytes and fibrin strands. Unless the pus is drained, a fibrous capsule will gradually be formed.

Disease Patterns.

Equine. Strangles is a highly contagious rhinopharyngitis caused by *S. equi* ssp. *equi* (*See*). After deposition on the mucous membranes of the upper respiratory tract, *See* adheres to epithelial cells by way of MSCRAMMs (M protein, fibronectin-binding protein, fibrinogen-binding protein, Psa) and hyaluronic acid capsule. Adherence triggers internalization and subsequent localization in the subepithelial spaces. Cell wall constituents as well as pyrogenic exotoxins (SPEH and SPEI) initiate an acute inflammatory response. Capsule, M protein, and Scp protect *S. equi* from opsonization and phagocytosis. Streptolysins may act to destroy host cells by damaging their membranes. Systemic clinical signs may be due to the superantigen effects of pyrogenic exotoxins (SPEH and SPEI). Other enzymes and toxins may contribute to the process by digesting DNA (DNases), fibrin (streptokinase), and hyaluronic acid (hyaluronidase). The disease is marked by a serous or purulent nasal discharge, diphasic temperature rise, local pain, cough, and anorexia. In regional lymph nodes, abscesses develop, which typically rupture and drain within 2 weeks. Recovery follows. The overall mortality rate is under 2%. Complications include bastard (malignant) strangles, which results from metastasis of *See* to bronchial, mediastinal, or mesenteric lymph nodes where they can drain internally. Pyemic dissemination to meninges, lungs, pericardium, and abdominal viscera, or extension to the guttural pouches can occur. Purpura hemorrhagica—a type III hypersensitivity manifested by subcutaneous swellings, mucosal hemorrhages, and fever—may follow the acute disease by about 3 weeks and is associated with significant (50%) mortality.

Bacterial pneumonia/pyothorax in horses is almost always associated with a β-hemolytic *Streptococcus* with *S. equi* ssp. *zooepidemicus* (*Sez*) being the most commonly isolated. In addition, a gram-negative microorganism (*Actinobacillus* is the most common) is frequently found along with *Sez*. The infectious process is endogenous. The microorganisms involved are part of the normal flora of the upper respiratory tract, which then contaminate a compromised lung (e.g., following viral pneumonia). *Sez* and the others are deposited in the lung and initiate or amplify a preexisting inflammatory process (cell wall constituents, pyrogenic exotoxins). The intensity of the inflammatory response is not as extreme as with the response initiated by *See*, nor are the constitutional signs as severe. However, the mechanisms involved in the pathogenesis are likely similar. Pyothorax is probably an extension of the pneumonic process just described. Like pneumonia, *Sez* is the most common isolate, combined with a gram-negative species. Unlike pneumonia, an obligate anaerobe (*Bacteroides* and *Fusobacterium* are the most common) is frequently found as well.

Genital tract diseases in horses are associated with *Sez*, which is frequently associated with cervicitis and metritis. Infections in newborn foals, which are often umbilical infections (navel ill, pyosepticemia, joint ill, and polyarthritis), disseminate via the bloodstream to joints and the renal cortex. The microorganisms originate from the genital tract of the dam (part of her normal flora).

β-Hemolytic streptococci (*Sez* is the most common) are associated with a variety of miscellaneous conditions in horses including osteomyelitis, arthritis, abscesses, and wounds. All are endogenous, with the infecting strain arising from the normal flora.

Swine. Cervical lymphadenitis of swine (jowl abscess) is a contagious disease affecting swine. This condition is associated with *Streptococcus porcinus* (previously known as "group E *Streptococcus*"). The disease is analogous to strangles but clinically less dramatic and frequently not diagnosed until slaughter. Its most damaging aspect is carcass condemnation.

Secondary pneumonias in swine are sometimes associated with *S. dysgalactiae* ssp. *equisimilis*.

Streptococcus suis, *S. dysgalactiae* ssp. *equisimilis*, and streptococci belonging to groups L and U cause neonatal septicemia, suppurative bronchopneumonia, arthritis, meningitis, polyserositis, endocarditis, reproductive problems, and abscesses. A "fading pig syndrome" has been reported in infected groups of pigs. Pigs usually have clinical signs and gross lesions referable to either the respiratory system or CNS, but not both. Transmission is from carrier pigs (upper respiratory tract and tonsils) with entry probably through the palatine tonsils. Disease is usually seen at 3–12 weeks of age, but all ages can be affected. Suilysin produced by *S. suis* may account for some of the tissue damage associated with this disease.

S. suis capsular type 2 has zoonotic potential. It causes serious infections in humans that may result in severe disability (deafness and ataxia). Association with swine is a predisposing factor.

Ruminants. The leading agent of streptococcal mastitis is *S. agalactiae*. Less frequent causes are *S. dysgalactiae* ssp. *dysgalactiae* and *S. uberis*. They produce a chronic subacute mastitis with periodic acute exacerbations.

S. agalactiae (group B streptococci) is a leading cause of sepsis and meningitis in human neonates and pregnant women. However, the strains that cause disease in cattle do not cause disease in humans.

Dogs and Cats. Secondary pneumonias affecting dogs are sometimes associated with *Streptococcus canis*. *S. canis* is associated with septicemia in newborn puppies and a toxic shock-like syndrome (streptococcal toxic shock syndrome, STSS) and necrotizing fasciitis (NF) in dogs. STSS is characterized by septic shock with multiple organ failure. NF may also be present. NF is a rapidly developing cellulitis of the soft tissues and fascia, usually in one limb, and characterized by necrosis of soft tissue. It is often followed by STSS.

Cats tend to be more resistant to streptococcal infections, and when they do occur, they are most common in young kittens or immunocompromised cats. The infections seen are the same as those seen in dogs.

Primates. *S. pneumoniae* is a leading cause of pneumonia, septicemia, and meningitis in primates. Pneumococcal pneumonia in monkeys runs an acute course with high mortality rates. The lesions are those of a fibrinous pleuropneumonia. Recent shipment and viral infection are common antecedents.

Miscellaneous Species. Cervical lymphadenitis in guinea pigs is caused by *Streptococcus zooepidemicus* ssp. *zooepidemicus*.

Septicemic disease in fish from freshwater aquaculture farms and saltwater environments has been associated with *Streptococcus iniae*, a β-hemolytic *Streptococcus* without a Lansfield designation. Handling (cleaning/necropsy)-affected fish is a risk factor for developing cellulitis, endocarditis, or arthritis presumably following self-inoculation.

Septicemic disease in seals is associated with *Streptococcus phocae*, a β-hemolytic *Streptococcus* that reacts to Lansfield group antisera C and F.

Septicemic disease and dermatitis in opossums are associated with *Streptococcus didelphis*, a β-hemolytic *Streptococcus* without affiliation with known Lansfield groups.

Epidemiology. Healthy individuals may carry all the streptococci discussed, and many infections are probably endogenous and stress-related. Neonatal infections are commonly maternal in origin.

Strangles and porcine lymphadenitis are contagious diseases preferably affecting young animals (past infancy). *S. equi* and *S. porcinus* are spread by contaminated food, drinking water, or utensils and by recovered animals, which may remain clinically healthy shedders for months. Milking equipment, unskilled attempts at intramammary medication, and unsanitary milking practices often spread *S. agalactiae* among dairy cows.

Immunologic Aspects

Immune Mechanisms of Disease. Human poststreptococcal diseases (rheumatic fever and acute glomerulonephritis) are attributed to immunopathogenic mechanisms. Similarly, equine purpura hemorrhagica following strangles is probably immune complex mediated.

Recovery and Resistance. The main defenses against streptococcal infections are phagocytic, and the antiphagocytic M protein elicits protective antibodies. Animals recovered from strangles and cervical lymphadenitis are at least temporarily immune to reinfection.

Polysaccharide capsules of *S. agalactiae* and *S. pneumoniae* evoke the formation of opsonizing antibody. In streptococcal pneumonia, their appearance determines recovery from infection. In bovine mastitis, no useful immunity develops; cows, unless treated, remain infected. Experimental evidence suggests that anticapsular IgG_2-type antibody is protective.

All immunity is serotype specific.

Artificial Immunization. A whole-cell bacterin and an M protein vaccine are available for vaccination against strangles. Neither is uniformly effective, and often elicits local reactions at the injection site. An intranasal avirulent live vaccine that stimulates essential local antibody responses is available. Feeding live avirulent cultures has produced immunity to porcine jowl abscesses.

Laboratory Diagnosis

Sample Collection. Aspirates from unopened lesions, in sterile syringes or sterile containers, are preferred. Swabs in transport media are acceptable. Milk is collected into containers under sterile precautions.

Direct Examination. Smears of exudates or sediments of suspect fluids are fixed and Gram stained. Streptococci appear as gram-positive cocci in pairs, short chains, and in some instances very long chains (typically seen in pus aspirated from cervical lymph nodes of horses infected with *S. equi*). Streptococci have a tendency to lose their gram-positivity and sometimes stain weakly gram-positive or gram-negative.

Culture. Exudates, milk, tissue, urine, transtracheal aspirates, and cerebrospinal fluid are cultured directly on cow or sheep blood agar. Incubation at 37 °C in 3–5% CO_2 is preferable. Streptococcal colonies, smooth or mucoid, will appear in 18–48 h.

Identification relies on a combination of classical techniques (e.g., determination of Lansfield grouping and biochemical tests), and molecular techniques (e.g., determination of the sequence of DNA encoding the 16S ribosomal DNA, or via PCR using species-specific primers). Commercial kits are available for both purposes. Other useful diagnostic tests include the following:

1. *The CAMP phenomenon (named after Christie, Atkins, and Munch–Petersen)*: It reflects hemolytic synergism between staphylococcal β-toxin (a sphingomyelinase) and an *S. agalactiae* toxin (CAMP protein sometimes referred to as cocytolysin). A β-toxin-producing staphylococcus is inoculated across a sheep or bovine blood agar plate. At right angles to

this line, and approximately 0.5 cm from it, a suspect *S. agalactiae* is inoculated. After incubation, hemolysis by CAMP-positive bacteria will be enhanced in the β-toxin zone (Figure 27.1). The combined action of these two toxins on sheep or bovine blood agar produces larger and clearer zones of hemolysis than either agent alone.

2. *Bacitracin sensitivity*: Bacitracin disks (0.04 units) inhibit growth of *S. pyogenes* on blood agar. This reaction is not entirely consistent or specific.
3. *Bile esculin agar test*: It tests the ability of 40% bile salt-tolerant bacteria to hydrolyze esculin, a characteristic of those belonging to Lansfield group D.
4. *Optochin sensitivity*: Growth of *S. pneumoniae*, but not other α-hemolytic streptococci, is inhibited around disks impregnated with optochin (ethyl hydrocuprein hydrochloride).

FIGURE 27.1. *(A)* S. equi *ssp.* zooepidemicus *on sheep blood agar plate showing β-hemolysis. (B) Gram stain of* S. equi *ssp.* zooepidemicus. *(C)* E. faecalis *showing typical α-hemolysis on sheep blood agar plate. (D) CAMP reaction on sheep blood agar. The vertical streak is growth of* S. aureus *flanked by a zone of β-toxin activity. Perpendicular to the* S. aureus *is a streak of* S. agalactiae. *Secretion of CAMP factor by the streptococci results in completion of the lysis of the β-hemolysin damaged erythrocytes, producing the characteristic arrowhead zone of lysis within the β-hemolysis zone of the* S. aureus *streak.*

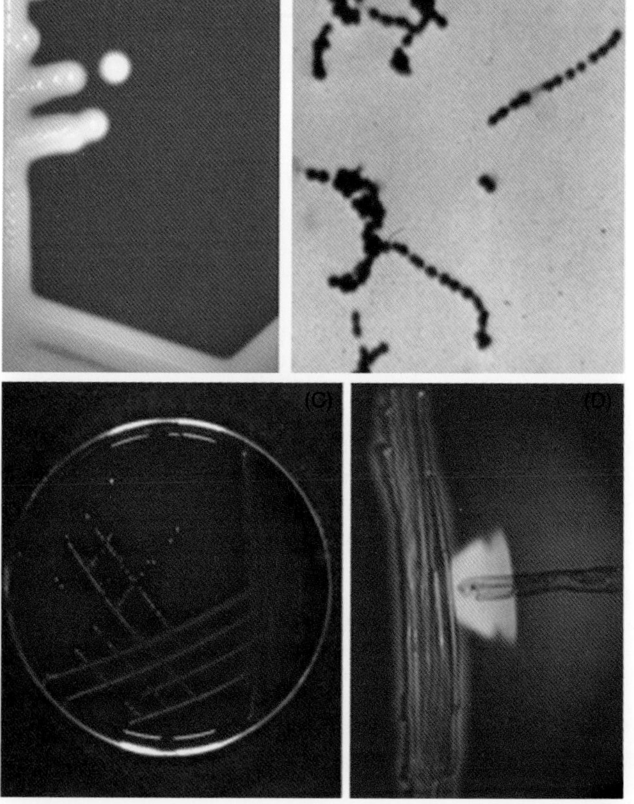

Treatment and Control

Localized suppurative conditions are drained of pus.

For systemic treatment, penicillin G and ampicillin are effective on most β-hemolytic and viridans streptococci. Cephalosporins, chloramphenicol, and trimethoprim-sulfas are alternatives. Streptococcal endocarditis is treated with combined penicillin and gentamicin. Susceptibility to fluoroquinolones is unpredictable. Streptococcal toxic shock and NF are treated with penicillin G and clindamycin (clindamycin decreases toxin production, and penicillin G is bactericidal).

Penicillins (intramammary) are effective for treating mastitis due to *S. agalactiae* and most other streptococci. For the many available alternatives, a specialty text should be consulted. Important aspects of mastitis control lie in the area of sanitation and herd management.

For strangles, it is most beneficial to treat exposed and affected animals prior to abscess formation and to continue treatment past the febrile stage. Inappropriate or inadequate therapy of strangles is blamed for prolonging the illness and causing "bastard strangles" (widespread abscess formation with systemic manifestations). Populations at risk may be vaccinated. Affected or suspected horses should be rigorously isolated.

Enterococcus

Enterococci were once classified as group D streptococci. Unlike most true members of the genus *Streptococcus*, these microorganisms possess phenotypic traits (resistance to salt, bile, methylene blue, and growth at increased temperatures) that set them apart. Molecular genetic analysis showed that they are unique, and prompted the establishment of a new genus, *Enterococcus*.

There are 41 species in the genus, most of which live in the intestinal tracts of mammals and birds. They are mainly opportunists that infect compromised sites to produce disease. There are some (*Enterococcus durans*, *E. hirae*, and *E. villorum*) that have been associated with intestinal disease in neonatal animals (piglets, foals, calves, puppies, and kittens) as well as adult dogs and cats. Enterococci are either α- or γ-hemolytic on sheep or cattle red blood cell-containing blood agar plates.

Descriptive Features

Morphology and Staining. Enterococci vary from spherical to short bacillary cells, about 1 μm in diameter. Division occurs in one plane, producing pairs and chains.

Structure and Composition. Enterococci have a typical gram-positive cell wall structure. Polysaccharide capsules are made by some species. Most enterococci possess Lancefield group D carbohydrate.

Cellular Products and Activities of Medical Interest. Much of what is known regarding cellular products and activities of medical interest comes from study of *Enterococcus faecalis* and *Enterococcus faecium*, the most common enterococci producing disease in human patients. Presumably, some of what is known about these two species also applies to the other members of the genus.

Aggregation Substance. Aggregation substance is a surface protein that promotes adherence of enterococci to each other (to form aggregates) and to epithelial surfaces (an adhesin). It is an important component of the pheromone-inducible transfer of conjugative plasmids.

Capsule. Some enterococci produce a polysaccharide capsule. The capsule discourages association with phagocytic cells by interfering with complement deposition and imparting a relative hydrophilicity to the microbe's surface.

Cell Wall. Cell wall peptidoglycan and lipoteichoic acids initiate an inflammatory response following their interaction with macrophages.

Pili. Pili of gram-positive bacteria have been implicated in adhesion to multiple types of human cells and in biofilm formation, two processes critical in the pathogenesis of many bacterial diseases. *E. faecalis* and *E. faecium* harbor pilin gene clusters.

Enterococcal MSCRAMMs. The publicly available genome sequences of *E. faecalis* V583 and *E. faecium* TX0016 revealed the presence of 17 and 15 MSCRAMMs, respectively. So far, 7 enterococcal MSCRAMMs have been characterized in detail: Ace (adhesion of collagen of *E. faecalis*), Fss1, Fss2, and Fss3 (*E. faecalis* surface protein), Acm (adhesin of collagen of *E. faecium*), Scm (second collagen adhesin of *E. faecium*), and EcbA (*E. faecium* collagen-binding protein A). Ace was shown to bind to collagen types I and IV, laminin, and dentin and was shown to be involved in the pathogenesis of experimental endocarditis. Fss1, Fss2, and Fss3 bind to fibrinogen.

Cytolysin. Cytolysin is a cytotoxin whose mechanism of cell destruction is not understood. It is also a hemolytic toxin, lysing human and horse red blood cells (but not sheep or bovine red blood cells, red blood cells most often used in blood agar plates). Cytolysin production is under the control of a quorum-sensing system.

Extracellular Superoxide. Some enterococci secrete a superoxide that appears to afford some protection against killing by phagocytic cells.

Gelatinase. Some enterococci produce a gelatinase that is expressed under the control of the *fsr* two-component regulatory system and is important in biofilm production and for virulence. Gelatinase specifically reduces Ace cell surface display and thus may affect cell adhesion properties.

Iron Acquisition. Enterococci produce a hydroxamate type of siderophore in response to low levels of iron.

Enterococcal Surface Protein. The enterococcal surface protein (*esp*) determinant is encoded on a pathogenicity island in the genome of both *E. faecalis* and *E. faecium*. It is important for biofilm formation, colonization of the urinary tract, and pathogenesis of endocarditis and urinary tract infections.

Growth Characteristics. Enterococci produce clear to gray colonies 1–2 mm in diameter (either α- or γ-hemolytic) after overnight incubation at 37 °C, though they will grow between 10 °C and 45 °C. Enterococci will grow in 6.5% sodium chloride, 40% bile, and in 0.1% methylene blue.

Biochemical Activities. Enterococci are catalase-negative facultative anaerobes, deriving energy from fermentation.

Resistance. Enterococci are hardy microorganisms able to survive in the environment for extended periods of time. They are able to grow in 6.5% sodium chloride and 40% bile, 0.1% methylene blue, and low (10 °C) and high (45 °C) temperatures. They are intrinsically resistant to the β-lactam antibiotics (including cephalosporins and penicillinase-resistant penicillins), aminoglycosides, clindamycin, fluoroquinolones, and trimethoprim–sulfonamides. (They are effective scavengers of thymidine found in exudates, thereby bypassing the effect of trimethoprim–sulfonamides.) They are able to acquire resistance to high levels of β-lactams, high levels of aminoglycosides, glycopeptides (vancomycin), tetracycline, erythromycin, fluoroquinolones, rifampin, and chloramphenicol.

Ecology

Reservoir. Enterococci live in the intestinal tract of mammals and birds as part of the normal flora of these species. Whether the enterococci associated with "primary" disease, *E. durans*, *E. hirae*, and *E. villorum*, as opposed to opportunistic-type disease, are members of the normal flora, is unknown.

Transmission. Enterococci that are associated with opportunistic disease are part of the normal flora of the host.

Pathogenesis

Except for *E. durans*, *E. hirae*, and *E. villorum*-associated disease, endogenous enterococci infect a compromised site (e.g., urinary bladder, moist external ear canal, and catheter). The cell wall peptidoglycan and lipoteichoic acids initiate an inflammatory response. Capsule, cytolysin, and superoxide potentate the inflammatory processes.

E. durans, *E. hirae*, and *E. villorum* associate with the villi (from tip to crypt) of the small intestine of affected animals. Associated diarrhea does not appear to be due to an enterotoxin or epithelial cell damage.

Disease Patterns

Dogs and Cats. Otitis externa is usually the result of infection (bacteria and a yeast, *Malassezia*) of a compromised external ear canal. The bacteria involved are usually an environmental species (e.g., *Pseudomonas* and *Proteus*) or a member of the patient's normal flora (e.g., *Enterococcus* and *Staphylococcus pseudintermedius*).

Enterococcus is a common isolate from dogs with lower urinary tract infections. *Enterococcus* spp. (*E. durans*, *E. hirae*, and *E. villorum*) are associated with diarrhea in puppies, kittens, and adult dogs and cats. Almost any compromised site may be contaminated with an *Enterococcus*.

Horse. *Enterococcus* spp. (*E. durans*, *E. hirae*, and *E. villorum*) are associated with diarrhea in foals. *Enterococcus* spp. should be expected in any condition that results from contamination of a compromised site with fecal material (e.g., street nail/sole abscess and wound).

Cattle. *Enterococcus* spp. (*E. durans*, *E. hirae*, and *E. villorum*) are associated with diarrhea in calves. *Enterococcus* spp. should be expected in any condition that results from contamination of a compromised site with fecal material (e.g., wound).

Swine. *Enterococcus* spp. (*E. durans*, *E. hirae*, and *E. villorum*) are associated with diarrhea in piglets. *Enterococcus* spp. should be expected in any condition that results from contamination of a compromised site with fecal material (e.g., wound).

Miscellaneous Species. *Enterococcus* spp. (*E. durans*, *E. hirae*, and *E. villorum*) are associated with diarrhea in infant rats.

Epidemiology. Most of the infectious processes from which enterococci are isolated are due to contamination with members of the normal flora. In hospital settings, nosocomial spread (e.g., fomites, hands of care givers, and soles of shoes) to compromised sites is an important issue. The epidemiology of the diarrhea-associated enterococci (*E. durans*, *E. hirae*, and *E. villorum*) is unknown.

Vancomycin-resistant strains of enterococci are a serious problem in human medicine because members of this genus (especially *E. faecalis* and *E. faecium*) are major contributors to nosocomially acquired disease. The vancomycin-resistance genes are encoded on a transposable element (Tn1546). Enterococci are very resistant to antimicrobial agents. Vancomycin (a glycopeptide antibiotic) is one of the few effective drugs for treatment of such infectious processes. Vancomycin-resistant strains of enterococci arose in Europe after the initiation of feeding of another glycopeptide avoparcin (a growth promoter) to food-producing animals. Although at first the vancomycin-resistant strains were limited to the intestinal tract of animals that fed this antibiotic, they soon spread, as did the genes encoding vancomycin resistance (*vanA*), to the human intestinal tract. In the United States (where avoparcin was not allowed), injudicious use of vancomycin in human hospitals resulted in the same effect, that is, an increase in selective pressure resulting in an increase in colonization by vancomycin-resistant enterococci (especially in hospitals).

Laboratory Diagnosis

Sample Collection. Aspirates from unopened lesions, in sterile syringes or sterile containers, are preferred. Swabs in transport media are acceptable. Urine samples are obtained by antepubic cystocentesis (bladder tap), catherization, or midstream catch.

Direct Examination. Stained (Gram's or Romanovsky-type such as Wright's or Giemsa) smears of exudates are examined. Urine can be examined unstained or stained (Gram's or Romanovsky-type). Histopathologic sections of small intestine obtained from animals with associated enterococcal enteritis are needed to demonstrate characteristic adherence of coccal forms to villi.

Culture. Samples are streaked onto the surface of blood agar plates and incubated at 37 °C overnight. Enterococci produce clear to gray colonies 1–2 mm in diameter (either α- or γ-hemolytic). Preliminary identification entails testing for the production of catalase (negative), and ability to grow in 6.5% sodium chloride and 40% bile. Most isolates can be speciated using commercially available kits, sequencing the gene encoding the 16S ribosomal RNA, or a combination of both.

Treatment and Control

Correction of the underlying condition is the most important aspect of treatment of most situations from which enterococci are isolated. In some instances, removal of the compromise is enough to initiate host elimination of enterococci (because they do not have potent virulence determinants). This is an important concept because enterococci tend to be quite resistant to antimicrobials. In those infectious processes that have a polymicrobic etiology (along with the compromise), success can be achieved by correction of the compromise and antimicrobic therapy aimed at the other (usually more susceptible) microorganisms.

Enterococci isolated from the lower urinary tract of dogs are usually susceptible to urine concentrations of amoxicillin–clavulanate, chloramphenicol, and tetracycline. Even though most urinary strains of enterococci test susceptible to trimethoprim–sulfonamides, care should be taken in interpreting *in vitro* test results because of the thymidine-savaging ability of this group of microorganisms.

Enterococci associated with otitis externa in dogs are dealt with by correcting the underlying compromise and use of any of the otic preparations that contain an antimicrobial. (Topical concentrations of most incorporated antimicrobics usually far exceed the minimal inhibitory concentration needed to inhibit growth of enterococci.)

Treatment options of diarrheal disease associated with *E. durans*, *E. hirae*, or *E. villorum* are undefined.

Abiotrophia and *Granulicatella* (Nutritionally Variant Streptococci)

Members of the genera *Abiotrophia* and *Granulicatella* were discovered as small colonies growing as satellites around other bacterial colonies when samples obtained from normal human mucosal surfaces (eyes, genital tract, mouth, and respiratory tract) were inoculated onto blood agar plates. The bacteria comprising these colonies were gram-positive, catalase-negative cocci requiring vitamin B_6 for growth (satisfied by the addition of 0.002% pyridoxal hydrochloride to media). These microorganisms were provisionally termed "nutritionally variant streptococci," but later placed into the genera *Abiotrophia* and *Granulicatella* based upon the sequence of the gene encoding the 16S ribosomal RNA.

Clinically, members of these genera have been isolated from the bloodstream, abscesses, dental plaque, joints, corneal ulcers, acute-onset postoperative endophthalmitis, and cardiac valve vegetations of human patients. They have been isolated from the genital tracts, respiratory tracts, abscesses, and eyes of horses and ruminants.

A fibronectin-binding protein, Cha, has been identified and characterized from *Granulicatella adiacens*.

Further Reading

Cole JN, Barnett TC, Nizet V, and Walker MJ (2011) Molecular insight into invasive group A streptococcal disease. *Nat Rev Microbiol*, **9**, 724–736.

Feng Y, Zhang H, Ma Y, and Gao GF (2010) Uncovering newly emerging variants of *Streptococcus suis*, an important zoonotic agent. *Trends Microbiol*, **18**, 124–131.

Moschioni M, Pansegrau W, and Barocchi MA (2010) Adhesion determinants of the *Streptococcus* species. *Microb Biotechnol*, **3**, 370–388.

Priestnall S and Erles K (2011) *Streptococcus zooepidemicus*: an emerging canine pathogen. *Vet J*, **188**, 142–148.

Sava IG, Heikens E, and Huebner J (2010) Pathogenesis and immunity in enterococcal infections. *Clin Microbiol Infect*, **16**, 533–540.

Waller AS, Paillot R, and Timoney JF (2011) *Streptococcus equi*: a pathogen restricted to one host. *J Med Microbiol*, **60**, 1231–1240.

28 Arcanobacterium

T.G. Nagaraja

Species of the genus *Arcanobacterium* (which means "secretive bacteria") are gram-positive rods, often pleomorphic, non-spore-forming and nonmotile. In shape, members of this genus are "diphtheroids," not filamentous, and many species were at one time included in the genus *Corynebacterium* (e.g., *Corynebacterium pyogenes*), and later in the genus *Actinomyces* (e.g., *Actinomyces pyogenes*). Sequence analyses of the gene encoding the 16S ribosomal RNA of several species in *Actinomyces* suggested placing of the species in a genus called *Arcanobacterium*.

The species of the genus *Arcanobacterium* include *A. bernardiae*, *A. bialowiezense*, *A. bonsai*, *A. haemolyticum*, *A. hippocoleae*, *A. phocae*, *A. pluranimalium*, and *A. pyogenes**. *Arcanobacterium bialowiezense* and *Arcanobacterium bonsai* have been isolated from the prepuce of European bison bulls suffering from balanoposthitis. *Arcanobacterium haemolyticum* and *Arcanobacterium bernardiae* are human pathogens, and involvement of *A. bernardiae* in infections is rare. *A. haemolyticum* is involved in pharyngitis, tonsillitis, and skin rash, most often in adolescents and young adults. *Arcanobacterium phocae*, *A. pluranimalium*, and *A. hippocoleae* have been isolated from the respiratory tract of seals, the spleen of a harbor porpoise and the lung of a deer, and from an equine vaginal exudate, respectively. A recent study suggests that sheep are most frequently affected by infection with *A. pluranimalium*, and most isolates were from aborted tissues. *Arcanobacterium pyogenes* is the main species of veterinary importance, being involved in suppurative processes in all animals, but more common in cattle, sheep, and swine.

A. pyogenes

Descriptive Features

Morphology and Staining. *A. pyogenes* is coccobacillary to short rods (0.5 μm by up to 2 μm) that occur singly or in pairs. Short diphtheroid forms with small clubs are also seen, particularly in young cultures. The organism lacks capsules and metachromatic granules. Cells from older cultures (>24 h) may be gram variable.

Structure and Composition. Its cell wall peptidoglycan contains lysine, rhamnose, and glucose. Unlike members of the genera *Corynebacterium* and *Rhodococcus*, it does not contain mycolic acids.

Cellular Products of Medical Interest

Cell Wall. The lipoteichoic acids and peptidoglycan of the gram-positive cell wall interact with macrophage cells, resulting in the release of proinflammatory cytokines.

A. pyogenes produces a number of extracellular products and surface-exposed proteins that contribute to adherence, colonization, and host damage:

1. *Pyolysin O*: A hemolytic exotoxin, designated as pyolysin O (PLO), produced by all strains of *A. pyogenes* is the primary virulence factor. The hemolysin is active against sheep, horse, human, rabbit, and guinea pig erythrocytes and is cytotoxic to polymorphonuclear neutrophils also, and in laboratory animals, it exerts dermonecrotic and lethal activities. It is a pore-forming toxin belonging to the thiol-activated family of cytolysins found in many gram-positive bacteria, such as streptococcal streptolysin O, listerial listeriolysin O, and clostridial perfringolysin O. The family is named for the sensitivity of their activity to oxygen and restoration of their activity by reducing compounds (thiol activation). The PLO is considered to be the major virulence factor in *A. pyogenes* infection.
2. *Neuraminidases*: Also called sialidases they cleave terminal sialic acid from carbohydrates or glycoproteins. *A. pyogenes* produces two neuraminidases. One is a cell wall-associated 107 kDa protein (NanH) encoded by the *nanH* gene. The nanH is produced in all strains of *A. pyogenes* that have been tested. The protein is similar to a number of other bacterial neuraminidases. The second neuraminidase (NanP) is a 186.8 kDa protein, encoded by *nanP*, is preferentially associated with bovine strains, and is not present in all the strains tested.

*It is now proposed that species *bernardiae, bialowiezense, bonasi,* and *pyogenes* should be reclassified as members of a new genus, *Trueperella*.

Veterinary Microbiology, Third Edition. Edited by D. Scott McVey, Melissa Kennedy and M.M. Chengappa.

3. *Extracellular matrix-binding proteins*: These are proteins on the surface of *A. pyogenes* that bind to host extracellular matrix composed of structural glycoproteins, such as fibronectin, collagen, fibrinogen, laminin, and elastin. A protein, CbpA, which binds to fibrinogen and fibrinonectin, has been described. This protein has 50.4% similarity to Cna, a protein that binds to collagen, of *Staphylococcus aureus*. A 20 kDa cell wall-associated, fibrinonectin-binding protein has been described.
4. *A. pyogenes* secretes at least four distinct proteases, possibly serine proteases, and a DNase. Although some aspects of these enzymes have been studied, there is no evidence to support a role for any these enzymes in the pathogenesis of *A. pyogenes* infections.

Growth Characteristics. *A. pyogenes* is a facultative anaerobe with a fermentative metabolism. They require increased CO_2 for optimal growth. On blood agar, the organisms form pinpoint colonies with distinct zone of β-hemolysis. The zone of hemolysis is typically two to three times the diameter of the colony.

Biochemical Activities. *A. pyogenes* is catalase-negative, ferments lactose, and digests protein (gelatin, casein, and coagulated serum).

Resistance. *A. pyogenes* is susceptible to drying, heat (60 °C), disinfectants, and β-lactam antibiotics. It is resistant to sulfonamides, and increasingly so to tetracycline.

Ecology

Reservoir. *A. pyogenes* is a normal inhabitant of the upper respiratory, urogenital, and gastrointestinal tracts of cattle, swine, and other domestic animals. In cattle, it has been isolated from the ruminal epithelium. The organism does not appear to be part of the normal flora in humans.

Transmission. Because *A. pyogenes* is a commensal on skin and mucous membrane, most infections are endogenous. In "summer mastitis," cow-to-cow spread, mediated by flies, has been reported.

Pathogenesis

Mechanisms. Entry of *A. pyogenes* into the deeper tissues requires an insult or a stress of some kind such as a wound or a primary viral or bacterial infection. The organism can get disseminated and even cause abortion, but more often it results in suppurative infections involving joints, skin, and visceral organs, usually complicated by other potentially pathogenic commensals, especially gram-negative, non-spore-forming anaerobes (*Bacteroides*, *Dichelobacter*, *Fusobacterium*, *Porphyromonas*, *Prevotella*, and *Peptostreptococcus*). The observation that *A. pyogenes* is almost always associated with *Fusobacterium necrophorum* has led to the suggestion of pathogenic synergy between the two species. Such synergistic interaction has been demonstrated in laboratory mice. The mechanisms involved in this synergism may be the supply of energy substrate (lactic acid by *A. pyogenes*), protection against phagocytosis (leukotoxin by *F. necrophorum*), and creation of anaerobiosis (oxygen use by *A. pyogenes*). Pyolysin is a major virulence determinant as evidenced by mutants deficient in production of the toxin have reduced virulence, and antibodies raised against the inactivated protein are host protective. The precise role of pyolysin in the pathogenesis of *A. pyogenes* infection is not known, but the membrane-damaging effect on host cells is probably a key mechanism. Neuraminidases play a role in bacterial adhesion to epithelial cells. The enzyme can also decrease viscosity of mucus, thus facilitating colonization. Neuraminidases can also impair host immune response by desialylation of IgA and increasing their susceptibilities to proteolysis. The ability of *A. pyogenes* to bind to extracellular matrix proteins, mediated by surface proteins, may promote adherence and subsequent colonization. The proteases may play a role in tissue invasion and destruction, evasion of host defenses, and modulation of the host immune system during infection and inflammation. DNAse may depolymerize viscous DNA released from lysed or disintegrating host cells in suppurative lesions. The exudate (pus) consists of bacteria, neutrophils (live or dead), and host cell debris.

Pathology. The lesions are abscesses, empyemas, or pyogranulomas. Abscesses are often heavily encapsulated. Any putrid odors are contributions of anaerobic bacteria.

Disease Patterns. *A. pyogenes* is involved in purulent infections, singly or in combination with other organisms, of traumatic or opportunistic origins, which may be local, regional, or metastatic. It is frequently isolated from a variety of pyogenic infections of the lung, pericardium, endocardium, pleura, peritoneum, liver, joints, uterus, renal cortex, brain, bones, and subcutaneous tissues of all animals, but most frequently in ruminants and swine.

The more common and economically significant infections are as follows:

Liver abscesses in cattle: *A. pyogenes* is the second most commonly isolated bacterium (next to *F. necrophorum*) from abscesses of the liver in feedlot cattle. The organism originates from the ruminal wall and reaches the liver via the portal vein. Generally, the occurrence of *A. pyogenes* ranges from 2% to 25% of liver abscesses, but in certain situations (cattle fed all-grain diet) the prevalence becomes noticeably high.

Summer mastitis in cows and heifers: *A. pyogenes* causes severe mastitis characterized by thick, purulent secretions, frequently in dry cows and heifers before or at the time of calving, and occasionally in lactating cows generally following teat or udder injury. The source of infection includes wound, abscesses, and the genital tract, and infection spreads in a herd because of contact of teats with a contaminated environment, such as calving area. In Europe, the disease is common in dry cows and heifers maintained on pasture, hence the name "summer mastitis." The seasonal prevalence is also associated with fly season because biting flies are involved in the entry of the organism into the teats and spread of the organisms between animals.

Septic arthritis in swine: Arthritis appears after farrowing, suggesting that the source of infection may be the uterus.

The other infections from which *A. pyogenes* is frequently isolated are umbilical infections in calves, traumatic reticulitis in cows, foot rot in cattle.

Epidemiology. Because *A. pyogenes* is part of the normal flora of susceptible species, disease prevalence is sporadic and governed by precipitating stress or trauma. Summer mastitis is most prevalent in northern Europe.

Immunologic Aspects

Immune responses to *A. pyogenes* are not well understood. There have been attempts to vaccinate mice, cattle, and sheep with bacterins or formalin-inactivated crude *A. pyogenes* supernatant. Results of such studies have not been very convincing. In mice, vaccination with purified recombinant PLO resulted in neutralizing antibodies, which protected mice against challenge with *A. pyogenes*. Because *A. pyogenes* infections are sporadic, vaccination is not a viable approach.

Laboratory Diagnosis

Gram-stained smears from tissues or exudates reveal gram-positive short to pleomorphic rods, often mixed with other bacteria. Material suspected of containing *A. pyogenes* should be cultured on blood agar in 5% CO_2 incubator. Generally, minute colonies on blood agar with distinct but narrow zone of hemolysis from a sample of pus are indicative of *A. pyogenes* involvement. Routine biochemical methods are used to identify this microorganism. Primers designed to amplify *A. pyogenes*-specific DNA by the polymerase chain reaction have been described.

Treatment and Control

Incision and drainage of abscesses are essential. *A. pyogenes* is susceptible to penicillin, ampicillin, chloramphenicol, erythromycin, sulfamethazine, tylosin, and tetracyclines. The *in vivo* response to antimicrobials is poor because of the capsulation of the abscesses and antibiotic-binding proteins in pus.

Further Reading

Billington SJ and Jost BH (2000) Thiol-activated cytolysins: structure, function and role in pathogenesis. *FEMS Microbiol Lett*, **182**, 197–205.

Billington SJ, Songer JG, and Jost BH (2001) Molecular characterization of the pore-forming toxin, pyolysin, a major virulence determinant of *Arcanobacterium pyogenes*. *Vet Microbiol*, **82**, 261–274.

Jost BH and Billington SJ (2005) *Arcanobacterium pyogenes:* molecular pathogenesis of animal opportunist. *Ant Van Leeuwenhock*, **88**, 87–102.

Ramos CP, Foster G, and Collins MD (1997) Phylogenetic analysis of the genus *Actinomyces* based on 16S rRNA gene sequences: description of *Arcanobacterium phocae* sp. nov., *Arcanobacterium bernardiae* com. nov., and *Arcanobacterium pyogenes* comb. *Nov Int J Syst Bacteriol*, **47**, 46–53.

Yassin AF, Hupfer H, Siering C, and Schumann P (2011) Comparative chemotaxonomic and phylogenetic studies on the genus Arcanobacterium Collins et al. 1982 emend. Lehnen et al. 2006: proposal for Trueperella gen. nov. and emended description of the genus Arcanobacterium. *Int J Syst Evol Microbiol*, **61**, 1265–1274.

29 Bacillus

George C. Stewart and Brian M. Thompson

Members of the genus *Bacillus* are gram-positive, endospore-forming, facultatively anaerobic rods that typically inhabit soil and water. They are ubiquitous in nature, and are commonly isolated from a wide variety of surfaces, soils, and animal byproducts. Average numbers of *Bacillus* spp. present in soil are between 10^6 and 10^7 per gram of soil. During periods of nutrient deprivation, a *Bacillus* cell undergoes a process known as sporulation by which it forms a dense, resistant endospore. Endospores are resistant to heat, desiccation, ultraviolet and ionizing irradiation, disinfectants, and a variety of other environmental stresses. They can remain viable in soil and water for decades, awaiting nutrients, or in the case of pathogenic members of *Bacillus*, entry of spores into their respective hosts.

Three species are considered pathogenic. *Bacillus anthracis* is a zoonotic pathogen and the causative agent of anthrax. *Bacillus cereus* is a causal agent of food poisoning, and *Bacillus thuringiensis* is a lepidopteran insect pathogen. Genomic studies, including DNA–DNA hybridization, 16S and 23S rRNA sequence comparisons, multilocus sequence typing, multilocus enzyme electrophoresis, and amplified fragment length polymorphism analysis, have revealed a high degree of relatedness among these organisms, leading to the proposal that *B. anthracis*, *B. cereus*, and *B. thuringiensis* may be viewed as a single species. Their virulence and host range are determined by their virulence gene-encoding plasmid content. For example, virulence of *B. anthracis* requires the presence of the pXO1 and pXO2 plasmids, required for production of the anthrax toxins and capsule, respectively.

Bacillus anthracis

Descriptive Features

Morphology and Staining. Cells of *B. anthracis* are gram-positive, nonmotile, roughly rectangular rods with square ends (about 1 μm by 3–5 μm) (Figure 29.1). Chains of rods are common. Chain formation is thought to contribute to the bacterium's ability to resist opsono-phagocytic killing. Spores are produced within the cells during conditions of nutrient deprivation and cause no cell swelling. A capsule is formed *in vivo*, or in bicarbonate-supplemented culture media and an elevated CO_2 atmosphere *in vitro*.

Cellular Composition. *B. anthracis* has a gram-positive cell wall structure. Covering the cell wall is a proteinaceous paracrystalline structure referred to as the S-layer. Although the S-layer has not been shown to be essential for virulence, S-layer deficient mutant strains were reported to be more sensitive to binding of the C3 component of the complement.

Spores are the infectious form of *B. anthracis*. Spores are immunogenic and the addition of inactivated spores has been shown to increase the degree of immunity against highly virulent strains of *B. anthracis* in animal models of infection. The spores consist of multiple layers (Figure 29.2). The core is the inert bacterial cell. It is surrounded by the cortex, a layer of modified peptidoglycan. This is surrounded by the inner and outer coat layers, protein layers that confer most of the resistance properties on the spore. The outermost layer of the spore is the exosporium layer that is separated from the coat by the interspace layer. The exosporium consists of a paracrystalline basal layer and its outer surface covered by filaments of the hair-like nap composed of the BclA collagen-like glycoprotein. Because the exosporium is the outermost structure of the spore, it is probable that it plays a major role in interactions with the environment and with the host immune system. The *B. anthracis* exosporium was reported to play a role in limiting access to inducers of cytokine responses *in vitro* in macrophages. The uptake of spores by macrophages has been shown to involve interactions between BclA and the integrin Mac-1 (CR3). Spores lacking the BclA glycoprotein do not specifically target these cells, but bind more generally to epithelial cells. Spores lacking BclA have been shown to bind to extracellular matrix components such as laminin and fibronectin. The spore-surface BclA fibers may act to promote uptake by professional phagocytes and to inhibit nonspecific interactions between *B. anthracis* spores with nonprofessional phagocytic cells in the early stages of infection.

Cellular Products of Medical Interest

1. *Lethal toxin (LeTx)*: Two virulence-associated, pXO1-encoded toxins are made by *B. anthracis*. LeTx is a binary toxin composed of "protective antigen" (PA) and "lethal factor" (LF). PA is responsible for

Veterinary Microbiology, Third Edition. Edited by D. Scott McVey, Melissa Kennedy and M.M. Chengappa.

FIGURE 29.1. *(A)* B. anthracis *colonies on a sheep blood agar plate; (B) Gram stain of* B. anthracis*; (C)* B. cereus *on a sheep blood agar plate with hemolysis evident; (D) string of pearls positive test with* B. anthracis*; and (E) spore stain of* B. anthracis.

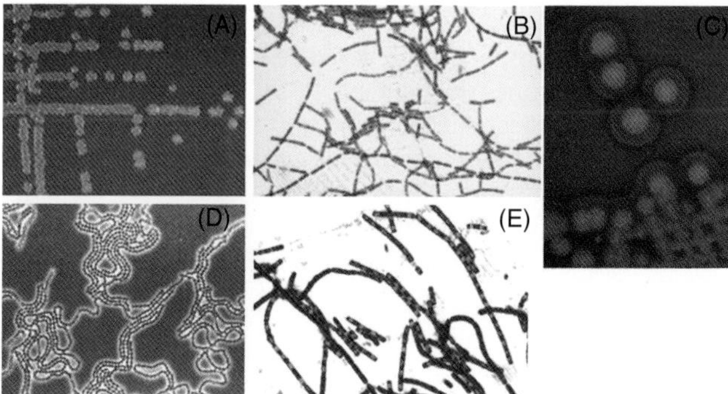

binding of LeTx to "target cells," while LF is responsible for its toxic activity. PA and LF associate only after PA has bound to its receptor and then proteolytically processed by endopeptidases of the furin family. Processed PA forms a homoheptameric (or homooctomeric) ring on the target cell surface. The PA can then serve as the binding component for the LF protein or the edema toxin. The toxin is endocytosed and when the reduction of pH in the endosome occurs, conformational changes ensue and the PA forms a transmembrane channel to deliver LF into the cytosol. LF is a zinc metalloprotease that inactivates mitogen-activated protein kinase kinases (MAPK kinases), by cleaving off their N-terminal sequences resulting in the disruption of signaling pathways within the affected cell and leads to inhibition of cell proliferation and ultimately to apoptosis of affected cells. Macrophages from numerous species have been shown to react to LeTx exposure by undergoing apoptosis. LeTx derives its name for its lethal effects in animal models of infection including guinea pigs, rats, and mice. LeTx induces vascular collapse (pleural edema and rapid shock) and yet exposure to purified LeTx often results in no observable histopathology. Activity of the toxin on heart tissue is thought to lead to the pulmonary edema. In certain mouse strains, LeTx exposure results in rapid lysis of macrophages and production of inflammatory cytokines. However, other strains do not show this property. Macrophage lysis is not a common feature in other animal models. LeTx exposure does result in apoptosis in a variety of cell types and a cell-death independent loss of barrier function in epithelial and endothelial cells *in vitro*. Production of LeTx is under control of the regulatory gene product, AtxA (for anthrax toxin activator), which responds to as yet unknown environmental cues AtxA is also encoded on pXO1. LeTx production by cells cultured *in vitro* is upregulated by the presence of bicarbonate in the medium and an elevated CO_2 atmosphere in an AtxA-dependent manner, suggesting this may be the cue recognized by AtxA. Lethal toxin is produced at levels five times greater than that of edema toxin.

FIGURE 29.2. *Transmission electron micrograph of a ruthenium red stained spore of* B. anthracis. *Ruthenium red enhances visualization of the BclA exosporium glycoprotein nap layer. Outer spore structures are labeled.*

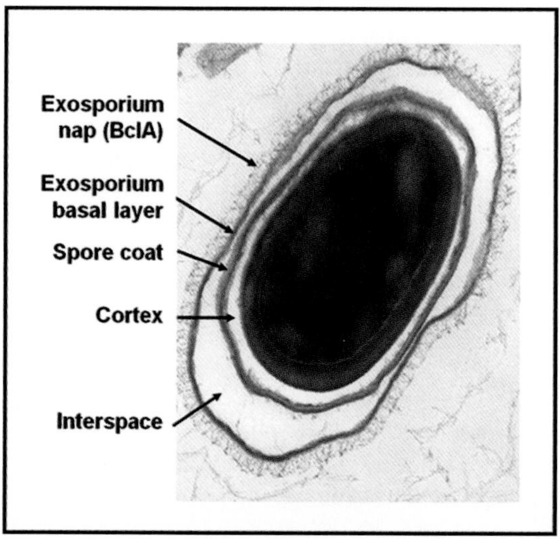

2. *Edema toxin*: Edema factor (EF), the enzymatically active component of edema toxin (EdTx), is also encoded on pXO1. EdTx is a binary toxin composed of the PA receptor binding subunit and EF. PA delivers EF to the target cells cytoplasm by the same mechanism as lethal toxin. EF is a calmodulin-dependent adenylyl cyclase that increases levels of cAMP within the affected cell. This disrupts cell-signaling pathways, resulting in cell type-specific physiologic changes. In animal models of infection, purified EdTx produces hemorrhagic lesions in multiple organs accompanied by hypotension and bradycardia. EdTx has not been shown to be cytotoxic for multiple cell types. EdTx has been reported to suppress thrombin-induced platelet aggregation and clotting function. Production of EdTx is also under AtxA control.
3. *Capsule*: The vegetative form of *B. anthracis* produces a capsule composed of a polymer of poly-γ-D-glutamic acid. The genes encoding this structure are on the pXO2 plasmid. The expression of the genes encoding the capsule are under control of two regulatory gene products, AtxA and AcpA (for anthrax toxin activator and anthrax capsule activator, respectively) that respond to environmental cues. The capsule enables the vegetative form to avoid phagocytosis. The Sterne vaccine strain is attenuated for virulence because it lacks the capsule-encoding pXO2 plasmid.
4. *Miscellaneous virulence-associated products*: Several homologs of proteins shown to be important in virulence of other microorganisms have been discovered in the DNA sequence of the genome of *B. anthracis*. These include genes encoding proteins important in survival within phagolysosomes

and on mucosal surfaces (InhA and MprF), and escape from phagolysosomes and phagocytic cells (anthrolysins).

a. *InhA*: Immune inhibitor A (InhA) is a metalloprotease similar to that produced by *B. cereus*. It contributes to pathogenicity through several mechanisms, including the cleavage of antibacterial proteins, escape of bacteria from macrophages, control of blood coagulation, and degradation of matrix-associated proteins. InhA recently has been postulated to play a role in increasing blood-brain barrier permeability and contributing to cerebral hemorrhages.
b. *MprF*: The genome of *B. anthracis* contains the gene encoding the homolog of MprF (for multiple peptide resistance factor) of *Staphylococcus aureus*. It has been shown to confer resistance to defensins (found within the phagolysosome, and in secretions bathing mucosal surfaces) by lysinylation of phospholipids in the bacterial cell membrane.
c. *Anthrolysins*: The genome of *B. anthracis* contains genes encoding anthrolysins (also referred to as anthralysins), three of which are phospholipase C homologs and anthrolysin O is a cholesterol-binding pore-forming cytolysin. Although each is dispensable for virulence, loss of all four results in attenuation. It is hypothesized that these are important in escape of the organism from the phagolysosome following germination of spores in macrophages. Anthrolysin O is poorly expressed by *B. anthracis* (which is why *B. anthracis* is nonhemolytic). The reason is that its regulator, PlcR, is inactive owing to a truncation of its coding sequence. Recombinant anthrolysin O is lethal to human monocytes, neutrophils, macrophages, and lymphocytes.
d. *Nitric oxide synthase*: *B. anthracis* bacilli and endospores exhibit nitric oxide synthase activity that may protect germinating spores from nitric oxide production by host macrophages by using up available substrate pools of arginine.

5. Regulation of the Cellular Products of Medical Interest.

There are two proteins AtxA and AcpA (for anthrax toxin activator and anthrax capsule activator, respectively) that are produced in response to environmental cues. What these cues are *in vivo* is unknown. Under the appropriate conditions, however, AtxA increases the production of LeTx, EdTx, and proteins involved in the "escape" from phagolysosomes and macrophages. AcpA production is amplified under increased amounts of CO_2 (5% or greater). AtxA acts synergistically with AcpA in this regard. The genes encoding AtxA and AcpA are on the plasmids, pXO1 and pXO2, respectively. The *B. anthracis* transcriptional regulator CodY activates toxin gene expression by posttranslationally regulating the accumulation of the AtxA virulence gene regulator. CodY is also required for heme utilization as an iron source.

Growth Characteristics. *B. anthracis* is a facultative anaerobe and grows on common media between 15 °C and 40 °C. Colonies reach a diameter of 2 mm or greater in 24 h at 37 °C (Figure 29.1). Colonies grown in air have a dull surface and wavy margin formed by strands of bacterial chains ("medusa-head"). Cells are nonencapsulated unless grown in greater than 5% carbon dioxide on media containing 0.7% bicarbonate, in which case the colonies are mucoid. No hemolytic zone is produced.

Sporulation occurs under conditions of nutrient deprivation *in vitro*. The process is oxygen requiring, and does not occur while inside a living animal host. Organisms in infected tissue or fluids exposed to air (i.e., rupturing of the carcass) sporulate after several hours.

Resistance. Although generally antibiotic sensitive, all sequenced strains of *B. anthracis* possess a latent β-lactamase gene, which is transcriptionally silent. Strains have been identified in which this gene is activated and inducible penicillin resistance is observed.

Vegetative cells in unopened carcasses may survive for up to 1–2 weeks, but spores can persist for decades in a stable, dry environment. Spores are killed by autoclaving (121 °C/15 min) and dry heat (150 °C/60 min), but not by boiling (100 °C) for less than 10 min. They are not highly susceptible to phenolic, alcoholic, and quaternary ammonium disinfectants. Aldehydes, oxidizing and chlorinating disinfectants, β-propiolactone, and ethylene oxide are more useful. Spores are efficiently inactivated by exposure to 10% bleach. Heat fixation of smears does not kill spores.

Variability. The peracute nature of the infectious process and spore-based life cycle mean that *B. anthracis* undergoes a limited number of divisions in infected hosts and do not replicate while dormant in the soil. Thus, these organisms have undergone far fewer replication cycles than other forms of pathogenic bacteria. This results in much less mutational alteration of their genomic sequences and very limited strain-to-strain variation. The genome is more homogeneous than is the case with other pathogens.

Ecology

Reservoir. The soil is the source of anthrax infection for herbivores. Other species, including humans, are exposed via infected animals and animal products.

Transmission. The spore is the infectious form. Infection usually takes place by ingestion of contaminated feed or water. Exposure via wound infection and arthropod bites can occur.

Human infections occur following exposure to spores on infected hides or other animal products, from soil, or exposure to infected animal blood or tissue.

Pathogenesis

Mechanisms. Spores are acquired from the environment (e.g., soil and animal products). They are phagocytosed by macrophages or dendritic cells (polymorphonuclear neutrophil leucocytes do not appear to play a role in the disease process). The spores germinate within the phagolysosome compartment. Vegetative bacteria escape from the phagolysosome and later from the phagocytic cell. During the intracellular replication process, the phagocytic cells traffic to the regional lymph nodes. Release of the bacteria permits access of the organisms to the bloodstream.

Pathology. In tissue, spores germinate and the vegetative form proliferates, producing gelatinous edema. Inflammatory reactions are minimal. Infection disseminates to reticuloendothelial sites. When these are saturated, a terminal bacteremia occurs, with enormous numbers of organisms in circulation. There are no consistent pathognomonic lesions and considerable similarities are seen to other infectious and toxic causes of acute death. Postmortem findings are widespread hemorrhages; a black, engorged, friable spleen; tarry, nonclotting blood; and absence of rigor mortis. Bleeding at body orifices is common.

Experimental transmission of *B. anthracis* has revealed that cattle are resistant to spores introduced parenterally, but sensitive to spores introduced by the oral route. The LD_{50} is likely to be $<10^7$ spores. With sheep, the LD_{50} is between 50 and 250 spores by the subcutaneous inoculation route. Swine are resistant to lethal infections by *B. anthracis* spores. Other species including dogs, rabbits, and chickens are highly resistant to anthrax infection as well.

Disease Pattern

Ruminants. The process described in the preceding text is typical for the most susceptible species—cattle and sheep. The course, following an incubation period of 1–5 days, ranges from a few hours to 2 days. Some animals die without overt clinical signs. Others develop high fever, agalactia, and they may abort. There is congestion of mucous membranes, hematuria, hemorrhagic diarrhea, and often-regional edema. These forms are regularly fatal. Occasional animals show just localized edema or an ulcerative skin lesion and recover.

Horses. Horses develop colic and diarrhea; edema also occurs, particularly of dependent parts and at the point of infection (e.g., the intestine or the throat) where it may cause death by asphyxiation. Alternatively, the course may be septicemic, as in ruminants.

Swine. In swine, localization in pharyngeal tissues is typical. An ulcerative lesion at the portal of entry is associated with regional lymphadenitis. Obstructive edema may cause death. Ulcerative hemorrhagic enteritis and mesenteric lymphadenitis sometimes occur.

Carnivores. Carnivores (including mink) are rarely affected; when they are, the disease pattern is similar to that in swine, although massive exposure through tainted meat may trigger septicemia.

Humans. Three distinct disease forms arise depending the route of spore entry into the patient. Exposure through skin wounds or abrasions results in cutaneous anthrax that constitutes 95% of naturally occurring human infections. The hallmark lesion is the malignant pustule, a local ulcerative inflammatory lesion covered by a black scab (eschar). Possible complications are subcutaneous edema and septicemia. The case fatality rate for cutaneous anthrax is 10–20%. Inhalation of spores leads to pulmonary anthrax or "wool-sorter's disease" which is highly fatal if untreated and 50% to >90% lethal even with antibiotic therapy. The poor prognosis is due to the initial nondescript influenza-like symptoms that delays correct diagnosis and the rapid time-course of the infection. Radiographic evidence of mediastinal widening is characteristic. Pulmonary edema, hemorrhagic pneumonia, and meningitis have been described in affected patients. Pulmonary anthrax is the form of human disease of concern from a bioterrorism standpoint.

Epidemiology. A soil rich in calcium and nitrate, with a pH range of 5.0–8.0, favors sporulation and bacterial proliferation at temperatures above 15.5 °C (60 °F), especially after flooding. The geography and seasonality of outbreaks reflect such circumstances. In cattle, sheep, and possibly horses, outbreaks begin with a few cases contracted from the soil. After excretions and postmortem discharges seed the area, secondary cases occur. Floods and industrial effluents from rendering works, tanneries, carpet mills, brush factories, or wherever else carcasses are salvaged may contaminate areas. Bone meal, an animal feed supplement, is a common vehicle in nonendemic areas. Carnivores (mink) are usually exposed via infected meat.

Human exposures are contracted in occupations dealing with animals and animal-derived material such as imported hides, wool, and bone. Anthrax occurring under industrial conditions is often the lethal airborne version. Nonindustrial exposures have recently been associated with products such as decorative drums. Cutaneous anthrax infections are the usual form of nonindustrial exposure.

Immunologic Aspects

Hyperimmune sera can prevent and alleviate disease. Antibacterial and antitoxic factors are thought to be involved. In most species, immunity is directed against the PA. Capsular polypeptide fails to stimulate protective antibody.

Immunization of livestock has utilized mostly modified live spore vaccines. Currently, these are derived from avirulent (noncapsulated) mutants. The most widely used is the Sterne vaccine (a strain of *B. anthracis* that lacks the pXO2 plasmid). A cell-free vaccine consisting of concentrated culture filtrate has been used on humans exposed to industrial anthrax, researchers working with *B. anthracis*, or victims of suspected bioterrorism events involving *B. anthracis*. Five intramuscular injections over an 18-month schedule are recommended. Recombinant PA-based vaccines show promise.

Laboratory Diagnosis

Sample Collection. During sample collection, precautions against contamination of the environment are important. Blood may be aspirated from a superficial vessel. Aqueous humor has the added advantage of remoteness from sources of early postmortem contamination. For direct examination, bloody discharges from orifices are sampled.

If the carcass has been opened, spleen material may be collected.

B. anthracis is categorized as a Select Agent and once identified is subject to strict regulations for possession or transport. Only registered facilities and individuals can possess or work with Select Agent pathogens or toxins. The regulations are available on the Center for Disease Control and Prevention web site (http://www.cdc.gov/phpr/dsat.htm, accessed January 11, 2013).

Direct Examination. Blood and organ smears are stained by Gram stain and a capsule stain such as McFadyean's methylene blue. Chains of encapsulated, gram-positive, nonspore-forming rods suggest *B. anthracis*. Contaminant *Bacillus* species are usually not encapsulated and lack the clipped, squared-off appearance of anthrax bacilli. Fluorescent antibody helps in the differentiation.

Isolation and Identification. *B. anthracis* grows on common laboratory media. No hemolytic zones are evident around the colonies, although this feature is true of certain other *Bacillus* contaminants, and the "string of pearls" test (the characteristic cell rounding that occurs when *B. anthracis* contacts penicillin producing a chain of spherical cells (Figure 29.1). Definitive identification is by sensitivity to the γ-bacteriophage.

Experimental animals (mice, guinea pigs) are injected subcutaneously with suspect material. Death from anthrax occurs after 24 h. Lesions include hemorrhages, gelatinous exudate near the inoculation site, and an engorged spleen. The encapsulated agent is demonstrable in blood and tissue.

Immunodiagnosis. *B. anthracis* antigens can be demonstrated in extracts of contaminated products by a precipitation test using antiserum prepared in rabbits by subcutaneous immunization with the Sterne strain (Ascoli test). The test lacks high specificity, in that the thermostable antigens of *B. anthracis* are shared by other *Bacillus* spp., and is dependent on the probability that only *B. anthracis* would proliferate throughout the animal and deposit sufficient antigen to give a positive reaction. Nowadays, it appears to be only used in Eastern Europe.

Molecular Techniques. PCR assays targeting pXO1, pXO2, and chromosome-specific gene targets have been developed.

Treatment, Prevention, and Control

B. anthracis does not normally exhibit antibiotic resistance. Treatment should continue for at least 5 days. In some areas, antiserum is given simultaneously. Antiserum is not available in the United States. In acute anthrax, antimicrobial treatment is often unsuccessful.

Populations at risk are vaccinated annually.

When an outbreak or a case of anthrax has occurred, animal health authorities are notified to supervise control measures. Carcass disposal involves incineration (preferred) or deep burial (>6.5 ft) under a layer of quicklime (anhydrous calcium oxide). Surviving sick animals are isolated and treated. Susceptible livestock are vaccinated. The premises are quarantined for 3 weeks subsequent to the last established case. Milk from infected animals is discarded under appropriate precautions. Barns and fences are disinfected with lye (10% sodium hydroxide). Boiling for 30 min will kill spores on utensils. Surface soil is cleared of spores by treatment with 3% peracetic acid solution at the rate of 8 l (2 gal) per square meter. Some other material can be gas-sterilized with ethylene oxide.

Prevention of anthrax exposure through animal products imported from endemic areas requires disinfection of such material as hair and wool by formaldehyde. Bone meal is sterilized by dry heat (150 °C/3 h) or steam (115 °C/15 min).

Bacillus cereus

B. cereus is a spore-former commonly found in soil and produces cells and colonies similar to that of *B. anthracis*. *B. cereus* cells tend to be motile and produce colonies with zones of complete hemolysis on sheep blood agar plates. Capsule formation is a variable trait in this species. Resistance to β-lactam antibiotics occurs frequently.

B. cereus can cause opportunistic infections, most notably abortions and bovine mastitis. This is often acutely gangrenous and rapidly fatal or destructive to entire quarters. Frequent initiators are udder surgery and intramammary medications.

B. cereus is also responsible for several forms of human food poisoning manifested by diarrhea or vomiting, the former being associated with various foods, the latter mostly with rice. Toxins are involved: an emetic toxin (cereulide) and three secretory enterotoxins (HBL, NHE, T). Spores survive cooking and are kept at temperatures that permit bacterial replication and toxin production.

B. cereus is responsible for endophthalmitis usually following traumatic eye injury. Spores introduced into the vitreous germinate and replicate. Severe pain accompanies a rapid decline in visual acuity, exacerbated by corneal ring abscess formation, periorbital edema, and proptosis. Systemic symptoms include fever, leukocytosis, and general malaise. Several clinical outcomes include the loss of all light perception and the need for enucleation or evisceration.

Anthrax-like disease (severe hemorrhage in the lungs, intestines and other internal organs, and characteristic edema and damage to the lungs) has been reported for *B. cereus* strains harboring *B. anthracis*-like plasmid-borne virulence factors. Strains were isolated from a deceased chimpanzees and a gorilla between 2001 and 2004 in the Taï National Park in Côte d'Ivoire and the Dja Reserve in Cameroon. Sequence analysis revealed a *B. cereus* that harbored pXO1 and pXO2 type plasmids. The isolate produced a capsule that was carbohydrate, rather than poly-γ-D-glutamic acid in composition.

Bacillus subtilis

Prior to the 1950s, aerobic spore-forming bacilli were frequently identified as *Bacillus subtilis*. As such, many of the early infections associated with *B. subtilis* were most likely the result of other members of the pathogenic *Bacillus* members. *B. subtilis* is a common contaminate of soil, water, animal byproducts, surgical instruments, and its occasional identification in human and animal wounds is not surprising. Rare cases of *B. subtilis* isolation from cases of bovine and ovine abortions as well as in mastitis have been reported, but *B. subtilis* has never been determined to be the actual causative agent. In humans, rare infections with *B. subtilis* have led to bacteremia, endocarditis, pneumonia, and septicemia, but each infection was associated with an immunocompromised individual.

Further Reading

Beierlein JM and Anderson AC (2011) New developments in vaccines, inhibitors of anthrax toxins, and antibiotic therapeutics for *Bacillus anthracis*. *Curr Med Chem*, **18**(33), 5083–5094. PMID: 22050756.

Beyer W and Turnbull PC (2009) Anthrax in animals. *Mol Aspects Med*, **30**(6), 481–489.

Driks A (2009) The *Bacillus anthracis* spore. *Mol Aspects Med*, **30**(6), 368–373.

Ndiva Mongoh M, Dyer NW, Stoltenow CL *et al.* (2008) A review of management practices for the control of anthrax in animals: the 2005 anthrax epizootic in North Dakota–case study. *Zoonoses Public Health*, **55**(6), 279–290.

Schwartz M (2009) Dr. Jekyll and Mr. Hyde: a short history of anthrax. *Mol Aspects Med*, **30**(6), 347–355.

Twenhafel NA (2010) Pathology of inhalational anthrax animal models. *Vet Pathol*, **47**(5), 819–830.

30 Corynebacterium

T.G. Nagaraja

Species of the genus *Corynebacterium* (from the Greek word *koryne*, meaning "club") are pleomorphic, non-spore-forming, nonmotile gram-positive rods. Microscopically, they appear coccoid to rods, with some appearing club shaped. Corynebacteria have characteristic cell arrangements described as a "V," stacked in packets of parallel, called "palisades," or crisscrossing cells that appear like "Chinese letters." The pattern (morphology and arrangement) is called "diphtheroid" after the type species *Corynebacterium diphtheriae*, a human pathogen that causes diphtheria in children and young adults. Cells also contain inclusion bodies, called metachromatic granules, which are composed of inorganic polyphosphates that can be visualized by staining with methylene blue.

Corynebacteria have some similarity with the genera *Mycobacterium* and *Nocardia* in that they have a high guanine and cytosine content and have specific cell wall organization composed of peptidoglycan, arabinogalactan, and mycolic acids. The chain lengths of mycolic acids are considerably shorter (28–40 carbons) than those of *Mycobacterium* (60–90 carbons) and *Nocardia* (40–56 carbons), and are usually saturated or have a single double bond.

Species of the genus *Corynebacterium* can be isolated from a variety of habitats, such as soil, water, plants, and animal surfaces. There are a number of species and only few are pathogenic. There are two species that are associated with diseases in animals: *Corynebacterium pseudotuberculosis*, a facultatively intracellular pathogen, which causes abscesses in ruminants and horses, and *Corynebacterium renale* that causes urinary tract infections in ruminants. Also, included in this chapter are *Actinobaculum suis* (previously called *Eubacterium suis* and *Corynebacterium suis*), the cause of urinary tract infection of sows, and *Corynebacterium auriscanis*, associated with otitis externa and dermatitis in dogs.

C. pseudotuberculosis

Descriptive Features

Morphology and Staining. *C. pseudotuberculosis* (Figure 30.1) is a typical diphtheroid that exhibits pleomorphic forms, ranging from coccoid to filamentous, and from 0.5 μm to >3.0 μm in length. They are nonencapsulated, nonmotile, often contain granules, and have fimbriae.

Structure and Composition. The cell wall is typical of gram-positive bacteria, with the addition of meso-diaminopimelic acid, arabinogalactan, and mycolic acids. The cell wall contains a high concentration of lipids.

Cellular Products of Medical Interest. Interestingly, no avirulent strains of *C. pseudotuberculosis* have been reported. Also, no plasmids have been identified in isolates of *C. pseudotuberculosis*. The two major virulence factors are phospholipase D (PLD) and cell wall lipids. PLD is a sphingomyelinase that hydrolyses sphingomyelins of host cell membranes, possibly contributing to spread of infection. The toxin has activity on endothelial cells, lyses erythrocytes of sheep and cattle, exhibits cytotoxicity to macrophages of goats, produces dermal necrosis, and is lethal to a number of laboratory animals. The gene, *pld*, has been cloned and sequenced. A mutant that lacks the *pld* gene does not induce the classic lymph node abscesses in sheep. Also, antitoxin to PLD limits the spread of infection. The PLD inhibits β-toxin of *Staphylococcus aureus* (Figure 30.2) and α-toxin of *Clostridium perfringens*, and its activity on erythrocytes is enhanced in the presence of extracellular factor of *Rhodococcus equi*.

Cell Wall Lipids. The waxy mycolic acid coat on the cell wall surface has well-established cytotoxic activities and is a major factor contributing to pathogenesis. The toxicity of extracted lipid material has been demonstrated by the induction of hemorrhagic necrosis by subcutaneous injection in mice and guinea pigs. The waxy coat provides the organism with mechanical, and possibly biochemical protection against lysosomal enzymes within phagocytic cells. The protection allows the organism to survive as a facultative intracellular pathogen and to facilitate spread of the organism from the site of entry to the eventual site of abscess formation. In fact, the toxicity of mycolic acid is a contributing factor in the formation of abscesses. There is direct relationship between the amount of mycolic acid in isolates and their ability to induce abscesses in mice.

Another factor contributing virulence may be the iron acquisition system.

Veterinary Microbiology, Third Edition. Edited by D. Scott McVey, Melissa Kennedy and M.M. Chengappa.

FIGURE 30.1. *C. pseudotuberculosis in pus from an equine chest abscess. Note club shapes, palisading, "Chinese letter" patterns, pleomorphism (Gram stain, 1000×).*

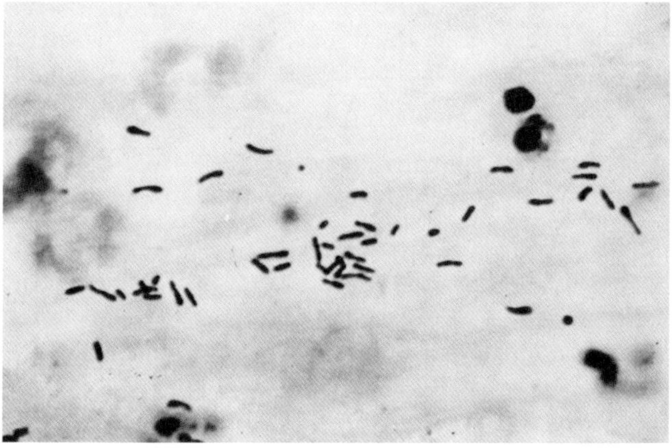

C. pseudotuberculosis possesses a cluster of four genes—*fagA*, *fagB*, *fagC*, and *fagD* (for Fe acquisition gene)—located downstream from the *pld* gene, which encode proteins involved with iron uptake. The uptake system is similar to the one used by enterobactin (a catechol-type of siderophore found in members of the family Enterobacteriaceae). Deletion of the *fagA–fagD* genes attenuates virulence. A secreted serine protease of 40 kDa (CP40) has been shown to be a protective antigen.

Growth Characteristics. *C. pseudotuberculosis* is a facultative anaerobe. It grows best on media containing blood or serum. At 48 h on blood agar (35–37 °C), colonies are off-white, dull, faintly β-hemolytic, and about 1 mm in diameter. They can be pushed across the agar without disintegrating (described as pushing a "hockey puck"), and disperse poorly in liquids because of the waxy coat.

FIGURE 30.2. *Inhibition of staphylococcal β-toxin (phospholipase C) activity on bovine blood agar by C. pseudotuberculosis exotoxin (phospholipase D).*

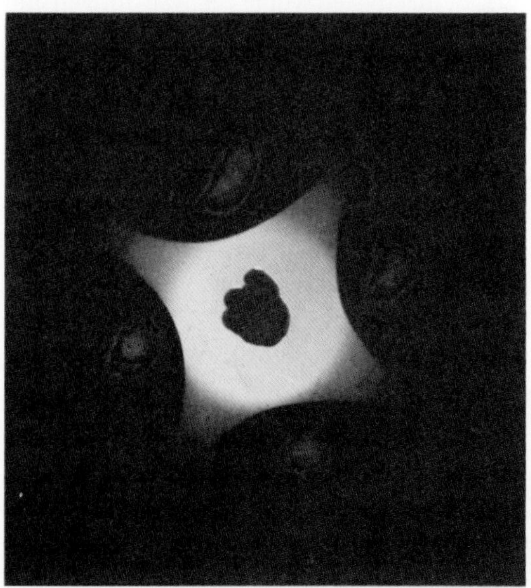

Biochemical Activities. The agent is catalase-positive. All strains produce acid but not gas from glucose, fructose, maltose, mannose, and sucrose.

Resistance. Disinfectants and heat (60 °C) kill *C. pseudotuberculosis*, but organisms survive well where moisture and organic matter abound. Penicillins (including ceftiofur), erythromycin, chloramphenicol, lincomycin, tetracycline, enrofloxacin, and trimethoprim–sulfonamide are inhibitory *in vitro*. The organism is resistant to aminoglycosides.

Variability. It is suggested that there may be "ovine/caprine" and "equine/bovine" biotypes of *C. pseudotuberculosis*, which are in other aspects (antigenic structure and virulence factors) are similar. Isolates from equine and most bovine sources reduce nitrates to nitrites (nitrate-positive); and the "ovine/caprine" isolates from ovine, caprine, and some bovine sources do not (nitrate-negative).

Ecology

Reservoir. The ovine biotype (see Section "Variability") *C. pseudotuberculosis* is found in lesions, the gastrointestinal tract of normal sheep, and the soil of sheep pens. The reservoir of the equine type is not known.

Transmission. Sheep become infected through breaks in the skin (e.g., wounds acquired during shearing, castration, ear tagging, and docking), goats probably following trauma related to butting, and horses following breaks in the skin (e.g., biting flies). The organism has the ability to survive for several weeks in the environment, which contributes to the spread within a herd or flock. In cattle, house flies have been shown to mechanically transmit the organism.

Pathogenesis

Mechanisms. *C. pseudotuberculosis* is a facultatively intracellular pathogen, and its survival within phagocytes is because of the protection afforded by surface lipids. The action of PLD includes increasing the permeability of vascular endothelial cells, activation of complementary pathway of the innate immune system, and impairment of chemotaxis of neutrophils. Following infection, abscesses form but remain localized when exotoxin and/or protease are absent or neutralized.

Pathology. Neutrophilic infiltration and endothelial damage characterize early changes. The lesions are abscesses. Distribution, progress, and appearance differ with species and routes of inoculation, but lymphatic involvement is consistent feature. The nature of the pus varies largely with the age of the lesion, which grossly appears creamy to dry and crumbly ("cheesy"). Old abscesses consist of dead macrophages with peripheral neutrophils, giant cells, and fibrous tissue. Lesions almost always contain just *C. pseudotuberculosis*.

Disease Patterns

Sheep and Goats. *C. pseudotuberculosis* causes caseous lymphadenitis, a chronic and contagious disease of sheep and goats in North America, Europe, Australia, and New Zealand. The disease causes significant economic losses to sheep and goat producers because of the reduction in wool, meat, and milk productions, decreased reproductive efficiencies of affected animals, and condemnation of skins in abattoirs. The disease is characterized by abscess formation in the skin, internal and external lymph nodes, and internal organs. The organism most commonly enters the body through breaks in the skin or mucous membranes. After entry, the organism elicits a diffuse inflammation, followed by the formation of an abscess that coalesces and undergoes encapsulation. Inflammatory cells traverse the capsule peripherally, adding a layer of suppuration and a new capsule. Several such cycles give the lesions, especially in sheep, an "onion ring" appearance. Old lesions acquire thick, fibrous capsules. There are two forms of the disease: an "external form" characterized by infection, at the site of entry, of the subcutaneous tissue and the regional lymph nodes (parotid, mandibular, superficial cervical, subiliac, popliteal, and mammary), and an "internal form" characterized by abscess development in internal organs such as lung, liver, kidneys, uterus, spleen, and internal organs (mediastinal, bronchial, and lumbar). Both forms can occur in the same animal. The internal form is subclinical and is commonly associated with progressive weight loss and ill thrift, a condition called, thin ewe syndrome. Most forms of infection are chronic.

Equine. *C. pseudotuberculosis* infections in horses can occur in three forms: ulcerative lymphangitis, external, and internal abscesses. In case of ulcerative lymphangitis, which is not very common, infection is cellulitis that ascends the lymphatics, usually of the hind limbs, starting at the fetlock. Its progress toward the inguinal region is marked by swelling and abscesses, which rupture to leave ulcers along its course. Hematogenous dissemination is rare. These horses are usually febrile, and exhibit pain and lameness of the affected limb. In the external abscess form, generally a single, often large abscess occurs underneath the abdomen or the pectoral region. The abscess tends to have a thick (few centimeters) capsule filled with a thick yellow to tan pus. The terms "pigeon fever" and "breast bone fever" are often used for the pectoral abscess because of pigeon breast appearance. The infective mechanism is not understood, but the seasonal peak (autumn) and geographic restriction (mainly California) suggest an arthropod vector. The lesions of cutaneous ventral habronemiasis and a midventral dermatitis due to horn fly (*Haematobia irritans*) activity are possible portals of entry. Contagious acne (Canadian horse pox) is an uncommon equine folliculitis due to *C. pseudotuberculosis* infection. The internal abscesses are difficult to recognize, and the most common symptoms are weight loss, fever, depression, and colic. The most common organ to have an internal abscess is the liver, but abscess can also occur on the kidneys, lungs, and spleen. Septicemia occurs rarely, but may result in abortions, renal abscesses, debilitation, and death. The superficial lesions resolve slowly after drainage.

Cattle. Cattle occasionally develop skin infections with lymph node involvement. Such episodes are often acute and can be epidemic. The most common site is the lateral body wall, suggesting that trauma initiates the disease by producing breaks in the skin.

Human Beings. Human infections with *C. pseudotuberculosis* occur rarely, and many of the reported cases are related to occupational exposure (e.g., sheep shearers). Infected humans generally have lymphadenitis and abscesses.

Epidemiology. The current view is that *C. pseudotuberculosis* is an animal parasite and only an accidental soil inhabitant. In sheep, shearing, docking, and dipping are significant factors in the spread of infection. In goats, direct contact, ingestion, and arthropod vectors must be considered. The prevalence of infection increases with age. Caseous lymphadenitis is one of the important bacterial infections of small ruminants.

The hypothesis concerning equine exposure has been considered. No age predilection has been noted. Ulcerative lymphangitis is thought to reflect poor management and is uncommon nowadays. "Pigeon fever" is limited to the far western United States. Annual prevalence varies, seemingly highest after a wet winter.

Immunologic Aspects

The roles of antibody and cell-mediated responses that occur during the infectious process are undefined. Antitoxin against PLD limits dissemination of abscesses.

Bacterins, culture supernatants, or combinations of both provide some protection from the disease. The efficacy of the culture supernatant is attributed to the protective effects of antibodies generated against the PLD exotoxin. Vaccination does not eliminate an established infection but prevents the establishment of infection and lessens the dissemination of an established infection. A vaccine composed of inactivated whole cell wall antigen and PLD toxoid is commercially available for use in sheep. The vaccine is given subcutaneously in sheep after 3 months of age followed by a booster dose in 4 weeks. Adult sheep are vaccinated annually. Most of the vaccines are generally combined with vaccines for other pathogens, particularly *Clostridium*. Experimental DNA vaccines have been evaluated and results have shown some promise.

Laboratory Diagnosis

Although the presence of external abscesses in sheep and goats is highly suggestive of caseous lymphadenitis, a bacteriologic culture is needed to confirm and rule out *Arcanobacterium pyogenes*, another abscess-causing pathogen. Intracellular or extracellular diphtheroid-shaped organisms may be demonstrable in stained direct smears of material from lesions (see Figure 30.1). Blood agar plates inoculated with abscess material and incubated for 24–48 h (35–37 °C) produce small, off-white, faintly hemolytic colonies

FIGURE 30.3. *Synergistic hemolysis by* C. pseudotuberculosis *(center) and* R. equi *(periphery). Hemolysis is maximal where the diffusion zones of the two organisms overlap.*

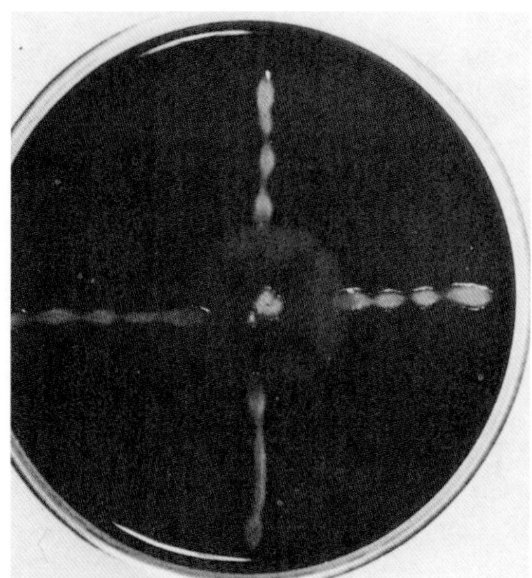

that can be pushed intact ("hockey puck effect") over the agar surface. Inhibition of staphylococcal β-toxin (see Figure 30.2) and synergistic hemolysis with *R. equi* (see Figure 30.3) confirm identification of *C. pseudotuberculosis*. Genus- and species-specific primers have been developed to amplify DNA by using the polymerase chain reaction.

Animals with internal abscesses are difficult to diagnose, although animals with lung abscesses can be diagnosed by radiography and transtracheal aspiration and abscesses in other organs can be visualized by ultrasonography. The synergistic hemolysin inhibition test to detect antibodies directed against the PLD exotoxin can be useful. High titers are highly correlated with internal abscesses. Several tests have been developed to detect anti-PLD antibodies, but most lack either sensitivity or specificity. The usefulness of many of those tests as diagnostic or culling tools is debatable. Some ELISA tests have been reported to be effective in control and eradication programs.

Treatment and Control

Generally, the caseous lymphadenitis abscesses are refractory to antibiotic therapy because of thick encapsulation. However, in sheep and goats, long-term (4–6 weeks) systemic antibiotic (penicillins or erythromycin, often in combination with lipid-soluble rifampin) treatment can be effective in treating internal abscesses and lessening the chance of recurrence of external abscesses. Control is aimed at limiting exposure by segregation or culling of affected animals and at scrupulous sanitary care during activities such as shearing, dipping, and surgical procedures.

Equine abscesses, if external, are handled surgically. Once the abscess is lanced and allowed to drain, the horse heals without complications. Prolonged penicillin therapy is used to prevent or treat ulcerative lymphangitis or the form with internal abscesses.

C. renale Group

The group consists of three species, *renale*, *pilosum*, and *cystitidis*, which were originally classified as serological types of *C. renale*, I, II, and III. All three species colonize the lower urogenital tract of cattle and sometimes sheep. They all cause bovine cystitis and pyelonephritis, but *C. renale* is the most common of the three species and causes the more severe infection. In sheep, *C. renale* can occasionally cause cystitis and pyelonephritis and osteomyelitis in goats. More often, *C. renale* causes ulcerative balanoposthitis ("pizzle rot") in sheep and goats.

Descriptive Features

Morphology and Staining. Members of the *C. renale* group are typical diphtheroids. The cells range from coccoid to filamentous, are non-acid-fast, nonencapsulated, and often contain granules.

Structure and Composition. The cell wall is typical of gram-positive bacteria, with the addition of meso-diaminopimelic acid, arabinogalactan, and mycolic acids (branched-chain fatty acids with a chain length for members of the genus *Corynebacterium* of C22–C38).

Cellular Products of Medical Interest

Pili. All three species of the *C. renale* group have pili.

Urease. All three species of the *C. renale* group produce urease, which is considered to be an important virulence factor. In a rat model, the enzyme has been shown to play a crucial role in establishment of pyelonephritis.

Cell Wall. The gram-positive cell wall contains polysaccharides, and lipids that are of medical interest. The lipoteichoic acids and peptidoglycan of the gram-positive cell wall interact with macrophage cells, resulting in the release of proinflammatory cytokines.

Growth Characteristics. Members of the *C. renale* group are facultative anaerobes capable of growing on most common laboratory media as nonhemolytic, opaque, off-white colonies that develop within 48 h at 37 °C on blood agar.

Biochemical Activities. Members of the *C. renale* group have potent urease activity, which is demonstrable in most strains within minutes of contact with urea. Glucose is slowly fermented, other carbohydrates variably so. All strains are catalase-positive. Members of the *C. renale* group produce an extracellular protein, renalin, which lyses erythrocytes in synergy with β-hemolysin of *S. aureus* (positive CAMP test; see *Streptococcus agalactiae*, Chapter 27).

Resistance. The agents are not particularly resistant to heat, disinfectants, or antimicrobial agents.

Ecology

Reservoir. Members of the *C. renale* group inhabit the lower genital tract, particularly of the vulval region, of apparently healthy cows and prepuce of steers and bulls, and sometimes other ruminants. Occasionally they are implicated in urinary tract infections of sheep, horses, dogs, and nonhuman primates. No human infections have been reported.

Transmission. Organisms pass between animals by direct and indirect contact. Many clinical cases are probably endogenous. They can survive in soil for a long time, and it is possible that pasture could be a source of infection or reinfection.

Pathogenesis

Infection begins with attachment of the bacteria to the epithelium of the lower urinary tract. Pili-mediated attachments to epithelium of the urinary bladder and ammonia production from urea hydrolysis are considered critical in the pathogenesis.

Pathology. A chronic inflammatory process successively involves the bladder, ureter(s), renal pelvis, and renal parenchyma in pyelonephritis in cattle. A similar inflammatory response occurs in small ruminants, but is usually localized to the distal urethra.

Disease Patterns

Cattle. Bovine pyelonephritis is an ascending urinary tract infection, beginning with hemorrhagic cystitis, proceeding to ureteritis and pyelonephritis. Rectal palpation reveals thickened bladder and ureteral walls, distended ureters, and enlarged kidneys with obscured lobulations. Clinical signs include fever, anorexia, with arched back. Urine is voided in small amounts at frequent intervals and contains large amounts of albumin, leukocytes, fibrin, and usually small blood clots. Chronic infections progress to debilitation and death due to uremia. *Corynebacterium cystitidis* causes severe hemorrhagic cystitis with ulceration of the bladder, also progressing to ureteritis and pyelonephritis. *Corynebacterium pilosum* is less pathogenic, and infection results in mild cystitis and rarely ascends to cause pyelonephritis.

Sheep and Goats. Ovine posthitis ("pizzle rot" or "sheath rot"), the more common form of infection in sheep, is a necrotizing inflammation of the prepuce and adjacent tissues in wethers or rams. Disease develops in the presence of the urease-producing bacteria in an area constantly irrigated with urine. Ammonia is thought to initiate the inflammatory process. A similar condition occurs in goats. Only *C. renale* and *C. pilosum* have been found in ovine posthitis.

Epidemiology. Bovine pyelonephritis is found mostly in cows near parturition, appearing as an opportunistic infection by a commensal organism. Bulls are rarely affected, but are commensal hosts of all three species and the sole commensal source of *C. cystitidis*. "Pizzle rot" occurs typically in animals on high-protein diets or grazing legume-rich pasture that is high in proteins, which increase urea excretion, which when hydrolyzed by the bacterial urease produces ammonia and causes irritation, inflammation, and ulceration of the skin. Preputial swelling and urine retention in the sheath may be seen. Pooled urine and purulent exudates inside the prepuce may lead to necrosis. In ewes, the disease is ulcerative vulvovaginitis.

FIGURE 30.4. C. renale *in urinary sediment of a cow with pyelonephritis. Note "diphtheroid" configurations, including palisades and "Chinese letters" (Gram stain, 3000×).*

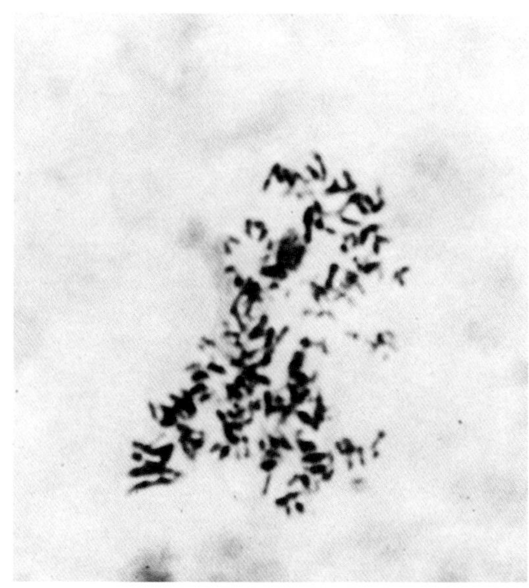

Immunologic Aspects

No useful immunity develops in the course of the infection. Serum antibody is present and antibody coating (mostly IgG) of bacteria in urine occurs in bovine pyelonephritis (not cystitis).

No immunizing agents exist.

Laboratory Diagnosis

Gross examination of urine may reveal the presence of red blood cells and high alkalinity (pH 9.0). Microscopically, packets of pleomorphic gram-positive diphtheroid rods are seen (Figure 30.4). The agent is readily cultured from sediment. A generous inoculum of colonial growth planted in one spot on a Christensen's urea agar slant will produce an alkaline shift, indicating urea hydrolysis, within minutes of inoculation. A diphtheroid isolate from urine capable of producing this reaction and fermenting glucose probably belongs to the *C. renale* group.

Treatment and Control

Members of the *C. renale* group are susceptible to penicillin, but antibiotic therapy is successful only in the early stage of the infection.

Ovine posthitis is treated by surgical care of lesions, local antiseptic applications, dietary restriction, and testosterone administration.

Corynebacterium ulcerans

This is the causative agent of several infections in a variety of animals, including mastitis in dairy cows and in other animals, respiratory infection in macaques, lymphadenitis in sheep and goats, and nasal discharge in cats and dogs. In humans, it is most often involved in pharyngitis, which in some cases has been reported in association with cow's milk. The organism produces exotoxin, PLD, similar to *C. pseudotuberculosis*. Some strains isolated from cases of diphtheria in humans have been shown to carry the prophage with the *tox* gene that encodes for diphtheria-like toxin. Other potential virulence factors include urease and iron-scavenging systems.

C. auriscanis

C. auriscanis is a typical diphtheroid isolated from various disease processes in dogs, mainly otitis externa and pyoderma. It has been isolated from the vagina of normal canines.

Actinobaculum suis

Actinobaculum suis, formerly *Corynebacterium suis*, *Actinomyces suis*, and *Eubacterium suis*, is a diphtheroid that is anaerobic. The new genus was warranted because *A. suis* displayed 10–14% 16S rRNA sequence divergence with the *Actinomyces bovis* cluster of species and 8–11% sequence divergence from species of *Arcanobacterium*.

Descriptive Features

Morphology and Staining. The organism is slender, pleomorphic rods (1–3 × 0.5 μm), arranged singly, in pairs (often at an angle to each other or in palisades), or in small clusters. The cells stain gram-positive, but old cultures are easily decolorized. It is not acid-fast, does not form spores, or has capsules.

Cellular Products of Medical Interest. The organism is piliated and produces urease.

Growth Characteristics. Colonies on blood agar plates are 0.5–3 mm in diameter after 48 h, and often show slightly raised centers (fried-egg appearance) and are non-hemolytic. After 1 week, colonies are slightly larger (3–5 mm) and flatter. The organism grows best at pH 7–8, but does not grow at pH 5 or below.

Biochemical Activities. The organism has a strictly fermentative metabolism. Of the carbohydrates, only maltose, starch, and glycogen are fermented. The organism is urease-positive but is negative for other common biochemical tests.

Transmission

The organism is a normal inhabitant of the preputial sac of the male pig. A high percentage of boars can be carriers.

Pathogenesis

The organism attaches to the epithelium of the urinary tract via pili. The ammonia production from ureolytic activity and subsequent elevation of urine pH may promote bacterial growth.

Disease Patterns

A. suis is a swine pathogen and causes cystitis and pyelonephritis in sows, producing acute or chronic renal failure (see Figure 74.3). The disease occurs worldwide and is recognized primarily not only in Britain and other European countries but also in North America, Australia, and Hong Kong. The disease is more prevalent in older sows housed in gestation stalls possibly because of increased chance for fecal contamination of the perineal region, lack of exercise, reduced water intake, and infrequent urination. Boars are frequent carriers. Urine stagnation promotes bacterial growth. Like bovine pyelonephritis, the disease is an apparently ascending infection. In the acute phase of the infection, the animal is anorexic and unwilling to rise. Pus or blood may be present in the urine. The urine is usually red-brown and has a foul odor. Mortality associated with untreated infections can be high, up to 100%. If the animal survives the infection, it can suffer weight loss and display polyuria and polydipsia. Typically, the sow becomes a repeat breeder with subsequent poor reproductive performance and is culled from the herd.

Diagnosis is generally based on clinical signs. Microscopic examination of purulent material from the urine or from bladder wall, ureter, and kidney pelvis will show a large number of organisms. The urine or other samples should be cultured under anaerobic conditions, and incubation should be for 48–72 h to see colonies.

The organism is susceptible to gram-positive or broad-spectrum antibiotics (penicillins, cephalosporins, erythromycin, clindamycin, and tetracyclines). However, treatment is rarely successful.

Further Reading

Baird GJ and Fontaine MC (2007) *Corynebacterium pseudotuberculosis* and its role in ovine caseous lymphadenitis. *J Comp Path*, **137**, 179–220.

Coyle MB and Lipsky BA (1990) Coryneform bacteria in infectious diseases: clinical and laboratory aspects. *Clin Microbiol Rev*, **3**, 227–246.

Dorellaa FA, Pachecoa LGC, Oliveirab SC *et al.* (2006) *Corynebacterium pseudotuberculosis*: microbiology, biochemical properties, pathogenesis and molecular studies of virulence. *Vet Res*, **37**, 201–218.

Williamson LH (2001) Caseous lymphadenitis in small ruminants. *Vet Clin North Am Food Anim Pract*, **17**, 359–371.

Yanagawa R (1986) Causative agents of bovine pyelonephritis: *Corynebacterium renale*, *C. pilosum*, and *C. cystitidis*. *Prog Vet Microbiol Immun*, **2**, 158–174.

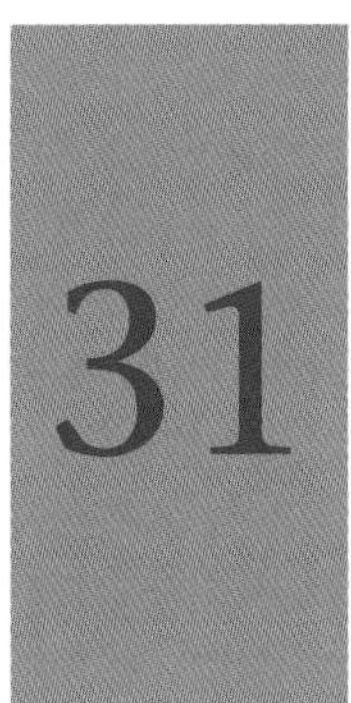

31 Erysipelothrix

TIMOTHY FRANA

Erysipelothrix rhusiopathiae causes erysipelas, an important disease of swine and poultry and a sporadic disease of sheep and lambs. Clinical presentations include septicemia, arthritis, vegetative endocarditis, and generalized skin lesions. The organism is commonly isolated from alimentary and lymphoid tissues of healthy animals as well as the exterior slime layer on fish. *E. rhusiopathiae* can survive for long periods without replication in soil and marine environments. In humans *E. rhusiopathiae* causes erysipeloid, an occupational disease of fish handlers, butchers, and veterinarians and generally results in a self-limiting infection of the hands.

A second species, *Erysipelothrix tonsillarum*, has been described for some strains previously designated as serotypes of *E. rhusiopathiae*. *E. tonsillarum* is biochemically and morphologically similar to *E. rhusiopathiae* but is genetically distinct by DNA–DNA homology. *E. tonsillarum* is only occasionally involved in clinical disease and is nonpathogenic for swine. An additional species, *E. inopinata*, and minor *Erysipelothrix* groups have been described.

Descriptive Features

Morphology and Staining

E. rhusiopathiae produces is a gram-positive, nonmotile, non-acid-fast, non-spore-forming bacillus, which measures 0.2–0.4 μm by 0.8–2.5 μm in size. On subculture, rough colonies may develop and produce filamentous forms ≥60 μm in length.

Structure and Composition

E. rhusiopathiae exhibits a cell wall typical of gram-positive organisms. It contains murein of the B1 delta type. The diamino acid of cell wall peptidoglycan is lysine. The DNA base composition is 35–40 mol% G+C. A polysaccharide capsule has been described and related to virulence. A protective protein, SpaA, shares similarities in the C-terminal region with choline-binding proteins of *Streptococcus pneumoniae.* To date, four different spa types have been identified in *Erysipelothrix* spp. (spaA, spaB1, spaB2, and spaC). Other surface proteins include a 16 kDa hemolysin and 64–66 kDa antigen. It has been suggested that antibody to the latter protein has protective activity.

Cellular Products of Medical Interest

Adhesion. Two adhesive surface proteins (RspA and RspB) have been identified and shown a high degree of binding to fibronectin and type I and IV collagens. It is believed that these proteins participate in initiation of biofilm formation and therefore enhance virulence.

Capsule. *E. rhusiopathiae* produces a heat-labile polysaccharide capsule, which provides resistance to phagocytosis. Capsule-deficient *E. rhusiopathiae* mutant organisms were susceptible to phagocytosis in murine polymorphonuclear leukocytes and did not cause disease in mice.

Cell Wall. The cell wall of the members of this genus is one typical of gram-positive bacteria. The lipoteichoic acids and peptidoglycan of the gram-positive cell wall interact with macrophage cells, resulting in the release of proinflammatory cytokines.

Neuraminidase. Neuraminidases are enzymes that cleave the terminal sialic acids from sialo-glycoconjugates on host cells, leading to a disruption in many functions as well as facilitating biofilm formation. Neuraminidase production varies between strains of *E. rhusiopathiae*, and virulence correlates directly with the amount of enzymes produced.

Hyaluronidase. It is thought that hyaluronidase destroys the polysaccharide matrix holding animal cells together, which allows spreading of a pathogen into tissues. Most strains of *E. rhusiopathiae* will produce hyaluronidase, but there does not appear to be a relationship between virulence and this enzyme.

Growth Characteristics

E. rhusiopathiae grows readily on most standard media. However, growth is enhanced in slightly alkaline media (pH of 7.2–7.6) with the addition of serum and glucose. *E. rhusiopathiae* is a facultative anaerobe preferring a reduced oxygen environment containing 5–10% CO_2. Optimal

Veterinary Microbiology, Third Edition. Edited by D. Scott McVey, Melissa Kennedy and M.M. Chengappa.

growth occurs in 24–48 h at 30–37 °C; however, it is capable of growing over a temperature range of 5–42 °C and a pH range of 6.7–9.2.

Resistance

E. rhusiopathiae is resistant to drying and withstands salting, pickling, and smoking. It survives for up to 6 months in swine feces and fish slime at cool temperatures. It is killed by moist heat (55 °C) in 15 min, but grows in the presence of potassium tellurite (0.05%), crystal violet (0.001%), phenol (0.2%), and sodium azide (0.1%). *E. rhusiopathiae* is susceptible to penicillin, cephalosporin, clindamycin, and fluoroquinolones, but is resistant to novobiocin, sulfonamides, and aminoglycosides. Resistance to erythromycin, oleandomycin, oxytetracycline, and dihydrostreptomycin has been observed. Resistance is apparently not plasmid mediated.

Variability

Common heat-labile antigens account for cross-reactions between strains. Heat-stable somatic antigens account for the existence of at least 25 serotypes. No relationship between host species and serotype has been recognized. Serotypes 3, 7, 10, 14, 20, 22, and 23 exhibit a higher degree of DNA–DNA homology with the type strain of *E. tonsillarum* than with the type strain of *E. rhusiopathiae*. Cultures dissociate on passage from convex, circular, smooth colonies with entire edges to rough colonies with undulate edges. L-forms have been reported.

Ecology

Reservoir

E. rhusiopathiae is widely distributed in nature and is often recovered from sewage effluent, abattoirs, surface slime of fresh and saltwater fish, and soil. It has been recovered from over 50 species of mammals including swine, sheep, lambs, cattle, horses, dogs, mice, and rabbits and 30 species of wild birds such as turkeys, chickens, geese, pheasants, and pigeons. *E. rhusiopathiae* can be isolated from the tonsils and gastrointestinal tracts of apparently healthy pigs, considered the most prominent reservoir.

Transmission

Transmission among animals is mostly by ingestion of contaminated material (food, soil, water, and feces). Wound infections and arthropod bites are other possible routes.

Pathogenesis

Mechanisms

Strains of *E. rhusiopathiae* vary in virulence for reasons not fully understood. Neuraminidase is considered an important virulent factor, and strains that produce high levels of this factor in the logarithmic growth phase are more likely to result in acute septicemic infections versus strains that do not. Neuraminidase cleaves sialic acid present on cell surfaces, leading to vascular damage and hyaline thrombus formation. Neuraminidase also plays a role in bacterial attachment and invasion into cells. Antibodies to neuraminidase are protective against experimental infections in mice. In addition, the presence of capsules has been described and appears to play a role in resistance to phagocytosis by polymorphonuclear leukocytes. Survival inside professional phagocytes is important for pathogenicity. In the presence of normal serum, acapsular mutants do not survive inside phagocytes, whereas encapsulated organisms survive and multiply. In the presence of immune sera, opsonized bacteria are readily eliminated by macrophages and polymorphonuclear leukocytes.

Cutaneous lesions may be seen in animals during the acute septicemia phase or following recovery. These are due to swelling of the endothelium leading to vasculitis, thrombosis, diapedesis, and fibrin deposition. Skin lesions may also appear with a nonsystemic infection due to partial immunity of the host and attack from low-virulence strains.

Localization of *E. rhusiopathiae* in joints of swine leads to fibrinous exudation and pannus formation. Subsequent proliferative changes are primarily due to an immunological response from the formation of immune complexes, activation of complement, and presence of neutrophils, which damages the auricular cartilage and synovial tissues. Joint deterioration becomes chronic and progresses for years. Although *E. rhusiopathiae* can no longer be cultured from joint fluid, the organism or bacterial antigens may persist. Valvular endocarditis is less common than joint involvement and is believed to be initiated by bacterial emboli and vascular inflammation, resulting in chronic changes and damage to the heart valves. Vegetative lesions can lead to valvular insufficiency and congestive heart failure or release emboli that may cause sudden death.

Pathology

Pigs dying from acute erysipelas infections exhibit hemorrhages of the gastric serosa, skeletal and cardiac muscles, and renal cortex. Congestion of lungs, liver, spleen, skin, and urinary bladder is frequent. Vascular damage with microthrombi is observed microscopically. A mononuclear infiltrate predominates in most cases. Raised, pink to purple cutaneous lesions result from vasculitis, thrombosis, and ischemia.

In joints, acute synovitis often proceeds to more chronic articular changes. Synovial membranes become hyperplastic and villous and are infiltrated with mononuclear cells. Spreading of granulation tissue over articular surfaces and erosion of articular cartilage may occur. Ankylosis of the joint may be the ultimate outcome. Localization to intervertebral disks leads to a destructive diskospondylitis.

In valvular endocarditis, the mitral valve is most commonly involved with development of large, valvular vegetations due to fibrin deposition and connective tissue proliferation. Emboli may produce infarcts in the spleen, kidney, and other internal organs.

In turkeys, the pathology associated with erysipelas infections is generally marked by congestion and

FIGURE 31.1. *Valvular endocarditis lesions sometimes seen with* Erysipelothrix *infection in pigs. (Courtesy of Iowa State University Veterinary Diagnostic Laboratory.)*

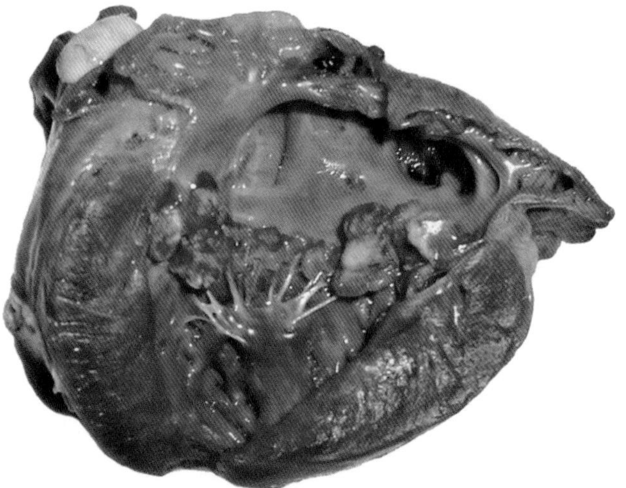

FIGURE 31.2. *Rhomboid, diamond-shaped skin lesions of erysipelas as seen in pigs. (Courtesy of Iowa State University Veterinary Diagnostic Laboratory.)*

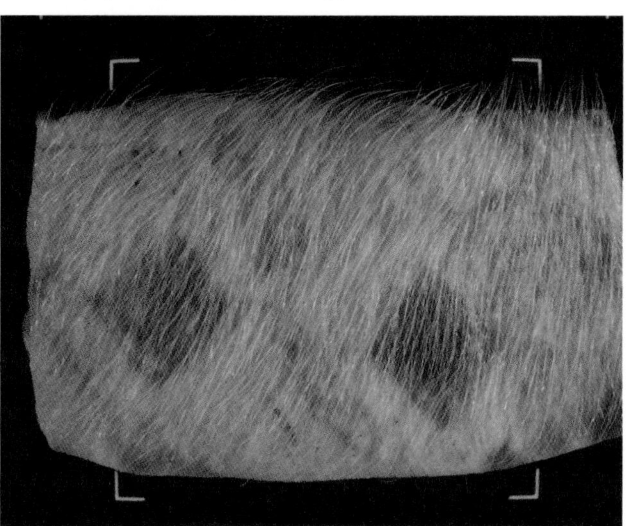

intramuscular and subpleural hemorrhages, particularly affecting breast and leg muscles (Figure 31.1). Hemorrhages are also found in the mucosa of the gizzard and small intestine as well as serosal surfaces of the heart. The liver and spleen are often swollen and the abdominal fat is petechiated. A swollen, cyanotic snood and diffuse reddening of the skin are frequent.

In lambs with polyarthritis, affected joints are swollen and thickened with granulation tissue present on the inner surface of the joint capsule. A clear to cloudy fluid is present with variable numbers of infiltrating polymorphonuclear leukocytes.

Disease Patterns

Swine. Swine with the septicemic form present with fever, anorexia, depression, vomition, stiff gait, and reluctance to walk. Urticarial lesions in the skin may be palpable before becoming visible. They may be pink or, in severe cases, purplish, especially on the abdomen, thighs, ears, and tail. In severe cases, the skin becomes necrotic and is sloughed. If untreated, this form has a high mortality rate.

In a less severe form of erysipelas in swine, lesions are limited to the skin but may be accompanied by a mild fever. Skin lesions are red to purple rhomboids ("diamond skin disease") (Figure 31.2). Lesions may progress to necrosis or resolve, leaving a mild scruffiness to the skin. Mortality is seldom associated with this form.

Localization to certain tissues leads to chronic forms, which may occur as sequelae to the acute stages or without previous illness. A vegetative endocarditis is manifested by signs of cardiac insufficiency or sudden death. Arthritis is the other chronic form seen in swine. Signs include limping, stiff gait, and enlargement of the affected joints. Infrequently, sows abort due to *Erysipelothrix* infection.

Birds. Erysipelas in birds, especially turkeys, is usually a septicemia. Turkeys develop a cyanotic skin, become droopy, and may subsequently die. A swollen cyanotic snood, if present, is considered almost pathognomonic. Mortality rates range from 2% to 25%. Chronic manifestations include vegetative endocarditis and arthritis. Turkeys with endocarditis appear weak and emaciated or die suddenly without prior signs. Other affected avian species include chickens, chukars, ducks, emus, geese, parrots, peacocks, pheasants, and pigeons.

Sheep. Polyarthritis is the most common presentation of *E. rhusiopathiae* infection in sheep. Entry is thought to be through the umbilicus or wounds associated with castration, docking, or shearing. Affected animals have a stiff gait and, often, swollen joints. Any joint may be affected, but most commonly the knee, elbow, hock, and stifle joints are involved. They may have trouble getting up and down. A cutaneous infection following dipping also occurs in sheep. Septicemia, pneumonia, and abortion have also been described in sheep.

Miscellaneous Species. *E. rhusiopathiae* causes arthritis and endocarditis in dogs. *E. tonsillarum* can also be a canine pathogen and has been isolated from dogs with endocarditis. Septicemia and urticaria due to *E. rhusiopathiae* have been reported in dolphins. Human infections of skin and subcutis are called erysipeloid and are seen mostly in animal and fish handlers. Septicemia, endocarditis, and polyarthritis are rare. Human "erysipelas" is a streptococcal infection.

Epidemiology

Pigs less than 3 months and over 3 years of age are least susceptible. Variable passive and active immunity probably accounts for age-related susceptibility. Predisposing factors include environmental stress, dietary change, fatigue, and subclinical aflatoxicosis.

In turkeys, the male is most frequently infected, possibly through fight wounds. Insemination of hens with contaminated semen is an important source of infection. Outbreaks have been reported after contact with sheep or sheep ranges.

In sheep, lambs between 2 and 6 months of age are most commonly affected. The condition is usually associated with poor hygiene at lambing, castration, or docking. A particular form of erysipelas associated with fecal contamination tank fluids used to dip sheep has been described.

Immunologic Aspects

Immune Mechanisms in Pathogenesis

Persistence of antigen in the joint tissue acts as a chronic stimulus for immune reaction and development of arthritis. In addition, an autoimmune process secondary to the erysipelas infection may be responsible for some of the chronic joint changes.

Mechanisms of Resistance and Recovery

Cell-mediated and humoral responses occur, directed at neuraminidase, protective surface protein, and other cell wall components. Serum opsonins apparently play a decisive role. Phagocytosis is carried out primarily by mononuclear phagocytes.

Artificial Immunization

Attenuated live vaccines and bacterins have been used for vaccination in swine and turkeys. The duration of immunity varies from 6 to 12 months for these vaccines and efficacy is variable. While effective against the acute forms, neither type appears to be highly protective against chronic erysipelas. Attenuated vaccines are given orally, parenterally, or, in some countries, by aerosol. Whole-cell bacterins and soluble antigen are given subcutaneously or intramuscularly. Most commercial vaccines are prepared from serotype 2. Cross-protection to acute disease caused by serotypes 1 and 2 has been demonstrated. However, certain strains have been refractory to vaccine-induced immunity. Formalin-inactivated, aluminum hydroxide-absorbed bacterins are available for turkeys and appear to be effective.

Recent studies have focused on the surface protection antigen (spa) as potential vaccine candidates, but to date no commercial products are available.

Passive Immunity

Temporary protection (<2 weeks) with administration of specific immune serum has been utilized in the past. However, treatment must be initiated early in the course of the disease, and antibodies may affect vaccine efficacy if given concurrently. This approach is seldom used any longer.

Laboratory Diagnosis

Specimens

Specimens are collected from appropriate sites according to signs. Blood cultures from several affected animals are useful in diagnosing septicemia. Necropsy specimens include liver, spleen, kidney, heart, and synovial tissue. Recovery of the organisms from skin lesions is also possible. In the more chronic forms, cultures from joints or heart valves are less successful.

Direct Examination

Specimens are examined by Gram stain for the presence of gram-positive rods. A negative result does not preclude infection.

Culture and Isolation

Culture methods for the isolation of *E. rhusiopathiae* have traditionally involved the use of selective and enrichment media. One commonly used enrichment broth is *Erysipelothrix* selective broth (ESB), which contains horse serum, kanamycin, neomycin, and vancomycin. Other enrichment broths described include Bohm's medium containing sodium azide, kanamycin, phenol, and water blue and Shimoji's enrichment broth containing tryptic soy broth, Tween 80, Tris-aminomethane, crystal violet, and sodium azide. In addition, selective agar media including sodium azide crystal violet, nalidixic acid medium, and a modified blood azide agar have been described. These media take advantage of the organism's resistance to various antimicrobials and chemicals. ESB is perhaps the most commonly used enrichment broth in conjunction with selective media. One study found that ESB combined with selective agar medium (colistin nalidixic acid or sodium azide crystal violet) markedly increased detection of *E. rhusiopathiae* from tissues versus direct culture. On blood agar incubated at 37 °C in 10% CO_2, colonies often appear nonhemolytic and pinpoint after 24 h incubation. At 48 h, a greenish hemolysis may be apparent. *E. rhusiopathiae* is catalase- and oxidase-negative and nonmotile. Inoculation of triple sugar iron agar slants will show an acid reaction and H_2S production along the stab line (Figure 31.3). A "pipe cleaner" type of growth occurs in gelatin stab cultures of rough colonies held at room temperature for 3–5 days. *E. rhusiopathiae* does not hydrolyze esculin or urea, reduce nitrates, or produce indole. Fermentative activity is weak. Fermentable carbohydrates include glucose, lactose, levulose, and dextrin. *E. tonsillarum* usually ferments saccharose while *E. rhusiopathiae* does not.

Serology

Serological tests to diagnose erysipelas have been developed. These include plate, tube, and microtitration agglutination, hemagglutination inhibition, complement fixation, enzyme-linked immunosorbent assay, and indirect immunofluorescence assay. However, none are conclusive in acute infections and may only be of value as herd tests in chronic infection cases. Serotyping is useful as a research tool and most commonly utilizes a double agar gel precipitation test. In swine, 76–80% of isolates either serotype 1 or 2 and serotype 1a has been associated with acute infections while serotype 2a more prevalent in chronic forms.

FIGURE 31.3. *Hydrogen sulfide production by* E. rhusiopathiae *along stab line in Kligler's iron agar slant. (Courtesy of Iowa State University Veterinary Diagnostic Laboratory.)*

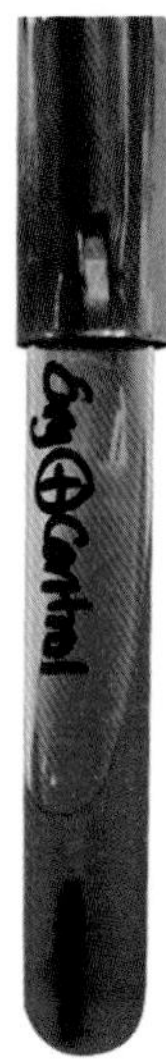

Molecular Identification

Various molecular methods have been described for detecting *E. rhusiopathiae*. Of these polymerase chain reaction (PCR) has the most utility in a diagnostic setting. Conventional PCR assays and real-time PCR assays have been developed. A genus-specific PCR targeting a region in the 16S rRNA gene is quite sensitive in that it can detect less than 20 bacteria from mouse spleen tissue. However, the test cannot differentiate *E. rhusiopathiae* from *E. tonsillarum*. An *E. rhusiopathiae*-specific PCR has been described, but the level of detection is about 1000 bacteria per reaction even with enrichment. Two conventional multiplex PCR assays, which can distinguish *Erysipelothrix* species and some serotypes, are described. These assays have multiple targets for identification but are not quantitative and require post-PCR processing. Recent multiplex real-time PCR assays with enrichment and without enrichment have been described with high sensitivity and specificity. Other molecular methods such as pulse-field gel electrophoresis, restriction fragment length polymorphism, randomly amplified polymorphic DNA, and spaA typing are described, but are mostly used for epidemiological studies or differentiating field and vaccine strains.

Treatment, Control, and Prevention

Treatment with penicillin for at least 5 days is effective against the acute forms of erysipelas in swine and usually results in dramatic improvement with 24–36 h. Other antimicrobials that *E. rhusiopathiae* appears highly sensitive include ampicillin, ceftiofur, clindamycin, enrofloxacin, erythromycin, tiamulin, tilmicosin, and tylosin. Intermediate sensitivity is seen with chlortetracycline, florfenicol, gentamicin, oxytetracycline, and trimethoprim. Resistance to apramycin, neomycin, sulfadimethoxine, sulfachlorpyridazine, and sulfathiazole appears very high. Antiserum (equine origin) is sometimes used in conjunction with antibiotic therapy. Treatment of chronic forms is much less successful.

Good sanitation and nutrition are beneficial in preventing outbreaks. Infected carcasses should be disposed of in a proper manner and replacement animals isolated for at least 30 days before introduction into the herd. A number of single or combination *E. rhusiopathiae* products are available. Immunization with live attenuated vaccines or killed bacterins is recommended in areas with previous history of erysipelas.

In turkeys, penicillin is the drug of choice. Subcutaneous injection of penicillin and vaccination with erysipelas bacterin are recommended, if practicable. Penicillin in the drinking water for 4–5 days has been effective in controlling some outbreaks. Injectable erythromycin is a recommended alternative treatment.

Good management practices including preventing fighting among toms, ensuring proper insemination practices of turkey hens, rotating turkey ranges away from contaminated areas, and using vaccination in areas with a history of erysipelas are useful preventive and control measures.

Further Reading

Bender JS, Irwin CK, Shen HG *et al.* (2011) *Erysipelothrix* spp. genotypes, serotypes, and surface protective antigen types associated with abattoir condemnations. *J Vet Diagn Invest*, **23**, 139–142.

Bender JS, Kinyon JM, Kariyawasam S *et al.* (2009) Comparison of conventional direct and enrichment culture methods for *Erysipelothrix* spp. from experimentally and naturally infected swine. *J Vet Diagn Invest*, **21**, 863–868.

Bender JS, Shen HG, Irwin CK *et al.* (2010) Characterization of *Erysipelothrix* species isolates from clinically affected pigs, environmental samples, and vaccine strains from six recent swine erysipelas outbreaks in the United States. *Clin Vaccine Immunol*, **17**, 1605–1611.

Nagai S, To H, and Kanda A (2008) Differentiation of *Erysipelothrix rhusiopathiae* strains by nucleotide sequence analysis of a hypervariable region in the spaA gene: discrimination of a live vaccine strain from field isolates. *J Vet Diagn Invest*, **20**, 336–342.

Opriessnig T, Hoffman LJ, Harris DL *et al.* (2004) *Erysipelothrix rhusiopathiae*: genetic characterization of midwest US isolates and live commercial vaccines using pulsed-field gel electrophoresis. *J Vet Diagn Invest*, **16**, 101–107.

Pal N, Bender JS, and Opriessnig T (2010) Rapid detection and differentiation of *Erysipelothrix* spp. by a novel multiplex real-time PCR assay. *J Appl Microbiol*, **108**, 1083–1093.

Riley TV, Brooke CJ, and Wang Q (2002) *Erysipelothrix rhusiopathiae*, in *Molecular Medical Microbiology*, vols 1–3 (ed. M Sussman), Academic Press, London, pp. 1057–1064.

Takahashi T, Fujisawa T, Umeno A *et al.* (2008) A taxonomic study on *Erysipelothrix* by DNA-DNA hybridization experiments with numerous strains isolated from extensive origins. *Microbiol Immunol*, **52**, 469–478.

Wang Q, Chang BJ, and Riley TV (2010) *Erysipelothrix rhusiopathiae*. *Vet Microbiol*, **140**, 405–417.

Listeria

SANJEEV NARAYANAN

Listeriosis is a sporadic disease affecting many species of animals and birds, and is of zoonotic importance. Of eight recognized species of *Listeria*—*L. grayi, L. innocua, L. ivanovii, L. marthii, L. monocytogenes, L. recourtiae, L. seeligeri,* and *L. welshimeri*—*L. monocytogenes* and *L. ivanovii* are pathogens of veterinary importance. Two subspecies of *Listeria ivanovii* are recognized—ssp. *ivanovii* and ssp. *londoniensis*.

Ruminants are the most frequently affected domestic species. Principal forms of listeriosis include septicemia, encephalitis, and abortion. In sheep and cattle, abortion is the usual manifestation of *L. ivanovii* infections. Listeriosis occurs worldwide, especially in temperate climates.

Descriptive Features

Morphology and Staining

Listeria is gram-positive, non-acid-fast, non-spore-forming, facultatively intracellular, acapsular rod-shaped bacteria, which measure 0.5–2 μm by 0.4–0.5 μm.

Structure and Composition

Listeria has a typical gram-positive cell wall. Meso-diaminopimelic acid is the major diamino acid. Cell wall polysaccharides determine O-antigen. Peritrichous flagella and motility are present at 22 °C. Motility is poor at 37 °C.

Cellular Products of Medical Interest

Adhesins. Many adhesins including *Listeria* adhesion protein (LAP) have been suggested to serve an important role in attachment and invasion. However, two protein adhesins are considered critical.

ActA. ActA protein is important in intracellular movement by actin polymerization and is also thought to play a role in cell trophism (adhesion) and invasion.

Internalins. Internalins A and B are surface proteins responsible for adhesion and entry into target cells.

Cell Wall. The cell wall of the members of this genus is one typical of gram-positive bacteria. The lipoteichoic acids and peptidoglycan of the gram-positive cell wall interact with macrophage cells, resulting in the release of proinflammatory cytokines. The peptidoglycan layer acts as an anchor for an array of surface-expressed proteins that have a conserved LPxTG motif in their C-terminus. A transpeptidase called sortase is essential for covalent immobilization of such proteins. Some surface adhesins including LAP (see under section on adhesins above) are anchored by this enzyme.

Hemolysin. See Section "Listeriolysin O."

Listeriolysin O. LLO (for listeriolysin O) is a pH-dependent pore-forming, cholesterol-dependent cytolysin that is a major virulence determinant for this species (mutants deficient in this protein have reduced virulence; antibodies to it are protective). The major role of LLO is in the release of *Listeria monocytogenes* from the phagosome into the cytosol following phagosome acidification, under which conditions LLO is most active. Other roles include lysis of ferritin vacuoles and its effect on secondary vesicles formed during *L. monocytogenes* movement from cell to cell. LLO induces apoptosis by modulating mitochondrial dynamics, and release of host cell granzymes. Ivanolysin, another cholesterol-dependent cytolysin, is the counterpart in *L. ivanovii*. (See also streptococcal streptolysin O, in Chapter 27; clostridial perfringolysin O, in Chapter 35; and arcanobacterial pyolysin, in Chapter 28.)

Phospholipases C. Phosphatidylinositol-specific phospholipase C and a lecithinase are important in mediating membrane lysis.

Miscellaneous Products. A bile salt hydrolase may promote survival and persistence of *Listeria* in the intestinal lumen. A protein, termed p60, may play a role in adherence to target cells.

Growth Characteristics

Listeria is facultative anaerobes that grow best under reduced oxygen and increased carbon dioxide concentration. Growth occurs at 4–45 °C, with an optimum at

Veterinary Microbiology, Third Edition. Edited by D. Scott McVey, Melissa Kennedy and M.M. Chengappa.

30–37 °C. Simple laboratory media support growth, preferably at an alkaline or neutral pH. On sheep blood agar, most strains of *L. monocytogenes* produce a narrow zone of hemolysis. Colonies are usually 1–2 mm in diameter and appear blue-green in obliquely transmitted light on solid media such as tryptose agar. Colonies of *L. ivanovii* typically produce a larger and more intense zone of hemolysis. Many commercial *Listeria* selective media are available. Most contain inhibitory compounds for nonlisterial organisms. The compounds include cycloheximide, colistin, acriflavine, amphotericin B, and cefotetan.

Listeria tolerates 0.04% potassium tellurite, 0.025% thallium acetate, 3.75% potassium thiocyanate, 10% NaCl, and 40% bile in media. Most strains grow over a pH range of 5.5–9.6. It has greater heat tolerance than other non-spore-forming bacteria; however, short-time high-temperature pasteurization is effective at killing *Listeria*.

Variability

There are 13 recognized serovars in the *L. monocytogenes* based on somatic (O) and flagellar (H) antigens. Most clinical isolates belong to serovars 1/2a, 1/2b, and 4b; and most food strains belong to serovar 1/2c. Although there is no correlation between serovars and species, strains of serovar 5 are *L. ivanovii*. No relationship between serovars and host specificity has been recognized. Various nucleic acid-based methods have been used to further discriminate between *Listeria* strains for epidemiologic analysis and strain tracking purposes. Whole genome sequencing of species within the genus has recently identified numerous genes found in virulent species but absent in avirulent species.

Smooth and rough colonial variants occur. In rough colonies, filaments of ≥20 μm in length may be observed. L-forms develop on media containing penicillin and have been isolated from clinical cases in humans.

Ecology

Reservoir

Listeria has a worldwide distribution, but more frequently in temperate and colder climates, and has been isolated from soil, silage, sewage effluent, stream water, and over 50 species of animals, including ruminants, swine, horses, dogs, cats, and various species of birds. In some areas, up to 70% of humans are reported to be asymptomatic fecal carriers. Many isolates from environmental samples, previously called *L. monocytogenes*, would now be identified as one of the nonpathogenic species based on current taxonomic criteria.

Transmission

Ingestion of contaminated feed and inhalation are the primary modes of transmission of *Listeria*. Poor-quality silage, with a pH greater than 5.5, is commonly implicated and accounts for listeriosis, often being referred to as "silage disease." An asymptomatic carrier can be a source for further contamination of the environment and, therefore, an indirect source of infection.

Pathogenesis

Mechanisms

Exposure to *Listeria* occurs via the oral or less commonly the nasal route. Most *Listeria* pathogens are destroyed by gastric acids. Use of antacids and H_2 blockers increases survival rate and are considered risk factors for developing listeriosis. Intestinal translocation appears to be a passive process that can involve both intestinal epithelial cells and M cells overlying Peyer's patches. Internalins A and B, two surface proteins, interact with host cell receptors to mediate entry. Internalin A interacts with cell adhesion molecule E-cadherin, and internalin B interacts with hepatocyte growth factor receptor Met. After passage through the intestinal barrier, *Listeria* can be observed in phagocytic cells within the lamina propria. Further dissemination occurs via the bloodstream. Various bacterial ligands have been identified for adherence and include internalin family, ActA and p60. Nonphagocytic cells can internalize listeriae through a zipper-type mechanism. After internalization, listeriae escape from the phagosome, become associated with actin filaments in the cytoplasm, and propel themselves to the cell's plasma membrane via polar assembly of actin filaments (ActA). In this way, they are able to pass to neighboring cells in plasma membrane protrusions and thus avoid host defense mechanisms.

An alternative route of entry into the host has been proposed for CNS infections through damaged oral, nasal, or ocular mucosal surfaces via the neural sheath of peripheral nerve endings, particularly the trigeminal nerve. It is postulated that centripetal migration along cranial nerves leads to infection of the central nervous system. Organisms have been demonstrated in the myelinated axons of the trigeminal nerve and cytoplasm of medullary neurons. The lack of visceral involvement supports a route other than hematogenous, although a primary hematogenous route cannot be discounted.

Pathology

The brain stem is the most commonly involved area in the encephalitic form of the infection. The cerebrospinal fluid may be cloudy and the meningeal vessels are congested. Occasionally, areas of softening (malacia) in the medulla are seen. Histologically, multifocal perivascular cuffing predominated by lymphocytes and histiocytes is commonly observed (Figure 32.1). Focal necrosis and microglial and neutrophilic infiltrates are seen in parenchymal tissue. Resulting microabscesses are characterized by liquefaction of the neuropil. Lesions may be present distributed throughout the brain stem or more frequently are present unilaterally, further supporting the neural migration to the brain.

In the septicemic form, multifocal to diffuse necrosis in the liver (Figure 32.2) and, less frequently, in the spleen may be noted.

In the aborted fetus of ruminants, gross lesions are minimal. Autolysis is usually present as a result of the dead fetus being retained for a period before being expelled.

FIGURE 32.1. *Section from the brain of a cow with the encephalitic form of listeriosis. Perivascular cuffing is present (H & E).* L. monocytogenes *was isolated.*

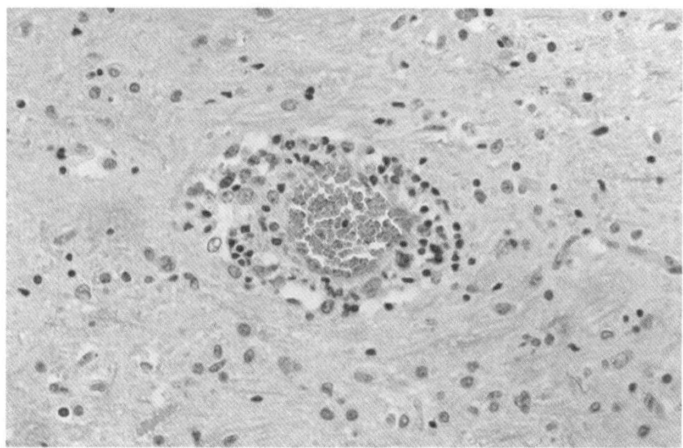

Disease Patterns

Clinical outcome depends on the number of organisms ingested, pathogenic properties of the strain of *Listeria*, and the immune status of the host. Septicemia, encephalitis, and abortion are the major disease forms.

Ruminants

Meningoencephalitis. The encephalitic form, sometimes called "circling disease", is the most common form in ruminants. In cattle, it is subacute to chronic. Signs include depression, anorexia, and tendency to circle in one direction, head pressing or turning of the head to one side, unilateral facial and trigeminal nerve paralysis, and bilateral keratoconjunctivitis. Similar signs are seen in sheep and goats, but the course is more acute and frequently fatal.

Abortion. Abortion is common in ruminants, but also occurs in other species. Abortion is usually late term—after 7 months in cattle and 12 weeks in sheep. The fetus may be macerated or delivered weak and moribund. Retained placenta and metritis may also be resulted. Systemic signs are rare in the cow unless the fetus is retained and triggers a fatal septicemia. Although abortion is usually sporadic, abortion rates of up to 10% have been noted. It is uncommon to find the encephalitic form and abortions occurring in a single outbreak.

FIGURE 32.2. *Section of liver from a 5-week-old foal that died of* L. monocytogenes *septicemia. A severe, diffuse necrotizing hepatitis was present.*

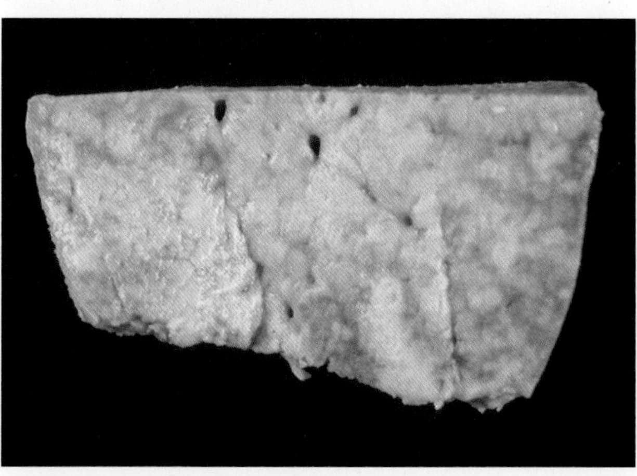

Conjunctivitis. Conjunctivitis in ruminants without associated abortions has been related to feeding on contaminated silage in elevated feed bunkers.

Localized infections such as acute or chronic mastitis are frequently subclinical, and their incidence may therefore be underestimated. Early diagnosis and treatment of listerial mastitis is an important measure to prevent transmission through milk.

Monogastrics and Neonates

The septicemic form marked by depression, inappetence, fever, and death is the most common in monogastric animals, preruminants, and neonates. Multifocal hepatic necrosis is the most common lesion in this form of the disease.

Chinchillas

Chinchillas are particularly susceptible to listerial septicemia.

Horses

Septicemia in neonates is the most common presentation in horses.

Humans

In humans, meningitis (or meningoencephalitis) is the most common form of listeriosis. Reproductive manifestations include abortion, stillbirth, premature birth, or septicemia in the newborn. Hydrocephalus is a frequent sequela of meningitis in newborns. Other clinical conditions include infective endocarditis, oculoglandular disease, and dermatitis.

Epidemiology

The widespread distribution of environmental and animal-associated occurrence of *Listeria* makes localizing the source of a particular outbreak difficult.

Contaminated silage is a classic source of infection. Other sources include particularly organic refuse (e.g., poultry litter). Stress factors predisposing to clinical disease include nutritional deficiencies, environmental conditions (including elevated iron concentrations), underlying disease, and pregnancy. Cases are usually sporadic and may involve up to 5% of cattle herds or 10% of sheep flocks over a 2-month duration. Listeriosis in animals usually occurs in the winter and spring.

Most human cases occur in urban environments in the summer. There are occasional reports of listerial dermatitis in veterinarians and others after handling tissues from listerial abortions. Otherwise, animals are unlikely direct sources of human infections. Human epidemics have been traced to food sources of animal origin, including milk, Latin-style cheeses, hot dogs, and liver paté. Coleslaw made from cabbage originating on a farm with recent history of ovine listeriosis was the source in one outbreak. Another recent outbreak was linked to consumption of whole cantaloupes. In many instances, postprocessing contamination is found to be the source of *Listeria* contamination. Frequently there is also opportunity for selective growth of *L. monocytogenes* to occur during long periods of refrigeration.

Immunologic Aspects

The majority of human cases of listeriosis are associated with immunosuppressed individuals, the elderly, the neonates, and pregnant women. Likewise in animals, neonates and pregnant animals are predisposed; however, in some cases a predisposing immunosuppressive factor is not apparent.

As a facultatively intracellular parasite, *Listeria* is primarily contained by cell-mediated responses. Humoral factors may play some limited role in host defense.

No immunizing preparations have met with significant success. Killed preparations have been ineffective, while live attenuated vaccines afforded some protection in sheep. The sporadic nature of the disease has not warranted vaccination as a primary medium for disease prevention.

Laboratory Diagnosis

Specimens

Laboratory diagnosis is based upon isolation of the organism. Spinal fluid, blood, brain tissue, spleen, liver, abomasal fluid, and/or meconium are cultured, depending on signs, lesions, and tissues available.

Direct Examination

A direct smear of infected tissue may reveal numerous gram-positive rods in septicemias and abortions; however, fewer numbers of organisms are typically observed in the encephalitic form (Figure 32.3). Negative findings are inconclusive. Immunohistochemical staining with specific antisera is also useful in diagnosing encephalitic listeriosis.

Isolation

Samples are plated on sheep blood agar and incubated at 35 °C in 10% CO_2. Isolation of *L. monocytogenes* from brain tissue may be enhanced by pour plate methods. After the initial isolation attempts, remaining tissue is stored at 4 °C for "cold enrichment." Such tissue is subcultured weekly for up to 12 weeks. Cold enrichment is not necessary for isolation from listerial abortions or septicemias.

For samples where contamination is likely, enrichment and the use of selective media (lithium chloride-phenylethanol-moxalactam medium, Oxford medium, or PALCAM *Listeria* selective medium) are advisable. Modified University of Vermont broth, MOPS-buffered *Listeria* enrichment broth, Fraser broth, and modified Oxford agar are essential components for USDA recommended isolation methods from food products. Various DNA-based and antigen-capture methods for detection of *Listeria* have been described, especially in food products.

FIGURE 32.3. *Gram-stained impression smear from the brain stem of a goat with listeriosis. Rare to small numbers of gram-positive, regular rods are present (arrows).*

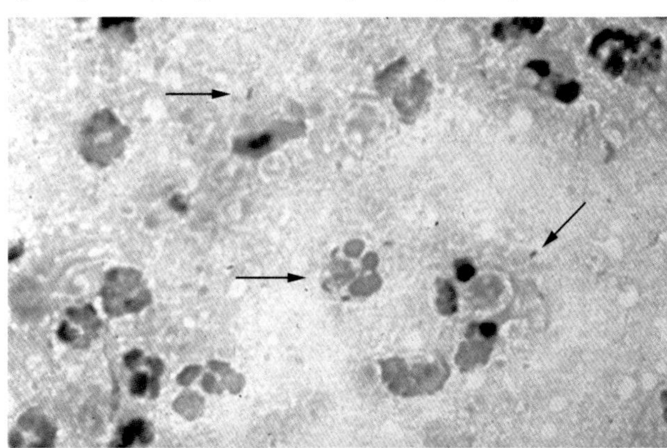

Identification

Typical colonies consisting of gram-positive, regular rods are suggestive. *Listeria* is catalase-positive, motile at 25 °C, and hydrolyzes esculin. *L. monocytogenes* is CAMP-positive when cross-streaked with a β-toxin-producing *Staphylococcus aureus* on 5% washed sheep blood agar. A similar phenomenon is observed when *L. ivanovii* is cross-streaked with *Rhodococcus equi*. A weak CAMP-like reaction is sometimes observed between *L. monocytogenes* and *R. equi* (Figure 32.4). In semisolid motility media incubated at

FIGURE 32.4. *Positive CAMP reactions of* L. monocytogenes *(LM) with* S. aureus *(SA) and* L. ivanovii *(LIV) with* R. equi *(RE). A weak reaction is seen between* L. monocytogenes *and RE. No reaction is detected with* Listeria innocua *(LIN). The variation in the degree of intensity of hemolysis of* L. monocytogenes *compared to* L. ivanovii *is apparent.* L. innocua *is not hemolytic.*

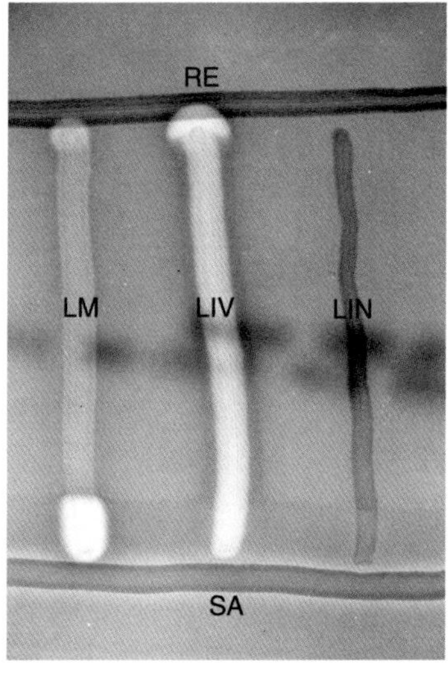

FIGURE 32.5. *Umbrella-type motility of* L. monocytogenes *in semisolid motility media incubated at room temperature.*

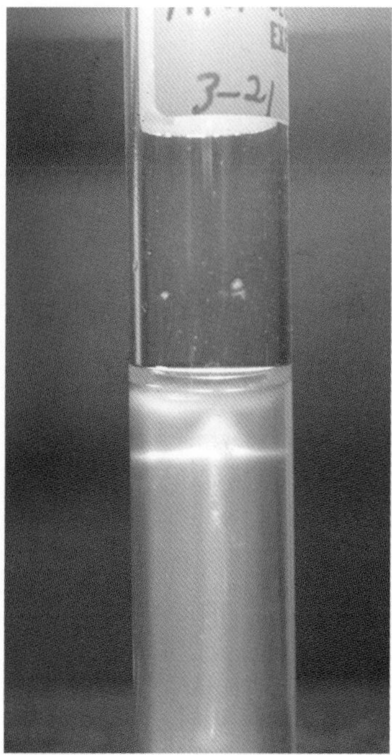

room temperature, a characteristic umbrella pattern of motility develops 3–4 mm below the surface, due to the microaerophilic nature of *Listeria* (Figure 32.5). An end-over-end tumbling type of motility with intermittent periods of quiescence is seen in hanging drop preparations. Acid is produced from glucose and L-rhamnose but not D-mannitol or D-xylose by *L. monocytogenes*. *L. ivanovii* differs by fermenting D-xylose but not L-rhamnose. Fluorescent antibody staining or agglutination with specific antiserum is helpful.

Mouse inoculation causes death within 5 days, with necrotic foci present in the liver. This procedure differentiates *L. monocytogenes* from nonpathogenic species of *Listeria*; however, it is rarely necessary for definitive identification.

Immunodiagnosis

Serology has not been useful for diagnosis due to the prevalence of positive titers in apparently normal animals and cross-reactions with *S. aureus*, *Enterococcus faecalis*, and *Arcanobacterium pyogenes*.

Treatment, Control, and Prevention

L. monocytogenes is susceptible *in vitro* to penicillin, ampicillin, chloramphenicol, erythromycin, enrofloxacin, lincomycin, nosiheptide, rifampin, salinomycin, tetracycline, vancomycin, and virginiamycin. Recent studies report that some isolates are resistant to tetracyclines and fluoroquinolones, and penicillin. Minimum inhibitory concentrations are on a rise. Chlortetracycline and penicillin may be effective in timely treatment of cattle with meningoencephalitis. Treatment of sheep has been less successful.

Control measures include reduction or elimination of feeding of silage, particularly poor-quality silage. All forms of stress should be minimized. Affected animals should be isolated and infected material disposed of properly.

Vaccination has not proven to be highly successful and may not be warranted due to the sporadic nature of the disease.

Further Reading

Maxie GM (ed.) (2007) *Pathology of Domestic Animals*, 5th edn, Saunders-Elsevier, vol. 1, pp. 405–408, vol. 3, pp. 492–493.

NCBI. *Bacterial Taxonomy*, http://www.ncbi.nlm.nih.gov/Taxonomy/ (accessed January 8, 2013).

Quinn PJ, Carter ME, Markey B, and Carter GR (1999) *Clinical Veterinary Microbiology*, Mosby, pp. 170–174.

Summers BA, Cummings JF, and de Lahunta A (1995) *Veterinary Neuropathology*, Mosby, pp. 133–135.

33 Rhodococcus

SETH P. HARRIS AND JOSHUA B. DANIELS

Rhodococcus is a genus of facultative intracellular bacteria that are classified within the Nocardiaceae family. Of the many species of bacteria within the genus *Rhodococcus*, *Rhodococcus equi* is the only one that is typically considered to be a pathogen. Clinical disease presents as pyogranulomatous pneumonia or enteritis in foals less than 6 months of age. Occasionally immunosuppressed adult horses and other animal species including humans can develop disease. The bacteria are found within the environment and foals are exposed within the first few days of life. Infection is seasonal and typically occurs during the dry summer months.

R. equi

Descriptive Features

Morphology and Staining. *R. equi* are strongly gram-positive pleomorphic coccobacilli (Figure 33.1). From solid growth media, cellular forms appear predominantly coccoid measuring approximately 1–5 μm. *R. equi* may stain weakly acid-fast with both the Ziehl–Neelsen and Kinyoun techniques, and the degree of acid-fast staining varies with the age of culture and growth medium. Direct visualization of the organism in tracheal aspirates and bronchoalveolar lavage specimens may be accomplished with Gram stain, Fite's acid-fast stain, and Grocott's methenamine silver stain. Colonies of *R. equi* have a characteristic salmon color.

Structure and Composition. The lipid-rich cell envelope of *Rhodococcus* is relatively resistant to drying, allows the bacterium to survive for months within soil, and confers the acid-fast staining characteristic. The basic cell wall structure is similar to other members of the suprageneric taxon Mycolata and consists of fatty acids and mycolic acids, which are perpendicularly linked to an arabinogalactan polysaccharide. The outer part of the wall contains a variety of lipids including mycolic acids, lipoarabinomannans, trehalose monomycolate, trehalose dimycolate, and cardiolipin. The *R. equi* mycolic acids are covalently bound to the cell wall. The VapA lipoprotein, which is associated with virulence in equine isolates, is located along the surface of the outer membrane. The structure of VapA allows it to anchor within the cell envelope. VapA can be isolated in conjunction with other surface antigens with sonication.

Cellular Products of Medical Interest

Virulence-Associated Proteins. Pathogenic strains of *R. equi* contain an approximately 85–90 kb virulence plasmid. Bacteria lacking this virulence plasmid are considered noninfectious to foals, even when experimentally infected with a high bacterial dose. Avirulent *R. equi* is effectively cleared by the immune system of adult horses and foals. Loss of the virulence plasmid can be induced by serial passage of the bacterium within culture.

The virulence plasmid contains genes for virulence-associated proteins (Vaps), of which VapA is immunodominant in virulent equine isolates. VapA is a 15–17 kDa lipoprotein, which is anchored to the cell wall, and functions to allow survival of the bacteria within macrophages. It does this by preventing fusion of phagosomes with lysosomes. The *vapA* gene requires expression of other virulence factors from the plasmid, such as the positive regulators *virR* and *orf8*. VapA is a ligand for Toll-like receptor 2 (TLR2) in macrophages and dendritic cells. Purified VapA has been shown to induce production of the proinflammatory cytokine tumor necrosis factor, IL-12p40, and nitric oxide in macrophages. Purified VapA in dendritic cells upregulates CD40 and CD86, which are surface-expressed costimulatory molecules.

VapB is a Vap protein related to VapA. However, VapB is slightly larger at approximately 20 kDa and typically isolated from pig strains instead of equine strains of *R. equi*. The *vapA* and *vapB* genes are never coexpressed in the same isolates of *R. equi* indicating that they represent distinct plasmid subpopulations.

Bovine isolates of *R. equi* were historically considered to lack a virulence plasmid as they express neither the *vapA* nor the *vapB* genes. However, recently it was discovered that the bovine isolates do in fact harbor a virulence plasmid, which lacks both the *vapA* and *vapB* genes, a finding consistent with a third unique plasmid subpopulation.

Additional *vapA* homologs, which have been discovered, include the functional *vapC*, *vapD*, *vapE*, *vapG*, and *vapH* and the nonfunctional pseudogenes *vapF*, *vapI*, and *vapX*. The proteins VapC, VapD, and VapE are secreted

Veterinary Microbiology, Third Edition. Edited by D. Scott McVey, Melissa Kennedy and M.M. Chengappa.

FIGURE 33.1. *Histopathology of pneumonia in a foal. Note the cytoplasm of this macrophage is distended by gram-positive coccobacilli (Gram stain, 600×).*

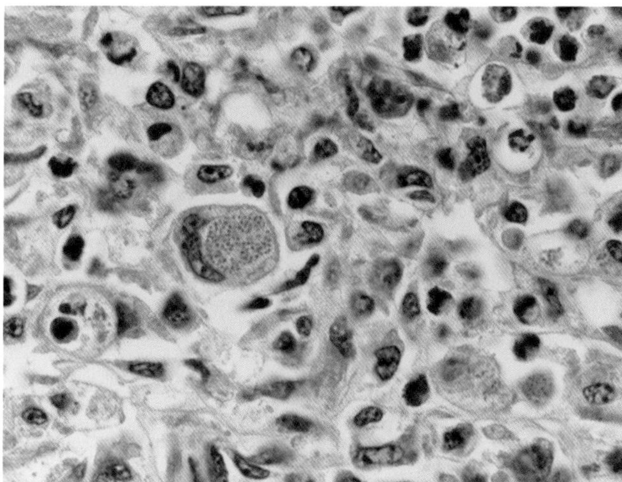

proteins, and similar to VapA have significantly elevated expression at a temperature of 38 °C and a pH <8. These conditions favoring expression of the Vap proteins are associated with the environment encountered inside a host phagosome.

Lipoarabinomannan. Lipoarabinomannan (LAM) is a cell envelope lipid that functions as a virulence factor. The LAM in *R. equi* is structurally unique compared to other Nocardiaceae such as *Mycobacterium tuberculosis* due to its smaller size and reduced arabinose content. While the exact *in vivo* function of *R. equi* LAM has not been determined, it is speculated that it influences the route of phagocytosis by macrophages and the subsequent production of early macrophage cytokines. With the related bacteria *M. tuberculosis*, LAM is needed for bacterial growth and viability and is recognized by the host innate immune system through TLRs. A similar function may occur with *R. equi.*

Cell Wall Lipids. Major extractable cell wall lipids of *R. equi* using a chloroform–methanol technique include trehalose monomycolate, trehalose dimycolate, and cardiolipin. Trehalose monomycolate has a chemical structure of $C_{48}H_{92}O_{13}$, trehalose dimycolate has a structure of $C_{84}H_{162}O_{15}$, and cardiolipin has a structure of $C_{79}H_{154}O_{17}P_2$. Of these cell wall lipids, cytotoxic T-lymphocytes have been shown to recognize and lyse blood-derived macrophages, which present trehalose monomycolate and cardiolipin, but not trehalose dimycolate. The presentation of these lipid antigens is not restricted by equine leukocyte antigen (equine major histocompatibility complex molecules) and is thought to occur through CD1 molecules. All three of these lipid fractions can induce upregulation of IFN-γ production in lymphocytes. This suggests that they may be recognized by CD4+ T cells, or possibly $\gamma\delta$ T cells or natural killer T cells, in addition to aforementioned cytotoxic T cells. The length of the carbon chains in cell wall lipids varies between *R. equi* and other

FIGURE 33.2. *"Milk-drop" appearance of R. equi colonies on culture plate.*

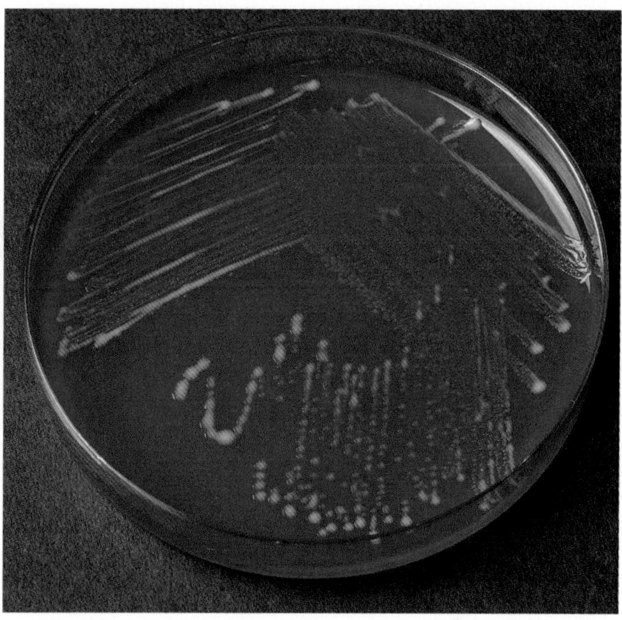

environmental *Rhodococcus* species, which may affect orientation of lipids within CD1 molecules and subsequent recognition by the immune system.

In-Vitro

Growth Characteristics. An obligate aerobe, *R. equi* grows readily on many types of nonselective growth media (e.g., trypticase soy agar with 5% sheep's blood) when incubated in ambient air. At 35–37 °C, pinpoint colonies will typically be visible at 24 h, but after 48 h develop a characteristic mucoid "milk-drop" appearance (Figure 33.2) with colonies that typically range 3–10 mm in diameter and frequently coalesce in areas of dense growth. Colonial growth of most *R. equi* isolates develops a salmon coloration after 3–4 days due to the production of γ-carotene pigment. In animal feces and soil, the organism may replicate at temperatures as low as 10 °C.

Biochemical Activities. The organism is catalase and urea-positive and typically reduces nitrate. *R. equi* does not ferment carbohydrates (asaccharolytic) and is oxidase-negative. An additional phenotypic characteristic that is helpful for laboratory identification is the activity of *R. equi* on a CAMP (Christie Atkins Munch-Petersen) test. *R. equi* produces phospholipases ("equi factors") that enhance the hemolytic activities of *Staphylococcus aureus* β-toxin and *Corynebacterium pseudotuberculosis* phospholipase C (Figure 33.3).

Resistance. *R. equi* is remarkably resistant to acid. This is consistent with the organism's ability to persist in phagolysosomes of alveolar macrophages—an environment with low pH and considerable oxidative stress. Its resistance to acid may be exploited when attempting to

FIGURE 33.3. *Phospholipases from R. equi enhance the hemolytic activities of S. aureus β-toxin and C. pseudotuberculosis phospholipase C (CAMP plate).*

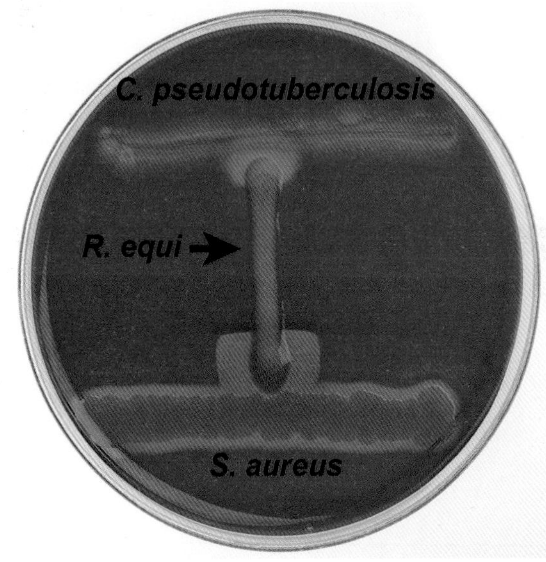

isolate the organism from a heavily contaminated substrate, such as soil or feces. *R. equi* also tolerates ultraviolet light exposure from direct sunlight and is resistant to desiccation, characteristics that help it to persist in equine environments.

In vitro, *R. equi* is susceptible to most antimicrobial agents with gram-positive spectra, with the exception of the β-lactams and tetracycline. *In vivo*, lipophilic antimicrobial agents are most effective particularly rifampin and the macrolides—erythromycin, clarithromycin, and azithromycin. Synergistic killing is achieved when rifampin is combined with a macrolide.

Variability. Over 27 antigenically distinct capsular types of *R. equi* have been described.

Ecology

Reservoir. *R. equi* is found within the soil wherever horses are present, and can become endemic in high-density horse farms. Infected foals are the major source of environmental contamination and can shed 10^6–10^8 bacteria per gram of feces. While adult horses can also shed the bacteria within their feces, it tends to occur sporadically and with a far lower quantity of bacteria. Adult shedding of less than 2000 colony-forming units per gram of feces is common. Bacteria shed by horses may be environmental strains, which lack a virulence plasmid encoding for the *vapA* gene. Pneumonic foals can exhale the bacteria, but it is questionable whether that is a significant route of environmental contamination.

Transmission. Acquisition of bacteria from the environment typically occurs via either ingestion or inhalation. As *R. equi* can survive within soil and foals are naturally coprophagic, it is likely that many foals are initially exposed following ingestion of manure within the first few days of life. However, ingested strains can encompass either virulent or avirulent bacteria, and the bacteria can become part of the normal enteric flora. Ingested *R. equi* from the environment can colonize the gastrointestinal tract rapidly and has been detected in foal feces during the first week of life. Inhalation is considered to be the major route of infection in foals, which leads to respiratory disease. Infection via inhalation normally occurs during the summer months when manure contaminated with virulent *R. equi* becomes desiccated, leading to aerosolization and subsequent inhalation. The route of infection (ingestion vs. inhalation) coupled with the infectious dose and immunological factors may help influence whether a foal will develop disease.

Pathogenesis

Mechanisms. *R. equi* is a facultative intracellular pathogen, which can survive within macrophages after phagocytosis. Phagocytosis is mediated by complement or antibody opsonization, and this plays a role in intracellular survival of the bacteria. Bacteria that are opsonized with antibody enter macrophages via the Fcγ-receptor and are killed as the phagolysosome matures. However, bacteria that are opsonized with the complement component C3b enter the cell through the Mac-1 receptor (CD11b/CD18) and are able to survive intracellularly by impeding phagosomal maturation and acidification. The ability to survive intracellularly is dependent on the presence of the virulence-associated plasmid expressing the VapA surface lipoprotein. Thus, *R. equi* pathogens that lack the virulence plasmid are avirulent in horses, and infections are cleared without pathology, even in foals. However, immunosuppressed animals can become infected with avirulent plasmid-cured bacterial strains.

Pathology. *R. equi* is a parasite of macrophages, which leads to the development of pyogranulomatous pneumonia (Figure 33.4). The severity of the disease can be highly variable with some naturally infected foals developing subclinical infections and others succumbing to disease. The abscesses and granulomas are characterized by centers of neutrophils and necrotic debris, which are surrounded by macrophages, multinucleate giant cells, lymphocytes, and a fibrous capsule. The more acute lesions are less organized, tend to have higher numbers of neutrophils, and lack a well-developed fibrous capsule. The chronic lesions are grossly visible and form well-defined granulomas with caseating centers. Abscesses that rupture can result in severe fibrinous pleuritis or peritonitis, septicemia, shock, and death.

Disease Patterns

Equine. Infected horses are almost always foals less than 6 months of age, with a majority of cases occurring in foals between 1 and 4 months. Affected foals develop pyogranulomatous bronchopneumonia as the most common lesion. The percentage of the lung affected

FIGURE 33.4. *Pyogranulomatous pneumonia from a foal. The lesions vary from caseating to solid. (Courtesy of Duncan Russell, Ohio State University.)*

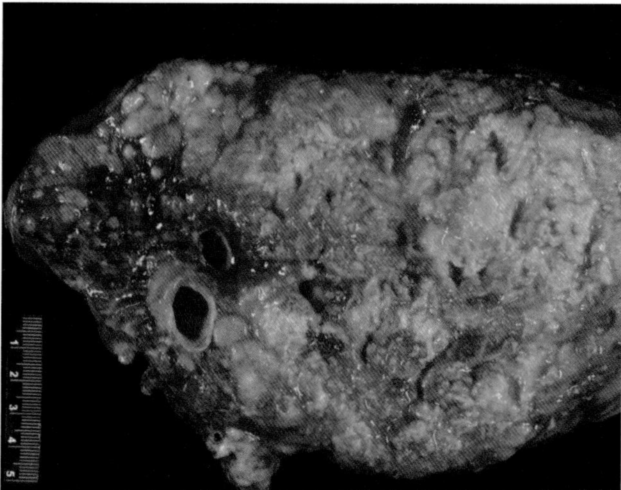

is highly variable. The reported survival rate for rhodococcal pneumonia can vary based on the age of the foal, interval between infection and diagnosis, and treatment protocol. Extrapulmonary infections are estimated to occur in approximately 74% of foals with rhodococcal infections. These can develop complementary to or independent of a respiratory infection. Many of the extrapulmonary infections are subclinical and are only diagnosed at necropsy in foals, which succumb to respiratory disease. The most common extrapulmonary manifestations include diarrhea, immune-mediated polysynovitis, ulcerative enterotyphlocolitis, intra-abdominal abscesses, and abdominal lymphadenitis. Other extrapulmonary disease such as uveitis, hepatitis, and osteomyelitis can rarely occur. Immunocompetent adult horses are nearly universally considered to be protected from disease and mount an effective immune response when experimentally infected, even when exposed to high bacterial challenges. Adult horses with no known immunological impairment rarely develop pneumonia. However, these horses may have an underlying undiagnosed immunodeficiency. Foal isolates from pneumonic animals contain a virulence plasmid encoding for VapA.

Swine. *R. equi* has been recovered from lymph nodes collected from wild and domestic swine. The submaxillary lymph node is the most common site. Swine isolates are considered to be of intermediate virulence and contain a virulence plasmid encoding for VapB.

Cattle. Bovine isolates of *R. equi* are rare and are associated with a low degree of pathogenicity. Cattle isolates typically cause granulomas in a single lymph node, which grossly resemble the lesion of bovine tuberculosis and should be distinguished with additional diagnostic testing. The retropharyngeal, bronchial, and mediastinal nodes are the most common lymph nodes affected. Cows have a lower incidence of infection than either steers or heifers, although an explanation for this epidemiological pattern is lacking. Cattle isolates were thought to not contain a virulence plasmid, although now are known to contain a plasmid that does not code for either VapA or VapB. This is in contrast to isolates from horses and pigs.

Goats. Infections in goats are rare. Multiple hepatic abscesses are the most common presentation. Other affected sites include the lung, lymph nodes, and rarely vertebral bodies. The pattern of abscesses in the liver and lung suggests that the bacterial pathogenesis in this species may involve accessing the enterohepatic circulation. This access may be due to damage within the gastrointestinal tract (e.g., compromised ruminal mucosal barrier due to ruminal acidosis). This has yet to be confirmed. Once within the blood supply, the bacteria can then disseminate to other organ systems. *C. pseudotuberculosis* is the main differential diagnosis as it is a common cause of abscesses in goats. Culture should be used for confirmation in suspected cases. No association with a virulence plasmid has been reported.

Humans. The incidence of *R. equi* in humans has increased with the growing numbers of immunosuppressed people. The AIDS epidemic, organ transplant recipients, and people undergoing chemotherapy are particularly at risk. Very rare reports of *R. equi* infections in immunocompetent people exist. However, immunocompetent individuals tend to have more localized infections and have a far lower mortality rate than the immunocompromised population. Pulmonary infections in humans can mimic tuberculosis. Culture can be used for differentiation of the organisms. Unlike some of the other animal species previously described, there is no required association of a virulence plasmid with human isolates of *R. equi*. Some human isolates contain a virulence plasmid coding for either VapA or VapB, while other isolates are plasmid free.

Others. *R. equi* infections are reported sporadically in a number of animal species including cat, dog, sheep, deer, llama, buffalo, koala, seal, marmoset, alligator, crocodile, and dromedary camels. *R. equi* may be an emerging disease in adult dromedary camels as all of their isolates have an association with the VapA-containing virulence plasmid. *R. equi* has been found in the feces of many clinically normal animal species and may represent part of their normal enteric flora or pass through of ingested environmental bacteria.

Epidemiology

R. equi is present in the environment wherever herbivore manure is present. High-concentration equine breeding farms have elevated bacterial concentrations within the soil. The disease is seasonally dependent, and dry, dusty condition during the late spring to summer predisposes to aerosolization of desiccated manure and soil leading to increased exposure to foals. Young foals are particularly susceptible due to their deficiency in mounting a protective type I immune response.

Immunological Aspects

Most of the features of a protective immune response to *R. equi* have been elucidated through studies in mice, as well as comparing the immune responses of adult horses to foals. These studies demonstrate that the type of immune response developed directly affects the course of infection. A type I immune response (leads to cell mediated immunity) is protective, while a type II immune response (leads to humoral immunity) is detrimental. The protective type I immune response encompasses both CD4+ and CD8+ T-lymphocytes. The CD4+ T-lymphocytes function as the predominant producers of IFN-γ, while CD8+ T-lymphocytes function as cytotoxic T-lymphocytes. Production of IFN-γ by CD4+ T-lymphocytes enhances phagosomal maturation and acidification, which kills intracellular bacteria without lysing the host macrophage. Cytotoxic T-lymphocytes kill intracellular bacteria by directly lysing *R. equi*-infected macrophages.

Rhodococcal pneumonia is considered to be an immune biased disease of which foals are uniquely susceptible. Foals and neonates, in general, are considered to have functionally impaired immune response during the neonatal period. This impairment is likely due to a combination of lack of previous pathogen exposure and subsequent memory response as well as quantitative and qualitative differences in the ability of their immune system to recognize and react appropriately to encountered pathogens. For example, under most circumstances neonates (as opposed to adult horses) develop a type II rather than a type I immune response, which is detrimental to *R. equi* infections. The difference in the neonatal immune system spans both antigen-presenting cells (macrophages and dendritic cells) and lymphocytes. Antigen-presenting cells lack expression of cytokines and costimulatory molecules, and are unable to properly prime lymphocytes during the neonatal period. Therefore, higher levels of surface molecules or differing antigen doses may be necessary to prime an early immune response. Likewise, neonatal CD4+ T-lymphocytes tend to produce lower levels of IFN-γ than adults, and *R. equi*-specific CD8+ cytotoxic T-lymphocytes are lacking early in life. The level of IFN-γ produced by CD4+ T-lymphocytes gradually increases as a foal ages, while *R. equi*-specific cytotoxic T-lymphocytes are absent and appear at adult levels when foals reach 6–8 weeks of age. Despite these impairments under select experimental conditions, foals are able to overcome some of their immune deficiencies. Foals intrabronchially challenged with virulent *R. equi* are able to produce IFN-γ at near adult levels. Foals orally inoculated with virulent *R. equi* during the first 2 weeks of life can develop *R. equi*-specific cytotoxic T lymphocytes by the time they reach 3 weeks of life. Therefore, a number of environmental factors (e.g., age when exposed, route of exposure, and bacterial dose) may influence the course of disease in individual animals.

While antibody is thought to play a role in protection, it alone is not considered to be sufficient to protect against disease. Antibody can function by altering the route of phagocytosis due to utilization of the Fc receptor. Phagocytosis via the Fc receptor is associated with poor bacterial survival in comparison to bacteria that are opsonized with complement that utilize the Mac-1 receptor. Based on this knowledge, hyperimmune plasma has been commercially marketed as a preventative for foals in high-risk areas. Hyperimmune plasma contains a variety of antibody types and other components that can function to enhance the humoral immune system. However, the efficacy of hyperimmune plasma can be highly variable. The variability may be attributed to product differences among the manufacturers as well as a lack of uniformity in product use by the consumers. Companies producing hyperimmune plasma use undisclosed proprietary techniques that impede independent evaluation of the quality of their product. Therefore, factors such as bacterial strain, adjuvant type and route of vaccination that could influence the effectiveness of hyperimmune plasma remain an unknown variable.

To date no effective commercial vaccine for *R. equi* in foals has been produced. It is possible that the immature neonatal immune system in conjunction with early exposure to environmental bacteria may be an obstacle that cannot be overcome with traditional vaccination techniques. Alternative means of vaccination have been attempted including the use of DNA vaccines, vaccination of mares to elevate antibody levels in colostrum consumed by neonatal foals, and oral vaccination. While DNA vaccinations show promise in inducing a type I immune response during the perinatal period in mice, they do not appear to be effective in foals. Likewise, utilization of triton X-extracted antigen to vaccinate mares results in elevation of opsonizing IgG antibody titers, but does not confer protection against *R. equi* pneumonia in foals that have consumed the colostrum. One technique that is currently showing the most promise is vaccination through the oral route. Oral vaccinations have been successfully utilized to protect against pathogens in other animal species such polio in humans. As foals are often initially exposed to environmental *R. equi* through ingestion, an oral vaccine could mimic natural exposure and induce a more appropriate immune response when compared to parenteral vaccination. Foals experimentally vaccinated orally during the first 2 weeks of life with live virulent *R. equi* were shown to not be susceptible to disease from a subsequent airborne challenge. Further safety studies will need to be performed, including specifically monitoring for extrapulmonary infections such as enteritis and lymphadenitis. At this point the oral vaccination strategy is not suitable for widespread use due to the potential risk of seeding the environment with virulent bacteria through the feces.

Laboratory Diagnosis

There is no gold standard for laboratory diagnosis. Transtracheal washes are considered the best means of diagnosis. Fluid from the wash may be examined with cytology, be cultured, or undergo PCR using *R. equi*-specific primers. With cytology the bacteria can be found predominately intracellularly within foamy macrophages and have a watermelon seed shape. In some instances, the shape of the bacteria can be difficult to differentiate from true cocci. Culture can have false-negative results depending on the quality of the specimen and results can be complicated if contaminating bacteria are present. Polymerase chain reaction (PCR) is a more sensitive means of detection than culture, although it carries a risk of false-positive results and needs to be evaluated in conjunction with the clinical history. In cases where transtracheal washes are negative, thoracic radiographs can be used to help make a diagnosis. Initial infections demonstrate an alveolar pattern with poorly defined regions of consolidation. Chronic infections may display nodular masses within the lungs and lymphadenopathy. Serological tests such as ELISA or AGID do not adequately differentiate between diseased and healthy foals.

Treatment and Control

The prognosis of *R. equi* pneumonia in foals is guarded. Approximately 44% of subclinically infected foals in endemic farms will recover without antimicrobial therapy. Foals with clinical disease are treated with a combination of a macrolide antibiotic and rifampin. Clarithromycin is a more effective macrolide than azithromycin or erythromycin, when combined with rifampin. Rare isolates of *R. equi* can be resistant to macrolides or rifampin, and foals infected with these isolates have a higher mortality rate. While there are reports that enrofloxacin has resulted in successful treatment, it carries a risk of articular cartilage toxicity and should not be used in young animals. In endemic farms attempts should be made at early detection and treatment of infection. Early signs of infection include pyrexia and hyperfibrinogenemia, which can be monitored with rectal temperate and a complete blood count with fibrinogen. Some foals display nonspecific clinical signs such as diarrhea and weight loss. Early cases can go undetected for weeks or longer.

Further Reading

Byrne BA, Prescott JF, Palmer GH *et al.* (2001) Virulence plasmid of *Rhodococcus equi* contains inducible gene family encoding secreted proteins. *Infect Immun*, **69**, 650–656.

Dawson TR, Horohov DW, Meijer WG, and Muscatello G (2010) Current understanding of the equine immune response to *Rhodococcus equi*. An immunological review of *R. equi* pneumonia. *Vet Immunol Immunopathol*, **135**, 1–11.

Flynn O, Quigley F, Costello E *et al.* (2001) Virulence-associated protein characterisation of *Rhodococcus equi* isolated from bovine lymph nodes. *Vet Microbiol*, **78**, 221–228.

Garton NJ, Gilleron M, Brando T *et al.* (2002) A novel lipoarabinomannan from the equine pathogen *Rhodococcus equi*. Structure and effect on macrophage cytokine production. *J Biol Chem*, **277**, 31722–31733.

Giguere S, Jacks S, Roberts GD *et al.* (2004) Retrospective comparison of azithromycin, clarithromycin, and erythromycin for the treatment of foals with *Rhodococcus equi* pneumonia. *J Vet Intern Med*, **18**, 568–573.

Harris SP, Hines MT, Mealey RH *et al.* (2011) Early development of cytotoxic T lymphocytes in neonatal foals following oral inoculation with *Rhodococcus equi*. *Vet Immunol Immunopathol*, **141**, 312–316.

Harris SP, Fujiwara N, Mealey RH *et al.* (2010) Identification of *Rhodococcus equi* lipids recognized by host cytotoxic T lymphocytes. *Microbiology*, **156**, 1836–1847.

Hooper-McGrevy KE, Wilkie BN, Prescott JF (2005) Virulence-associated protein-specific serum immunoglobulin G-isotype expression in young foals protected against *Rhodococcus equi* pneumonia by oral immunization with virulent *R. equi*. *Vaccine*, **23**, 5760–5767.

Kinne J, Madarame H, Takai S *et al.* (2011) Disseminated *Rhodococcus equi* infection in dromedary camels (*Camelus dromedarius*). *Vet Microbiol*, **149**, 269–272.

Meijer WG and Prescott JF (2004) *Rhodococcus equi*. *Vet Res*, **35**, 383–396.

Ocampo-Sosa AA, Lewis DA, Navas J *et al.* (2007) Molecular epidemiology of *Rhodococcus equi* based on *traA*, *vapA*, and *vapB* virulence plasmid markers. *J Infect Dis*, **196**, 763–769.

Patton KM, McGuire TC, Hines MT *et al.* (2005) *Rhodococcus equi*-specific cytotoxic T lymphocytes in immune horses and development in asymptomatic foals. *Infect Immun*, **73**, 2083–2093.

Reuss SM, Chaffin MK, and Cohen ND (2009) Extrapulmonary disorders associated with *Rhodococcus equi* infection in foals: 150 cases (1987–2007). *J Am Vet Med Assoc*, **235**, 855–863.

Sutcliffe IC (1997) Macroamphiphilic cell envelope components of *Rhodococcus equi* and closely related bacteria. *Vet Microbiol*, **56**, 287–299.

Venner M, Rodiger A, Laemmer M, and Giguere S (2012) Failure of antimicrobial therapy to accelerate spontaneous healing of subclinical pulmonary abscesses on a farm with endemic infections caused by *Rhodococcus equi*. *Vet J*, **192**, 293–298.

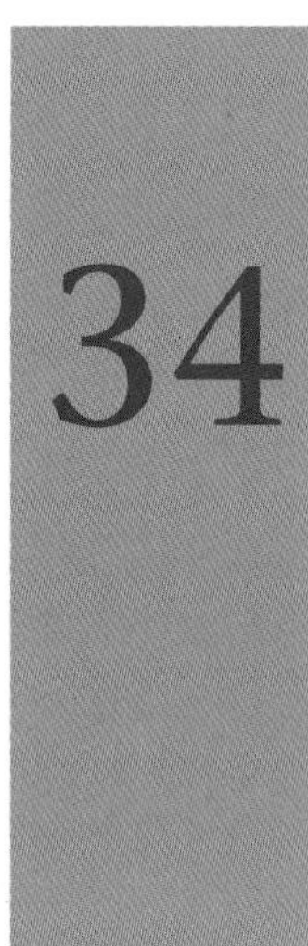

Gram-Negative, Non-spore-Forming Anaerobes

T.G. NAGARAJA

Gram-negative, non-spore-forming anaerobes are commonly encountered in a variety of clinical samples of animals. Most of these species are part of the normal flora of the mucosa lining the mouth, intestine, and upper respiratory, urinary, and genital tracts of animals. Therefore, these organisms are opportunistic pathogens and generally cause infections following the breakdown in mucosal barriers and the entry of the bacteria into normally sterile sites of the body. For example, breakdown in the barrier of the ruminal epithelium allows *Fusobacterium necrophorum*, a member of the ruminal flora, to reach liver via portal circulation to set up abscesses. In recent years, gram-negative, non-spore-forming anaerobes have undergone pronounced reorganization in the taxonomy and nomenclature because of phylogeny-oriented taxonomy approaches, primarily based on 16S rRNA nucleotide sequences. Clinically important gram-negative, non-spore-forming anaerobic bacilli, other than those under *Fusobacterium*, were once grouped primarily in the genus *Bacteroides*, and the genus was regarded as phenotypically heterogeneous. In fact, the taxonomy of gram-negative anaerobes is in a state of constant revision with new genera and species being described. Existing taxa have been reclassified and old species have been renamed. Presently, gram-negative, non-spore-forming bacilli of clinical importance in animals belong primarily to the genera *Bacteroides*, *Dichelobacter*, *Fusobacterium*, *Porphyromonas*, and *Prevotella*.

Descriptive Features

Morphology and Staining

Gram-negative, non-spore-forming anaerobes include rods, cocci, filaments, and spiral organisms. The rods are the most common.

Cellular Anatomy and Composition

The cell wall structure and composition are similar to facultative and aerobic gram-negative bacteria.

Cellular Products of Medical Interest

The ability of pathogenic anaerobes to create an anaerobic microenvironment (low redox potential) or to tolerate oxygen exposure is a prerequisite to their ability to establish infection. Anaerobic microenvironment may be created by the action of certain virulence factors (e.g., endotoxic lipopolysaccharide (LPS), hemolysin, and platelet aggregation factor) or because of synergy with facultative bacteria. Oxygen tolerance allows anaerobes to survive in infected tissues until conditions become more conducive for multiplication and invasion. Many pathogenic gram-negative anaerobes are aerotolerant. *Bacteroides fragilis* and *F. necrophorum*, for example, not only survive but can grow at low oxygen tensions. Superoxide dismutase, and in some instances catalase, protects against the toxic effects of oxygen. Variable amounts of superoxide dismutase are present in gram-negative anaerobes.

The virulence factors of gram-negative, non-spore-forming anaerobes are poorly understood. Although various virulence factors have been identified, the precise mechanisms by which gram-negative anaerobes cause disease are not well defined. However, similar to facultative bacteria, gram-negative anaerobes contain cell structures (e.g., capsule, fimbriae, flagella, agglutinins, adhesins, LPS, and outer membrane proteins) and produce exotoxins (e.g., enterotoxin, hemolysin, and leukotoxin) and extracellular enzymes (e.g., neuraminidase, proteases, DNases, and lipases) that facilitate adherence, colonization, invasion, and tissue destruction. In addition, some fermentation products of anaerobic bacteria (e.g., lactic acid, butyric acid, succinic acid, and ammonia) have inflammatory and cytotoxic effects and contribute to pathogenesis.

The hallmark of infection caused by gram-negative, non-spore-forming anaerobes is abscesses, although septicemic conditions can occasionally be observed. Generally, abscesses are formed closer to the mucosal surfaces or at sites of direct contact, although distant abscesses can be formed because of hematogenous spread. Suppurative infections caused by anaerobic gram-negative bacilli are

Veterinary Microbiology, Third Edition. Edited by D. Scott McVey, Melissa Kennedy and M.M. Chengappa.

often polymicrobial, including both anaerobic and facultative bacteria, suggesting that anaerobic gram-negative bacteria may be of low virulence and that the virulence factors may be of low potency. For example, gram-negative anaerobes possess "conventional" LPS based on chemical structure and biological activity. However, several studies have shown that gram-negative anaerobic bacterial LPSs are biologically less potent than LPS of *Salmonella* or *Escherichia coli*. Association of certain organisms may contribute to synergy, resulting in some cases enhanced infectivity of anaerobes. The mechanisms involved in this synergism may be the supply of energy substrate and essential growth factors, or in the case of facultative bacteria, creation of low redox potential. The frequent association of *F. necrophorum* or *Dichelobacter nodosus* with *Arcanobacterium pyogenes* provides a classic example of synergistic interaction.

Capsule. Capsular substances protect the outer membrane from the membrane attack complex of the complement cascade (in the case of gram-negative anaerobes) and inhibit the bacterium from attachment to, and ingestion by, phagocytic host cells. The capsules of *B. fragilis*, pigmented *Prevotella*, and *Porphyromonas* incite an intense inflammatory response. Capsular polysaccharide of *B. fragilis* can produce abscesses even in the absence of live cells.

Cell Wall. Gram-negative anaerobes contain a typical wall composed of lipoteichoic acids, peptidoglycan, LPS, and protein. The LPS in the outer membrane is an important virulence determinant. The LPS of gram-negative anaerobes has always been considered to be biologically less potent than typical LPS of Enterobacteriaceae. Several conflicting explanations have been suggested, including differences in lipid A composition. However, the LPS of *Fusobacterium* sp. has been reported to be as potent as that of *E. coli* LPS. The interactions of lipoteichoic acids and peptidoglycan with macrophage cells have been shown to release proinflammatory cytokines. The composition of inner and outer membrane proteins of certain gram-negative anaerobes (*B. fragilis*) has been described.

Fimbriae. The fimbriae, if present on anaerobes, play an important role in adhesion, an initial event in the bacteria–host interaction. An example of a fimbriated gram-negative anaerobe is *D nodosus*, a primary causative agent of foot rot in sheep.

Extracellular Products. Exotoxins, enzymes, and metabolic fermentation products with toxic activity have been demonstrated. The two well-characterized exotoxins are leukotoxin produced by *F. necrophorum* and an enterotoxin secreted by *B. fragilis*. Many produce proteolytic and other enzymes that may play a role in their pathogenic activities. IgA proteases, which have been shown to be produced by highly pathogenic species of facultative gram-negative bacteria, are also produced by *Porphyromonas levii*. Short-chain fatty acids, which are produced in great quantities by anaerobes and accumulate at the infected site (contribute to putrid smell), have been shown to impair host phagocytic functions.

Growth Characteristics

Anaerobes do not use oxygen as a final electron acceptor and are able to generate adenosine triphosphate without the use of oxygen. Some are "obligate" anaerobes because molecular oxygen may be toxic and the degree of sensitivity varies with species and even strains. When exposed to molecular oxygen, obligate anaerobes form powerful oxidants, such as hydrogen peroxide, superoxide anions, singlet oxygen, and other oxygen radicals. These oxygen radicals interact with cell macromolecules, proteins, and nucleic acids to cause lethal damage to the cells. Obligate anaerobes lack mechanisms and enzyme systems, such as superoxide dismutase, and catalase, to neutralize the toxic products. Gram-negative anaerobes of clinical importance are generally aerotolerant because many of them do contain superoxide dismutase and can resist exposure to oxygen and the duration of resistance varies with species. Generally, clinical anaerobes can grow in medium that is not prereduced and are able to grow on agar surfaces as long as incubation is carried out under oxygen-free atmosphere.

Ecology

Reservoir and Transmission

The non-spore-forming, gram-negative anaerobes implicated in pyonecrotic lesions are usually part of the normal flora, but they are sometimes transmitted by bites or other trauma involving contaminated fomites.

Pathogenesis

Disease results from the extension of the normal flora (both obligate and facultative anaerobic bacteria) into a compromised site, either by contamination of a wound with nearby normal flora or from inoculation into tissue with biting or contaminated instruments. The kinds of anaerobes found in samples of such material reflect the site of injury or the bacterial population of the source of inoculation. Initiation of infection requires proliferation of anaerobes, which would be facilitated by the establishment of anaerobic conditions by trauma, vascular breakdown, or coinfection with facultative or aerobic bacteria. Synergistic interactions occur between facultative aerobic and anaerobic bacteria. The facultative species scavenge oxygen, curtail phagocytosis of the anaerobic component, provide nutrients (e.g., lactic acid), and may produce enzymes (e.g., β-lactamase) that might protect a penicillin-susceptible facultative or obligate anaerobic partner (and vice versa). Also, in compromised tissue, inflammatory cells and coinoculated facultative bacteria lower the redox potential (Eh) sufficiently for anaerobes to grow. Some anaerobes produce capsules that, due to their chemistry, are potent inducers of abscess formation.

Laboratory Diagnosis

Clinical conditions that are indicative of anaerobic infections include putrid-smelling lesions and discharges, gas in the tissue, deep infections of mucosal or skin surfaces, and necrotic or gangrenous tissues. Specimens that exhibit bacteria on direct examination but are culture-negative by routine cultivation and infections that do not respond to aminoglycoside therapy are also suggestive of anaerobic bacterial involvement.

Sample Collection

Anaerobic culture is time-consuming, expensive, and would require some degree of expertise in handling samples and in isolation and identification. Samples obtained from sites that possess a normal anaerobic flora (feces, oral cavity, and vagina) are not usually cultured anaerobically. Routine anaerobic culture of urine specimens or ear, conjunctival, or nasal swabs is rarely justified. Suppurative and necrotic processes are the most promising sources of clinically significant anaerobic bacteria.

Samples of fluids for anaerobic culture are collected in containers containing little if any air space or oxygen. The easiest way is to collect the sample directly into a syringe and expel all the air. Materials collected onto swabs or bronchial brushes must be placed in culture immediately or into an anaerobic environment (anaerobic transport medium). A number of commercial sample collection or transport systems for anaerobic bacteria are available.

Direct Examination

Examination of stained smears prepared directly from the collected material may give valuable clues regarding the presence of anaerobic bacteria, particularly if aerobic culture comes out negative. Many obligate anaerobes have typical, unique morphologies: rods are usually narrow and thread-like in appearance; some having pointed ends or bulges. Most of the gram-negative species stain poorly with the safranine used in the Gram stain (thus will be pale staining in gram-stained smears). The material may have a putrid odor if anaerobes are present.

Isolation

Generally, anaerobic techniques for bacteriological analysis are based on the following principles:

1. Specimens and samples should be shielded from oxygen (exposure to air should be minimized) prior to bacteriological analysis.
2. Culture media used should have low redox potential. The media generally used include cooked meat broth, sodium thioglycollate medium, and brain-heart infusion (BHI) or *Brucella* medium containing reducing agents (prereduced, anaerobically sterilized medium).
3. Cultures should be incubated in oxygen-free atmosphere. The two most commonly used incubation methods are anaerobic jar and anaerobic glove box. The anaerobic environment is established by the interaction of a hydrogen-containing gas with the oxygen found in air in the presence of a palladium catalyst in a closed container, such as in an anaerobic jar or in a glove box. A major advantage of an anaerobic glove box with a built-in incubator is that inoculated plates can be examined at any time without being exposed to oxygen.

It is always prudent to process samples intended for anaerobic culture with minimal delay. If the sample is not processed immediately after collection, it should be held in a container free from oxygen, usually a container into which oxygen-free gas (e.g., O_2-free CO_2) is flowing. The sample is plated onto a blood agar (usually with a BHI or *Brucella* agar base) that has been stored in an anaerobic environment. After the plate has been inoculated, it is placed into an anaerobic environment and incubated at 37 °C.

Most obligate anaerobes grow slowly, especially during the early stages, and plates are not examined for the first 48 h unless they can be examined in an O_2-free environment (e.g., in a glove box). Because facultative species can grow anaerobically, colonies growing in an anaerobic environment must be tested for aerotolerance.

Identification

After an isolate has been shown to be an obligate anaerobe, the genus to which it belongs is determined by shape, gram-staining characteristics, growth in the presence of various antibiotics, and metabolic by-products formed from an assortment of substrates, as determined by liquid–gas chromatography. Reactions in prereduced, anaerobically sterilized media containing different substrates help determine the species. Rapid and miniaturized systems are commercially available for identification of anaerobes of clinical importance.

Treatment, Control, and Prevention

Treatment of infectious processes caused by anaerobes typically involves drainage of abscesses and the use of antimicrobial agents. Susceptibility data are usually not available for at least 48–72 h after the sample is collected. Prior to this time, if the presence of anaerobes is suggested by the clinical presentation, direct smear, and other circumstances (odor), one of the following can be used: penicillin (ampicillin and amoxicillin), chloramphenicol, tetracyclines, metronidazole, and clindamycin. Although most anaerobes will test "susceptible" to trimethoprim–sulfonamides *in vitro*, this combination has unpredictable activity *in vivo* due to the presence of thymidine in necrotic material. The obligate anaerobes are resistant to all of the aminoglycoside antimicrobial agents as well as to most of the fluoroquinolones (trovafloxacin is the exception). Approximately 10–20% of the isolates, usually members of the *B. fragilis* group, will be resistant to the penicillins (penicillin G, ampicillin, and amoxicillin) and first- and second-generation cephalosporins due to the production of a cephalosporinase, and often to tetracycline as well. Resistant isolates are susceptible to clavulanic acid–amoxicillin, clindamycin, metronidazole, and chloramphenicol. Antimicrobial therapy should be aimed at both the facultative and obligate anaerobic bacteria.

D. nodosus

The organism, formerly *Bacteroides nodosus*, is the primary etiologic agent of foot rot in sheep and goats. Foot rot is a contagious and debilitating hoof disease that begins as an interdigital dermatitis, which progresses into formation of lesions on the interdigital wall of the hoof, leading to separation of the keratinous hoof from the underlying tissue. The obvious clinical signs are lameness and loss of body condition because of reduced feed intake and in some cases death from a combination of starvation, thirst, and systemic bacterial infections in sheep that are recumbent for prolonged periods. In addition to *D. nodosus*, another gram-negative anaerobe, *F. necrophorum* (described later), and a gram-positive, facultative bacterium, *A. pyogenes*, are implicated. In pen trials, *F. necrophorum* has been shown to be required for infection of foot to be initiated by *D. nodosus* and a strong association of the two bacteria has been shown in field cases of foot rot in New Zealand. There is indication that *F. necrophorum* associated with sheep foot rot may be a distinct variant of *F. necrophorum* involved in bovine foot rot.

Descriptive Features

Structure. *D. nodosus* is a straight or slightly curved rod measuring 1–1.7 to 3–10 μm. In smears from lesions, the rods exhibit terminal swellings giving the appearance of "dumbbell" (Figure 34.1); however, the feature is less discernible when clinical isolates are subcultured in broth. The organism is not flagellated but possesses long filamentous appendages, called type IV fimbriae, because of their polar location and the conserved structure of the major fimbrial subunit protein (similar to type IV of *Moraxella bovis*, *Neisseria gonorrhoeae*, *Pasteurella multocida*, and *Pseudomonas aeruginosa*). Type IV fimbriae confer flagella-independent motility, called twitching motility. The fimbrial proteins are highly immunogenic and are the basis of serotyping of *D. nodosus*.

FIGURE 34.1. *Exudate from ovine foot rot. Mixture of bacterial species, with* D. nodosus *recognizable as large rods with swollen ends: "dumbbells" (arrows) (Gram stain, 1000×).*

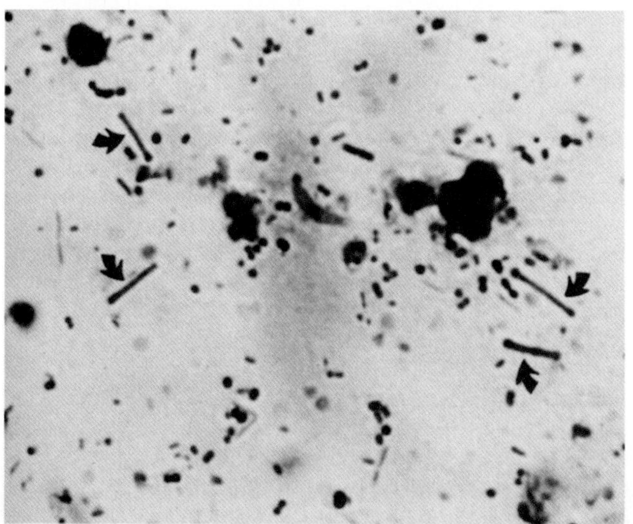

Cellular Products of Medical Interest

Fimbriae. The fimbriae are involved with adherence of *D. nodosus* to epithelial cells of interdigital epidermis. The role of fimbriae in causing foot rot involves initially the promotion of close contact between *D. nodosus* and host cells. The twitching motility then enables translocation of the organism into a more anaerobic microenvironment, which is required for the bacterial growth and extracellular protease production, ultimately leading to lesion formation. Therefore, the twitching motility and production of extracellular proteases are key processes for virulence.

Cell Wall. The physicochemical and biological characteristics of LPS of *D. nodosus* are similar to LPS of other gram-negative bacteria.

Outer Membrane Proteins. These are not known to play a direct role in the pathogenesis but are thought to interfere with the host's immune response. The outer membrane proteins are highly antigenic and phase variant as a result of site-specific inversions within the outer membrane protein genes. The phase variance allows *D. nodosus* to undergo antigenic shifts to evade the immune system during the course of infection.

Serine Proteases. Strains of *D. nodosus* secrete three closely related serine proteases that have been postulated to be responsible for the tissue damage in foot rot infections. All proteases have a similar structure, and are synthesized with a preproregion at the N-terminus of the mature protease and a C-terminal extension. The cleavage of both of these regions results in the active proteases. Highly virulent strains produce two acidic proteases, AprV2 and AprV5, and one basic protease, BprV. The AprV2 has been shown to be essential for virulence because a mutant lacking the *aprV2* does not cause the disease. Strains that cause benign lesions produce similar proteases designated as AprB2, AprB5, and BprB, which only show minor differences in amino acid sequences compared to the proteases of the virulent strains. The protease genes are located on pathogenicity islands (a cluster of genes encoding virulence determinant(s), an integrase protein, a specific insertion site, and mobility), which suggests that they may have originated from extrachromosomal sources.

The strains of *D. nodosus* have a wide range of virulence and are categorized as virulent, benign, and intermediate. The virulence can be tested *in vitro* for the presence and activity of certain virulence factors (e.g., proteases and twitching motility). Certain genes, such as *intA* (formerly *vap*) and *vrl* (virulence-related locus), have been associated with virulence. These genes do not encode any known virulence factors. Possibly, they may play a regulatory role in gene expressions.

Growth Characteristics. *D. nodosus* requires carbon dioxide and a rich medium, preferably containing protein for growth. Although colonies may be visible on plates after 2 days, at least 4–5 days of incubation are required to see smooth colonies of about 1–2 mm in diameter.

Resistance. Although described as a "strict" anaerobe, the organism is highly aerotolerant and can survive on plates exposed to air for up to 10 days. *D. nodosus* survives in the environment for 2–3 days and is killed by disinfectants and many antibiotics. The organism can survive in and transmitted via soil and can also persist for months as a subclinical infection in the interdigital skin or in small cryptic lesions within the hoof.

Variability. Colony morphological variation and virulence are related to abundance of fimbriae. Virulence also varies with proteolytic activities of strains. Ten major serogroups (A–I and M) are recognized, and are based upon differences in the antigenic constitution of the fimbrial adhesins. Based on the structural variation within the fimbrial protein FimA and the genetic organization of the *fimA* gene, the isolates of *D. nodosus* from the 10 serogroups are divided into two major classes. The isolates in serogroups A–C, E–G, I, and M that have the *fimB* gene (downstream to *fimA* gene), which is not required for fimbrial synthesis, belong to class I. The isolates in serogroups D and H that contain three genes adjacent to *fimA*, *fimC*, *fimD*, and *fimZ* of unknown functions belong to class II. The fimbrial subunits of class II isolates have more in common with *P. aeruginosa* and *M. bovis*.

Ecology

Reservoir. The significant reservoir is the infected foot of sheep or goats. Cattle and swine strains are of low virulence.

Transmission. Transmission is by direct or indirect contact. The brief environmental survival time of the agent requires prompt colonization of new hosts.

Pathogenesis. Pathogenic mechanisms include the fimbriae-mediated attachment to host cells, proteolytic activity, and synergy with *F. necrophorum*, to which *D. nodosus* supplies growth factors.

Disease Patterns. Foot rot is characterized by an exudative inflammation, followed by necrosis, of the epidermal tissues of the hoof. Three different forms of the disease have been recognized: virulent, intermediate, and benign. The virulence of a specific outbreak is governed by the population type of *D. nodosus* and the various factors that affect the infections, including environmental factors. The virulent form of foot rot is characterized by destruction of the horn, erosion of the skin–horn junction that penetrates the underlying tissues causing delamination. The virulent form is also highly contagious and has significant impact on productivity. The benign form has inflammation of the interdigital skin with dermatitis but no destruction of the underlying tissues and delamination. The sequence of events is typically as follows:

1. The interdigital epidermis is softened and easily damaged because of persistent soaking.
2. *F. necrophorum*, a soil organism, infects the damaged skin and produces superficial inflammation, hyperkeratosis, parakeratosis, and necrosis.
3. *D. nodosus* colonizes (with the aid of fimbriae) and proliferates in the lesion initiated by *F. necrophorum*, producing interdigital swelling. Invasion of epidermal structures begins at the medial aspect of the claw and, probably with the help of secreted proteases, advances to the epidermal matrix of the hoof, eventually separating it from the underlying dermal tissues ("underrunning").

Secondary invaders help maintain or aggravate the process. The result is extreme lameness, which becomes immobilizing when two or more feet are involved.

Epidemiology. Although *D. nodosus* is specific to sheep and goats, the organism is reported in foot lesions of other animals, including cattle, horses, pigs, deer, and so on. The disease occurs on all continents. It is most serious in regions with a mild climate and periods of abundant rainfall (>20 inches (500 mm)). Dissemination of *D. nodosus* essentially ceases at ambient mean temperatures of less than 50 °F (10 °C), and foot rot does not occur in arid regions and improves during dry periods in endemic areas. All ages of animals beyond nursing stages are susceptible, but genetic differences in susceptibility exist. Fine wool breeds are most severely affected. The agent is eliminated from contaminated pastures within 2 weeks.

Immunologic Aspects. Resistance is related to circulating antifimbrial antibody; it is serogroup specific. Natural infection produces no immunity. Even sheep that have recently recovered from foot rot are susceptible to reinfection.

Laboratory Diagnosis

Diagnosis is usually based on obvious clinical signs. Direct smears from the foot lesion may reveal stout rods with terminal swellings (see Figure 34.1). Culture-based diagnosis is not routinely done because of fastidious growth requirements and slow growth of the organism. A test that determines digestion of elastin (elastase activity) has shown a good correlation with virulence. A rapid alternative to the elastase test is the gelatin gel test, which is based on the thermostability of the secreted proteases. Molecular techniques utilizing the gene probes, polymerase chain reaction (PCR) (genes encoding the fimbrial adhesins or *intA* gene), and monoclonal antibodies (against proteases) have improved diagnosis and determination of the association of virulent strains.

Treatment and Control

Treatment begins with removal and exposure of diseased tissue by hoof trimming (foot paring), followed by topical application of disinfectants or antibiotics, such as repeated treatment with 5–10% formalin, 5% copper sulfate, 10–20% zinc sulfate, or 5% tetracycline tincture. Formalin, copper sulfate, and zinc sulfate are used in footbaths. Three 1 h 20% zinc sulfate soaks at weekly intervals have proven effective without foot paring. Systemic treatment with large doses of penicillin and streptomycin has been successful in the absence of topical therapy.

Vaccines have been shown to be effective in treating and preventing foot rot. Vaccination is extensively used in sheep-producing countries, particularly Australia and New Zealand, and is an integral part of the eradication programs. Vaccination also has some therapeutic benefit in accelerating healing. The effective vaccines are based on fimbrial proteins as the protective antigen. There is reasonable correlation between serum antifimbrial agglutinin titers and resistance of vaccinated sheep to homologous infection. The limitation of the vaccine is the need to protect multistrain infections, and inclusion of multistrains in a vaccine reduces the effectiveness because of antigenic competition. Commercially available vaccines contain 8–10 strains of the common serogroups. Use of monovalent vaccine is useful, but requires isolation and identification of the serogroup.

Control is achieved by a combination of repeated examination, vaccination, treatment of active cases, and segregation of active cases from the healthy flock. Care must be taken to avoid adding infected animals to the flock. Contaminated lots should not be restocked for 2 weeks. Control programs should be instituted during dry weather.

F. necrophorum

The name, *Fusobacterium*, comes from the Latin word *fusus* meaning "spindle." However, not all fusobacterial species have the characteristic spindle-shaped cells. A common biochemical feature of members of the genus is the production of butyric acid as a major fermentation product. Although fusobacteria stain gram-negative, the organisms are related more to the gram-positive phylum. For example, fusobacterial species are susceptible to typically gram-positive antibacterial spectrum antibiotics such as penicillins, tylosin, and virginiamycin. Currently, the genus *Fusobacterium* includes the following species: *F. canifelinum*, *F. equinum*, *F. gonidiaformans*, *F. mortiferum*, *F. naviforme*, *F. necrogenes*, *F. necrophorum*, *F. nucleatum*, *F. perfoetans*, *F. periodonticum*, *F. plautii*, *F. polysaccharolyticum*, *F. russi*, *F. simae*, *F. ulcerans*, and *F. varium*. Of these *F. nucleatum* and *F. necrophorum* are the two most prevalent species of *Fusobacterium* in clinical samples. Both species are further categorized into two or more subspecies.

Fusobacterium canifelinum, *F. mortiferum*, *F. naviforme*, *F. nucleatum*, *F. periodonticum*, *F. ulcerans*, and *F. varium* have been isolated mainly from human clinical samples. *F. canifelinum* and *F. russi* are members of the canine and feline flora and have been isolated from infected dog and cat bite wounds in humans. *Fusobacterium nucleatum* is one of the predominant organisms involved in gingivitis and periodontal diseases, particularly in children and young adults. *Fusobacterium equinum*, *F. necrogenes*, and *F. simiae* are isolated mainly from animal infections. *F. equinum* is relatively a new species, which is phenotypically similar to *F. necrophorum*, and has been isolated from the normal oral cavity and oral-associated diseases of horses.

F. necrophorum is a major human and animal pathogen and is part of the bacterial flora of the oral cavities, gastrointestinal tracts, and genitourinary tracts of animals and humans. The species name is derived from the organism's frequent association with necrotic lesions in humans and animals. In humans, *F. necrophorum* is an important cause of pharyngitis, especially in young adults, being second only to group A streptococci. Occasionally, it is associated with a condition called Lemierre's syndrome that primarily affects young and healthy persons. The infection starts out as an acute sore throat with purulent exudate, high fever, cervical, and submandibular lymphadenopathy that rapidly leads to disseminated metastatic abscesses, frequently involving septic thrombophlebitis of the internal jugular vein. In animals, *F. necrophorum* is considered as a major bovine pathogen because of its involvement in certain economically important diseases. It is one of the most common anaerobes isolated from abscesses in the abdominal area and respiratory tract infections in animals.

Descriptive Features

F. necrophorum is classified into three biotypes or biovars: A, B, and AB. Biotype AB has been isolated from sheep foot abscesses and has characteristics, including 16S ribosomal RNA sequence, of both biotypes A and B. Currently, the taxonomic status of biotype AB is unresolved. The biotypes have been assigned subspecies status; biotype A is ssp. *necrophorum* and biotype B is ssp. *funduliforme*. These two subspecies differ in cell morphology, colony characteristics, growth patterns in broth, extracellular enzymes, hemagglutination properties, hemolytic activities, leukotoxin activities, chemical composition of LPS, and virulence in laboratory mice (Table 34.1). Strains of *F. necrophorum* causing human infections appear to be distinct from the ssp. *necrophorum* of animal infections and seem to resemble ssp. *funduliforme* more closely.

Morphology and Staining. *F. necrophorum* is a gram-negative, nonmotile, nonsporulating, rod-shaped (pleomorphic) bacterium. Microscopically, the two subspecies can easily be distinguished. The ssp. *necrophorum* is highly pleomorphic and many of the rods are filamentous (2–100 μm), whereas ssp. *funduliforme* is typically more uniform and short rods. The presence of a mucopolysaccharide wall in *F. necrophorum*, as visualized by electron microscopy, has been described.

Growth Characteristics. The organism is anaerobic but aerotolerant. Clinical isolates grow well on blood agar or *Brucella* agar, as long as incubation is under anaerobic conditions. Colony morphologies of the two subspecies are different. The colonies of ssp. *necrophorum* are smooth, opaque, umbonate with irregular edges, and grayish to white in color, and those of ssp. *funduliforme* are small, waxy, raised, and yellow in color. Although the organism secretes a hemolysin, a zone of hemolysis is usually not observed. When cultured in a broth (grows well in BHI broth that is prereduced and anaerobically sterilized), cells

Table 34.1. Growth and Biochemical, Biological, and Molecular Characteristics of Subspecies of *F. necrophorum* ssp. *necrophorum* and ssp. *funduliforme* of Liver Abscess Origin of Cattle

Characteristics	Ssp. *necrophorum*	Ssp. *funduliforme*
Growth in broth, sedimentation	−	+
Biochemical characteristics		
Indole production	+	+
Phosphatase	+	−
Proteases	++	+
DNAse	+	−
Lipase	+	−
Virulence in mice, % mortality	92–97	8–10
Biological activities		
Leukotoxin production	+++	+ or −
Hemagglutinin titer	+++	+ or −
Lipid A, % of LPS	15	4
Molecular characteristics[a]		
RpoB gene	+	+
Hemagglutinin (*hem*) gene	+	−
lkt operon promoter length (bp)	548	337

[a]PCR amplification methods.

of ssp. *necrophorum* sediment to the bottom of the tube. The growth of ssp. *funduliforme* is uniformly turbid in a broth. The organism generally does not ferment any carbohydrates, although some strains ferment glucose weakly. The major energy substrate is lactic acid, which is fermented mainly to acetate, butyrate, and small amounts of propionate. An important biochemical characteristic that is useful in the identification is thc production of indole from tryptophan.

Cellular Products of Medical Interest. Cellular products (virulence factors) implicated in the pathogenesis of *F. necrophorum* include leukotoxin (or leukocidin), endotoxic LPS, hemolysin, hemagglutinin, capsule, adhesins, platelet aggregation factor, dermonecrotic toxin, and several extracellular enzymes, including proteases and deoxyribonucleases. These factors contribute to entry, colonization, proliferation, and establishment of the organism, and to the development of pyonecrotic lesions. Similar to other gram-negative bacteria, the outer membrane of *F. necrophorum* contains endotoxic LPS. The chemical composition of *F. necrophorum* LPS varies depending on the subspecies. Also, LPS from ssp. *necrophorum* has been shown to biologically more potent than that from ssp. *funduliforme.* Leukotoxin is considered to be the major virulence factor involved in fusobacterial infections in animals.

Leukotoxin. *F. necrophorum* leukotoxin is a secreted protein that has been shown to exert cytotoxic activity to neutrophils, macrophages, hepatocytes, and possibly to ruminal epithelial cells. The toxin is a high-molecular-weight (336 kDa) and heat-labile protein and is somewhat unique in lacking the amino acid cysteine, being considerably larger than leukotoxins of other bacteria with no significant sequence similarity to any other bacterial toxin. The leukotoxin operon consists of three genes—*lktB, lktA,* and *lktC*—of which *lktA* is the structural gene. The LktB protein is probably involved in secretion, and the function of LktC is not known. The importance of leukotoxin as a virulence factor is indicated by a correlation between toxin production and ability to induce abscesses in laboratory animals, an inability of leukotoxin-negative strains to induce foot abscesses in cattle following intradermal inoculation, and a relationship between antileukotoxin antibody titers and protection against infection in experimental challenge studies. *F. necrophorum* ssp. *necrophorum* produces more leukotoxin than ssp. *funduliforme,* which may explain why ssp. *necrophorum* is frequently associated with infections, particularly in liver abscesses of cattle, than the ssp. *funduliforme*. The role of leukotoxin in the pathogenesis includes thwarting attempts to contain the infection, modulation of the host immune system by its toxicity, including cellular activation of polymorphonuclear neutrophils and apoptosis-mediated killing of phagocytes and immune effector cells. The release of inflammatory mediators and the activated immune effector cells end up playing the central role in the pathophysiology of fusobacterial infections.

Ecology

Reservoir. *F. necrophorum* is a normal inhabitant of the gastrointestinal tract of animals and humans. The bacterium is frequently isolated from healthy hosts, although at a relatively low concentration. Normal human feces contain relatively high concentrations of *Fusobacterium*, of which *F. necrophorum* is the most predominant species. The organism is also a member of the normal flora of the oral cavity and female genital tract of animals and humans. In cattle, *F. necrophorum* is a normal inhabitant of the rumen and has been isolated from ruminal contents of cattle fed a variety of diets. The concentration in the rumen ranges from 10^5 to 10^7/g of ruminal contents, with concentrations higher in grain-fed cattle compared to forage-based diet. Because *F. necrophorum* uses lactate as its major substrate and not sugars, the increased population in cattle fed high-grain diet is probably due to increased lactate availability. Both subspecies of *F. necrophorum* have been isolated from ruminal contents.

In the rumen, fusobacteria are either present as free-floating organisms or attached to the ruminal epithelial wall. Fusobacteria are ideally suited to the ruminal wall niche because of their aerotolerance and ability to grow best at physiological pH (7.4). Possibly, the attachment is mediated via cell surface proteins, called hemagglutinins, which are responsible for agglutinating erythrocytes from various species. Reports on isolations of *F. necrophorum* from the ruminal wall are limited and are always in association with ruminal lesions

Transmission. Fusobacterial infections in animals are endogenous, generally initiated by entry into compromised tissues, such as oral mucosa or ruminal wall. In case of foot rot, the source of infection could be soil, which probably got contaminated from feces.

Pathogenesis

Disease Patterns in Animals. *F. necrophorum* is commonly associated with numerous clinically significant anaerobic infections. However, the prevalence of *F. necrophorum* infection is still believed to be underestimated. *F. necrophorum* is associated with numerous necrotic disease conditions, generally termed "necrobacillosis," and most often the infection is common in the liver (hepatic abscesses), feet (interdigital necrobacillosis or foot rot), mammary gland (mastitis), uterus (metritis and pyometra), and oropharyngeal mucosa (necrotic laryngitis or calf diphtheria in cattle and mandibular abscesses in antelopes, marsupials, and wild animals). Most often fusobacterial infections are polymicrobial, with multitude of facultative and anaerobic species involved, but the most common ones are *A. pyogenes*, *D. nodosus*, and *P. levii*.

F. necrophorum is considered to be a major pathogen of cattle. It causes three economically important diseases in cattle: liver abscesses, interdigital necrobacillosis, and necrotic laryngitis.

Liver Abscesses (Hepatic Necrobacillosis). Liver abscesses occur in all ages and in all types of cattle and in different parts of the world, but are most common in intensively fed beef cattle in the United States, Canada, Japan, and South Africa. Abscesses in the liver are secondary to the primary foci of infection on the ruminal wall. Because of the close correlation between the incidence of ruminal pathology and liver abscesses in cattle, the term "rumenitis–liver abscess complex" is often used. Although the precise pathogenesis is not proven, it is accepted that rapid fermentation of grain by ruminal microbes and the consequent accumulation of organic acids result in ruminal acidosis. Acid-induced rumenitis and damage of the protective surface, often aggravated by foreign objects (e.g., sharp feed particles and hair), predispose the ruminal wall to invasion and colonization by *F. necrophorum*. The organism causes ruminal wall abscesses, which subsequently shed bacterial emboli into the portal circulation. Bacteria from the portal circulation are filtered by the liver, resulting in infection and abscess formation (Figure 34.2). Abscesses found in the liver at the time of slaughter are often well encapsulated, possessing thick fibrotic walls (Figure 34.3). Histologically, a typical abscess is pyogranulomatous, with a necrotic center, encapsulated, and often surrounded by an inflammatory zone. Of the two subspecies of *F. necrophorum*, the ssp. *necrophorum* is more frequently encountered in liver abscesses than the ssp. *funduliforme*. The difference in prevalence is reflective of the difference in virulence, particularly with regard to leukotoxin production. In most liver abscesses, *A. pyogenes* is the second most frequent pathogen isolated. The origin of *A. pyogenes* is also the rumen, and there is evidence of pathogenic synergy between *A. pyogenes* and *F. necrophorum*.

Necrotic Laryngitis (Calf Diphtheria). The infection occurs in cattle up to 3 years of age and is characterized by necrosis of the mucous membrane of the larynx, particularly in the lateral arytenoid cartilage, and adjacent structures. The lesions appear as erosions progressing to ulcers and abscesses. Because *F. necrophorum* is a normal inhabitant of the respiratory tract of cattle, the source of infection is endogenous. The infection can be acute or chronic and is noncontagious. Clinically, an initial fever is followed by dyspnea that causes a roaring noise on inspiration ("hard breathers") and, in severe cases, painful swallowing and cough. Necropsy lesions include necrosis of the larynx and vocal cords and a mucous membrane covered by inflammatory exudate. Occasionally, bronchopneumonia may be evident.

Interdigital Necrobacillosis (Interdigital Phlegmon or Foot Rot). This form of necrobacillosis (foot rot or foot abscesses) is characterized by acute or subacute necrotizing infection, involving the skin and adjacent underlying

FIGURE 34.2. *Pathogenesis of liver abscesses in cattle fed high-grain diet.*

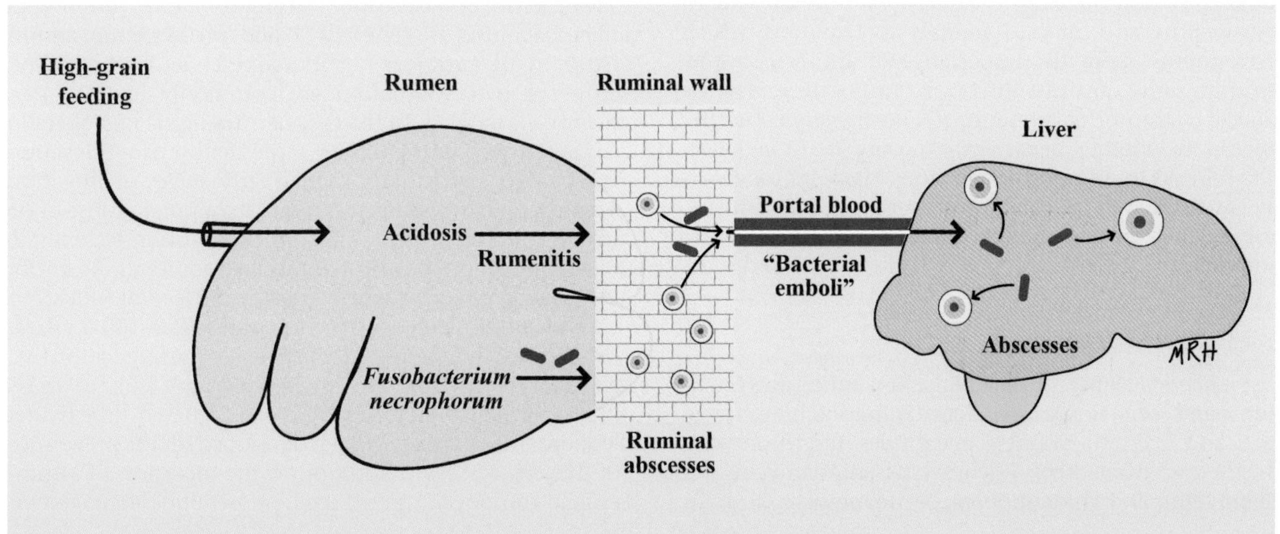

FIGURE 34.3. *An abscessed liver at the time of slaughter.*

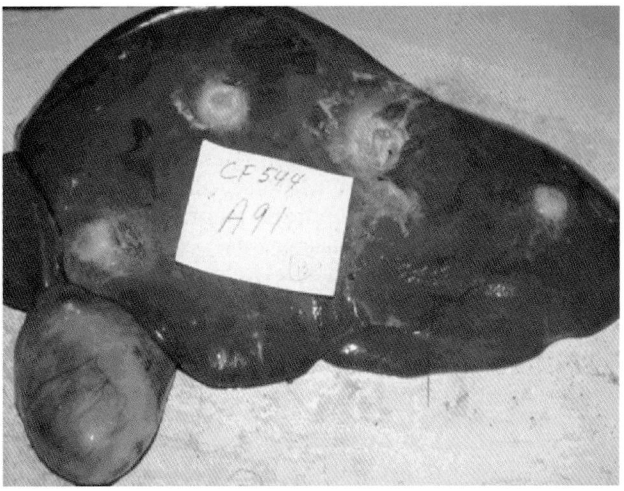

soft tissues of the feet. The infection is the major cause of lameness in dairy and beef cattle. The economic impact is from loss in productivity (milk production and weight gain). Predisposing factors involved in the pathogenesis of foot rot are damp soil and injury to the skin of the interdigital area. Fecal excretion of *F. necrophorum* is believed to provide the primary source of infection in foot rot and abscesses. In addition to *F. necrophorum*, *P. levii*, *Porphyromonas asaccharolytica*, *Prevotella melaninogenica*, and *Prevotella intermedia* are commonly isolated foot rot lesions. The lesions are characterized initially by mild cellulitis and swelling between the digits. Within a few days, fissuring with scabby exudate that eventually becomes pus in the margin of the fissure is observed. Fever and lameness are common clinical signs. Usually, healing is rapid once the abscess has discharged. Diagnosis is based on recognition of the characteristic interdigital necrotic lesion accompanied by foul-smelling discharge.

Immunologic Aspects

Serum antibodies against *F. necrophorum* are present in both healthy and infected animals and humans, which raises doubts about the importance of anti-*F. necrophorum* immunity against infection. Antibodies may be induced by the normal presence of *F. necrophorum*. Another concern is whether persistent exposure to *F. necrophorum* will lead to immunosuppression. Many investigators have attempted to induce protective immunity against *F. necrophorum* by using bacterins, toxoids, or other cellular components.

Antimicrobial Susceptibility

F. necrophorum is susceptible to β-lactam antibiotics (penicillins and cephalosporins); tetracyclines (chlortetracycline and oxytetracycline); macrolides (erythromycin, tylosin, and tilmicosin); lincomycins (clindamycin and lincomycin); and chloramphenicol, novobiocin, and virginiamycin. The organism is insensitive to aminoglycosides (gentamicin, kanamycin, neomycin, and streptomycin, which are less active against anaerobes in general), ionophore antibiotics (monensin). The *in vitro* activity of penicillins and cephalosporins against *F. necrophorum* isolates is interesting considering that the organism is gram-negative, even based on the cell wall architecture. The susceptibility of *F necrophorum* to virginiamycin and tylosin does not conform to the generality because both are principally active against gram-positive bacteria.

Laboratory Diagnosis

Necrobacillosis, particularly foot rot and necrotic laryngitis, can be diagnosed based on clinical signs. However, liver abscesses are detected only at the time of slaughter because cattle, even those that carry multitude of small abscesses or several large abscesses, seldom show any clinical signs. Moreover, hematology and liver function tests have not proved to be good indicators of liver abscesses. The usefulness of serum enzymes as indicators of liver dysfunction in cattle with naturally developed abscesses is minimal, because of lack of specificity as well as large variation in serum activity in clinically normal cattle. Ultrasonography that permits visualization of the liver has limited application because the scanning cannot visualize the whole liver, particularly of the visceral side, and parts of lobes that are covered by lungs and kidneys. The involvement of *F. necrophorum* requires isolation and identification. *F. necrophorum* is one of the gram-negative anaerobes that can easily be isolated and identified from clinical samples. The presumptive identification can be made based on the sample source and colony morphology on blood agar. Commercial rapid identification kits (e.g., RapID ANA II, Innovative Diagnostic Systems, Atlanta, GA) have proven to be useful in identification of the species and even of the subspecies of *F. necrophorum*.

Treatment and Control

Treatment of necrotic laryngitis and interdigital necrobacillosis is generally based on systemic administration of antibiotics. Sulfonamides and tetracyclines alone or in combination are commonly used to treat necrotic laryngitis. In the case of interdigital necrobacillosis, systemic administration of penicillin or tetracyclines is effective, particularly in the early stages of infection. Treatment of liver abscesses is not an option because of the insidious nature of the infection. Prevention is generally based on the use of antimicrobial feed additives. An antibiotic that is most commonly used in the feedlot industry is tylosin, administered at 10 g/ton of feed (90–100 mg/head per day). The extent of reduction in prevalence of liver abscesses varies from 30% to 70%. Because leukotoxin is a major virulence factor, a leukotoxoid-based (inactivated leukotoxin) vaccine has been developed for the prevention of liver abscesses. In addition to the inclusion of antimicrobial compounds in the feed, proper bunk management to minimize ruminal imbalance is well accepted as a key factor for effective control of liver abscesses

F. equinum

F. equinum is indistinguishable from *F. necrophorum* (both subspecies) based on morphological and biochemical characteristics. A PCR-based assay has been developed to distinguish between *F. equinum* and *F. necrophorum*. *F. equinum* is a normal inhabitant of the gastrointestinal, respiratory, and genitourinary tracts of horses. It is an opportunistic pathogen and is generally associated with abscesses and various necrotic infections in horses, particularly oral, paraoral, and lower respiratory tract infections. Very little is known about the virulence factors associated with *F. equinum* infections in horses, but the species does contain leukotoxin genes and exhibit leukotoxic activity.

Bacteroides

The genus *Bacteroides* includes several species, but only one species, *B. fragilis*, is clinically important. *B. fragilis* is part of the normal colonic flora of humans and animals and is the most common anaerobe isolated from human clinical samples. It is associated with abscesses, generally intraabdominal, soft tissue infections in animals. The capsular polysaccharide is a major virulence factor in the cause of abscesses. An abscess can be induced in laboratory animals by injecting purified capsular polysaccharide in the absence of bacteria. Some strains of *B. fragilis* produce an enterotoxin that have been shown to cause diarrhea in lambs, calves, piglets, foals, and infant rabbits. The strains have also been associated with diarrhea in humans, particularly in children.

Enterotoxigenic *B. fragilis*

Strains of *B. fragilis* that are enterotoxigenic (stimulate secretion in ligated ileal loops of lamb) were first identified in a diarrheic disease of newborn lambs. Subsequently enterotoxigenic *B. fragilis* (ETBF) has been isolated from cases of enteritis in calves, foals, and piglets. The enterotoxin, called *B. fragilis* toxin or fragilysin, is a heat-labile, approximately 20 kDa, protein that causes fluid secretion in intestinal loops, increases bacterial internalization in enterocytes, and modulates epithelial permeability. The toxin is in fact a zinc metalloprotease, suggesting that the toxic properties are due to the proteolytic activity. The enterotoxigenic strains can be identified by amplifying the *bft* gene (by PCR), and diagnosis of ETBF infections can also be made by direct detection of the *bft* gene in DNA extracted from feces.

Prevotella and *Porphyromonas*

These two genera of gram-negative, non-spore-forming anaerobes include saccharolytic (*Prevotella*) and asaccharolytic (*Porphyromonas*), pigmented and nonpigmented species, previously included in the genus *Bacteroides*. Members of both genera are part of the normal flora of the oral cavity and gastrointestinal tract of animals and humans.

The genus *Prevotella* currently includes about 50 species, and the species associated with human or animal infections are recovered mainly from the oral cavity and the upper respiratory and urogenital tracts. A majority of *Prevotella* spp. have been isolated from the human oral cavity. About 6 species found in animals have been isolated from the rumen or oral cavity.

The genus *Porphyromonas* includes 17 species, many of them are of animal origin. The strains isolated from the gingival sulcus of various animals, which are distinct from related human strains of *Porphyromonas gingivalis*, are now included under a new species *Porphyromonas gulae*. The organism is asaccharolytic and forms black-pigmented colonies and, similar to *P. gingivalis*, contains a 41 kDa fimbrial protein, which is an important colonizing factor in the periodontal disease. In addition to *P. gulae*, other *Porphyromonas* species that have been identified include *P. canoris*, *P. cangingivalis*, *P. canis*, *P. cansulci*, *P. gingivicanis*, and *P. crevioricanis*.

Diseases

Because *Prevotella* and *Porphyromonas* species are members of the oral flora of all animals, they have a prominent role in oral and bite wound infections. Periodontal disease is the most common oral disease of adult animals, and includes gingivitis, periodontitis, and periodontal abscesses initiated by bacteria in the dental plaque. Periodontal diseases affect a wide range of animals, such as dogs, cats, sheep, cattle, and captive and free-roaming wild animals. It is estimated that approximately 80% of dogs and cats have some degree of periodontal disease by 4 years of age. Periodontitis in dogs and cats can be a serious infection that could lead to anorexia, weight loss, swollen gums, tooth decay, loose teeth, breakage, or loss of teeth and even breakage of the mandibular bone. If left untreated, periodontal bacteria may spread to other sites in the body and lead to renal, coronary, or hepatic infections. Not surprisingly, *Prevotella* and *Porphyromonas* are frequently isolated anaerobes from infected dog and cat bite wounds in humans.

P. levii is often the predominant organism associated with cases of bovine foot rot. However, whether isolated strains fulfill Koch's postulates has not been determined. Not much is known about the source of the organism and virulence factors involved. It is believed that the organism works in synergy with *F. necrophorum* to produce the infection.

Further Reading

Bennett GN and Hickford JGH (2011) Ovine foot: New approaches to an old disease. *Vet Microbiol*, **148**, 1–7.

Botta G, Arzese A, Minisini R, and Train G (1994) Role of structural and extracellular virulence factors in gram-negative anaerobic bacteria. *Clin Infect Dis*, **18**, S260–S264.

Duerden BI (1994) Virulence factors in anaerobes. *Clin Infect Dis*, **18**, S253–S259.

Kennan RM, Han X, Porter CJ, and Rood JI (2011) The pathogenesis of ovine footrot. *Vet Microbiol*, **153**, 59–66.

Nagaraja TG and Chengappa MM (1998) Liver abscesses in feedlot cattle: a review. *J Anim Sci*, **76**, 287–298.

Nagaraja TG, Narayanan SK, Stewart GC, and Chengappa MM (2005) *Fusobacterium necrophorum* infections in animals: Pathogenesis and pathogenic mechanisms. *Anaerobe*, **11**, 239–246.

Tadepalli S, Narayanan SK, Stewart GC *et al.* (2009) *Fusobacterium necrophorum:* A ruminal bacterium that invades liver to cause abscesses in cattle. *Anaerobe*, **15**, 36–43.

Tan ZL, Nagaraja TG, and Chengappa MM (1996) *Fusobacterium necrophorum* infections: virulence factors, pathogenic mechanism and control measures. *Vet Res Comm*, **20**, 113–140.

Clostridium

John F. Prescott

Members of the genus *Clostridium* are gram-positive, spore-forming, anaerobic rods characterized also by production of powerful extracellular toxins. In this chapter, the diseases produced by members of this genus (Table 35.1) are discussed under three categories: enterotoxic, including the enterotoxemias and diarrheas, produced by *C. perfringens*, *C. colinum*, *C. difficile*, *C. piliforme*, *C. septicum*, *C. spiroforme*, and *C. sordellii*; histotoxic, produced by *C. perfringens*, *C. chauvoei*, *C. haemolyticum*, *C. novyi*, *C. septicum*, and *C. sordellii*; and neurotoxic, produced by *C. botulinum* and *C. tetani*.

Clostridial infections are serious infections because of the powerful toxins produced by these organisms. Many have been controlled successfully by immunization almost since the dawn of bacteriology. However, other clostridial infections are emerging as ever more common and important, perhaps partly because their ability to form resistant spores gives them selective advantage in growing in the intestinal tract whenever antibiotics are administered. Much remains to be discovered.

Descriptive Features of the Genus *Clostridium*

Morphology and Staining

Members of the genus *Clostridium* are gram-positive rods measuring 0.2–4 μm by 2–20 μm. Location and shape of endospores are consistent within a species. Their ability to form spores is crucial to persistence in the intestine and the environment, and contributes to difficulties in their control.

Structure and Composition

Little of medical relevance is known of the ultrastructure and composition of clostridia. A surface-associated structure characterized by orderly paracrystalline protein arrays (S-layer) in the cell wall of *Clostridium difficile* may contribute to the ability of this bacterium to resist antimicrobial peptides in the intestine. Some clostridia produce pili (*Clostridium perfringens* and *C. difficile*) and others produce adhesive structures, presumably cell wall proteins, but their role in disease is not well defined. Considerable cellular intraspecific antigenic diversity and interspecific cross-reactivity exist but are of less interest than the antigenic properties of toxins because these latter are crucial in immunity. Those that are motile have peritrichous flagella or pilus-mediated "twitching motility." Of the pathogenic species, *C. perfringens* and *C. difficile* may form capsules.

Original chapter written by Drs. Dwight Hirsh and Ernie Biberstein.

Growth Characteristics

Clostridia are anaerobes, but the strictness of anaerobic requirements varies among species. For example, *C. difficile* is far more readily killed by exposure to air than is *C. perfringens*. In general, clostridia are characterized by simplicity of their growth requirements, though some require relatively rich and complex media; blood is beneficial. A temperature of 37 °C is optimal. Growth is visible within 1 or 2 days. Colonies are often irregular in shape and contour. Several clostridia swarm across moist agar media without forming colonies. Most clostridia produce hemolysis on blood agar. In liquid media, clostridia often grow in air provided a reducing agent is present (cooked meat pieces and thioglycolate), though growth occurs only in the anaerobic portions of the medium.

Biochemical Activities

Most clostridia are metabolically highly active and masters at attacking carbohydrates, proteins, lipids, and nucleic acids. Clostridial cultures typically emit putrid odors due to production of volatile fatty acids and hydrogen sulfide during the fermentative degradation of carbohydrates and proteins. Biochemical reactions and their end products furnish a basis for species identification.

Resistance

The vegetative form is as susceptible to environmental stresses and disinfectants as other bacteria. Endospores impart resistance to drying, heat, irradiation, and disinfectants (Figure 35.1).

Veterinary Microbiology, Third Edition. Edited by D. Scott McVey, Melissa Kennedy and M.M. Chengappa.

Table 35.1. Selected Members of the Genus *Clostridium* and Their Usual Source or Associated Condition

Clostridium Species	Usual Source or Associated Condition
C. botulinum	Botulism
C. chauvoei	Blackleg in ruminants; iatrogenic myositis of horses
C. colinum	Ulcerative enteritis and hepatitis in birds
C. difficile	Antibiotic-associated typhlocolitis in guinea pigs, hamsters, horses, humans, pigs, rabbits, and other species
C. haemolyticum	Bacillary hemoglobinuria in ruminants
C. novyi	Gas gangrene and "pseudoblackleg," "big head" in rams, "black disease" in ruminants; iatrogenic myositis of horses
C. perfringens	Enteric disease and enterotoxemias including necrotic enteritis of chickens, lamb dysentery, hemorrhagic and necrotizing gastroenteritis in neonatal and sometimes older farm animals and other species, "pulpy kidney" disease of ruminants, food poisoning in humans and possibly dogs; gas gangrene; gangrenous mastitis of cows
C. piliforme	Tyzzer's disease
C. septicum	Gas gangrene in ruminants and pigs; "pseudoblackleg"; gangrenous dermatitis of poultry; severe abomasitis ("braxy") of lambs; iatrogenic myositis of horses
C. sordellii	Gas gangrene and "pseudoblackleg"; severe abomasitis of lambs; equine atypical myositis
C. spiroforme	Antibiotic-induced and spontaneous typhlocolitis of rabbits
C. tetani	Tetanus

Enterotoxic Clostridia

C. perfringens

Descriptive Features. *C. perfringens* is a gram-positive, usually spore-forming, nonmotile, encapsulated anaerobic rod that produces a variety of toxins. Four of these toxins are used to type members of this species. There are five toxinotypes, designated A through E (Table 35.2), although the toxinotyping scheme is now widely recognized as inadequate to describe the range of enteric diseases caused by this organism.

FIGURE 35.1. *Gram stain of* Clostridium *species, showing the spores that are a characteristic of the genus.*

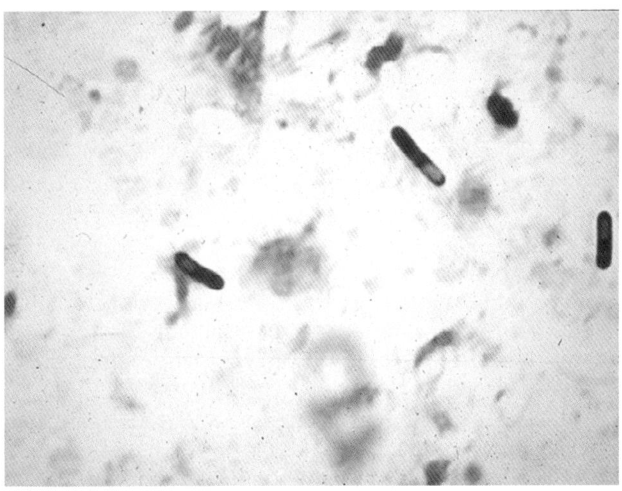

Table 35.2. Major Toxinotypes of *Clostridium perfringens* in Animal Disease

Type	Major Toxin Produced: α	β	ε	ι	Diseases Produced
A	+				Gas gangrene; gangrenous mastitis in cows; sporadic hemorrhagic and necrotizing gastroenteritis in numerous species; hemorrhagic abomasitis in calves; avian necrotic enteritis (NetB toxin-associated); enterotoxin-associated food-borne infection (humans, possibly other species). The full range of enteric disease associated with type A infections, and their toxin-associated basis, remains to be characterized.
B	+	+	+		Lamb dysentery
C	+	+			Neonatal hemorrhagic and necrotizing enteritis of farm animals (calves, foals, lambs, and piglets), "struck" adult sheep
D	+		+		Ovine enterotoxemia (rarely calves); enterotoxemia and enterocolitis in adult goats
E	+			+	Bovine hemorrhagic gastroenteritis

C. perfringens is associated with enterotoxic and other enteric disease including diarrhea in a variety of species, as well as histotoxic infections such as wound infections (gas gangrene) and serious mastitis. Understanding of the role of *C. perfringens* in enteric disease in animals, particularly in serious hemorrhagic or necrotizing enteric disease, resembles that of understanding of *Escherichia coli* in enteric disease 50 years ago, when it was thought to be exclusively normal microflora. *C. perfringens* is as dynamic a bacterium as *E. coli*, increasingly recognized as having, like *E. coli*, the ability to adapt to cause disease in different host species. One important base of its adaptability is its possession of different conjugative plasmids that can move readily between *C. perfringens* in the intestine and that can also acquire mobile genetic elements carrying virulence determinants, and likely to change these through DNA recombination.

Cellular Products of Medical Interest

Adhesins. *C. perfringens* possesses genes encoding fibronectin-binding and collagen-adhesion proteins. These proteins are thought to be involved in binding to the extracellular matrix during infection.

Capsule. The capsule probably acts as a deterrent to phagocytosis. Encapsulation is an important virulence determinant in wounds (e.g., gas gangrene), but probably not in the intestinal tract.

Toxins. *C. perfringens* produces a large variety of protein toxins and tissue-degradative enzymes consistent with its adaptation to break down tissue quickly and efficiently. It is auxotrophic for 15 amino acids, which it requires to obtain intact rather than being able to synthesize. Under optimal conditions, it divides every 10 min, the fastest known multiplication rate of any bacterium. It has been aptly described as an "anaerobic flesh-eater." Most toxins are regulated by a global regulatory system ("VirR/VirS," discussed in Section "Regulation of Toxin Genes"), which is itself under the control of a "quorum sensing" system. The "major toxins" are the mouse-lethal α-, β-, ε-, and ι-toxins. The others are currently described as "minor." Some are described here.

α-Toxin. α-Toxin (Cpa) also sometimes called Plc (for phospholipase C) is produced by all *C. perfringens*. It is a mouse-lethal phospholipase C (a lecithinase) that hydrolyses host cell membranes as part of its action in breaking down tissues to extract nutrients.

β-Toxin. The genes encoding β-toxin (Cpb) are located on a conjugative plasmid. β-Toxin is a mouse-lethal pore-forming toxin, which damages host target cells (intestinal epithelial cells and endothelial cells). In addition, β-toxin affects nervous tissue by influencing the distribution of calcium ions across their membranes, thereby disrupting normal nerve conduction. It is susceptible to the proteolytic activity of trypsin.

ε-Toxin. The gene encoding the mouse-lethal ε-toxin (Etx) is also located on a conjugative plasmid. ε-Toxin targets lipid (cholesterol and sphingolipids) rafts found in eukaryotic cell membranes, though the toxin concentrates in brain and kidney. It is a permease that acts by affecting the cellular cytoskeleton resulting in an increase in the permeability of epithelial and endothelial cells (both in the intestine but especially in the microvasculature of the brain, leading to leakage of toxin into that organ). The toxin seems to target neuronal granule cells in the cerebellum and elsewhere in the brain to release the neurotransmitter glutamate. Etx is secreted as a protoxin that is activated in the intestine by proteolytic enzymes. The toxin may delay intestinal transit time in affected animals.

ι-Toxin. ι-Toxin (Itx) is a binary mouse-lethal toxin composed of a binding portion (Ib) that binds the toxin to target epithelial cells, and an enzymatically active portion (Ia). After the toxin binds to specific receptors on the cell surface, Ia gains entry into the cytoplasm. Although it is not clear precisely how entry occurs, it seems that a pore (composed of Ib) is formed in the cell membrane through which Ia traverses. Ia is an adenosine diphosphate (ADP)-ribosylating toxin that ribosylates actin within the host cell, resulting in disorganization of the cellular cytoskeleton and death of the affected cell.

Enterotoxin. The genes encoding *C. perfringens* enterotoxin (Cpe) are either chromosomal (isolates from cases of human food-related gastrointestinal disease), or conjugative plasmid-based (isolates from dogs with diarrhea, or from human patients with non-food-related and sometimes antibiotic-associated diarrhea). Enterotoxin is produced during sporulation of *cpe*-containing *C. perfringens* ($<5\%$ of type A strains, the strains in which *cpe* is most commonly found). When the endospore is released, enterotoxin is also released into the surrounding milieu. Enterotoxin is a bifunctional toxin, first forming a pore in the apical portion of small intestinal epithelial cells resulting in fluid and electrolyte abnormalities, as well as providing access to tight junction proteins (specifically claudins and occludins). Interactions of Cpe with tight junction proteins result in further losses in control of fluid and electrolytes.

Necrotic Enteritis Toxin B. Necrotic enteritis toxin B (NetB) is a recently described VirR/VirS-regulated pore-forming toxin related to the *C. perfringens* Cpb toxin that is essential for the production of necrotic enteritis in chickens. Like almost all the major toxins (Cpb, Etx, and Itx) of *C. perfringens*, it is found on a conjugative plasmid.

Examples of Minor Toxins. κ-Toxin (Col for collagenase) is a collagenase. Col is thought to aid spread of clostridial cells through the tissue. μ-Toxin (Nag for *N*-acetylgalactosaminidase) is a hyaluronidase. Nag aids spread of clostridial cells through the tissue. Perfringolysin O (Pfo, θ-toxin) is a cholesterol-binding cytolysin (like novyilysin and chauveolysin, described later; and streptolysin O, Chapter 28; listerial listeriolysin O, and Chapter 32). Perfringolysin binds to cholesterol-containing rafts in the eukaryotic cell membrane, and forms a pore, which results in the death of the cell. Sialidase (neuraminidase, or Nan) removes sialic acid residues from glycoconjugates on cell walls of eukaryotic cells, resulting in disruptions of the intercellular matrix. The β-2 toxin (Cpb2) is newly described weakly mouse-lethal pore-forming toxin that occurs in two variants, but its role in disease is not well characterized. The gene encoding this toxin is also on a plasmid, and is controlled by the VirR/VirS system.

Regulation of Toxin Genes. *C. perfringens* globally synchronously regulates its toxin production and production of major metabolic enzymes by the two-component regulatory system, VirR/VirS. VirS is a histidine kinase that acts as a "sensor" of environmental cues resulting in autophosphorylation of one of its histidine residues. This phosphate is then transferred to an aspartate residue, then to another histidine before being used to phosphorylate VirR, the "regulator." Phosphorylated VirR is a transcriptional activator of the genes encoding the proteins mentioned earlier. The environmental cues sensed by *C. perfringens* include microcolony formation ("quorum sensing") *in vivo*.

Reservoir and Transmission. Type A *C. perfringens* occurs in intestinal tracts of humans and other animals and in most soils. Types B, C, D, and E are found mostly in the intestinal tracts of animals, and their survival in soil is variable. Transmission is by ingestion and wound infection.

Pathogenesis and Disease Patterns. *C. perfringens* causes both serious enteric diseases, including important enterotoxemias, and histotoxic infections.

Enterotoxemias and Enteric Disease. Most animal diseases due to *C. perfringens* are intestinal and involve all toxinotypes.

Type A. Type A *C. perfringens* has been implicated in enteritis, notably hemorrhagic or necrotizing forms, in numerous species, but understanding of the molecular basis of these infections (and hence of optimal microbiological diagnosis) is in some cases poor. For example, type A *C. perfringens* causes necrotic enteritis of chickens and other birds (Figure 35.2). It has only recently been recognized that strains that cause this infection are characterized by production of the NetB toxin, the gene for which is on one of three pathogenicity loci that are characteristic of chicken necrotic enteritis strains. This unexpected discovery illustrates the largely unrecognized likely ability of this bacterial pathogen to adapt to cause distinct diseases in different animal species. Type A *C. perfringens* is important causes of necrotizing and emphysematous abomasitis in young calves (Figure 35.3), as well as sporadic hemorrhagic gastroenteritis in numerous species including dogs and foals, although the basis of these diseases is still unclear. Tissue destruction is usually attributed to the virulence determinants important in gas gangrene, but this assumption is probably incorrect. Cpb2-producing *C. perfringens* may be associated with fatal typhlocolitis in adult horses following gentamicin treatment. Extraordinarily, the *cpb2* toxin gene is usually out-of-frame and therefore unread in horse isolates, but treatment with gentamicin may cause ribosomal distortion such that the mRNA transcript is read in frame, and the toxin produced. Type A isolates are also involved in nonenterotoxemic food poisoning in humans (strains of which possess the chromosomally encoded Cpe enterotoxin as well as being more resistant to heat) and antibiotic-associated diarrhea in humans (associated with plasmid-borne carriage of the *cpe* and *cpb2* genes). There is a suspicion that type A *C. perfringens* encoding the Cpe enterotoxin may be involved in watery diarrheal illness in dogs and cats, but this is not proven. There is also a suspicion that Cpb2-positive type A strains can cause a mild diarrheal illness and growth setback in neonatal swine, but again this is unproven.

FIGURE 35.2. *Necrotic enteritis caused by type A* C. perfringens *in a chicken. (Courtesy of Department of Pathobiology, University of Guelph.)*

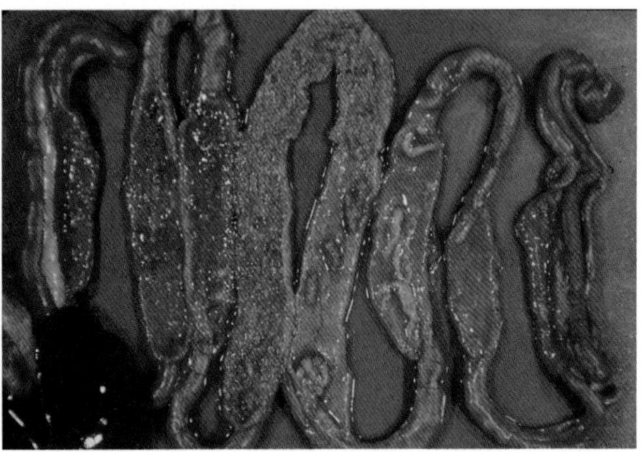

FIGURE 35.3. Necrotizing *and emphysematous abomasitis in a young calf caused by type A* C. perfringens. *(Courtesy of Department of Pathobiology, University of Guelph.)*

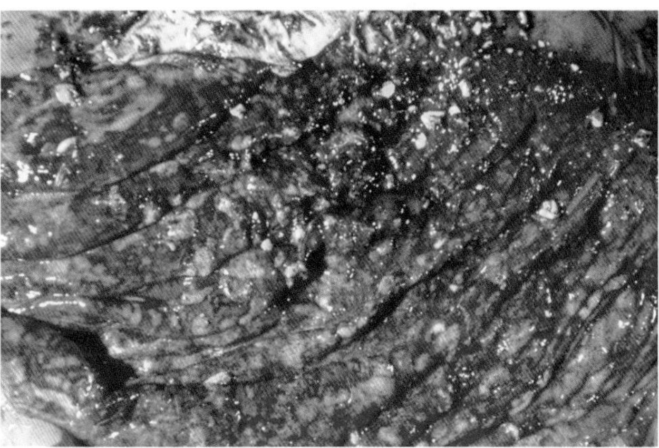

Type B. Type B *C. perfringens* is an "old world" infection usually causing "lamb dysentery" in newborn lambs. β-Toxin is the principal factor producing hemorrhagic enteritis, affecting the entire small intestine. Its trypsin susceptibility explains in part the predilection of the disease for the newborn, since colostrum contains antitrypsin substances. The signs are depression, anorexia, abdominal pain, and diarrhea. The course is rapid, with mortality rates approaching 100%. A chronic form occurs in older animals. Extraintestinal lesions include congestion, edema, serosal effusions, and hemorrhages in various organs. The signs and pathology associated with this disease are due to the action of the membrane-active toxins (β and ε). ε-Toxin, being a permease, increases intestinal permeability, ensuring its absorption into the circulation where it affects vascular endothelium, leading to fluid loss and edema, as well as damage to kidney function. β-toxin and ε-toxin also affect the nervous system, and the severe depression, lack of response to corrective therapy, and high mortality may be due in part to this activity. Since ε-toxin requires activation by proteolytic enzymes, its role in disease caused by type B strains is less important than that played by β-toxin.

Type C. Type C *C. perfringens* causes hemorrhagic enteritis in neonatal calves, foals, piglets, and lambs worldwide (Figure 35.4). In some other species, including humans and rarely chickens, the organism can also produce a necrotic enteritis. An often rapidly fatal intestinal toxemia of older sheep is called "struck" (as in "struck dead," because the associated sudden death might suggest lightning strike). β-Toxin is the principal factor producing hemorrhagic

FIGURE 35.4. *Hemorrhagic enteritis in a piglet caused by type C C.* perfringens.

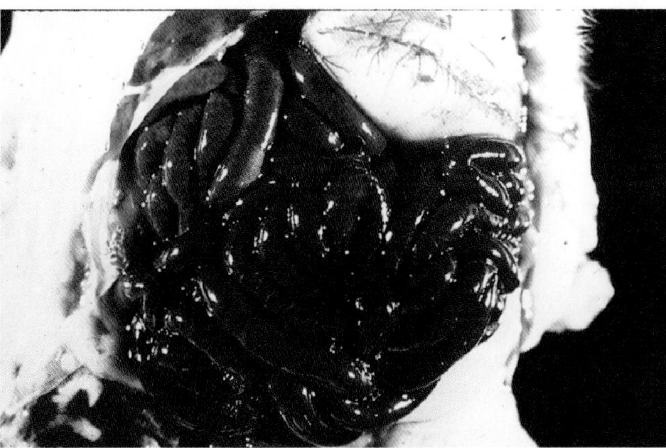

FIGURE 35.5. *"Pulpy kidney" changes in kidney at necropsy associated with autolysis of ε-toxin-damaged kidney tissue. Kidney on left is affected, and on right is a normal kidney. (Courtesy of Department of Pathobiology, University of Guelph.)*

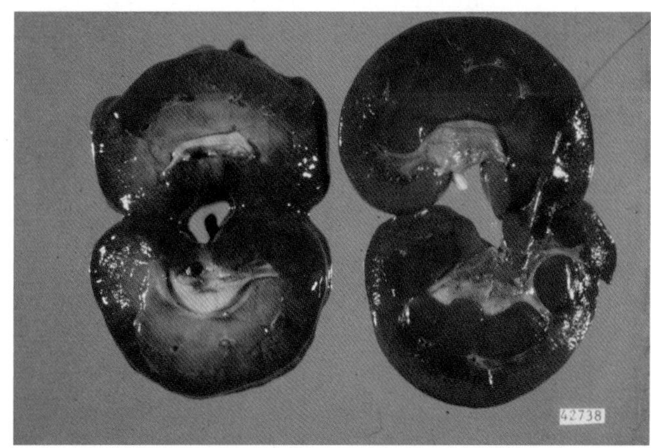

enteritis, affecting the small intestine. Its trypsin susceptibility explains in part the predilection of the disease for the newborn, since colostrum contains antitrypsin substances. The signs are depression, anorexia, abdominal pain, and diarrhea. The course is rapid, with mortality rates near 100%. The signs and pathology associated with this disease are due to the action of the membrane-active β-toxin. In humans in New Guinea, type C enteritis ("pig bel") has been associated with feasting on undercooked and contaminated pork as well as on cassava; the trypsin-inhibiting properties of cassava prevent the breakdown of β-toxin produced by type C organisms in the small intestine.

Type D. Type D *C. perfringens* produces an enterotoxemia ("overeating disease" or "pulpy kidney disease") in older lambs (<1 year), in goats of all ages, and occasionally in calves. ε-Toxin is secreted as protoxin activated by intestinal proteases, explaining the predilection of this disease for older animals since colostrum contains antitrypsin activity. ε-Toxin increases intestinal permeability, ensuring its absorption into the circulation where it damages vascular endothelium, leading to fluid loss and edema. When toxin levels are high, affected capillary endothelial cells in the brain are damaged, and the resultant edema greatly increases the intracranial pressure. When the amount of toxin is lower, however, as might be the case in a partially immune animal or when the amount of toxin produced in the intestinal tract is less, it damages the capillary endothelial cells in the brain so that toxin levels are increased in that organ. This results in a focal symmetrical encephalomalacia. In addition to these changes (which are toxin dose related), ε-toxin triggers catecholamine release, resulting in adenylyl cyclase activation, cAMP-related hyperglycemia, and glycosuria, a frequent finding in enterotoxemia.

Gross lesions may be absent and death rates may be high in lambs. Postmortem autolysis is rapid because of vascular endothelial damage (Figure 35.5). Subserous and subendocardial hemorrhages and excess fluid in the body cavities are sometimes seen in lambs. Cerebral hemorrhage and degenerative lesions are common in less acute cases. Histopathology may reveal enteritis. Lambs may die without premonitory signs, but convulsions may occur in agonal stages and diarrhea in protracted cases. Cattle and older sheep show neurological manifestations. In adult goats, local necrotizing enteritis with diarrhea is common. In calves and goats, nonfatal subacute and chronic cases occur.

Type E. Type E *C. perfringens* produces a relatively uncommon form of hemorrhagic enteritis in calves, and sometimes of lambs. The membrane-active ι-toxin produces this disease. Hemorrhagic enteritis and ulcerative abomasitis are the pathologic lesions. Type E disease was erroneously described in rabbits since the *Clostridium spiroforme* toxin is neutralized by ι-toxin antiserum.

Nonenterotoxemic Diarrhea. The role of *C. perfringens* in nonenterotoxemic and mild diarrhea in animals remains to be confirmed. For example, neonatal piglets may have a syndrome of weight loss, failure to thrive, and diarrhea associated with β2-toxin-producing type A strains. It is possible that nonenterotoxemic diarrhea occurs in other species subsequent to the interaction of the Cpe enterotoxin (with epithelial cells of the small intestine following sporulation of the microorganism in that environment). Although any type of *C. perfringens* can harbor the genes encoding Cpe, type A is the most common. This disease is one of the most commonly occurring food-related diseases in human patients. In addition to altering fluid and electrolyte flow of the epithelium, Cpe damages epithelial cells and tight junctions leading to sloughing with accompanying inflammatory changes.

Histotoxic Infections. *C. perfringens* type A, alone or with other bacteria, causes wound infections (gas gangrene, sometimes called malignant edema in animals), a gangrenous anaerobic cellulitis following inoculation into a normally sterile site. *C. perfringens* is also an occasional cause of severe and fatal necrotizing mastitis in newly calved cows.

The membrane-active toxins (α- and perfringolysin O) account for the major tissue destruction. Spread of the infection is aided by collagenases, sialidases, and hyaluronidases. The numerous powerful degradative proteases, glycosidases, lipases, and other enzymes upregulated by the VirR/VirS system assist in the tissue destruction and nutrient assimilation, while encapsulation helps the organism resist phagocytosis. The disease is a necrotizing cellulitis and myonecrosis with edema, hemorrhage, gas production, and an often fatal toxemia. This type of *C. perfringens* infection in animals is rare, and follows introduction of clostridia from the environment into usually severely traumatized tissue, where trauma assists in production of an anoxic environment suitable for the establishment of clostridia.

Epidemiology. Many healthy animals commonly carry *C. perfringens* in their intestinal tracts, probably as frequently as they carry *E. coli*. During outbreaks of diarrheal disease, pathogenic strains survive in soil long enough to infect other animals.

The determinant of enterotoxemic (type D) disease is the intestinal environment, which is influenced by diet and age. Overeating, especially on protein and energy-rich food (milk, legume forage, and grain), is almost a prerequisite. In young animals, the excess feed is often passed, inadequately digested, into the intestine, where it provides a rich medium for proliferation and toxinogenesis by ingested or resident bacteria. Overloading slows intestinal motility, thereby favoring retention of bacteria and absorption of their toxins. In addition, there are likely to be bacterial factors promoting intestinal colonization, but these are not well described. In broiler chickens, necrotic enteritis is predisposed by concurrent coccidiosis, as well as by wheat-based diets, and diets containing trypsin inhibitors (such as unheated soybean meal).

The age predilection of many of these enteric diseases is due to the diet and the infantile digestive tract, which often lacks enzymes to inactivate the toxins. In particular, colostral antitrypsin activity exacerbates this aspect. Type D proliferation, for which the ε-toxin requires trypsin activation, in older lambs appears to be favored by high-carbohydrate intake.

Seasonal prevalence relates to the seasonal abundance of susceptible populations and rich forage, with warm temperatures favoring proliferation of bacteria in the environment.

Type A-associated conditions occur worldwide. Type B lamb dysentery occurs in Europe and South Africa, while type B enteritis of sheep or goats is reported from Iran. Type C occurs worldwide, and type D is prevalent wherever sheep are raised. Type E is found in Britain, the United States, and Australia. A toxin similar to its ι-toxin is also produced by *C. difficile* and *C. spiroforme*.

Immunologic Aspects. Immunity is antibody-mediated and correlates with antitoxin levels. Immunizing preparations often include bacterial components as well. Active immunization is important in the control of the diseases (see Section "Treatment and Control").

Laboratory Diagnosis. *C. perfringens* is relatively aerotolerant, and is easy to isolate and to identify in the diagnostic laboratory. Spores are rarely demonstrable in exudates obtained from normally sterile sites.

Isolation follows inoculation of blood-containing agar media, and incubation in an anaerobic environment. If *C. perfringens* is to be isolated from a contaminated environment (e.g., intestinal contents), the sample can first be heated to 80 °C for 15 min since endospores will resist this treatment, whereas vegetative forms will not, and then placed into or onto isolation media. Diagnostic features include the characteristic double zone of hemolysis on blood agar (Cpa, Pfo toxins) and the clotting of milk followed by gaseous disruption ("stormy fermentation"). In cases of enterotoxemia, stained (e.g., Gram's, Wright's, and Giemsa) contents of the small intestine often contain large numbers of fat gram-positive rods typical of *C. perfringens*. However, this test is of limited value due to rapid postmortem bacterial overgrowth in all parts of the gut. DNA primers specific for the various genes encoding the toxins have been developed for detection in feces or cultures by the polymerase chain reaction (multiplex PCR).

Demonstration of toxin in the contents of the small intestine is definitive and involves injecting small amounts of clarified intestinal contents into the tail vein of mice. Death after more than a few minutes postinjection constitutes presumptive evidence of enterotoxemia, and the toxin can be neutralized using specific antitoxins. Such a procedure, or guinea pig intradermal toxin testing, is now generally regarded as barbaric, and therefore most diagnostic laboratories rely on PCR testing. Lambs with type D enterotoxemia usually test positively for glycosuria.

Cpe is detected immunologically in feces of affected dogs or cats by enzyme-linked immunosorbent assay. Although sporulation and Cpe production are coregulated, there is disagreement regarding the usefulness of determining the presence of spores in stained smears of feces as a method of diagnosis.

Treatment and Control. Most cases of enterotoxemia are too acute for successful treatment. The best method of preventing enterotoxemia is active immunization of dams with two injections of bacterin-toxoid combinations prior to parturition. Commercial immunizing products usually cover types C and D. This ensures nurslings passive protection for the first weeks of life. During outbreaks, antitoxin and toxoid are sometimes given and a second dose of toxoid is administered some weeks later. Protection of lambs against type D enterotoxemia requires two vaccinations at a monthly interval. The course should be completed 2 weeks before the lambs are placed on full feed. Milking goats respond poorly to immunization with pulpy kidney (type D) vaccines, and therefore, vaccination is often repeated several times a year.

Antitoxin of appropriate type may be given to sick animals and to those at risk. Protection lasts 2–3 weeks. Prophylactic dosages, given subcutaneously, can be doubled and given intravenously for therapy. However, antibiotics now usually replace antitoxins because of the cost and unavailability of antiserum.

Ensuring against overeating is a worthwhile preventive measure where practicable. Feeding broad-spectrum antibiotics reduces the prevalence of enterotoxemia of lambs, but creates other problems (see Chapter 4). Feeding antibiotics to poultry prevents mortality and illness in chickens due to necrotic enteritis caused by type A *C. perfringens*. Diarrhea in dogs and cats associated with type A Cpe-producing *C. perfringens* responds to metronidazole, macrolides (tylosin), or ampicillin.

Clostridium colinum

C. colinum causes quail disease, an ulcerative enteritis and necrotizing hepatitis of several species of poultry. The agent is fastidious nutritionally and forms spores sparingly. Its life cycle is unknown, and a toxin has not been identified. The untreated disease is usually fatal.

C. difficile

C. difficile is a gram-positive, motile, encapsulated, spore-forming anaerobic rod. This species produces adhesins (pili or fimbria), and its cell wall contains paracrystalline arrays (S-layer) visible with the electron microscope.

C. difficile is an important cause of serious diarrheal disease in humans, commonly associated with antibiotic use that may progress to fatal pseudomembranous colitis. It has become a scourge in human hospitals, particularly in older patients (>65 years of age), associated with the difficulty of controlling spores by disinfection in the hospital environment and with other features that include use of certain antibiotics and of gastric antacids. It may also cause non-antibiotic-associated diarrheal disease in people. *C. difficile* is increasingly recognized as an important cause of fatal diarrheal disease in animals, notably horses, hamsters, guinea pigs, and piglets, but its significance in other animals is only now being established. Other species in which *C. difficile* diarrheal disease has been described include dogs, cats, rabbits, and ratites. The microorganism has been isolated from symptomatic diarrheic as well as asymptomatic dogs and cats. Disease commonly follows broad-spectrum antibiotic use (e.g., third-generation cephalosporin and clindamycin). Pathological findings in horses, hamsters, and guinea pigs include hemorrhagic necrotizing enterocolitis, typhlocolitis, and pseudomembranous colitis, and in piglets necrotizing typhlocolitis and mesocolonic edema. There is usually a history of association with antimicrobial agents, though *C. difficile*-associated disease has been reported in previously normal, unmedicated foals.

Descriptive Features

Cellular Products of Medical Interest

Adhesins. *C. difficile* produces pilus adhesins that probably play a role in adhesion to target cells in the large intestine. *C. difficile* also produces a cell wall protein (Cwp66, for cell wall protein of 66 kDa in size) with affinity for intestinal epithelial cells.

Capsule. *C. difficile* produces a carbohydrate capsule that protects it from phagocytic cells.

Toxins. *C. difficile* produces three toxins that are responsible for enteritis observed with this microorganism: toxin A ("enterotoxin"), toxin B ("cytolysin"), and ADP-ribosyltransferase.

C. difficile toxin A (TcdA) is a glycosyltransferase that glucosylates Rho GTPases, rendering them ineffectual in interacting with their substrates (i.e., they become biologically inactive). In addition, glycosylation blocks interaction of Rho GDP with guanine exchange factor, and the interaction of Rho GTP with GTPase-activating factor, thereby preventing membrane cycling. Several signaling pathways are disrupted, resulting in a breakdown of the cytoskeletal components of the affected cell including disruption of the tight junctions between intestinal epithelial cells. These changes result in death of the cell. The enterotoxic property of TcdA, in addition to the cytotoxic effects just described, is due to its ability to stimulate influx of polymorphonuclear neutrophils (PMNs) by way of the enteric nervous system (through the release of substance P and mast cell degranulation). Prostaglandin synthesis by the recruited PMNs (and perhaps by affected host cells), as well as activation of various inositol-signaling pathways within affected host cells, results in the secretion of chloride ions and water (diarrhea).

C. difficile toxin B (TcdB), like TcdA, is a glycosyltransferase that glucosylates Rho GTPases. However, TcdB has little enterotoxic activity but far more cytotoxic activity than TcdA.

C. difficile also produces an ADP-ribosyltransferase (Cdt, for *C. difficile* transferase). Cdt is a binary toxin (see *C. perfringens* ι-toxin, described earlier, and *C. spiroforme*, described later), composed of a binding portion (Cdtb) that binds to the target intestinal epithelial cells and an enzymatically active portion (Cdta). After the toxin binds to specific receptors on the cell surface, Cdta gains entry into the cytoplasm. Although it is not clear precisely how entry occurs, it seems that a pore (composed of Cdtb) is formed in the cell membrane through which Cdta traverses. Cdta is an ADP-ribosylating toxin that ribosylates actin within the host cell, resulting in disorganization of the cellular cytoskeleton and death of the affected cell.

Reservoir and Transmission. *C. difficile* is found in the large intestine of normal as well as clinically affected animals. The spores are resistant to most environmental stresses, which results in their widespread distribution in locations where animals are housed. There is some overlap between those strains that produce disease in human patients and those that are associated with animals.

Pathogenesis. *C. difficile* adheres to mucus or epithelial cells of the large intestine by pili as well as the surface protein Cwp66. Disease most often follows a "trigger" event (e.g., antibiotics, nonsteroidal drugs, and chemotherapeutic agents) that results in relaxation of the control the

FIGURE 35.6. *Fatal necrotizing colitis in a horse caused by* C. difficile. *The large colon and cecum of the horse can result in severe and often fatal disease caused by this bacterium. (Courtesy of Department of Pathobiology, University of Guelph.)*

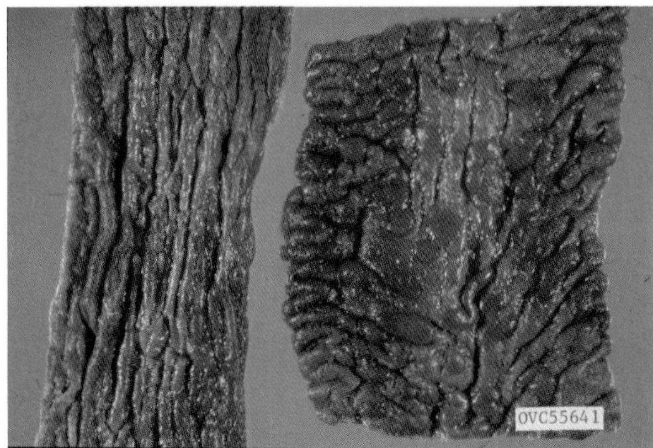

FIGURE 35.7. *Gram stain of* C. difficile. *Like many clostridia, some organisms appear gram-negative; spores are not readily visible in this smear.*

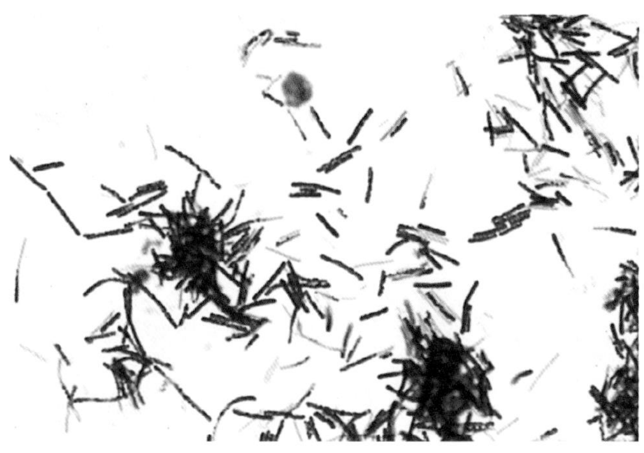

normal intestinal flora has on the numbers of *C. difficile*. In some cases these antibiotics may temporarily control *C. difficile*, but once they are removed, the organisms, which have survived the antibiotic as spores, can rapidly proliferate to produce disease. In addition, the reduced activity or quantity of antimicrobial peptides found as part of the innate defenses of the large intestine of elderly human patients also predisposes to infection. Toxins are produced (TcdA, TcdB, and Cdt), resulting in death of the epithelial cells, which follows disruption of their actin cytoskeleton and tight junctions. Prostaglandin along with the products of the inositol pathway stemming from the intense inflammatory response (TcdA) results in fluid and electrolyte secretion (Figure 35.6). Diarrhea, with or without blood, results.

Epidemiology. *C. difficile*-associated diarrhea is often linked to administration of antibiotics, stress, chemotherapeutic agents, or nonsteroidal anti-inflammatory drugs. For this reason, disease appears to be more frequent and worse in those species with expanded large intestines (colon and cecum) such as horses, rabbits, and swine. Newborn foals have been shown to develop disease without a recognizable "trigger" event, but the diagnosis is complicated by the presence of toxin in the intestine of some healthy neonatal foals, presumably protected against disease by maternal antibodies. Spread occurs through contamination of the environment by spores; the numbers shed in the feces of animals treated with antibiotics can be massive, and therefore, spores can commonly be found in hospital environments. The spore form is resistant to usual disinfection and cleaning procedures.

C. difficile isolated from dogs and cats with diarrhea does not commonly contain the genes encoding Cdt.

Immunologic Aspects. Immunity is probably antitoxic, although the role of antibodies to *C. difficile* is unknown. Orally administered antitoxin (made in bovines) is protective for human patients.

Laboratory Diagnosis. The genes encoding the toxin(s) can be detected in feces by assays based on PCR. Immunologically based tests are available for the detection of the toxin (TcdA and TcdB) in fecal specimens. *C. difficile* can also be isolated from feces by using a selective medium, CCFA (cycloserine, cefoxitin, and fructose agar), and the presence of toxigenic types confirmed by PCR (Figure 35.7). Perhaps surprisingly, an optimal approach to laboratory diagnosis is still being developed in human medicine because enzyme immunoassays (EIA) for toxin A and toxin B are not as sensitive as direct toxicity assays and in addition are not always specific. The current "algorithm" for diagnosis in human medicine involves EIA for glutamate dehydrogenase (GDH) and toxins. If both are negative the diagnosis is reported as negative, and if both are positive the diagnosis is regarded as positive. However, if the more sensitive GDH assay is positive while the toxin assay is negative, a cell cytotoxicity assay or real-time PCR for toxin genes is recommended as the second stage of testing. Enzyme assays are currently preferred over alternates because of speed of diagnosis, although real-time PCR is increasingly used because it is fast, though expensive. Ideal algorithms for diagnosis of disease in animals have not been developed, although toxin testing remains a method of choice. Culture is slow and sometimes also hampered by the death of the organism in air during transport to the laboratory.

Treatment and Control. Diarrhea-associated *C. difficile* responds rapidly to metronidazole. Unfortunately, metronidazole-resistant strains exist. The alternative antibiotic used in humans is vancomycin. There are no vaccines available. However, the use of orally administered yeast, *Saccharomyces boulardii*, has been shown to be useful in preventing the disease in human patients. In pigs, colonization with a nontoxigenic strain has prevented infection by toxigenic bacteria. Probiotics administered at the time of antibiotic use appear to reduce the incidence of *C. difficile* infection. In human hospitals, hand washing by health care personnel is an efficient mechanism for curtailing spread. Disinfectants are not effective against the spores.

Clostridium piliforme ("Bacillus piliformis")

An acute fatal diarrheal disease of laboratory mice with focal liver necrosis (Tyzzer's disease) is associated with a spore-forming organism, *C. piliforme*, which occurs in bundles within hepatocytes. It is unable to grow on cell-free media. *C. piliforme* is linked to identical diseases in rabbits, hares, gerbils, rats, hamsters, muskrats, dogs, cats, snow leopards, foals, and rhesus monkeys. Tyzzer's disease has been reported in a human patient infected with the human immunodeficiency virus, but not in immunocompetent persons.

Descriptive Features. *C. piliforme* is a large, gram-variable, spore-forming rod that is motile by peritrichous flagella. Giemsa and silver stains are preferable to hematoxylin–eosin and Gram stains. Growth has been obtained in embryonated hen's eggs and on cultured mouse hepatocytes.

Vegetative cells die even when deep-frozen or freeze-dried. Spores survive moderate heating, freezing, and thawing. Litter remains infective for months. Strains are pathogenically and morphologically uniform.

Reservoir and Transmission. The source of the agent is the infected animal. The agent spreads by the fecal–oral route and transplacentally. Many infections are believed to be endogenous and stress triggered.

Pathogenesis. Lesions suggest hepatic invasion from the intestine via lymphatics and blood vessels. Foci of coagulation necrosis are periportal (Figure 35.8). There may be dissemination to the myocardium. Parasitized cells include hepatocytes, myocardial cells, smooth muscle, and epithelial cells of the intestine, in which a dysentery-like condition may develop. Lymphadenitis, especially of hepatic nodes, is seen in foals. The course of disease is usually under 3 days.

FIGURE 35.8. *Tyzzer's disease in a foal, showing extensive focal hepatic necrosis. (Courtesy of Department of Pathobiology, University of Guelph.)*

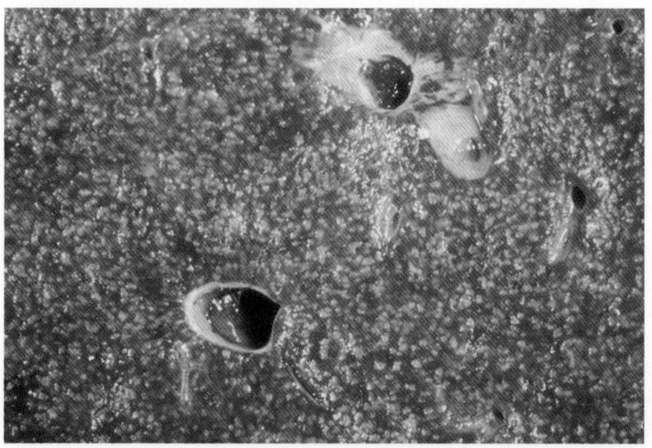

FIGURE 35.9. *Tissue Gram stain of Tyzzer's disease, showing accumulations of* C. piliforme. *(Courtesy of Department of Pathobiology, University of Guelph.)*

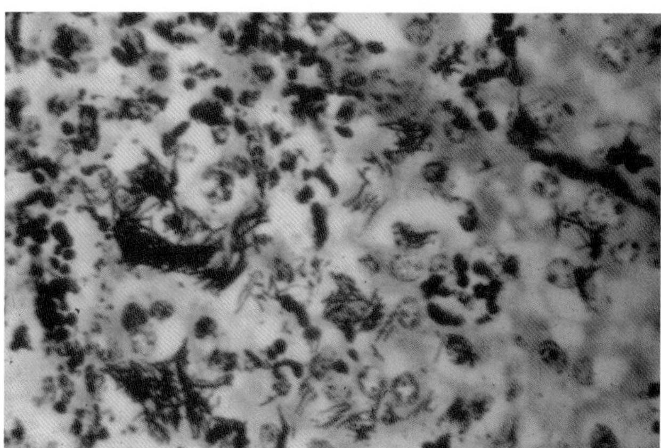

Epidemiology. Outbreaks are often stress related (crowding, irradiation, steroid administration). Morbidity is high in laboratory animal colonies. Case fatality rates reach 50–100%, especially among young stock. In many colonies, subclinically infected individuals are evidently present; these are often identifiable serologically.

Laboratory Diagnosis. Laboratory diagnosis rests on the demonstration of typical bundles of intracellular bacilli (0.5 μm by 8.0–10 μm), especially in hepatocytes surrounding lesions (Figure 35.9). Fluorescent antibody aids diagnosis.

A complement fixation test that utilizes an infected mouse liver extract as antigen has been used to determine the degree of infection in mouse colonies.

Treatment and Control. Treatment of clinical cases is usually unsuccessful. Prophylactically effective antimicrobial drugs include erythromycin and tetracycline.

C. spiroforme

C. spiroforme is isolated frequently from rabbits with typhlocolitis. Like *C. difficile* infection, it may also be predisposed by antibiotic use. Its exotoxin is identical to the ι-toxin of *C. perfringens* type E and the ADP-ribosyltransferase of *C. difficile*. It acts by ADP-ribosylating cellular actin.

Other Clostridia Causing Enteric Disease

Enteric disease caused by *Clostridium septicum* and *Clostridium sordellii* is described in Section "Histotoxic Clostridia."

Histotoxic Clostridia. Histotoxic clostridia are characterized by their ability to cause serious soft tissue including muscle infections, associated with the presence of anaerobic environments including those caused by severe traumatic events. Histotoxicity associated with *C. perfringens* has been briefly described earlier. Some of the histotoxic clostridia also cause enterotoxic infections.

Clostridium chauvoei

C. chauvoei is a gram-positive, motile, obligately anaerobic rod that produces subterminal or subcentral spores. *C. chauvoei* produces an endogenous, emphysematous, necrotizing myositis ("blackleg") in cattle.

Descriptive Features

Cellular Products of Medical Interest. Like other clostridia, *C. chauvoei* produces a number of powerful protein exotoxins that are responsible for the diseases it causes. α-Toxin is an oxygen-stable hemolysin similar to the pore-forming, lethal α-toxin of *C. septicum*. Other extracellular products thought to be important in the pathogenesis if the infection include a DNAase ("β-toxin") and a neuraminidase (sialidase) that removes sialic acid residues from glycoconjugates on cell walls of eukaryotic cells, resulting in disruption of the intercellular matrix. Chauveolysin ("δ-toxin") is a cholesterol-binding cytolysin similar to perfringolysin O, described earlier, that binds to cholesterol-containing rafts in the eukaryotic cell membrane to form a pore that results in the death of the cell.

Reservoir and Transmission. *C. chauvoei* inhabits the intestine, liver, and other tissues of susceptible and resistant species. Blackleg occurs in endemic regions of the world, where the infection is thought to be acquired from soil including soil contaminated with the feces of carrier animals. Infection of the intestinal tract is followed by seeding of the organism into tissues via the liver, with survival of the bacterium in the form of spores in muscle throughout the body. The organism can also be introduced into traumatic wounds from soil, in which case it may cause gas gangrene.

Pathogenesis. Seeding of tissues, especially skeletal muscle, with spores from the intestine precedes disease in cattle. Conditions favoring spore germination, with subsequent bacterial growth and toxin production, cause formation of local lesions marked by edema, hemorrhage, and myofibrillar necrosis, and toxemia systemically. It is usually not clear what factor triggers the spores to germinate, but any local anoxic condition including bruising or injection with irritating products will cause germination. It is suspected that the flight ("gadding") of groups of well-fed and probably physically slightly unfit young cattle to escape the vicious biting flies common in the summer is the major stimulus that causes local muscle anoxia and activates the spores. The necrotizing α-toxin, together the other exotoxins mentioned, is responsible for the initial lesions. Bacterial metabolism producing gas from fermentation may be contributory. The centers of lesions become strikingly dry, dark, and emphysematous because of the necrotizing infection, while the periphery is edematous and hemorrhagic (Figure 35.10). A rancid butter odor is typical. Microscopically, there are degenerative changes in muscle fibers disrupted by edema, emphysema, and hemorrhage. Leukocytic infiltration is minor.

FIGURE 35.10. *"Blackleg" in a cow, showing the characteristic blackened color of the affected muscle, with emphysema due to gas production by* C. chauvoei *in the center of the necrotic muscle. (Courtesy of Department of Pathobiology, University of Guelph.)*

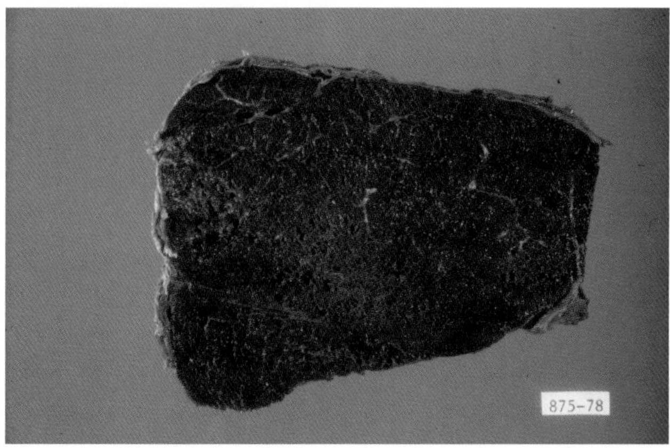

Clinically, there are high fever, anorexia, and depression. Rapidly developing lameness is common. Superficial lesions cause visible swellings, which crepitate on being handled. Although blackleg characteristically affects the focus in one of the major limb muscles, the site of infection sometimes involves more minor muscles such as those of the diaphragm, myocardium, or tongue. Some animals die suddenly, others within 1 or 2 days.

Activation of endogenous spores by injection of irritant chemicals has sometimes produced iatrogenic fatal myositis in horses.

Epidemiology. "Blackleg" occurs worldwide at rates that differ between and within geographic areas, which suggests a soil reservoir or climatic or seasonal factors yet to be defined. Young, well-fed cattle (<3 years) are preferentially attacked. As noted, exertion or bruising is suspected triggering events.

In sheep and some other species, *C. chauvoei* typically causes wound infections resembling malignant edema or gas gangrene. Other clostridia (*Clostridium novyi, C. septicum*, and *C. sordellii*) may be present.

Immunologic Aspects. Circulating antibody to toxins and cellular components apparently determines resistance to *C. chauvoei*. Commercial formalinized adjuvant vaccines include components from up to six other clostridial species (*Clostridium haemolyticum, C. novyi*, type C and type D *C. perfringens, C. septicum*, and *C. sordellii*).

Laboratory Diagnosis. Sporulated gram-positive rods can be demonstrated in smears of infected tissues and identified with immunofluorescent reagents.

C. chauvoei requires strict anaerobic conditions and media rich in cysteine and water-soluble vitamins. The agent resembles *C. septicum* and is frequently recovered with it. Unlike *C. septicum* it ferments sucrose but not salicin and will not grow at 44 °C. The use of DNA primers to amplify the 16S–23S DNA spacer regions (by PCR) will differentiate *C. septicum* from *C. chauvoei*. This assay can also be used to detect the microorganism in tissue.

Detection in tissue or identification in culture can also be accomplished by using DNA primers designed to amplify species-specific portions of the gene encoding the flagellar protein flagellin by PCR, and have been used successfully to differentiate the histotoxic clostridia.

Treatment and Control. Treatment is often disappointing. Penicillin should be given intravenously at first, followed by repository forms intramuscularly.

Cattle are vaccinated against blackleg in endemic regions at 3–6 months of age and annually thereafter. Vaccination should precede exposure by at least 2 weeks. During an outbreak, all cattle are vaccinated and given long-acting penicillin. Pregnant ewes are vaccinated 3 weeks prior to parturition, when infection often occurs. Lambs may require vaccination during their first year. Because of the infectious nature of the disease, a change of pasture is often advisable when cases are first observed.

C. haemolyticum

C. haemolyticum is a nonencapsulated, motile, strict anaerobe, producing large, oval, highly heat-resistant spores. *C. haemolyticum* (previously known as type D *C. novyi*) resembles type B *C. novyi* in practically all phenotypic traits. Its toxin, a phospholipase C, is identical to that of the type B *C. novyi* β-toxin, but is produced in much larger amounts. Serologic and toxigenic variants of *C. haemolyticum* have been noted.

C. haemolyticum produces bacillary hemoglobinuria ("red water") disease of ruminants.

Reservoir and Transmission. *C. haemolyticum* exists in the ruminant digestive tract, in the liver, and in soil. Appearance of the disease in new, widely separated regions suggests that movement of cattle plays a part in its dissemination. Transmission is by ingestion.

Pathogenesis. The pathogenesis of bacillary hemoglobinuria involves ingestion of spores, colonization of the liver, liver injury, spore germination, and toxinogenesis (see *C. novyi* type B "black disease," in Section "Infectious Necrotic Hepatitis"). The exotoxin is a powerful phospholipase C that produces a hemolytic crisis and death within hours or days. Other pathological effects include serosal effusions and widespread hemorrhages. The diagnostic lesions are circumscribed areas of liver necrosis (misnamed "infarcts"), which are the effects of β-toxin (Figure 35.11). Clinically there are fever, pale, icteric mucous membranes, anorexia, agalactia, abdominal pain, hemoglobinuria ("red water"), and hyperpnea. Pregnant cows may abort.

Epidemiology. Bacillary hemoglobinuria occurs in North America in the Rocky Mountain and Pacific Coast states and along the Gulf of Mexico, and in Latin America, parts of Europe, and New Zealand. Although swampy lowlands are associated with endemic disease and flooding with the spread of infection, little is known of the agent's persistence in soil. Shedder animals may have a role in dissemination.

FIGURE 35.11. *Histological section of liver of a cow with bacillary hemoglobinuria, showing coagulation necrosis at the top of the figure, bordered by a zone of intense inflammation. (Courtesy of Department of Pathobiology, University of Guelph.)*

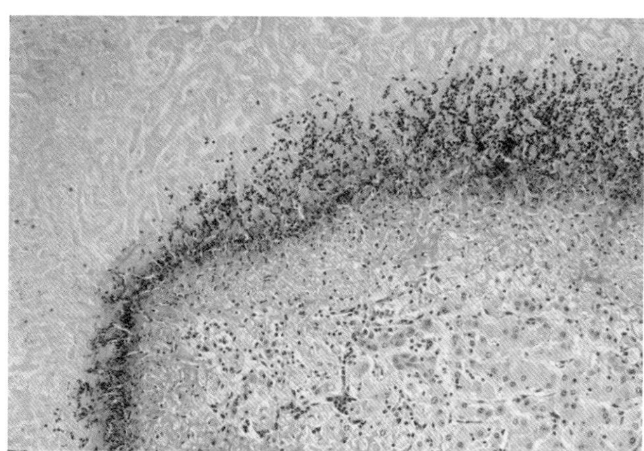

Cases are clustered in the summer and fall, typically among well-nourished animals a year or more of age. Correlation with fluke infection is less consistent than in "black disease" (see *C. novyi* type B, in Section "Infectious Necrotic Hepatitis").

Immunologic Aspects. Immunity is antitoxic. Animals in endemic areas develop some immunity. Whole culture bacterin–toxoids are effective prophylactically.

Laboratory Diagnosis. Liver lesions are the best source of positive smears for Gram stains and immunofluorescence tests. Cultivation requires freshly poured blood agar and strict anaerobic conditions.

Detection in tissue or identification in culture can be accomplished by using PCR as noted for other histotoxic clostridia.

Treatment and Control. Early treatment of sick animals with a broad-spectrum antibiotic (e.g., tetracycline), antitoxin (if available), and blood transfusion produces good results. Animals in endemic areas are vaccinated minimally every 6 months and preferably 3–4 weeks before anticipated exposure.

C. novyi

Descriptive Features. *C. novyi* is a nonencapsulated, motile, gram-positive, obligately anaerobic rod, producing large, oval, highly heat-resistant spores. There are two pathogenic types (A and B), which differ biochemically, epidemiologically, and pathogenically. A different species, *C. haemolyticum*, discussed earlier, used to be known as type D *C. novyi*. *C. novyi* produces gas gangrene, "big head," and "black disease" of ruminants, and, rarely, blackleg of cattle.

Cellular Products of Medical Interest

Toxins. *C. novyi* produces a number of extracellular protein toxins that are responsible for the diseases associated with it. Of these, the α- and β-toxins and the cholesterol-binding cytolysin novyilysin have proven roles in the diseases produced by this species.

α-Toxin. α-Toxin is produced by *C. novyi* types A and B. It is a glycosyltransferase that glucosylates Rho GTPases, rendering them ineffectual in interacting with their substrates and therefore as cell signaling systems. In addition, glycosylation blocks interaction of Rho GDP with guanine exchange factor, and the interaction of Rho GTP with GTPase-activating factor, thereby preventing membrane cycling. As a consequence, several signaling pathways are disrupted, resulting in a breakdown of the cytoskeletal components of the affected cell, followed by its death.

β-Toxin. β-Toxin is produced by *C. novyi* type B. It is a phospholipase C (a lecithinase) that hydrolyzes the phosphatidylcholine and sphingomyelin constituents of host cell membranes, resulting in death of the cell. This toxin is also hemolytic.

δ-Toxin (Novyilysin). δ-Toxin or novyilysin is produced *by C. novyi* type A, and is a cholesterol-binding cytolysin (see also perfringolysin O, mentioned earlier). Novyilysin binds to cholesterol-containing rafts in the eukaryotic cell membrane. Once bound, it forms a pore resulting in the death of the cell.

Miscellaneous Toxins. *C. novyi* produces a number of other extracellular protein enzymes or minor toxins with uncertain roles in the pathogenesis of disease. These include lecithinases, lipases, and myosinases.

Reservoir and Transmission. Type A is common in soil. Types A and B occur in the healthy intestine and liver of herbivores, and may also be found as spores persisting in muscle. All enter their hosts by ingestion or by wound infection.

Pathogenesis. Of several toxins produced by *C. novyi*, α-, β-, and novyilysin toxins are lethal and necrotizing, and are of established pathogenic significance. The pathogenic roles of the minor nonlethal toxins are uncertain.

Gas Gangrene and Blackleg. *C. novyi* type A is implicated in gas gangrene ("clostridial wound infection") of humans and animals. One unique form of these, "bighead of rams," starts as a fight injury at the top of the head of rams, and may result from the activation of spores endogenously present in muscles of the head. Toxic endothelial damage produces edema involving head, neck, and cranial thorax. Death occurs in 2 days. The yellow tinge of the edema fluid, which is clear and gelatinous with little hemorrhage, is a postmortem change. *C. novyi* may also rarely cause a blackleg-like disease of cattle, sometimes known as "pseudoblackleg" to distinguish it from the identical disease caused by *C. chauvoei*. Activation of endogenous spores by injection of irritant chemicals has sometimes produced iatrogenic fatal myositis in horses.

Infectious Necrotic Hepatitis. *C. novyi* type B causes infectious necrotic hepatitis ("black disease") of sheep and cattle, and rarely horses, swine, and other species. Spores originating in the intestine reach the liver and remain there dormant within Kupffer cells. When liver cells are injured, as commonly follows fluke migration, the resulting anaerobic conditions cause the spores to germinate. Vegetative growth results in toxin production and dissemination. Death may be sudden or within 2 days of clinical onset. Signs include depression, anorexia, and hypothermia. Necropsy reveals edema, serosal effusion, and one or more areas of liver necrosis, containing bacteria. Subcutaneous venous congestion secondary to pericardial edema darkens the underside of the skin, hence the name "black disease." The occasional outbreak in swine might be associated with ascarids migrating through the liver.

Epidemiology. The agent occurs worldwide. "Bighead" is recognized in Australia, South Africa, and North America. Distribution of "black disease" largely coincides with that of the liver fluke *Fasciola hepatica*. Both diseases occur mostly in adult sheep, during summer and fall. "Black disease" affects notably well-nourished animals.

Immunologic Aspects. Circulating antitoxins (antibodies to α-, β-, and novyilysin toxins) and antibodies to cellular components of the organism are presumably the basis of immunity to *C. novyi* infections. Whole culture bacterins and toxoids have prophylactic value.

Laboratory Diagnosis. Liver lesions contain large gram-positive to gram-variable rods with oval subterminal, large spores, which are identifiable by fluorescent anti-*C. novyi* conjugates.

Isolation of the bacteria requires the strictest anaerobic conditions, especially for type B, which is also nutritionally fastidious. *C. novyi* may be demonstrable in normal livers of herbivores within hours after death, and therefore, postmortem invaders need to be differentiated from genuine pathogens.

Increasingly, detection in tissue or identification in culture is accomplished by using PCR, including real-time PCR, that allows quantitation of the bacterial load. DNA primers designed to amplify species-specific portions of the gene encoding the flagellar protein, flagellin, have been used successfully to differentiate histotoxic clostridia

Treatment and Control. There is no effective treatment. Control is directed at eliminating flukes and other hepatopathic agents. Prophylactic vaccination with a bacterin–toxoid combination is generally effective.

C. septicum

Descriptive Features. *C. septicum* is a short, stout, and pleomorphic gram-positive, motile, spore-forming obligately anaerobic rod. In some exudates, long filaments are found.

C. septicum is the leading cause of wound infections (gas gangrene = malignant edema) of farm animals and gangrenous dermatitis in poultry, but may also cause a fatal abomasitis in sheep and, unusually, blackleg ("pseudoblackleg") in ruminants.

Cellular Products of Medical Interest. *C. septicum* produces a number of protein exotoxins that are purportedly responsible for the diseases associated with it. However, only α-toxin has been definitively shown to be a virulence factor. The α-toxin is a pore-forming, lethal toxin. Following secretion, it is bound to glycosylphosphatidylinositol-anchored proteins on the eukaryotic cell surface (mainly endothelial cells). There, the cell-bound proteolytic enzyme, furin, cleaves it, resulting in fragments that insert into the membrane forming pores leading to death of the cell. *C. septicum* also produces a DNAase ("β-toxin") with leukocytotoxic activity, a hyaluronidase ("γ-toxin"), a cholesterol-binding cytolysin (septicolysin O) (with activity similar to that of perfringolysin O and novyilysin, and so on), and miscellaneous extracellular products (chitinases, neuraminidases, lipases, sialidases, and hemagglutinins) with undefined roles in the pathogenesis of disease.

Reservoir and Transmission. *C. septicum* occurs in soils worldwide and in the animal and human intestines. It is acquired by wound infection and ingestion.

Pathogenesis. Wound infection caused by *C. septicum* is often called "malignant edema," but the term "gas gangrene" is probably better understood. All of the toxic products outlined earlier probably play a role in this serious necrotizing infection, but only the α-toxin has been shown to be definitively involved. Systemic effects are thought to be the result of endothelial damage throughout the body, leading to severe fluid and electrolyte imbalances as well as for the edema seen locally. Membrane-active toxins, dissolution of connective tissue components, along with destruction of polymorphonuclear leukocytes and release of their digestive enzymes may account for the tissue destruction observed. The infectious process radiates from the point of inoculation within hours to days of exposure. A hemorrhagic, edematous, necrotizing process frequently follows fascial planes as adjacent muscle is darkened (Figure 35.12). With muscular involvement and emphysema, there may be close resemblance to "blackleg" (Section "*Clostridium chauvoei*"). Crepitant swellings change from painful and hot to painless and cold. Signs include fever, tachycardia, anorexia, and depression. The course may be rapid and fatal within a day. Wounds include traumatic wounds, but may include the postparturient uterus of animals.

C. septicum causes a blackleg-like disease of cattle, sometimes known as "pseudoblackleg" to distinguish it from the identical disease caused by *C. chauvoei*. Activation of endogenous spores by injection of irritant chemicals has produced iatrogenic fatal myositis in horses.

C. septicum also causes gangrenous dermatitis, a fatal necrotizing cellulitis and myonecrosis of poultry including turkeys and broiler chickens. *C. perfringens* may be concurrently involved. The factors precipitating the sometimes devastating infection are unclear, but include poor hygiene, overcrowding, and likely fecal contamination of pressure sores.

FIGURE 35.12. *Gas gangrene in a young piglet, likely associated with injection or castration. The necrotizing process has followed fascial planes. (Courtesy of Department of Pathobiology, University of Guelph.)*

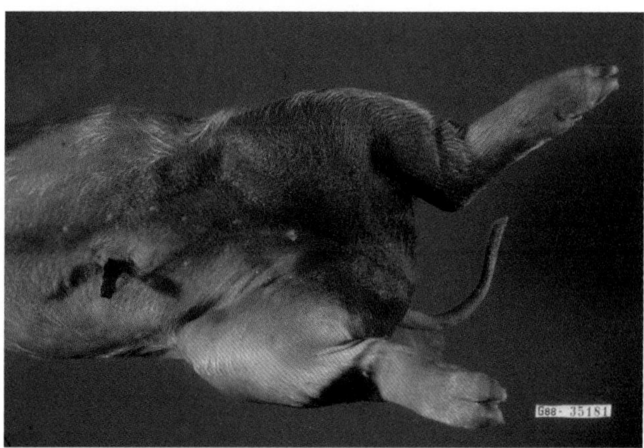

Severe and fatal abomasitis (*braxy* in Scottish or *bradsot* in Danish) is a fatal *C. septicum* cold weather disease of sheep in which *C. septicum* produces a necrotizing lesion in the abomasal wall comparable to the subcutaneous one described earlier. Clinical signs are mostly toxemia and gastrointestinal distress. Most aspects of the pathogenesis of this unusual, dramatic, and generally fatal disease are poorly understood. The association of the infection with ingestion of frozen food including hay might suggest traumatic damage of the abomasal mucosa (Figure 35.13).

Human wound infections due to *C. septicum* may develop into serious cellulitis and gas gangrene, and are associated with illegal intravenous drug injection, abortion (producing septic metritis) under unhygienic conditions, malignancies, skin infections, the peripheral vasculopathy associated with diabetes, and severe trauma. The organism also causes a "spontaneous" non-wound-associated myonecrosis ("gas gangrene") in humans with pathogenesis likely similar to that of blackleg in cattle.

Epidemiology. Gas gangrene may follow such procedures as castration, docking, shearing, tagging, and injections. Postparturient genital infections are sometimes linked to dystocia and unskilled obstetrical assistance. "Braxy" or "bradsot" occurs mostly in colder countries such as Canada, Scotland, and Scandinavian countries.

Immunologic Aspects. Immunity is probably antitoxin dependent.

Laboratory Diagnosis. Sporulated rods may be demonstrable in exudates by Gram stain or immunofluorescence.

C. septicum grows readily on blood agar under anaerobic conditions, producing hemolytic colonies up to 5 mm in diameter within 48 h, with rhizoid contours and a frequent tendency to swarm. Although recovery and identification of this agent by culture are not difficult, positive results

FIGURE 35.13. *"Braxy" in the abomasum of a lamb, showing extensive hemorrhage, edema, gas formation, and areas of focal necrosis. (Courtesy of Department of Pathobiology, University of Guelph.)*

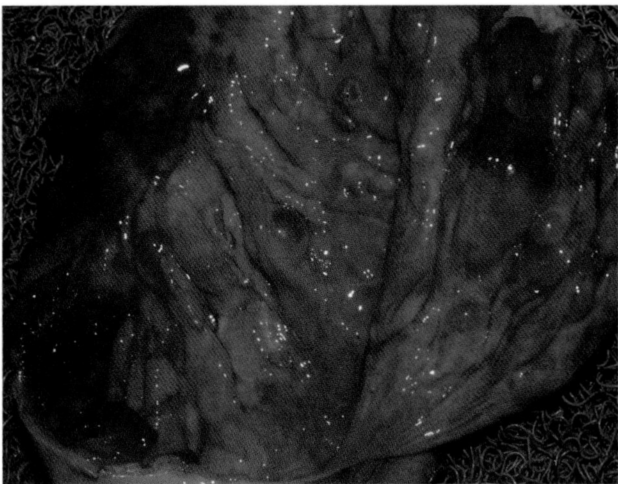

should be interpreted with caution since *C. septicum* is an aggressive postmortem invader. Its presence may therefore be unrelated to the problem at hand and may obscure that of more significant pathogens, such as *C. haemolyticum* and *C. chauvoei*.

Demonstration in tissue or identification of isolates is possible by fluorescent antibody staining or by PCR amplification of the α-toxin. PCR amplification of species-specific portions of flagellin gene has been to differentiate the organism from other clostridia causing severe tissue necrosis.

Treatment and Control. Prognosis is guarded. Possible therapy includes penicillin or tetracycline given systemically, incision and drainage of the wounds, and their irrigation with antiseptics.

Calves are vaccinated at 3–4 months of age, sheep and goats at weaning. Hygienic precautions at times of likely exposure are helpful.

C. sordellii

The role of *C. sordellii* in serious infections of animals and humans may have been underestimated, or infections may be increasing. The agent produces numerous toxins and is experimentally pathogenic for many species of animals.

C. sordellii is associated with a fatal myositis and hepatic disease in ruminants and horses, although the precise pathogenic process is not known. "Acute pasture myopathy" ("equine atypical myopathy," "seasonal pasture myopathy"), associated with acute and usually fatal rhabdomyolysis, has become an increasing problem in recent years in European countries. It occurs especially in young adult grazing horses under frosty and stormy, fall-like, conditions. The disease is associated with sudden onset of muscle weakness, the result of generalized myodegeneration, although the focus of infection is unclear. It may be the intestine. The presence of the lethal toxin of *C. sordelliii* (TcsL) has been demonstrated in myofibers of affected horses by immunohistochemistry.

C. sordellii has caused fatal disease in perinatal foals following infection of the umbilical remnants as well as fatal uterine infections in postparturient sheep. It is also emerging as a pathogen of humans, associated with very serious and often fatal infections following abortion and "spontaneous" non-wound-associated myonecrosis ("gas gangrene") similar to blackleg.

There is increasing evidence that the organism can cause severe enteric disease including a disease identical to *C. septicum* abomasitis ("braxy") in lambs. The organism has been isolated from fatal enteric disease in lions.

Mixed clostridial bacterin–toxoids for blackleg and gas gangrene usually contain *C. sordellii*.

Neurotoxic Clostridia

Clostridium botulinum (the cause of botulism) and *Clostridium tetani* (the cause of tetanus) produce disease strictly through the action of neurotoxins, botulinum and tetanus toxins, respectively. Although botulinum and tetanus toxins have the same mechanism of action, they produce different diseases with remarkably different manifestations because they affect different sites in the nervous system.

Botulinum and tetanus toxins block neurotransmitter release. Both toxins are zinc endopeptidases that interfere with the fusion of neurotransmitter-containing vesicles with the membrane lining the presynaptic cleft. Interference is due to hydrolysis of the proteins involved with "docking," which precedes fusion of neurotransmitter-containing vesicles with the membrane lining the cleft. Hydrolysis of these proteins leads to degeneration of the synapse and to the blockage of neurotransmission. Regeneration of the synapse takes several weeks to months.

C. botulinum

C. botulinum is a gram-positive, spore-forming, obligately anaerobic rod, which produces the disease botulism, a neuroparalytic intoxication characterized by flaccid paralysis. The intoxication is caused by any of seven protein neurotoxins (A to G) (Table 35.3) that are identical in action but differ in potency, antigenic properties, and distribution. They are produced by a heterogeneous group of clostridia, called *C. botulinum* (*C. botulinum* group G has been renamed *C. argentinense*) on the basis of the toxins, which in some types (C and D) are bacteriophage encoded.

Botulism is seen mainly in ruminants, horses, mink, and birds, particularly waterfowl, though the infection is increasingly diagnosed in commercial poultry. Swine, carnivores, and fish are rarely affected.

Descriptive Features

Morphology. *C. botulinum* is a gram-positive, spore-forming obligately anaerobic rod. At a pH near and above neutrality, it produces subterminal oval spores.

Table 35.3. Classic Botulinum Toxin Types: General Distribution, Origin, and Pathogenicity

Type (Toxin Present)	Geographic Distribution	Source	Species Affected
A (A)	Western North America, former Soviet Union	Vegetables, fruits (meat, fish)	Humans (chicken, mink)
B (B)	Eastern North America, Europe, former Soviet Union	Meat, pork products (vegetables, fish)	Humans (horses, cattle)
Cα (C_1)	New Zealand, Japan, Europe	Vegetation, invertebrates, carrion	Waterfowl
Cβ (C_1, D)	Australia, Africa, Europe, North America	Spoiled feed, carrion	Horses, cattle, mink (humans)
D (D)	Africa, former Soviet Union, Southwestern United States, Europe	Carrion, chicken manure	Cattle, sheep, chickens (horses, humans)
E	North America, North Europe, Japan, former Soviet Union	Raw fish, marine mammals	Humans, fish, fish-eating birds
F	United States, North Europe, former Soviet Union	Meat, fish	Humans
G	Argentina	Soil	Humans

Cellular Products of Medical Interest

Toxin. *C. botulinum* produces several proteins with "toxic" activity (botulinum toxin, C2 toxin, and C3 exoenzyme), but only botulinum toxin has a central role in the production of botulism.

There are seven types of botulinum toxins (BoNT for botulinum neurotoxin), differentiated by antigenic differences, although new "mosaic" toxins have recently been described. Letters A through G depict the types (Table 35.3). The type of neurotoxin characterizes the strain of *C. botulinum* producing it. Thus, a strain of *C. botulinum* producing type A BoNT would be described as *C. botulinum* type A.

All seven types of BoNT are zinc endopeptidases with identical activity, that is, hydrolysis of the docking proteins required by neurotransmitter-containing vesicles to fuse with the presynaptic membrane. Although the end result is the same (blockage of the release of neurotransmitter), the various types of BoNT hydrolyze different docking proteins. Types A and E hydrolyze SNAP (synaptosomal-associated protein); types B, D, F, and G hydrolyze VAMP (vesicle-associated membrane protein also known as synaptobrevin), and type C hydrolyzes SNAP and syntaxin. Once hydrolyzed, the synapse degenerates, taking weeks to months to regenerate.

BoNT is a "di-chain" molecule consisting of a light chain (with zinc endopeptidase activity), a heavy chain composed of a translocation domain (responsible for forming a pore through which the light chain passes), and a binding domain (responsible for binding to nerve cells). Several "accessory" proteins thought to aid the survival of the toxin in the gastrointestinal tract are secreted with BoNT.

BoNT binds to cholinergic nerve cells, each type of BoNT binding to a different receptor. After binding, the toxin is internalized by way of receptor-mediated endocytosis. Vesicles containing BoNT remain at the neuromuscular junction. Following a cleaving event, the light chain (the zinc endopeptidase) translocates across the vesicle membrane into the cytosol of the nerve cell where it hydrolyzes the docking proteins.

Both the C2 toxin and C3 exoenzyme are ADP-ribosyltransferases. C2 toxin and C3 exoenzyme ribosylate G-actin and Rho, respectively, resulting in disruptions in the cytoskeleton. Neither enzyme appears to play a role in the disease process.

Resistance. Although heat resistance of spores varies between culture groups, toxin types, and strains, moist heat at 120 °C for 5 min is generally lethal. Exceptions exist. Low pH and high salinity enhance heat sterilization. Salt, nitrates, and nitrites suppress germination of spores in foods. Heating to 80 °C for 20 min inactivates the toxin. The seven types of toxins differ in antigenicity, heat resistance, and lethality for different animal species (probably related to receptor density on the surface of the motor neuron). Four culture groups are also recognized.

Reservoir and Transmission. Reservoirs of *C. botulinum* are soil and aquatic sediments. Vehicles of intoxication are animal and plant material contaminated from these sources. When animals die, *C. botulinum* spores, which are common in gut and tissues, germinate and generate toxin. This may contaminate the immediate local environment. An example of this is an animal killed during hay making and rolled into a "big bale" hay bale. In rotting vegetation, a similar process occurs. Apart from toxin ingestion, spore ingestion and wound contamination may lead to botulism. Spore ingestion is important in human infant botulism. Wound infection botulism is seen rarely in humans and horses.

Pathogenesis. Botulinum toxin is the most toxic protein known; 1 μg can kill a person. Ingested BoNT is absorbed from the glandular stomach and anterior small intestine and distributed via the bloodstream. It binds to receptors and enters the nerve cell after receptor-mediated endocytosis. How BoNT gets from the bloodstream to the surface of nerve cells is not understood. Toxin-containing vesicles remain at the myoneural junction. A fragment of the toxin (light chain) translocates across the vesicle membrane into the cytosol of the nerve cell and subsequently hydrolyzes a "docking" protein (which protein depends upon which botulinum toxin). The synapse degenerates and flaccid paralysis results due to the lack of neurotransmitter (acetylcholine). When this affects muscles of respiration, death due to respiratory failure occurs. No primary lesions are produced.

Clinical signs include muscular incoordination leading to recumbency, extrusion of the tongue, and disturbances in food prehension, chewing, and swallowing. No changes in consciousness occur. The temperature remains normal unless secondary infections such as aspiration pneumonia supervene. In nonfatal cases, recovery is slow and residual signs may persist for months. There is still an unproven but plausible suggestion that equine grass sickness, a commonly fatal dysautonomia, affecting the enteric nervous system is associated with the ingestion of BoNT secreted by *C. botulinum* type C living in association with blades of grass (as a biofilm).

In birds such as ducks, the disease has been named "limberneck" after the characteristic drooping head posture, which often causes waterfowl to drown.

Epidemiology. Types A and B are found in all soils, including virgin soils; types C, D, E, and F are linked with wet environments—that is, muddy soils or aquatic sediment. In animals, types C and D predominate. Type C living in biofilms on the surface of blades of grass may be the source of BoNT seen in equine grass sickness, although whether equine grass sickness is truly the result of botulism remains to be definitively demonstrated. Type E is associated with aquatic environments, so is characteristically associated with eating affected or contaminated fish.

Dead animals (birds, rodents, and cats) in feed can be sources of outbreaks, as can chicken litter (which may contain dead chickens) when used as a cattle and sheep feed supplement, as bedding, or is spread as a fertilizer onto pastures to which ruminants have access. The increasing use of "big bale silage" and round hay baling in recent years, in which grass is ensiled without acidification in large plastic airtight bags or wrapped in tight round bales, has been associated with increased botulism in horses and cattle. It is likely that this is a combination of the cutting of grass very close to the ground, so that baby grassland nestling birds or rodents are collected, as well as the anaerobic conditions of ensilage or of tightly wrapped hay. Outbreaks on mink ranches are usually due to tainted meat, and those in fish hatcheries to fish food containing *C. botulinum* type E spores that germinate in bottom sludge. Decaying vegetation triggers outbreaks in waterfowl. As lakes recede in summer leaving muddy shores or shallow pools, rotting plant material becomes accessible. *C. botulinum* and its toxin are ingested and after death permeate the carcass, which is fed upon by blowfly larvae that absorb the toxin. Waterfowl ingesting these larvae become intoxicated. Type C and type D botulism is increasing in commercial laying and broiler chickens, apparently as a result of production of toxin within the intestine ("toxicoinfectious" botulism), although the reason for this increase is unclear. This intestinal infection may be related to the increased botulism observed in ruminants exposed to chicken litter.

Type B botulism has been seen in cattle and mules. In "toxicoinfectious botulism" of foals ("shaker foal syndrome") and adult horses, no toxin has been demonstrated, but the agent has been isolated consistently from tissue.

Type D botulism is classically linked to phosphorus-deficient ranges, where grazing animals feed on carcasses and bones that often contain botulinum toxin. In South African cattle, the condition is called *lamziekte* ("lame disease"), which describes the lameness associated with phosphorus deficiency. Type D botulism is increasingly identified in ruminants in the United Kingdom exposed to broiler chicken litter.

Type E botulism has emerged in fish-eating birds in the Great Lakes of North America, the result of complex ecological changes induced in the aquatic environment by various invasive species. Migrating fish-eating birds catch fish with botulism, which makes them easier to catch, and succumb to intoxication.

Human botulism is usually traced to improperly processed meat, seafood, or canned vegetables. Infant botulism involves clostridial growth and toxinogenesis in the intestinal tract, producing the "floppy baby syndrome," and may be associated with ingestion of honey, since this frequently contains large numbers of *C. botulinum* spores. Wound infection botulism results from contaminated external injuries.

Immunologic Aspects. Resistance to botulism depends on circulating antitoxin. Some carrion-eating animals, such as vultures, apparently acquire immunity through repeated sublethal exposure.

Laboratory Diagnosis. Diagnosis of botulism requires demonstration of toxin in plasma or tissue before death or from a fresh carcass. Isolation of the organism, especially from intestinal contents, or postmortem demonstration of toxin is not definitive. Demonstration of toxin in feedstuffs, fresh stomach contents, or vomitus supports a diagnosis of botulism.

Toxin is extracted from suspect material (unless fluids) overnight with saline. The mixture is centrifuged and the clear portion filter-sterilized and trypsinized (1% at 37 °C for 45 min). Guinea pigs or mice are injected intraperitoneally with the extract, mixtures of extract and antitoxins, and extract heated to 100 °C for 10 min. Death due to botulism occurs within 10 h to 3 weeks (average is 4 days) preceded by muscular weakness, limb paralysis, and respiratory difficulties. To confirm that animals die of intoxication rather than peritonitis, any toxin must be neutralizable by one of the *C. botulinum* antitoxins.

Isolation of *C. botulinum* from suspect feeds or tissue begins with heating suspect material at 65–80 °C for 30 min to induce germination. Type E spores require, in addition, treatment with lysozyme (5 mg/ml of medium). Culture is anaerobically on blood agar plates. Identification is by biochemical reactions and toxin production. Immunofluorescence is used to identify some cultural groups. Primers designed to amplify the genes encoding the various toxins (by the PCR) can be used to support the demonstration that *C. botulinum* has been isolated.

Treatment and Control. If recent ingestion is suspected, evacuation of the stomach and purging are helpful. Antitoxin treatment following onset of signs is sometimes beneficial, especially for mink and ducks, but prevention by vaccination is infinitely preferred. Mink and other animals at risk should be vaccinated with toxoid (types A, B, C, and D). Clinical trials to prevent equine grass sickness with a botulinum toxoid vaccine are ongoing. Removal of affected waterfowl to dry land, if feasible, saves many from exposure and drowning. Placing food on dry ground may lure birds from contaminated areas. It is mandatory that farmers in the United Kingdom remove carcasses from chicken litter before selling it as fertilizer.

Guanidine and aminopyridine stimulate acetylcholine release, and germine intensifies neural impulses. Clinical reports on their use are few and mixed.

C. tetani

C. tetani is a gram-positive, spore-forming, obligately anaerobic rod, which produces the disease tetanus, a neuroparalytic intoxication characterized by tetanic spasm of muscle and tonic–clonic convulsions. The intoxication is due to a protein neurotoxin.

All mammals are susceptible to varying degrees to tetanus, with horses, ruminants, and swine being more susceptible than carnivores and poultry. In all animals, the mortality rate is high. Humans and horses are the most susceptible species.

Descriptive Features

Morphology. *C. tetani* is a gram-positive, spore-forming, obligately anaerobic rod. A distinguishing morphologic feature of *C. tetani* is the spherical shape and terminal position of its spores ("drumstick" or "tennis racket"; Figure 35.1).

Cellular Products of Medical Interest. *C. tetani* produces two toxins (tetanolysin and tetanus toxin), though only tetanus toxin is of clinical significance.

The genes encoding tetanus toxin (TeNT for tetanus neurotoxin, also called tetanospasmin) are located on a large plasmid. TeNT is released upon lysis of the clostridial cell. There is only one type of TeNT, a zinc endopeptidase, which hydrolyzes the docking proteins required by neurotransmitter-containing vesicles to fuse with the presynaptic membrane. TeNT hydrolyzes the docking protein VAMP (vesicle-associated membrane protein, also known as synaptobrevin). Once the docking proteins are hydrolyzed, the synapse degenerates, taking weeks to months to regenerate.

TeNT is a "di-chain" molecule consisting of a light chain (with zinc endopeptidase activity), a heavy chain composed of a translocation domain (responsible for forming a pore through which the light chain passes), and a binding domain (responsible for binding to nerve cells).

TeNT binds to cholinergic nerve cells by virtue of receptors that are different from those recognized by BoNT. These receptors are composed of lipid-containing rafts and glycosylphosphatidylinositol-anchored proteins. After binding, the toxin is internalized by way of receptor-mediated endocytosis. Vesicles containing TeNT travel by retrograde axonal transport to the inhibitory interneurons in the ventral horn of the spinal cord. Following a cleaving event, the light chain (the zinc endopeptidase) translocates across the vesicle membrane into the cytosol of the nerve cell where it hydrolyzes the "docking" proteins involved with vesicles containing the neurotransmitters γ-aminobutyric acid and glycine.

The other toxin, tetanolysin is a cholesterol-binding cytolysin but has no known pathogenic significance in the production of tetanus.

Growth Characteristics. *C. tetani* grows on blood agar under routine anaerobic conditions. There may be swarming. Its differential reactions (carbohydrate fermentation, proteolysis, and indole production) vary with the medium used. Spores resist boiling up to 1.5 h, but not autoclaving (121 °C for 10 min). Disinfection by some halogen compounds (3% iodine) can be effective within several hours, but phenol, lysol, and formalin in the usual concentrations are ineffective.

Reservoir and Transmission. *C. tetani* is widely distributed in soil and is often a transient in the intestine. Spores are introduced into wounds.

Pathogenesis. Spore germination requires an anaerobic environment as is found in tissues devitalized by crushing, burning, laceration, breakdown of blood supply (e.g., umbilical stump or placental remnants), or bacterial infection. Under these circumstances, *C. tetani* proliferates and its toxin diffuses via vascular channels or peripheral nerve trunks. The toxin attaches to receptors on the nearest cholinergic nerve and is internalized within a vesicle, which travels retrograde inside the axons to the cell bodies in the ventral horns of the spinal cord. The light chain of the toxin translocates across the vesicle membrane into the cytosol where it hydrolyzes "docking" proteins and suppresses release of afferent inhibitory messenger substances (glycine and γ-aminobutyric acid), causing the innervated muscles to remain in sustained clonic or tonic spasms. The toxin also travels within the cord to other levels affecting additional muscle groups. Synapses degenerate following hydrolysis of the vesicular docking proteins, taking several weeks to regenerate.

The process described ("ascending tetanus") is typical of animals not highly susceptible to tetanus toxin (e.g., dogs and cats). Only nerve trunks near the toxigenic site absorb sufficient toxin to produce overt signs.

"Descending tetanus" (a generalized toxemia) is typical of highly susceptible species (horses and humans) in which effective toxin quantities are disseminated via vascular channels to nerve endings in areas remote from the toxigenic site. Toxin enters the central nervous system at many levels producing generalized tetanus, frequently beginning cranially since the cranial nerves have short distances into the central nervous system. The sequence reflects susceptibility of various neurons.

Disease Patterns. Early signs, following an incubation period of a few days to several weeks, are stiffness, muscular tremor, and increased responsiveness to stimuli.

In horses, ruminants, and swine, which usually develop descending tetanus, retraction of the third eyelid (because of spasm of ophthalmic muscles), erectness of ears, grinding of teeth, and stiffness of the tail are observed. Bloat is common in ruminants. Feeding becomes impossible ("lockjaw"). Rigidity of extremities causes "sawhorse" attitudes and, eventually, recumbency. Tetanic spasms occur first in response to stimuli, but later become permanent. There are fecal and urinary retention, sweating, and high fever. Consciousness persists. Death, due to respiratory arrest, occurs in lambs and piglets within the first week, in adult animals in 1–2 weeks. Full recovery requires weeks to months. Mortality is at least 50% and highest in the young.

In carnivores, the incubation period tends to be longer, and local (ascending) tetanus (stiffness and tremors) is frequently seen near the original wound. Progression may be slower than in ungulates, but signs and course are comparable.

Epidemiology. Occurrence of tetanus is linked to the introduction of *C. tetani* spores into traumatized tissue (see Section "Pathogenesis"). Penetrating nail wounds of the foot, barnyard surgery, the use of rubber bands for castrating and docking sheep, ear tagging, injections, shearing wounds, postpartum uterine infections, perinatal umbilical infections, and small animal fights and leghold traps all predispose to the type of injury and the soil or fecal contamination associated with tetanus.

Immunologic Aspects. TeNT is antigenically uniform. Acquired resistance to tetanus depends on circulating antitoxin. Small amounts have been demonstrated in normal ruminants. Surprisingly, but because of its great toxicity, survivors of tetanus with the possible exception of dogs and cats are susceptible to reinfection. The amount of toxin needed to result in tetanus in dogs and cats is sometimes large enough to elicit an antitoxin response. Passive and active protection is provided by administration of antitoxin or immunization with toxoid, respectively (see Section "Treatment and Control").

Laboratory Diagnosis. A Gram-stained smear from a suspect wound may reveal the typical "drumstick" type of bacteria (see Figure 35.1). Their absence does not exclude tetanus, and their presence is merely suggestive as the morphology is not unique. Wound exudate is plated on blood agar for anaerobic culture. Increased agar content (up to 4%) inhibits swarming, and a drop of antitoxin will inhibit hemolysis on that portion of the plate.

Traditionally, replicate cooked meat broth cultures were incubated and some were heated at 80 °C for varying periods (up to 20 min) to kill bacteria other than spores. All were incubated at 37 °C for 4 days and subcultured to blood agar periodically during that time. Previously unheated ones were heated before subculture. Suspect isolates were identified by differential tests and confirmed as tetanus toxin producers by intramuscular injection of a 48 h broth culture into two mice, one of which had received antitoxin. It is actually now rare for this to be done because the disease is so characteristic that laboratory diagnosis is not required.

Primers designed to amplify the gene encoding tetanus toxin (by the PCR) can also be used to support the demonstration that *C. tetani* has been isolated.

Treatment and Control. Therapy aims at neutralization of circulating toxin, suppression of toxin production, and life support and symptomatic relief to the patient. The first objective is pursued by injection of adequate doses of antitoxin, 10 000–300 000 units for horses. Some suggest intrathecal administration since this can be beneficial

Wound care and parenteral penicillin or metronidazole are aimed at stopping toxin production. Supportive treatment includes use of sedatives and muscle relaxants and exclusion of external stimuli. Artificial feeding by a stomach tube or intravenously may be necessary after the hyperesthetic phase. Nursing care is most important.

Wounds should be properly cleaned and dressed. During surgical procedures, especially on a mass scale under farm conditions, appropriate hygienic precautions should be observed. Horses, unless actively immunized, are given antitoxin after injury or surgery, and depot penicillin.

Active immunization employs formalinized toxoid, given twice at 1- to 2-month intervals and often annually thereafter, although it is increasingly common to immunize less frequently. All highly susceptible species, especially horses, humans and sheep, should be vaccinated against tetanus. Package insert directions should be followed. Passive immunity passes from immunized mare to nursing foals and provides protection for about 10 weeks, when toxoid can be given.

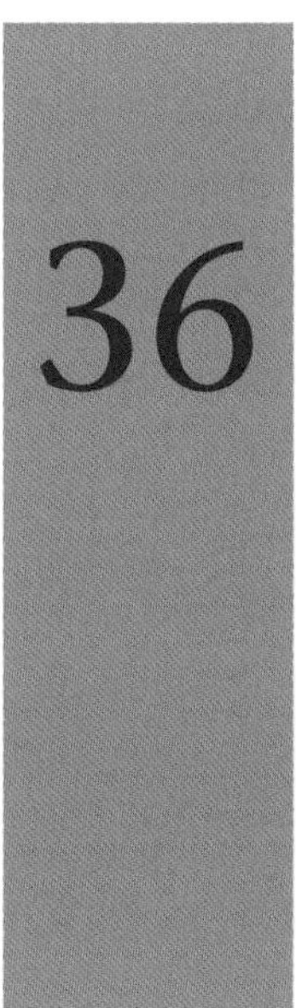

Filamentous Bacteria: *Actinomyces, Nocardia, Dermatophilus,* and *Streptobacillus*

MEGAN E. JACOB

Members of the genera *Actinomyces, Nocardia, Dermatophilus,* and *Streptobacillus* are associated by their ability to appear in filamentous forms. Apart from this characteristic, and a common manifestation of pyogranulmatous inflammation, these organisms have little in common. Table 36.1 summarizes their differential characteristics.

Actinomyces

Actinomyces organisms are anaerobic or facultative anaerobic, gram-positive, branching rods considered normal flora in the oral, gastrointestinal, and urogenital tracts of humans and animals. They are most commonly associated with oral cavity colonization, where they can subsequently result in pyogranulomatous inflammation after disruption of the mucus membrane. The genus is composed of multiple species and clinical manifestations may resemble other morphologically similar organisms like *Nocardia* species.

Descriptive Features

Morphology and Staining. Members of the genus *Actinomyces* are gram-positive, non-acid-fast, diphtheroid or filamentous rods. These organisms do not form spores. Branching filaments, often beaded due to uneven staining, are most readily observed in pathologic specimens. In culture, diphtheroid forms predominate.

Structure and Composition. *Actinomyces* species have distinctive cell wall constituents, differentiating them from morphologically similar species including *Nocardia*. Surface fibrils in *A. viscosus* may be adhesins for host cells or other bacteria ("coaggregation"). Surface antigens are related to chemotactic and mitogenic activities.

Original chapter written by Drs. Ernst L. Biberstein and Dwight C. Hirsh.

Growth Characteristics. *Actinomyces* species are facultative or strict anaerobes that require a rich media, preferably containing serum or blood for growth *in vitro*. The organisms tend to be capnophilic, so growth is enhanced with carbon dioxide. Development of macroscopic colonies may require several days (2–3) of incubation at 37 °C. Colonial morphology varies between and within species and hemolysis is rare.

Resistance. *Actinomyces* species are readily killed by heat and disinfectants and require frequent passage to survive in culture. The antimicrobial susceptibility patterns of *Actinomyces* are predictable, particularly with regard to penicillin, and resistance is not widely reported. Resistance to fluorquinolones has been noted.

Ecology

Reservoir. Members of the genus *Actinomyces* are normal flora, most often present on the oral mucous membranes or tooth surfaces; however, they can colonize the mucous membranes of the urogenital tract and be found secondarily in the gastrointestinal tract of many animal species. They are not associated with the environment.

Transmission. Most *Actinomyces* infections are endogenous; that is, they are caused by introduction of a commensal organism into susceptible tissue of its host. Although rare, bites are another means of transmission.

Veterinary Microbiology, Third Edition. Edited by D. Scott McVey, Melissa Kennedy and M.M. Chengappa.

Table 36.1. Differential Characteristics of *Actinomyces*, *Nocardia*, *Dermatophilus*, and *Streptobacillus* Genera

	Actinomyces	*Nocardia*	*Dermatophilus*	*Streptobacillus*
Gram reaction	+	+	+	−
Acid-fast reaction	−	Partial +	−	−
Motility	−	−	Motile zoospores	−
Atmospheric preference	Strict or facultative anaerobe	Aerobe	Facultative anaerobe	Facultative anaerobe
Primary reservoir	Oral mucosa	Soil	Skin	Pharynx of rodents

Pathogenesis

Members of the genus *Actinomyces* typically evoke pyogranulomatous reactions by largely unknown mechanisms. Bacterial colonies form in tissue, triggering suppurative responses in the immediate vicinity. Peripheral to this, granulation, mononuclear infiltration, and fibrosis furnish the granulomatous elements. Sinus tracts carry exudate to the outside; the exudate often contains characteristic yellow "sulfur granules." These sulfur granules can be greater than 5 mm in size and have also been referred to as rosettes or club colonies. *Actinomyces* species are often part of a polymicrobial infection.

Disease Patterns

Ruminants. In cattle, *Actinomyces bovis*, or rarely, *Actinomyces israelii* typically present as "lumpy jaw" when they are introduced from an oral reservoir by a traumatic event (e.g., poor-quality feed) into the alveolar or paralveolar region of the jaw initiating a chronic rarefying osteomyelitis. This leads eventually to replacement of normal bone by porous bone, which is laid down irregularly and honeycombed with sinus tracts containing pus. There may be dislodgement of teeth, inability to chew, and mandibular fractures. The lesion expands but has little tendency for vascular dissemination. Similar infections occur in humans and marsupials. *A. bovis* also has been associated with pulmonary infection in cattle.

Horses. Reports of *Actinomyces* isolated from abscesses, corneal swabs, and skin pustules have all been described in horses. Organisms have been associated with fistulous withers, often accompanying a *Brucella* species. In addition, because horses can develop a lymphadenitis, *Actinomyces* infection may mimic *S. equi* ssp. *equi* or "strangles" infections.

Dogs and Cats. *Actinomyces* have been associated with thoracic and abdominal infections in companion animals. In dogs, actinomycosis may be associated with foreign bodies (e.g., by licking), particularly migrating grass awns. If these are lodged near vertebrae they can cause an actinomycotic discospondylitis. Cutaneous actinomycosis in dogs is a rare noduloulcerative lymphangitis.

Swine. Clinically, *Actinomyces* infection in swine, usually *A. suis*, is associated with mastitis, likely initiated from suckling piglets. *Actinomyces* has also been recovered from lung lesions and aborted fetuses.

The similarity of clinical signs of *Actinomyces* infection with other disease patterns (e.g., strangles in horses) makes these organisms important differentials clinically.

Epidemiology. Actinomycosis are noncommunicable, except via bites (which is a rare form of transmission). Contamination of bursae or body cavities may be hematogenous or result from perforations of the alimentary tract, or body wall. Actinomycosis associated with plant awns have been reported in outdoor dogs in semiarid areas. *Actinomyces*-associated disease has been reported in goats, sheep, wild ruminants, monkeys, rabbits, squirrels, hamsters, marsupials, and birds throughout the world.

Immunologic Factors

Infected humans show cell-mediated and humoral immune responses. Circulating antibody, produced during infection, confers no protection. Specific resistance, if any, is probably cell-mediated. Phagocytes kill *Actinomyces*. No commercial vaccine is available.

Laboratory Diagnosis

Aspirates from unopened lesions or tissues, preferably including granules, are optimal for laboratory diagnosis. Suspected exudates are examined for "sulfur granules"—yellowish particles, varying in firmness, up to several millimeters in diameter. Granules are washed, crushed and observed under the microscope. Rosettes are suggestive of actinomycosis, especially if bacterial-sized filaments extend into the clubbed fringe.

Crushed granules, exudate, or tissue impressions can be stained with Gram and acid-fast stains. Branching, gram-positive, beaded, non-acid-fast filaments suggest *Actinomyces* species. Most *Actinomyces* strains obtained from animals do not require anaerobic incubation but benefit from increased carbon dioxide. Granules offer the best chance of isolation from the usually mixed flora. Colonies can develop within 48–72 h after incubation at 35–37 °C. Organisms of suggestive morphology and staining characteristics can be evaluated biochemically to aide in identification. Different species can react differentially on most common biochemical tests. Colonies are typically nonhemolytic and white and can appear either smooth or rough; colonies tend to adhere to the surface of the media. Meaningful species identification is improved with molecular techniques. DNA primers based upon the sequence of genes encoding the 16S ribosomal RNA have been designed for speciation of *Actinomyces* members.

Treatment and Control

In bovine actinomycosis, iodine compounds have been used for treatment, however, must be stopped when signs of toxicity appear. Accessible soft tissue lesions can be drained or excised. Antimicrobials including penicillin and aminoglycoside combinations are often administered concurrently. Treatment of lumpy jaw will not restore normal bone structure, but the process can be arrested by systemic medication aided by drainage, lavage (iodine), and debridement of lesions.

In other species, surgery (drainage, lavage, excision, removal of foreign bodies) is controversial but may be used and supplemented by long-term antimicrobial therapy. A penicillin derivative (e.g., ampicillin) is the drug of choice. Alternatives are erythromycin, clindamycin, doxycycline or amoxicillin-clavulanic acid. Relapses are common, especially with short-term therapy or thoracic involvement. It is important to note that many *Actinomyces* infections are polymicrobial and may require modified treatment strategies.

Nocardia

Nocardia species are aerobic, saprophytic, gram-positive, filamentous bacteria ubiquitous in the environment including the soil and water. The list of recognized species is rapidly expanding, currently consisting of more than 80 members, with approximately half of veterinary or human medical importance. Infections attributed to *Nocardia* species have been reported in mammals, fish, mollusks, and birds. Because of the opportunistic nature of these organisms, they are frequently found in immunocompromised individuals. *Nocardia* infections often begin as suppurative or pyogranulomatous processes that can become chronic; however, species can differ in their ability to cause disease. *Nocardia asteroides*, historically the species most often associated with diseases, is now designated as the *N. asteroides* complex with several member species and types. For this reason, in the discussion that follows, a species designation will not be given to the nocardial agents associated with the various diseases ascribed to members of this genus, unless isolates were identified by techniques (mostly DNA-based analyses) currently accepted for identification of this group of bacteria.

Descriptive Features

Morphology and Staining. *Nocardia* species are nonmotile, gram-positive bacteria that when gram-stained are difficult to distinguish from *Actinomyces* species. They often appear as branching, beaded filaments that can fragment into pleomorphic rods or cocci. They are partially acid-fast due to the presence of mycolic acids in their cell wall, which can distinguish them from morphologically similar genera.

Structure and Composition. The cell wall is typical of gram-positive bacteria, with the addition of meso-diaminopimelic acid (DAP), arabinogalactan, and mycolic acids. The cell wall contains a high concentration of lipids.

Growth Characteristics. Pathogenic *Nocardia* species are obligate aerobes, capable of growing on simple (e.g., Sabouraud's) or enriched (blood agar) media over a wide temperature range (10–50 °C). Small, indiscriminate colonies can appear after 48 h. Older colonies can vary phenotypically, appearing opaque or variously pigmented. The colony surface has been described as waxy, powdery, and velvety depending on the abundance of aerial growth. The formation of aerial hyphae aides in differentiating *Nocardia* species from related genra. Colonies may develop a wrinkled appearance with age. In broth, a surface pellicle or sediment is produced, but little turbidity.

Resistance. Nocardiae thrive in the environment yet are susceptible to disinfectants. *Nocardia* species exhibit varying resistance patterns to antimicrobials, which have traditionally been used in the differentiation of species. *Nocardia farcinica* have been reported to be particularly resistant to antimicrobials. Resistance to trimethoprim-sulfamethoxazole has been reported in a large proportion of human *Nocardia* isolates, where it is considered the drug of choice.

Ecology

Reservoir. *Nocardia* species are common inhabitants of the environment including soil, water, decaying vegetation, and can also be shed in the feces of animals. The organisms have a worldwide distribution; however, species can cluster geographically. Because of the nature of these organisms, they can be environmental contaminants or rarely asymptomatically colonize humans or animals; when isolated from a clinical specimen they are generally considered pathogens.

Transmission. Three main routes of infection are inhalation, direct contact through trauma, and ingestion. Dust, soil, and plant material can serve as vehicles. *Nocardia* associated with bovine mastitis can be introduced and disseminated by equipment and personnel. The route of transmission is associated with the clinical presentation of disease.

Pathogenesis

Pathogenic *Nocardia* strains are facultative intracellular organisms that survive within phagocytic vacuoles initially by preventing phagolysosome formation. The cell wall content and mycolic acids exhibited during the growth phase of the bacteria facilitate intracellular survival. Superoxide dismutase and lysosomal enzyme inhibition protect against phagocytic killing. Other cell wall lipids may trigger granulomatous reactions. Variations between strains and growth phases in cell envelope constituents are paralleled by changes in virulence and infectivity.

Nocardiosis is a predominantly suppurative process with variable granulomatous features. Lymph nodes are consistently involved, particularly in wound cases. Lesions, particularly in the lung, can erode into blood vessels and result in dissemination and widespread abscess formation. Central nervous involvement is rare in animals, though fairly common in human patients. In dogs, the common form is thoracic empyema with granulomatous serositis. Exudates are sanguinopurulent and sometimes contain small (<1 mm diameter), soft granules consisting of bacteria, neutrophils, and debris ("sulfur granule-like"). They usually lack the microstructure of sulfur granules sometimes seen with *Actinomyces* infections (see Section "*Actinomyces*").

Disease Patterns. Nocardiosis is frequently overlooked because of its ability to co-exist with or masquerade as other familiar diseases. Infection due to a *Nocardia* species may be difficult to distinguish from mycobacterial and *Actinomyces* infections without laboratory diagnosis. Infections can be regional or disseminated. Human and animal cases of nocardiosis are almost always associated with the immune status of the individual.

Ruminants. Bovine mastitis is the most common manifestation of *Nocardia* infection in cattle. This infection is generally associated with the hygiene of the herd. Onset is sudden with fever, anorexia, and abnormal milk secretion. The affected gland is swollen, hot, and painful. Discharging fistulous tracts may develop. Lymphadenopathy is common, and there is occasional dissemination. The affected gland usually becomes nonfunctional. Rarely, pneumonia, abortion, and lymphadenitis associated with *Nocardia* species have been reported in ruminants.

Horses. In horses, local or disseminated infections with *Nocardia* have been reported, including *Nocardia*-induced mycetomas, pulmonary infection and abortion. "Nocardioform placentitis" is a relatively uncommon condition of mares that can result in late-term abortion, still birth, or premature birth. Although morphologically similar, gram-positive, branching, and filamentous, the causative agent, *Crossiella equi*, is unrelated to *Nocardia*.

Dogs and Cats. Dogs and cats often develop debilitating, febrile illness with depression and anorexia. Pneumonia and suppurative pleuritis with empyema is the common finding in dogs. Dissemination occurs to liver, kidneys, bones, joints, and, rarely, the central nervous system. Co-infection with canine distemper virus is common. Cutaneous subcutaneous abscess formation is the more common clinical manifestation in cats, although pulmonary or systemic disease can also occur. There is a high mortality rate in these animals, although that may be related to predisposing factors such as being immunosuppressed or co-infection status.

Swine. Pneumonia, abortion, and lymphadenitis associated with *Nocardia* have rarely been reported.

Other Species. Nocardiosis observed in birds (rare), whales, and dolphins are mostly respiratory in nature with signs of dissemination. In fish, granulomas within the muscle or associated with internal organs have been reported.

Epidemiology. The distribution of *Nocardia* species in the environment is worldwide; however, some species cluster geographically. In animals and humans, disease is associated largely with immunodeficiency. Bovine nocardial mastitis is most often traceable to unsatisfactory hygienic practices. Typically infection is introduced during the "dry period" with intramammary mastitis therapy.

Immunologic Aspects

Antibody and cell-mediated immune responses, including hypersensitivity, commonly develop during nocardial infections. Yet severe nocardiosis is commonly associated with immunosuppression, particularly of cell-mediated responses. Antibody apparently confers little protection. Specific resistance is largely cell-mediated. No practical immunization method is presently available.

Laboratory Diagnosis

Branching, gram-positive, filaments and or shorter, coccobacillary forms are found in smears made from *Nocardia*-infected samples, impressions, or sections. The presence of these organisms is not definitive for *Nocardia* diagnosis because of the morphological similarities with other genera. For confirmation, samples should be submitted for culture or molecular identification.

Nocardial colonies on blood agar, incubated at 37 °C, will initially appear small and indistinct; older cultures will vary phenotypically, ranging between dull opaque to orange or yellowish. The colony surface may appear velvety or powdery depending on the abundance of aerial growth. Colonies may be hard to dislodge by loop or needle, adhering to the surface of the medium. Stains confirm nocardial morphology that may be pleomorphic rods, coccobacilli or branching filaments. Acid-fastness may be lost on culture. Biochemical activities include catalase production, nitrate reduction, and acidification of various carbohydrates. Biochemical properties and susceptibility to various antimicrobial agents have traditionally been used in identification of specific *Nocardia* species, however, are now considered insufficient to differentiate members of the *N. asteroides* complex.

Serological tests are not widely available for *Nocardia* detection and their reliability is uncertain. Molecular methods are gaining popularity for identification of *Nocardia* species. Determination of restriction enzyme patterns from a heat shock protein gene, *hsp*65, had been used to differentiate species; however, the discriminative ability of this test has been challenged. Sequencing of the DNA encoding the 16S rRNA or *hsp*65 gene has been proposed as useful identification tools for *Nocardia* species. The usefulness of these techniques in clinical settings in not established.

Treatment and Control

Antimicrobial therapy of nocardial mastitis may produce temporary clinical relief and cessation of shedding, but no permanent cures. Control involves removal of infected animals, thorough disinfection of premises and equipment, and scrupulous stabling and milking hygiene.

In other forms of nocardiosis, trimethoprim-sulfonamide combinations have been considered the therapy of choice. Amikacin, linezolid and some beta-lactam compounds (imipenem, cefotaxime) have also been used effectively in humans and animals. Fluoroquinolones are reported to have limited therapeutic value. Therapy of nocardial infections is typically prolonged (months) with relapses common in short-term courses. Abscesses or empyema are often treated surgically and or drained, in combination with administration of antimicrobials. Antimicrobial resistance has been observed during the course of treatment, and there are species-associated susceptibility profiles.

Dermatophilus

Dermatophilus species are generally associated with exudative dermatitis or skin lesions in animals and occasionally humans. The most predominant and type species of the genus is *Dermatophilus congolensis* that is responsible for dermatophilosis or streptothricosis (cattle and other species), rain scald or rain rot (horses), grease heal (horses), lumpy wool (sheep), and strawberry footrot (sheep). *Dermatophilus chelonae* is also rarely isolated from skin lesions of more exotic animals, although the taxonomy this organism has recently been challenged. *Dermatophilus* species are gram-positive, branching, filamentous rods that exhibit a unique bacterial life cycle. In temperate climates, dermatophilosis is often a cosmetic problem controllable by management practices. In sheep and cattle of tropical areas, it can severely affect productivity and may be a disposing factor for other problems including myiasis. *Dermatophilus* organisms are rarely found at sites other than the skin.

Descriptive Features

Morphology and Composition. *D. congolensis* are gram-positive bacteria that exhibit a unique life cycle that includes the germination of a motile coccoid "zoospore," forming a germ tube. Next, transverse and longitudinal septa formation occurs, forming a strand several layers thick. Binary fission of constituent cells become coccoid in shape and appears in parallel rows. Mature, motile (flagellated) zoospores are released, completing the life cycle. The cell wall of *Dermatophilus* contains meso-DAP, but lacks galactose and arabinose.

Growth Characteristics. *D. congolensis* grows well on blood agar media, but not on Sabouraud dextrose agar. It is a facultative anaerobe and capnophilic. Colonies, which develop in 48 h, vary from mucoid to viscous and waxy, whitish-gray to yellow, and smooth to wrinkled. There is large phenotypic variation, including hemolytic and enzymatic activity between *D. congolensis* isolates. Generally, *D. congolensis* is highly hemolytic on blood agar plates. In addition, antigenic variation has been reported in field isolates. Genotyping work suggests that the variation between isolates is correlated to host species and not geographical location.

Ecology

Reservoir. *D. congolensis* does not multiply saprophytically, it is an obligate parasite. Cattle, sheep, and horses are common hosts; however, it has been diagnosed in goats, swine, dogs and cats, turkeys, primates (including humans), and wild mammals, including marine mammals. The distribution of *D. congolensis* is worldwide, but its greatest economic significance is in tropical regions in Africa. Younger animals appear to be more susceptible than older animals, possibly related to an immature immune system.

Transmission. Spread of *D. congolensis* is by direct physical contact of animals or indirect contact via arthropods. Injury by thorny range plants and shearing cuts may create portals of infection or inoculate the agent. Transmission is exacerbated in moist conditions.

Pathogenesis

D. congolensis results in an exudative epidermitis. Its primary activity is confined to the living epidermis. Infection results after soaking or trauma occur to this area. Deposited zoospores respond to a CO_2 gradient and penetrate deeper cell layers. Upon germination, germ tubes and filaments arborize within the epidermis and colonize hair follicles. A layer of inflammatory cells (largely neutrophils) forms under the infected epidermis, which keratinizes. Beneath the neutrophils new epidermis forms, which can be invaded. The eventual result is a scab consisting of layers of neutrophilic exudate and infected keratinizing epidermis. The scabs are easily lifted by the hair, which protrudes from both surfaces. Virulence factors of *D. congolensis* including phospholipase and proteolytic enzymes aide by increasing the permeability of the epidermis and interacting with the inflammatory response.

The primary lesions from *D. congolensis* are painless and nonpruritic. Wetting favors their expansion. Biting arthropods can infect areas protected from soaking rain. Soaking provides the preparatory step for lesions on the back (equine "rain scald"), feet, and legs (ovine "strawberry footrot," equine "grease heel"). The extent varies from a few scabby areas of roughened hair or "lumpy wool" to widespread loss of epidermis, causing secondary parasitisms or infections and eventual loss of the animal. More severe disease is generally associated with infestation with the *Amblyomma variegatum* tick that promotes an immunosuppression. The genetic makeup of the animal may also contribute to the severity of disease. Dermatophilosis in nonepidermal tissue including the tongue and lymph nodes has only been rarely reported in cats.

Epidemiology. Infection with *D. congolensis* is strongly correlated to environmental conditions, and as such, prevalence can vary significantly. The prevalence of dermatophilosis depends on (1) infected animals; (2) dissemination, for example, by arthropods or thorny plants; and (3) susceptible hosts' epidermis rendered accessible by trauma or wetting.

Immunologic Aspects

Antibody is widespread among cattle in endemic areas. Its protective role is not well understood.

Laboratory Diagnosis

Gram or Giemsa stains of crushed scab or scab flakes usually show typical phases of the *D. congolensis* life cycle and provide a strong presumptive diagnosis. In subacute and chronic cases, bacterial elements may be rare and lack, for example, multicellular branching filaments. Zoospores resemble large cocci. They and other *Dermatophilus* fragments in skin debris may be identified by fluorescent antibody. Impression smears from the base of recently removed scabs may also be useful in identification.

D. congolensis is cultured from the undersurface of fresh, uncontaminated scabs on blood agar under 5–10% carbon dioxide at 35–37 °C. Small, grayish yellow hemolytic colonies typically appear within 24–48 h. Colonies typically adhere to the media and after an extended incubation (3–4 days) appear larger (3 mm), rough, and wrinkled. When colonies are gram-stained, branching filaments or coccoid forms are seen. A wet mount may reveal motile zoospores. The organisms are not acid-fast and catalase and urease positive, indole and nitrate negative.

Treatment and Control

Acute cases of *D. congolensis* infection are often self-limited. Mild cases respond to grooming and removal of the animal from the moist environment. Severe cases can be treated with antimicrobials including penicillin and streptomycin, tetracycline, and chloramphenicol. Control should be aimed at minimizing skin trauma and exposure to rain and arthropods. Multiple live and killed vaccines have been investigated for *D. congolensis* control in sheep and cattle; however, there has not been widespread implementation of a vaccine do to their effectiveness.

Streptobacillus

Streptobacillus moniliformis is the only known species in a genus renamed numerous times, and now taxonomically placed in the family *Fusobacteriaceae*. The organism is the more common of two zoonotic agents (the other is *Spirillum minus*) associated with rat-bite fever.

Descriptive Features

S. moniliformis is a nonmotile, non-spore-forming gram-negative, pleomorphic rod. There is no capsule. The organisms often grow in culture as long, beaded filaments bearing knobby irregularities. Its cellular proteins vary with geographic and pathologic sources. Cell wall deficient L-forms, which can be more difficult to grow, can form readily. Very little is known about specific virulence factors or cellular products; however, antigens expressed by the two forms may not be identical.

Ecology

The primary reservoir for *S. moniliformis* is the pharynx of rodents, particularly rats. Wild mice are not considered a primary reservoir and *S. moniliformis* has been associated with severe clinical disease in these animals. Other carnivores that feed on or mouth rats may also be a source of the organism. Infection is generally attributed to being bit by an infected animal reservoir; however, oral ingestion of contaminated material also can result in infection. Oral-related infection in humans, usually from rat excrement contamination of water, milk, or food is referred to as "Haverhill fever."

Bite lesions are inflammatory and often purulent or necrotic. Reports of clinical disease in rodents range from swelling of the joints and lymph nodes to bronchopneumonia, abscess formation in the liver, and septicemia. In turkeys and mice, septicemic infections lead to polyarthritis or synovitis and often death. Clinical infection of *S. moniliformis* in dogs has resulted in vomiting, diarrhea, and arthritis in the hindlegs. Other animals associated with the rat reservoir may become infected and develop a range of clinical signs.

In humans, an abrupt fever, accompanied by a headache, vomiting and a rash on the extremities precede localization in joints in 50–70% of *S. moniliformis* patients. Other complications including endocarditis, pneumonia, abscess formation on organs, and meningitis may occur. Mortality rates may approximate 10% in untreated cases. Treatment may induce the L-form of *S. moniliformis*, which may persist in the body and cause relapses, including recurrent fever, after therapy is completed.

Immunologic Aspects

Although antibodies against *S. moniliformis* are produced during infection, the role of immunity is not understood.

Laboratory Diagnosis

S. moniliformis is fastidious yet can be cultured in the laboratory using a blood or serum-enriched media. Proper diagnostic submissions include blood or joint fluid, abscess aspirates, synovial fluid and wound cultures. Some anticoagulants from blood culture systems may impede growth. The organism is a facultative anaerobe and in enriched liquid media, *S. moniliformis* forms a characteristic "puff-ball" appearance. On enriched plates, incubation for 48 h or more at 35–37 °C produces visible gray, mucoid colonies. Subsequent identification is by morphologic and biochemical characteristics. Although *S. moniliformis* is relatively unreactive, including catalase, oxidase, indole, urease, and nitrate negative, it can produce acid from select carbohydrates including glucose. In culture, the production of L-form colonies may be favored by special media, forming mycoplasma-like colonies that are recognizable among the conventional colonies.

Direct fluorescent antibody tests and molecular methods including PCR and sequencing have been used more recently for diagnostic identification of this organism, and in rodents, ELISA and immunoblot tests have been used.

Treatment and Control

Penicillin is the antibiotic of choice; however, tetracycline is also effective in treating *S. moniliformis* infections in penicillin-allergic individuals. Although antimicrobial resistance is not thought to be a large problem, resistance to cephalosporins and aminoglycosides have been reported. The most obvious preventive measure is avoidance of direct and indirect contact with likely carriers.

Further Reading

Burd EM, Juzych LA, Rudrik JT, and Habib F (2007) Pustular dermatitis caused by *Dermatophilus congolensis*. *J Clin Microbiol*, **45**, 1655–1658.

Gaastra W, Boot R, Ho HTK, and Lipman LJA (2009) Rat bite fever. *Vet Microbiol*, **133**, 211–228.

Larrasa J, Garcia A, Ambrose NC *et al.* (2002) A simple random amplified polymorphic DNA genotyping method for field isolates of *Dermatophilus congolensis*. *J Vet Med B: Infect Dis Vet Public Health*, **49**, 135–141.

Larruskain J, Idigoras P, Marimon JM, and Perez-Trallero E (2011) Susceptibility of 186 *Nocardia* sp. isolates to 20 antimicrobial agents. *Antimicrob Agents Chemother*, **55**, 2995–2998.

Norris BJ, Colditz IG, and Dixon TJ (2008) Fleece rot and dermatophilosis in sheep. *Vet Microbiol*, **128**, 217–230.

Rodriguez-Nava V, Couble A, Devulder G *et al.* (2006) Use of PCR-restriction enzyme pattern analysis and sequencing database for *hsp65* gene-based identification of *Nocardia* species. *J Clin Microbiol*, **44**, 536–546.

Saubolle M and Sussland D (2003) Nocardiosis: Review of clinical and laboratory experience. *J Clin Microbiol*, **41**, 4497–4501.

Sullivan DC and Chapman SW (2010) Bacteria that masquerade as fungi: Actinomycosis/Nocardia. *Proc Am Thorac Soc*, **7**, 216–221.

Wauters G, Avesani V, Charlier J *et al.* (2005) Distribution of *Nocardia* species in clinical samples and their routine rapid identification in the laboratory. *J Clin Microbiol*, **43**, 2624–2628.

Mycobacterium

Raul G. Barletta and David J. Steffen

Members of the genus *Mycobacterium* are aerobic, acid-fast rods with high guanine-cytosine (GC) content (approximately 65%) in their genomes. There are approximately 100 species and subspecies within this genus, and most of their members are saprophytic organisms that live in the environment. However, the genus also includes some of the most dreaded pathogens such as the agents of bovine and human tuberculosis, leprosy, and various types of granulomatous diseases in normal or compromised mammals, birds, reptiles, and fish.

Based on growth rate, mycobacteria can be classified in fast (colonies develop in agar plates in 7 days or less; e.g., *Mycobacterium smegmatis* and *Mycobacterium fortuitum*) and slow growers (colonies take more than 7 days to develop in agar plates; e.g., *Mycobacterium tuberculosis* and *Mycobacterium avium*). Most of the pathogenic species are slow growers with generation times of 12 h and upward. It is to be noted that even the fast growers have a considerable longer generation time as compared to typical *Escherichia coli* strains that may develop colonies in agar plates upon overnight incubation. Another property useful in the classification of mycobacteria is the presence of carotenoid pigments in some species ("chromogens" vs. "nonchromogens") and their light dependence ("photochromogens" vs. "scotochromogens").

Morphology and Staining

Mycobacteria are nonflagellated, predominantly rod-shaped, about 0.5 μm wide, and variable in length. Cytochemically, these microorganisms are gram-positive, but often resist staining with the Gram stain. However, mycobacteria can be stained with carbolfuchsin (Ziehl–Neelsen stain, Figure 37.1) or fluorescent dyes (e.g., auramine-rhodamine). Their most noted staining property is their acid-fastness (i.e., once stained, they resist discoloration with 3% hydrochloric acid in ethanol). Growth in agar media leads to colonies of variable morphology, but typically they are dry and crumbly. Colonies of *M. avium* ssp. *hominissuis* are usually dome shaped with most virulent strains assuming a smooth, transparent appearance, gradually changing to rough and opaque as virulence may be lost upon repeated culturing.

The presence of an outer layer (capsule) of loosely bound carbohydrates and proteins has been demonstrated by cryoelectron microscopy. This material is shed during growth in liquid medium, but is readily visible *in vivo*. Some experiments indicate that mycobacteria may form spores. These findings, highly dependent on microscopic examination of aged cultures, remain highly controversial.

Structure and Composition

Mycobacteria are characterized by lipid-rich cell walls. Lipids account for acid-fastness and some pathogenic and immunologic properties. The surface mycosides (mostly glycolipids and peptidoglycolipids) determine colonial characteristics, serologic specificities, and bacteriophage susceptibilities. Subsurface layers of long-chain branched mycolic acids and their esters make up the bulk of cell wall lipids. Mycolic acids are linked to the innermost peptidoglycan layer by way of arabinogalactans (see also Chapters 30 and 36). Determination of mycolic acid chain length has diagnostic relevance for genus and species identification as mycobacteria have longer chains of 60–90 carbon atoms. Some mycolic acids are loosely bound to the disaccharide trehalose in the form of trehalose monomycolates (TMM) and dimycolates (TDM). One of the capsular antigens (antigen 85) carries the enzyme activity responsible for the formation of TMM and TDM. TDM has recently been identified as "cord factor," the mycobacterial component that determines the characteristic serpentine-like appearance observed upon culture in certain liquid media. TDM is associated with multiple activities in the mechanisms of pathogenesis, both protecting mycobacteria from phagocytic killing and contributing to disease pathology of host cells within the granuloma.

The mycobacterial peptidoglycan has also an unusual structure as the muramyl dipeptide subunit component has a 50% mixture of *N*-acetylated and *N*-glycosylated moieties that departs from the typical 100% *N*-acetylated moiety of most eubacteria. This particular composition seems

Original chapter written by Drs. Dwight C. Hirsh and Ernst L. Biberstein.

Veterinary Microbiology, Third Edition. Edited by D. Scott McVey, Melissa Kennedy and M.M. Chengappa.

FIGURE 37.1. *Acid-fast staining. The procedure demonstrates numerous rods in the cytoplasm of the macrophages of the lamina propria in the jejunum of a bovine with Johne's disease (Ziehl–Nielsen acid-fast stain, 60×). (Specimen from the University of Nebraska Veterinary Diagnostic Center.)*

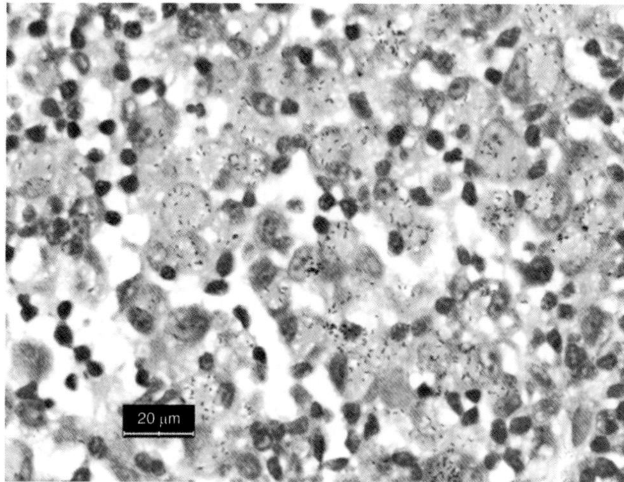

directly linked to the ability of this component to potentiate humoral and cellular immune responses (adjuvanticity) and the basis for its inclusion as the active component of Freund's complete adjuvant.

Mycobacteria possess typical cell membranes composed by lipid bilayers, but they have the salient characteristic that one major cell wall glycolipid (lipoarabinomannan, LAM) is covalently attached to this membrane. LAM is also involved in mycobacterial pathogenesis (phagocytosis and inhibition of phagolysosome fusions see Section "The Immune Response to Mycobacterial Infections"), especially in *M. tuberculosis* as LAM is capped with mannose residues (ManLAM). Other mycobacterial lipids (glycolipids, phospholipids, sulfolipids, and waxes) may also play some role in these processes.

The mycobacterial cell wall architecture is completed by the presence of porins and other proteins such as transporters involved in nutrient acquisition. Some of the proteins are antigenic and can be readily isolated in large amounts from broth culture supernatant fluids. In addition to the already mentioned antigen 85, mycobacteria "secrete" superoxide dismutase, L-alanine dehydrogenase, and glutamate synthetase.

Overview of Pathogenic Species, Epidemiology, and Microbial Evolution

The group of closely related mycobacteria causing tuberculosis in humans and animals is denominated the *M. tuberculosis* complex. In medical terms, a complex is a group of microorganisms producing similar disease, but the term does not have taxonomic implications. The microorganisms *Mycobacterium bovis* and *M. tuberculosis* were discovered to be the agents of tuberculosis in animals and human beings by Robert Koch in his 1882 pioneering studies. These studies provided the basis to develop the Koch's postulates of disease causation. Rodents, especially mice and guinea pigs, are especially susceptible to experimental infection with *M. bovis* and *M. tuberculosis*. However, *M. tuberculosis* is a human-adapted pathogen and rarely infects other animals. Transmission occurs from one individual to another by infected aerosols. In contrast, *M. bovis* is a zoonotic agent that can be transmitted by aerosols bidirectionally from (to) animals to (from) humans, though the most frequent case is mediated by unpasteurized milk from infected animals (cattle and other ruminants) that serve as a main source of infection. The work of Koch involved samples from both humans and animals. Thus, Koch worked with both *M. bovis* and *M. tuberculosis*, at a time when the subtle distinctions between these microorganisms had not been defined. There are two closely related host-adapted mycobacteria that have been given special names based on the infected hosts: *Mycobacterium pinnipedii* (seals) and *Mycobacterium caprae* (goats). Latest citations refer *M. caprae* as a subspecies of *M. bovis*. The antituberculosis vaccine BCG (bacillus Calmette–Guerin) is an attenuated strain of *M. bovis*. The original isolate was sent to different locations around the world, and each isolate underwent independent mutations during passage and maintenance and was defined as BCG substrains (e.g., BCG Copenhagen, BCG Pasteur, BCG Tokyo, and BCG Russia).

Another related human-restricted pathogen is the African version of the tubercle bacillus designated *Mycobacterium africanum*. Another microorganism, *Mycobacterium canettii* has also been described in North Africa. The host range of *M. canettii* remains unknown. *Mycobacterium microti* is another member of the complex identified as the agent of tuberculosis in voles and more recently isolated from some human cases. Molecular and genomic studies established that mycobacterial genomes were generated by reductive evolution involving both single-nucleotide polymorphisms and serial deletions of genetic materials. The deletions gave rise to regions of difference in the corresponding genomes and defined major speciation events. This analysis leads to the conclusion that an ancestral strain of *M. canettii* is the precursor of *M. tuberculosis* and *M. bovis*. Thus, the old paradigm that *M. tuberculosis* evolved from *M. bovis* (e.g., human tuberculosis has its origin in bovine tuberculosis) is no longer tenable. Interestingly, *M. bovis*, the species with the smaller genome, has a greater host range than *M. tuberculosis*. This has been attributed to deletions of "avirulence" islands (e.g., encoding regulatory elements that modulate the expression of virulence determinants) from the genome, allowing *M. bovis* to have a greater host range.

Mycobacterium leprae is a peculiar human pathogen that is considered an obligate intracellular pathogen as it has never been grown *in vitro*. The nine-banded armadillo is one of the few experimental hosts that can be used to grow the microorganism under laboratory conditions. Both in experimental infections of armadillos and in human infections, *M. leprae* has a favorite niche in bodily areas of lower temperature, such as the extremities (feet and hands) followed by spreading to the face. Transmission of leprosy occurs by contact and may be mediated by aerosols. Very few cases of zoonotic transmission have been observed.

M. leprae attacks the peripheral nervous system, but does not affect the central nervous system. These features result in mentally normal patients with characteristic disfigurements due to these peripheral lesions. This disease was well documented in biblical times both in the Old Testament and the New Testament. This disease was popularized in theaters in the 1959 epic movie "Ben-Hur." From the ancient times until the early years of the twentieth century, leprosy patients were confined in isolation; nowadays the disease is readily treatable and only progresses to the worst scenario, if patients are left untreated or if complications in therapy occur.

M. avium complex (MAC) infections were once considered the most common opportunistic bacterial infections of AIDS patients. Advances in AIDS therapy have resulted in patients maintaining a higher, yet less than normal, level of T cell CD4 counts, and thus in better control of MAC infections. *M. tuberculosis*, the most virulent mycobacterial species, has now overtaken MAC as the main cause of complicating coinfections in AIDS patients. However, MAC infections are still of concern in patients that do not undertake proper AIDS therapy. The MAC complex includes related but distinct species: *Mycobacterium intracellulare* and *M. avium* (these two usually grouped as the MAI complex, a term without taxonomical relevance), and the fast growers *Mycobacterium chelonae* and *M. fortuitum*. As a result of biochemical and genetic analysis, the species *M. avium* is now divided in four subspecies: *M. avium* ssp. *avium*, the agent of a tuberculosis-like disease in birds; *M. avium* ssp. *hominissuis*, the classical *M. avium* in the medical literature that affects humans and swine, and the main example of "environmental mycobacteria"; *M. avium* ssp. *paratuberculosis*, the agent of Johne's disease in ruminants and associated with Crohn's disease in humans; and *M. avium* ssp. *silvaticum* found colonizing wild life such as wood pigeons, whose status as a pathogen has not been well defined. Both aerosols and contaminated water have been associated with infection, especially with the ssp. *hominissuis*. In the case of the ssp. *paratuberculosis*, the main route of infection in ruminants is oral. Calves are usually infected by drinking contaminated milk from their dams or by the ingestion of fecal material from contaminated manure. An environmental exposure of susceptible individuals or consumption of unpasteurized or incompletely pasteurized (adulterated) milk has been mentioned as a potential source of infection in humans. Regarding evolutionary lineage, it has been suggested that an ancestral strain of the MAC leads to two subspecies—*M. avium* ssp. *avium* and *M. avium* ssp. *hominissuis*—and the species *M. intracellulare*. The ssp. *paratuberculosis* seems to have been originated from the ssp. *hominissuis*.

Another species of relevance is *Mycobacterium kansasii*, a species related to the MAC complex that may cause disseminated infections in AIDS patients and pulmonary diseases in patients with noninfectious lung disease. *Mycobacterium marinum*, a pathogen of fish, has also been related to human skin granulomas in swimming pools. *Mycobacterium ulcerans* is an emerging pathogen associated with severe skin ulcerations prevalent in tropical regions. Other mycobacteria such as *Mycobacterium aurum* and *M. smegmatis* are usually saprophytic environmental species, but from time to time may cause opportunistic infections in human and animal hosts.

Primary Interaction with Phagocytic Cells and Disease Onset

Upon entry via the bronchial or the intestinal mucosa, resident alveolar or intestinal macrophages are mobilized to engulf the pathogenic mycobacteria. This phagocytic process is receptor mediated and antibody independent with the involvement of complement receptors, the mannose receptor, and/or integrins. *Mycobacterium* avoids antibody-dependent receptors that normally trigger, as it is the case with many bacterial pathogens, macrophage activation, and a bactericidal response. In this way, mycobacteria remain in phagocytic vacuoles preventing phagosome activation (production of bactericidal reactive intermediates) and maturation (e.g., phagosome acidification and fusion with lysosomes). In this way, mycobacterial bacilli are able to survive and multiply within resident phagocytic cells. There are some reports that highly virulent strains of *M. tuberculosis* could even escape from the phagosome into the cytosol where they can replicate faster.

Monocytes (blood phagocytic cells) are then recruited to the site of infection that finally evolves into a granuloma or tubercle. This focal rounded structure is evident in gross pathology as yellow nodulations near the entry/exit of blood vessels from affected organs (e.g., the Ghon complex in lungs). The tubercle contains infected macrophages at its center encircled by enlarged phagocytic cells (epithelioid cells), lymphocytes, and fibroblasts surrounded by a collagen layer. At the center of the lesion, caseation necrosis develops. Depending upon disease outcome, this lesion may either calcify if the disease is contained, or liquefy if disease worsens. Tubercles may enlarge, coalesce, and eventually occupy sizable portions of organs. Such tubercles consist mostly of caseous material.

In the case of human *M. tuberculosis* infections, a favorable host immune response may prevent disease altogether or keep bacilli in check within granulomas that eventually calcify. However, live bacilli still remain in a nonreplicating state, the so-called latent state. If the host response is weak from the start, or the host response wanes after 40–50 years, infectious centers may become necrotic and release infectious bacilli that are spread by coughing. This latter process is known as reactivation from latency. This clear sequence of latency and reactivation is not well documented in nonhuman hosts. Certainly, granulomas are formed in animal hosts, but it is unclear whether a true process of latency and reactivation takes place. Possibly, as a result of a shorter life span and a weaker host response, in many nonhuman animal hosts, mycobacterial infections may progress from subclinical to overt disease in absence of drug therapy.

Immune Response to Mycobacterial Infections

Mycobacteria possess numerous antigenic macromolecules including proteins, lipids, glucan, and glycolipids that induce humoral immunity. However, as mycobacteria are intracellular pathogens, the humoral response is ineffective to control the infection and appears at medium or late stages of disease. Thus, the humoral response has only diagnostic significance as a way to determine whether a host is infected as well as a marker of disease progression. However, research in the last few years has implicated a role for humoral immunity in the host defense against mycobacterial pathogens. For example, antibodies against surface virulence determinants preventing the entry of mycobacterial into phagocytic cells may have a protective effect if timely administered.

The major host defense against mycobacterial pathogens is nonetheless the acquired cellular immune response that results in macrophage activation and the production of cytotoxic T cells. Mycobacteria may activate macrophages to a first level of responsiveness via an innate immune process mediated by the interaction of mycobacterial products with Toll-like receptors present on the phagocytic cells. This process results in dendritic cells and macrophages producing the polypeptide messenger interleukin-12 (IL-12, a type of cytokine) and presentation of mycobacterial antigens to helper CD4+ T cells. This antigen presentation process requires antigen degradation in the phagosome and association of degraded peptides with class II major histocompatibility complex (MHC) molecules. In presence of IL-12, and possibly other cytokines such as IL-17, these cells undergo a differentiation process and become T_{H1} cells with the property of producing γ-interferon that further activates macrophages undergoing a respiratory burst. This process leads to the increased production of highly bactericidal products known as reactive oxygen (superoxide anion and hydrogen peroxide) and nitrogen (nitric oxide (NO) and nitrite) intermediates. It seems that NO and a combined product of nitrogen and oxygen intermediates (peroxynitrite) exert the most important bactericidal action. Still, mycobacteria partially resist these actions by producing catalase—superoxide dismutase and alkyl hydroperoxidase—enzymes that detoxify these reactive intermediates by a redox mechanism. NO has also an immunostimulatory role that results in further cytokine secretion and the activation of macrophage apoptosis that further reduces the number of host cells that can be used for mycobacteria to replicate. Activated macrophages also undergo maturation with phagosome acidification and phagolysosome fusion events, thus complementing the bactericidal action of NO and other reactive intermediates.

IL-12 (IL-17)-activated T_{H1} cells also secrete IL-2 that triggers the differentiation of CD8+ T cells into cytotoxic T cells. Their role is to lyse infected macrophages that then release the intracellular bacilli. These microorganisms can be further phagocytosed and cleared by activated macrophages. Thus, the effective control of mycobacterial infections requires both branches of the acquired cellular response: macrophage and cytotoxic T cell activations upon antigen presentation. It is to be noted that activation of CD8+ cells requires antigen presentation with the assistance of class I MHC molecules. This process requires antigen presentation via secretion of mycobacterial antigens from the phagosome into the cytosol, escape of mycobacteria into the cytosol, and/or an effective crosstalk of the antigen presentation pathways.

Depending upon the immune status of the host, differentiation of CD4+ cells into the T_{H1} pathway does not occur. Infected macrophages secrete IL-10 and IL-4 instead of IL-12. This process leads to the maturation of CD4+ cells via the T_{H2} pathway. T_{H2} cells secrete more IL-4 that stimulates B cells to mature into antibody-secreting cells. Unfortunately, this delayed humoral response dependent on T_{H2} cells is completely nonprotective and it has devastating consequences for the host. For example, in tuberculosis infections it can lead to disseminated (miliary) tuberculosis and high number of bacilli with many organs compromised in addition to the lung. In leprosy, cases of disfigurement occur upon activation of the T_{H2} response.

Overview of Disease Patterns in Veterinary Medicine

Birds. Birds are naturally susceptible primarily to *M. avium* ssp. *avium*. Most poultry infections occur via the alimentary canal and disseminate to liver and spleen. Bone marrow, lung, and peritoneum are often affected. Although the agent has been isolated from eggs, transovarian infection of chicks is rare. Although *M. avium* ssp. *avium* affects many species of birds, psittacines are resistant but are susceptible to *M. tuberculosis*. Canaries are also more susceptible to mammalian than to avian bacilli.

Cattle. Cattle are usually infected with *M. bovis*, and the infection is centered on the respiratory tract and adjacent lymph nodes and serous cavities. The disease is commonly progressive via air spaces and passages. Hematogenous dissemination involving liver and kidney occurs. The uterus may serve as portal for fetal infection, a pattern virtually unknown in other domestic animals. Surviving calves commonly develop liver and spleen lesions. Udder infection is rare (<2% of cases) but has obvious public health implications. Infection with *M. avium* ssp. *hominissuis* is generally subclinical. Abortions resulting apparently from localization of bacilli in the uterine wall occur, in some instances repeatedly. In experimental infections, *M. tuberculosis* causes minor, nonprogressive lesions in cattle.

Cervidae. *M. bovis* readily infects free-ranging and domesticated cervidae and is problematic in captive herds and maintained in some wild populations. Disease progression and lesions are similar to those in cattle, although species variations exist among cervidae particularly at the histologic level. Lesions are, in some species, more suppurative, varied in numbers of acid-fast bacteria, giant cell numbers, and in degree of encapsulation.

Dogs and Cats. Dogs and cats are readily infected with *M. bovis* but rarely with *M. avium* spp. Dogs are also susceptible to *M. tuberculosis*. Intestinal and abdominal localization of infection is more common in cats than in dogs, reflecting a likely alimentary route of exposure. Ulcerative skin lesions are more common in cats than in other hosts, as is eye involvement, with tuberculous choroiditis leading to blindness. Lesions, especially in dogs, often more closely resemble a foreign body reaction than tubercles, since they may lack typical epithelioid and giant cells, and neither caseate and calcify, nor liquefy. The course is usually progressive.

Horses. Horses are rarely infected, but relatively more often with *M. avium* ssp. *hominissuis* than with *M. bovis*. Infection enters usually by the alimentary tract, with primary complexes related to pharynx and intestine. Secondary lesions may be in lung, liver, spleen, and serous membranes. Lesions in cervical vertebrae may be due to a secondary, nonspecific hypertrophic periostitis. Gross lesions are tumor-like. They lack caseation and gross calcification and contain few lymphocytes. There is fibroblast proliferation but usually no firm encapsulation.

Primates. Nonhuman primates are susceptible to *M. tuberculosis* and *M. bovis*, but resistant to *M. avium* unless severely compromised, as by simian immunodeficiency virus infection or preexisting bronchopulmonary disease. These individuals also become infected with nontuberculous mycobacteria.

Sheep and Goats. Sheep and goats are susceptible to *M. bovis* and perhaps slightly less so to *M. avium* ssp. *hominissuis*, but they are resistant to progressive infection by *M. tuberculosis*. Disease patterns resemble those described in cattle.

Swine. Swine can be infected by tubercle bacilli, usually via the alimentary route, but only *M. bovis* causes progressive disease with classical lesions. *M. tuberculosis* infections do not advance past regional lymph nodes. *M. avium* ssp. *hominissuis* infections, the predominant form in many countries, may disseminate to viscera, bone, and meninges. The lesions lack the organization of tubercles, but contain granulomatous elements. Caseation, calcification, or liquefaction is negligible. Bacteria may be abundant.

Wild Life and Infection Reservoirs. With near-eradication of bovine tuberculosis in North America and Europe, the traditional reservoir in domestic mammals might be of diminished concern. However, resurgence is a problem where efforts toward eradication are losing support and consolidation of livestock enterprises makes elimination of large infected herds cost prohibitive. Game farms, animal parks, zoos, and isolated wildlife pockets of infection can serve as reservoirs of *M. bovis*. Tuberculosis is typically a disease of captivity and domestication. Clinical improvement and more limited spread in free-living animals contrast with high communicability in confined domestic groups. *M. bovis*, probably originating from cattle, is endemic in badgers of southern England and in brush-tailed opossums of New Zealand, both of which are considered sources of infection for livestock. Infections in raccoons, opossums, foxes, and coyotes can also be important as transmission to and from cattle in shared environments may frustrate infection control measures. Coyote–deer interaction is also common, and coyote sampling has been proposed as a way to monitor infection spread in wild deer. Farming of exotic animals comingling with ruminants has also significantly increase risks of bovine tuberculosis transmission, as captive cervidae are highly susceptible to *M. bovis*. Sporadic cases of canine tuberculosis often prove to be *M. tuberculosis* infections traceable to human contacts—"reverse zoonoses"— that are also found in nonhuman primates in laboratory colonies and zoos.

In commercial poultry establishments, rapid population turnover (<1 year) and eliminating transgenerational transmission has eradicated *M. avium* ssp. *avium* from that population. Mycobacteria remain a problem in barnyard flocks, aviaries, and zoological parks, particularly since the agent can survive in soil for several years. It has been hypothesized that amoeba may be involved in the transmission process of *M. avium* ssp. Support for this hypothesis has been provided by experiments indicating that bacilli grown in amoeba have increased infectivity and pathogenicity than those microorganisms grown in broth or agar cultures.

Effects on Age, Breed, and Sex. In general, across all animal species, immature individuals often develop more severe lesions than older ones to a given mycobacterial infection. Breed susceptibilities differ: zebu cattle are more resistant than European breeds, and fox terriers and Irish setters are more often infected than dachshunds and Doberman Pinscher dogs. The higher prevalence in dairy than beef cattle may reflect closer confinement and greater productivity stress among dairy cows. Exemption from pregnancy and lactation may explain the lower disease prevalence in bulls than in cows, although in dogs the reverse sex ratio is observed.

Laboratory Diagnosis

Sample Collection

Collection of sputum and serum samples is more common in human cases. In animals, especially ruminants, samples include aspirates or biopsies of active lesions, tracheobronchial and gastric lavages, lymph nodes (thoracic and abdominal), urine or feces, and biopsy specimens. Lung and lymph nodes associated with the respiratory tract including pharynx and lymph nodes of the intestinal tracts are common sites for lesions and are selectively sampled at necropsy when gross lesions are not obvious. Freezing samples during transit or preserving tissue in sodium borate is effective, preserving mycobacterial viability and diminishing growth of microbial contaminants.

Direct Examination

Fluids are concentrated by centrifugation in tightly capped containers. Smears of sediment or tissue are processed using the acid-fast staining procedure, or with auramine-rhodamine where fluorescence microscopy is available. Histologic sections are stained with hematoxylin–eosin and acid-fast stains. Positive acid-fast staining results should be confirmed by culture or nucleic acid detection.

Culture and Identification

Digestion and selective decontamination are advisable especially with specimens likely to contain a mixture of microorganisms. Identification is based upon growth characteristics (fast vs. slow), pigmentation (in the presence or absence of light), and biochemical reactions. DNA probes, specific for the main groups, are commercially available. Tests for the amplification of mycobacteria-specific DNA fragments by use of the polymerase chain reaction (PCR) have become methods of choice to demonstrate or identify members of this genus.

Immunodiagnosis

Tuberculin Test. The Mantoux tuberculin skin test consists in the intradermal application of tuberculin (tuberculin-purified protein derivative, tuberculin PPD) that is a cell-free extract of proteins and peptides released by *M. tuberculosis* into the culture medium. This inoculation, in infected individuals, results in swelling characterized by an induration area 48–72 h postapplication (delayed-type hypersensitivity reaction). In cattle, a 0.2–0.3 mg/dose of bovine PPD (PPD from *M. bovis*) is injected intradermally in the caudal, vulvar, or anal skin or, in some situations, the neck region. In positive cases, a swelling (>5 mm) develops within 72 h. While tuberculin cannot induce the hypersensitive state, it may desensitize animals for weeks or months. A positive test implies past or present infection, requiring the reacting animal to be slaughtered and necropsied. False-positive reactions occur and are explained by hypersensitivity to nontuberculous (e.g., *M. avium*), and related agents such as *Nocardiae*. Simultaneous use of avian "tuberculin" (*M. avium* PPD) often helps to decide, by comparative size assessment of the two reactions, whether sensitivity is due to *M. bovis* or other mycobacteria. False-negatives occur in animals too recently infected and in advanced cases in which anergy (lack of reactivity) develops due to antigen excess or immunosuppression. Nonspecific factors, such as malnutrition, stress, and impending or recent parturition, are alternative causes of anergy. "Tuberculins" of appropriate specificity are used on swine and poultry. In swine the ears are injected, in poultry the wattles. The reliability of tuberculin tests on horses, sheep, goats, dogs, and cats is not established. The ease and the sensitive and inexpensive nature of the skin test establish it as the most effective antemortem screening test in ruminants.

γ-Interferon Assays. These tests are based on the release of γ-interferon from whole blood of infected animals when mixed with mycobacterial antigens (e.g., PPD) as the result of the activation of the cell-mediated immune response. Recent studies have demonstrated increases in specificity by altering the antigens used to stimulate the interferon response. Other studies suggest that adding cytokines to the analysis such as interleukin 1β may increase test sensitivity as well.

Serology. Serologic tests have been moderately useful. These assays are sensitive but are produced late in the disease process. The greatest success has been in the detection of animals infected with *M. avium* ssp. *paratuberculosis.*

Treatment and Control

First-line drugs for tuberculosis therapy are isoniazid (INH), rifampin, pyrazinamide, streptomycin, and ethambutol. Second-line drugs are para-aminosalicylic acid, kanamycin, cycloserine, capreomycin, and ethionamide. Since resistance often develops under a single-drug regimen, a combination is commonly used; a favored one in human medicine is INH–ethambutol–rifampin given for at least 9 months.

Because of the public health hazards inherent in the retention of tuberculous animals, antituberculous chemotherapy for animals is discouraged. Prophylactic treatment with INH may be considered for pets recently exposed to tuberculosis. Some experimental successes with INH for prophylaxis and treatment of calves have been reported. In countries with eradication programs, treatment is generally discouraged or illegal.

Bovine tuberculosis is controlled by identification and elimination of infected animals. This approach has resulted in near-eradication of the infection in many countries. Continued surveillance is required to prevent resurgence. These efforts have changed tuberculosis from a clinical disease in cattle and a frequent source of zoonotic infection to an often subclinical disease and rare source of human infection.

Vaccination of humans with BCG produces temporary immunity and hypersensitivity. The benefits of vaccination have been greatest where exposure is most intense, and negligible where prevalence is low. Vaccination in humans is focused on infants and tuberculin-negative individuals anticipating exposure.

BCG has been used in calves. This practice is inappropriate in countries attempting to eradicate tuberculosis because it interferes with the interpretation of the tuberculin test. Vaccines of moderate efficacy are available against *Mycobacterium paratuberculosis*, but most of these vaccines also interfere with diagnostic tests. New approaches include the development of new and more effective vaccines capable of distinguishing infected from vaccinated animals (DIVA formulation).

M. *Avium* Ssp. *paratuberculosis*, the Agent of Johne's Disease

M. avium ssp. *paratuberculosis* (MAP) is the causative agent of a chronic, irreversible wasting disease of ruminants called Johne's disease. Young animals are the most susceptible to infection. Older animals can be infected, but with larger inocula. Economic losses are traced to reduced milk production and breeding problems (e.g., longer calving intervals), and an increased incidence of mastitis (not caused by MAP), and to general ill thrift.

Like the rest of the genus *Mycobacterium*, MAP is aerobic but grows extremely slowly (8–12 weeks of incubation at 37 °C) in Herrold's egg yolk medium. Primary clinical isolates require the addition of the siderophore mycobactin (an iron-binding compound derived from hydroxamic acid). This growth dependency on mycobactin is of diagnostic value to identify and confirm MAP in clinical samples.

The reservoir for MAP is the intestinal tract of infected animals, both the clinically affected and, more importantly, those infected but asymptomatic. In an affected herd, infected, asymptomatic fecal shedders may be

FIGURE 37.2. *Typical histopathology of the jejunum of a bovine infected with Johne's disease. Lamina propria is expanded by abundant epithelioid macrophages; crypts are rarified and contain some debris (hematoxylin and eosin staining, 10×). (Specimen from the University of Nebraska Veterinary Diagnostic Center.)*

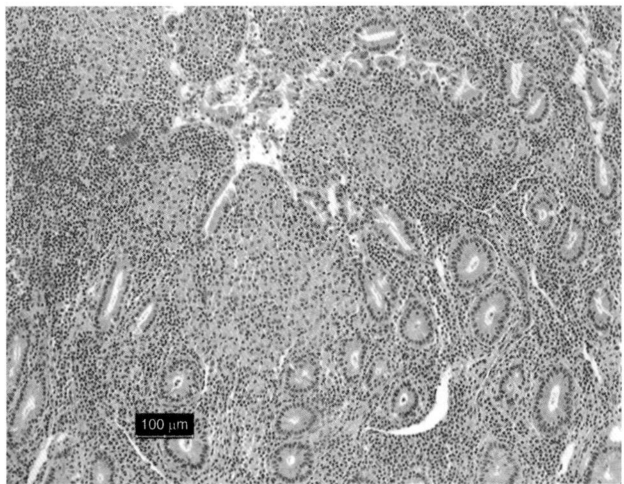

FIGURE 37.3. *Large epithelioid macrophages. Epithelioid macrophages dominate the superficial lamina propria and separate crypts in the jejunum of a bovine with Johne's disease. A few degenerate cells are evident in crypts (hematoxylin and eosin staining, 20×). (Specimen from the University of Nebraska Veterinary Diagnostic Center.)*

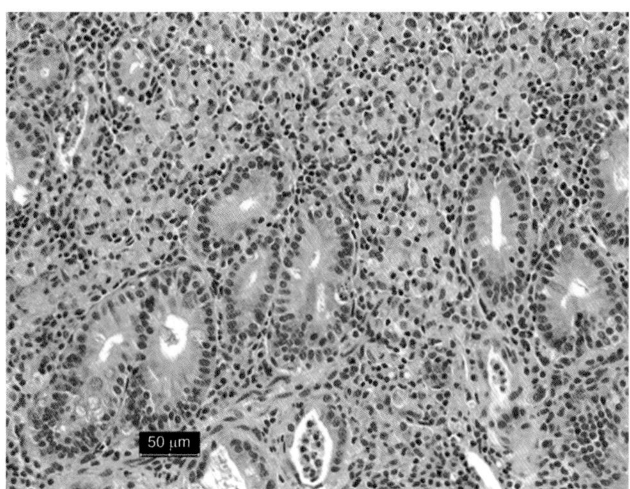

20 times more numerous than those showing clinical signs. An infected animal may also shed MAP into colostrum and milk, and may pass the organism to her fetus in utero. MAP has been isolated from semen, seminiferous tubules, and the prostate glands of infected bulls. The infection is usually acquired through the ingestion or contact with fecally contaminated materials (food and fomites). In utero infection and ingestion of contaminated colostrum or milk are also possible routes.

MAP probably enters into the intestinal mucosa through M cells and is later found within macrophages in the submucosa of the ileocecal area and the adjacent lymph nodes (ileocecal) following ingestion (Figure 37.2, 37.3, and 37.4). The establishment of the primary focus of infection is the intestine. Initially the animal shows no signs of disease. The incubation period before overt clinical disease is 12 months or longer. Disease progression follows the course of other mycobacterial infection as described earlier with the formation of slowly progressing granulomatous lesions.

The disease in some affected animals progresses to malabsorption, protein-losing enteropathy, and overt clinical disease. However, only 3–5% of the animals in an infected herd progress to this terminal phase. The mucosal epithelium displays a characteristic appearance (corrugated mucosa) that underlies the malabsorption syndrome. Diarrhea is not a common clinical sign of the disease in sheep and goats. Herd unthriftiness, however, should prompt examination for MAP. Intestinal lesions in sheep and goats are less obvious than in cattle. Weight loss has been a consistent finding in affected goats.

A number of DNA tests have been developed for the demonstration of the presence of MAP. These assays utilize a specific sequence for the development of probes or for the design of primers needed to amplify DNA by using the PCR. Specific sequences that have been exploited are those found in the gene encoding the 16S ribosomal RNA, the insertion sequence IS900 (proper primer selection is crucial since there are segments within this genetic element shared with insertion sequences found in other subspecies).

At present there are no economically useful antimicrobial agents that are effective against MAP *in vivo*. The newer macrolides, such as clarithromycin, and some experimental fluoroquinolones are effective *in vitro*, but are too expensive to use clinically. As mentioned earlier, live attenuated

FIGURE 37.4. *Large epithelioid macrophages. These cells are seen among the crypts in the jejunum of a bovine with Johne's disease. Nuclei are eccentric and cytoplasm slightly vacuolated and sometimes granular (hematoxylin and eosin staining, 40×). (Specimen from the University of Nebraska Veterinary Diagnostic Center.)*

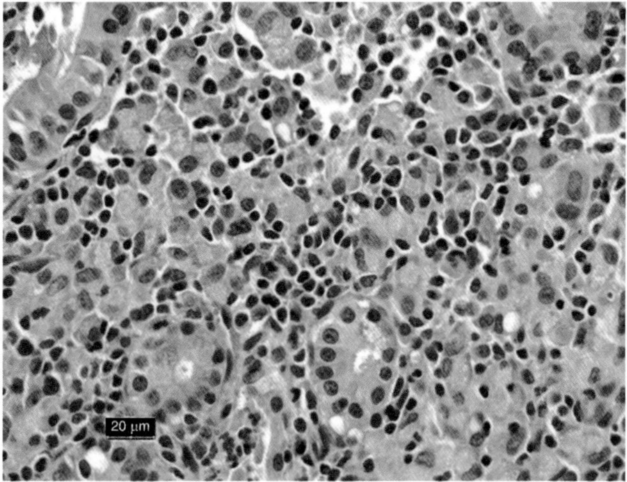

and killed vaccines are used in some countries, but are not universally available.

Eliminating infected animals and preventing possible spread within the herd is an effective means of disease control. Husbandry procedures that must be implemented include segregating the neonate from the dam and other adult animals, ensuring that parturition takes place in noncontaminated areas, and taking precautions against feeding neonates potentially infectious, unpasteurized colostrum or milk. Immunologic and cultural tests are applied to promptly identify those animals that are infected and shedding.

Pasteurization is an important step in control on dairies in assuring that calves receive milk or colostrum that is free of MAP. Given the potential relationship between MAP and Crohn's disease, this process has also significance from a public health perspective. High-temperature, short-time pasteurization has been shown not to be 100% effective in killing MAP in naturally infected milk, but only if the numbers of microorganisms in the milk are large. This probably has little public health consequence in areas where large quantities of milk are mixed together from several dairies, thereby diluting any infected milk. However, this may become important for producers that process milk from a single farm. Environmental contamination of water reservoirs may be another source of MAP infection in Crohn's disease cases.

Feline Leprosy Syndrome

There is no true leprosy in domestic animals. Since a disease of cats is called feline leprosy, it is appropriate to contrast key features of the prototype (human) condition with disease in animals.

In leprosy, the disease picture ranges between two extremes. In lepromatous leprosy, bacterial proliferation is profuse. Poorly circumscribed nondestructive lesions develop, dominated by a monocytic response, but little other inflammatory reactivity. Cell-mediated immunity is suppressed, but circulating immunoglobulins are high. In tuberculoid leprosy, bacteria are scarce. Lesions are granulomatous, and cell-mediated inflammatory responses are well developed. They cause neural damage, leading to anesthesia, paralysis, dystrophy, disfigurement, and mutilation.

Feline leprosy syndrome is a chronic noduloulcerative, mycobacterial infection of the skin. It exists in two histomorphologic forms, lepromatous (organism rich) and tuberculoid (paucibacillary). *Mycobacterium lepraemurium*, the rodent leprosy bacillus, has been identified in tuberculoid and occasionally lepromatous lesions. The causative agent varies and new mycobacterial species named *Mycobacterium visibile* and *Mycobacterium* sp. strain Tarwin are proposed to define organisms detected by PCR in several cats in independent reports of the lepromatous form. Several other mycobacterial species are described in individual case reports. Many studies do not clearly separate leprosy syndrome from other forms of mycobacteriosis, and in some instances the possibility of surface epidermal mycobacterial contaminants cannot be excluded. Sources, mode of spread, and pathogenic mechanisms are not well defined. The location of lesions on the head, neck, and forelimbs suggests transmission by rodent bite or arthropods. Nodules occur in cutis or subcutis in many sites, and are freely movable and painless. Ulceration and lymph node involvement are frequent. Disease is more common in older cats and is slowly progressive. The form of disease does not consistently predict rate of progression. The general health of the cat may be unaffected. Microscopically, the lesions are granulomas largely of monocytic with variable neutrophilic, lymphocytic, plasmacytic, and giant cell admixtures. Caseation necrosis and irregular neural involvement occur. Neurotropism has not been a feature. Acid-fast bacteria abound within histiocytes. Routine culture for rapidly growing mycobacteria or for mycobacteria causing tuberculosis is negative. PCR technology may aid in making a definitive diagnosis.

Treatment includes surgical excision of affected sites coupled with antibiotics. Clofazimine, fluoroquinolones, doxycycline, and clarithromycin individually or in combination have been tried with varied success. Treatment as long as 3–6 months is required to prevent relapse.

Canine Leproid Granuloma Syndrome

Canine leproid granuloma syndrome is caused by an uncultured, saprophytic species of *Mycobacterium* (based on sequence comparisons of DNA obtained from infected tissue with other members of this genus as regards the gene encoding the 16S ribosomal RNA). Diagnosis is based upon demonstration of numerous acid-fast organisms in stained (Ziehl–Neelsen) biopsies or smears of affected tissue or sites. The condition affects the subcutis and skin of the outer pinnae, face, and forelimbs. Lesions can be single, but multiple lesions are common. Large lesions may ulcerate. Histologic features are of pyogranulomatous inflammation with necrosis and limited numbers of giant cells. Nerve bundles are not involved, and thus leproid refers only to the mycobacterial etiology rather than pathologic similarity to human disease. The disease can be self-limiting and is cured by surgical excision or antibiotic therapy. A combination of rifampicin and clarithromycin has been effective as has enrofloxacin. The disease was described first in Africa and has been well characterized in Australia and Brazil and is present in North America. Boxers may be predisposed. The disease is most common in large breed, short-haired, outdoor dogs during summer months. This summer occurrence and a strong predilection for lesions on the pinnae suggest arthropod injury may contribute to transmission. Cases in the United States, Brazil, and Australia all share common mycobacterial 16S ribosomal sequence identity.

Ulcerative Dermatitis of Cats and Dogs due to Rapidly Growing Mycobacteria

The most common cases of ulcerative dermatitis are chronic (months to years), nonhealing skin lesions. There is a tendency for lesions to occur on the ventral and inguinal regions and for disease to be progressive and requiring protracted treatment. Histopathologic evaluation of biopsies of affected tissue reveals pyogranulomatous inflammation. Microorganisms may stain poorly ("ghosts" or "speckled" structures, thought to represent nonstaining or poorly staining mycobacteria, respectively) when stained with Gram's or a Romanovsky-type stain (e.g., Wright's and Giemsa). When samples are stained by the acid-fast method (Ziehl–Neelsen), microorganisms are not often seen. Cavitated nonstaining areas may contain clusters of bacteria.

Culture on standard blood agar medium will result in the isolation of rapidly growing (48–72h incubation) colonies. Isolates are identified by biochemical traits and DNA tests. The most commonly isolated in western North America is *M. fortuitum*. A wide array of opportunistic mycobacteria have been identified and each clinical case needs careful evaluation if etiologic diagnosis is sought. Other species identified in cases of dermatitis and panniculitis include *M. smegmatis*, *M. chelonae*, *M. abscessus*, *M. microti*, *M. flavescens*, *M. massiliense*, *M. ulcerans*, and *Mycobacterium* sp. strain Tarwin. *M. bovis* and *M. avium* have also been identified in individual cases of feline dermatitis. Geographic location of studies varied on common isolates, suggesting the distribution of opportunistic mycobacteria in the environment is the critical factor in anticipating what agent might be infecting cats in a particular location.

Percutaneous wound infection is the likely portal of entry. Mycobacteria that can be isolated from soil and water are likely to lead to opportunistic infections of skin wounds. Treatment includes surgical excision of affected sites coupled with antibiotic treatment. Clofazimine, fluoroquinolones, doxycycline, and clarithromycin, individually or in combination, have been tried with varied success. Antimicrobial resistance patterns vary between species in the limited studies published and, thus, etiologic diagnosis can be critical for proper medical management. Treatment as long as 3–6 months is required to prevent relapse.

Special topic

Is the paradigm changing on *M. tuberculosis* intracellular localization? Prior and latest research suggest this may be the case and a mechanism has been proposed.

Further Reading

Chacon O, Bermudez LE, and Barletta RG (2004) Johne's disease, inflammatory bowel disease, and *Mycobacterium paratuberculosis*. *Annu Rev Microbiol*, **58**, 329–363.

Cole ST and Riccardi G (2011) New tuberculosis drugs on the horizon. *Curr Opin Microbiol*, **14**, 570–576.

Conceição LG, Acha LM, Borges AS *et al.* (2011) Epidemiology, clinical signs, histopathology and molecular characterization of canine leproid granuloma: a retrospective study of cases from Brazil. *Vet Dermatol*, **22**, 249–256.

De Leon J, Jiang G, Ma Y, *et al.* (2012) *Mycobacterium tuberculosis* ESAT-6 exhibits a unique membrane-interacting activity that is not found in its ortholog from non-pathogenic *Mycobacterium smegmatis*. *J Biol Chem*, **287**, 44184–44191.

Dhama K, Mahendran M, Tiwari R *et al.* (2011) Tuberculosis in birds: Insights into the *Mycobacterium avium* infections. *Vet Med Int*, 2011, 712369. Epub July 4, 2011.

Fyfe JA, McCowan C, O'Brien CR *et al.* (2008) Molecular characterization of a novel fastidious *Mycobacterium* causing lepromatous lesions of the skin, subcutis, cornea, and conjunctiva of cats living in Victoria, Australia. *J Clin Microbiol*, **46**, 618–626.

Gengenbacher M and Kaufmann SH (2012) *Mycobacterium tuberculosis:* Success through dormancy. *FEMS Microbiol Rev*. doi:10.1111/j.1574-6976.2012.00331.x.

Hunter RL, Olsen MR, Jagannath C, and Actor JK (2006) Multiple roles of cord factor in the pathogenesis of primary, secondary, and cavitary tuberculosis, including a revised description of the pathology of secondary disease. *Ann Clin Lab Sci*, **36**, 371–386.

Kalscheuer R, Syson K, Veeraraghavan U *et al.* (2010) Self-poisoning of *Mycobacterium tuberculosis* by targeting GlgE in an alpha-glucan pathway. *Nat Chem Biol*, **6**, 376–384.

Kaufmann SH (2011) Fact and fiction in tuberculosis vaccine research: 10 years later. *Lancet Infect Dis*, **11**, 633–640.

Kaur D, Guerin ME, Skovierová H *et al.* (2009) Chapter 2: Biogenesis of the cell wall and other glycoconjugates of *Mycobacterium tuberculosis*. *Adv Appl Microbiol*, **69**, 23–78.

Kaur D, McNeil MR, Khoo KH *et al.* (2007) New insights into the biosynthesis of mycobacterial lipomannan arising from deletion of a conserved gene. *J Biol Chem*, **14**, 282, 27133–27140.

Mishra AK, Driessen NN, Appelmelk BJ, and Besra GS (2011) Lipoarabinomannan and related glycoconjugates: structure, biogenesis and role in *Mycobacterium tuberculosis* physiology and host-pathogen interaction. *FEMS Microbiol Rev*, **35**, 1126–1157.

Niederweis M, Danilchanka O, Huff J *et al.* (2010) Mycobacterial outer membranes: in search of proteins. *Trends Microbiol*, **18**, 109–116.

Palmer MV, Waters WR, and Thacker TC (2007) Lesion development and immunohistochemical changes in granulomas from cattle experimentally infected with *Mycobacterium bovis*. *Vet Pathol*, **44**, 863–674.

Palmer MV, Waters WR, and Whipple DL (2002) Lesion development in white-tailed deer (*Odocoileus virginianus*) experimentally infected with *Mycobacterium bovis*. *Vet Pathol*, **39**, 334–340.

Russell DG (2007) Who puts the tubercle in tuberculosis? *Nat Rev Microbiol*, **5**, 39–47.

Takayama K, Wang C, and Besra GS (2005) Pathway to synthesis and processing of mycolic acids in *Mycobacterium tuberculosis*. *Clin Microbiol Rev*, **18**, 81–101.

Tsai MC, Chakravarty S, Zhu G *et al.* (2006) Characterization of the tuberculous granuloma in murine and human lungs: cellular composition and relative tissue oxygen tension. *Cell Microbiol*, **8**, 218–232.

van der Wel N, Hava D, Houben D, *et al.* (2007) *M. tuberculosis* and *M. leprae* translocate from the phagolysosome to the cytosol in myeloid cells. *Cell* **129**, 1287–1298.

Chlamydiaceae

Roman R. Ganta

Descriptive Features

The family Chlamydiaceae includes obligate, intracellular pathogenic bacteria that can only survive and multiply inside a host cell. They also have a cell wall like most other Gram-negative organisms, respond to antibiotics (tetracyclines and chloramphenicol), and possess ribosomes, DNA, and RNA. Members of the order Chlamydiales are transmitted primarily by inhalation of dust particles, droplets, and through interpersonal contact, all of which containing chlamydial organisms (known as the elementary bodies). These microorganisms infect the host epithelial cells and mucous membranes. The cell tropism of Chlamydiales to epithelium is similar to that by several *Mycoplasma* species; therefore, the infections in target tissue and the diseases caused by *Chlamydia* and *Mycoplasma* are very similar. Based on the clinical symptoms, sometimes it is difficult to distinguish a *Chlamydia* infection from a *Mycoplasma* infection. Taxonomically members of Chlamydiales are classified in the order, Chlamydiales having only one family, Chlamydiaceae, with the genera, *Chlamydophila* and *Chlamydia*. Four known pathogens are *Chlamydophila psittaci*, *Chlamydophila pecorum*, *Chlamydia trachomatis*, and *Chlamydia pneumoniae*. *C. psittaci* has been reclassified into two species: *C. psittaci* and *C. abortus*. *C. psittaci*, *C. trachomatis*, and *C. pneumoniae* cause infections in people. Veterinarians and workers in poultry and slaughterhouses are at the highest risk of acquiring the infections from birds and farm animals.

Morphology and Staining

Members of Chlamydiales are short cocci bacteria with a size of the organisms ranging from 0.2 to 1.0 μm that is similar to Rickettsiales. Giemsa or other polychromatic stains are used to stain these organisms.

Life Cycle and Growth Characteristics

Infectious organisms called elementary bodies, 0.2–0.4 μm in size, enter susceptible cells by receptor-mediated endocytosis. The phagosome containing the organism is not fused with lysosomes, and the elementary body changes into a noninfectious and replicating form that is metabolically active. The replicating form is called reticulate body, which is larger in size (0.6–1.0 μm) compared to elementary bodies. The reticulate bodies replicate by binary fission, which later transform to elementary bodies, and are released upon complete lysis of the infected host cell or by exocytosis.

Members of the order Chlamydiales do not grow in standard bacteriological media or on media plates. They require eukaryotic cells or yolk sacs of chicken embryos for their growth under *in vitro* conditions. Members of Chlamydiales undergo replication inside a phagosome of a host cell by binary fission that is very similar to Anaplasmataceae pathogens of the genera *Ehrlichia*, *Anaplasma*, and *Neorickettsia*. Members of Chlamydiales also have a broad host preference that is similar to Rickettsiales.

Diagnosis, Immunity, and Control

Diagnosis is almost always established by serological methods to detect chlamydial antibodies. Diagnosis is based on clinical signs and demonstration of the organism by Giemsa or other polychromatic-stained impression smears of an infected animal tissue, immunological assays, and/or molecular techniques. An enzyme-linked immunoadsorbent assay (ELISA) technique is also used to detect chlamydial antigens from a sample. Serological tests include complement fixation and ELISA to detect antibodies in the serum of an infected animal. Molecular methods are also available to detect nucleic acids derived from infection-associated chlamydial organisms. Many different and most sensitive molecular methods have been developed *in vitro* to amplify a target of chlamydial nucleic acids, mostly representing the 16S and 23S ribosomal DNA or ribosomal RNA. Molecular methods allow the most sensitive means of rapidly detecting an infection in a tissue sample from clinically ill animals or people or from a sample collected from a persistently infected patient. Chlamydial organisms can also be detected in an impression smear of an infected tissue sample stained with a Diff-Quick stain (Figure 38.1).

As in Rickettsiales, an infected host induces cell-mediated and humoral immune responses resulting in the rise of antibody titers, but the immune response does not eliminate the infectious agents, nor does it help in preventing reinfection. Members of Chlamydiales establish

Veterinary Microbiology, Third Edition. Edited by D. Scott McVey, Melissa Kennedy and M.M. Chengappa.

FIGURE 38.1. C. abortus *inclusions identified from an impression smear sample prepared from an aborted placenta collected from an infected sheep. The smear is stained with Diff-Quick stain (magnification, 1000×). (The slide prepared by Dr Jerome C. Nietfeld, Department of Diagnostic Medicine/Pathobiology, College of Veterinary Medicine, Kansas State University.)*

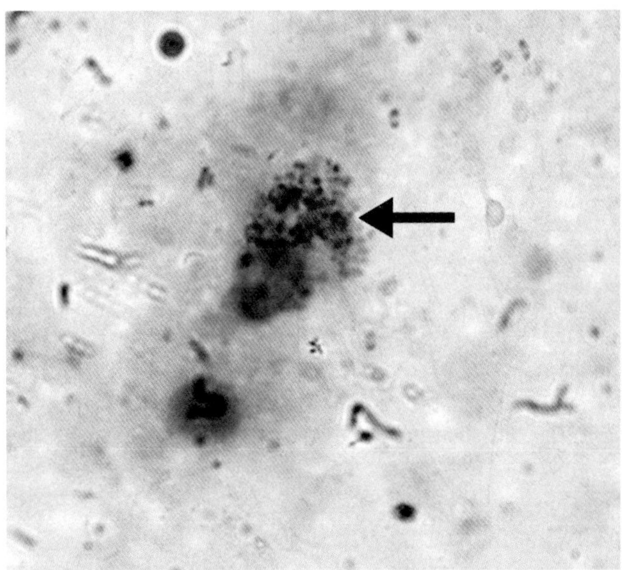

persistent infections in the infected host. Tetracycline is the drug of choice in the treatment of chlamydial infections. It is offered as part of the feed additive or to treat clinically ill animals. The dose for controlling infections is moderate, whereas higher dose is used to treat active infections. Vaccination against chlamydial infections has a variable success, and vaccines are constituted of modified or killed organisms.

Pathogenicity and Toxins

Members of the order Chlamydiales infect epithelial cells and mucous membranes. These bacteria possess hemagglutinin that facilitates attachment to cells. The cell-mediated immune response is largely responsible for tissue damage during inflammation. Chlamydial cell wall lipopolysaccharides and low-density lipoprotein oxidation by chlamydial heat shock proteins are implicated in the pathogenicity.

Diseases Caused by Chlamydiales

Because chlamydial infections are primarily in the epithelium, they infect the respiratory tract, eyes, urogenital tracts, and joints, thus causing respiratory disease, conjunctivitis, urogenital infections, and polyarthritis, respectively. With respect to the host cell preference, the mode of transmission, and the diseases they cause, chlamydial infections resemble many *Mycoplasma* infections.

C. psittaci/C. abortus Infections

C. psittaci has been reclassified into two species, *C. psittaci* and *C. abortus*. *C. abortus* is the causative agent of abortions in sheep and goats in many countries. It is also responsible for abortions in cattle, pigs, and women. *C. psittaci* is responsible for the majority of infections in various vertebrate animals. This species infects birds, goats, sheep, pigs, cattle, and humans.

Birds. *C. psittaci* infections in birds are referred to as avian chlamydiosis (AC), psittacosis, and parrot fever in parrots, and ornithosis in all other bird species. It is an important cause of systemic illness in companion birds and poultry and can cause large economic losses in the poultry industry throughout the world. A great variation in pathogenicity exists for this species resulting from strain-specific variations. AC could be asymptomatic, acute, subacute, or chronic clinical disease. Clinical signs and mortality depend on the species of birds, virulence of a strain, infective dose, stress factors, age, and extent of treatment or prophylaxis. Birds infected with *C. psittaci* typically exhibit clinical signs such as lethargy, anorexia, and ruffled feathers. Other signs include ocular or nasal discharge, diarrhea, and excretion of green to yellow-green urates. Infected birds may die soon after the onset of the illness or may become emaciated and dehydrated before death.

Cattle. *C. psittaci* is well recognized in many countries as an important bovine pathogen. The infection in neuroepithelium is implicated to cause the neurological disease, sporadic bovine encephalomyelitis (SBE), also known as Buss disease. SBE is more common in cattle less than 3 years of age and is characterized by encephalitis, fibrinous pleuritis, and peritonitis. It is manifested with profound depression, and is usually associated with fever that lasts until recovery or death. A staggering gait is often seen and some infected animals tend to walk or stagger in circles. The disease can be transmitted to calves through the milk of infected dams. In addition to SBE, *C. psittaci* infections can lead to polyarthritis, pneumonitis, conjunctivitis, abortion, and infertility. *C. psittaci* infections can result in great economic losses. *C. pecorum* is also isolated from cattle and sheep. It is responsible for various diseases, including sporadic encephalitis, polyarthritis, pneumonia, and diarrhea.

Sheep. *C. psittaci* infections in sheep cause pneumonitis, polyarthritis, and conjunctivitis. *C. abortus* causes abortion.

Goats. Pneumonitis, abortion, enteritis/diarrhea, and arthritis in goats are caused by *C. psittaci/C. abortus*.

Horses. Chlamydial infections by *C. psittaci* also cause pneumonitis, arthritis, abortion, and infertility in horses.

Cats. *C. psittaci* infections in cats may begin with conjunctivitis and nasal discharge, followed by interstitial bronchopneumonia.

Swine. Infections in swine are associated with pneumonitis, conjunctivitis, and polyarthritis.

Other Animal Species. *C. psittaci* also infects guinea pigs, rabbits, and mice, causing conjunctivitis and fertility problems.

C. pecorum Infections

C. pecorum infects cattle, sheep, and pigs. Clinical signs of a *C. pecorum* infection vary from no clinical symptoms to severe disease, involving the central nervous, respiratory, and digestive systems, joints, and conjunctiva. After recovery from a clinical disease, many animals remain as the carriers of infection and excrete elementary bodies for a long time.

Chlamydiosis: A Zoonotic Disease

C. psittaci

Infections in people with *C. psittaci* are reported worldwide. The disease is referred to as psittacosis, which can cause fatal pneumonia. Most human cases are acquired from the organisms shed from parrots, pigeons, turkeys, sheep, and goats. The disease agent can also be transmitted from person to person. Infected birds and animals shed elementary bodies in their feces, urine, saliva, ocular and nasal secretions, and feather dust. These infectious particles are inhaled or ingested by other birds, animals, and people. Humans are usually infected by the inhalation of infective particles in the air. The incubation period is 1–2 weeks. Symptoms are generally like those of the flu, such as fever, diarrhea, chills, conjunctivitis, and sore throat. *C. psittaci* infections in both people and birds are treated with doxycycline or tetracycline. People are treated for 3 weeks, while birds are treated for 45 days.

C. trachomatis

C. trachomatis is the most common sexually transmitted pathogen of humans in the United States. It is responsible for approximately 3–4 million cases each year. Pelvic inflammatory disease (PID), a serious complication of chlamydial infection, has emerged as the leading cause of infertility among childbearing age-group women. Infection may be passed on from a pregnant mother to her newborns during delivery, which can also cause neonatal conjunctivitis and/or pneumonia. *C. trachomatis* cases are five times more in females compared to males. Clinical symptoms are also often milder in males although some infected females can be asymptomatic. Chlamydiosis in both sexes can lead to a serious disease, and can cause sterility due to the scarring of the tubes. *C. trachomatis* infections can also cause blindness in people. *C. trachomatis* infections are also reported in pigs, monkeys, and laboratory mice.

C. pneumoniae

C. pneumoniae is responsible for causing a respiratory disease in people (Figure 38.2). This is very similar to pneumonia caused by *Mycoplasma*. The mode of transmission of the organism is by inhalation. *C. pneumoniae* infections are also implicated in causing atherosclerosis.

FIGURE 38.2. C. pneumoniae *infection in HEp-2 cells (A and B) containing typical inclusions inside phagosomes of the infected cells. EB, elementary bodies; RB, reticulate bodies; im, inclusion membrane. (Reproduced from Kutlin et al. 2001 with the permission from the American Society for Microbiology.)*

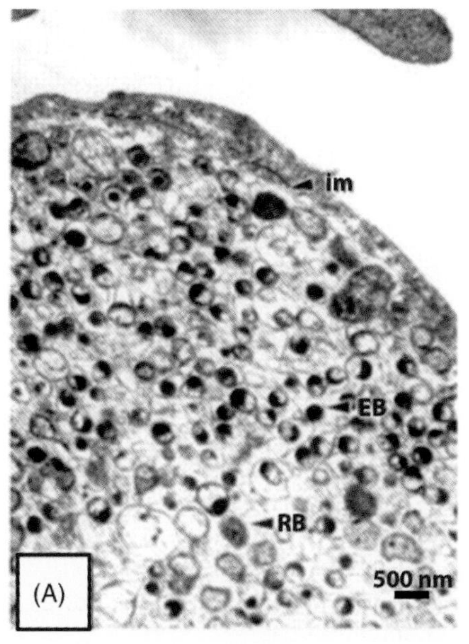

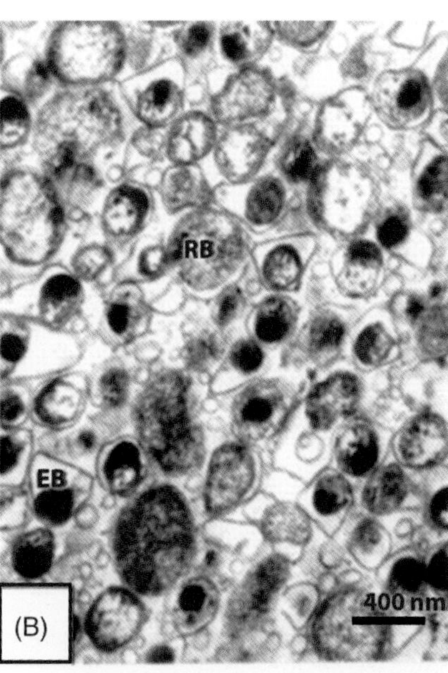

Reference

Kutlin A, Flegg C, Stenzel D *et al.* (2001) Ultrastructural study of *Chlamydia pneumoniae* in a continuous model. *J Clin Microbiol*, **39**, 3721–3723.

Further Reading

Bavoil PM and Wyrick PB (2006) *Chlamydia: Genomics and Pathogenesis*, Horizon Scientific Press.

Harvey JW (2012) *Veterinary Hematology: A Diagnostic Guide and Color Atlas*, Elsevier Inc.

Raskin RE and Meyer DJ (2010) *Canine and Feline Cytology, A Color Atlas and Interpretation Guide,* Elsevier Inc.

Stephens RS (1999) *Chlamydia: Intracellular Biology, Pathogenesis, and Immunity*, ASM Press.

Stuen S and Longbottom D (2011) Treatment and control of chlamydial and rickettsial infections in sheep and goats. *Vet Clin North Am Food Anim Pract*, **27** (1), 213–233. Epub December 13, 2010.

39 Mollicutes

ERIN L. STRAIT AND MELISSA L. MADSEN

The mollicutes are members of the order Mycoplasmatales and class Mollicutes (Latin: *mollis*, soft; *cutis*, skin). Only the genera *Mycoplasma* and *Ureaplasma* have pathogenic species important in veterinary medicine. Members of the *Acholeplasma* are sometimes encountered, but usually as contaminants. "Mollicutes" is the correct term to use when collectively referring to members in this order; however, the trivial name "mycoplasma(s)" is also used for this purpose. Mollicutes are ubiquitous in nature. Species have been found in mammals, reptiles, fish, arthropods, insects, and plants. They are also common tissue-culture contaminants. It is likely that only a small portion of the total number of mollicutes have yet been identified as it seems that wherever one looks a new species can be found. Over 113 animal mycoplasmas and 5 ureaplasmas have been identified with many more at the "candidatus" stage, and of these more than 45 complete genomes have been sequenced. In addition, hemotrophic rickettsial species of the genera *Haemobartonella* and *Eperythrozoon* were reclassified to the genus *Mycoplasma* in 2001, based on 16S ribosomal RNA gene sequence analysis. They have collectively been given the common name "hemoplasmas."

Infections with mollicutes are parasitic in nature. They are most often subclinical to mild but severely debilitating and sometimes fatal diseases can also be observed. Most pathogenic mycoplasmas and ureaplasmas infect the mucosa of the respiratory and/or urogenital tract, but are also found in other body sites such as the conjunctiva, synovial surfaces, and mammary glands. The hemoplasmas infect red blood cells and most commonly cause hemolytic anemia.

Descriptive Features

Morphology and Staining

The cell morphology of the mollicutes is extremely pleomorphic. Cell shapes include spherical, ring-shaped, pear-shaped, spiral-shaped, and filamentous forms. Cells sometime appear as chains of beads, the result of asynchronized genomic replication and cell division. Ring forms found in red blood cells infected with hemoplasmas have also been observed. The diameter of the spherical form ranges from 0.3 μm to 0.8 μm. Due to the size and shape of these organisms, they are able to pass through 0.22 μm and 0.45 μm membrane filters commonly used to filter sterilize liquid media; therefore, it is difficult to rid tissue culture cell lines of these organisms.

Mollicutes stain poorly by the Gram method due to their lack of a cell wall. Giemsa, Castaneda, Dienes, cresyl-fast violet, orcein, and acridine orange stains are preferred.

Structure and Composition

The mollicutes lack the genetic capacity to produce a cell wall. Instead, they are bound by a single trilaminar membrane composed of proteins, glycoproteins, lipoproteins, phospholipids, and sterols. Cholesterol in the membrane provides osmotic stability. Carbohydrate capsules have been described for some species.

The mollicutes have a small genome (ranging from 540 to 1380 kb) relative to other bacteria and are the smallest self-replicating organisms that have yet been described. Their base composition is poor in guanine and cytosine content, with their G+C mol% content of DNA ranging from 24% to 40%. They are related most closely to the *Clostridium–Streptococcus--Lactobacillus* group from which it is presumed the mollicutes evolved through a process of reductive or degenerative evolution. Transposons, plasmids, and bacteriophages have been demonstrated in some species.

Nonhemotrophic Mollicutes

The "nonhemotrophic" mollicutes include members of the genus *Ureaplasma* and those of the genus *Mycoplasma* that do not colonize red blood cells. Unlike the "hemotrophic" mollicutes (see Section "Hemotrophic Mollicutes"), they can be grown *in vitro* on axenic (lifeless) media. Clinical manifestations include respiratory and urogenital tract infections, conjunctivitis, arthritis, mastitis, septicemia, and otitis media. Most species exhibit a high degree of host specificity, but infections across host species are also observed, most commonly in immunocompromised individuals (Table 39.1).

Original chapter written by Richard L. Walker.

Veterinary Microbiology, Third Edition. Edited by D. Scott McVey, Melissa Kennedy and M.M. Chengappa.

Table 39.1. Pathogenic Mycoplasma Species and Their Primary Host(s)

Animal Species	Agent	Common Clinical Manifestations
Cats	*M. felis*	Conjunctivitis
	M. feliminutum	Respiratory disease
	M. gatae	Arthritis
Cattle	*M. alkalescens*	Arthritis, mastitis
	M. bovigentialium	Infertility, mastitis, seminal vesiculitis
	M. bovis	Abscesses, arthritis, mastitis, otitis, pneumonia
	M. bovoculi	Keratoconjunctivitis
	M. californicum	Arthritis, mastitis
	M. canadense	Arthritis, mastitis
	M. dispar	Alveolitis, bronchiolitis
	M. diversum	Infertility, pneumonia, vulvovaginitis
	M. mycoides ssp. *mycoides* (SC)	Arthritis, pleuropneumonia
	M. wenyonii	Anemia
Chickens	*M. gallisepticum*	Respiratory disease
	M. synoviae	Airsacculitis, sternal bursitis, synovitis
Dogs	*M. canis*	Urogenital tract disease
	M. cynos	Pneumonia
	M. spumans	Arthritis
Felids	*M. felifaucium*	Respiratory disease
	M. leocaptivus	Respiratory disease
	M. leopharyngis	Respiratory disease
	M. simbae	Respiratory disease
Goats	*M. agalactiae*	Agalactiae, arthritis, conjunctivitis
	M. capricolum ssp. *capricolum*	Arthritis, mastitis, pneumonia, septicemia
	M. capricolum ssp. *capripneumoniae*	Pleuropneumonia
	M. conjunctivae	Keratoconjunctivitis
	M. mycoides ssp. *mycoides* (LC)	Abscesses, arthritis, mastitis, septicemia
	M. mycoides ssp. *capri*	Pneumonia
	M. putrefaciens	Arthritis, mastitis
Horses	*M. equigenitalium*	Infertility
	M. equirhinis	Respiratory disease (suspected)
	M. fastidiosum	Respiratory disease (suspected)
	M. felis	Pleuritis
	M. subdolum	Infertility
Mice	*M. neurolyitcum*	Conjunctivitis, neurological disease
	M. pulmonis	Respiratory disease
Rats	*M. arthritidis*	Arthritis
	M. pulmonis	Respiratory disease, genital tract disease
Sheep	*M. agalactiae*	Agalactiae
	M. conjunctivae	Keratoconjunctivitis
	M. ovipneumoniae	Pneumonia
Swine	*M. hyopneumoniae*	Enzootic pneumonia
	M. hyorhinis	Arthritis, pneumonia, polyserositis
	M. hyosynoviae	Arthritis
Turkeys	*M. gallisepticum*	Sinusitis, respiratory disease
	M. iowae	Embryo mortality, leg deformities
	M. meleagridis	Airsacculitis, decreased egg hatchability, perosis
	M. synoviae	Sternal bursitis, synovitis

Growth Characteristics

The nonhemotrophic mollicutes are generally slow-growing and often require 3–10 days (or more) of incubation before colonies are apparent on agar. *In vitro* growth is generally best at 33–38 °C in an atmosphere of increased CO_2. Mollicutes lack many biosynthetic pathways. They are unable to synthesize any amino acids and have either a complete or partial inability to synthesize fatty acids. Exogenous sterols are required by mycoplasmas that they acquire from serum. Because of the high nutritional demands of the mollicutes, media supporting growth of the various mycoplasmas and ureaplasmas are often highly enriched and complex. Most are based on beef heart infusion, peptone, yeast extract, and serum along with various other supplements. Optimal pH for growth ranges from 6.0 to 8.0 for mollicutes depending on the normal host environment in which they are found. Mollicute colonies are small and difficult to visualize with the unaided eye. Colony sizes vary from 0.01 to 1.0 mm. When observed with a dissecting microscope, many species exhibit a "fried-egg" morphology (Figure 39.1). This umbonate appearance

FIGURE 39.1. *"Fried-egg" colony morphology that is typical of many* Mycoplasma *species.*

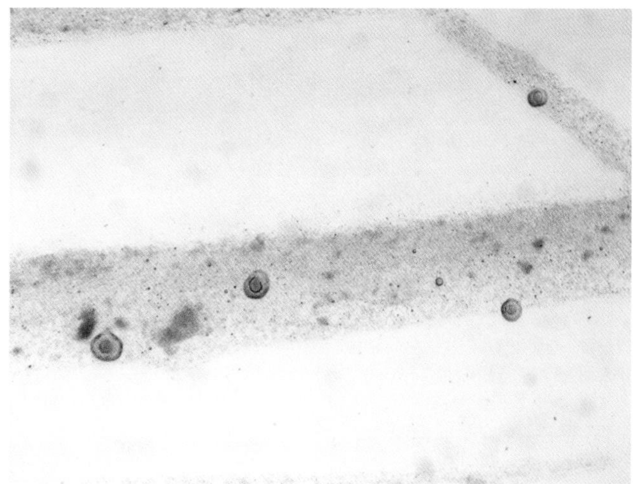

is the result of the central portion of the colony embedding into the agar with a peripheral zone of surface growth. Some species produce film spots, which are composed of cholesterol and phospholipids and appear as a wrinkled film on the media surface. Differences in colony morphology and size can be used to distinguish some of the mollicutes. For example, the colony size of *Mycoplasma mycoides* ssp. *mycoides* isolates from goats is consistently larger than those isolated from cattle. This size difference is used to distinguish between the two variants. *Ureaplasma* species produce substantially smaller colonies than other mollicutes and often lack the fried-egg colony morphology.

Ecology

Reservoir. The major reservoir for the nonhemotrophic mollicutes is the host they infect. Subclinically infected animals carry organisms on mucosal surfaces, including upper and lower respiratory tracts, the urogenital tract, conjunctiva, alimentary canal, mammary glands, and/or joints. In general, mollicutes can survive outside the host for substantial lengths of time in moist, cool environments. They are very susceptible to heat and most detergents (tween) and disinfectants (quaternary ammonium, iodine, and phenol-based compounds).

Transmission and Epidemiology. While there are several clinically and economically important species of mollicutes, primary pathogens such as *M. mycoides* ssp. *mycoides*, small colony (SC) variants in cattle are the exception rather than the rule. Mollicutes most often cause mild to moderate disease that can be exacerbated by cofactors including age, genetic predisposition, environmental conditions, crowding, and concurrent infections. These are all involved in contributing to resistance to infection or lack thereof. Minimizing predisposing stresses will minimize disease. Virulence varies not only among species but also among strains within species of mollicutes. This also accounts for some of the observed variations in disease manifestation.

Transmission occurs predominately by spread from animal to animal through direct contact and is mediated by aerosolization of respiratory secretions or venereal transmission. Introduction of an infected animal into an uninfected population is a common route for dissemination of infection. Asymptomatic carriers, usually colonized on mucosal surfaces, serve as the source for maintaining organisms within a population. Long-distance spread of infectious *Mycoplasma* can occur through wind under optimal conditions. For instance, viable *Mycoplasma hyopneumoniae* has been recovered >9 km from an infected swine herd source. Mechanical transmission through milking machinery is a means for spreading bovine and caprine mycoplasma mastitis, and contaminated milk can be a source of infection for calves and goat kids. In poultry, vertical transmission through hatching eggs is an important means of spread for many of the pathogenic avian species. Little is known regarding the role of ectoparasites and/or flying insects in transmission; however, pathogenic caprine species have been isolated from ear mites of goats.

Pathogenesis and Immunity. Mollicutes employ a variety of strategies in order to occupy such a wide range of host niches and to maintain themselves as chronic, parasitic infections. These organisms have a complex relationship with their host(s) especially with regard to immunity, making it difficult to separate the pathogenesis of the organism from the host's own immune response against them. In fact, the immune response of the host is intimately involved in the pathogenesis of disease (immunopathology).

The chronicity of mollicute infections suggests that the immune response is not effective at eliminating infection once established, and latent infections are common. In the face of an intense inflammatory response in the acute stage of infection, mycoplasmas generally appear able to avoid elimination and at least a portion of hosts maintain long-term infections. Antigenic variability is a mechanism employed by some mollicutes to evade host defenses. The pMGA gene family, which accounts for 16% of the entire genome of *Mycoplasma gallisepticum*, generates antigenic variants of a major surface protein. Incorporation of host antigens by mycoplasmas, a condition referred to as capping, further aids some mollicutes in escaping detection by the immune system. Phase shift in *Mycoplasma hyorhinis* aids in eluding the host immune response by varying the length of surface proteins, so they are less accessible to immune cells. Alternatively, antigens shared between *Mycoplasma* species and the host tissues may result in a biological mimicry, whereby the host recognizes the *Mycoplasma* as self, leading to persistent infections. Similarly, shared host and *Mycoplasma* antigens, such as the galactans found in the lungs of cattle and in *M. mycoides* ssp. *mycoides*, can also result in autoimmune disease. Another mechanism to achieve carrier state in a host is to form biofilms that are a community of individual organisms living in a matrix of extracellular polymeric substance as a means of avoiding the host immune response and antibiotic therapies. Several mycoplasmas readily form biofilms (Figure 39.2). Underlying factors such as age,

FIGURE 39.2. *Mycoplasma colony forming a biofilm attached to an air saccule surrounded by leukocytes (A) and an in vitro grown Mycoplasma biofilm on glass wool (B). (Courtesy of Dr D. Trampel and Dr F.C. Minion, respectively.)*

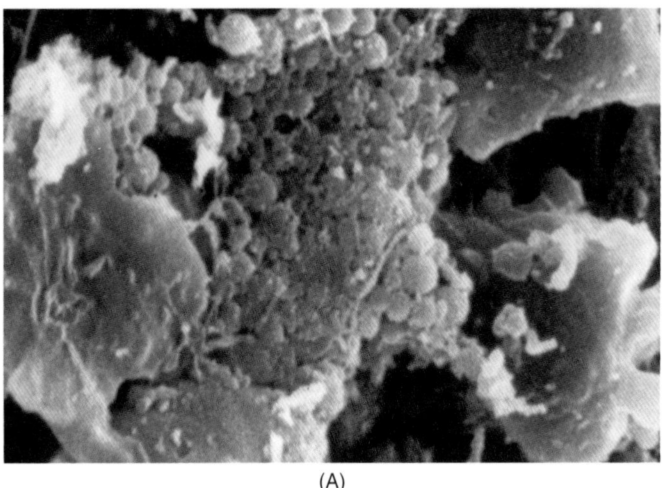

(A)

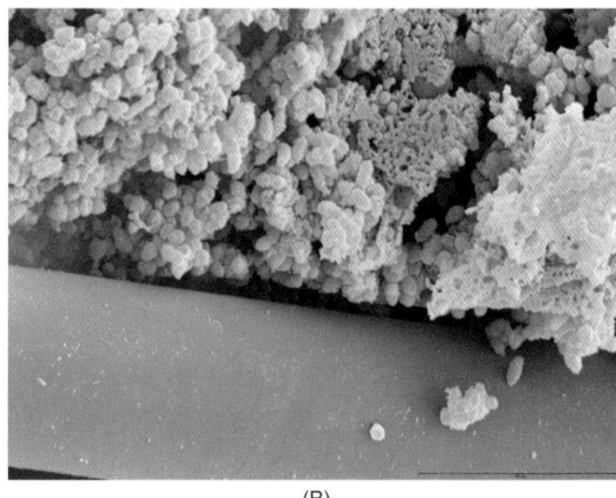

(B)

overcrowding, concurrent infections, and transportation stresses lead to overt disease.

Attachment to host cells is the first step in establishing infection and is facilitated by the anionic surface layer on most mycoplasmas (Figure 39.3). Host receptors for attachment are surface proteins, especially glycoconjugates that allow colonization of mucosal surfaces. In some species such as *M. gallisepticum*, attachment is mediated through a specialized tip structure. A polar bleb has been demonstrated in some species, including *M. gallisepticum*, and also has a role in adherence to host cell surfaces. These blebs aid in the motility of mycoplasmas that possess them, which is referred to as gliding motility. There is evidence that some *Mycoplasma* and *Ureaplasma* species can penetrate and exist inside nonphagocytic cells, protecting them from the immune system and facilitating their dissemination within the host. Some mycoplasmas that cause pneumonia are able to induce ciliostasis, which damages and impedes the effectiveness of the mucociliary escalator, aiding colonization.

FIGURE 39.3. *Scanning electron micrograph of M. hyopneumoniae attached to cilia of the respiratory epithelia. (Courtesy of Dr F. C. Minion.)*

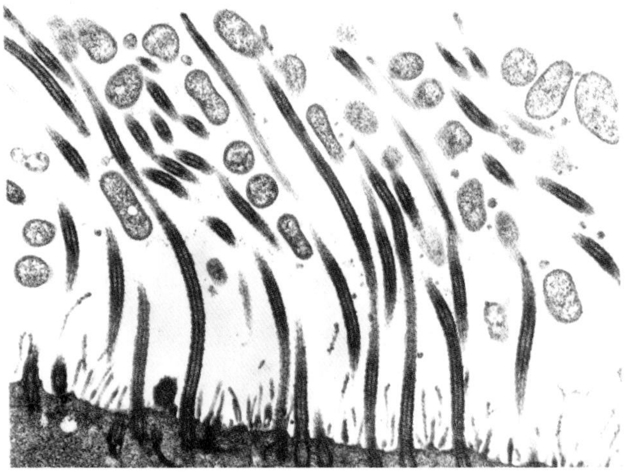

Downregulation of the innate immune response, such as inhibition of macrophage phagocytic activity, has been associated with some *Mycoplasma* infections. Alternatively, lipoproteins abundant in the plasma membrane of mollicutes activate the innate immune system through Toll-like receptors 2 and 6 and stimulate a proinflammatory response mediated by the production of cytokines and various other factors. In addition, mycoplasmas activate the complement cascade by the classical pathway, which contributes to the inflammatory response. The inflammatory response results in damage to bystander host cells that may benefit the mycoplasmas by freeing nutrients from host cells that these parasitic organisms require for growth while the ensuing immune response does not effectively clear the organisms.

Injury to host tissue may also be induced through other mechanisms. Products of metabolism such as hydrogen peroxide and superoxide radicals in mycoplasmas result in local host cell damage. Ureaplasmas have potent enzymes as well, including phospholipases and urease. Persistence of antigen in selected sites, such as joints, allows for further damage due to development of an immune complex-mediated inflammatory response. Induction of interleukin 1 (IL-1), IL-6, IL-12, IL-18, and tumor necrosis factor from activated macrophages leads to activation of cytotoxic T-lymphocytes and results in an endotoxin-like effect in the host. Acute, septicemic forms of disease can result in a coagulopathy and widespread vascular thrombosis, which resembles a gram-negative septicemia and is, at least in part, mediated through induction of cytokines.

Both the cellular and humoral immune systems respond to infection by mollicutes, and each has been demonstrated to have a role in controlling the number of *Mycoplasma* organisms present in the host. Yet similar to the innate immune response, mollicutes are able to subvert these host response mechanisms as well. For example, *Mycoplasma bovis* has been shown to suppress lymphocyte responses; conversely many *Mycoplasma* species have been shown to possess unique mitogenic factors that induce nonspecific polyclonal B and/or T cell stimulation. *Mycoplasma arthritidis* possesses a small peptide, MAM, which acts as a superantigen and stimulates a broad population of T-lymphocytes. While the mechanism of action has not been elucidated for all suppressive and mitogenic factors utilized by mollicutes, it is clear that they are important in the pathogenesis of these organisms.

Disease Patterns. Infections can manifest in a variety of ways including septicemias, disseminated infections involving multiple sites, or localized infections. Common manifestations caused by the different pathogenic species in major animal species are listed in Table 39.1. In addition to specific effects related to *Mycoplasma*, generalized effects on the immune system may increase susceptibility to secondary infections with other bacterial and viral pathogens.

The lesions associated with *Mycoplasma* infections vary from acute to chronic and are dependent on the agent involved and the site affected. In acute infections, there is an inflammatory reaction with an infiltration of neutrophils, macrophages, and lymphocytes and an accumulation of fibrin. An infiltration of lymphocytes and plasma cells is often observed in *Mycoplasma* infections, particularly around vessels, airways, and in the submucosa. Peribronchial, peribronchiolar, and perivascular lymphoplasmacytic cuffing is a characteristic finding in respiratory tract infection. The profound perivascular and peribronchiolar lymphoid hyperplasia observed in many infections is due to nonspecific mitogenic effects as well as to a specific antimycoplasmal immune response.

Generalized infections lead to a fibrinopurulent exudate on serosal surfaces and synovial membranes. In persistent localized infections, tissue destruction can be substantial. Abscesses may develop at pressure sites in calves and are characterized by an eosinophilic coagulative necrosis with peripheral fibrosis. In cases of mycoplasma mastitis, pockets of purulent exudate may develop in affected mammary tissue. Eventually the affected gland becomes fibrosed. In the acute stage of *Mycoplasma* infections of the joint, the joint becomes distended with fluid containing fibrin. As infections become chronic, there is villus hypertrophy of the synovia and a proliferative and erosive arthritis develops.

Avian. Mycoplasmosis in poultry has important economic consequences. *M. gallisepticum* causes a chronic respiratory disease in chickens and infectious sinusitis in turkeys, and infects a number of other domestic avian species. Clinical signs include coughing, nasal discharge, and tracheal rales. Turkeys can develop sinusitis with production of a thick, mucoid exudate that results in severe swelling of the infraorbital sinuses (Figure 39.4). Occasionally, clinical signs related to brain and joint involvements are recognized. Decrease in egg production also occurs. *Mycoplasma synoviae* also infects a wide range of

FIGURE 39.4. *Infraorbital sinusitis in a turkey caused by* M. gallisepticum. *(Courtesy of Dr D. Trampel.)*

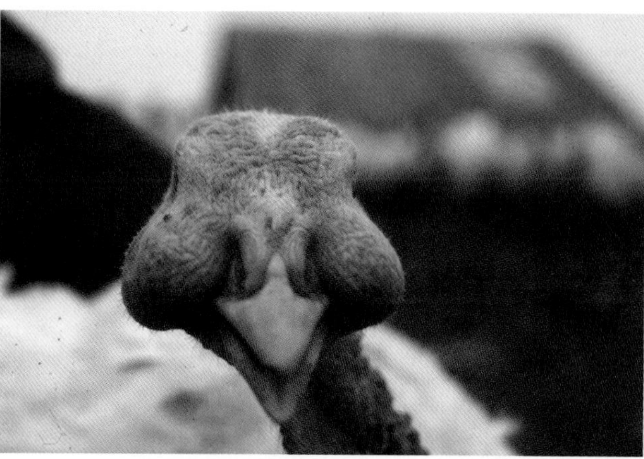

avian species. Synovitis resulting in lameness, swelling of joints and tendon sheaths, and retarded growth are common presentations. Sternal bursitis is also frequently observed in turkeys. Airsacculitis, which is usually subclinical, is another manifestation. *Mycoplasma meleagridis* and *Mycoplasma iowae* infections are mostly limited to turkeys. *M. meleagridis* causes respiratory disease, predominately an airsacculitis, which is often clinically mild or inapparent. Skeletal deformities, including bowing or twisting of the tarsometatarsal bone and cervical vertebrae, are occasionally detected. Decreased egg hatchability is a serious consequence of *M. meleagridis* infections. Airsacculitis, leg deformities, and stunting in poults have been demonstrated with *M. iowae*. Decreased egg hatchability has also been noted with *M. iowae* infections. Natural outbreaks of conjunctivitis in house finches due to *M. gallisepticum* have caused substantial reductions in the finch population on the eastern coast of the United States.

Bovine. *M. mycoides* ssp. *mycoides* SC variant is considered the most virulent of the bovine mycoplasmas. It causes a respiratory disease, contagious bovine pleuropneumonia (CBPP), in cattle that ranges from a persistent, subclinical infection to an acute, sometimes fatal disease. Clinical signs include respiratory distress, coughing, nasal discharge, and reluctance to move. In severe cases, the animal will stand with its neck extended and mouth open to facilitate breathing. Subclinically affected animals serve as a source for maintaining and spreading infection in the herd. Most infections are limited to the respiratory tract, although arthritis occurs in calves.

Mycoplasma mastitis is caused by a number of species. *M. bovis* is the most common cause and results in the most severe disease. *Mycoplasma californicum* and *Mycoplasma canadense* are also frequently involved. *Mycoplasma alkalescens* and *Mycoplasma bovigenitalium* have also been implicated as etiologic agents on occasion. Typically, there is a drop in milk production. The milk becomes thick and intermixed with a watery secretion and may progress to a purulent exudate. The udder is often swollen, although not painful. Sometimes all four quarters are involved. It is a

FIGURE 39.5. *Pneumonia in a cow caused by* M. bovis. *(Courtesy of Dr R. Rosenbusch.)*

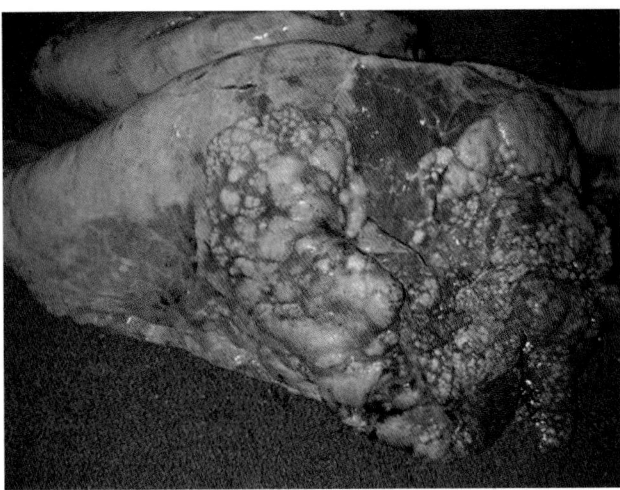

destructive mastitis and often refractory to treatment. Most infections are limited to the mammary gland; however, arthritis subsequent to bacteremia occurs. In some cases disseminated infection results in periarticular involvement and fasciitis. Spread from cow to cow is directly related to inadequate management and sanitation practices.

Mycoplasma respiratory tract infections in calves often present as pneumonia in association with other bovine respiratory pathogens (Figure 39.5). *M. bovis* is the predominant species recovered. *Mycoplasma dispar* causes a mild respiratory disease characterized by bronchiolitis and alveolitis and is usually precipitated by environmental stresses or a primary viral infection. Both *M. bovis* and *M. dispar* can be recovered as commensals from the upper respiratory tract.

Urogenital tract infections are caused by *M. bovigenitalium* and *Ureaplasma diversum*. Seminal vesiculitis in bulls and granular vulvitis, vaginitis, endometritis, infertility, and abortion in cows are associated with both of these organisms. Both are found as normal commensals in the lower urogenital tract.

Arthritis in calves occurs sporadically. While a number of different species can cause arthritis, *M. bovis* is most frequently recovered. Other less common presentations include otitis media and decubital abscesses. Otitis media usually occurs in conjunction with respiratory disease. Decubital abscesses have been associated with confined housing conditions. *M. bovis*, again, is the usual agent.

Canine. A number of *Mycoplasma* species have been isolated from dogs; however, little is known regarding their role in disease. Experimental and clinical evidence suggests that *Mycoplasma canis* can cause urogenital tract disease including prostatitis, cystitis, endometritis, orchitis, and epididymitis. The role of *Mycoplasma* in reproductive disorders of the bitch is uncertain although infertility has been associated with mycoplasmal infections, especially in kennels with poor hygiene. Canine infectious respiratory disease (CIRD) is a common respiratory infection found mostly in kenneled animals. *Mycoplasma cynos* is the primary *Mycoplasma* associated with the disease and is found to exacerbate the pathogenesis of CIRD. *Mycoplasma spumans* has been reported to cause arthritis.

Caprine. *Mycoplasma* infections in goats are economically important and can result in disease of epizootic proportion. *M. mycoides* ssp. *mycoides* (large colony variant) infections present as a mastitis, pneumonia, bursitis, or arthritis in adult animals. Some develop a generalized toxic disease that can be fatal. A rapidly fatal septicemia is common in kids. Those that survive develop a chronic, destructive arthritis and/or bursitis. *M. mycoides* ssp. *capri* causes a pleuropneumonia similar to that of goat strains of *M. mycoides* ssp. *mycoides*. It has been proposed that *M. mycoides* ssp. *mycoides* (large colony variant) be combined with *M. mycoides* ssp. *capri* as a single subspecies *capri* based on the high DNA homology they share. Septicemia, arthritis, and mastitis occur with *Mycoplasma capricolum* ssp. *capricolum* infections. *M. capricolum* ssp. *capripneumoniae* (formerly *Mycoplasma* sp. F-38) causes contagious caprine pleuropneumonia (CCPP), which is similar to CBPP in cattle. Both *Mycoplasma agalactiae* and *Mycoplasma putrefaciens* cause mastitis. The mastitis due to *M. putrefaciens* is purulent in nature, while infections with *M. agalactiae* result in a decrease or total cessation in milk production. Both species can cause arthritis. *Mycoplasma conjunctivae* causes a keratoconjunctivitis that presents with lacrimation, conjunctival hyperemia, and keratitis. Pannus is sometimes evident.

Equine. *Mycoplasma felis* is the only species that has been solidly associated with disease in the horse. It is recovered from the upper respiratory tract as a commensal, but can cause a pleuritis, usually related to some exertional activity. The pleuritis is self-limiting and frequently resolves spontaneously. *Mycoplasma equirhinis* and *Mycoplasma fastidiosum* have been suspected of causing respiratory disease, but this has not been confirmed. *Mycoplasma equigenitalium* and *Mycoplasma subdolum* have been identified in the genital tract of both stallions and mares and are implicated as a cause of infertility in mares.

Feline. A variety of commensal mycoplasmas have been recovered from mucosal surfaces of cats. Relatively few are associated with disease. *Mycoplasma gatae* has been recovered from cats with arthritis. *M. felis* has been associated with a serous to mucoid conjunctivitis. Typically the conjunctiva is edematous; however, the cornea is not involved. A *Mycoplasma*-like organism has been associated with subcutaneous abscesses, but neither the disease nor the organism has been well characterized. *Mycoplasma* spp. have been isolated as part of the polymicrobial component from pyothorax exudates.

Murine. *Mycoplasma pulmonis* causes a low-grade respiratory disease in rats. Infections involve the nasal cavity, middle ear, larynx, trachea, and lungs. The most common clinical sign is a low-pitched wheezing or snuffling resulting from the purulent nasal exudate. In mice, clinical signs are often inapparent, although a chattering sound and continued rubbing of the eyes and nose may suggest infection in the colony. Mortality is low and when it occurs is related to pneumonia. Genital tract infections with *M. pulmonis* are also recognized in rats. *M. arthritidis* causes a polyarthritis in rats and mice, although many infections are subclinical. Experimental infections in mice result in joint swelling and, in some cases, posterior paralysis. Natural infections with *Mycoplasma neurolyticum* generally do not cause disease, although conjunctivitis has been reported. Experimental inoculation with *M. neurolyticum* or cell-free filtrates causes a neurologic syndrome referred to as rolling disease.

Ovine. Compared to other ruminant species, *Mycoplasma* infections in domestic sheep are generally mild. Wild populations of big horn sheep appear to be quite susceptible to *Mycoplasma ovipneumoniae* infection and can be severely affected. The disease in big horn sheep is often fatal when previously naïve populations become infected. *M. ovipneumoniae* is associated with pneumonia and is usually found in conjunction with other common bacterial pathogens of the ovine respiratory tract. Outbreaks of keratoconjunctivitis have been attributed to *M. conjunctivae*. Agalactic mastitis caused by *M. agalactiae* is similar to that observed in goats. Sheep can also be infected with many of the other species that affect goats.

Porcine. A number of clinical entities are associated with *Mycoplasma* infections in swine. *M. hyopneumoniae* causes a chronic respiratory disease referred to as "porcine enzootic pneumonia." There is high morbidity but low mortality associated with this disease. The principal clinical sign is a chronic nonproductive cough, and pigs exhibit ill-thrift and impaired weight gain. *M. hyopneumoniae* is a significant contributor to the porcine respiratory disease complex (PRDC). The PRDC has a severe negative impact on swine production, and *M. hyopneumoniae* has been shown to potentiate the disease caused by other agents in this complex, such as the porcine reproductive and respiratory syndrome virus. *M. hyorhinis* causes a systemic infection in pigs between 3 and 12 weeks of age. Initial signs include fever, inappetence, and listlessness. Arthritis and lameness frequently follow. There is a characteristic polyserositis that involves pleural, peritoneal, and pericardial serosa. *Mycoplasma hyosynoviae* causes arthritis in growing pigs 12–24 weeks of age (Figure 39.6). Lameness and associated difficulty with mobility are the principal clinical signs.

Laboratory Diagnosis

Sample Collection. The appropriate sample for isolation attempt is determined by the clinical presentation and includes exudates, swabs from affected sites, affected tissues, and milk. Because of the mollicutes' fastidious nature, samples should be submitted to the laboratory as soon as possible after collection. During transportation, samples should be kept cool and moist. Various commercially available media (Stuart's and Amies' without charcoal) are suitable for transporting swabs. If a prolonged transport time

FIGURE 39.6. *Arthritis in a pig with villous synovial tissue proliferation caused by M. hyosynoviae. (Courtesy of Dr J.C.G. Neto.)*

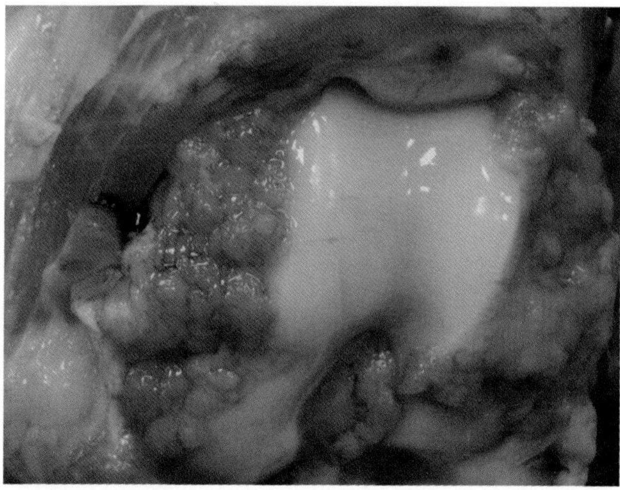

(>24 h) is expected, samples should be shipped frozen and preferably on dry ice or in liquid nitrogen.

Direct Examination. The variability in microscopic morphology and poor staining with the Gram method make direct examination for most mollicutes unrewarding. Direct fluorescent antibody tests and DNA fluorochrome staining have been described, particularly for diagnosing conjunctivitis and mastitis, but they are not widely used.

Immunoperoxidase, immunofluorescent, and immunohistochemistry staining of histopathologic sections has been used successfully for identification of some species in tissues, including *M. bovis* in cattle tissues, *M. hyopneumoniae* in pig lungs, and some of the poultry mycoplasmas.

Isolation. No one media formulation is suitable for growth of all of the mollicutes. The media selected should be based on the specific species or group of species of interest. In general, a fairly complex and enriched medium is required. Serum is the usual source of sterols and is required by most species. Different species, however, grow better with different sources of serum. Yeast extract is also included as a source of growth factors. Growth of some species is enhanced or requires incorporation of specific substances such as vaginal mucus (*M. agalactiae*) and nicotinamide adenine dinucleotide (*M. synoviae*). Some goat mycoplasmas grow on sheep blood agar as small colonies with an α-type ("greening") hemolysis. Mollicutes are resistant to a number of antibiotics and growth inhibitors such as nafcillin, bacitracin, cefobid, thallium acetate, and amphotericin B are commonly added to media to inhibit contaminating bacteria and fungi. Specific immune sera directed against commensal mycoplasmas can be incorporated in media to allow for selective isolation for pathogenic species. For optimal recovery, samples are inoculated into both a liquid and a solid media and incubated at 36–38 °C in 5–10% CO_2 for at least 7 days. Some species require

FIGURE 39.7. *Immunoperoxidase staining method used for typing* Mycoplasma *isolates directly on agar media. Two different types of* Mycoplasma *are present in the sample. One type* (M. hyorhinis) *stains when anti-*M. hyorhinis *antisera is used (darkly stained colonies); the other colonies of* M. hyosynoviae *do not significantly react with that antisera.*

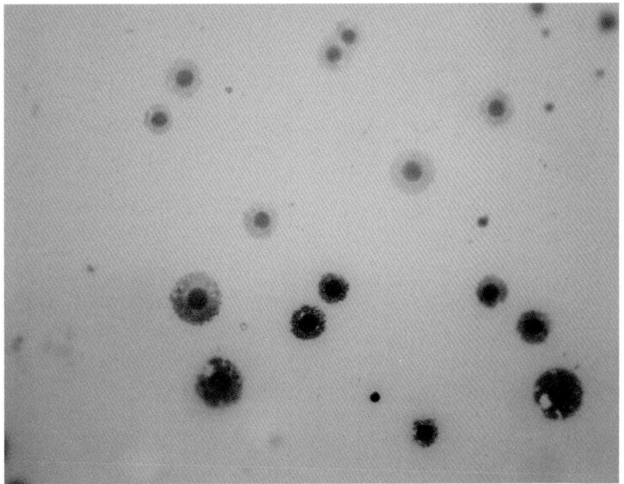

longer incubation times. Semen and joint fluids may contain inhibitory factors and should be diluted prior to culture to enhance recovery. Blind passages from broth to broth for up to three passages may enhance the recovery. *Ureaplasma* species are susceptible to pH changes as a result of hydrolysis of urea included in the media and must be subcultured frequently to maintain their viability when isolation attempts are made. None of the hemoplasmas are cultivable.

Identification. Agar cultures must be examined with the aid of a dissecting microscope. Colonies with the typical umbonate morphology can be stained directly on the agar to differentiate them from other bacteria (Figure 39.7) or can be smeared on a glass slide. Mollicutes stain poorly by the Gram method due to their lack of a cell wall. Dienes is a commonly used stain. The mollicutes stain blue because of their inability to reduce methylene blue in the stain. Other bacteria reduce methylene blue by using it as a hydrogen acceptor in maltose oxidation, and therefore appear colorless with the Dienes stain. The exceptions are L-form bacteria, which exhibit a similar colony morphology and staining reaction as the mollicutes. L-forms must be differentiated from mollicutes by demonstrating reversion of the L-form bacteria back to a walled form. Other stains used to detect mollicutes include Giemsa, Castaneda, Wright's, cresyl-fast violet, orcein, and acridine orange.

Digitonin sensitivity can be used to distinguish *Mycoplasma* and *Ureaplasma* from *Acholeplasma*. A large zone of inhibition around paper disks saturated with 1.5% digitonin will be present with *Mycoplasma* and *Ureaplasma*, but only a small or no zone is observed with *Acholeplasma*. Commonly used biochemical tests to further characterize isolates include detection of phosphatase activity, fermentation of glucose, and hydrolysis of arginine or urea.

While some antigens are shared among the mollicutes, antigenic differences are usually sufficiently specific to allow for species identification. A number of identification methods have been employed based on either the ability of specific antisera to inhibit growth or metabolism or the demonstration of reactivity with specific antisera using either a fluorescence or chromogen-based detection system. Growth inhibition tests employ antisera-impregnated disks or antisera placed in wells in media and demonstrating a zone of inhibition. Metabolic inhibition tests use growth inhibition in liquid media and a color change based on pH as an indicator system. Other test procedures that have been used to demonstrate specific reactivity are direct or indirect immunofluorescence on colony impressions, colony epifluorescence, and immunoperoxidase staining of colonies on agar plates.

A number of immunodiagnostic tests have been developed for many of the important *Mycoplasma* diseases, although problems with sensitivity, especially related to asymptomatic carriers, are common and can complicate interpretation of results. Lack of specificity as a result of cross-reacting antibodies is also a problem.

Enzyme-linked immunosorbent assays, plate agglutination, and hemagglutination inhibition tests are routinely used to detect flock infections with *M. gallisepticum*, *M. meleagridis*, and *M. synoviae* in poultry and are an important part of overall eradication programs used by commercial poultry operations.

Fast replacing the traditional assays described earlier are molecular assays, primarily based on the polymerase chain reaction (PCR). Amplification of specific DNA sequences by PCR, or less frequently restriction endonuclease analysis of PCR products, has been used for identification and characterization of isolates. A number of PCR methods have been described for identification of pathogenic species directly from clinical material that bypasses the need for culture.

Treatment, Control, and Prevention

Current understanding of the immunology related to *Mycoplasma* and *Ureaplasma* infection(s) is very incomplete, and the necessary components of a protective immune response to these organisms are not well-defined. Both killed and attenuated vaccines have been shown to be at least partially protective against *Mycoplasma*-induced disease, but do not provide complete immunity. Vaccinated animals demonstrate fewer lesions and have a reduced number of organisms present relative to nonvaccinated animals, but disease is still observed in both groups. Some vaccine preparations have actually resulted in increased disease after subsequent infection. The mechanism by which this occurs is not known.

An attenuated vaccine is used to protect cattle in areas where CBPP is enzootic. Protection lasts for approximately 18 months. Attenuated and killed, adjuvanted vaccines have been used with variable success to control some caprine infections, specifically those caused by *M. agalactiae*, *M. mycoides* ssp. *capri*, and *M. capricolum* ssp.

capripneumoniae. Killed vaccines for *M. hyopneumoniae* in swine reduce the severity of mycoplasmal pneumonia, but do not prevent disease or colonization. In poultry, live (attenuated strain) and inactivated vaccines are employed to control egg production losses and respiratory disease associated with *M. gallisepticum* infections. No vaccines for ureaplasmas or hemoplasmas are currently available.

Antibiotics are used to treat *Mycoplasma* and *Ureaplasma* infections. The lack of a cell wall renders mollicutes resistant to the action of antimicrobial agents that target the cell wall or its synthesis, such as the glycopeptides and β-lactams, but are sensitive to compounds that interfere with protein and nucleic acid synthesis. Mycoplasmas show sensitivity to the following antibiotics: tetracyclines, macrolides, lincosamides, ketolides, aminoglycosides, cephalosporins, pleuromutilins, and fluoroquinolones. Treatment success varies depending on the species involved, the affected site, and the time course of the disease. Isolates of mycoplasmas and ureaplasmas have been identified with resistance to many of these antibiotics, which is mediated through a variety of mechanisms. The incidence of antibiotic resistance is not well-documented because of the difficulties in culturing these organisms that is necessary for most antibiotic susceptibility assays, and this testing is only performed by specialized laboratories.

Control measures depend on the disease status of the country, specific disease, and animal species infected. Diseases such as CBPP and CCPP, which affect large populations of animals, are controlled by test and slaughter of affected herds in countries attempting to maintain a disease-free status. Vaccination, culling of infected animals, and management changes to prevent dissemination are employed in countries where the disease is enzootic. In general, because of the poor success in treating infected animals, culling of clinically ill animals is often employed as a control measure in infected populations where test and slaughter are not feasible. Routine culturing of bulk tanks is used to monitor for *Mycoplasma*-induced mastitis in cow and goat herds. Animals identified as shedding organisms in the milk are usually culled. Industry-driven efforts, particularly for poultry, have outlined measures to eliminate or prevent infection. Attempts to eradicate infections, particularly in breeding flocks, include serologic testing and elimination of positive flocks and antibiotic treatment of hatching eggs to produce *Mycoplasma*-free chicks. Treatment of eggs involves immersing warmed eggs in a chilled antibiotic solution, which promotes antibiotic penetration into the egg.

Preventing infection should be based on following strict biosecurity practices to preclude introduction of infected animals into a *Mycoplasma*-free herd. New animals should be quarantined and tested before being mixed with the herd, but subclinically infected animals can be difficult to identify. Taking animals to shows and fairs and returning them to the herd may also serve as a source for introducing infection. Good hygiene and management practices are important in preventing spread among animals where infections are enzootic. Because milk can be a source of infection, especially in goats and cattle, it should be pasteurized to prevent infecting young animals in the herd.

Table 39.2. Hemotrophic Mycoplasma Species and Their Primary Host

Animal Species	Agent	Common Clinical Manifestations
Cat	*M. haemofelis*	Anemia (feline infectious anemia)
Cattle	*M. wenyonii*	Anemia
Dog	*M. haemocanis*	Anemia
Mice	*M. coccoides*	Anemia
	M. haemomuris	Anemia
Sheep	*M. ovis*	Anemia
Swine	*M. suis*	Anemia

Hemotrophic Mollicutes

The hemotrophic mollicutes include microorganisms previously included in the genera *Haemobartonella* and *Eperythrozoon* (Table 39.2). All are parasites of red blood cells (Figure 39.8), and produce hemolytic anemia, which can be observed in animals of any age, but is often observed in immunocompromised or otherwise stressed individuals. Subclinically infected animals are the source for hemoplasmas, and they are spread by blood-to-blood contact. Several members of this group are transmitted by ectoparasites. Unlike the nonhemotrophic mollicutes, they have not been cultivated on axenic media.

Infections with the hemoplasmas may cause icterus, splenomegaly, and/or bone marrow hyperplasia. Diagnosis is based upon clinical signs, demonstration of the agent in stained (e.g., Wright's, Giemsa, or acridine orange) smears of peripheral blood, or detection by PCR. Treatment includes correction of the hemolytic anemia and antibiotic treatment, usually with tetracyclines.

FIGURE 39.8. Mycoplasma haemofelis *on feline erythrocytes (modified Wright's stain, 1000×). (Courtesy Dr S. Hostetter.)*

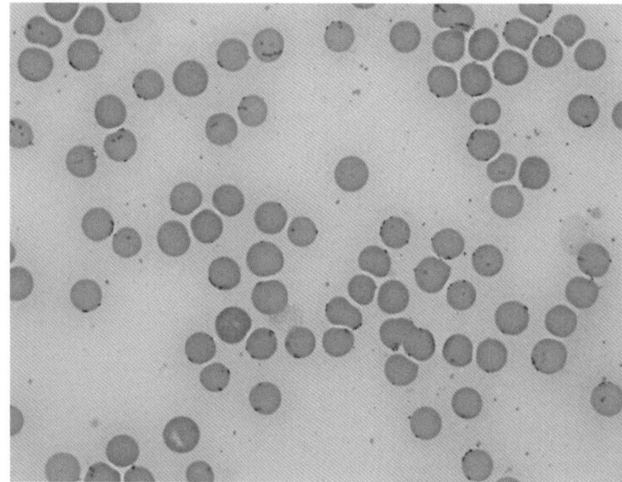

Further Reading

Dybvig K and Voelker LL (1996) Molecular biology of mycoplasmas. *Ann Rev Microbiol*, **50**, 25–57.

Herrmann R and Razin S (eds) (2002) *Molecular Biology and Pathogenicity of Mycoplasmas*, Springer, New York, NY.

Krieg NR, Staley JT, Brown DR *et al.* (eds) (2010) Division (= Phylum) III. Tenericutes, in *Bergey's Manual of Systematic Bacteriology*, Vol. **4**, 2nd edn, *The Bacteroidetes, Spirochaetes, Tenericutes (Mollicutes), Acidobacteria, Fibrobacteres, Fusobacteria, Dictyoglomi, Gemmatimonadetes, Lentisphaerae, Verrucomicrobia, Chlamydiae, and Planctomycetes*, Springer, New York, NY, pp. 567–723.

Miles R and Nicholas R (1998) *Mycoplasma Protocols, Methods in Molecular Biology*, Vol. **104**, Humana Press, New York, NY.

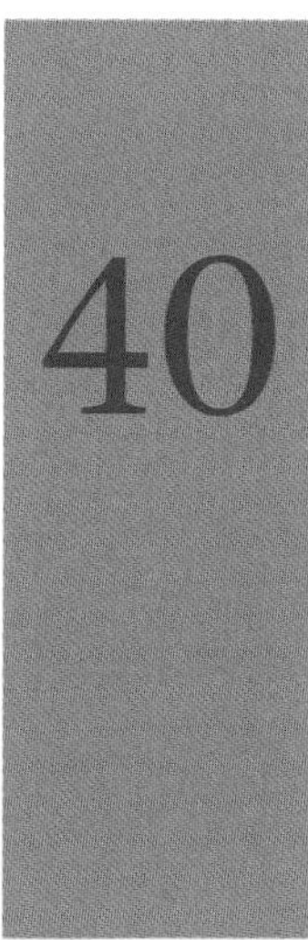

Rickettsiaceae and Coxiellaceae: *Rickettsia* and *Coxiella*

Roman R. Ganta

Descriptive Features

The order Rickettsiales includes small obligate intracellular gram-negative bacteria. Two families within this order are Anaplasmataceae and Rickettsiaceae, both of which include several important pathogens causing diseases in various vertebrate animals and people. The family Anaplasmataceae of the class Alphaproteobacteria includes intraphagosomal pathogens of the genera *Anaplasma, Erlichia*, and *Neorickettsia*. These organisms look very similar under the microscope, as they reside within a phagosome of an infected host cell. The cell tropism is a major distinguishable feature for identifying the organisms in a vertebrate host. The family Rickettsiaceae includes pathogens of the genus *Rickettsia* that invade vascular endothelium. The family Coxiellaceae of the class Gammaproteobacteria includes one pathogen, *Coxiella burnetii* which infects macrophages.

The Rickettsiales are like viruses in that they multiply only inside a host cell (intracellular). Most of the Rickettsiales, except *Ehrlichia* and *Anaplasma* species, have a cell wall like most other gram-negative organisms, respond to antibiotics (such as tetracycline derivatives and chloramphenicol), and possess ribosomes, DNA, and RNA. They are small coccid to short rod shaped bacteria. The size of the organisms ranges from 0.2 to 0.5 μm in diameter and 0.8 to 2 μm in length. Giemsa or other polychromatic stains stain the organisms the best. These aerobic pathogenic bacteria are responsible for many fatal and chronic infections in animals and people. They do not grow in standard bacteriological media. *In vitro* growth requires the close association with eukaryotic cells such as yolk sacs of chicken embryos, macrophages, or epithelial cells of vertebrate or arthropod vectors. The pathogens replicate by binary fission inside a phagosome or in the cytoplasm. They heavily depend on their host for energy (ATP) and other nutrients. Some pathogens (e.g., *Rickettsia* species) have an ATP/ADP translocase with which they obtain ATP molecules from the host in exchange for ADPs.

Pathogenicity of Rickettsiales is not well defined and may be complex because they represent organisms belonging to multiple genera having widely different host specificities and host cell associations. Virulence may be due to release of endotoxins (lipopolysaccharides), production of immune complexes, and hypersensitivity reactions. The pathogens mostly damage vascular endothelium or hematopoietic cells and severely weaken the host defense mechanisms. Rickettsiales are highly pathogenic and are responsible for high mortality rates in humans and animals. Typical diagnosis is based on the clinical presentation, detection of organisms in specific host cell types and cell organelles, serology, and molecular techniques. Culture isolation methods are available for some bacteria, but are time-consuming and are not practical for routine diagnosis. However, *in vitro* culture methods serve as excellent research tools for studies on these pathogens. Vertebrate hosts produce antibodies and several species share extensive antigen similarity. Antibodies cross-react between species; thus, it is difficult to use antibody tests as specific diagnostic tools. Inactivated or live attenuated vaccines are available for some pathogens, but appear to lose effectiveness rapidly, probably due to continuous changes in their outer membrane expressed proteins. Control may be best achieved by controlling vector burden for some of the pathogen infections.

The pathogens of veterinary importance of the family Rickettsiaceae are discussed in this Chapter. Anaplasmataceae family pathogens are discussed in Chapters 41 and 42. Two major pathogens of the genus *Rickettsia* are *R. rickettsii* (the disease causing agent of Rocky Mountain spotted fever in dogs and people) and *R. prowazekii* (epidemic typhus disease agent in people). The parasitic bacteria of the genus *Rickettsia* infect vascular endothelium. Transmission from arthropod vectors to vertebrate hosts is achieved when arthropods take a blood meal. The capillary endothelium is damaged, thus producing hemorrhagic skin rashes. Hallmark symptoms of acute disease are fever, petechial rashes, and intractable headache. The organisms escape

Veterinary Microbiology, Third Edition. Edited by D. Scott McVey, Melissa Kennedy and M.M. Chengappa.

FIGURE 40.1. *(A)* R. rickettsii *showing long actin tails that are frequently comprised multiple, twisting, distinct F-actin bundles. (B) High magnification of an* R. rickettsii *actin tail in panel A comprised of two F-actin bundles. (Reproduced with permission from the American Society for Microbiology; Van Kirk* et al. *2000.)*

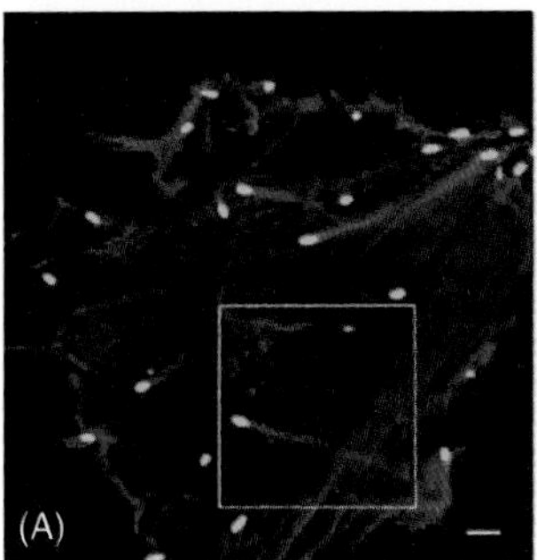

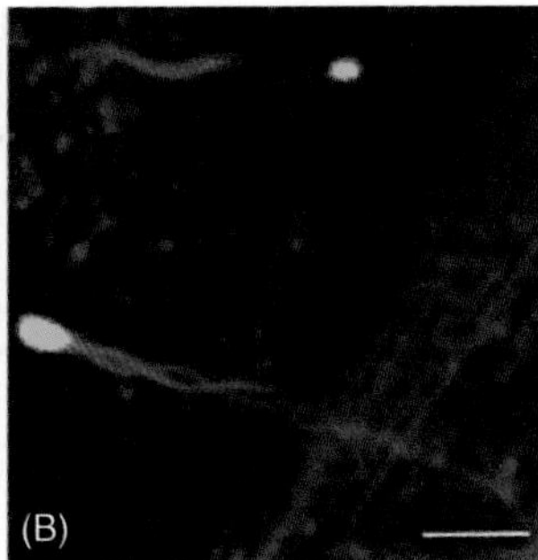

the phagosome and multiply freely in the cytoplasm or nucleus. The genus *Coxiella* includes one major pathogen, *C. burnetii*. This organism is transmitted from one host to another, primarily by means of aerosol transmission and does not require an invertebrate host for completing its lifecycle. This organism differs from *Rickettsia* species by its way of growth in a host cell cytoplasm. It replicates within the cytoplasmic phagocytic vacuoles of under acidic conditions.

Rickettsia rickettsii

Ecology

R. rickettsii is responsible for the century old disease, Rocky Mountain spotted fever (RMSF), in dogs and people. RMSF is common in both North and South America but has a worldwide occurrence. *R. rickettsii* is transmitted by *Dermacentor andersoni* and *D. variabilis* ticks. Cell-to-cell migration of *R. rickettsii* from within the cytoplasm of infected cells occurs as a result of polymerization of host cell actin induced by the pathogen (Figure 40.1). Infection may result in a spectrum of diseases ranging from subclinical to severe or fatal multiorgan collapse. The disease agent is maintained in nature in small mammals and ticks. Canines and humans are infected following bites from infected ticks.

Pathogenesis

Early clinical signs in dogs are often nonspecific. Laboratory testing generally indicates thrombocytopenia, but serologic testing is necessary to confirm infection. Differentiation of RMSF cases by clinical signs from canine ehrlichiosis (described in Chapter 41) is often difficult. Both diseases resulting from tick-borne rickettsial agents are characterized by fever, depression, lymphadenopathy, and signs of neurologic dysfunction. Distinctive red rashes, particularly in people, are one of the important symptoms of the RMSF. RMSF and most other tick-borne illnesses tend to be seasonal as they result from tick bites. Younger dogs and children develop more rapid and severe clinical disease with RMSF.

R. rickettsii replicates in the epithelium of an infected tick, and is transferred to salivary glands and ovarian tissue. After an infected tick bites a suitable host, the pathogen enters into the blood stream of that animal and infects vascular endothelium cells by endocytosis and subsequently escapes from the phagosome and multiplies within cell cytoplasm and nucleus. Rickettsial phospholipase and proteases damage endothelial cell membranes, leading to necrosis, vasculitis, hemorrhage, edema, perfusion inadequacies, thrombosis, and dyspnea. The infected dogs present clinical signs that include high fever (40 °C), anorexia, vomiting, diarrhea, petechiated or ecchymotic mucous membranes, and tenderness over lymph nodes, joints, and muscles. Central nervous system disturbances may also occur. In some instances, heart and kidney involvement leads to fatal outcomes. Immune complexes are suspected in the pathogenesis of late vascular manifestations of RMSF. Humoral and cell-mediated responses occur. The latter especially is significant for removal of the agents by activated macrophages. No vaccine is available for RMSF.

Laboratory Diagnosis

Indirect fluorescent antibody (IFA) and enzyme-linked immunosorbent assay (ELISA) are most commonly performed to detect antibodies specific to rickettsial antigens and the detectable antibody response may take at least two weeks following the rickettsial infection. The organisms may also be detected in the host endothelial cells by direct immunofluorescence assays. The molecular methods such as the polymerase chain reaction are available to evaluate for *R. rickettsii* DNA in ticks and dogs.

Treatment and Control

Treatment with tetracycline, doxycycline, and chloramphenicol for 14–21 days is effective against *R. rickettsii* infections. Infected dogs with clinical signs must also receive aggressive supportive therapy. Control of RMSF disease is also better achieved by reducing the tick burden and exposure.

Epidemic typhus fever

Epidemic typhus, caused by *Rickettsia prowazekii*, is a highly fatal human disease. The disease is responsible for more than 3 million deaths during the last century (considerable number of fatalities resulted during wars, such as during the World Wars I and II). This louse-borne typhus spreads rapidly in crowded areas under cold weather and unhygienic conditions. The mortality rate with this agent is very high (~30%). The organism persists in wild animals such as wild squirrels.

Coxiella burnetii

Ecology

Coxiella burnetii is distributed globally and is responsible for the zoonotic disease, Q fever, in people. This organism differs from other Rickettsiales, as it is transmitted by aerosol.

This pathogen, however, can also be hosted by vectors, such as ticks. Cattle, sheep, and goats are the primary reservoirs of *C. burnetii* infection. This pathogen does not usually cause clinical disease in these animals, although abortions in goats and sheep have been implicated to *C. burnetii* infections. The organisms in infected animals are excreted in the milk, urine, and feces. During birth, the organisms are shed in high numbers within the amniotic fluids and the placenta. *C. burnetii* is resistant to heat, drying, and to many common disinfectants, which enable it to survive for long periods in the environment. Moreover, inhalation of a single organism can cause the disease in a person.

Human infections usually occur by inhalation airborne organisms from barnyard dust contaminated by dried placental material, birth fluids, and excreta of infected herd animals. Humans, particularly those in close contact with the animals shedding the organisms, are often very susceptible to this disease, and as few as one organism is sufficient to cause infection and disease. About one-half of all people infected with *C. burnetii* show signs of clinical illness. Most acute cases of Q fever begin with the sudden onset of one or more of the following: high fevers, severe headache, general malaise, myalgia, confusion, sore throat, chills, sweats, nonproductive cough, nausea, vomiting, diarrhea, abdominal pain, and chest pain. Fever usually lasts for 1–2 weeks. Weight loss can occur and persist for some time. *C. burnetii* is a highly infectious agent that is also resistant to heat and drying. It can become airborne and inhaled by humans. Because, a single *C. burnetii* organism may cause disease in a susceptible person, it could be developed for use in biological warfare and is considered a potential bioterrorism agent. However, as the fatality rate is low, it is not a serious cause of concern.

Pathogenesis

C. burnetii is acquired through inhalation, ingestion, or arthropod bite and gains access to lung macrophages. It replicates within the phagosome of a macrophage, similar to *Ehrlichia canis, E. chaffeensis* and *Neorickettsia* species. About 50% of people acquiring the pathogen exhibit no clinical signs or show mild, self-limiting infection. Less than 10% may develop severe disease with signs including vasculitis, pneumonitis, splenomegaly, fever, and lymphocytosis. Mortality in human cases is primarily due to pneumonia, hepatic infection, or endocarditis.

Immunologic Aspects

A vaccine is available in some countries but is reported to have a poor efficacy. A whole cell killed vaccine may be protective. There is considerable interest in the development of a Q fever vaccine, as it is classified as a select agent.

Laboratory Diagnosis

C. burnetii can be isolated following injection into guinea pigs and mice, cultured in chicken eggs, or grown in cell cultures. This is not a useful diagnostic tool. Indirect immunofluorescence, complement fixation, or ELISA tests are used to detect antibodies. In cell culture, eggs, and experimental animal tissues, direct immunofluorescent staining aids in identifying the organisms. Polymerase chain reaction–based assays are also established in detecting the *Coxiella* DNA from a sample. In culture, *C. burnetii* replicates inside a phagosome. Two forms of the organism are the replicating large variants and infectious form, referred to as the small variant (Figure 40.2).

FIGURE 40.2. *Transmission electron micrograph image showing a typical vacuole in J774A.1 cells infected with* C. burnetii *(100 nm). (Reproduced with permission from the American Society for Microbiology; Howe and Mallavia 2000).*

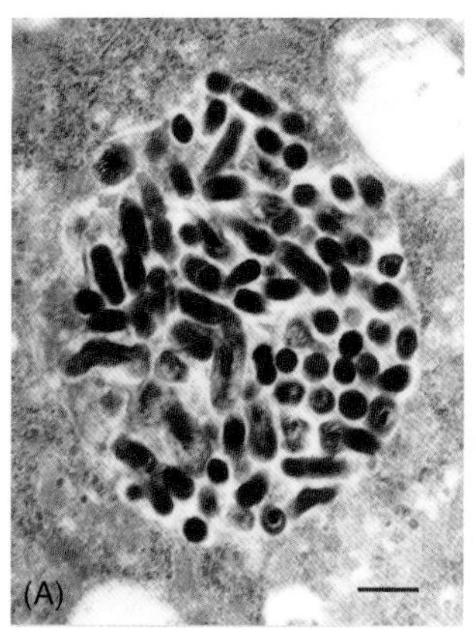

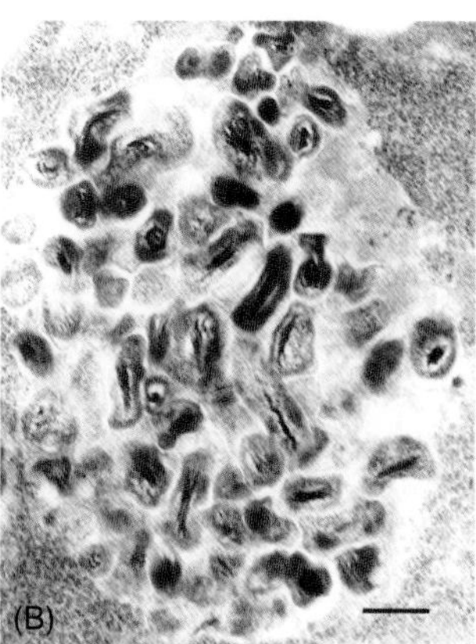

Treatment and Control

The major challenge for successful therapy is that the phagosome where *C. burnetii* persists is highly acidic, and most antimicrobial agents are not effective at low pH. Alkalinizing cells by using chloroquine has been shown to improve clinical efficacy of tetracycline. Drugs with moderate efficacy for *C. burnetii* infection include tetracycline, chloramphenicol, clarithromycin, enrofloxacin, and trimethoprim-sulfa. Long-term tetracycline feeding is considered as an attempt to control excretion of *C. burnetii* organisms from animals. Pregnant sheep and goats may be treated with tetracycline to reduce the risk of abortions.

References

Van Kirk LS, Stanley FH, and Robert AH (2000) Ultrastructure of Rickettsia rickettsii actin tails and localization of cytoskeletal proteins. *Infect Immun*, **68**, 4706–4713.

Howe D and Mallavia LP (2000) Coxiella burnetii exhibits morphological change and delays phagolysosomal fusion after internalization by J774A.1 cells. *Infect Immun*, **68**: 3815–3821.

Further Reading

Dumler JS, Barbet AF, Bekker CP *et al.* (2001) Reorganization of genera in the families Rickettsiaceae and Anaplasmataceae in the order Rickettsiales: unification of some species of Ehrlichia with Anaplasma, Cowdria with Ehrlichia and Ehrlichia with Neorickettsia, descriptions of six new species combinations and designation of Ehrlichia equi and "HGE agent" as subjective synonyms of Ehrlichia phagocytophila. *Int J Syst Evol Microbiol*, **51**(Pt 6), 2145–2165.

Harvey JW (2012) *Veterinary Hematology: A Diagnostic Guide and Color Atlas*. Elsevier Inc. ISBN: 978-1-4377-0173-9.

Raskin RE and Meyer DJ (2010) *Canine and Feline Cytology: A Color Atlas and Interpretation Guide*, Elsevier Inc. ISBN: 978-1-14160-4985-2.

Renvoisé A, Merhej V, Georgiades K, and Raoult D (2011) Intracellular Rickettsiales: Insights into manipulators of eukaryotic cells. *Trends Mol Med*, **17**(10), 573–583. Epub July 15, 2011.

Rikihisa Y (2006) New findings on members of the family Anaplasmataceae of veterinary importance. *Ann N Y Acad Sci*, **1078**, 438–445.

Stuen S and Longbottom D (2011) Treatment and control of chlamydial and rickettsial infections in sheep and goats. *Vet Clin North Am Food Anim Pract*, **27**(1), 213–233. Epub December 13, 2010.

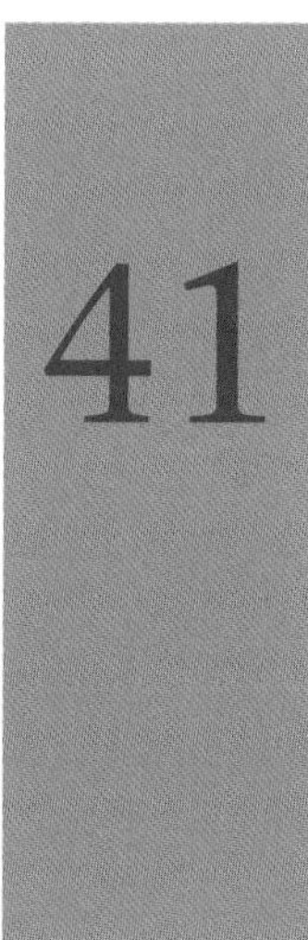

Anaplasmataceae: *Ehrlichia* and *Neorickettsia*

Roman R. Ganta

Descriptive Features

The order Rickettsiales includes small, obligate intracellular gram-negative bacteria. Two families within this order are Anaplasmataceae and Rickettsiaceae, both of which include several important pathogens causing diseases in various vertebrate animals and people. The family Anaplasmataceae of the class Alphaproteobacteria includes intraphagosomal pathogens of the genera *Anaplasma*, *Ehrlichia*, and *Neorickettsia*. These organisms look very similar under the microscope as they reside within a phagosome of an infected host cell. The cell tropism is a major distinguishable feature for identifying the organisms in a vertebrate host. The family Rickettsiaceae includes pathogens of the genus *Rickettsia* that invade vascular endothelium.

Members of the Rickettsiales are like viruses in that they multiply only inside a host cell (intracellular). Most of the Rickettsiales, except *Ehrlichia* and *Anaplasma* species, have a cell wall like most other gram-negative organisms, respond to antibiotics (such as tetracycline derivatives and chloramphenicol), and possess ribosomes, DNA, and RNA. They are small coccoid to short rod-shaped bacteria. The size of the organisms ranges from 0.2 to 0.5 μm in diameter and 0.8–2 μm in length. Giemsa or other polychromatic stains stain the organisms the best. These aerobic pathogenic bacteria are responsible for many fatal and chronic infections in animals and people. They do not grow in standard bacteriological media. *In vitro* growth requires the close association with eukaryotic cells such as yolk sacs of chicken embryos, macrophages, or epithelial cells of vertebrate or arthropod vectors. The pathogens replicate by binary fission inside a phagosome or in the cytoplasm. They heavily depend on their host for energy (ATP) and other nutrients. Some pathogens (e.g., *Rickettsia* species) have an ATP/ADP translocase with which they obtain ATP molecules from the host in exchange for ADPs.

Pathogenicity of Rickettsiales is not well defined and may be complex because they represent organisms belonging to multiple genera having widely different host specificities and host cell associations. Virulence may be due to release of endotoxins (lipopolysaccharides), production of immune complexes, and hypersensitivity reactions. The pathogens mostly damage vascular endothelium or hematopoietic cells and severely weaken the host defense mechanisms. Rickettsiales are highly pathogenic and are responsible for high mortality rates in humans and animals. Typical diagnosis is based on the clinical presentation, detection of organisms in specific host cell types and cell organelles, serology, and molecular techniques. Culture isolation methods are available for some bacteria, but are time-consuming and are not practical for routine diagnosis. However, *in vitro* culture methods serve as excellent research tools for studies on these pathogens. Vertebrate hosts produce antibodies, and several species share extensive antigen similarity. Antibodies cross-react between species; thus, it is difficult to use antibody tests as specific diagnostic tools. Inactivated or live attenuated vaccines are available for some pathogens, but appear to lose effectiveness rapidly, probably due to continuous changes in their outer membrane-expressed proteins. Protection may be best achieved by controlling vector burden for some of the pathogen infections.

The Anaplasmataceae family pathogens of the genera *Ehrlichia* and *Neorickettsia*, which are of veterinary importance, are discussed in this chapter. Pathogens of the genus *Anaplasma* are discussed in Chapter 42, and the Rickettsiaceae family pathogens are discussed in Chapter 40. *Ehrlichia* species are transmitted from infected ticks to vertebrate hosts, while *Neorickettsia* species are fluke transmitted. The major pathogens of the *Ehrlichia* genus causing diseases in animals include *Ehrlichia canis* (an important monocyte/macrophage tropic canine pathogen), *Ehrlichia ruminantium* (ruminant heartwater disease agent, which infects vascular endothelium of a wide range of domestic and wild ruminants), *Ehrlichia ewingii* (mostly a canine granulocytic pathogen), and *Ehrlichia chaffeensis* (the human monocytic

Veterinary Microbiology, Third Edition. Edited by D. Scott McVey, Melissa Kennedy and M.M. Chengappa.

ehrlichiosis agent, which also infects dogs, goats, and coyotes). Two species of the *Neorickettsia* causing diseases in animals are *Neorickettsia risticii* (Potomac horse fever agent) and *Neorickettsia helminthoeca* (canine salmon poisoning agent). Both the *Neorickettsia* species infect monocytes and macrophages.

E. canis (Figure 41.1), *E. chaffeensis* (Figures 41.2 and 41.3), *E. ewingii* (Figure 41.4), and *E. ruminantium*

Ecology

Reservoir and Transmission. *E. canis* is the major pathogen responsible for causing the disease canine monocytic ehrlichiosis. It is transmitted by *Rhipicephalus sanguineus* tick, commonly referred to as the brown dog tick. The organism causes a clinical disease within first 2 weeks following infection. The pathogen persists in recovered animals for the rest of the life with high titers of antibody response, but the organism is often undetectable in the blood. The infected and carrier status animals are also a major source of infection for ticks. Young and German shepherd breed dogs are the most severely affected and exhibit clinical signs. *E. canis* infection is prevalent in tropical and subtropical regions of the world and occurs on all continents except Australia. A few cases of human monocytic ehrlichiosis caused by *E. canis* infection are reported in Venezuela.

The vector for *E. ewingii*, the agent of canine granulocytic ehrlichiosis, is *Amblyomma americanum*, which is commonly referred to as the lone star tick *E. ewingii* infections are more common in central North America; however, as the tick is more widely distributed throughout the southeastern part of the United States, the disease occurrence is also reported from coastal areas. *E. ewingii* infections in people, also transmitted from the lone star tick, are reported from the mid-western region of the United States.

FIGURE 41.1. E. canis *cultured in canine macrophage cell line, DH82. Inclusions within the cytoplasm contain many organisms. In vitro cultures transferred to a slide and stained with polychromatic stain.*

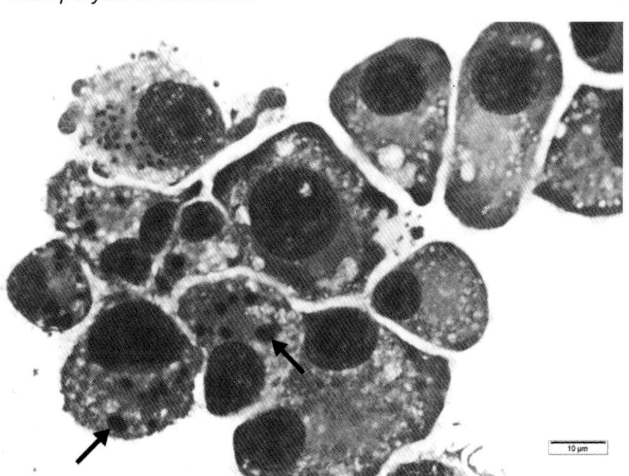

FIGURE 41.2. E. chaffeensis *cultured in canine macrophage cell line, DH82. Inclusions within the cytoplasm contain many organisms. In vitro cultures transferred to a slide and stained with polychromatic stain.*

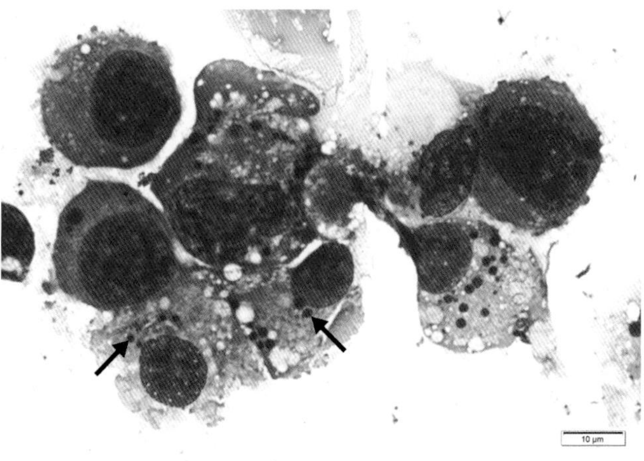

E. ruminantium (formerly *Cowdria ruminantium*) is an important tick-borne pathogen in sub-Saharan Africa, as it is responsible for causing the heartwater disease in domestic and wild ruminants. This organism infects vascular endothelium and causes a severe neurological disease in cattle, sheep, and goats. The pathogen is vectored by several exotic ticks of the genus *Amblyomma*. The importation of this pathogen together with the *Amblyomma* ticks onto the Caribbean islands resulted in a significant concern that the pathogen might be introduced onto the American mainland. In particular, if the pathogen is introduced into a nonendemic region, the mortality rates can reach up to 90% in domestic and wild ruminants.

E. chaffeensis is first identified as the pathogen causing the human monocytic ehrlichiosis. Subsequently, infections with this organism are also reported in dogs,

FIGURE 41.3. *Transmission electron micrographs (TEM) of E. chaffeensis infection (morula) in the cytoplasm of cultured canine macrophages (DH82) (A) and tick cells (B). The TEM images with morulae containing multiple Ehrlichia organisms can be seen in the figure. (Reproduced with permission from Ganta et al. 2009.)*

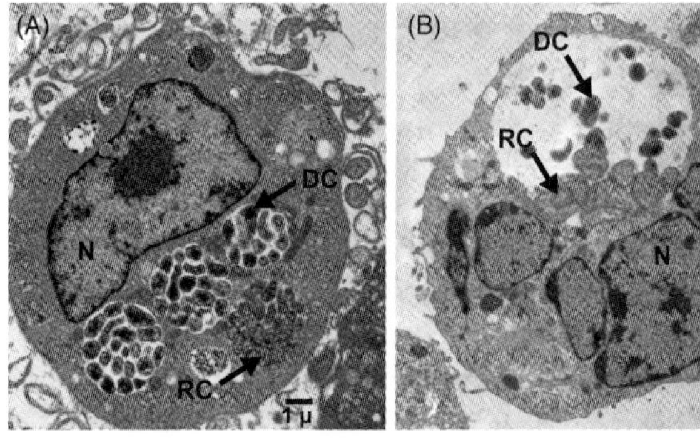

FIGURE 41.4. *E. ewingii infection (morula) in the cytoplasm of a neutrophil in blood from an infected dog (Wright–Giemsa stain). (Reproduced with permission from Harvey 2012.)*

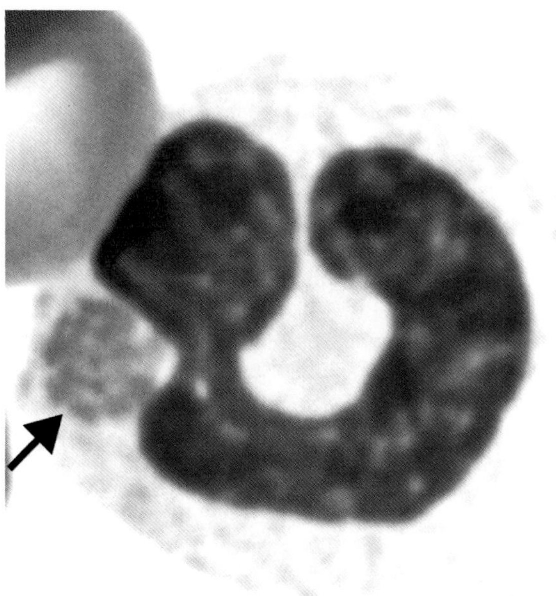

coyotes, and goats. All four *Ehrlichia* species have close genetic similarity, and thus antibodies against one pathogen have extensive cross-reactivity against other members of the *Ehrlichia*. The extensive genetic similarity, establishment of persistent infections, and serological cross-reactivity, together with the shared cell tropism for some pathogens, pose a challenge in the accurate diagnosis of clinical diseases and in initiating a treatment. The white-tailed deer and other wildlife animals play a major role in maintaining the pathogens' persistence in nature.

FIGURE 41.5. *N. helminthoeca inclusions in canine lymph node peripheral aspirate (Romanowsky; HP oil) (Reproduced with permission from Raskin and Meyer 2010.)*

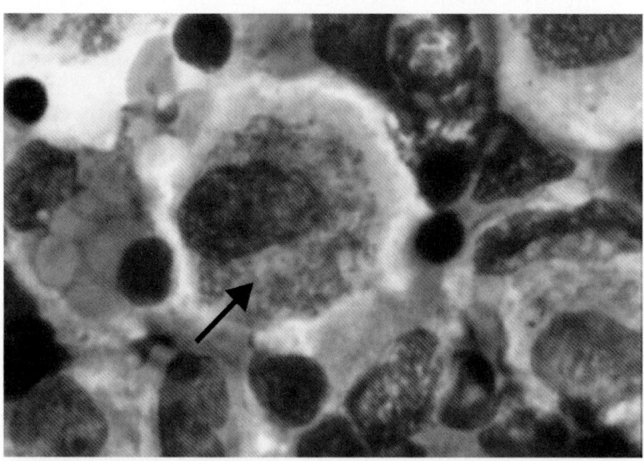

Pathogenesis. Acute onset of disease is more common within 2–3 weeks following the tick transmission of *Ehrlichia* species pathogens to an animal, during which time the organisms replicate within a phagosome of an infected host cell by binary fission. In severe acute cases where the disease may be lasting up to several weeks, there may be several clinical symptoms that may be undistinguishable for some of the pathogens. For example, clinical symptoms significantly overlap for *E. canis*, *E. chaffeensis*, and *E. ewingii*. They may include high fever, muscle aches, vomiting, anorexia, and lethargy. Leukopenia and anemia are common, as the blood cell count drops due to *Ehrlichia* species infections. Other clinical signs include malaise, depression, loss of appetite, weight loss, lymphadenopathy, and joint pains (joint pain is more common in dogs and people with *E. ewingii* infections). Canine monocytic ehrlichiosis is characterized by three stages: acute, subclinical, and chronic. Dogs with *E. canis* infection remain infected for their entire life, and the persistent presence of the pathogen occurs even after the animals treated with the antibiotic doxycycline. Chronic phase with canine ehrlichiosis persists for several months to several years, may cause reduction of all blood cell types, which may accompany hemorrhages, edema, dyspnea, interstitial pneumonia, anemia, and secondary infections, and may be coupled with enlarged spleen, liver, and lymph nodes.

Heartwater disease caused by *E. ruminantium* is an acute and fatal disease of ruminants. Goats and sheep are more susceptible than cattle. Clinical symptoms of the disease include a sudden increase of high fever, depression, and neurological signs, which may lead to mortality. Hydropericardium and hydrothorax and lung edema are commonly associated with the mortality. Animals recovered from a clinical disease, including both domestic and wild ruminants, become carriers of infection that is similar to canine ehrlichiosis.

Immunologic Aspects

Infection with *E. canis* induces strong humoral and cellular immune responses. Antibodies are raised by an infected host against several outer membrane proteins, and the antibody titers increase with time postinfection. Despite the strong humoral and cellular response, and even after treating the animals with an antibiotic, such as doxycycline, the pathogen remains in the host virtually for the life. Upon challenge with live *E. canis*, rapid anamnestic humoral responses were detected in the serum of immunized dogs, and primary antibody responses were detected in the serum from control dogs. The immune response against *E. ruminantium* is also associated with the development of high antibody titers developed against major outer membrane proteins. The response also includes strong cell-mediated response. Immune responses against *E. ewingii* and *E. chaffeensis* are also very similar to *E. canis* and *E. ruminantium*.

Laboratory Diagnosis

Giemsa-stained blood smears of buffy coat or total blood are typically evaluated for the presence of intracellular inclusions (commonly referred to as morulae). The inclusions, however, are most likely to be visible during the acute phase of infection. The morulae with all species of *Ehrlichia*, *Neorickettsia*, and *Anaplasma* are very similar in their appearance. Thus, the distinguishing features of infection with a specific pathogen may depend on the host cell tropism and vector and host associations with the pathogen. All *Ehrlichia* species, except *E. ewingii*, can be cultivated under *in vitro* conditions using a canine macrophage cell line or using tick cell cultures. Serodiagnosis by indirect immunofluorescence antibody or enzyme-linked immunosorbent assay (ELISA) to detect antibodies against outer membrane-expressed proteins is a commonly used diagnostic tool. This method, however, often results in serological cross-reactions among different *Ehrlichia* species antigens. Molecular methods such as the polymerase chain reaction assays are developed for the specific pathogen diagnosis, and this method is most useful for detecting active infection in blood during the early clinical phage of infection and prior to initiating the antibody treatment.

Treatment and Control

Tetracycline derivatives are the most effective in treating the early clinical phase of infections with *Ehrlichia* species, but less effective against clearing chronic infections. Controlling the tick burden and live infection vaccination in younger animals or infection and treatment vaccination protocol are important steps for reducing the heartwater disease caused by *E. ruminantium* in sub-Saharan African countries. Although several inactivated whole-cell or subunit vaccines are under evaluation, their value to protect against *Ehrlichia* infections remains to be established.

N. risticii

In the late 1970s, Potomac horse fever in the Potomac River Valley of Maryland is recognized as an epidemic in horses. The Anaplasmataceae pathogen, *N. risticii* (previously known as *Ehrlichia risticii*) is the agent responsible for this disease. Clinical signs with this disease in animals include depression, fever, poor appetite, and diarrhea, and are often accompanied by laminitis (founder). Diarrhea is fairly common and can vary from being profuse and watery to scant and cow-like in consistency. Death occurs in 5–30% of untreated horses and can result in toxemia, colic, or euthanasia due to severe founder.

Ecology

Reservoir, Transmission Pathogenesis. The infection was initially recognized in North America. Later it was reported also from Canada and Europe. *N. risticii* infects equine monocytes, intestinal epithelium, and colonic mast cells and is transmitted by cercaria that is released from the infected snails into the water, which are taken up by the horses when drinking the contaminated water. Clinically, Potomac Horse Fever resembles ehrlichioses with fever, listlessness, anorexia, and variable leukopenia. Diarrhea and laminitis are the symptoms associated with the disease at later stages and can lead to mortalities up to 30%.

Immunologic Aspects

Immunologic factors are not fully understood, but the infected animals induce humoral response. Recovered horses appear to be immune to disease, suggesting that the cellular immune response may be a major contributing factor.

Laboratory Diagnosis

Microbiologic diagnosis involves demonstration of the agent in monocytes in Wright-stained blood smears. Serologic diagnosis is made by an indirect fluorescent antibody test or by ELISA. Nucleic acid assays such as the polymerase chain reaction are described for the pathogen diagnosis.

Treatment and Control

Tetracycline, if given early, is considered important in reducing mortality. Supportive care is also necessary. An effective bacterin is commercially available, but appeared to be less effective against infections resulting from strain variations.

N. helminthoeca

Descriptive Features

N. helminthoeca causes salmon poisoning in dogs. This pathogen multiplies in the cytoplasm of monocytes and macrophages. This infection is very similar to *E. canis* and *E. chaffeensis* in dogs, except that the organism is not transmitted by ticks. After staining a sample with a Giemsa stain, the organism may be visible as cytoplasmic inclusions in the macrophages of a lymph node tissue or in the monocytes from a blood smear made from a clinically ill animal.

Ecology

Reservoir and Transmission. The reservoir of infection for *N. helminthoeca* is the fluke, *Nanophyetus salmincola*. The life cycle of the fluke includes passage through a fish and a snail. Dogs eating raw fish infested with a fluke containing *N. helminthoeca* are likely to acquire infection and the disease. The geographical distribution of salmon poisoning pathogens is limited by the range of the snail, intermediate hosts of the fluke. In particular, the distribution of the snail includes North American coastal regions, such as northern cost of California, Oregon, Washington, and British Columbia. Dogs are the definitive hosts of the fluke, harboring the adults in their intestine. If *N. helminthoeca* fluke gains entry into a dog as a result of eating fluke-infected fish, the pathogen infection establishes in the dog. Fluke eggs are shed in canine feces and hatch miracidia, which reach to a snail in the environment. Cercaria emerges from the fluke-infected snail and invades a fish.

Pathogenesis. Exposure to an infected raw fish in an endemic area is the primary cause for acquiring the *N. helminthoeca* infection by dogs as a result of fluke gaining entry from the fish. The fluke then matures in the dog's gastrointestinal tract where *N. helminthoeca* organisms are released, which enters into the canine bloodstream and lymph nodes. In blood, the organism infects monocytes. The replication of the organism in the dog results in the clinical signs associated with the disease. Within 1–2 weeks of exposure, dogs develop fever, anorexia, depression, weight loss, swollen lymph nodes, and often hemorrhagic enteritis. Vomiting and diarrhea are also common clinical signs. Mortality can be up to 90% in untreated animals, which can occur within 2 weeks.

Immunologic Aspects

Dogs recovered from the clinical disease appear to be protected from the disease.

Laboratory Diagnosis

The presence of organisms within the cytoplasmic vacuoles of monocytes in a stained blood smear or in lymph node aspirates is an evidence of the disease. The organisms may be cultured, but it is a time-consuming method. Molecular methods can be used to detect the rickettsial nucleic acids from a blood or lymph node sample.

Treatment and Control

Tetracycline, chloramphenicol, and sulfonamides are effective in treating *N. helminthoeca* infections. Supportive treatment is also necessary. The best preventive measure is the exclusion of infected salmon from the canine diet. Flukes and *N. helminthoeca* are killed by cooking at high temperatures or by freezing for 24 h.

References

Ganta RR, Peddireddi L, Seo GM *et al.* (2009) Molecular characterization of *Ehrlichia* interactions with tick cells and macrophages. *Front Biosci*, **14**, 3259–3273.

Harvey JW (2012) *Veterinary Hematology: A Diagnostic Guide and Color Atlas*, Elsevier Inc.

Raskin RE and Meyer DJ (2010) *Canine and Feline Cytology, A Color Atlas and Interpretation Guide*, Elsevier Inc.

Further Reading

Dumler JS, Barbet AF, Bekker CP *et al.* (2001) Reorganization of genera in the families Rickettsiaceae and Anaplasmataceae in the order Rickettsiales: unification of some species of *Ehrlichia* with *Anaplasma*, *Cowdria* with *Ehrlichia* and *Ehrlichia* with *Neorickettsia*, descriptions of six new species combinations and designation of *Ehrlichia equi* and "HGE agent" as subjective synonyms of *Ehrlichia phagocytophila*. *Int J Syst Evol Microbiol*, **51** (6), 2145–2165.

Renvoisé A, Merhej V, Georgiades K, and Raoult D (2011) Intracellular Rickettsiales: Insights into manipulators of eukaryotic cells. *Trends Mol Med*, **17** (10), 573–583. Epub July 15, 2011.

Rikihisa Y (2006) New findings on members of the family Anaplasmataceae of veterinary importance. *Ann N Y Acad Sci*, **1078**, 438–445.

Stuen S and Longbottom D (2011) Treatment and control of chlamydial and rickettsial infections in sheep and goats. *Vet Clin North Am Food Anim Pract*, **27** (1), 213–233. Epub December 13, 2010.

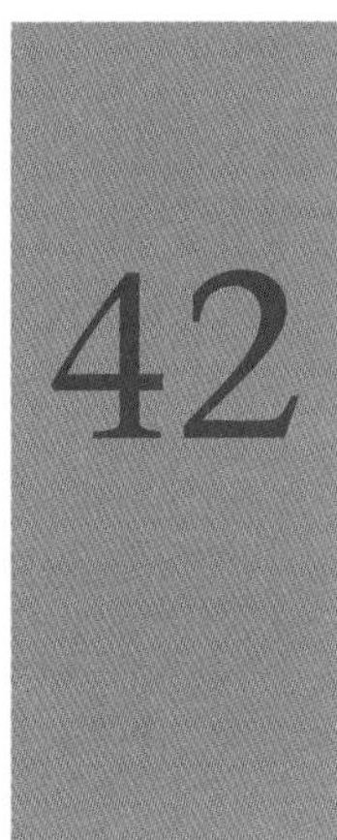

Anaplasmataceae: *Anaplasma*

Roman R. Ganta

Descriptive Features

The order Rickettsiales includes small, obligate intracellular gram-negative bacteria. Two families within this order are Anaplasmataceae and Rickettsiaceae, both of which include several important pathogens causing diseases in various vertebrate animals and people. The family Anaplasmataceae of the class Alphaproteobacteria includes intraphagosomal pathogens of the genera *Anaplasma*, *Ehrlichia*, and *Neorickettsia*. These organisms look very similar under the microscope as they reside within a phagosome of an infected host cell. The cell tropism is a major distinguishable feature for identifying the organisms in a vertebrate host. The family Rickettsiaceae includes pathogens of the genus *Rickettsia* that invade vascular endothelium.

Members of the Rickettsiales are like viruses in that they multiply only inside a host cell (intracellular). Most of the Rickettsiales, except *Ehrlichia* and *Anaplasma* species, have a cell wall like most other gram-negative organisms, respond to antibiotics (such as tetracycline derivatives and chloramphenicol), and possess ribosomes, DNA, and RNA. They are small coccoid to short rod-shaped bacteria. The size of the organisms ranges from 0.2 to 0.5 μm in diameter and 0.8–2 μm in length. Giemsa or other polychromatic stains stain the organisms the best. These aerobic pathogenic bacteria are responsible for many fatal and chronic infections in animals and people. They do not grow in standard bacteriological media. *In vitro* growth requires the close association with eukaryotic cells such as yolk sacs of chicken embryos, macrophages, or epithelial cells of vertebrate or arthropod vectors. The pathogens replicate by binary fission inside a phagosome or in the cytoplasm. They heavily depend on their host for energy (ATP) and other nutrients. Some pathogens (e.g., *Rickettsia* species) have an ATP/ADP translocase with which they obtain ATP molecules from the host in exchange for ADPs.

Pathogenicity of Rickettsiales is not well defined and may be complex because they represent organisms belonging to multiple genera having widely different host specificities and host cell associations. Virulence may be due to release of endotoxins (lipopolysaccharides), production of immune complexes, and hypersensitivity reactions. The pathogens mostly damage vascular endothelium or hematopoietic cells and severely weaken the host defense mechanisms. Rickettsiales are highly pathogenic and are responsible for high mortality rates in humans and animals. Typical diagnosis is based on the clinical presentation, detection of organisms in specific host cell types and cell organelles, serology, and molecular techniques. Culture isolation methods are available for some bacteria, but are time-consuming and are not practical for routine diagnosis. However, *in vitro* culture methods serve as excellent research tools for studies on these pathogens. Vertebrate hosts produce antibodies, and several species share extensive antigen similarity. Antibodies cross-react between species; thus, it is difficult to use antibody tests as specific diagnostic tools. Inactivated or live attenuated vaccines are available for some pathogens, but appear to lose effectiveness rapidly, probably due to continuous changes in their outer membrane-expressed proteins. Protection may be best achieved by controlling vector burden for some of the pathogen infections.

The pathogens of veterinary importance of the genus *Anaplasma* from the family Anaplasmataceae are discussed in this chapter. Pathogens of the genera *Ehrlichia* and *Neorickettsia* are discussed in the Chapter 41 and the Rickettsiaceae family pathogens are discussed in Chapter 40. The genus *Anaplasma* includes the species *Anaplasma marginale* and *Anaplasma centrale* (bovine erythrocytic pathogens), *Anaplasma ovis* (the causal agent of ovine anaplasmosis infecting erythrocytes), *Anaplasma platys* (canine cyclic thrombocytopenia agent, which infects thrombocytes), and *Anaplasma phagocytophilum* (granulocytic pathogen causing a disease in a broad range of hosts, including cattle, horses, dogs, and people).

Veterinary Microbiology, Third Edition. Edited by D. Scott McVey, Melissa Kennedy and M.M. Chengappa.

FIGURE 42.1. *A. marginale in bovine erythrocytes (Wright–Giemsa stain, 1000×).*

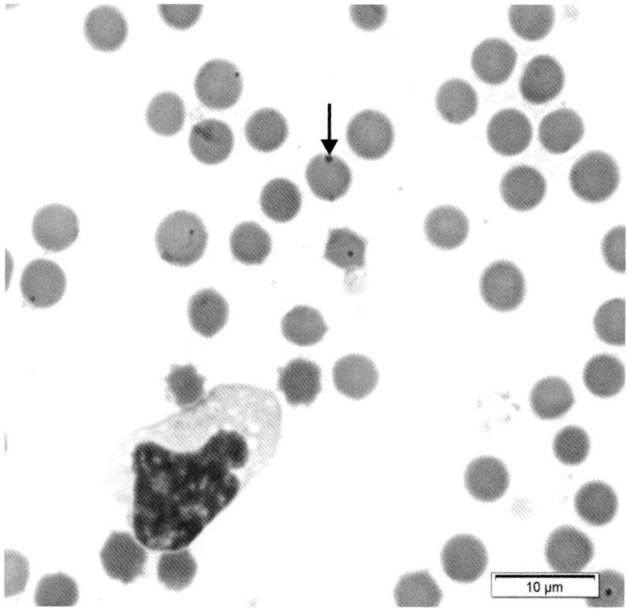

A. marginale

Descriptive Features

In Giemsa- or polychromatic-stained blood smears, *A. marginale* organisms appear as purple inclusions within the cytoplasm of bovine erythrocytes and are typically located near to the periphery of erythrocytes (Figure 42.1). These marginal (inclusion) bodies are membrane-bound phagocytic vacuoles containing up to 10 organisms. The organism can be serially propagated by needle inoculation of infected blood from one animal to the other. Recent studies also allowed the establishment of *in vitro* cultivation and serial passaging of the organism *Ixodes scapularis* in tick cell culture under aerobic conditions.

Ecology

Reservoir and Transmission. Infected ruminants are the primary reservoirs of infection with *A. marginale*. Although many vertebrate animals can be infected, the infection with this organism is the major cause of illness in cattle as a result of tick-borne and mechanical transmission. Bovine anaplasmosis is reported from all continents. Transmission through the use of contaminated needles, dehorning procedures, or from the use of other surgical instruments is a major source of the disease spread from an infected animal. In nature, most often transmission occurs from infected ticks, such as *Dermacentor variabilis*, when taking blood meals on naïve animals. Other means of transmission include the mechanical transmission by blood-sucking flying insects, such as horseflies.

Pathogenesis. Infectious organisms enter erythrocytes by endocytosis after adhering to the cell surface by way of its cell surface-expressed proteins and replicate within a phagosome by binary fission. New infectious organisms are released from the infected erythrocytes by lysing the cells. Erythrocyte destruction can also occur following an immune response against phagocytized erythrocytes, resulting in indiscriminate erythrocyte removal by the macrophage system. Clinical sings of bovine anaplasmosis vary from diarrhea, fever, anemia, increased heartbeat, anorexia, depression, constipation, abortion, muscle weakness, myocardial hypoxia, and finally to cardiac arrest.

Severity of the disease varies and depends on the age of an infected animal. Typically, infected calves of less than 6 months old exhibit no clinical signs, whereas cattle ages ranging from 6 months to 3 years may develop a serious illness. Cattle over 3 years old have a 30–50% mortality rate. However, animals that recover from the disease establish persistent, chronic infections with no apparent signs of illness. The chronically infected animals serve as the source of infection for ticks and for naive animals. In mature cattle (>3 years), mortality may reach 50%. Disease is generally seen in cattle 1 year of age or more.

Immunologic Factors. *A. marginale*-infected animals induce both humoral and cell-mediated responses. Several major surface proteins are expressed by the pathogen during its growth in erythrocytes. During the organism's persistent growth in cattle, some of its major antigenic surface proteins' expression is varied. The antigenic variation is likely to aid in the pathogen's escape from host immune clearance. Animals that recover from the early clinical stage of infection appear normal, but the infection persists with the possibility of serving as the reservoirs of infection for transmission to ticks and naïve animals. Thus, immunity developed against the clinical disease is not an indication that the pathogen is cleared.

Infection with *A. centrale* causes a mild disease. Animals infected with *A. centrale* are also protected against infection with *A. marginale*. Cattle can be protected against *A. marginale* infection with an inactivated whole-cell vaccine that produces immunity for several months. A modified live vaccine is also known to induce protective immunity for a long period of time. Infection followed by treatment with tetracyclines is also considered a good method in conferring protection against bovine anaplasmosis clinical disease, but this type of vaccine does not induce sterile immunity.

Laboratory Diagnosis

A. marginale is demonstrable in erythrocytes of a blood smear following the staining with polychromatic stain (Figure 42.1). Immunofluorescence can be performed using the polyclonal sera against the pathogen. Blood smear staining may not detect infection beyond the first few weeks following the infection. Molecular techniques such as the polymerase chain reaction, utilizing a gene-specific primer set, are most valuable for the sensitive detection of *A. marginale*.

FIGURE 42.2. *A. phagocytophilum infection (morula) in the cytoplasm of a neutrophil in blood from an infected dog (Wright–Giemsa stain). (Reproduced with permission from Harvey 2012.)*

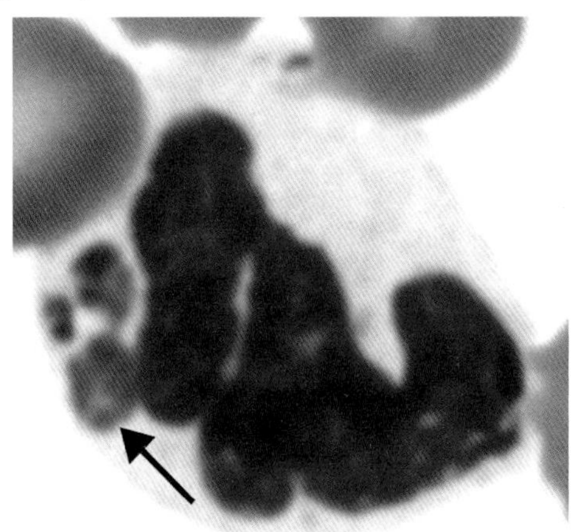

Treatment and Control

Tetracycline is the most effective antibiotic against *A. marginale* infection in cattle. Vaccination and vector control are effective in reducing the disease in animals.

A. phagocytophilum (Figure 42.2) and *A. platys* (Figures 42.3 and 42.4)

Descriptive Features

In polychromatic stained thick blood smears, *A. phagocytophilum* appears in neutrophils as membrane-bound morulae consisting of several organisms. The infection is common among ruminants, horses, dogs, and humans. *A. platys* infection occurs within the canine platelets and causes a cyclic thrombocytopenia. This organism may be visible in the think blood smear as well. Blood smear positives may be seen during the early clinical phages of infection for both of the organisms. Clinical diseases with these Rickettsiales, like most other tick-borne illnesses, are most likely reported during summer months. *A. phagocytophilum* is transmitted to vertebrate hosts as a result of *Ixodes* species ticks, whereas the tick association for *A. platys* remains to be established. Much can be understood about the disease from clinical picture and the patient history in predicting that the animals are likely suffering with *A. phagocytophilum* and *A. platys* infection.

FIGURE 42.3. *A. platys infection (morula) in the cytoplasm of platelets in blood from an infected dog (Wright–Giemsa stain). (Reproduced with permission from Harvey 2012.)*

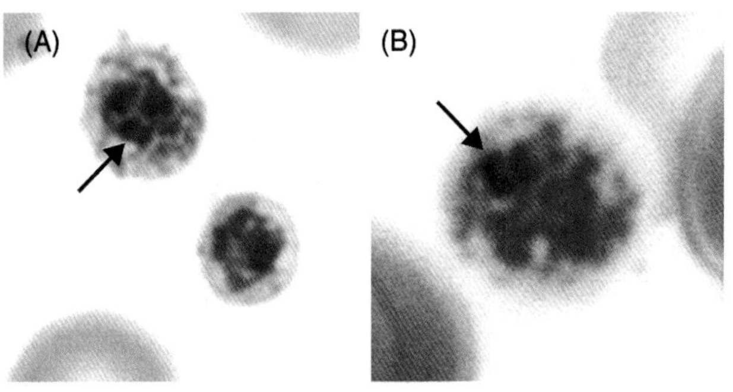

Ecology, Reservoir, and Transmission

Rodents are considered the primary reservoirs of *A. phagocytophilum* infection. The reservoirs of infection may also be significantly different in different geographical regions. In eastern region of the North America, the white-footed mouse (*Peromyscus leukopus*) and the *I. scapularis* tick are the primary reservoir host and vector, respectively. In the US West Coast, the *Ixodes pacificus* may be the important vector. In Europe, the primary transmitting vector is *Ixodes ricinus* tick, and various rodent species are implicated as the reservoirs of infection. The reservoir host(s) and vector(s) for *A. platys* remain to be determined, although the pathogen transmission to dogs is suspected to be via tick bites.

Pathogenesis. The primarily granulocytic infection with *A. phagocytophilum* was originally documented in ruminants in Europe where it was commonly referred to as the tick-borne fever. Later, the pathogen infections were reported in North American horses (earlier, it was called the equine ehrlichiosis agent, *Ehrlichia equi*). The pathogen also infects humans and dogs in North America. All hosts develop vasculitis associated with thromboses, thrombocytopenia, edema, and hemorrhage. Vascular changes are more noticeable in testes and ovaries of ruminants. Lesions as a result of the *A. phagocytophilum* infection may include splenomegaly and hemorrhages. Clinical symptoms may include fever, depression, accelerated breathing, lack of apatite, edema, anemia, icterus, and ataxia. Ataxia appears to be more common in horses. The infection in cows may also result in the drop in milk yield. The disease is milder in young animals. As a result of depressed neutrophil count, the infected animals are also more susceptible to a secondary infection. More serious complication of the disease can occur in some animals, which may include respiratory infections and/or laminitis. Canine *A. platys* infection results in developing cyclic thrombocytopenia.

Immunologic Aspects

Host immune response against the pathogens includes cellular and humoral responses. Antigenic variation in both *A. phagocytophilum* and *A. platys* may contribute to the pathogens' persistence and immune evasion. Although considerable research has been carried out in support of understanding of the variation in some of the outer surface-expressed antigens of *A. marginale* and *A. phagocytophilum*, little is known about the mechanism of antigenic

FIGURE 42.4. *Transmission electron micrograph of* A. platys *infection (morula) in the cytoplasm of platelets in blood from an infected dog, with morulae containing multiple (A) and four visible organisms (B). (Reproduced with permission from*Harvey et al. *1978.)*

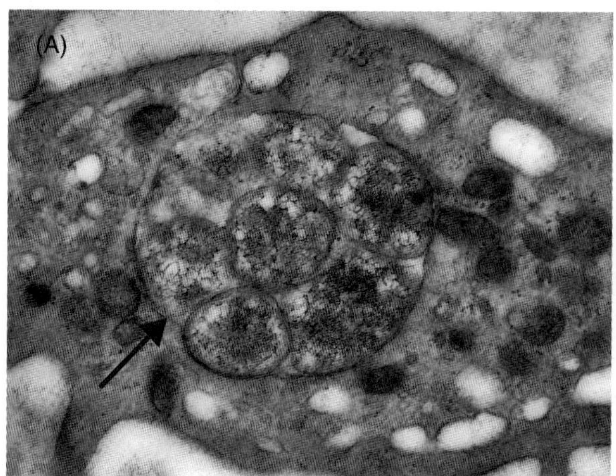

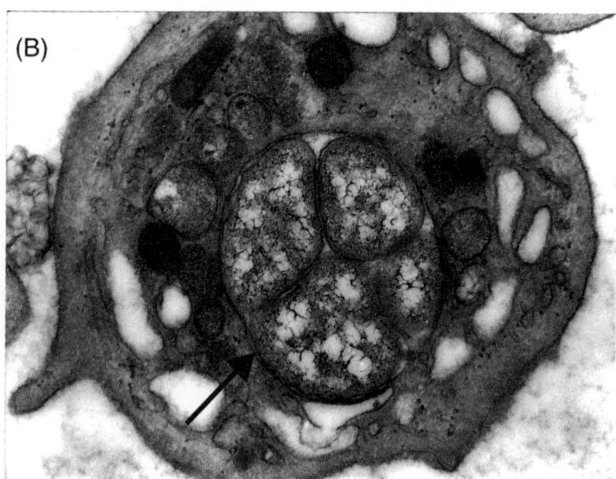

variation for *A. platys*. However, cyclic thrombocytopenia in *A. platys* may be caused as a result of cyclical changes in the bacteremia levels, leading to cyclical changes in platelet counts. Significant diversity in the expressed major surface proteins is also reported for *A. phagocytophilum* and *A. marginale* strains.

Laboratory Diagnosis

Inclusions in the cytoplasm (replicating organisms in phagosomes) of granulocytes may be detected during the early clinical phage of infection following the polychromatic (such as the Giemsa stain) stained thick smear of a blood or buffy coat sample (Figure 42.2 and 42.3). Indirect immunofluorescent antibody and enzyme-linked immunosorbent assay (ELISA) tests have been developed using infected neutrophils of a host. Recombinant antigens are typically used for an ELISA. Molecular methods such as the polymerase chain reaction are used to detect the pathogens during the clinical phase of the disease. Similarly, *A. platys* organisms may be detected in the polychromatic stained platelets of infected dogs.

Treatment and Control

As with other Rickettsiales, tetracycline is the most effective antibiotic against *A. phagocytophilum* and *A. platys*. Vector control may be effective in reducing the disease in animals. Currently, there are no vaccines available for use in controlling *A. phagocytophilum* or *A. platys* infections in animals.

References

Harvey J (2012) *Veterinary Hematology: A Diagnostic Guide and Color Atlas*, Elsevier Inc.

Harvey JW, Simpson CF, and Gaskin JM (1978). Cyclic thrombocytopenia induced by a rickettsia-like agent in dogs. *J Infect Dis*, **137**, 182–188.

Further Reading

Dumler JS, Barbet AF, Bekker CP *et al.* (2001) Reorganization of genera in the families Rickettsiaceae and Anaplasmataceae in the order Rickettsiales: unification of some species of *Ehrlichia* with *Anaplasma*, *Cowdria* with *Ehrlichia* and *Ehrlichia* with *Neorickettsia*, descriptions of six new species combinations and designation of *Ehrlichia equi* and "HGE agent" as subjective synonyms of *Ehrlichia phagocytophila*. *Int J Syst Evol Microbiol*, **51** (6), 2145–2165.

Raskin RE and Meyer DJ (2010) *Canine and Feline Cytology, A Color Atlas and Interpretation Guide*, Elsevier Inc.

Renvoisé A, Merhej V, Georgiades K, and Raoult D (2011) Intracellular Rickettsiales: Insights into manipulators of eukaryotic cells. *Trends Mol Med*, **17** (10), 573–583. Epub July 15, 2011.

Rikihisa Y (2006) New findings on members of the family Anaplasmataceae of veterinary importance. *Ann N Y Acad Sci*, **1078**, 438–445.

Stuen S and Longbottom D (2011) Treatment and control of chlamydial and rickettsial infections in sheep and goats. *Vet Clin North Am Food Anim Pract*, **27** (1), 213–233. Epub 2010 December 13, 2010.

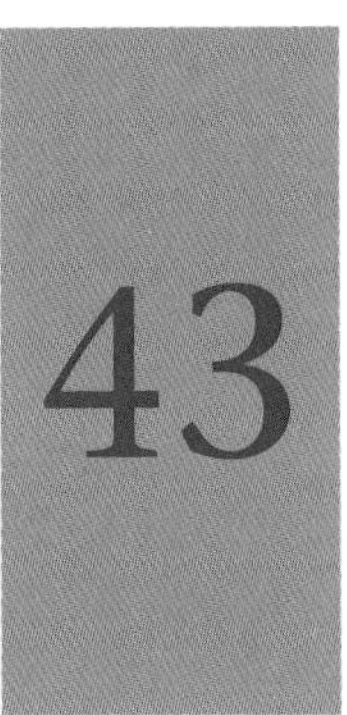

43 Bartonellaceae

Bruno B. Chomel and Rickie W. Kasten

Members of the Family Bartonellaceae are small gram-negative rods. Until the early 1990s, the genus *Bartonella* consisted of only one species, *Bartonella bacilliformis*. The genus now contains all the species that were once included in the genera *Bartonella*, *Rochalimaea*, and *Grahamella*. The genus *Bartonella* has been placed into the family Bartonellaceae (which has also been removed from the order Rickettsiales). Members of the genus *Bartonella* belong to the α-2 subgroup of the α-proteobacteria. Most of these bacteria are erythrocyte-adherent bacilli.

The present family consists of more than 20 species or subspecies and many *Candidatus* species, of which 14 species, subspecies, or *Candidatus* species are human pathogens:

1. *Associated with disease in human patients*: *B. bacilliformis* is the etiologic agent of Oroya fever, an acute bacteremic infection characterized by sepsis and hemolysis, and of verruga peruana, mainly a cutaneous nodular vascular eruption representing chronic infection.

   Bartonella quintana, the agent of trench fever, has also been found to be one of the agents of bacillary angiomatosis (BA), a vascular proliferative lesion observed in immunocompromised individuals, mainly with acquired immunodeficiency syndrome (AIDS). BA caused by *B. quintana* usually occurs in homeless people infested with body lice. BA can also be caused by *Bartonella henselae*.

   B. henselae causes mainly cat scratch disease (CSD) in immunocompetent individuals.

   Bartonella elizabethae, *B. koehlerae*, *B. alsatica*, and *Candidatus* B. mayotimonensis have been associated with endocarditis in immunocompetent patients.

   Bartonella vinsonii ssp. *berkhoffii* and *B. washoensis* are associated with endocarditis or myocarditis.

   Bartonella grahamii has been associated with neuroretinitis.

   B. vinsonii ssp. *arupensis* was isolated from the blood of a rancher with fever and mild neurological symptoms and detected in a patient with endocarditis.

   B. melophagi has been associated with pericarditis and fatigue.

   Bartonella tamiae has been isolated from febrile people in Thailand.

   Bartonella clarridgeiae is suspected to also be a minor agent of CSD.
2. *Associated with animal patients*: Some of the Bartonella species that are pathogenic to humans (*B. vinsonii* ssp. *berkhoffii*, *B. clarridgeiae*, *B. henselae*, *B. elizabethae*, *B. quintana*, *B. washoensis*, *B. elizabethae*, *B. grahamii*, *B. taylorii* and new BK1, KK1, and KK2) have recently been associated with various clinical entities, including endocarditis, in domestic dogs. Several other species have been diagnosed in dogs without report of specific clinical entity, such as *B. vinsonii* ssp. *arupensis*, *B. volans*-like, *B. bovis* or strain HMD (proposed *Candidatus* B. merieuxii). Cases of endocarditis have been described also in cats caused by *B. henselae* and in cattle caused by *B. bovis*.

   Several other *Bartonella* species, such as *B. vinsonii* ssp. *vinsonii*, *B. doshiae*, *B. taylorii*, *B. peromysci*, *B. birtlesii*, *B. tribocorum*, *B. talpae*, *B. bovis*, *B. schoenbuchensis*, and *B. capreoli*, have only been isolated from the blood of various animal species, including various wild rodents, squirrels, rabbits, felids, canids, bovids, and cervids. At present, these species are not known to induce any specific disease in the infected animal.

Descriptive Features

Morphology and Staining

Bartonellaceae are fastidious, aerobic, short, pleomorphic gram-negative coccobacillary or bacillary rods (0.6 μm by 1.0 μm) that take from 5 to 15 days and up to 45 days on primary culture to form visible colonies on enriched blood-containing media, as they are highly hemin dependent (Figure 43.1). In infected tissues, Warthin–Starry silver impregnation stain reveals small bacilli, which tend to appear as clumps of tightly compacted organisms. Similarly, small organisms can be identified in red blood cells by May-Grünwald Giemsa coloration. Bartonellae have a close evolutionary resemblance with members of the genera *Brucella*, *Agro bacterium*, and *Rhizobium*.

Veterinary Microbiology, Third Edition. Edited by D. Scott McVey, Melissa Kennedy and M.M. Chengappa.

FIGURE 43.1. *B. henselae colonies on blood culture on 5% rabbit blood agar.*

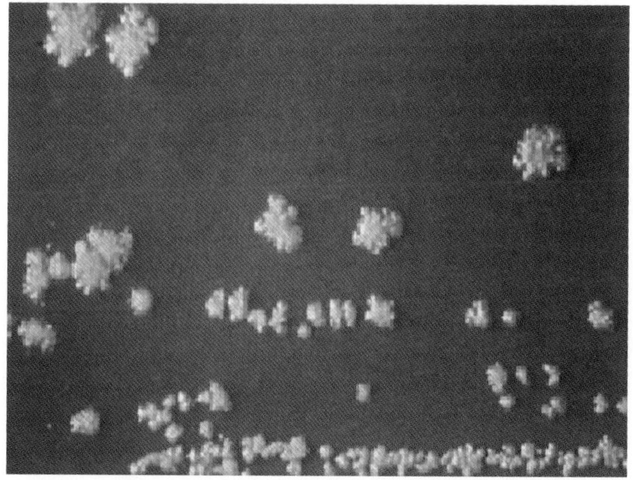

Cellular Composition

B. bacilliformis and *B. clarridgeiae* are the only members of the genus that are motile by means of unipolar flagella. *B. quintana* and *B. henselae* have a twitching motility associated with fimbriae or pili. Because of their slow growth, standard biochemical methods for identification are not as useful for identification. The bartonellae are oxidase and catalase-negative. Measurements of preformed enzymes and standard testing have revealed differences between species. Most species are biochemically inert except for the production of peptidases. The MicroScan Rapid Anaerobe Panel (Baxter Diagnostics, Deerfield, IL) has been reported to provide species identification. Whole cell fatty acid (CFA) analysis for the genus has proven useful for identification because Bartonellae have a unique and characteristic whole CFA composition. The Bartonellae have gas–liquid chromatography fatty acid profiles consisting mainly of $C_{18:09}$, $C_{18:19}$, and $C_{16:0}$. Molecular genetic methods such as restriction fragment length polymorphism (RFLP) of genes encoding citrate synthase, 16S ribosomal RNA (rRNA) or 16S-23S rRNA spacer region, and more recently analysis based on polymerase chain reaction (PCR) of random, repetitive extragenic palindromic sequences have been used to distinguish strains and species of *Bartonella*. RFLP or sequence analysis of DNA encoding 16S rRNA, citrate synthase genes after PCR amplification both directly from specimens or pure cultures have been largely used for detecting and characterizing *Bartonella*. Identification is mainly performed with the amplification of the DNA encoding the 16S-23S rRNA intergenic spacer region (ITS) or protein-encoding genes. The genes most widely used are those encoding the citrate synthase (gltA), the heat shock protein (groEL), the riboflavine (ribC), a cell division protein (ftsZ), and a 17-kDa antigen.

Growth Characteristics

Traditionally, members of the genus *Bartonella* are cultivated in semisolid nutrient agar containing fresh rabbit blood (or sheep or horse blood) at 35 °C (except for *B. bacilliformis*, which grows best at 28 °C) in 5% CO_2. On primary isolation, some *Bartonella*, such as *B. henselae*, *B. clarridgeiae*, *B. vinsonii*, or *B. elizabethae*, have colonies with a white, rough, dry, raised appearance and pit the medium. They are hard to break up or transfer. Other bartonellae such as *B. quintana* have colonies that are usually smaller, gray, translucent, and somewhat gummy or slightly mucoid. A novel pre-enrichment liquid medium *Bartonella*/alpha-Proteobacteria growth medium (BAPGM) has been developed and used successfully to detect *Bartonella* in biological products.

Ecology

Reservoir, Transmission, and Geographic Distribution

Most members of the genus *Bartonella* species are vector-borne organisms. The reservoirs, vectors, and geographic distribution are shown in Table 43.1.

Pathogenesis

Mechanisms

B. quintana and *B. henselae* are clinically associated with proliferative neovascular lesions (Figure 43.2). The pathogenesis of BA involves injury and proliferation of the vascular endothelium both with *B. henselae* and *B. quintana*. These organisms induce endothelial cell proliferation and migration *in vitro*, and a protein fraction was identified as the angiogenic factor. *Bartonella* infection (*in vitro*) stimulated endothelial cell proliferation and induced obvious morphological changes due to modifications of the cytoskeleton. *B. henselae* has been shown to induce infected cells to produce vascular endothelial growth factor, which in turn stimulated the proliferation of endothelial cells and the growth of *B. henselae*.

B. henselae seems to share with *B. bacilliformis*, a common mechanism for mediating pathogenesis. A bacteriophage-like particle similar to the bacteriophage observed in *B. bacilliformis* has been found in culture supernatant from *B. henselae*. This particle has at least three associated proteins and contains 14 kbp linear DNA segments that are heterogeneous in sequence. It has been speculated that an ancestor of *B. henselae* and *B. bacilliformis* acquired the ability to mediate angioproliferation as a means of enhancing its dissemination or its acquisition of nutrients within the host. It is possible that a common transducting phage may be the mechanism of genetic exchange by which the two organisms acquired this pathogenic trait.

All *Bartonella* species multiply and persist in red blood cells. *B. bacilliformis* possess polar flagella that have been shown to mediate erythrocyte adhesion. For nonflagellated *Bartonella*, bundle-forming pili as well as surface proteins may play a role in erythrocyte adhesion. Until recently, mechanisms of persistence of *Bartonella* bacteremia in mammals were not well understood. Recent reports have revealed the intraerythrocytic localization of these bacteria, which is a unique strategy for bacterial persistence. Nonhemolytic intracellular colonization of erythrocytes would preserve the organisms for efficient vector

Table 43.1. *Bartonella* Species or Subspecies Presently Described, Their Main Reservoir, Confirmed or Possible Vectors

Bartonella spp.	Main Reservoir	Vectors or Potential Vectors
B. alsatica[a]	Rabbits (*Oryctolagus cuniculus*)	Fleas (*Spilopsyllus cuniculi*)
B. bacilliformis	Humans	Pheblotomines (sand flies) (*L. verrucarum*)
B. quintana[a]	Humans	Human body lice (*Pediculus humanis corporis*)
B. henselae[a]	Cats (*Felis catus*)	Fleas (*Ctenocephalides felis*) Ticks?
B. clarridgeiae	Cats (*Felis catus*)	Fleas (*Ctenocephalides felis*)
B. koehlerae[a]	Cats (*Felis catus*)	Fleas (*Ctenocephalides felis*)
B. vinsonii ssp. *vinsonii*	Meadow voles (*Microtus pennsylvanicus*)	Ear mites (*Trombicula microti*)?
B. vinsonii ssp. *arupensis*[a]	White footed mice (*Peromyscus leucopus*)	Fleas?
B. vinsonii ssp. *berkhoffii*[a]	Coyotes (*C. latrans*) Dogs (*Canis familiaris*)	Ticks? Fleas?
B. talpae	Moles (*Talpa europaea*)	Fleas?
B. peromysci	Field mice (*Peromyscus* spp.)	Fleas?
B. birtlesii	Wood Mice (*Apodemus* spp.)	Fleas?
B. grahamii[a]	Bank voles (*Clethrionomys glareolus*)	Fleas (*Ctenophthalmus nobilis*)
B. taylorii	Wood mice (*Apodemus* spp.)	Fleas (*Ctenophthalmus nobilis*)
B. doshiae	Meadow voles (*Microtus agrestis*)	Fleas?
B. elizabethae[a]	Rats (*Rattus norvegicus*)	Fleas
B. tribocorum[a]	Rats (*Rattus norvegicus*)	Fleas?
B. rochalimae[a]	Gray and red foxes, (*Urocyon cinereoargenteus, Vulpes vulpes*) Raccoons (*Procyon lotor*)	Fleas (*Pulex irritans, P. simulans*)
B. bovis (*weissii*)	Domestic cattle (*Bos taurus*)	Biting flies? Ticks?
B. chomelii	Domestic cattle (*Bos taurus*),	Biting flies? Ticks?
B. capreoli	Roe deer (*capreolus capreolus*)	Biting flies? Ticks?
B. schoenbuchensis	Roe deer (*capreolus capreolus*)	Deer keds (*Lipoptena cervi, Lipoptena mazamae*)
B. aff. *schoenbuschensis*	Rusa deer (*Cervus timorensis russa*)	Deer keds?
B. volans	Southern flying squirrel (*Glaucomys volans*)	Fleas?
B. japonica	Small Japanese field mouse (*Apodemus argenteus*)	Fleas?
B. silvatica	Large Japanese field mouse (*Apodemus speciosus*)	Fleas?
B. tamiae	Rat (*Rattus* spp.)?	chigger mites? (*Leptotrombidium, Schoengastia, Blankarrtia*), ticks?
B. rattimassiliensis	Rats (*Rattus norvegicus*)	Fleas?
B. phoceensis	Rats (*Rattus norvegicus*)	Fleas?
B. australis	eastern grey kangaroos (*Macropus giganteus*)	Fleas? Ticks
Candidatus B. melophagi[a]	Sheep (*Ovis aries*)	Sheep ked (*Melophagus ovinus*)
Candidatus B. washoensis[a]	California ground squirrel (*Spermophilus beecheyi*)	Fleas (*Oropsylla montana*)
Candidatus B. thailandensis	Rodents	Fleas?
Candidatus B. mayotimonensis[a]	Rodents? (mice)?	Fleas?
B. rattaustraliani	Australian rodents	Fleas?
B. queenslandensis	(*Melomys* sp., *Uromys caudimaculatus Rattus tunneyi, R fuscipes, R. conatus, R leucopus*)	
B. coopersplainsensis	*Rattus leucopus*	
Candidatus B. antechini	Yellow-footed Antechinus (*Antechinus flavipes*)	Fleas (*Acanthopsylla jordani*) Ticks (*Ixodes antechini*)
Candidatus B. bandicootii	Western barred Bandicoot (*Perameles bougainville*)	Flea (*Pigiopsylla tunneyi*)
Candidatus B. woyliei	Woylie (*Bettongia Penicillata*)	Flea (*Pygiopsylla hilli*) Tick (*Ixodes australiensis*)
Candidatus B. merieuxii (HMD strain)	jackal (*Canis aureus*)	Ticks, fleas?

[a] *Bartonella* species or subspecies reported to be zoonotic.
? - Indicates most likely vector species.

FIGURE 43.2. *Canine endocarditis caused by* B. clarridgeiae. *(Used with permission from Chomel* et al. *2001.)*

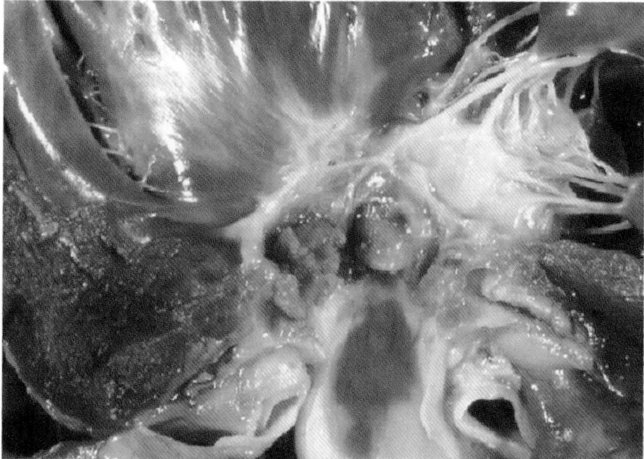

transmission, protect *Bartonella* from the host immune response and contribute to decreased antimicrobial efficacy. Persistence of infection was demonstrated in a rat model using *B. tribocorum*. After a 5-day "hidden/silent" phase following experimental infection, the organism multiplied until there were an average of eight *Bartonella* per red blood cell. Thereafter, the organisms remained within the cell for the life of the erythrocyte. Nonhemolytic intracellular colonization of erythrocytes is likely a bacterial persistence strategy that preserves the *Bartonella* species for potential transmission by arthropods, because the reservoir host would serve as a source of infection for blood-feeding arthropods, which could then subsequently infect a new host.

Bacterial type IV secretion systems, which are supramolecular transporters ancestrally related to bacterial conjugation systems, represent crucial pathogenicity factors that have contributed to a radial expansion of the *Bartonella* lineage in nature by facilitating adaptation to unique mammalian hosts. On the molecular level, the type IV secretion system VirB/VirD4 is known to translocate a cocktail of different effector proteins into host cells, which subvert multiple cellular functions to the benefit of the infecting pathogen. Furthermore, bacterial adhesins mediate a critical, early step in the pathogenesis of the bartonellae by binding to extracellular matrix components of host cells, which leads to firm bacterial adhesion to the cell surface as a prerequisite for the efficient translocation of type IV secretion effector proteins. The best-studied adhesins in bartonellae are the orthologous trimeric autotransporter adhesins, BadA in *B. henselae* and the Vomp family in *B. quintana*. Genetic diversity and strain variability also appear to enhance the ability of bartonellae to invade not only specific reservoir hosts but also accidental hosts, as shown for *B. henselae*.

Disease Patterns and Epidemiology

Human Patients

Cat Scratch Disease. CSD is caused by *B. henselae*. In CSD, 1–3 weeks elapse between the scratch or bite of a cat and the appearance of clinical signs. In 50% of the cases, a small skin lesion, often resembling an insect bite, appears at the inoculation site, usually the hand or forearm, and evolves from a papule to a vesicle and partially healed ulcers. These lesions resolve within a few days to a few weeks. Lymphadenitis develops approximately 3 weeks after exposure and is generally unilateral. It commonly appears in the epitrochlear, axillary, or cervical lymph nodes. Swelling of the lymph node is usually painful and persists for several weeks to several months. In 25% of the cases, suppuration occurs. The large majority of the cases show signs of systemic infection: fever, chills, malaise, anorexia, headaches. In general, the disease is benign and heals spontaneously without sequelae. Atypical manifestations of CSD occur in 5–10% of the cases. The most common of these is Parinaud's oculoglandular syndrome (periauricular lymphadenopathy and palpebral conjunctivitis), but also meningitis, encephalitis, osteolytic lesions, and thrombocytopenic purpura may occur. Encephalopathy is one of the most serious complications of CSD, which usually occurs 2–6 weeks after the onset of lymphadenopathy. However, it usually resolves with complete recovery and few or no sequelae.

There were an estimated 22 000 human cases of CSD in the United States in 1992, some 2000 of whom were hospitalized. The estimated annual health cost of CSD was more than $12 million. From 55% to 80% of CSD patients are under the age of 20 years. There is a seasonal pattern, with most cases seen in autumn and winter.

New clinical presentations associated with *B. henselae* infection have been reported in immunocompetent persons, including neuroretinitis or bacteremia as a cause of chronic fatigue syndrome, and cases of *B. henselae* endocarditis in a cat owner. *B. henselae* was also recently determined as a frequent cause of prolonged fever and fever of unknown origin in children. Rheumatic manifestations of *Bartonella* infection have been described in children, including a case of myositis and a case of arthritis and skin nodules. Arthritis has also been described in a very limited number of cases. Other rheumatic manifestations related to *Bartonella* infection in humans include erythema nodosum, leukocytoclastic vasculitis, fever of unknown origin with myalgia, and arthralgia. Chronic infection and bacteremia have been reported in humans, especially in the United States.

Endocarditis. Several *Bartonella* spp. have also been recognized as causative agents of blood culture-negative endocarditis or myocarditis in humans, including *B. henselae*, *B. quintana*, *B. elizabethae*, *B. vinsonii* ssp. *berkhoffii* and *B. vinsonii* ssp. *arupensis*, *B. alsatica*, and *Candidatus* B. mayotimonensis. *Bartonella* spp. account for approximately 3% of all human cases of endocarditis, a percentage similar to endocarditis cases caused by *Coxiella burnetii*, the agent of Q fever (see Chapter 40).

Bacillary Angiomatosis. For BA in immunocompromised persons, the signs and symptoms are very different from CSD. BA, also called epithelioid angiomatosis, is a vascular proliferative disease of the skin characterized by multiple, blood-filled, cystic tumors. It is usually characterized by violaceous or colorless papular and nodular skin lesions that clinically may suggest Kaposi's sarcoma, but histologically resemble epithelioid hemangiomas. When visceral parenchymal organs are involved, the condition is referred to as bacillary peliosis hepatis, splenic peliosis, or systemic BA. Fever, weight loss, malaise, and enlargement of affected organs may develop in people with disseminated BA. Endocarditis has also been reported in patients with BA.

Cats. No major clinical signs of CSD have been reported in cats under natural conditions, but infection is very common, especially in young kittens. It is estimated that about 10% of pet cats and up to 30–50% of stray cats are *Bartonella* bacteremic at a given time. In western North America (California), a 40% prevalence of bacteremic cats was found in the San Francisco–Sacramento area. Minor clinical signs, including fever, enlarged lymph nodes, uveitis, and mild neurological symptoms have been reported in experimentally infected cats. However, several cases of uveitis and a few cases of *B. henselae* endocarditis were diagnosed in pet cats. Potential association between either seropositivity or bacteremia and presence of oral lesions (gingivitis, stomatitis) has been reported, too. Additionally, reproductive disorders (lack of pregnancy or pregnancy only after repeated breedings and stillbirths) have been observed in experimentally infected queens. Bacteremia usually lasts a few weeks to a few months. The organisms have been reported to be intraerythrocytic, and pili may be a pathogenic determinant for this *Bartonella* species. Cats can yield more than 1 million colony-forming units (CFU) per milliliter of blood. Direct transmission from cat to cat, as well as vertical transmission from bacteremic female cats to kittens, was unsuccessful in various experiments. Transmission from cat to cat was successfully achieved by depositing infected fleas collected from bacteremic cats onto noninfected kittens. It was shown that flea feces are the likely infectious material that transmits infection when inoculated by a cat scratch. The role of saliva as a possible source of infection still needs to be fully demonstrated. Presence of *B. henselae* DNA was found in infected fleas. Epidemiological studies clearly demonstrate that antibody prevalence and bacteremia prevalence is the highest in stray cat populations living in warm and humid areas where flea infestation is usually higher.

Dogs. *B. vinsonii* ssp. *berkhoffii* has been identified as an important cause of canine endocarditis, especially in large breed dogs. In a 2-year prospective study of endocarditis cases, almost one-third of the 18 cases were caused by *Bartonella* species. *B. clarridgeiae, B. washoensis, B. rochalimae, B. quintana, B. koehlerae*, and *B. henselae* have been associated with dog endocarditis cases. The clinical spectrum of this infection in dogs has also been expanding, as it has been associated with cardiac arrhythmias, endocarditis and myocarditis, granulomatous lymphadenitis, and granulomatous rhinitis. In some dogs, intermittent lameness, bone pain, or fever of unknown origin can precede the diagnosis of endocarditis for several months. *B. clarridgeiae* DNA was detected in a dog with lymphocytic hepatitis. *B. henselae* DNA was initially detected in a dog with peliosis hepatis, and in a dog with hepatopathy and in three dogs with various clinical entities. These three *B. henselae*–DNA-positive dogs presented nonspecific clinical abnormalities, such as severe weight loss, protracted lethargy, and anorexia. A fourth dog was diagnosed as being infected with *B. elizabethae* by PCR amplification and sequencing, increasing the number of *Bartonella* species identified in infected dogs. Serological studies in North America and Europe indicate that *Bartonella* infection in domestic dogs is quite rare (less than 5%), whereas high seroprevalence has been reported from dogs living in tropical countries (up to 65% of dogs tested from Sudan). In North America, especially in the Southeast, high seroprevalence has been reported in dogs also seropositive for various tick-borne pathogens (mainly Erlichia, Babesia, Anaplasma). A high seroprevalence (35%) has been reported in coyotes from California, and in one specific California county, 28% of the coyotes tested were bacteremic.

Rodents. Experimental infection of pregnant laboratory mice with *B. birtlesii* showed pathogenic effects on the reproductive function of these mice. Bacteremia was significantly higher in virgin females than in males. In mice infected before pregnancy, fetal loss and resorption was higher in infected mice than controls, and the weight of viable fetuses was significantly lower for infected than for uninfected mice. Transplacental transmission was also demonstrated, since 76% of the fetal resorptions were culture-positive for *B. birtlesii*. The histopathological analysis of the placentas of infected mice showed vascular lesions in the maternal placenta, which could explain the reproductive disorders observed. The isolation and characterization of the complete virB homolog (virB2–11) and a downstream-located virD4 gene in *B. tribocorum* has been described. An essential role for this VirB/VirD4 T4SS in establishing intraerythrocytic infection was demonstrated.

Immunologic Aspects

Infection by *Bartonella* organisms stimulates both the cellular and the humoral responses. *B. henselae* and *B. quintana* induce proliferation and migration of endothelial cells. These effects are due to a trypsin-sensitive factor that appears to be associated with the bacterial cell wall or membrane or intracellular molecules. *B. henselae* infects and activates endothelial cells. *B. henselae* outer membrane proteins are sufficient to induce NFκß activation and adhesion molecule expression, followed by enhanced rolling and adhesion of leukocytes.

In infected individuals, specific antibodies can be detected a few days to a few weeks after infection. Most of the clinical cases of CSD or BA are associated with elevated titers against *B. henselae* or *B. quintana*. Immunity is usually long lasting in cases of CSD. Human cases of endocarditis are frequently associated with very high indirect fluorescent antibody (IFA) titers (>1 : 800).

In a murine model, spleen cells from infected C57BL/6 mice proliferated specifically upon stimulation with heat-killed *Bartonella* antigen and CD4 T-lymphocytes mainly mediate proliferative responses. These responses increased during the course of infection and peaked at 8 weeks postinfection. Gamma interferon, but not interleukin-4, was produced *in vitro* by spleen cells from infected animals upon stimulation with *Bartonella* antigens. As described also in humans, cats, and dogs, *Bartonella*-specific IgG antibodies were detectable in the serum of the infected mice by the second week, and the antibody concentration peaked at 12 weeks postinfection. IgG_{2b} was the prominent isotype among the *Bartonella*-specific serum IgG antibodies. Therefore, *B. henselae* induces cell-mediated immune responses with a T_{H1} phenotype in immunocompetent C57BL/6 mice.

In cats, *B. henselae* antibodies detected by IFA or enzyme-linked immunosorbent assay (ELISA) appear 2–3 weeks after experimental inoculation and usually persist for several months. Most infected cats are bacteremic for several weeks despite high antibody titers. Chronic bacteremia, despite a humoral immune response, is commonly observed among cats. There is no direct correlation between antibody titer and the magnitude of bacteremia; however, cats with IFA serologic titers of 512 or more are more likely to be bacteremic than cats with lower titers.

Dogs with endocarditis often show high antibody titers. In experimentally infected dogs, *B. vinsonii* ssp. *berkhoffii* establishes chronic infection, which may result in immune suppression, characterized by defects in monocytic phagocytosis, an impaired subset of CD8 T-lymphocytes, and impaired antigen presentation within the lymph node.

Laboratory Diagnosis

For years, the diagnosis of CSD was based on clinical criteria, history of exposure to a cat, failure to isolate other bacteria, and/or histologic examination of biopsies of lymph nodes. A skin test using antigen prepared from pasteurized exudate from lymph nodes of patients with CSD was also used in diagnosing CSD, but this test was not standardized and elicited concerns about the safety of such a product.

Serologic tests, such as IFA or ELISA, and techniques to isolate the organism from human, dog, and cat specimens have been developed since the mid-1990s. Because Bartonellae are intraerythrocytic bacteria, cell lysis using a lysis-centrifugation technique greatly facilitates bacterial isolation from the blood. However, blood isolation is seldom obtained from human cases of CSD and from domestic dogs. On the contrary, isolation is more commonly successful from human BA cases, for which serology is often negative. Isolation from the blood of natural reservoirs is also quite common with bacteremia prevalence ranging from 10% to 20% (such as for wild felids or coyotes) to up to 95% (beef cattle and deer).

For blood culture from cats, 1.5 ml of blood is drawn into lysis-centrifugation tubes (Isostat Microbial System, Wampole Laboratories) or more commonly, cat blood collection in EDTA tubes kept frozen at 270 to −70 °C for a few days or weeks has been a preferred alternative because of easier handling and lower cost. For dogs or cattle a larger volume of blood can be collected (3–5 ml). The tubes are centrifuged and the pellet spread onto infusion agar plates containing 5% fresh rabbit blood, which are maintained at 35 °C in a high humidity chamber with 5% CO_2 for 3 or 4 weeks. Colonies usually will develop in a few days from cat blood, although some strains may require a few weeks (Figure 43.1).

Bacterial isolation, ELISA or IFA detection of *Bartonella* spp. antibodies and PCR amplification of *Bartonella* spp. DNA directly from patient samples all have substantial diagnostic limitations. As antibodies to *B. vinsonii* ssp. *berkhoffii* antigens are infrequently detected (<4%) in a sick referral or healthy (<1%) dog population. Detection of *B. vinsonii* ssp. *berkhoffii* antibodies in a sick dog provides strong clinical evidence for prior exposure to and potentially active infection with this organism.

Other means of isolation of *Bartonella* have been by using Bactec blood-culture system or BacT/Alert blood-culture system. Identification of isolates as *Bartonella* can be performed by using enzyme-based identification systems, but is usually confirmed by DNA amplification using PCR-RFLP analysis. Several restriction endonucleases, such as TaqI and HhaI for citrate synthase gene, are used to digest the single product amplified by specific primers. PCR has also been used to identify *Bartonella* spp. in tissues, in absence of culture. Diagnosis of *Bartonella* endocarditis relies heavily on this method in humans and dogs in conjunction with high antibody titers.

Evidence of infection can be detected in humans or animals by detection of antibodies by IFA or ELISA. An IFA titer of at least 1 : 64 is considered positive. *B. henselae* antibodies can be detected despite concurrent bacteremia in cats and sometimes in humans.

In 2005, Maggi *et al.* described a novel, chemically modified, insect-based liquid culture medium (BAPGM) that supports the growth of at least seven *Bartonella* spp. This medium also supported co-cultures consisting of different *Bartonella* spp. Subsequently, a unique diagnostic platform that combines pre-enrichment culture utilizing BAPGM, followed by a highly sensitive PCR assay (which has a sensitivity of 0.5 bacterial genome copies per microliter of sample DNA template) targeting the 16S-23S ITS region or Pap31, a bacteriophage-associated gene was developed. This approach has allowed to characterize and quantify *Bartonella* infection in blood, CSF, aqueous, and joint fluids in addition to seroma fluids, transudates, and modified transudates from dogs with idiopathic cavitary effusions and tissue biopsy samples obtained at surgery.

Treatment

In humans, antimicrobial treatment is generally indicated for patients with BA, bacillary peliosis, or relapsing bacteremia. BA patients respond dramatically to macrolide antibiotics. Treatment with erythromycin, rifampicin, or doxycycline for at least 2–3 months in immunocompromised people is recommended, but relapses can occur. In such cases, patients should receive lifelong treatment with one of these antibiotics. For CSD, antimicrobial treatment is not generally indicated, because most typical cases do not respond to antimicrobial administration. Intravenous administration of gentamicin and doxycycline and oral administration of erythromycin have been used successfully in the treatment of disseminated CSD and therapy of patients with neuroretinitis. In cases of *Bartonella* endocarditis, patients receiving an aminoglycoside were more likely to fully recover, and those treated with aminoglycosides for at least 14 days were more likely to survive than those with shorter therapy duration.

Treatment with azithromycin is recommended for dogs with microbiologic documentation of active *Bartonella* spp. infection. A standard treatment regimen using azithromycin (5–10 mg/kg daily for 7 days followed by every other day administration for an additional 5 weeks) has proven effective for most, but not all cats and dogs. Fluoroquinolones alone, or in combination with amoxicillin, have also elicited a positive therapeutic response in dogs, which is accompanied by a progressive decrease in *B. vinsonii* antibody titers. Doxycycline may or may not be effective for treatment of *B. vinsonii* ssp. *berkhoffii*, but data from cats experimentally or naturally infected with *B. henselae* or *B. clarridgeiae* indicate that a high dose of doxycyline (10 mg/kg, q 12 h, for 4–6 weeks) may be necessary to eliminate *Bartonella* infection in cats, dogs, or other animal species.

Various antibiotics (doxycycline, erythromycin, enrofloxacin) have been shown to reduce the level of bacteremia in experimentally infected cats but do not eliminate infection, and the level of bacteremia may surpass the initial level a few weeks after the cessation of treatment.

Prevention

A large reservoir for *B. henselae* and possibly for *B. clarridgeiae* exists among the 68.9 million pet cats residing in one-third of homes in North America. Consequently, negative publicity about the perceived hazards of cat ownership is likely, especially for immunocompromised people. Seronegative cats are likely not to be bacteremic, but young kittens, especially impounded kittens and flea-infested kittens, are more likely to be bacteremic. Therefore, people who want to acquire a pet cat, especially if they are immunocompromised, should seek a cat raised in a cattery or an adult cat coming from a flea-controlled environment. Unfortunately, there is no correlation between seropositivity and bacteremia. Bacteremia can also be transient with relapses. Declawing cats has also been suggested but has a limited value, because fleas can transmit infection from cat to cat. Flea control, therefore, appears to be one of the major control measures to prevent cat infection and its spread from cat to cat. The most effective means of preventing *B. henselae* infection are common sense, hygiene, flea control, and, possibly, modification of behavior of the cat owners themselves. Wash hands after handling pets and clean any cuts, bites, or scratches promptly with soap and water.

For dog bartonellosis, where tick infestation could be a risk factor for acquiring infection, tick and flea control measures should be used during the tick and flea season. Systematic inspection of the dog for the presence of ticks after a walk in infested areas is highly recommended.

Reference

Chomel BB *et al.* (2001) Aortic valve endocarditis in a dog due to *B. clarridgeiae*. *J Clin Microbiol*, **39**(10), 3548–3554.

Further Reading

Billeter SA, Levy MG, Chomel BB, and Breitschwerdt EB (2008) Vector transmission of *Bartonella* species with emphasis on the potential for tick transmission. *Med Vet Entomol*, **22**(1), 1–15.

Breitschwerdt EB, Maggi RG, Chomel BB, and Lappin MR (2010) Bartonellosis: an emerging infectious disease of zoonotic importance to animals and human beings. *J Vet Emerg Crit Care (San Antonio)*, **20**(1), 8–30.

Chomel BB, Boulouis HJ, Breitschwerdt EB *et al.* (2009) Ecological fitness and strategies of adaptation of *Bartonella* species to their hosts and vectors. *Vet Res*, **40**(2), 29.

Chomel BB and Kasten RW (2010) Bartonellosis, an increasingly recognized zoonosis. *J Appl Microbiol*, **109**(3), 743–750.

Tsai YL, Chang CC, Chuang ST, and Chomel BB (2011) *Bartonella* species and their ectoparasites: selective host adaptation or strain selection between the vector and the mammalian host? *Comp Immunol Microbiol Infect Dis*, **34**(4), 299–314.

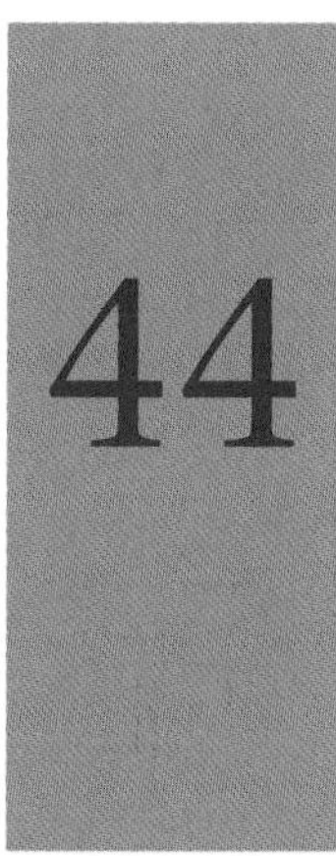

Yeasts—*Cryptococcus*, *Malassezia*, and *Candida*

LISA M. POHLMAN AND M.M. CHENGAPPA

Whether a fungus is categorized as mold or yeast is based upon the microscopic appearance in tissue or on routine culture media (the asexual stage). Microscopically, if hyphal structures are observed, the fungus is termed a mold; if single-celled, budding structures are observed, the fungus is termed a yeast. On routine culture media, molds will have a "fuzzy" or wooly appearance, and a yeast will be bacteria-like in its colonial morphology and consistency. Some pathogenic fungi will produce either hyphal-like structures or yeast-like structures, depending upon the conditions in which they are growing. Such fungi are called dimorphic fungi (Chapters 46 and 47).

In this chapter, three important representatives of yeast fungi are discussed: *Cryptococcus neoformans*, *Malassezia pachydermatis*, and *Candida albicans*.

C. neoformans

C. neoformans is typically associated with ulcerative lesions affecting the mucous membranes of the upper respiratory tract (including nasal sinuses), the central nervous system (meninges), and eyes (chorioretinitis) and has been reported in many veterinary species including cats (the domestic animal most commonly affected), dogs, ferrets, horses, sheep, goats, cattle, llamas, parrots, and elk. It is the most common systemic mycosis of cats, an uncommon cause of mastitis in cattle and has been, in rare instances, associated with intestinal disease, endometritis, and abortion in horses. However, this yeast has the potential to affect all animals, including humans. It is an opportunistic pathogen of humans, especially immunocompromised patients all over the world. In all species, there is the tendency for the central nervous system to become involved.

Original chapter written by Drs. Dwight C. Hirsh and Ernst L. Biberstein.

Descriptive Features

Morphology. *C. neoformans* is a yeast. The spherical cells (2–20 μm in diameter) produce single (usual) buds attached by slender stalks and surrounded by polysaccharide capsules (Figure 44.1). It is a monomorphic fungus with only one morphology in infected tissue and in the environment. It has a very thick capsule that is very characteristic of this fungus.

Cellular Products of Medical Interest

Capsule. The polysaccharide capsule (composed primarily of a glucuronoxylomannan) is a major virulence factor in that it mediates many deleterious effects on the host immune response. These harmful effects include, but are not limited to, the following: prevention of effective antibody-mediated phagocytosis, stimulation of T-regulatory (formerly known as suppressor) lymphocytes, inhibition of leukocyte migration, alteration of cytokine production, blockage of costimulatory molecules, and limitation of complement activation to the alternate pathway. Capsule size is significantly affected by environment.

Melanin. Melanin (which is produced from phenols by phenol oxidase via the laccase pathway) is a powerful antioxidant (free radical scavenger) and thus reduces the toxicity of hydroxy radicals, superoxides, and singlet oxygen radicals found within the phagolysosome. Melanin also provides temperature tolerance and protects the organism against enzyme degradation, radiation, and heavy metals, and while allowing acquisition of nutrients, the packing of melanin granules within the cell wall decreases entrance of antifungal compounds.

Phospholipase. Phospholipase is important for survival within macrophages, and is needed for the systemic spread of the yeast from the respiratory tract to the central nervous system. Phospholipase is believed to be involved in the membrane disruption process in the host.

Veterinary Microbiology, Third Edition. Edited by D. Scott McVey, Melissa Kennedy and M.M. Chengappa.

FIGURE 44.1. *Impression smear of an oral lesion from a cat caused by* C. neoformans. *Note the narrow-based budding (arrow) (modified Wright's stain, 1000×).*

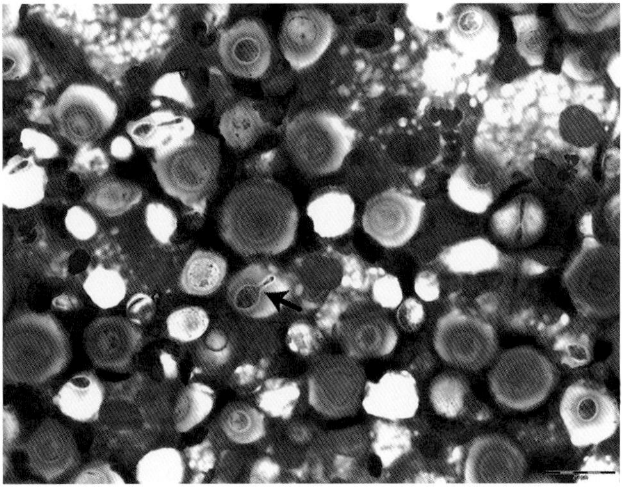

Sialic Acids. Sialic acids found within the cell wall direct complement proteins toward the degradative pathway, rather than generating effective opsonizing fragments and anaphylatoxins.

Growth Characteristics. *C. neoformans* grows on common laboratory media at room temperatures or at 30 °C. Encapsulation is optimal on chocolate agar plates (see Chapter 13) incubated under 5% carbon dioxide at 37 °C. Colonial growth may be apparent within 2 days. Colonies are convex, grayish white to white and mucoid and can reach diameters of several millimeters.

Biochemical Reactions. *Cryptococcus* spp. hydrolyze urea. Their carbohydrate assimilation patterns are utilized in identification procedures. *C. neoformans* (but few other *Cryptococcus* spp.) utilizes creatinine and produces melanin-pigmented colonies on media containing diphenolic and polyphenolic compounds. These substances are used in media for selective recovery of *C. neoformans*.

Resistance. Cycloheximide concentrations found in some fungal isolation media inhibit *C. neoformans*. Replication ceases above 40 °C. Highly alkaline environments kill the agent.

Variability. Four antigenic types A, B, C, and D based on the antigenic makeup of the capsular polysaccharides have been described. Phenotypic, genetic, and epidemiological differences between the antigenic types have resulted in the establishment of three varieties of *C. neoformans*: var. *grubii* (serotype A), var. *gattii* (serotypes B and C), and var. *neoformans* (serotype D). Varieties *grubii* and *neoformans* predominate in the temperate zone except for an area in Southern California, where variety *gattii* is prominent.

Ecology

Reservoir. *C. neoformans* (var. *grubii* and *neoformans*) lives in surface dust and dirt. In soil it does not compete well with resident microbiota. *Acanthamoeba*, an ameba, phagocytoses and destroys some strains of cryptococci. Interestingly, there are other strains that are capable of surviving within ameba by using the same intracellular survival strategies that are used for their survival within macrophages. Thus, some strains are destroyed, while others are endosymbionts using amebae as an environmental niche. In dried pigeon droppings (rich in creatinine, which inhibits other microorganisms), the fungus reaches high concentrations and survives for more than a year at much reduced capsular and cell size. *C. neoformans* var. *gattii* is now considered a distinct species, *Cryptococcus gattii*. This species lives mainly in association with decaying wood of the red river gum group of eucalyptus trees. *C. neoformans* var. *neoformans* and var. *grubii* are occasionally isolated from decaying wood in hollows of a variety of different species of trees.

Transmission. The route of infection is usually respiratory, rarely percutaneous. Cryptococcosis is noncontagious.

Pathogenesis

In an environment where moisture and nutrients are plentiful, *C. neoformans* makes little if any capsular material. In arid conditions, the capsule collapses and protects the yeast from dehydration. In either case, the size (approximately 3 μm) is small enough to make it to the lung alveoli. At physiologic concentrations of bicarbonate, CO_2, and free iron, a capsule is produced. The cryptococcal capsule is a very efficient activator of the alternate complement pathway, resulting in the deposition of C3b on its surface. Although opsonized, even in the presence of anticapsular antibody, the yeast is poorly phagocytosed, as capsular components block the binding of IgG via interference of the interaction between the Fc portion of bound antibodies and receptors on host phagocytes. Capsular polysaccharide increases participation of regulatory T-lymphocytes (formerly known as suppressor T-lymphocytes) and decreases antigen processing, leading to a poor antibody response. Capsular polysaccharide also diminishes the chemoattractive effects of the anaphylatoxins C3a and C5a generated by activation of the alternate complement pathway. In the event phagocytosis occurs, the production of melanin and mannitol by the yeast scavenges free radicals and reduces the hostile environment within the phagolysosome by inactivating superoxides, hydroxyl, and singlet oxygen radicals. In addition, phospholipase is produced, further diminishing the ability of phagocytic cells in eliminating the fungus. Thus, inflammatory responses are minimal and cryptococci grow into large space-occupying "myxomatous" masses, consisting of capsular slime, yeast cells, and few inflammatory cells. Eventually these masses acquire histiocytes, including epithelioid and multinucleated macrophages.

Development of pulmonary lesions is erratic. Infections often localize in the central nervous system (perhaps due to lower complement concentrations in the central nervous system and high concentrations of catechols, a substrate for phenol oxidase, the enzyme the yeast uses to produce melanin) following dissemination from the lungs and are manifested by neurologic signs (see Figure 71.3). Eye involvement, leading to chorioretinitis and blindness, is relatively common.

Disease Patterns

Cats and Dogs. Cats and dogs are most often clinically affected. Signs include ulcerative lesions of the mucous membranes in nose, mouth, pharynx, and sinuses or myxomatous nasal masses. Central nervous system involvement is common. These lesions may arise from local infections. Most skin lesions are probably hematogenous. Infection in dogs is less common than in cats. Infection in cats is generally seen between 3 and 7 years of age.

Cattle. Cattle acquire cryptococcosis during administration of contaminated material of intramammary medication. There are gross swelling, hardening of the gland, and gradual changes in the secretions. Destruction of the lactiferous epithelium is extensive. Several glands may be irreversibly damaged. The disease rarely advances beyond regional lymph nodes.

Horses. *C. neoformans* causes meningitides, nasal granulomas, and occasionally rhinitis and granulomatous pneumonia in horses. In rare instances, it has been associated with intestinal disease, endometritis, and abortion.

Cryptococcosis has been reported in other animals such as chickens, pheasants, goats, sheep, koalas, opossums, and a cheetah. Cryptococcosis is not common in sheep and goats.

Epidemiology. *Cryptococcus* can probably affect any mammal. Its occurrence is sporadic and worldwide. Birds, particularly pigeons, often carry the agent in their intestinal contents and contribute to its reservoir. They are rarely affected clinically, and then mostly on mucosal surfaces.

Human cryptococcosis is often associated with immunosuppression (organ transplants, Hodgkin's disease, pregnancy, acquired immunodeficiency syndrome, and malignancy) or intensive exposure. Attempts to relate animal infections to similar circumstances have been speculative.

Bovine cryptococcal mastitis usually starts as an iatrogenically induced inoculation infection.

Immunologic Aspects

Immunosuppression is a predisposing factor. The capsular polysaccharides produce immune paralysis, complement depletion, and antibody masking.

Humoral and cell-mediated phenomena (T_{H1} subset resulting in macrophage activation) evidently contribute to defense against cryptococcal infection. Macrophages participate in disposal of the agent. There is some evidence that T-lymphocytes (CD4 and CD8) as well as natural killer cells kill or inhibit *C. neoformans* directly.

Results of experimental immunization have been equivocal. No vaccines are available.

Cryptococcosis is not more common in cats with retroviral infections (e.g., feline immunodeficiency virus (FIV) and feline leukemia virus (FeLV)), whereas it is much more common in human patients infected with human immunodeficiency virus (HIV). FIV- or FeLV-positive cats may or may not respond to appropriate antifungal therapy; human HIV-positive patients respond poorly if at all.

Laboratory Diagnosis

Direct Examination. In the clinical setting, cytologic preparations stained with Romanowsky-type stains (Wright's and Giemsa) are frequently used to diagnose infection of *Cryptococcus* spp. via visualization of the pale blue/purple or clear capsule surrounding the blue-stained yeast that may exhibit narrow-based budding (see Figure 44.1). To enhance visualization, a small amount of sediment from exudates, tracheobronchial washes, and cerebrospinal fluids can also be mixed with an equal amount of India ink on a slide; a cover slip is placed on top and the sample is viewed under a microscope. The encapsulated organisms appear as bright circular lacunae in a dark field, containing the yeast cells in their centers. Yeast cells with or without budding cells are visible. With hematoxylin and eosin stain, the organism appears as a round to oval yeast body within a clear (unstained) capsule. Fungal stains—for example, periodic acid Schiff and Gomori methenamine silver—delineate the cell wall but not the capsule, which is stainable by mucicarmine.

In sections processed by the usual histologic methods, the capsules are unstained halos separating the yeast cells from tissue constituents or from each other.

Culture. Blood agar and Sabouraud's agar cultures (without cycloheximide) are incubated, respectively, at 30 °C and room temperature (see Chapter 46). Suggestive colonies are examined by India ink wet mount. If found to consist of encapsulated yeasts, *C. neoformans* is confirmed by demonstration of urease activity, absence of lactose, melibiose, and nitrate assimilation. Commercial test kits are available for identification of *C. neoformans*.

Selective media incorporating antibacterial and antifungal drugs, creatinine and diphenyl, are used for environmental sampling.

Some normal dogs and cats harbor small numbers of *C. neoformans* in their nasal cavities. Therefore, care should be taken when interpreting culture results from samples obtained from this site. Examination of direct smears (the numbers of yeast in smears from clinically normal animals are too low to see) and/or analysis of serum for capsular antigen are helpful adjuncts to culture. Capsular antigen is not detectable in serum of normal dogs, regardless of whether they harbor *C. neoformans* in their nasal passages.

Immunodiagnosis. Antigen demonstration in serum and cerebrospinal fluid is attempted in diagnosis and assessment of patient progress. Latex particle suspensions coated with anticapsular antibody are marketed as slide agglutination test kits.

Antibody is irregularly demonstrable because of the "sponging" action of circulating capsular antigens. Its presence (demonstrated by indirect fluorescent antibody tests or by latex particles coated with capsular polysaccharide) is a favorable sign of decreasing antigen levels.

An enzyme immunoassay is also available for the serodiagnosis of cryptococcosis in cats and dogs.

Treatment and Control

The treatment of choice is fluconazole and itraconazole. Alternative therapy is 5-fluorocytosine, but its efficacy should be tested periodically as strains may be resistant or become resistant. Amphotericin B is used in severe disseminated cases. It is used sometimes in combination with flucytosine.

Therapy should be continued until clinical signs are resolved and antigen disappears from serum and cerebrospinal fluid.

Contaminated surfaces (pigeon lofts, attics) can be disinfected with lime solution (1 lb hydrated lime/3 gal water) prior to physical cleanup. Dirt removed is placed in containers and covered with hydrated lime powder, which can also be used on exposed floors and beams. Masks are worn during the operation.

M. pachydermatis

M. pachydermatis is commonly associated with animal disease, most often otitis externa, and dermatitis in dogs. However, this lipid-dependent yeast has been isolated from skin and external ear canals of normal and clinically affected dogs, cats, ruminants, and horses. Thus, the reason why *M. pachydermatis* is more commonly found may be due to the relative ease in which this species is demonstrated. It is believed to be an opportunistic pathogen of animals and humans. There are numerous other species of *Malassezia* believed to be associated with diseases in animals. However, these diseases or conditions are rare and in many instances not diagnosed with proper identification procedures.

Descriptive Features

Morphology and Composition. *M. pachydermatis* is an oval budding yeast (2 μm by 5 μm). In direct smears (and from colonies obtained from culture), there will be a single bud attached by a broad base (0.9–1.1 μm) (Figure 44.2). Filaments are not usually observed, regardless of culture conditions. The cell wall is composed of glycoproteins (75–80%), lipids (15–20%), and chitin (1–2%).

Growth Characteristics. Although not requiring lipids for growth, *M. pachydermatis* is lipophilic, and growth is improved when lipids are added to the medium. Most strains of *M. pachydermatis* grow on blood agar plates, though the colonies will be very small (<1 mm in diameter, and sometimes only a "greenish" tint will be seen on the surface of the plate) after several days of incubation (optimum temperature is 37°C, although it will grow at temperature ranging from 25 to 41 °C). The yeast will grow in either an aerobic or microaerophilic atmosphere (it does not grow well anaerobically).

FIGURE 44.2. *Exudate of canine otitis externa containing many* M. pachydermatis *yeasts. Note characteristic "shoe print" pattern of budding yeasts (arrow) (modified Wright's stain, 1000×).*

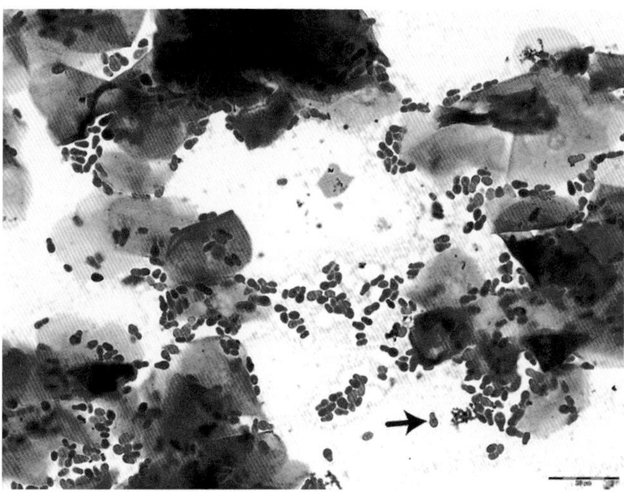

Biochemical Reactions. *M. pachydermatis* assimilates the carbon of glucose and D-mannitol, but does not ferment carbohydrates. Urea hydrolysis is strain dependent. However, *M. pachydermatis* strains produce enzymes such as proteinase, chondroitin sulfatase, hyaluronidase, and phospholipase, which are believed to contribute to the disease process. Immune-mediated hypersensitivity reaction is also believed to be a contributing factor of the disease.

Resistance. *M. pachydermatis* is resistant to cycloheximide.

Variability. There are a number of biotypes of *M. pachydermatis* as reflected in variability in D-mannitol and sorbitol assimilation, hydrolysis of urea, and cell wall fatty acid concentration.

Seven genetic types (Ia through Ig) have been described using the sequence of DNA, encoding the large ribosomal subunit as the basis for comparison. Others have delineated four genetic types (A through D) after using the random amplification of polymorphic DNA method, together with sequence comparisons of the gene encoding chitin synthase.

Ecology

Reservoir. *M. pachydermatis* lives on the skin and external ear canal of healthy animals, including dogs, cats, ferrets, pigs, and rhinoceros (from which it gets its name). The surface of *M. pachydermatis* has mannose-containing glycoproteins that are responsible for binding to mannose receptors on the surface of corneocytes, thus allowing adherence in this niche. It is rarely isolated from human skin, or the environment.

Transmission. *M. pachydermatis* is an opportunistic fungus, contributing to disease processes already in progress (e.g., allergic dermatitis). The source of the yeast is endogenous (i.e., a member of the patient's normal flora). Iatrogenic disease has been reported for the transmission of the yeast from a dog with otitis externa to a human patient via the hands of a caregiver (the dog's owner) who handled a lipid-rich intravenous solution (for total parenteral nutrition) subsequently administered to the patient.

Pathogenesis

M. pachydermatis plays a secondary, but significant, role in otitis externa and dermatitis in a variety of animals, but most commonly in dogs and, to a lesser extent, in cats. The exact role played by *M. pachydermatis* remains unclear, and what causes the yeast to change from a harmless commensal to one that contributes to disease is unknown. However, it is believed that the disease may be associated with immunosuppression and other predisposing conditions. If its presence is ignored when formulating a treatment regimen, however, resolution of the disease process is problematic.

Epidemiology. *M. pachydermatis* is a parasite of skin (including the external ear canal) of nonhuman animals. *M. pachydermatis*-associated dermatitis is more commonly reported in Australian silky terriers, basset hounds, cocker spaniels, dachshunds, poodles, and West Highland white terriers. The yeast has worldwide distribution.

Immunologic Aspects

M. pachydermatis is an opportunistic yeast, contributing to preexisting compromises of the skin and external ear. It is unknown how *M. pachydermatis* contributes to disease. However, *M. pachydermatis* strains produce enzymes such as proteinase, chondroitin sulfatase, hyaluronidase, and phospholipase, which are believed to contribute to the disease process. Immune-mediated hypersensitivity reaction is also believed to be a contributing factor of the disease.

Laboratory Diagnosis

Direct Examination. The numbers of yeasts on normal skin or in the normal external ear canal are usually too low to visualize in samples taken from such sites. Thus, determining whether *M. pachydermatis* is a contributing factor to otitis externa or to a dermatological condition is relatively easy, because the numbers of yeasts will be high enough to be seen in samples taken from affected areas. However, some atopic dogs have been shown to have increased numbers of *M. pachydermatis* in normal as well as affected areas.

Samples taken with cotton-tipped swabs are the easiest to obtain from cases of otitis externa. Swabs are "rolled" over the surface of a microscope slide; the smear is air-dried, then stained with a Romanowsky-type stain (Wright's and Giemsa). Examination of smears will reveal yeasts with characteristic "bottle-shaped" or "shoe print" morphology (see Figure 44.2). If the swabs are also streaked onto the surface of a blood agar plate, small colonies (or a greenish coloration) will appear within 24–48 h after incubation of the plate at 37 °C incubator. *M. pachydermatis* grows well on fungal selective media such as Mycosel or Sabouraud dextrose agar plates incubated at 37 °C.

Molecular Techniques. Polymerase chain reaction amplification of DNA, encoding either the large or the small ribosomal subunit together with the internal transcribed spacer region, may be used to detect *Malassezia* spp. The same technology has been applied to speciation of the yeast.

Culture. As a means of determining whether *M. pachydermatis* is a contributor in otitis externa, culture is not worth the effort because most samples taken from such conditions contain bacteria (e.g., *Pseudomonas*) that quickly overgrow the slower growing yeast. The determination that *M. pachydermatis* is involved can be made quicker by microscopic examination of samples.

Culture plays a role in assessing the microbiological makeup of dermatological conditions, as well as formulating a treatment regimen. Media that have proven useful include Mycosel or Sabouraud's dextrose agar. Plates are incubated at 37 °C.

Treatment and Control

Correction of the underlying condition is the most important aspect of treatment of *M. pachydermatis*-associated otitis externa or dermatitis. Almost all commercially available topical preparations that contain an antifungal agent (nystatin, clotrimazole, or miconazole) are effective in treating the fungal component of otitis externa. Medicated shampoos (e.g., miconazole + chlorhexidine), along with systemic antifungal administration (ketoconazole or itraconazole), are effective in reducing the influence of *M. pachydermatis* upon dermatological diseases. Griseofulvin is not effective.

C. albicans

Candidiasis is usually due to the parasitic yeast *C. albicans*, which inhabits mucous membranes of most mammals and birds. Of the more than 200 other species of *Candida* that are associated with many diverse habitats, few are associated with animal disease and *C. albicans* is the most important pathogen of animals and humans. Disease produced by *C. albicans* usually occurs in an immunocompromised host. Overuse of antibiotics and prolonged use of steroids and hormonal therapy could disrupt the normal cutaneous defense mechanisms, leading candidiases in animals and humans.

Descriptive Features

Cell Morphology and Composition. On routine laboratory media and mucous membranes, *C. albicans* typically grows as oval budding yeast cells (blastoconidia), 5–8 μm in size. Under certain conditions of temperature, pH, nutrition, and atmosphere, yeast cells sprout germ tubes (Figure 44.3) that develop into septate-branching mycelium. "Pseudohyphae" are produced by elongation

FIGURE 44.3. *C. albicans* in peritoneal fluid from a dog. Note the yeast cells (blastoconidia and pseudohyphae) (modified Wright's stain, 1000×).

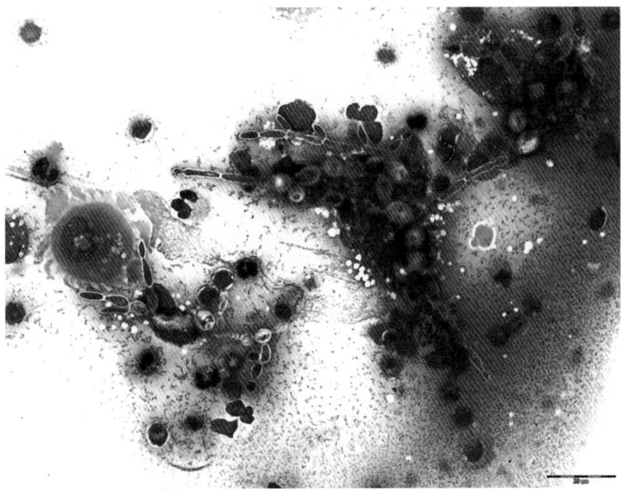

of the blastoconidia and their failure to separate. *In vivo*, mycelial (a collection of hyphae) or pseudomycelial growth is associated with active proliferation and invasiveness.

The so-called chlamydospore (chlamydoconidium) is a thick-walled sphere of unknown function, attached by a suspensor cell to (pseudo)mycelium and essentially confined to *in vitro* growth (Figure 44.4) of *C. albicans* (rarely other *Candida* spp.).

The cell wall contains glycoproteins; the polysaccharide portions are glucans and especially mannans. Lipids and chitin are also present. Mannoproteins are found on the cell surface. Cellular products include peptidolytic enzymes, which may be virulence factors. Two major cross-reacting serogroups are recognized. These are termed A and B, and are identifiable with absorbed sera.

Candida can be visualized under light microscopy when stained with Romanowsky-type stains (Wright's and Giemsa) (Figure 44.3), periodic acid Schiff, Gomori methenamine silver, and other fungal stains, but is usually

FIGURE 44.4. *C. albicans* culture on chlamydospore agar, showing blastoconidia (arrow).

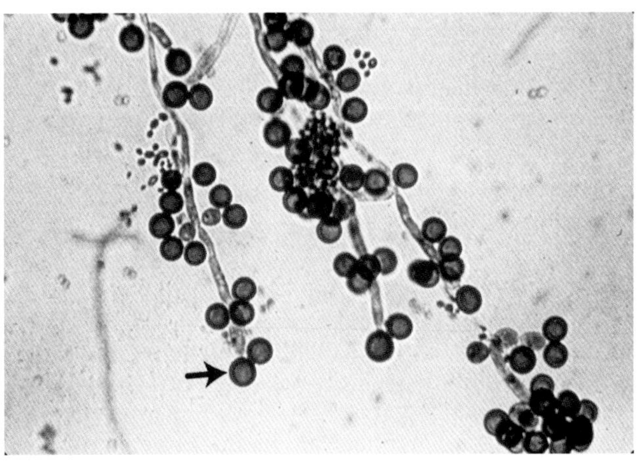

studied in culture unstained. With Gram stain, *Candida* cells are gram-variable.

Cellular Products of Medical Interest

Adhesins. Various cell wall components (chitin, mannoproteins, and lipids) have been associated with adherence to extracellular matrix proteins.

Miscellaneous Products. Proteases and neuraminidases have been proposed to play a role in pathogenesis. Cell wall glycoproteins have endotoxin-like activity (see Chapters 7 and 8). Virulence factors such as phospholipases and proteases have been demonstrated in *C. albicans*. These enzymes seem to promote tissue invasion and adherence of yeasts to host cells, respectively.

Growth Characteristics. *C. albicans*, an obligate aerobe, grows on ordinary media over a wide range of pH and temperature. At 25–30 °C, creamy to pasty white colonies consisting predominantly of yeast cells appear in 24–48 h. Incubation temperatures above 35 °C, a slightly alkaline pH, and a rich, carbohydrate-free fluid medium are often recommended. It grows well on a variety of nonselective fungal and bacterial media including Sabouraud's dextrose or blood agar plates.

Differential ability to ferment or assimilate carbohydrates is the basis of species identification.

C. albicans cells are killed by heat above 50 °C, ultraviolet light, chlorine, and quaternary ammonium-type disinfectants. They withstand freezing and survive well in the inanimate environment. They are susceptible to polyene antimycotics, and usually to flucytosine and the azoles.

Ecology

Reservoir. *C. albicans* is associated with mucocutaneous areas, particularly of the alimentary and lower genital tract, of mammals and birds. However, *C. albicans* can invade any organ of the body and cause disease.

Transmission. Most *Candida* diseases arise from an endogenous source; that is, they are caused by a commensal strain. The bovine udder becomes infected via the teat canal by way of administered medication, during milking, by cow-to-cow spread, or from the environment. Hematogenous spread has also been reported leading to systemic infections with this yeast.

Pathogenesis

Mechanisms. Chitin, mannoprotein, and lipids are possible adhesins, in human candidiasis; several extracellular matrix proteins have been shown to be the receptor. Germ tube formation is correlated with experimental pathogenicity, but the role of mycelium formation in virulence is under dispute. Proteases and phospholipases are believed to be virulence factors. Cell wall glycoproteins have endotoxin-like activity.

Pathology. Candidiasis most frequently affects the mucous surfaces on which the agent is normally found, possibly the anterior digestive tract from mouth to stomach; it typically remains confined to areas of squamous epithelium. The genital tract, skin, and claws can be involved as well. Occasional respiratory, intestinal, and septicemic infections occur.

On epithelial surfaces, candidiasis forms whitish to yellow or gray plaques, marking areas of ulceration with varying degree of inflammation. Diphtheritic membranes may form in the gut or respiratory tract, and abscesses may form in the viscera. Granulomatous lesions are rare. Inflammatory responses are predominantly neutrophilic.

Disease Patterns

Birds. Avian candidiasis affects chickens, turkeys, pigeons, and other birds. Crop mycosis (thrush) in avian species is caused by *C. albicans*. The existing digestive tract of birds can be affected; and mortality is very high with this disease condition.

Swine. In the alimentary tract of pigs, candidiasis is seen as ulcerative lesions that may lead to rupture.

Equine. In the alimentary tract of foals, candidiasis is seen as ulcerative lesions that may lead to rupture. Equine genital infections cause infertility, metritis, and abortions.

Cattle. Pneumonic, enteric, and generalized candidiasis affects calves on intensive antibiotic regimens. *Candida* mastitis in dairy cows is typically mild and self-limiting, ending in spontaneous recovery within about a week. Bovine abortions have been reported.

Dogs and Cats. Localized infections in dogs and cats are characterized by nonhealing, ulcerative lesions of the oral, upper respiratory, gastrointestinal, and/or genitourinary mucosae. Rarely, dogs and cats may develop disseminated disease; clinical signs on presentation will typically reflect involvement of a specific organ system.

Other. Lower primates and marine mammals may acquire mucocutaneous candidiasis.

Epidemiology. The common agents of candidiasis are commensal with most warm-blooded species. Disease is linked to immune and hormonal inadequacies, reduced colonization resistance (a measure of the "health" of the normal flora), or intensive exposure of weakened hosts or vulnerable tissues. These conditions account for susceptibility of infants, diabetics, subjects on antibiotic and steroid regimes, patients with indwelling catheters, and mammary glands of lactating cows.

Immunologic Aspects

Immunoincompetent individuals are preferred targets for infection.

Polymorphonuclear neutrophil leukocytes and activated macrophages form the chief defense against candidiases. The role played by opsonins (antibody, complement) is to facilitate phagocytosis. Macrophages are activated by γ-interferon secreted by T_{H1} cells stimulated by interleukin 12 from macrophages actively engaged in phagocytosis.

There is no vaccine for candidiasis.

Laboratory Diagnosis

In exudate, *Candida* appears as yeast cells (blastoconidia) or (pseudo)hyphae. All forms are demonstrable in unstained wet mounts, or in fixed smears stained with Gram's stain, Romanowsky-type stains (Wright's and Giemsa) or fungal stains (e.g., periodic acid Schiff and Gomori methenamine silver).

C. albicans grows well on blood or Sabouraud's agar, with or without inhibitors (see Chapter 46). Other *Candida* spp. may be inhibited by cycloheximide. Yeast isolates producing (pseudo)mycelium can be considered *Candida* spp. Isolation of *Candida* spp. from mucous membranes (even in large numbers) suggests a diagnosis of candidiasis only in the presence of compatible lesions, and abundant (pseudo)hyphal forms in direct smears.

Incubation at 37 °C for ≥2 h of a lightly inoculated tube of serum will produce germ tubes if the isolate is *C. albicans* (see Figure 44.3), which also produced chlamydospores on cornmeal-Tween 80 agar (see Figure 44.4). Yeast identification kits are commercially available.

Molecular and serologic methods for diagnosis of candidiasis are not routinely done in the diagnostic laboratories. However, DNA-based tests are available in the reference laboratories.

Treatment, Control, and Prevention

Correcting conditions underlying clinical candidiasis may, in itself, lead to recovery.

In poultry, copper sulfate in drinking water is a traditional treatment. Nystatin can be given in feed or water. It is also used topically in mucosal and cutaneous forms of candidiasis of mammals, as are amphotericin B, itraconazole, and miconazole. Fluconazole (preferred) or flucytosine is useful for treating dogs or cats with lower urinary tract candidiasis.

In disseminated forms, oral fluconazole and flucytosine are drugs of choice. Susceptibility testing is advisable. Combined flucytosine–amphotericin B is sometimes used in humans and occasionally in animals.

Other Yeasts

Geotrichum candidum

This yeast-like fungus occurs widely in nature and causes an uncommon disease in animals called geotrichosis. Diagnostic relevance of this fungus in clinical samples is always questionable. However, it is known to cause infections of mucous membranes of alimentary tract, respiratory tract, and mammary glands of animals including cattle, pigs, horses, dogs, avian species, and humans. The organism grows rapidly on fungal growth medium and is identified based on colony characteristics and microscopic examinations of culture. It is susceptible to amphotericin B and flucytosine.

Trichosporon beigelii

It is a soil-borne, yeast-like, imperfect fungus that causes trichosporonosis. It is an opportunist fungus that causes deep-seated and superficial infections in immunocompromised animals and humans. Colonies are initially creamy, smooth on Sabouraud's agar and may take 5–7 days of incubation at 37 °C. Definitive identification is based on assimilation tests, growth characteristics, and microscopic appearance. Treatment is like other yeast infections.

Further Reading

Bond R (2006) Malassezia dermatitis in cutaneous fungal infections, in *Infectious Diseases of the Dog and Cat*, 3rd edn, Saunders Elsevier, pp. 565–569.

Greene CE and Chandler FW (2006) Candidiasis and rhodotorulosis, in *Infectious Diseases of the Dog and Cat*, 3rd edn, Saunders Elsevier, pp. 627–633.

Malik R, Krockenberger M, O'Brian CR *et al.* (2006) Cryptococcosis, in *Infectious Diseases of the Dog and Cat*, 3rd edn, Saunders Elsevier, pp. 584–598.

Quinn PJ, Markey BK, Carter ME *et al.* (2002) Veterinary microbiology and microbial diseases, in *Yeast and Disease Production*, Blackwell Publishing Ltd, pp. 233–239.

Songer JG and Post KW (2005) *Veterinary Microbiology: Bacterial and Fungal Agents of Animal Diseases*, Elsevier Saunders.

Dermatophytes

M.M. Chengappa and Lisa M. Pohlman

Whether a fungus is categorized as mold or yeast is based upon the microscopic appearance in tissue or on routine culture media (the asexual stage). If hyphal structures are observed, the fungus is termed a mold; if a single-celled, budding structure is observed, the fungus is termed a yeast. On routine culture media, molds will have a "fuzzy" or wooly appearance, and a yeast will be bacteria-like in its colonial morphology and consistency. Some pathogenic fungi will produce either hyphal-like structures or yeast-like structures, depending upon the conditions in which they are growing. Such fungi are called dimorphic fungi (Chapters 46 and 47).

Dermatophytes are molds capable of parasitizing only keratinized epidermal structures: superficial skin, hair, feathers, horn, hooves, claws, and nails. Those that have a sexual reproductive phase belong to the ascomycetes. Dermatophyte infections are called ringworm or dermatophytoses. Occasionally, yeast and saprophytic fungi cause cutaneous infections mimicking infections caused by dermatophytes; hence, the generic term dermatomycoses is used to represent all fungal Infections of skin.

Descriptive Features

Morphology

In their nonparasitic state, including culture, dermatophytes produce septate, branching hyphae collectively called mycelium. The asexual reproductive units (conidia) are found in the aerial mycelium. These units may be either macroconidia: pluricellular, podlike structures up to 100 μm long; or microconidia: unicellular spheres or rods less than 10 μm in any dimension. Shape, size, structure, arrangement, and abundance of conidia are diagnostic criteria. Hyphal peculiarities—spirals, nodules, rackets, chandeliers, and chlamydoconidia (chlamydospores)—are more common in some species than others, but they are rarely diagnostic. Colony characteristics and pigmentation are useful in dermatophyte differentiation.

Original chapter written by Drs. Ernst L. Biberstein and Dwight C. Hirsh.

In the parasitic state, only hyphae and arthroconidia (arthrospores), another asexual reproductive unit, are seen. Except in size ranges, which overlap among dermatophyte species, arthroconidia are indistinguishable from species to species.

Sexual spores (ascospores) are absent in the parasitic phase.

The distinguishing features of the three genera of dermatophytes—*Microsporum, Trichophyton*, and *Epidermophyton*—are shown in Table 45.1. Only *Microsporum* and *Trichophyton* affect animals consistently. *Epidermophyton* is seen primarily in humans.

Growth Characteristics

The traditional medium for propagating dermatophytes (and other pathogenic fungi) is Saboraud's dextrose agar containing 2% agar, 1% peptone and 4% dextrose. Its acidity (pH 5.6) renders it mildly bacteriostatic and selective. The selectivity is enhanced by addition of cycloheximide (500 μg/ml), which inhibits saprophytic fungi, and gentamicin and tetracycline (100 μg/ml of each) or chloramphenicol (50 μg/ml), which inhibit bacteria. Dermatophytes are aerobes and nonfermenters. Some attack proteins and deaminate amino acids. They grow optimally at 25–30 °C and require several days to weeks of incubation.

Some dermatophytes in skin and hair (but not in culture) produce a green fluorescence due to a tryptophan metabolite that is visible under ultraviolet light (366 nm), sometimes referred to as a Wood's light. Of animal dermatophytes, only *Microsporum canis* produces this reaction.

Resistance

Dermatophytes are susceptible to common disinfectants, particularly those containing cresol, iodine, or chlorine. They survive for years in the inanimate environment.

Variability

There are a number of strains of each species of *Microsporum* and *Trichophyton*, making construction of effective immunizing products difficult.

Veterinary Microbiology, Third Edition. Edited by D. Scott McVey, Melissa Kennedy and M.M. Chengappa.

Table 45.1. Features of Dermatophyte Genera

	Microsporum	Tricophyton	Epidermophyton
Macroconidia	Usually present	Variable; often absent	Present
Walls	Thick	Thin	Thick
Surface	Rough	Smooth	Smooth
Shape	Spindle, cigar	Club (slender)	Club (broad)
Microconidia	Variable, often absent	Usual	Absent
Sexual form	Nannizzia	Arthroderma	None known

Ecology

Reservoir

One speaks of geophilic, zoophilic, and anthropophilic dermatophytes when discussing dermatophytes having a soil, animal, or human reservoir, respectively. Table 45.2 shows the important dermatophytes of animals. Animal dermatophytes can infect humans through direct contact, whereas human dermatophytes rarely infect animals.

Transmission

Dermatophytes are disseminated by direct and, owing to their persistence on fomites and premises, indirect contact.

Pathogenesis

Mechanisms

Proteolytic enzymes (elastase, collagenase, keratinase) may determine virulence, particularly in severe inflammatory disease. Localization in the keratinized epidermis has been attributed to the lack of sufficient available iron elsewhere. This may account for the frequent arrest of dermatophytoses by inflammatory responses (through the influx of iron-binding proteins) and by enzyme inhibitors.

The infectious unit, a conidium, enters via a defect in the stratum corneum. Germination is triggered by unknown cues. The germ tube develops into hyphae branching among cornified epithelium. Portions of hyphae differentiate into arthroconidia. This growth pattern in the hairless skin predominates with some dermatophytes (*Microsporum nanum* and *Trichophyton rubrum*). Hair invasion, which is prominent in most animal ringworm, begins with germination of a spore near a follicular orifice. Hyphal strands grow into hair follicles along outer root sheaths and invade growing hairs near the living root cells. Hyphae grow within the hair cortex, in the outer parts of which arthroconidia form and accumulate on the surface of the hair. The pattern of accumulation of arthroconida outside the hair shaft is called ectothrix, whereas, the accumulation of arthroconida inside the hair shaft is called endothrix formation.

Table 45.2. Important Dermatophytes of Animals

Dermatophyte Species	Affected Animal Hosts	Humans Affected
Microsporum canis[a]	Cat, dog, (horse, sheep, cattle, pig, others)	+
M. gallinae	Poultry (cat, dog)	+
M. gypseum	Dog, horse (cattle, pig, others)	+
M. nanum	Pig	+
Trichophyton equinum	Horse (dog)	+
T. mentagrophytes	Dog (horse, cattle, sheep, cat, pig, others)	+
T. verrucosum	Cattle (cat, dog, sheep, horses, others)	+
T. simii	Monkey, poultry	+

[a]Occasionally reported in cattle, sheep, horses and pigs.
() uncommon host.

Pathology

The pathogenic process begins with colonization, during which the events just described occur but evoke little host response. There may be hypertrophy of the stratum corneum with accelerated keratinization and exfoliation, producing a scurfy appearance and hair loss. In dogs with *M. canis* infections, this is often the main effect. In adult cats there may be no signs. Adult cats are known to carry *M. canis* spores on their skin without exhibiting any clinical signs or lesions of ringworm.

The second phase begins at about the second week with inflammation at the margin of the parasitized area. Manifestations range from erythema to vesiculopustular reactions and suppuration. Mild forms are seen in *Trichophyto verrucosum* infection of calves. Severe reactions are typical in *T. mentagrophytes* infection of dogs and *Microsporum gypseum* infection of horses. Local plaques ("kerion") may resemble certain skin tumors, especially in dogs. The inflammatory reaction may arrest the mycotic infection but become the primary problem through secondary suppurative bacterial infection.

The circular pattern of the lesions and their inflamed margins suggested the terms ringworm and tinea (Latin for worm).

Disease Patterns

The patterns of dermatophytosis in domestic animals are summarized in Table 45.3.

Ringworm generally regresses spontaneously within a few weeks or months, unless complicated by secondary bacterial infections or constitutional factors. The agents may persist after clinical cure.

Epidemiology

Dermatophytoses often affect the young. Extent and severity are influenced by environmental factors. Crowding of animals or assembling of large numbers is often associated with increased prevalence. Improvement in calves often

Table 45.3. Important Dermatophyte Infections in Domestic Animals

Host	Agent	Nature of Lesions
Horse	*T. equinum*	Dry, scaly usually noninflammatory (unless secondarily infected)
	M. gypseum	Often suppurative under alopecic thickened areas
	M. equinum	Not more than mildly inflammatory, resembling *T. equinum* lesions
Cattle	*T. verrucosum*	Painless, thick, white, "asbestos" plaques, local alopecia
Swine	*M. nanum*	Tannish, crusty, spreading centrifugally on trunk; painless, margins slightly inflamed. No hair loss.
Dog	*M. canis*	Typically noninflammatory, scaly, alopecic patches, occasional kerion
	T. mentagrophytes	Often spreading, extensively scaling to inflammatory lesions, secondary suppuration
	M. gypseum	As *T. mentagrophyes*
Cat	*M. canis*	Often subclinical in adults. Generally noninflammatory, except in young kittens, may become generalized in debilitated kittens. Occasional mycetoma (Persian cats).
	T. mentagrophytes	As in dogs
Chicken	*M. gallinae*	Generally affects unfeathered portions. Whitish chalky scaling on comb and wattles, noninflammatory.
	T. simii	Superficially similar to *M. gallinae* but often inflammatory and even necrotizing. A poultry problem only in India.

follows their release from damp, dark, crowded winter quarters to the outdoors.

Infected individuals of the same species perpetuate the important dermatophytoses of animals. Sporadic occurrence of the soil-derived *M. gypseum* infections contrasts with endemic to epidemic but bland infections of swine with geophilic *M. nanum*.

The major agents of animal ringworm are globally distributed.

Immunologic Aspects

Immune Mechanisms of Disease

The major antigens associated with dermatophyte infections are the keratinases (elicit cell-mediated responses) and glycoproteins (carbohydrate moieties stimulate antibody; protein moieties stimulate cell-mediated responses).

Antibody-mediated and cell-mediated hypersensitivities occur in the course of dermatophytoses. Their onset generally coincides with that of the inflammatory phase of infection and may contribute to its manifestations. Production of skin lesions is facilitated due to the release of interferon gamma in the host.

Sterile inflammatory skin lesions (phytids) occur in human ringworm infections. They are allergic reactions to circulating fungal antigens.

Recovery and Resistance

Antibodies play at best a limited role in resistance. Evidence favors cell-mediated mechanisms as decisive in protection and recovery.

Recovered individuals resist reinfection, although local reactions may be more acute and intense than on primary exposure. Acquired resistance varies in degree and duration with host, dermatophyte species, and possibly anatomical area.

Artificial Immunization

Mycelial *T. verrucosum* vaccines, inactivated and live avirulent, are used in Europe in cattle. They are credited with reducing the number of infected herds and new infections. Mixtures of *Microsporum* and *Trichophyton*—either as a live, attenuated vaccine, or a killed product—have been disappointing in protecting cats from developing dermatophytosis, though they do appear to restrict spread upon individual cats. Although live vaccines appear to elicit a better immune (protective) response, the presence of numerous strains of *Microsporum* and *Trichophyton* make concocting such products difficult.

Laboratory Diagnosis

Direct Examination

In 50–70% of cases, hairs and skin scales infected with *M. canis* or *M. audouinii* may emit a bright greenish-yellow fluorescence under ultraviolet light, for example, a Wood's lamp ($\lambda = 366$ nm).

Microscopic Examination

Skin scrapings and hair are examined microscopically for the presence of hyphae and arthroconidia. The scraping should include material from the margins of any lesion and the full thickness of the keratinized epidermis. The hair is plucked, so as to include the intrafollicular portion. The sample is placed on a slide, flooded with 10–20% potassium hydroxide, covered with a cover slip, and heated gently. The treatment clears the sample (makes it "transparent") while leaving fungal structures and enough of the hair and epidermis intact to reveal the agent in its relation to the parasitized structures.

Microscopic examination should begin under low power (100×) and subdued light. At higher magnification (400×) of such hairs, individual, spherical arthroconidia are recognizable.

Stains and penetrating and wetting agents (permanent ink, lactophenol cotton blue, dimethylsulfoxide) improve visualization. Calcofluor white reagent imparts fluorescence to fungal structures and facilitates diagnosis where a fluorescent microscope is available.

FIGURE 45.1. Microsporum canis. *Lactophenol cotton blue mount from Sabouraud's dextrose agar culture. Spindle-shaped macromedia, 400×.*

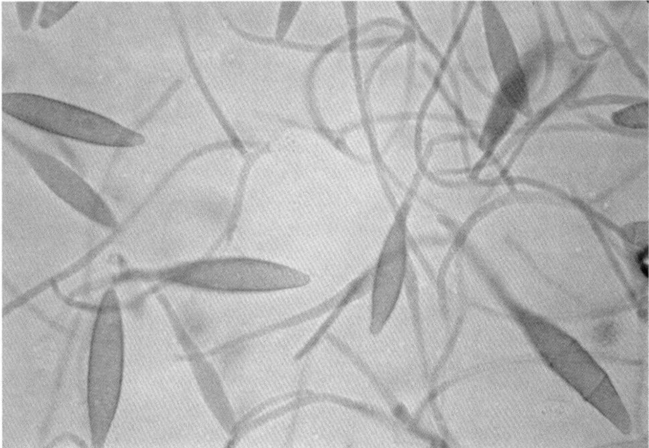

FIGURE 45.2. Trichophyton verrucosum. *Lactophenol cotton blue mount from Sabouraud's dextrose agar culture grown at 37 °C. Macromedia, 400×.*

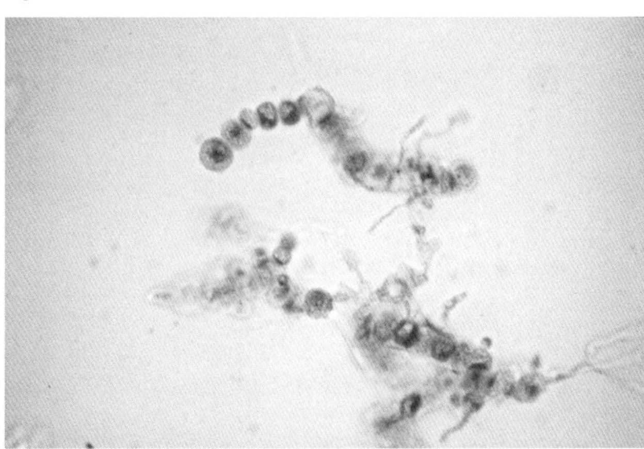

Culture

Scrapings are planted onto and into the surface of selective media (Sabouraud's agar with chloramphenicol and cycloheximide, Dermatophyte Test Medium (DTM), Rapid Sporulation Medium (RSM)), which are incubated at 25 °C (room temperature) for up to 4 weeks. Samples suspected of containing *T. verrucosum* are incubated at 37°C. On DTM and RSM, an alkaline reaction suggests presence of a dermatophyte. (Dermatophytes, if given a choice of glucose and protein, will usually digest the protein first, leading to alkaline products; saprophytic fungi will most often utilize glucose, leading to acid by-products. Caution: After the preferred substrate is utilized, the microorganism will make use of the other, shifting the pH in the other direction.)

Suspicious growth is examined microscopically. The adhesive side of a clear cellophane tape strip is pressed gently on the suspect colony (taken from RSM, or Sabouraud's agar with chloramphenicol and cycloheximide—dermatophytes do not sporulate well on DTM) and mounted in a drop of lactophenol cotton blue on a slide and examined microscopically (see Table 45.1, Figure 45.1, 45.2, and 45.3). Colony color (front and back), texture, and rate of growth are important for identification of dermatophytes. Also important are the size and shape of macro- and microconidia of dermatophytes. With *Trichophyton* spp., in the absence of diagnostic conidia, auxotrophic tests are used for speciation.

Knowledge of source (host species and type of lesion) aids significantly in provisional identification of animal dermatophytes.

Molecular Techniques

There are a number of DNA-based techniques that are available for direct examination of clinical samples, or for use in identification of an isolated dermatophyte. These techniques include determination of the sequence of DNA encoding specific products (e.g., chitin synthase 1 gene), determination of the sequence of the internal transcribed spacer region, determination of the sequence of the DNA encoding large ribosomal subunit (28S), and generation of unique DNA fragments following arbitrary or randomly primed polymerase chain reactions. These both are not routinely used in the diagnostic laboratories.

Treatment and Control

Combined topical and systemic treatment is often preferable. Topical antifungal agents include, but are not limited to, products containing miconazole, econozole, ketoconazole, itraconazole and thiobendazole. Terbinafine (an allylamine antifungal that inhibits ergosterol biosynthesis, and concentrates in skin and nails), fluconazole and itraconazole (especially effective in cats) are drugs of choice may be a useful alternative.

Antifungal orchard spray is effective on ringworm of large and small animals (Captan 45% powder, 2 tablespoons/gal). Affected areas are first clipped. In large

FIGURE 45.3. Microsporum nanum. *Lactophenol cotton blue mount from Sabouraud's dextrose agar culture. Pear-shaped macromedia, 400×.*

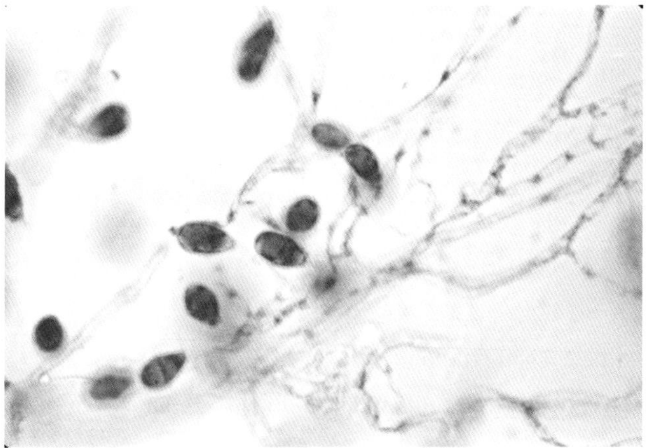

animals, two applications at biweekly intervals are recommended. With dogs, weekly dips can be repeated to effect. Contact with human skin should be avoided. Thiabendazole is used on small and large animals. Lime sulfur dips in combination with systemic miconazole or other azoles is effective.

Povidone-iodine (Betadine) and chlorhexidine (Nolvasan), available as lotions and ointments, are general antiseptics with antifungal action.

A thorough cleanup of premises involving use of an iodine, chlorine, or phenol-containing disinfectant is essential. Utensils and equipment are disinfected with Captan or Bordeaux orchard spray.

Identification of carriers in kennels and catteries can be attempted by culture of brushings. The Wood's lamp is useful in population screening of cat colonies where *M. canis* is the only concern. Infected individuals should be isolated and treated. Exposed animals are treated prophylactically.

Successful vaccination is widely practiced on European cattle. A live attenuated strain (*T. verrucosum*) appears to be most immunogenic. Neither live attenuated vaccines nor killed products have been effective in preventing dermatophytosis in cats.

Further Reading

Songer JG and Post KW (2005) *Veterinary Microbiology: Bacterial and Fungal Agents of Animal Diseases*. Elsevier Saunders.

Agents of Subcutaneous Mycoses

Lisa M. Pohlman and M.M. Chengappa

Whether a fungus is categorized as mold or yeast is based upon the microscopic appearance in tissue or on routine culture media (the asexual stage). If hyphal structures are observed, the fungus is termed a mold; if a single-celled, budding structure is observed, the fungus is termed a yeast. On routine culture media, molds will have a "fuzzy" or wooly appearance, and yeast will be bacteria-like in its colonial morphology and consistency. Some pathogenic fungi will produce either hyphal-like structures or yeast-like structures, depending upon the conditions in which they are growing. Such fungi are called dimorphic fungi, which are discussed here and in Chapter 47.

This chapter deals with dimorphic fungi and fungus-like microorganisms affecting skin and subcutis. To be discussed are *Sporothrix schenckii*, which is the cause of sporotrichosis in a variety of animal species, but more frequently in humans, horses, dogs, and cats; *Histoplasma capsulatum* var. *farciminosum*, the cause of epizootic lymphangitis in equids (horses, donkeys, and mules); the agents of oomycosis (*Aphanomyces*, *Lagenidium*, *Pythium*, and *Saprolegnia*), which cause a variety of diseases in fish and mammals; and miscellaneous conditions involving the skin and subcutis, including chromoblastomycosis, phaeohyphomycosis, and mycetoma. Systemic mycoses, of which skin lesions may be one manifestation, are described in Chapter 47.

S. schenckii

Sporotrichosis is a relatively rare disease caused by *Sporothrix* species (usually *S. schenckii*, although several other causative species have recently been reported) that are saprophytic, dimorphic fungi. In immune-competent people, this disease usually manifests as a chronic, ulcerative lymphangitis of skin and subcutis. Systemic (disseminated) disease occurs occasionally in immunocompromised human patients (e.g., alcoholics; individuals affected with the human immunodeficiency virus). In immune-competent horses and dogs, the disease is usually limited to the cutaneous or cutaneolymphatic form, and organisms are typically sparse or rare within the lesions. Disseminated disease is very rare in horses and dogs unless the patient is immunosuppressed. Conversely, most cats with sporotrichosis will develop cutaneolymphatic or disseminated disease regardless of their immune status at the time of infection. Further, in cats, organisms are typically abundant and found easily within the lesions and exudates.

Descriptive Features

Morphology and Staining. *S. schenckii* is a dimorphic fungus; that is, it exhibits a different morphology depending upon the conditions of growth. At room temperature (25 °C, on Sabouraud's agar), *S. schenckii* grows as a mold. This so-called saprophytic phase consists of septate hyphae, with oval or tear-shaped conidia (2–3 μm by 3–6 μm) in clusters on conidiophores and along hyphae. At 35–37 °C (in tissue or on rich media, e.g., blood agar, incubated at that temperature), it exists as budding pleomorphic yeasts (characterized typically by the unique "cigar bodies" but yeasts can also be round shaped) measuring up to 10 μm in the longest dimension. The yeast phase stains with the Gram's stain, and either phase accepts Romanowsky-type stain (e.g., Wright's or Giemsa) (Figure 46.1) or fungal stains (periodic acid Schiff, Grocott methenamine silver, and Gridley).

Cellular Constituents and Products. *S. schenckii* possesses a typical fungal cell wall containing chitin, and ergosterol. Various glycoconjugates found upon the wall have adhesive properties (see Section "Cellular Products of Medical Interest").

Cellular Products of Medical Interest

Adhesins. The cell wall of *S. schenckii* contains glycoconjugates with affinity for extracellular matrix proteins

Original chapter written by Drs. Dwight C. Hirsh and Ernst L. Biberstein.

Veterinary Microbiology, Third Edition. Edited by D. Scott McVey, Melissa Kennedy and M.M. Chengappa.

FIGURE 46.1. *Exudate from a cutaneous sporotrichosis lesion in a cat. Note the pleomorphism of the yeast cells; shapes vary from round- to oval- to cigar-shaped (cigar bodies) (modified Wright's stain, 1000×).*

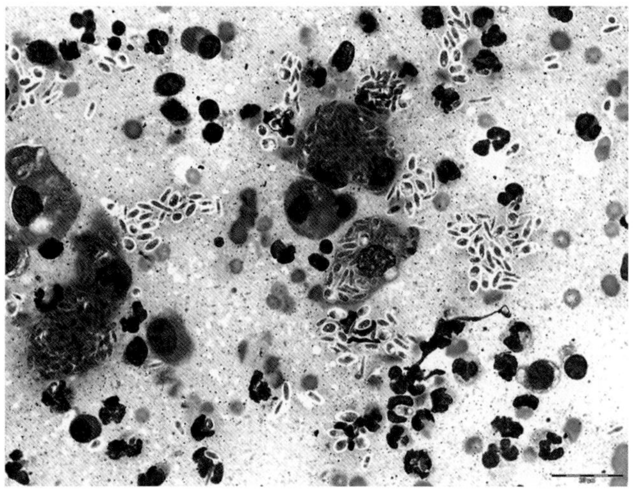

(fibronectin, laminin, and type II collagen). This interaction does not involve an "Arg–Gly–Asp" sequence.

Cell Wall. The cell wall of *S. schenckii* contains several substances that may play a role in the virulence of this microorganism. These include lipid, melanin, peptide-rhamnomannan, and sialic acid:

1. *Lipid*: The lipid portion of the cell wall of *S. schenckii* inhibits phagocytosis by monocytes and macrophages.
2. *Melanin*: Melanin found in the cell wall protects *S. schenckii* from the effects of reactive oxygen intermediates within phagolysosomes of phagocytic cells. Melanin is a free radical scavenger (reduces the toxicity of hydroxy radicals, superoxides, and singlet oxygen radicals found within the phagolysosome).
3. *Peptide-rhamnomannan*: The peptide-rhamnomannan fraction of the cell wall acts as an immunosuppressive substance by suppressing the liberation of proinflammatory cytokines by phagocytic cells.
4. *Sialic acids*: Sialic acids found in the cell wall inhibit uptake of *S. schenckii* by phagocytic cells. Sialic acid directs complement proteins toward the degradative pathway, rather than generating effective opsonizing fragments and anaphylatoxins needed to generate an effective inflammatory response.

Proteinases. *S. schenckii* produces two proteinases: I and II. The significance of these enzymes in the pathogenesis of sporotrichosis is unclear. However, these enzymes are believed to hydrolyze human stratum corneum cells *in vitro*.

Growth Characteristics. After several days on Sabouraud's agar at room temperature, initially moist, off-white to black colonies develop that become wrinkled and fuzzy. On blood agar at 35–37 °C, whitish, smooth yeast colonies appear within a few days. Colonies at room temperature on potato dextrose agar are black and wrinkled.

Variability. Examination of mitochondrial DNA (by restriction length polymorphism analysis) shows that there are at least 20 different types or strains of *S. schenckii* (1–20).

Ecology

Reservoir. The organism prefers soil rich in decaying and organic matter; it has also been isolated on many live plants throughout the world. Occasionally it is isolated from claws of clinically healthy cats, mucous membranes of healthy animals and animal products. Disease has been reported in people, dogs, cats, horses, mules, donkeys, goats, cattle, rats, mice, hamsters, foxes, birds, camels, dolphins, armadillos, and chimpanzees. The disease is most common in the cat, dog, and horse where it occurs in multiple forms. Human infections are often associated with rose gardening (and often called a "rose gardener's disease") since infection usually occurs via a traumatic puncture wound after handling plants and plant materials. More correctly, however, any thorny plant should be regarded as a possible source of infection. Infection via inhalation of spores has also been reported, but this is much less common.

Transmission. The mycelial form of the organism enters the tissue via traumatic inoculation and then converts to the yeast form where local proliferation of the organism occurs to result in ulcerated, exudative, cutaneous nodules that involve the dermal and subcutaneous tissues. These discharging lesions may be contagious, especially in cats where the numbers of microorganisms in the exudates from this species are quite large. The organism has also been isolated from nails of affected cats, and from clinically healthy cats in contact with infected individuals. Rare cases of internal infection are due to inhalation or ingestion.

Pathogenesis

Postinoculation, local proliferation of the organism and the associated inflammatory reaction results in draining wounds that first appear similar to cat-bite abscesses or cellulitis. These wounds, that are refractory to antibiotic therapy, progress to become ulcerated cutaneous nodules that involve the dermal and subcutaneous tissues. Subsequently the affected area becomes ulcerated and forms large crusts. The typical inflammatory reaction is pyogranulomatous, with a purulent center surrounded by epithelioid and multinucleated macrophages, and, peripherally, lymphocytes and plasma cells. However, upon removal of the crusts there is often a purulent exudate. The infectious process follows subcutaneous lymph channels, producing suppurating ulcers at intervals. These heal slowly but often re-erupt. Lymphatics often become thickened. In immune-competent patients (except cats), the disease is usually limited to the cutaneous or cutaneolymphatic form. Again, with the exception of cats, disseminated disease is very rare unless the patient is immunosuppressed. Conversely, most cats will develop cutaneolymphatic or disseminated disease regardless of their immune status at the time of infection, and thus dissemination to viscera, joints, bones, and the central nervous system is common in cats.

Proteinases are possible virulence factors, and proteinase inhibitors have been shown to suppress nodule formation. Cell wall constituents and adhesins delay elimination of the microorganism.

Epidemiology. Sporotrichosis is acquired from the nonliving environment, but transmission from suppurating lesions is possible. The zoonotic potential of infection from cats to people is well established. The occurrence of infection transmission from dogs and horses to people is not as well documented. It is reported that the abundance of organisms in the lesions, exudates, feces, and under the nails of infected cats and the relative lack of organisms in the lesions of dogs is the reason for this difference. However, transmission from cats to people has been reported even when the cat's lesions have had very few organisms, and transmission from dogs has not occurred when owners have been exposed to lesions with abundant organisms. Therefore, it is likely that there are other factors that affect zoonotic potential, and not simply the number of organisms in a lesion. Transmission from person to person does not occur.

Immunologic Aspects

Cell-mediated reactivity is significantly related to resistance. No artificial immunization procedures exist.

Laboratory Diagnosis

Direct examination of exudates is often unrewarding except with feline specimens or specimens from immune compromised patients, which generally contain abundant yeast cells (round-shaped organisms and cigar bodies) (Figure 46.1). If organisms are present in the cytologic preparation, identification of the organism is straightforward assuming the classic oval to cigar-shaped yeast forms (cigar bodies) are seen. However, in rare instances when only the round-shaped yeast forms are present, these organisms can be difficult to distinguish from *H. capsulatum*. In tissue sections, *S. schenckii* has also reportedly been misidentified as *Cryptococcus neoformans*. This error is likely due to an artifact of sample preparation in which there is contraction of the cytoplasm from the cell wall resulting in the impression of a large clear capsule. With other hosts, fungal stains and immunofluorescence may help detect yeast cells.

The agent grows readily in culture. Definitive diagnosis requires demonstration of both phases. Serologic tests (yeast cell and latex agglutination, agar gel diffusion) have had limited use in animals. Molecular techniques utilizing the polymerase chain reaction (PCR) with primers designed to amplify segments of the gene encoding the chitin synthase 1 have been used to demonstrate the fungus in clinical samples, as well as identification of isolates (useful when an isolate resists the mold–yeast conversion).

Treatment and Control

The cutaneous form responds generally to the oral administration of sodium or potassium iodides. The azole drugs, especially itraconazole and ketoconazole, are effective. Terbinafine (an allylamine antifungal agent, which inhibits ergosterol biosynthesis) has shown some success in treating human patients with the cutaneous form of sporotrichosis. Amphotericin B and flucytosine are used on deep and disseminated forms.

H. capsulatum var. *farciminosum*

H. capsulatum is a dimorphic fungus existing as a mold at 25–30 °C (saprophytic phase) and as a yeast at 37 °C (parasitic phase). This fungus has three varieties: *H. capsulatum* var. *capsulatum*, *H. capsulatum* var. *duboisii*, and *H. capsulatum* var. *farciminosum*. Varieties *capsulatum* and *duboisii* cause histoplasmosis, a systemic fungal disease that is discussed in Chapter 47. Variety *farciminosum* causes epizootic lymphangitis (pseudoglanders), a chronic pyogranulomatous disease typically involving the skin and lymphatics that mainly affects horses, donkeys, and mules but has also been reported in camels, cattle and dogs. In mice, guinea pigs, and rabbits, experimental infections have been established. Rarely, internal organs may be involved.

Descriptive Features

Morphology and Staining. *H. capsulatum* var. *farciminosum*, a dimorphic fungus, produces budding yeasts (2–3 μm by 3–4 μm) in tissue, and usually sterile hyphae in its mycelial form when grown at 25 °C or room temperature. Exceptionally, arthroconidia, chlamydoconidia, and spherical, thick-walled macroconidia are seen.

The yeast phase is best demonstrated with a Romanowsky-type stain (e.g., Wright's or Giemsa) or fungal stains (periodic acid Schiff, Grocott methenamine silver, and Gridley).

Growth Characteristics. *H. capsulatum* var. *farciminosum* grows on common laboratory media (Sabouraud's glucose, infusion, and blood-supplemented media with or without cycloheximide and antibacterial agents) over a broad temperature range. The optimum for mycelial growth is 25–30 °C, taking several weeks to form a cottony, white to brown colony. Pigmentation parallels abundance of macroconidia. The yeast phase requires rich media (e.g., glucose cysteine blood agar and brain–heart infusion blood agar) and temperatures of 34–37 °C, taking several days to form a cream to tan, yeast-like colony. Conversion of mold to yeast on blood-containing agar requires incubation at 37 °C under 15–20% CO_2. Several passages may be needed to convert the mold to the yeast phase.

Resistance. *H. capsulatum* var. *farciminosum* is quite resistant to physical and chemical agents. It survives in soil at ambient temperatures for months (several weeks in corrals and stables) and at refrigerator temperature or in a desiccated form for years.

Ecology

Reservoir. The primary reservoir for *Histoplasma* species is nitrogen-rich soil.

Transmission. Infection is thought to occur through skin wounds. Infective organisms may be in the yeast form and come from skin lesions, or nasal and/or ocular exudates of infected animals, or they may be in the mycelial from the environment (e.g., soil). Fomites such as grooming or harness equipment are also a source of infection. Organisms spread most readily where large numbers of equids are assembled in high concentrations in tropical and subtropical climates since warm, moist conditions allow the organism to survive in the soil for months. Arthropods may play a part. Respiratory and localized gastrointestinal infections, which are rare, likely develop subsequent to inhalation or ingestion of the organism, respectively. However, experimental studies have not reliably been able to establish gastrointestinal disease with oral administration of organisms.

Pathogenesis

The first symptom is a painless, freely moveable skin nodule, which overtime enlarges, becomes abscessed, and eventually bursts resulting in an ulcerated lesion. Although some lesions seem to heal spontaneously, more commonly they continue to ulcerate and grow, with periods of granulation, and partial healing, followed by the development of new lesions. Typically, adjacent lymphatics develop nodules along their course, showing the same alternating activity. Regional lymph nodes develop abscesses, which drain by sinus tracts to the outside, but fever is uncommon. Hematogenous spread and visceral involvement is possible. Histologically, the process evolves from suppurative to granulomatous (pyogranulomatous), marked by lymphocytes, macrophages, and giant cells, to eventual fibrosis. Yeast cells occur extracellularly and intracellularly, especially in macrophages.

Skin lesions, chiefly on head, neck, and limbs, are the predominant signs. The general condition is usually unaffected except in the primary respiratory tract or disseminated infections. Mild cases do not progress beyond the local stage.

Epidemiology. Endemic areas include parts of Africa, much of Asia including India, Japan, and Pakistan, and the Mediterranean littoral. The epidemiology of *H. capsulatum* var. *farciminosum* infection is unclear. Manifestations vary with geographic area. Seasonal peaks suggest arthropod transmission.

The disease mainly affects equids but cattle, camelids, and dogs may also be affected. Young horses (less than 6 years of age) are most susceptible.

Immunologic Factors

The role of immune mechanisms in pathogenesis or resistance is not known, but cell-mediated immunity is probably the key host defense. Skin sensitivity develops following exposure, even in the absence of disease. Circulating antibodies, demonstrable by indirect fluorescent antibody, agar gel diffusion, an enzyme-linked immunosorbent assay, or by the serum agglutination tests, are indicative of infection.

Laboratory Diagnosis

Differential diagnosis includes sporotrichosis (see Section "*S. schenckii*") and ulcerative lymphangitis produced by *Corynebacterium pseudotuberculosis* (see Chapter 30). The agent must be demonstrated. Direct examination of stained exudates (Wright's or Giemsa stained) or biopsy material (hematoxylin–eosin, periodic acid Schiff, and Grocott methenamine silver) may reveal intracellular (within macrophages) or extracellular characteristic yeasts.

H. capsulatum var. *farciminosum* grows on Sabouraud's glucose agar with inhibitors (cycloheximide and chloramphenicol). Mycelial extracts contain genus-specific antigens demonstrable by agar gel diffusion or by the serum agglutination test. Growth patterns and microscopic morphology differentiate *H. capsulatum* var. *farciminosum* from *H. capsulatum* var. *capsulatum* (Chapter 47).

Treatment and Control

Intravenous iodides (with or without griseofulvin) have been relatively successful. Amphotericin B has been used with some success. Itraconazole and fluconazole may also be used. In nonendemic areas, destruction of infected animals is advisable.

Oomycosis

Oomycosis is caused by a member of a group of eukaryotic microorganisms belonging to the kingdom Stramenopiles (which also contains the diatoms and brown algae). They are saprophytic microbes that usually live in water and moist soil. Although they are morphologically similar to fungi (they produce hyphae in tissue and grow as mold-like colonies on media *in vitro*), they are not members of the kingdom Fungi. Members of this group are the agents of several plant and animal diseases. Historically, the most notorious is *Phytophthora*, the cause of the Irish potato famine, which at present is responsible for killing oak trees along the Pacific coast of North America. The following genera are associated with disease in animals: *Aphanomyces* (ulcerative disease of fish and crustaceans), *Lagenidium* (pyogranulomatous disease of dogs and cats identical clinically to pythiosis), *Pythium* (pyogranulomatous disease, called pythiosis, of a variety of animal species), and *Saprolegnia* (systemic disease of cultured salmonids). The discussion that follows is focused on *Pythium insidiosum*, the cause of pyogranulomatous conditions (pythiosis) of dogs ("swamp cancer"), horses ("Florida horse leeches"), cattle, cats, and people.

Cutaneous Pythiosis ("Swamp Cancer"—"Florida Horse Leeches")

The genus *Pythium* contains over 85 species, and only *P. insidiosum* is associated with disease in animals.

P. insidiosum causes ulcerative fibrogranulomatous or pyogranulomatous and eosinophilic cutaneous and subcutaneous lesions in horses, cattle, dogs, and cats, and gastrointestinal disease in dogs. It has also been reported as a cause of arteritis, keratitis, or periorbital cellulitis in people. It is mainly seen in tropical or subtropical areas—in North America this disease is seen most frequently diagnosed along the Gulf Coast. Dogs and horses are the species most commonly affected. The agent is an aquatic oomycete with wide (4 μm), sparsely septate hyphae. Lesions in horses are typically large, exudative swellings, usually on extremities, ventral trunk, or head. The nasal mucosa may be involved. Hyphae are demonstrable within granulomatous coagula (termed "kunkers" or "leeches" in horses) consisting of necrotic macrophages (including epithelioid and multinucleated macrophages), eosinophils.

Diagnostic methods include cytology (in which the broad, poorly septate, and branching hyphal elements are seen among the pyogranulomatous and eosinophilic inflammation), serology (an enzyme-linked immunosorbent assay), molecular techniques (utilizing primers designed to amplify *P. insidiosum*-specific DNA by means of the PCR), immunohistochemical examination of exudates, and culture. Cultural techniques are tedious and time-consuming and entail growth of a mold-like microorganism on Sabouraud's dextrose agar or brain–heart infusion agar after 24–48 h at 30 °C. Identification requires demonstration of motile zoospores and/or reaction of extracts of the isolate with reference antisera. The PCR-based assay mentioned is used to establish the presence of *P. insidiosum* in clinical samples as well as for identification of isolates. The PCR assay also successfully identifies members of the genus *Lagenidium* (another oomycete), which produces a similar clinical picture in dogs and cats.

Early diagnosis is the key to successful treatment. Treatments include surgery and antifungal therapy (amphotericin B). Immunotherapy utilizing killed whole organisms or extracts has shown promise.

Chromoblastomycosis and Phaeohyphomycosis

Chromoblastomycosis and phaeohyphomycosis are caused by dark-pigmented (dematiaceous) fungi. Most of the roughly 70 species implicated belong to the genera *Alternaria, Bipolaris, Cladosporium, Cladophialophora, Curvularia, Exophiala, Fonsecaea, Phaeoacremonium,* and *Phialophora*. In chromoblastomycosis, the fungal elements in tissue are large (<12 μm), pigmented, "sclerotic bodies." Infections in which hyphae are present are called phaeohyphomycosis.

Chromoblastomycosis is rare in nonhuman mammals, but occurs in frogs and toads. Phaeohyphomycosis is seen sporadically in cats, dogs, horses, cattle, and goats and may be systemic. *Cladophialophora bantiana* is the fungus most commonly seen in dogs and cats, with central nervous system localization frequently observed.

The agents, soil- and plant-associated saprophytes, enter through skin and multiply subcutaneously, causing pyogranulomatous reactions. No tissue colonies or granules are seen. Nodular or larger swellings develop, which may ulcerate and discharge pus.

Diagnosis is made by biopsy and culture. Sclerotic bodies (chromoblastomycosis) and hyphae (phaeohyphomycosis) are seen in stained (hematoxylin–eosin, periodic acid Schiff, and Grocott methenamine silver) biopsy sections. Culture, on Sabouraud's agar without inhibitors, often requires lengthy incubation. The resulting colonies range from olive to brown to black, depending on the color of species of fungus involved

Lesions are excised, but may recur. Medical treatment (flucytosine, itraconazole, amphotericin B, and ketoconazole) has given mixed results.

Eumycotic Mycetoma

Swelling, granule formation, and discharging sinus tracts are characteristics of mycetoma. They may be associated with bacteria, most notably an actinomycete such as members of the genus *Nocardia* or *Actinomyces* (actinomycotic mycetoma, see Chapter 36) or a fungus (eumycotic mycetoma). Mycetomas are occasionally reported in cattle, horses, dogs, and cats. The cutaneous form is often nodular and is associated with similar nasal lesions.

Fungi associated with eumycotic mycetoma include *Pseudallescheria boydii, Cochliobolus spiciferus* (the sexual forms of *Scedosporium apiospermum* and *Bipolaris spicifera*, respectively), and *Curvularia geniculata*. All are saprophytes that presumably enter via a wound. It is not clear what triggers this course of pathogenesis because the same agents can cause other pathologic patterns.

Fungal colonies are surrounded by suppuration bordered by granulomatous reactions. Sinus tracts carry pus and granules, consisting of microorganisms and inflammatory components, to the surface. The color and the texture of granules vary depending on the species of fungus involved in the mycetoma. The processes are slowly progressive, involving adjacent tissues.

Treatment is excision if possible. Antifungal agents (azoles and amphotericin B) have been disappointing.

Rhinosporidiosis

The cause of this disease is *Rhinosporidium seeberi*. This fungus occurs in nature and has not been cultivated on fungal media, but has been propagated in cell culture. It causes chronic granulomatous type of infection at mucocutaneous junction in horses, cattle mules, dogs, goats, and wild waterfowls. Infection, though rare, occurs in humans. Formation of cauliflower-like growths, also known as polyps, is very characteristic of infection caused by this fungus. The disease occurs mostly in tropical and subtropical countries; however, sporadic cases have been reported in the United States. Diagnosis is based on gross lesion and microscopic examination of tissue sections or discharge from polyps. On tissue section, presence of large sporangia (200–300 μm) filled with endospores is sufficient to make a

FIGURE 46.2. *Impression smear of cauliflower-like growth in the nasal cavity of a dog. Note the central clump of endospores among the pyogranulomatous inflammation (modified Wright's stain, 1000×).*

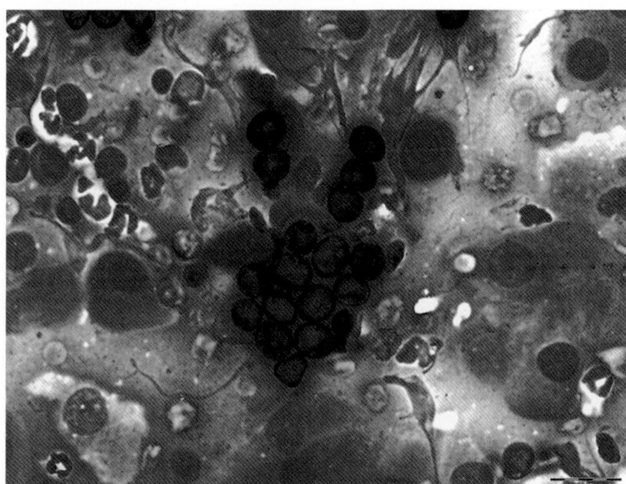

definitive diagnosis of this disease. On cytologic preparations, however, sporangia are rarely seen and the numerous endospores are the typical finding (Figure 46.2). Treatment is not effective. Surgical excision is practiced, but many lesions recur.

Further Reading

Ginn PE, Mansell JEKL, and Rakich PM (2007) *Skin and Appendages in Jubb, Kennedy, and Palmer's Pathobiology of Domestic Animals*, vol. 1, 5th edn, Elsevier Saunders.

Greene CE (2006) *Infectious Diseases of the Dog and Cat*, 3rd edn, Elsevier Saunders.

Gross TE, Ihrke PJ, Walder EJ, and Affolter VK (2006) *Skin Diseases of the Dog and Cat: Clinical and Histopathologic Diagnosis*, 2nd edn, Blackwell Science.

Raskin R and Meyer D (2009) *Canine and Feline Cytology: A Color Atlas and Interpretation Guide*, 2nd edn, W.B. Elsevier Saunders Company.

Songer JG and Post KW (2005) *Veterinary Microbiology: Bacterial and Fungal Agents of Animal Diseases*, Elsevier Saunders.

Agents of Systemic Mycoses

M.M. Chengappa and Lisa M. Pohlman

Whether a fungus is categorized as mold or yeast is based upon the microscopic appearance in tissue or on routine culture media (the asexual stage). Microscopically, if hyphal structures are observed, the fungus is termed a mold; if single-celled, budding structures are observed, the fungus is termed a yeast. On routine culture media, molds will have a "fuzzy" or wooly appearance, and yeast will be bacteria-like in its colonial morphology and consistency. Some pathogenic fungi will produce either hyphal-like structures or yeast-like structures, depending upon the conditions in which they are growing. Such fungi are called dimorphic fungi. These fungi are discussed here and in Chapter 46.

The agents of most systemic (or "deep") mycoses are saprophytic fungi. Morphologically and ecologically diverse, they share disease-related features:

1. Many are dimorphic; that is, their saprophytic and parasitic phases differ morphologically. *Coccidioides*, *Histoplasma*, *Blastomyces*, and *Paracoccidioides* grow as molds in their inanimate habitat. In tissue, *Coccidioides* produces sporangia, whereas the others grow as budding yeasts.
2. Infection is usually by inhalation.
3. Host factors are often the decisive disease determinants. Some mycoses (aspergillosis and zygomycosis) are seen primarily in immunocompromised animals.
4. Lesions tend to be granulomatous to pyogranulomatous. After primary pulmonary infection, the course of disease is determined by the effectiveness of cell-mediated immune responses. If these are inadequate, dissemination may occur to bone, skin, central nervous system, or abdominal viscera.
5. Systemic mycoses are noncontagious. Although the agent is often demonstrably shed, it fails to infect individuals on contact.
6. Since the inflammatory lesions are granulomatous to pyogranulomatous, all have the potential to cause hypercalcemia in the patient. This hypercalcemia occurs as a result of the response to granulomatous inflammation in which activated macrophages are stimulated to convert vitamin D precursors to the active form of vitamin D (i.e., calcitriol) in an unregulated manner. This chapter discusses the dimorphic fungi *Coccidioides immitis*, *Histoplasma capsulatum*, and *Blastomyces dermatitidis*, together with the mold *Aspergillus*. The fungus *Pneumocystis* and the alga *Prototheca* are briefly mentioned.

Original chapter written by Drs. Dwight C. Hirsh and Ernst L. Biberstein.

Coccidioides

Members of the genus *Coccidioides* are dimorphic fungi. The genus *Coccidioides* contains two species: *immitis* and *posadasii*. The disease, coccidioidomycosis, is caused by both. *C. immitis* and *C. posadasii* differ in their preferred geographic habitats. Both species occur only in the Western Hemisphere in the Lower Sonoran Life Zone, apparently as a result of the area's peculiar soil properties and temperature and rainfall patterns. *C. immitis* is found in the Central Valley of California in the United States (mainly the San Joaquin Valley), whereas *C. posadasii* is found in non-California locations (Texas, New Mexico, and Arizona in the United States, and in South America). Of domestic animals, dogs are most frequently affected, and horses are occasionally affected. Less commonly infections are also reported in cats, swine, sheep, cattle, human and non-human primates, and some 30 species of nondomestic mammals.

Descriptive Features

Morphology, Structure, and Composition. In the soil, *Coccidioides* is a mold made up of slender septate hyphae that give rise, on thicker secondary branches, to chains of infectious arthroconidia (arthrospores, arthroaleuriospores, and arthroaleurioconidia). These are bulging, barrel-shaped, thick-walled cells, 2–4 μm by 3–6 μm,

Veterinary Microbiology, Third Edition. Edited by D. Scott McVey, Melissa Kennedy and M.M. Chengappa.

FIGURE 47.1. *Tissue section from a skin lesion on a dog. A large* C. immitis *spherule containing endospores (arrow) surrounded by pyogranulomatous inflammation (hematoxylin–eosin stain, 1000×).*

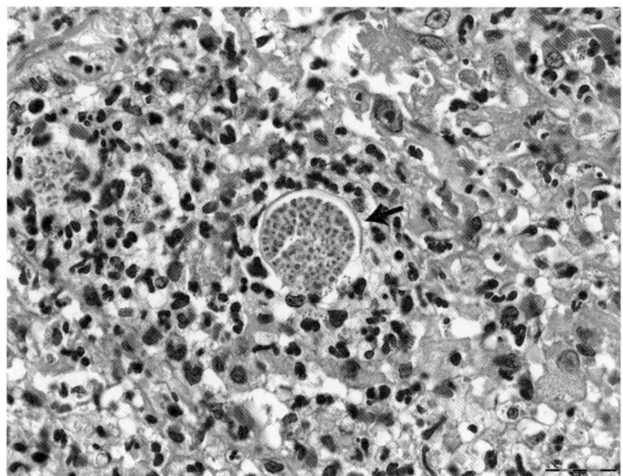

separated by empty cells (disjunctors), through which breaks occur when arthroconidia are dispersed.

In tissue, arthroconidia grow into spherical sporangia with birefringent walls, "spherules" (10–100 μm in diameter), which by internal cleavage produce several hundred "endospores" (2–5 μm in diameter) (Figure 47.1). The walls disintegrate, allowing dissemination of endospores, each of which may repeat the cycle or, on a nonliving substrate, give rise to mycelial (a collection of hyphae) growth. Although only arthroconidia are naturally infectious, endospores can experimentally initiate disease. Sexual spores are not known.

"Coccidioidin" in supernatants of mycelial *Coccidioides* broth cultures is largely polysaccharide, but contains some amino acid nitrogen. It is used in cutaneous hypersensitivity and serologic tests. "Spherulin," a lysate of cultured spherules, is also used in skin tests.

Cellular Products of Medical Interest

Adhesins. SOWgp (for spherule outer wall glycoprotein) is a proline-rich glycoprotein adhesin on the surface of spherules. SOWgp has affinity for extracellular matrix proteins (laminin, fibronectin, and collagen). SOWgp stimulates a strong T_{H2} lymphocyte response, resulting in elevated levels of antibody and suppression of the protective cell-mediated immune response. Mutants unable to produce SOWgp have greatly reduced virulence.

Miscellaneous Products

1. *β-Glucosidase 2*: Bgl2 (for β-glucosidase 2) is an enzyme secreted by the endospores of *Coccidioides* that most likely plays a role in endospore morphology. Antibodies (IgM isotype) to Bgl2 are made early in the infectious process, and are useful diagnostically (detected by the precipitin test) to signal that a recent infection has occurred.
2. *Chitinase 1*: Cts1 (for chitinase 1) is one of several chitinases that are involved with the formation of, and release of, endospores from the spherule. An important target for the Cts enzymes is the "segregation apparatus" (a weblike mesh of chitin-containing structures within the spherule). Antibodies (IgG isotype) to Cts1 are made late in the infectious process (in disseminated disease), and are useful diagnostically (detected by the complement fixation, CF, test).
3. *β-1,3-glucanosyltransferase*: Gel (for glucan-elongating glucanosyltransferase) is located on the surface of endospores. Gel elicits a strong T_{H1} lymphocyte response, resulting in elevated levels of γ-interferon followed by protection against disseminated disease (activates macrophages).
4. *Serine proteases*: These enzymes play a role in the stimulation of the inflammatory response elicited by *Coccidioides*. These enzymes digest elastin, collagen, and immunoglobulins
5. *Urease*: Although its role in virulence is unknown, the enzyme urease (Ure) elicits a strong protective immune response following stimulation of T_{H1} lymphocytes (activates macrophages).

Growth Characteristics. *Coccidioides* grows on simple media over a broad temperature range. On Sabouraud's or blood agar, growth is mycelial. Over several days, initially dull gray colonies develop with sparse aerial mycelium, which gradually becomes more abundant. Arthroconidia are produced in 5–7 days.

Spherules (sporangia) can be demonstrated *in vitro* by growth at 40 °C in media containing casein hydrolysate, glucose, biotin, glutathione, and a salt mixture (spherule medium).

Ecology

Reservoir. *Coccidioides* inhabits the soil in the Lower Sonoran Life Zone, including parts of California in North America (*C. immitis*) and the southwestern portion of the United States, Mexico, Central America, the northern and western rim states of South America, Argentina, and Paraguay (*C. posadasii*). High prevalence is associated with an annual rainfall of 5–20 inches and mean summer and winter temperatures of over 80 °F and 45 °F, respectively.

Arthroconidia resist drying and tolerate heat and salinity better than do competing soil organisms. In summer heat, *Coccidioides* survives in soil layers nearer the surface than its competitors. When conditions favor growth again after rains, *Coccidioides* repopulates the superficial soil layers first, ensuring its widespread dispersal. Arthroconidia are dispersed by wind. Rodent burrows are heavily concentrated with arthroconidia in endemic areas. Dogs are frequently exposed to the fungus by sniffing the burrows.

Transmission. Infection is caused mainly by inhalation of arthroconidia. The organism is highly infectious and very few arthroconidia need to be inhaled to produce disease. Primary cutaneous infections are rare.

Pathogenesis

Mechanisms and Pathology. Following inhalation, the barrel-shaped arthroconidia round into spherical-shaped endospores, which, following enlargement and internal cleavage, differentiate into multinucleate spherules (10–100 μm) containing hundreds of endospores (2–5 μm), a process that takes several days. Spherules rupture, releasing endospores, and the cycle is repeated. Arthroconidia, endospores, and spherules trigger an inflammatory response in the lung (serine proteases are partly responsible). Arthroconidia and endospores are engulfed but not killed by phagocytes, and are conveyed to the hilar lymph node, where another inflammatory focus develops (as well as more spherules). Inflammation is stimulated in part by serine proteases, which are liberated during the growth of the fungus. Normally, cell-mediated immune responses arrest the process at this stage following stimulation of T_{H1} lymphocytes that activate macrophages, permitting destruction of the endospores. Antibodies to Bgl2 are made during this phase of the infectious process. With inadequate cell-mediated immunity (caused by SOWgp-directed immunomodulation, genetic makeup, and infectious dose), dissemination can occur to bones, skin, abdominal viscera, heart, genital tract, and eyes (and rarely in animals to brain and meninges). Gross lesions are white granulomas varying from miliary nodules to irregular masses. Peritoneal, pleural, and pericardial effusions occur. Antibodies to Cts1 are made during this phase of the infectious process. Microscopically, the predominant response is pyogranulomatous: to arthroconidia and endospores, the response is suppurative; and to spherules, the response is granulomatous, with epithelioid macrophages the chief component, admixed with multinucleated giant cells, lymphocytes, and neutrophils (Figure 47.1).

Disease Patterns

Dogs. Disseminated disease of dogs is the pattern seen most commonly by veterinarians. The complaints are lassitude, anorexia, and loss of condition. There may be respiratory signs (including cough), fever, and lameness due to bone involvement or arthritis, or discharging sinuses from deep lesions.

Cats. Disseminated disease in cats presents with less osseous and more visceral involvement. Skin lesions are the most frequent reason for presentation to the veterinarian.

Horses. As with cats, there is usually less osseous and more visceral involvement.

Cattle, Sheep, and Swine. In these species, the disease is usually asymptomatic, limited to lungs and regional lymph nodes, and undiagnosed until slaughter.

Human Beings. Naturally occurring, asymptomatic coccidioidomycosis occurs frequently in humans. Clinical symptoms range from a flu-like illness to severe pneumonia. It is fatal in immunocompromised patients.

Epidemiology. In all species, overt disease is the exception. Highest prevalence of canine systemic coccidioidomycosis is observed in male dogs, 4–7 years of age, with peak occurrence of illnesses from January to March and May to July. These peaks may represent seasonal stress and increased exposure, respectively. Geographic and climatic factors have been mentioned. Young Boxer dogs and Doberman Pinschers appear particularly susceptible.

Immunologic Aspects

Cell-mediated hypersensitivity, as determined by skin tests, develops within one or more weeks of exposure and can persist indefinitely. Its presence is an indicator of resistance to progressive disease. Its absence is the rule in disseminated infections, and its return is a favorable sign.

IgM antibody (specific for Bgl2), demonstrable by tube precipitin or latex particle test, appears temporarily after infection and usually disappears. IgG antibody titers (specific for Cts1), which are detectable by CF and immunodiffusion tests, rise in disseminated disease and remain high (1 : 16) until the process is brought under control.

No vaccine is presently available.

Laboratory Diagnosis

Direct Examination of Specimens. Animal fluids and tissues are examined for spherules by wet mount in saline containing 10% KOH. Spherules are 10–100 μm in diameter, have a thick wall (<2 μm), and contain endospores when mature (see Figure 47.1). Free endospores look indistinct in wet mounts but are recognizable in fixed smears stained by a fungal stain (e.g., periodic acid Schiff, Gridley, or Gomori methenamine silver stains).

Cytologic preparations, such as aspirates or imprints of lesions, stained with Romanowsky-type stains, typically reveal the pyogranulomatous inflammation and may have the characteristic large (diameter of 10–100 μm), double-contoured, clear to blue spheres that have variably visible round endospores inside. It is the presence of endospores and the extreme variation in size of the spheres that differentiates this organism from *B. dermatitidis*. Stained tissue sections (hematoxylin and eosin, Figure 47.1, Gomori methenamine silver, or Gridley) show both the agent and the characteristic lesion.

Culture. Blood agar and Sabouraud's agar with or without antibiotics are inoculated, tape-sealed, and incubated at 37 °C and 25 °C, respectively. All processing of cultures is done under a microbiological safety hood. Mycelial growth should be evident within a week and is examined for presence of barrel-shaped arthroconidia in a lactophenol cotton blue wet mount. Colonies are white and cottony with tan, brown, pink, or yellow pigmentation. The isolate can be reconverted to the sporangial phase by animal inoculation or cultivation in a spherule medium (see Section "Growth Characteristics"). Culturing and handling of culture should be avoided if a proper biocontainment facility is not available. Contamination of the laboratory with arthrospore could easily occur if the culture is not handled with the proper procedure.

A commercially available "exoantigen" test kit furnishes prepared antisera to *Coccidioides*, *H. capsulatum*, and *B. dermatitidis* to be tested against extracts of suspect cultures in an immunodiffusion agar plate, where precipitation lines develop between extracts and their homologous antisera.

Immunodiagnosis. The CF and immunodiffusion tests detect disseminated disease. Because it is quantifiable, the CF test gauges progress and cure of infection more accurately.

The coccidioidin skin test has been used in animal surveys.

Molecular Methods. Most molecular methods used to identify or detect *Coccidioides* make use of primers specific for sequences contained within the DNA encoding ribosomal RNA. These sequences are amplified using the polymerase chain reaction.

Treatment and Control

Amphotericin B has been the mainstay of anticoccidioidal therapy in human patients. Limitations are its toxicity and the intravenous route of administration, requiring hospitalization or frequent visits. Liposomal preparations of amphotericin B show promise because of lower toxicity, which makes possible higher doses. Fluconazole (drug of choice) ketoconazole and itraconazole are also used in small animals. Given orally over a period of months, they have affected permanent cures. Toxic effects are relatively minor except during pregnancy, when fetal deaths may occur. The CF titer is used to monitor the effect of treatment.

Vaccines are not available.

H. capsulatum var. *capsulatum*

H. capsulatum is a dimorphic fungus existing as a mold at 25–30 °C (saprophytic phase) and as a yeast at 37 °C (parasitic phase). This fungus has three varieties: *H. capsulatum* var. *capsulatum*, *H. capsulatum* var. *duboisii*, and *H. capsulatum* var. *farciminosum*. Variety *farciminosum* causes epizootic lymphangitis (pseudoglanders), a chronic pyogranulomatous disease of equine skin and is discussed in Chapter 46. Varieties *capsulatum* and *duboisii* cause histoplasmosis, a systemic fungal disease of mammals. Variety *duboisii* is found only in Africa, whereas variety *capsulatum* is found worldwide, and is the most common cause of histoplasmosis. In this chapter, histoplasmosis is discussed without regard to this varietal distinction; that is, *H. capsulatum* var. *capsulatum* and *H. capsulatum* var. *duboisii* are regarded as *H. capsulatum*.

Descriptive Features

Morphology, Structure, and Composition. The free-living form of *H. capsulatum* consists of septate hyphae bearing spherical to pyriform microconidia 2–4 μm in diameter, and "tuberculate" macroconidia, thick-walled spheroidal cells, 8–14 μm in diameter, studded with fingerlike projections (Figure 47.2). In animal hosts or appropriate culture, the mold becomes a yeast consisting of round or oval, singly budding cells that measure 2–4 μm in diameter. A sexual, ascomycetous state, *Ajellomyces capsulatus*, has been described.

FIGURE 47.2. H. capsulatum, *mycelial phase. Lactophenol cotton blue mount of a culture grown at 25 °C. "Tuberculate" macromedia studded with finger-like projections, 400×.*

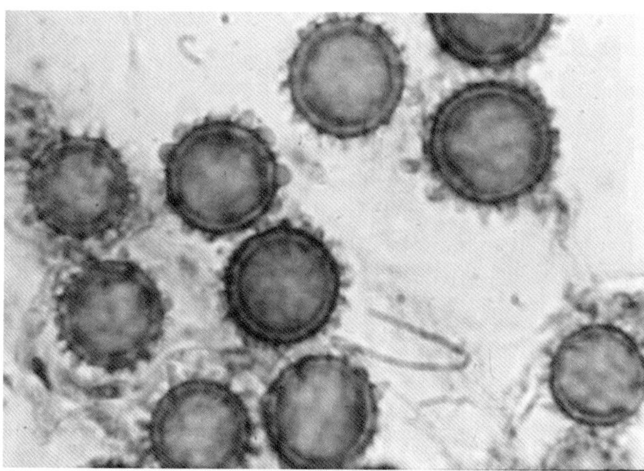

Histoplasmins, which are used in immunodiagnosis, are obtained from mycelial culture filtrates. They contain polysaccharides, with variable admixtures of glycoproteins and cellular breakdown products. Mycelial and yeast phases differ in cellular constituents, some of which (e.g., cell wall glucan) have been related to virulence.

Cellular Products of Medical Interest

Adhesins. Inhaled microconidia and yeast-phase parasitic forms are recognized by, and bind to, β-2 integrins on the surface of neutrophils and macrophages. It is unknown what fungal structure is involved. Likewise, an unknown adhesin is responsible for the adherence of *H. capsulatum* to fibronectin receptors on dendritic cells. Adherence in this fashion to neutrophils, macrophages, or dendritic cells allows the fungus to enter the cell without triggering an effective oxidative burst and the generation of reactive oxygen and nitrogen intermediates.

Miscellaneous Products. *H. capsulatum* produces a variety of products that may play a role in histoplasmosis:

1. *Calcium-binding protein*: The yeast (parasitic) phase of *H. capsulatum* produces a calcium-binding protein (Cbp) that permits the yeast phase to grow in low-calcium environments (the phagolysosome) by efficiently chelating calcium and delivering it to the fungus. In addition, since Cbp chelates available calcium within the phagolysosome, this impedes effectiveness of several calcium-requiring lysosomal enzymes. Normal acidification of the phagolysosome is also a calcium-dependent event. *H. capsulatum* mutants unable to produce Cbp are avirulent.
2. *H antigen*: Host immune responses to H-antigen were originally used as a diagnostic tool in the diagnosis of

histoplasmosis. Subsequently, H-antigen was found to be a β-glucosidase that elicited a cell-mediated (protective) immune response to the yeast (parasitic) phase of *H. capsulatum*.

3. *Iron acquisition*: Iron is an absolute growth requirement for *H. capsulatum* (as it is for all life forms). *H. capsulatum* acquires iron in several ways: production of hydroxamate siderophores capable of removing iron from host iron-binding proteins (transferrin and lactoferrin); expression of a hemin-binding receptor on the surface of yeast (parasitic) forms; glutathione-dependent ferric reductase, which reduces Fe(III) to Fe(II), thereby releasing it from host iron-binding proteins; and several poorly defined iron reductases on the surface of the yeast phase.
4. *M-antigen*: Host immune response to M-antigen was originally used as a diagnostic tool in the diagnosis of histoplasmosis. Subsequently, M-antigen was found to be a catalase enzyme, which played a role in the survival of the yeast phase within the phagolysosome.
5. *Melanin*: Melanin is produced by *H. capsulatum*. Melanin is a free radical scavenger (reducing the toxicity of hydroxy radicals, superoxides, and singlet oxygen radicals found within the phagolysosome).
6. *Phagolysosome acidification*: Normal phagolysosomes have a pH <5, a pH that optimizes the activity of many of the digestive enzymes found in this environment. *H. capsulatum* raises the pH of the phagolysosome to 6.0–6.5, thereby reducing the activity of these lysosomal enzymes. How the fungus does this is unknown.

Growth Characteristics. *H. capsulatum* grows on common laboratory media over a broad temperature range. The optimum temperature for mycelial growth is 25–30 °C. The cottony aerial mycelium is white, brown, or intermediate. Pigmentation parallels abundance of macroconidia. The yeast phase requires richer media (e.g., glucose cysteine blood agar) and temperatures of 34–37 °C. Growth may take a week or more before characteristic colonies are seen.

H. capsulatum survives at ambient temperatures for months and at refrigerator temperature for years. It withstands freezing and thawing and tolerates heating for more than 1 h at 45 °C.

Variability. *H. capsulatum* exists as three varieties: *capsulatum*, *duboisii*, and *farciminosum*. Varieties *capsulatum* (worldwide) and *duboisii* (Africa) produce histoplasmosis, and variety *farciminosum* causes epizootic lymphangitis (pseudoglanders) of equids (see Chapter 46). Although *H. capsulatum* var. *capsulatum* is found worldwide, its central focus is in the Americas. Genetically, variety *capsulatum* is divided into six classes: class 1 and class 2 are found in North America; class 3 is found in Central and South America; class 4 is found in Florida (North America); and class 5 and class 6 are found in human patients with acquired immunodeficiency syndrome from New York (North America) and Panama (Central America), respectively.

Ecology

Reservoir. Although most are concentrated in the Mississippi and Ohio River watersheds of North America, *H. capsulatum* occurs sporadically worldwide. It is found in the topsoil layers, especially in the presence of bird (mainly starlings in North America and chickens in South America) and bat guano, which provide both enrichment (nitrogen) and inoculum. Birds are mainly passive carriers, whereas bats undergo intestinal infectious processes. *H. capsulatum* is favored by neutral to alkaline soil environments with annual rainfall between 35 and 50 inches and mean temperatures between 68 °F and 90 °F.

Transmission. Transmission is mostly by inhalation of microconidia or hyphal fragments, possibly by ingestion, and, rarely, by wound infection.

Pathogenesis

Mechanisms and Pathology. Microconidia, hyphal fragments (from the environment), or yeast cells (from an intraphagocytic cell environment) attach to macrophages in the lung by way of a β-2 integrin. It is immediately phagocytosed, a minimal respiratory burst occurs, and a phagolysosome results following fusion with lysosomes. Microconidia and hyphal elements differentiate into yeast. Survival within the phagolysosome is related to modulation of phagolysosome pH (around 6.0–6.5), secretion of M-antigen (a catalase), secretion of Cbp, melanin, and successful acquisition of iron from intracellular iron stores. The yeast multiplies within the phagolysosome, ultimately killing the cell and the release of yeast cells (which continue the cycle). Intracellular multiplication continues until an effective cell-mediated immune response occurs resulting in activated macrophages, which effectively control the multiplication of the yeast.

Early events and lesions resemble those of tuberculosis. Thoracic lymph nodes become enlarged, and lungs may contain grayish-white nodules. The histologic response varies from suppurative to granulomatous inflammation. Caseation necrosis and calcification are common.

In disseminated disease, lymph nodes and parenchymatous organs are enlarged and may contain gross nodular lesions. There may be ulcerations of skin and mucous membranes, abdominal and pleural effusions, and involvement of the central nervous system (including eyes), skin, and bone marrow. The inflammatory exudate consists of macrophage elements colonized by yeast cells (Figure 47.3).

Disease Patterns. Histoplasmosis can occur in almost any animal species, but dogs and cats are the most commonly affected. Most affected dogs and cats have disseminated disease by the time they present to the veterinarian. A wide range of nonspecific clinical signs are seen in these patients including depression, fever, lethargy, anorexia, weight loss, diarrhea, dehydration, and anemia. Hepatomegaly, splenomegaly, mesenteric lymphadenitis, and ascites may cause abdominal distention. Coughing is relatively common in dogs but not in cats; however, both species often

FIGURE 47.3. *Rectal scraping from a dog with systemic histoplasmosis. Note the numerous intraphagocytic yeast cells that are round to oval and ~2 μm in diameter (modified Wright's stain, 1000×).*

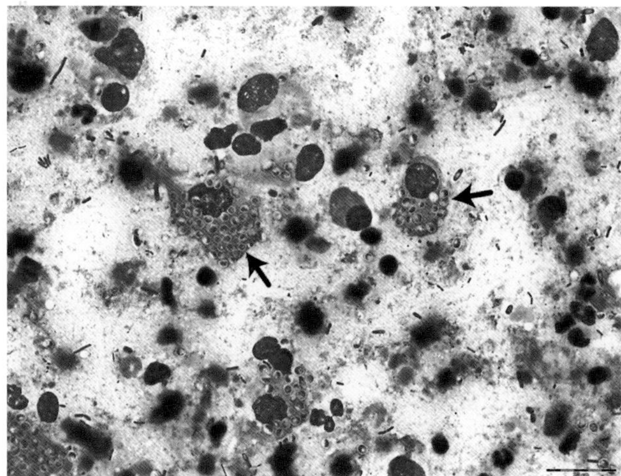

exhibit dyspnea and have abnormal lung sounds. Clinical signs resulting from gastrointestinal involvement are very common in affected dogs, but rare in affected cats.

Disease patterns in human patients parallel those described.

Epidemiology. Subclinical infections with histoplasmosis are common in dogs and cats—and humans—in endemic areas. Clinical disease is most prevalent in dogs aged 2–7 years, in early autumn (September to November) and later winter to early spring (February to April). No sex predilection is reported, but the pointing breeds, Weimaraners, and Brittany spaniels have the greatest risk. Disseminated histoplasmosis in people, dogs, and cats is found in association with immunosuppression.

Immunologic Aspects

Recovery and resistance are governed by cell-mediated immune responses, while circulating antibodies have no apparent protective function. Recovery from histoplasmosis appears to confer immunity.

No vaccines are available. However, certain antigens of *H. capsulatum* appear to protect mice against experimental challenge.

Laboratory Diagnosis

Direct Examination. Blood films, buffy coat smears and cytologic preparations such as aspirates, and tissue impressions are stained with a Romanowsky-type (e.g., Giemsa or Wright's) and examined for intraphagocytic yeast cells that are round to oval (not cigar shaped) and approximately 2–4 μm in diameter (approximately one-fourth to half the size of a RBC) (Figure 47.3). The yeasts stain light blue and have a pink to purple-staining, eccentrically placed nucleus. Organisms are observed primarily within macrophages, but may also be seen within neutrophils, as well as in monocytes in peripheral blood. Fungal stains (periodic acid Schiff, Gridley, or Gomori methenamine silver) may be used to aid visualization, but are not routinely used on cytologic preparations.

In sections stained with hematoxylin–eosin, *H. capsulatum* appears as tiny dots surrounded by haloes. A duplicate fungal stain (e.g., periodic acid Schiff, Gridley, or Gomori methenamine silver) can be helpful.

Immunofluorescence has been used to identify the yeast in tissue and exudates.

Culture. Specimens are inoculated onto blood agar and Sabouraud's agar, with and without inhibitors) and incubated in jars or plastic bags at room temperature for up to 2 months.

Colonial growth may look reddish-wrinkled before the appearance of cottony brownish to white mycelium.

Microconidia and macroconidia are demonstrated in lactophenol cotton blue wet mounts. Dimorphism must be proven by conversion to the yeast phase by incubating plates at 37 °C or by intravenous injection of mice. Mice will die within a few weeks. Their macrophages will contain the yeast forms.

A commercially available "exoantigen" test kit furnishes prepared antisera to *Coccidioides*, *H. capsulatum*, and *B. dermatitidis* to be tested against extracts of suspect cultures in an immunodiffusion agar plate, where precipitation lines develop between extracts and their homologous antisera.

Immunodiagnosis. Histoplasmin skin and CF tests using antigens of either mycelial or yeast origins have not been reliable diagnostic aids in animal infections. The position of the precipitin band in immunodiffusion tests differentiates early and recovered human cases (near serum well) from active and progressive ones (near antigen well). Limited use of these tests on animals has given erratic results.

A radioimmunoassay for antigen detection has been described.

Molecular Techniques. Molecular methods used to identify or detect *H. capsulatum* make use of primers for specific sequences contained within the DNA, for example, genes encoding ribosomal RNA, or those encoding the M protein. These sequences are amplified using the polymerase chain reaction. These tests are not used routinely in the diagnostic laboratory.

Treatment and Control

Azoles (ketoconazole, itraconazole, and fluconazole) and amphotericin B have been used successfully in the treatment of some cases of canine and feline histoplasmosis.

The duration of treatment is variable depending on the severity of the infection and the patient's response. Response to therapy is monitored by frequent evaluation for resolution of clinical signs and radiographic lesions and abnormalities in hematologic and biochemical profiles. When treatment is not continued for the appropriate length of time (at least 4–6 months), relapses are common. The prognosis for disseminated cases is guarded to grave.

Applications of formalin (3%) or phenol (5%) seem to help control the fungus in the environment. Elimination of starling and pigeon roots may also help control the fungus.

B. dermatitidis

B. dermatitidis is a dimorphic fungus existing as a mold in the soil (saprophytic stage) and as a yeast in tissue (parasitic stage). It causes the systemic fungal disease called "blastomycosis," which occurs most commonly in the eastern third of North America. Cases of the disease arise sporadically in Africa, Asia, and Europe. People and dogs are the species most frequently affected by blastomycosis. However, the disease has been reported in many animals including horses, cats, ferrets, and numerous wildlife species.

Descriptive Features

Morphology, Structure, and Composition. In the saprophytic phase (in soil or on artificial media at 25–30 °C), the hyphae of *B. dermatitidis* produce conidiophores with spherical or oval smooth-walled conidia, 2–10 μm in diameter. In tissue or on blood agar at 37 °C, the agent is a thick-walled yeast, 5–20 μm in diameter, that reproduces by single buds attached by a broad base. The fungus has a sexual form *Ajellomyces dermatitidis*.

Cell wall extracts contain 3–10 parts of polysaccharide to 1 part of protein. Protein is highest in the mycelial phase, while chitin is highest in the yeast phase. The lipid content of *B. dermatitidis* is higher than in other fungi. Lipid, protein, and chitin levels vary directly with virulence.

Cellular Products of Medical Interest

Adhesin. The yeast phase of *B. dermatitidis* produces a protein adhesin termed Bad1 (for *Blastomyces* adhesin 1), formally called WI-1. Bad1 has two functions related to virulence of the fungus: (1) Bad1 adheres to β-2 integrins on the surface of phagocytic cells, triggering uptake of the yeast, invoking a minimal respiratory burst, resulting in little generation of reactive oxygen and nitrogen intermediates; (2) Bad1 downregulates the production of proinflammatory cytokines (particularly tumor necrosis factor) by affected macrophages. The amino acid sequence of Bad1 is homologous to the invasion protein produced by *Yersinia* (see Chapter 10). *B. dermatitidis* mutants that do not produce Bad1 are avirulent.

Miscellaneous Products. *B. dermatitidis* produces a variety of extracellular enzymes and products that may be involved with disease production. These include proteases, phosphatases, esterases, and glycosidases. Culture filtrates are leukotactic for human neutrophils. The role played by these products in the production of disease is unknown.

Growth Characteristics. *B. dermatitidis* grows on most media at room temperature and 37 °C. Colonies develop from within 2 to over 7 days. Mold colonies, formed at ambient temperatures (25–30 °C), are cottony white to tan depending on the abundance of conidia. Yeast colonies develop on blood agar at 37 °C. They are opaque off-white to tan, with rough surface and a pasty consistency.

Variability. The two recognized serotypes are related to geographic origin of the strains. Similar geographic relationships are seen when polymerase chain reaction-based fingerprinting systems are used.

Ecology

Reservoir. Soil is believed to be the reservoir for *Blastomyces*. Moisture, low pH, animal wastes, and decaying vegetation appear to favor colonization. Humidity promotes release of conidia.

Transmission. Blastomycosis most commonly begins by inhalation of microconidia. Percutaneous infection probably occurs in dogs with organisms entering tissue via traumatic inoculation, but generally, solitary lesions should be considered part of a systemic disease.

Pathogenesis

Microconidia or hyphal fragments are inhaled and convert to the yeast form within the alveolar spaces of the respiratory tract. The yeast expresses Bad1, which is followed by uptake (with minimal respiratory burst) by phagocytic cells. Downregulation of tumor necrosis factor production by affected macrophages delays stimulation of cell-mediated immunity (which is necessary to kill the yeast). In dogs, an inflammatory response involving macrophages and neutrophils and resulting in pyogranulomatous lesions occurs in the terminal bronchioles, followed by similar reactions in satellite lymph nodes. Blastomycosis is more often progressive than histoplasmosis and coccidioidomycosis. Dissemination is believed to occur via vascular and lymphatic routes. Preferred sites in the dog are the lymph nodes, skin, bones, bone marrow, eyes, subcutaneous tissue, brain, testes, and external nares. Less common sites of dissemination are mammary glands, prostate, liver, heart, mouth, vulva, and urogenital tract. Although organisms usually enter the body via the lungs, occasionally lung lesions have resolved by the time the animal is presented to the veterinarian. The nodular lesions can be tubercle-like, with mononuclear cell types predominating, or there may be numerous neutrophils admixed. Liquefaction and caseation occur, but calcification and encapsulation are exceptional.

Signs include skin lesions and respiratory distress with fever, depression, anorexia, and weight loss. Locomotor disturbances result from bone or joint infection or—rarely—central nervous system involvement. Ocular disease is common in disseminated blastomycosis. Most dogs with multiple organ system involvement die within months. Evidence for a benign form is uncertain. Although much less common, the disease in cats resembles that in dogs.

Epidemiology. The highest prevalence in dogs is from spring to fall. Male dogs less than 4 years of age are most often affected. In general, large breed dogs are more often affected than small breed dogs. No sex, age, or breed predisposition has been identified in cats. Although generally noncontagious, one human infection resulted from a dog bite.

Immunologic Aspects

Impaired cell-mediated responsiveness may explain canine-disseminated blastomycosis.

Humoral and cell-mediated responses occur as a result of infection. Cell-mediated immunity is decisive in determining resistance. Artificial immunization is not available.

Laboratory Diagnosis

Direct Examination. *B. dermatitidis* can be demonstrated in wet mounts of exudates and tissue smears as thick-walled yeast cells with single buds attached by a broad base. In section, intracellular yeasts may be found. Cytologic preparations, such as aspirates, and tissue impressions are stained with a Romanowsky-type (e.g., Giemsa or Wright's) and examined for yeast cells that are approximately 5–20 μm in diameter, have a thick, retractile, double-contoured cell wall (Figure 47.4 and 47.5). Broad-based budding of organisms may be seen in some preparations; however, most organisms are singular. *Blastomyces* organisms are differentiated from *Cryptococcus* species by their lack of a clear capsule, their deeply basophilic cell wall, and by the presence of broad-based budding. Fungal stain (periodic acid Schiff, Gridley, or Gomori methenamine silver) can also be applied to aid visualization of the organisms but is not routinely done on cytology.

FIGURE 47.4. B. dermatitidis. *Yeast phase, skin scraping of dog (hematoxylin–eosin stain, budding yeast cell, 1000×).*

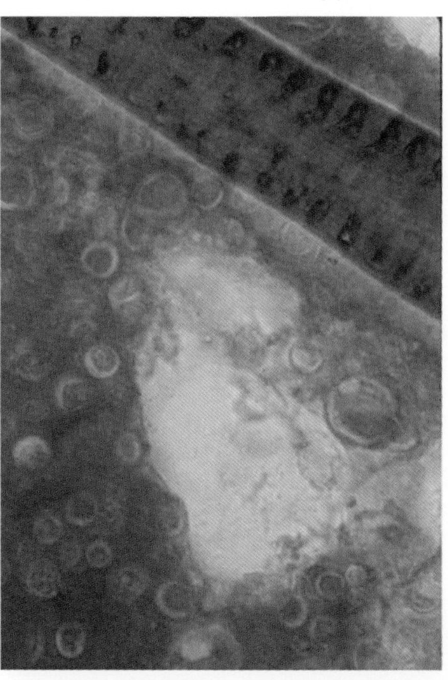

FIGURE 47.5. *Exudate from the center of a necrotic lymph node from a dog with blastomycosis. Note the dark staining* B. dermatitidis *yeasts characterized by the thick, double-contoured cell wall (arrow) (modified Wright's stain, 1000×).*

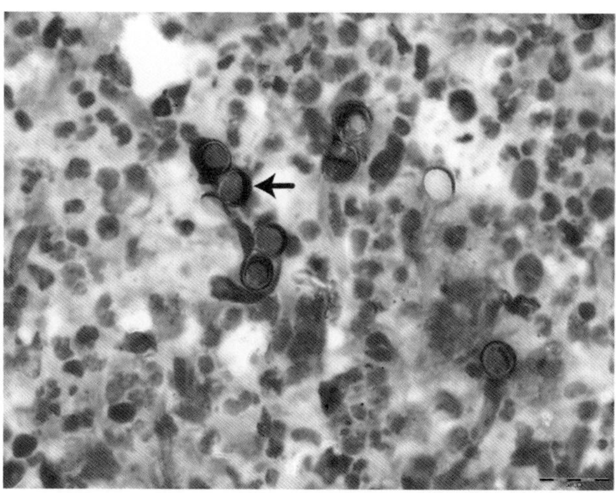

In sections stained with hematoxylin–eosin, *B. dermatitidis* appears as thick-walled yeast cells with single buds attached by a broad base. A duplicate fungal stain (e.g., periodic acid Schiff, Gridley, or Gomori methenamine silver) can be helpful.

Culture. Cultures on Sabouraud's agar (with or without inhibitors) are incubated at ambient temperature (25–30 °C) for up to 3 weeks. It is difficult to obtain the yeast form on primary isolation, but it is relatively easy to convert the mold to the yeast phase by increasing the temperature to 37 °C.

A commercially available "exoantigen" test kit furnishes prepared antisera to *Coccidioides*, *H. capsulatum*, and *B. dermatitidis* to be tested against extracts of suspect cultures in an immunodiffusion agar plate, where precipitation lines develop between extracts and their homologous antisera.

Immunodiagnosis. Blastomycin skin and CF tests lack acceptable sensitivity and specificity. The commercially available agar gel double diffusion test (making use of antigens composed of a cell wall autolysate called "antigen A") appears to be specific (96%) and sensitive (91%), but titers remain after successful treatment. Antibodies to Bad1 detected by various means (e.g., radioimmunoassay) increase during disease, and decline with successful treatment, making detection of antibodies with specificity to Bad1 more useful clinically. An enzyme-linked immunosorbent assay using a commercially available antigen has been effective in diagnosis of blastomycosis.

Molecular Methods. Molecular methods used to identify or detect *B. dermatitidis* make use of primers for specific sequences contained within DNA encoding ribosomal RNA (e.g., 28S RNA; the internally transcribed spacer region). These sequences are amplified using the polymerase chain reaction.

Treatment and Control

Blastomycosis responds to amphotericin B and ketoconazole (or both together), and to itraconazole (drug of choice). Fluconazole is moderately effective. Precaution must be taken to avoid exposure when handling animals or tissues suspected of blastomycosis; even though transmission from animals to humans is extremely rare.

Aspergillus spp.

Members of the genus *Aspergillus* are ubiquitous saprophytic molds with opportunistic pathogenic patterns that depend on impaired, overwhelmed, or bypassed host defenses. Of some 900 species, *Aspergillus fumigatus* is most frequent in animal and human infections.

Descriptive Features

Morphology and Composition. *Aspergillus* spp. are molds consisting of septate hyphae and characteristic asexual fruiting structures that are borne on conidiophores. Conidiophores are hyphal branches originating by a foot cell in the vegetative mycelium and ending in an expanded vesicle. The vesicle is covered by a layer or layers of flask-shaped phialides, from which chains of pigmented conidia (the asexual reproductive units) arise (Figure 47.6). They give the fungal colony its color.

In tissue, only hyphae are seen. In aerated cavities (e.g., nasal passages, air sacs, and cavitary lesions), fruiting structures may be found.

Fruiting bodies are important diagnostic features of *Aspergillus* spp. by which species are identified.

Cellular Products of Medical Interest

Adhesins. Members of the genus *Aspergillus* produce a number of surface proteins (conidial and hyphal) that bind to extracellular matrix proteins (collagen, fibronectin, fibrinogen, and laminin).

FIGURE 47.6. A. fumigatus. *Lactophenol cotton blue mount from Sabouraud's dextrose agar culture, 400×.*

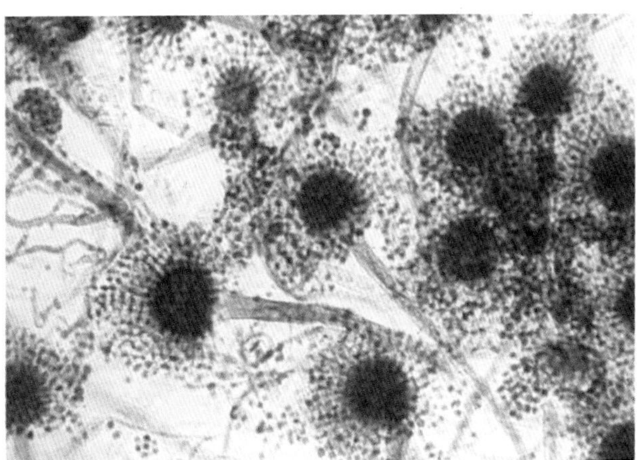

Cell Wall. The cell wall of *Aspergillus* displays a "pathogen-associated molecular pattern" that is recognized by Toll-like receptors (see Chapter 2) on the surface of host macrophages. Binding to these receptors leads to the secretion of proinflammatory cytokines.

Extracellular Enzymes. *Aspergillus* produces a number of enzymes that have the potential to function *in vivo* to break down host tissue. These include elastase, proteases, and phospholipases. In addition, members of this genus produce catalases that reduce the effectiveness of peroxides generated by phagocytic cells.

Iron Acquisition. *Aspergillus* produces several hydroxamate siderophores (a ferrichrome and a fusarinine) needed to acquire iron from host iron-binding proteins (transferrin and lactoferrin).

Pigment (Melanin). Conidia of *Aspergillus* are pigmented. The pigment, melanin, is a free radical scavenger (reducing the toxicity of hydroxy radicals, superoxides, and singlet oxygen radicals found within the phagolysosome).

Growth Characteristics. Aspergilli grow on all common laboratory media over a wide range of temperatures (up to 50 °C). Their biochemical activities have not been clearly related to virulence or utilized diagnostically.

Aspergilli thrive in the environment. Some are highly resistant to heat and drying. Most do not grow in cycloheximide-containing fungal media.

Ecology

Reservoir. Aspergilli are present in soil, vegetation, feed, and secondarily in air and water and objects exposed to them. *A. fumigatus* becomes predominant over competing microbiota in fermented plant material (e.g., hay, silage, and compost). Animal disease outbreaks are often traced to such sources.

Transmission. Aspergillosis is acquired from environmental sources, generally by inhalation or ingestion. Most *Aspergillus* mastitis follows intramammary inoculation. Intrauterine infections in cattle result from dissemination of subclinical lung or intestinal infections.

Pathogenesis

Mechanism. Following their deposition in tissue or on a surface (adhesins hinder removal), recognition (by way of "pathogen-associated molecular pattern") by phagocytic cells triggers an inflammatory response. Inflammation, along with release of fungal elastase, proteases, and phospholipases, results in tissue damage. Pigment and catalase delay destruction by phagocytic cells.

Allergenic factors, which are recognized in human aspergilloses, are insufficiently documented in animal disease.

Pathology. In pulmonary infection, suppurative exudate accumulates in bronchioles and adjacent parenchyma. It surrounds colonies of mycelial growth, which may extend into blood vessels and produce infected thrombi and vasculitis, leading to dissemination. Infection may also spread directly into adjacent air spaces. Granulomas develop; they are grossly visible as grayish white nodules and consist of mononuclear cells and fibroblasts. In older lesions, colonies are fringed by acidophilic clubs (asteroid bodies), which resemble actinomycosis (see Figure 37.2).

Lesions in avian lungs are caseous nodules. On serous membranes, caseous foci are covered by macroscopic mold colonies, accompanied by thickening of the membranes (e.g., air sacs). The cellular response is acute suppurative to chronic granulomatous.

Bovine abortion results from hematogenous seeding of placentomes, which is possibly a response to a growth factor in placental tissue. There is hyphal invasion of blood vessels producing vasculitis and a necrotizing, hemorrhagic placentitis. The fetus undergoes disseminated infection with signs of emaciation and dehydration. Lymph nodes, viscera, and brain may be involved. Ringworm-like plaques on the fetal skin are often seen.

On mucosal surfaces (e.g., nasal passage and trachea), mold colonies form on top of necrotic tissue, which is surrounded by a hemorrhagic zone.

Disease Patterns. Pulmonary and disseminated infections, frequently involving kidneys and the central nervous system, occur in most species.

Avian. Avian aspergillosis, which affects many species of birds, sometimes in epidemics, reflects heavy exposure or severe stress on domestic flocks or pet bird operations, or the effects of oil spills on marine birds. The disease is usually a respiratory tract infection, sometimes with hematogenous dissemination. The disease is also called "brooder pneumonia" in chicks and poults. The young bird acquires the disease by inhaling a massive dose of spores in the brooder. Signs are inappetence, listlessness, weight loss, dyspnea, sometimes diarrhea, and abnormal behavior and posture. The eyes are often affected. Mortality may approach 50%, especially in young birds. In mild cases, only gasping and hyperpnea may be seen. The course varies from a day to several weeks.

Ruminant. Bovine abortions usually occur late in pregnancy and resemble abortions due to other causes. Fetal skin plaques occur also in other mycotic abortions.

Mastitis due to *A. fumigatus* is reported at an increased rate, especially from Europe. It is usually chronic progressive, producing abscesses in the udder. Occasionally it causes diarrhea in calves.

Dogs and Cats. Aspergillosis of mucous membranes occurs commonly in dogs, rarely in cats, in nasal passages or paranasal sinuses. It is manifested by sneezing and unilateral or bilateral persistent nasal discharge that is unresponsive to medical treatment. Purulent nasal discharge may be seen due to secondary bacterial infection.

Aspergillus terreus and *Aspergillus deflectus* cause disseminated aspergillosis in dogs, particularly in German shepherd dogs. Osteomyelitis is a common feature.

Intestinal aspergillosis presenting as diarrhea has been reported in cats.

Horses. *Aspergillus* infection of the cornea is the leading cause of keratomycosis.

Vague upper respiratory signs may point to an aspergillosis of the equine guttural pouch. Intestinal aspergillosis may cause diarrhea in foals.

Human Beings. *Aspergillus* spp. could be a primary or secondary pathogen in humans, depending on the immune status of the individual. Tissues involved include lungs, bones, sinuses, ear skin, and meninges.

Miscellaneous Species. Infrequent infections involving the lungs occur in other animals as well.

Epidemiology. Intensity of exposure is a significant feature in animal aspergillosis. Bovine abortion outbreaks are often related to moldy fodder. Aspergillosis in chicken flocks commonly coincides with the use of heavily contaminated litter.

Stress aspects are usually recognizable in outbreaks. Avian aspergillosis is seen under conditions of poor husbandry. In oiled seabirds, there is severely impaired thermal regulation. In pregnant cattle, advanced gestation combined with low-quality feed and poor weather and housing add up to severe challenge.

Canine nasal aspergillosis occurs especially in young dogs of dolichocephalic breeds.

Some T-lymphocyte deficiency may exist.

In keratomycosis of horses, the frequent history of topical antibacterial and steroid treatment suggests immunosuppression and impaired colonization resistance.

Immunologic Aspects

Circulating antibody with no demonstrably protective role may be present in dogs with nasal aspergillosis (see Section "Treatment, Control, and Prevention"). Cell-mediated immunity is believed to be the major factor in limiting the dissemination of infection.

Immunization procedures are not available.

Laboratory Diagnosis

Direct Examination. Hyphae, fruiting heads, and conidia can often be demonstrated in samples either in wet mounts in 10% KOH or with calcofluor white. For fixed-stained smears, fungal stains (periodic acid Schiff, Gridley, or Gomori methenamine silver) are best; Romanowsky-type stains (e.g., Wright's and Giemsa) are satisfactory, and Gram stains are of limited use. Septate branching hyphae constitute strong evidence of aspergillosis. Other fungi (*Penicillium*, *Pseudallescheria*, and *Paecilomyces*) present a similar picture but rare. Conidia may occur in air passages or other exposed sites in the absence of infection.

In stained cytologic preparations and tissue sections, septate hyphae dividing dichotomously at acute angles are the only structures seen.

Isolation and Identification. *Aspergillus* is readily cultured. Because it is a ubiquitous contaminant, interpretation of positive cultures is often problematic. Presence of the agent must always be correlated with pathologic and clinical findings. Identification of agents rests upon morphologic features and growth characteristics of isolates.

Immunodiagnosis. Serologic tests are useful adjuncts to the diagnosis of aspergillosis. Because the tests that are available are species specific, it is necessary to know which *Aspergillus* to expect. For example, *A. fumigatus* is most commonly seen in nasal aspergillosis of dogs, whereas disseminated aspergillosis in that species is either *A. deflectus* or *A. terreus*. An immunodiffusion kit is commercially available for detection of antibodies to *A. fumigatus*. An enzyme-linked immunosorbent assay and a counterimmunoelectrophoresis test are also available for the serodiagnosis of aspergillosis in humans.

Molecular Methods. Primers designed to amplify DNA encoding ribosomal RNA (including the "internal transcribed spacer" region) are available for demonstration or identification of members of the genus. Amplification of DNA is by the polymerase chain reaction.

Treatment, Control, and Prevention

The nasal form in dogs is treated topically with instillation of clotrimazole or enilconazole into the nasal passages and sinuses. Itraconazole (given orally) has been successfully used to treat nasal aspergillosis when topical treatment is not possible.

Itraconazole has been beneficial in treating disseminated aspergillosis.

There is no established treatment for mammary aspergillosis.

For intestinal infections in pigs, foals, and calves, oral nystatin is recommended.

Keratomycosis is treated topically with antimycotic ointments and solutions.

Avoidance of massive exposure requires elimination of cattle feed, particularly hay and silage that has undergone noticeable deterioration. *A fumigatus* only reaches high concentrations under conditions of "biologic heat" generation, after other microbiota are eliminated. With poultry litter, proper storage and frequent changes of litter can prevent such buildup.

Other Saprophytic/Opportunistic Fungal Pathogens

Rhizopus spp., *Rhizomucor* spp., *Absidia* spp., *Mucor* spp., and *Mortierella* spp. cause mycotic bovine abortion, gastrointestinal infections, marked by ulcerative lesions and mesenteric lymphadenitis, in ruminants, swine, and dogs, as well as respiratory and hematogenous infections affecting various viscera and the central nervous system. They are secondary to stress, such as dietary changes and inadequacies, antibiotic suppression of the gastrointestinal flora, concurrent infections, recent parturition, or trauma. Several cases of infections caused by these agents have been reported in humans and nonhuman primates. These agents grow rapidly on Sabouraud's agar at room temperature. Amphotericin B is the preferred drug for treatment in both animals and humans.

Paecilomyces spp. are associated with disseminated canine, and feline paecilomycosis with bone involvement and a respiratory epidemic in captive turtles have been reported. *Conidiobolus* spp. and *Basidiobolus* spp. cause nasal granulomas and subcutaneous infections in horses, mules, dogs, sheep, nonhuman primates, and humans. Agents are identified by direct examination of clinical samples and by cultural techniques. Considerable expertise is needed for species identification in the laboratory. Amphotericin B is the drug of choice. Other agents such as fluconazole and 5-flurocytosine are also effective. *Diplorhinotricum gallopavum* causes dactylariosis in turkeys and chickens. It is a central nervous system disease with high morbidity and approximately 20% mortality. Treatment is not practical, but good sanitation of the poultry house and the hatchery is essential for control of this disease.

Pneumocystis

Members of the genus *Pneumocystis* are fungi capable of causing pneumonia in immunocompromised individuals. They have only been isolated from affected hosts (e.g., humans, dogs, cats, horses, pigs, goats, ferrets, mice, rats, chimpanzees, and monkeys). At present there are two species: *jiroveci* (affecting human patients) and *carinii* (affecting all the rest). The taxonomy of members of the genus *Pneumocystis* is still not clear and needs further studies. *Pneumocystis carinii* is composed of at least 30 varieties or "special forms," with each "special form" affecting a particular host. For example, *P. carinii* f. sp. *ratti* affects rats, while *P. carinii* f. sp. *muris*, only mice. Thus, *Pneumocystis* is a host-specific fungus, which is contagious between members of the same species but is not zoonotic.

Spread is by way of aerosol. Affected hosts are usually immunocompromised, though there are reports of healthy animals (with no evidence of immunosuppression or underlying condition) developing pneumocystis pneumonia when housed with known infected animals.

The fungus has not been grown in a cell-free culture system. Diagnosis is made by examination of material from the alveolar spaces, which is usually concentrated by cytocentrifugation and stained with Romanowsky-type stains (e.g., Giemsa or Wright's). On these cytologic preparations, intracellular (within alveolar macrophages) and extracellular round-shaped cysts (approximately 4–7 μm in diameter) that contain four to eight basophilic bodies arranged in a circle are observed. Numerous ovoid to crescent-shaped trophozoites (approximately 1–2 μm) are also typically seen. Silver stain (e.g., Gomori methenamine silver) can also be used to aid visualization of the organism. DNA primers have also been designed to amplify specific segments of the fungal genome, so that detection and identification is possible using the polymerase chain reaction.

Treatment includes one or more of the following: trimethoprim–sulfonamides, carbutamide, dapsone, atovaquone, pentamidine, clindamycin, or trimetrexate/leucovorin.

Protothecosis

Prototheca is an alga lacking chlorophyll. It multiplies by endosporulation, producing roughly spherical cells that are 8–25 μm in diameter. *Prototheca zopfii* and *Prototheca wickerhamii* (which probably belongs to the genus *Auxenochlorella*) are occasionally pathogenic. They grow on fungal media (without cycloheximide) at 25 °C and 37 °C, respectively, into white to tannish dull colonies in less than a week and are differentiated serologically and by carbohydrate assimilation tests.

Prototheca spp. are widespread in nature. Exposure is by ingestion, percutaneously, or, in dairy cows, by intramammary injection.

Disease occurs in dogs, cats, cattle, deer, bats, snakes, fish, and humans. In dogs, it is usually disseminated and accompanied by hemorrhagic diarrhea. Central nervous system involvement and eye lesions are frequent. In cats and humans, cases to date have been cutaneous. Immunodeficiency is suspected. In cattle, chronic progressive mastitis develops. Tissue reactions are pyogranulomatous.

The agent is easily cultured and can be demonstrated in unstained wet mounts from specimens or in fixed smears stained with a Romanowsky-type (Wright's or Giemsa) or fungal (periodic acid Schiff, Gridley, or Gomori methenamine silver) stain.

Amphotericin B and ketoconazole are used in humans. The agents are susceptible to the aminoglycosides *in vitro*. Treatment of animals has not been effective, although liposomal formulations of amphotericin B show promise.

Further Reading

Greene CE (2006) *Infectious Diseases of the Dog and Cat*, 3rd edn, Elsevier Saunders.

Raskin R and Meyer D (2009) *Canine and Feline Cytology: A Color Atlas and Interpretation Guide*, 2nd edn, W.B. Elsevier Saunders Company.

Songer JG and Post KW (2005) *Veterinary Microbiology: Bacterial and Fungal Agents of Animal Diseases*, Elsevier Saunders.

PART III

Viruses

48 Pathogenesis of Viral Diseases

MELISSA KENNEDY

Pathogenesis can be defined as the process(es) by which a virus produces disease in the host. The term "virulence" is used to describe the degree of pathogenicity of a virus—a virulent virus being the one that results in a significant disease. The pathogenesis of viral infections is a multifactor process and involves both the status of the host and properties of the infecting virus. The outcome of viral infection (i.e., the severity of disease or death) is, therefore, determined by the virulence of virus and susceptibility of the host. Susceptibility of a host to a viral infection is determined by many factors including the genetic background of the host, species of the host animal affected, level of immunity, immune competency of the host, nutritional status, age, and presence of concurrent infection(s). Some of the viral virulence-related properties include production of cytotoxic effects by the virus (direct or indirect), replication strategies, tissue tropism, dose of the infecting virus, and route of exposure. The host-virus interaction, as determined by these factors, can be examined at the cellular level and at the level of the host animal. The former relates to the ability of a virus to infect and replicate in a cell and effects of virus replication on that cell, while the latter is related to the cumulative effects of cellular infection on the animal host. Thus, what is seen at the host level is a reflection of the cellular effects of the virus.

Virus–Host Relationships

The outcome of any virus-host interaction can differ, depending on critical factors such as virus-cell interactions, species of the animal host, route of exposure, mode of virus dissemination, and host resistance. Most virus-infected animals that present to veterinarians do so because they exhibit clinical signs of their infection. However, it is very important to recognize that microbial infections of animals often do not result in clinical disease. In fact, the majority of virus-animal interactions result in asymptomatic or subclinical infection, and viruses, however virulent, will not infect animals that are resistant to them. The potential consequences of virus-animal relationships are shown in Table 48.1.

There are several major routes of viral entry into a host: the respiratory, alimentary, and urogenital routes and direct transmission (such as by an insect or animal bite). Successful establishment of viral infection depends on the presence of appropriate cell receptors and the physicochemical nature of the viral agent. In order to successfully initiate infection in the host, the virus must be able to survive until a susceptible host is encountered and gain access to cells/tissues in which it can replicate (permissive cells). This requires the virus to overcome the host's defense mechanisms at these sites. For example, viruses that infect animals through the alimentary tract are typically resistant to the low pH and potent enzymes that occur in the digestive tract.

Modes of Dissemination of Viruses within the Hosts

Viruses cause two basic patterns of infection: localized and generalized (Figure 48.1). In localized infections, viral multiplication and cellular damage remain localized near the site of entry (e.g., the skin or the mucous membranes of the respiratory, gastrointestinal, or genital tract), so that the infecting virus spreads only to neighboring cells immediately adjacent to the original site of infection. For example, rhinovirus infections of animals are often restricted to the nasal epithelium and do not even spread to the lower respiratory tract. Other respiratory viruses, such as parainfluenza and respiratory syncytial viruses, replicate within the lungs of infected animals, but tissue injury induced by these viruses typically remains restricted to the respiratory tract. Generalized infections develop through several sequential steps: (1) the virus undergoes primary replication at the site of entry and in regional lymph nodes, (2) progeny virus spreads through blood (primary viremia) and lymphatics to additional tissues, where (3) further virus replication takes place, (4) the virus is disseminated to the other target organs via a secondary viremia, and (5) it multiplies further in these target tissues where it causes cellular degeneration and/or necrosis, tissue injury, and clinical disease.

The incubation period is the asymptomatic period after infection and prior to expression of clinical disease. In

Veterinary Microbiology, Third Edition. Edited by D. Scott McVey, Melissa Kennedy and M.M. Chengappa.

Table 48.1. Potential Consequences of Virus-Animal Relationships

1. Animal is resistant to viral infection–no relationship established
2. Asymptomaic or subclinical infection–recovery or persistent infection
3. Acute viral infection–death, recovery, or persistent infection
4. Chronic viral infection–recurrent clinical disease, or persistent infection
5. Tumor formation

generalized viral infections, overt disease begins only after the virus becomes widely disseminated in the body and has attained maximum titers. It is at this stage of the infection that the veterinarian is usually first alerted. Canine distemper illustrates a generalized viral infection of animals. The canine distemper virus initiates the infection at the site of entry, but then disseminates through the blood or the lymphatic system to produce generalized infection with involvement of a variety of target organs (Figure 48.2). The sequence of events during the incubation period and development of signs of disease in experimental canine distemper infections indicate that the different clinical signs that occur in individual animals depend on which of the various organ systems are infected by the virus. The virus is disseminated to these organs during viremia, which may be characterized by the presence of free virus particles in the blood or, as with the canine distemper virus, blood cells can also serve as carriers to disseminate the virus to target organs (cell-associated viremia). Cell-associated viremias typically involve blood leukocytes, but some viruses, such as bluetongue virus, hog cholera virus, or parvovirus, can associate with red blood cells of the infected host. The dissemination of virus to the central nervous system can occur by viremia or, in the case of rabies, by transmission along peripheral nerves.

Viral Tropism

The restriction of viral infection and/or replication to certain cells or tissues is referred to as tropism. Some viruses have a very broad-spectrum of tropism, infecting a variety of cell types, organs, and even host species. *Pseudorabies* virus, a herpesvirus, can infect the respiratory tract, central nervous system, and fetus in swine. In addition, this virus causes fatal infection in most mammals except primates. The virus of malignant catarrhal fever, also a herpesvirus, infects only a subpopulation of T-lymphocytes in some ruminant species, including cattle and wildebeests. Viral tropism is integral to understanding the disease that results from infection with a particular virus.

The tropism of a virus, though it manifests at the host level, is largely determined at the cellular level. The presence or absence of certain cellular factors governs whether a virus can infect and/or produce infectious progeny in a cell. The cell must express an appropriate cellular receptor for virus attachment, the first step in virus replication. Viruses exploit these normal cell surface molecules to enter the cell. A particular cell surface molecule/receptor may be utilized by more than one virus. Conversely, a virus may be able to utilize multiple cellular receptors for attachment. The expression of appropriate cell receptor is a major factor in determining the susceptibility of cells to a specific

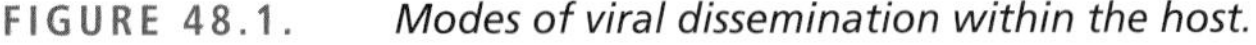

FIGURE 48.1. *Modes of viral dissemination within the host.*

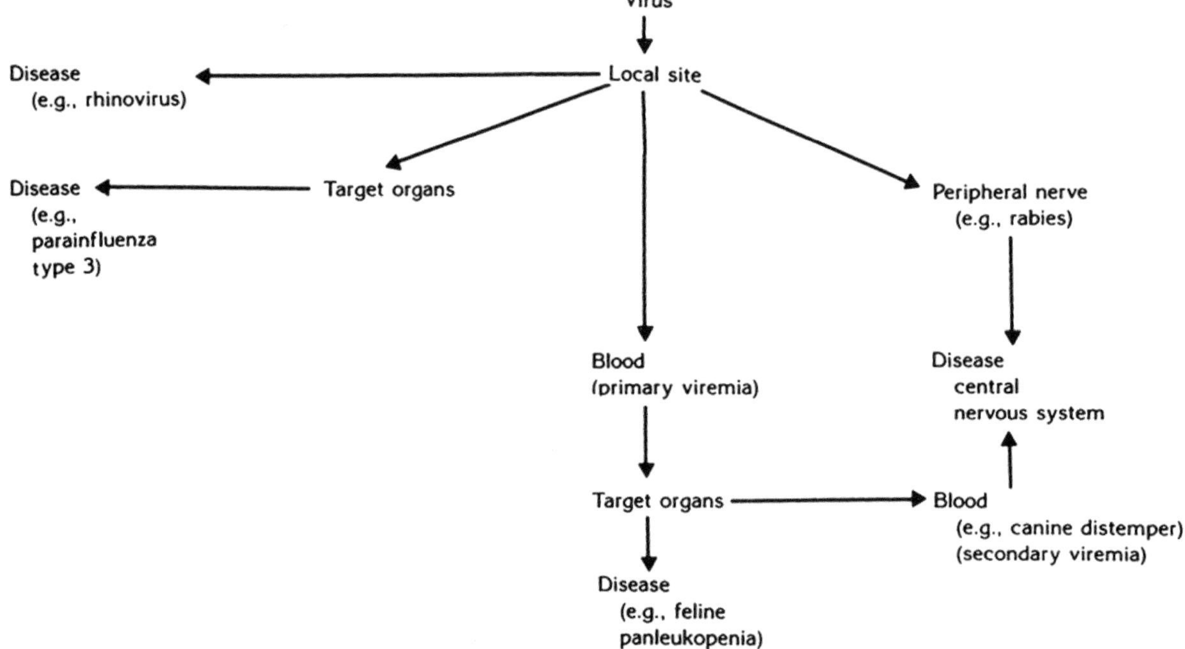

FIGURE 48.2. *Pathogenesis of canine distemper viral infection in dogs.*

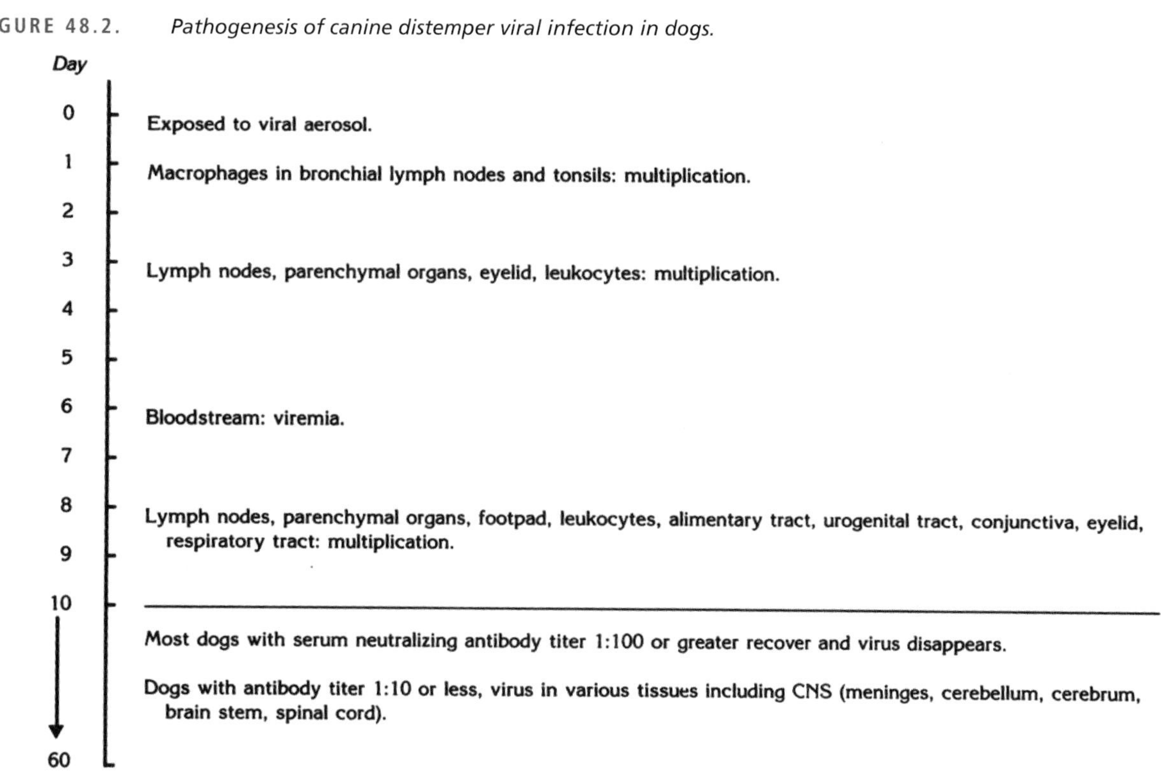

virus. In order for a virus to complete its replicative cycle after entry into a cell, the cell must provide certain factors. The absence of these factors prevents production of infectious progeny by the virus. The cellular factors required by viruses vary. Some of these cellular factors are available only during certain stages of cell growth cycle. For example, parvoviruses require cellular DNA polymerase for synthesis of their genome. This enzyme is expressed in abundance in actively dividing cells (i.e., cells in S phase of their growth cycle). Thus, parvoviruses replicate in cells with high mitotic index, such as hemopoietic cells in the bone marrow and intestinal crypt cells where the cell turnover rate is very high. Viruses that infect cells of the immune system are especially dependent upon the stage of differentiation of the cell. Activated lymphocytes and macrophages are usually better able to support productive virus replication than resting cells, though the mechanisms are unclear. The progeny of papillomaviruses is produced only in the differentiated keratinocytes.

Local environmental factors can also determine the tissue tropism for a given virus. These include temperature and pH. *Feline herpesvirus*-1 (FHV-1) prefers temperatures of 33–35 °C for replication—temperature of the upper respiratory tract. Thus, FHV-1 is associated with disease of the upper respiratory tract, rhinotracheitis. The enteroviruses of the family Picornaviridae are quite resistant to acidic pH and can survive transit through the stomach to the intestine, the target organ. Rhinoviruses, which are also members of the Picornaviridae, are degraded by the acidic pH of the stomach and therefore remain confined to the upper respiratory tract.

The severity of the outcome of a viral disease in an animal is determined largely by organ(s) targeted. Infection of organs that do not tolerate even minimal tissue damage, such as the nervous tissue, can be life-threatening. In other tissues, particularly those that are capable of regeneration such as the intestine, the infection may result in mild or short-lived, self-limiting disease. In pregnant animals, viruses that may cause little disease in adult animals may be lethal to the gestating fetus.

Viral infections that occur without producing overt disease are very common and are potentially important in the dissemination of viruses. Significantly, inapparent infections can confer protective immunity against subsequent challenge with virulent strains of the same agent. Several factors are involved in producing inapparent infections: (1) the nature of the virus (e.g., virulent or attenuated strains), (2) degree of host immunity, (3) appearance of viral interference, and (4) failure of the virus to reach the target organ (e.g., due to the blood–brain barrier).

Host Responses to Viral Infections

The resistance of animals to viral infection is dependent in part on factors that act indiscriminately on most viruses and are therefore called nonspecific or innate resistance factors. These include anatomical barriers, physiologic conditions (e.g., pH and temperature), hormonal factors, inhibitors other than antibodies, and phagocytes. Phagocytosis is an important defense mechanism in bacterial infections. However, many viral agents are capable of infecting lymphocytes and/or monocytes/macrophages, and thus these cells can actually serve as a vehicle to spread the virus through the host.

Interferon

An important component of viral defense is the production and secretion of interferon. Interferons are a group of cell proteins (cytokines) that can modulate the immune system, regulate the differentiation of certain cells, confer antiviral resistance on sensitive cells, and exert anticancer effects. Many viruses will induce interferon synthesis in infected cells, and many cell types have the ability to synthesize interferon after appropriate stimulation. At least three different types of interferon can be produced in the course of a viral infection: α, β, and γ. Two distinct mechanisms have been identified in interferon-treated cells (Figure 48.3). The first involves the production in interferon-treated cells of a protein kinase (P1/eIF2α kinase), which, in the presence of double-stranded RNA, blocks initiation of protein synthesis by phosphorylating the protein synthesis initiation factor eIF-2. The other mechanism involves an enzyme, 2–5A synthetase, which, in the presence of adenosine triphosphate and dsRNA, synthesizes a group of oligoadenylates collectively known as 2–5A. In turn, 2–5A activates a specific endonuclease that degrades viral and cellular RNA and so inhibits protein synthesis.

Besides its action on virus replication, interferon exerts other effects on cells, including effects on cell multiplication and regulation of such cellular functions as phagocytosis, production of antibodies and lymphokines by lymphocytes, expression of cell surface antigens, and cytotoxicity of cellular immunity. Interferon plays an important role in host resistance to viral infection.

Humoral and Cellular Immunity

Viruses are antigenic and typically induce a strong specific immune response after infection. Humoral immune responses involve the production of antibodies that can be demonstrated by the usual serologic procedures, such as complement fixation, agglutination, precipitation, and gel diffusion techniques. Antibodies, when bound to a virus or viral protein, mediate several antiviral events, including viral neutralization, virus agglutination, activation of complement, and antibody-dependent cell-mediated immune responses. These effects play an important role in terminating primary viral infection, limiting viremia, and preventing disease and reinfection. The neutralizing antibody is of

FIGURE 48.3. *Mechanisms of interferon action on protein synthesis.*

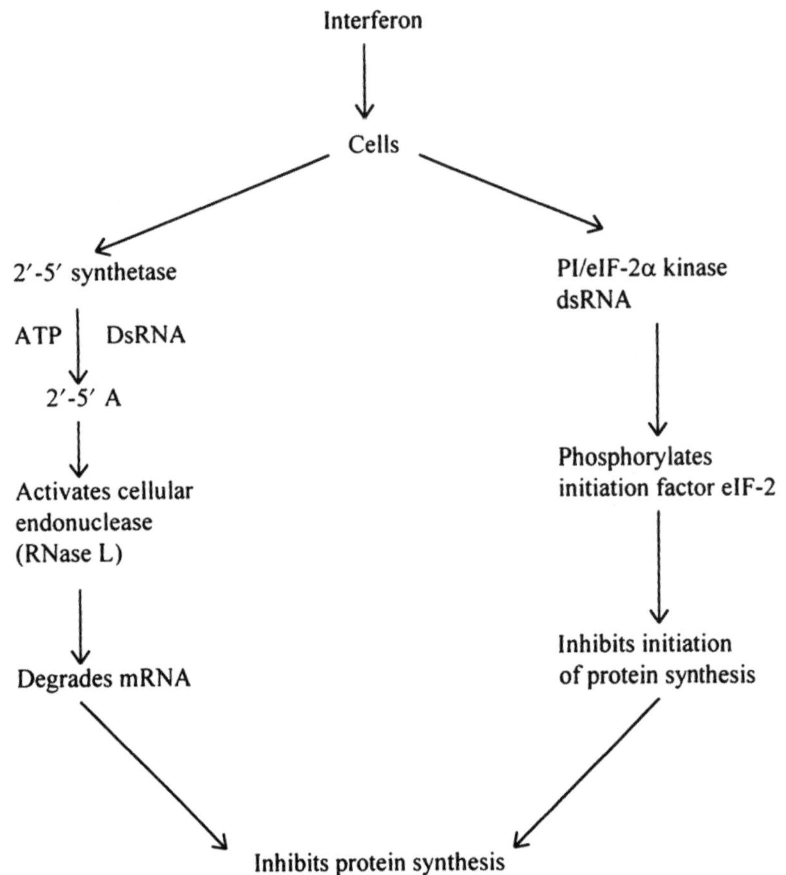

particular importance in viral infections—when preparations of viruses are mixed with appropriate antisera and the mixtures are inoculated in susceptible hosts, infection will not occur if the antisera contain the virus-neutralizing antibody. Three classes of immunoglobulins—IgG, IgM, and IgA—can serve as neutralizing antibodies. The interaction of a virus and an antibody, particularly antibodies specific to the viral antigens responsible for attachment to specific cell receptors, results in a virus–antibody complex formation that prevents attachment of the virus to cell receptors, and to a lesser extent prevents the penetration of the virus into the susceptible cell. It is possible to recover the infectious virus from such apparently inert virus–antibody mixtures by simple dilution or centrifugation, suggesting that the virus and the antibody may be linked in a loose combination in the initial stages of reaction. The interaction between the virus and the antibody does not physically alter viral structure; however, the complement system and antiviral antibody can induce lysis of enveloped viruses as well as destroy virus-infected cells.

Cellular immunity, discussed in Chapter 2, is another important factor in host resistance to some viral infections. The destruction of virus-infected cells by cytotoxic lymphocytes can limit the infection and dissemination of the virus, particularly in instances where the virus is transmitted from infected to noninfected cells. Recent evidence also indicates that macrophages play a role in host resistance to viral infections. Macrophages are key participants in the inflammatory response, and they can be activated either by interaction with viruses or by the soluble products produced by the virus reacting with lymphocytes. Activated macrophages have been shown to participate in a wide range of host responses to viral infections, including phagocytosis of virus–antibody complexes, production of interferon, cytotoxicity for virus-infected cells, and immunoregulatory functions.

In viral infections, cellular and tissue damage result not only directly from the viral infection but also from the host's immune response generated against the invading pathogen as well. Cellular and humoral responses target the virus as well as virus-infected cells. In addition, "bystander" destruction of nearby uninvolved cells occurs. Cytotoxic mediators released from neutrophils, cytotoxic T-lymphocytes, and natural killer cells may affect uninfected cells in close proximity. In most cases, this damage is minimal and is a necessary component of the recovery process in viral diseases because virus-infected cells must be destroyed. However, in some instances such as persistent infections, the immune response may be responsible for the disease. The prolonged presence of antigens continually stimulates immunocompetent cells, leading to an excessive inflammatory response. The excessive response can be humoral and cell mediated. The end result is cellular, tissue, and organ damage that manifests as disease.

Viral Immunosuppression

Several viruses of veterinary importance can infect lymphocytes, including canine distemper virus, feline panleukopenia virus, feline leukemia virus, bovine viral diarrhea virus, hog cholera virus, Newcastle disease virus, and infectious bursal disease virus of chickens. The destruction of lymphocytes and resultant atrophy of lymphoid tissues by the viruses can suppress or compromise immune response, predisposing the affected host to other opportunistic bacterial or viral infections. Less commonly, a variety of inherited primary immune deficiencies are possible in animals that can predispose them to infectious diseases. A good example is the fatal respiratory tract infection of Arabian foals with combined immunodeficiency disorder (lack of production of functional T- and B-lymphocytes) by equine adenovirus.

Persistent Viral Infection

Persistent and latent viral infections are characterized by the fact that the virus is not eliminated from the host. Disease may or may not occur in such chronically infected animals. Potential mechanisms of viral persistence include noncytocidal infection of host cells, destruction of immune effector cells or growth within these cell types, evasion of protective host responses including cytokines and antibodies, and integration of the viral genome into that of the host cell. Persistent infections are those in which the virus is continuously present, with or without expression of disease. Disease, when it does occur in persistently infected animals, often is a result of immunopathologic mechanisms. Latent infections are those in which the virus is demonstrable only when reactivation (recrudescence) occurs; this is highly characteristic of herpesvirus infections.

Viral Shedding

The final stage of a viral infection is the shedding of the virus by the host into the environment. This may occur from the same body surface where the virus gained entrance into the host, even if systemic dissemination occurs. For example, many viruses infecting the respiratory tract are shed via respiratory secretions. Viruses that do not disseminate within the host are generally shed from the site of entry. Papillomaviruses enter through traumatic openings in the skin, replicate in the layers of epidermis, and are shed from the differentiated keratinocytes on the skin surface. Viruses that infect multiple tissues may be shed from a variety of locales. *Canine distemper virus*, which infects many epithelial cells throughout the host during generalized disease, may be shed in feces, respiratory secretions, ocular secretions, and urine. Viruses that infect the gastrointestinal tract are usually shed in the feces. Semen and milk can be the source of some viruses, particularly those that infect leukocytes. Viruses that infect hematopoietic cells or that cause a significant viremia can spread via blood. Blood is the source of infection for the arthropod-borne viruses as well as for viruses that spread iatrogenically via the contaminated needles, through blood transfusions, and so on.

In certain viral infections, no shedding of virus may occur from the host. This happens most often in viruses infecting an aberrant or a "dead-end" host. For example, *Eastern equine encephalitis virus*, a togavirus, normally cycles between birds and mosquitoes. When horses, which are not the natural host of this virus, are bitten by infected mosquitoes, a transient viremia leads to the infection of the central nervous system. Because the viremia is so transient, horses are not normally a source of virus for mosquitoes and there is no virus shedding.

Further Reading

Flint JS, Racaniello VJ, Krug R *et al.* (1999) *Principles of Virology: Molecular Biology, Pathogenesis, and Control*, ASM Press.

Norkin LC (2009) *Virology: Molecular Biology and Pathogenesis*, ASM Press.

MacLachlan NJ and Dubovi EJ (2010) *Fenner's Veterinary Virology*, 5th edn, Academic Press.

Parvoviridae and Circoviridae

RICHARD A. HESSE, BENJAMIN R. TRIBLE, AND RAYMOND R. ROWLAND

Parvoviridae

Members of the genus *Parvovirus* in the family Parvoviridae are the causative agents of specific diseases in animals but not in humans. They tend to be species specific, but this is not always the case. For example, some strains of canine parvovirus infect not only dogs but also cats, wolves, and foxes. The name parvovirus is derived from the Latin term *parvus*, which means small. Parvoviruses are some of the smallest viruses known (18–26 nm). These viruses are nonenveloped, have icosahedral symmetry, and contain a linear single-stranded DNA genome of approximately 5000 nucleotides that typically codes for two open reading frames. One open reading frame codes for proteins that mediate the functions required for transcription and DNA replication, while the other open reading frame codes for the capsid proteins that enclose a single-stranded minus-sense DNA genome. A useful characteristic of these viruses is that they hemagglutinate (HA) red blood cells and an antibody response following infection results in the generation of hemagglutination inhibition (HAI) antibodies, which correlate with viral neutralization. HA and HAI are useful assays for the study of pathogenesis, protection, and prevalence. The icosahedral virion confers great stability to the virus particles that are resistant to inactivation by pH, organic solvents, and temperatures up to 60 °C. They are among the most stable viruses known and are resistant to environmental factors and many commercial disinfectants. A 5% solution of household bleach (sodium hypochlorite) is an effective and practical virucidal disinfectant for these viruses

Because of the simplicity of these viruses, actively dividing cells are a strict requirement for productive viral replication. Virus replication occurs within the nucleus of host cells, and because the virus lacks its own DNA polymerase, replication of parvoviruses requires cells that are cycling (late S phase or early G2 phase of the cell cycle) so that they can utilize host cell enzymes for their own replication.

Infections with feline parvovirus, canine parvovirus, porcine parvovirus, and mink parvovirus cause the most common diseases of economic significance in pets and production animals, which are discussed in detail. A variety of other animal parvoviruses have been identified, including chicken parvovirus, mink enteritis virus, mice minute virus, mouse parvovirus 1, and raccoon parvovirus, as well as a number of uncharacterized parvoviruses from a variety of species.

Feline Panleukopenia

Disease. Feline panleukopenia, also known as feline distemper and feline infectious enteritis, is a highly contagious, acute viral disease of cats. The disease is characterized by high fever, anorexia, depression, and vomiting, followed by dehydration, diarrhea, and death due to the loss of small intestinal crypts cells, which results in villus atrophy and subsequent prevention of the absorption of nutrients and fluids. Leukopenia is also a prominent characteristic of feline panleukopenia. The clinical severity of disease is often linked directly to the severity of leukopenia; secondary bacterial infections often occur as a result of a compromised immune system. Cats of all ages are susceptible to infection, but mortality is highest among kittens. Infection can occur by either oral or respiratory routes, and the incubation period following infection is short. Pregnant queens may experience intrauterine infection with the feline panleukopenia virus, which leads to neonatal death or congenital abnormalities of the central nervous system manifested by cerebellar ataxia in kittens after birth. This syndrome has also been observed in kittens infected with the virus before 2 weeks of age. Infection of healthy seronegative mature cats usually results in mild or no apparent disease.

Etiologic Agent. Feline panleukopenia virus (FPV) is a typical parvovirus in regard to virion structure, genomic organization, replication requirements, and physical/chemical properties as previously described. FPV is closely related to the canine parvovirus and mink enteritis virus. Although all three viruses are antigenically related,

Veterinary Microbiology, Third Edition. Edited by D. Scott McVey, Melissa Kennedy and M.M. Chengappa.

they can be distinguished by sequence analysis. A very closely related virus that is antigenically indistinguishable from FPV causes enteritis in mink and can produce disease in raccoons and coatimundi. Canine parvovirus type 2 (CPV2) is ancestrally closely related to FPV (discussed in detail in Section "Canine Parvovirus"). Canine parvoviruses types 2a, 2b, and 2c are capable of infecting felines and causing a disease indistinguishable from feline panleukopenia. FPV grows in primary or continuous feline kidney cell cultures but not in canine cell cultures.

Host–Virus Relationship

Distribution, Reservoir, and Transmission. All members of the family Felidae, as well as mink, ferrets, and raccoons, are likely to be susceptible to infection with FPV and recently evolved canine variants. Feline panleukopenia occurs worldwide with infected cats being the principal reservoir. Both infected cats suffering from acute disease and those having clinically inapparent infection excrete the virus in their urine, feces, and various secretions. Physical contact with FPV-contaminated utensils, cages, and bedding results in infection and subsequent transmission that rapidly spreads in contained housing situations. The virus is highly stable in the environment making it more difficult to control.

Pathogenesis and Pathology. Inhalation or ingestion of secretions from animals infected with the virus is the most common means of transmission. The virus replicates in tissues and then travels via the bloodstream, resulting in a generalized infection. Cell-free viremia occurs for several days in kittens experimentally infected intranasally or orally with FPV. The virus disseminates throughout the body and infects cells with the correct receptors. Feline parvovirus requires actively dividing cells that are in S phase of the cell cycle, particularly hematopoietic cells located within the bone marrow and lymphoid tissues (thymus, spleen, and lymph nodes), or cells of the intestinal crypts. Infection of hematopoietic and lymphoid cells leads to severe and protracted leukopenia, affecting all white blood cell types and leading to atrophy of lymphoid tissues, whereas infection of crypts cells leads to marked destruction of the intestinal epithelium with resultant malabsorption diarrhea. Severe infections often result in death of the animal due to secondary infections or severe dehydration. Histologic lesions of acutely infected animals are characterized by necrosis of the epithelium of the intestinal crypts and marked destruction and depletion of lymphocytes in the lymph nodes, thymus, and spleen. Animals that survive a mild infection undergo regenerative lymphoid hyperplasia followed by recovery.

In utero infection of late-term fetuses and very young kittens results in the destruction of the cells within the external granular layer of the cerebellum. This leads to cerebellar hypoplasia, degeneration, loss of Purkinje cells, and atrophy as a consequence of failure of the internal granular layer to develop. Kittens that develop this condition experience tremors of the head and have difficulty walking and maneuvering. In utero infections of rats, hamsters, ferrets, and mice at critical stages of gestation with the appropriate species of parvovirus result in congenital lesions similar to those observed in kittens.

Host Responses to Infection. Following infection, hemagglutination-inhibiting and neutralizing antibodies appear in cats approximately 1 week after infection. High levels of antibodies are generally present after 10–12 days, and these antibodies can persist in cats for several years. Lactogenic immunity based on maternal antibodies with neutralizing HAI titers of more than 80 against FPV protects kittens against viral infection; however, these antibodies also interfere with active immunization by modified live or inactivated FPV viral vaccines. Cellular immune responses are also generated during infection and likely are important in limiting virus replication during acute infection.

Laboratory Diagnosis. Kittens or young cats presenting with the clinical signs of high fever, anorexia, depression, vomiting, diarrhea, and dehydration or the presence of severe leukopenia should be considered for the presumptive diagnosis of feline panleukopenia. The diagnosis can be confirmed by one of the following laboratory methods:

1. The viral antigen may be detected in feces from live animals by antigen-capture enzyme-linked immunosorbent assay (ELISA), polymerase chain reaction (PCR) amplification of viral nucleic acid, or electron microscopy.
2. The virus may be detected in tissues from dead animals by antigen-capture ELISA, immunofluorescence staining or immunohistochemistry with an FPV-specific antisera conjugate, or PCR.
3. The virus may be isolated in cell culture from filtered feces or tissue samples, using cultured feline kidney cells.

Serodiagnosis of FPV following acute disease or for monitoring vaccine antibody levels may be accomplished by HAI testing (HAI titers of >80 are considered protective). Other antibody tests that are useful to monitor exposure include ELISA or indirect immunofluorescence. Paired sera and a fourfold rise in titer are required to confirm the diagnosis or "vaccine take."

Treatment and Control. Supportive therapy directed to restoration of fluid and electrolyte balance will increase the survival rate of clinically affected animals; however, there is no specific treatment that eliminates FPV from the infected animal. Prevention of infection is the key to controlling this disease. Vaccination, isolation of cats that survive infection, and meticulous decontamination of premises that have housed affected cats are critical for containment of this highly transmissible virus. Household bleach at a 5% solution is (1 : 20 dilution) or commercial products labeled for use against parvovirus provide effective virucidal activity against FPV and should be used extensively. Numerous efficacious inactivated and modified live FPV vaccines are commercially available. Maternal antibodies can interfere with the immunization of young kittens, and this needs to be considered as part of the vaccination regime. The passive antibody typically wanes around 4–12 weeks of age, and multiple vaccinations are required in order to immunize kittens immediately prior to the "susceptibility window" and ensure uniform protection.

Canine Parvovirus

Disease. Parvoviral disease in dogs is a relatively new disease of canines. It is somewhat similar to FPV disease in felines, characterized by sudden onset of diarrhea, vomiting, anorexia, fever, depression, lymphopenia, and dehydration. Mortality is higher in puppies than in adults, and very young puppies sometimes develop myocarditis without clinical signs of enteritis.

Canine parvovirus disease (CPD) was first recognized in North America in 1978, but retrospective serological studies indicate that the virus was rapidly spreading around the world in the early 1970s and caused a global pandemic. CPD is caused by CPV2, which is a variant of FPV. CPV2 has continued to evolve since it first emerged in dogs. New variants of CPV seem to have arisen through point mutations in the capsid protein and are designated as CPV type 2a, type 2b, and most recently type 2C. Another parvovirus capable of infecting canines is the minute virus of canines also known as canine parvovirus type 1 (CPV1), which does not cause clinical disease.

Etiologic Agent. CPV2 is clearly a variant of FPV that has acquired the ability to infect canines through a small number of mutations in the capsid protein VP2. Those mutations resulted in modifications of surface-exposed residues and allowed for binding to the transferrin receptor type I molecule of dogs. CPV2 was replaced in 1979–1980 by CPV2a, which has different antigenicity and receptor binding than its parent. CPV2a has an extended host range and is capable of infecting a number of carnivores including felines. CPV2a is the common ancestor of the CPV2b and CPV2c variants that currently circulate in dogs worldwide. Recent cross-species transmission data suggest that raccoon parvoviruses and subsequent canine–raccoon passages may have served as intermediates to the evolution of the CPV2a lineage and their extended host range.

Resistance to Physical and Chemical Agents. CPV is a typical parvovirus and is very stable in the environment. It is resistant to environmental factors, such as extremes of temperature, pH, and most disinfectants. The virus can persist for long periods in premises where infected dogs are kept and can be transmitted to other areas by fomites. Household bleach at a 1 : 20 dilution (5%) or commercial products labeled for use against parvovirus provide effective virucidal activity against CPV and should be used extensively.

Infectivity for Other Species and Culture Systems. CPV2 infects dogs of all breeds and other members of the family Canidae, such as wolves, foxes, and coyotes. Domestic cats without antibodies to the virus are susceptible to experimental infection but remain asymptomatic. CPV2a, CPV2b, and CPV2c also infect all breeds of dogs and members of Canidae family, but unlike CPV2, these viruses are capable of infecting felines and causing panleukopenia.

Canine parvoviruses can be isolated and propagated in primary cell cultures of canine or feline fetal lung and kidney, as well as continuous cell lines such as canine cell line A72, and feline cell lines NLFK and CRFK.

Host–Virus Relationship

Distribution, Reservoir, and Transmission. CPV infection of dogs, other members of the family Canidae, as well as most carnivores, is prevalent throughout the world. Parvovirus-infected dogs continue to excrete the infectious virus in their feces for up to 10 days after the onset of infection, and the virus is readily transmitted between dogs by the fecal–oral route.

Pathogenesis and Pathology. The pathogenesis of CPV infection of dogs is similar to that of panleukopenia virus infection of cats, although cerebellar hypoplasia and atrophy are not recognized as a consequence of in utero infection of dogs. Myocarditis is a potential consequence of parvovirus infection of young pups, whereas it is not described in panleukopenia virus-infected kittens.

Inhalation or ingestion of secretions from animals infected with the virus is the most common means of transmission. The virus replicates in tissues and then travels via the bloodstream and can result in a generalized infection. Virus replication requires infection of rapidly dividing cells in the intestinal epithelium and lymphoid tissues, including thymus, tonsils, retropharyngeal and mesenteric lymph nodes, and spleen. Widespread infection of the intestinal mucosa occurs on about the sixth day following experimental inoculation. Fecal excretion of virus begins as early as the third day postexposure and peaks soon thereafter. Most dogs stop excreting the virus by the twelfth day postinfection.

Hemorrhage is the most striking lesion of parvovirus enteritis in dogs, occurring in the lumen of the small bowel and accompanying enlargement and edema of the mesenteric lymph nodes. Gross myocarditis lesions that appear as mottled white streaks within the myocardium are indicative of cardiac involvement in young puppies.

Histological lesions resulting from CPV infection are confined to organs with large populations of rapidly proliferating cells, such as the small intestine, lymph nodes, and bone marrow. Necrosis of crypt epithelium and atrophy of epithelial villi are the most frequent findings in the small intestine. Regeneration of intestinal epithelium occurs in dogs surviving the acute phase of enteric infection. CPV infects lymphocytes in the thymic cortex and germinal centers of lymph nodes, which results in lymphocytolysis and cellular depletion in lymphoid tissue. The myocardial form of CPV infection of the ventricular myocardium results in myofiber degeneration and necrosis that is accompanied by infiltration of mononuclear cells.

Host Response to Infection. The immune response of canines following CPV infection is similar to that of felines. HAI and neutralizing antibodies appear in dogs approximately 1 week after infection. High levels of antibodies are generally present after 10–12 days, and these antibodies can persist for the life of the animal. Lactogenic immunity based on maternal antibodies with neutralizing/HAI titers of more than 80 against CPV protects a puppy against viral infection; however, these antibodies also interfere with active immunization by modified live or inactivated CPV viral vaccines. Cellular immune responses are also generated during infection, and are likely important in limiting virus replication during acute infection.

Laboratory Diagnosis. Laboratory diagnosis of CPD is very similar to feline parvovirus disease. Puppies or young dogs presenting with the clinical signs of high fever, anorexia, depression, vomiting, diarrhea, and dehydration, or the presence of severe leukopenia should be considered for the presumptive diagnosis of CPD. The diagnosis can be confirmed by one of the following laboratory methods:

1. The viral antigen may be detected in feces from live animals by antigen-capture ELISA, PCR amplification of viral nucleic acid, or electron microscopy.
2. The virus may be detected in tissues from dead animals by antigen-capture ELISA, immunofluorescence staining or immunohistochemistry with a CPV-specific antisera conjugate, or PCR.
3. The virus may be isolated in cell culture from filtered feces or tissue samples using cultured feline or canine cells.

Serodiagnosis following disease or tracking vaccine antibody levels may be accomplished by HAI testing (HAI titers of >80 are considered protective). Other antibody tests that are useful to monitor exposure include ELISA or indirect immunofluorescence. Paired sera and a fourfold rise in titer are required to confirm the diagnosis or "vaccine take."

Treatment and Control. Severe cases of canine parvoviral disease are characterized by marked dehydration and metabolic acidosis. Supportive therapy directed to restoration of fluid and electrolyte balance will increase the survival rate of clinically affected animals; however, there is no specific treatment that eliminates CPV from the infected animal. Prevention of infection is the key to controlling this disease. Vaccination, isolation of dogs that survive infection, and meticulous decontamination of premises that have housed affected animals are critical for containment of this highly transmissible virus. Household bleach at a 1 : 20 dilution or commercial products labeled for use against parvovirus provide effective virucidal activity against CPV and should be used extensively. Antibody levels correlate directly with the degree of protection against CPV infection. Numerous efficacious inactivated and modified live CPV vaccines are commercially available. Maternal antibodies can interfere with the immunization of young puppies, and this needs to be considered as part of the vaccination regime. The passive antibody typically wanes around 4–12 weeks of age, and multiple vaccinations are required in order to immunize puppies immediately prior to the "susceptibility window" and ensure uniform protection.

Porcine Parvovirus Infection Disease. Porcine parvovirus (PPV) is ubiquitous among swine throughout the world and is enzootic in most herds in the United States. Infection of pregnant dams with PPV causes reproductive failure or SMEDI syndrome, which is characterized by stillbirth, mummification, embryonic death, and infertility. Typically, the virus infects seronegative pregnant dams resulting in transplacental infection of developing fetuses. If fetal infection occurs prior to the development of immunocompetency, generalized infertility, embryonic death, mummification, and stillborn pigs are observed. Infection of nonpregnant swine with PPV results in the development of a rapid and lifelong immune response to the virus with no apparent clinical disease.

Etiologic Agent

Physical, Chemical, and Antigenic Properties. PPV is a typical parvovirus and has similar appearance and genome organization to FPV and CPV. To date, four different genotypes of porcine parvovirus (1–4) have been described, however, genotype 1 is the most common PPV found in North America. Like other parvoviruses, PPV is very stable because viral infectivity, hemagglutinating activity, and antigenicity are resistant to a wide range of heat, pH, and enzyme treatments. Assuming proper pen management, the virus can be inactivated by a 5% household bleach solution and commercial disinfectants that have been "parvo approved." Only one serotype has been identified, and all isolates of PPV that have been compared have been found to be antigenically similar to each other. PPV is antigenically distinct from other parvoviruses.

Infectivity for Other Species and Culture Systems. The host range for PPV appears to be limited to swine. The virus can replicate in fetal or neonatal swine kidney cells as well the established PK-15 (porcine kidney) and ST (swine testicle) cell lines.

Host–Virus Relationship

Distribution, Reservoir, and Transmission. PPV is ubiquitous in swine herds throughout the world, and serosurveillance data indicate that infection is very common. PPV is maintained in the environment due to shedding of the virus in oral secretions and feces following infection. There is evidence that in utero infection and immunotolerance may occur and persistently infected animals can shed the virus for prolonged periods of time. In one study, gilts were inoculated with PPV prior to 55 days of gestation. As a result, seronegative, live-born offspring carried the virus in a variety of tissues up to 8 months of age when the study was terminated. PPV can persist in the environment for extremely long periods of time, making contaminated premises a major reservoir for infection of naïve swine. Venereal transmission through infected semen is also a mechanism of PPV transmission. Immunotolerant, persistently infected boars can harbor the virus for at least 8 months and acutely infected seronegative boars can maintain the virus for at least 35 days postinfection.

Since most herd sows have experienced PPV infection, they are solidly immune to the virus and have high antibody levels that are then passed to their offspring through colostrum. Young pigs are resistant to PPV infection until the maternal antibody wanes, typically around 3–6 months of age. Gilts infected prior to pregnancy mount a vigorous immune response with no clinical disease and are refractal to subsequent exposure and infection. Infection of gilts or sows during the first half of pregnancy often results in generalized infertility, embryonic death, mummification, and stillborn pigs.

Pathogenesis and Pathology. PPV infection of nonpregnant, seronegative swine results in no apparent clinical disease and is accompanied by a vigorous antibody response. Most herd sows have experienced PPV infection, causing them to remain immune to the virus and maintain very high antibody levels that are then passed to their offspring through colostrum. Young pigs are resistant to PPV infection until maternal antibody wanes, typically around 3–6 months of age. Gilts infected prior to pregnancy mount a vigorous immune response with no clinical disease and maintain immunity to subsequent exposure and infection. Infection of gilts or sows during pregnancy often results in generalized infertility, embryonic death, mummification, and stillborn pigs.

PPV infection occurring early in gestation (<30 days) is not always apparent as it often results in embryonic death and fetal resorption, which may be misinterpreted as generalized infertility and return to service. However, if the fetus becomes infected between 30 and 70 days of gestation, death and mummification generally occur. If the fetus becomes infected between 70 days of gestation and term, an immune response is generated and although live birth generally occurs, often times these late-gestation infections result in offspring that fail to thrive.

Gross lesions of PPV-infected pregnant dams have not been reported. Microscopic lesions following experimental infection include extensive cuffing of myometrial and endometrial vessels with mononuclear cells and focal accumulation of lymphocytes in the uterus. Microscopic changes in the fetus are often nonspecific, but can include foci of necrosis and mononuclear cell infiltration in organs such as the liver, heart, kidney, and cerebrum.

Host Responses to Infection. No clinical disease is observed when PPV infection of seronegative, nonpregnant swine occurs. Following infection, the animals become viremic and mount a vigorous antibody response that provides lifelong immunity in most cases. Immune dams provide high levels of lactogenic immunity to their offspring through colostrum. Young pigs remain resistant to infection with PPV until the maternal antibody wanes, usually around 3–6 months of age. Reproductive disease may occur if seronegative gilts become infected while pregnant.

Laboratory Diagnosis. PPV should be considered in the differential diagnosis of reproductive failure when there is evidence of embryonic or fetal deaths. This is especially true if gilts but not sows are affected. Direct detection of PPV antigens or nucleic acid from tissues of mummified or stillborn pigs will result in a solid diagnosis of PPV-induced reproductive failure. Immunofluorescence staining or immunohistochemistry with a PPV-specific antiserum conjugate, and/or PCR are the most common diagnostic techniques used to confirm PPV. Isolation of the virus in cell culture from tissue samples can sometimes be accomplished using cultured swine cells as the substrate; however, this is not a very reliable method of detection as isolation attempts are not always successful.

Serodiagnosis following infection or tracking vaccine antibody levels in adult swine may be accomplished by serum neutralization or HAI testing (HAI titers of >40 are considered protective). Detection of PPV antibodies in thoracic fluids of mummified or stillborn pigs is indicative of in utero infection.

Treatment and Control. There is no treatment for reproductive failure caused by PPV infection. Vaccination is the preferred method of controlling PPV infection in the breeding herd. Controlled infection and acclimation during gilt development will induce infection in nonpregnant gilts, resulting in subsequent protection against reproductive failure. Both vaccination and acclimation must be carefully timed to ensure that animals are immunized and/or infected after passive antibodies wane but before breeding occurs.

Aleutian Disease in Mink Disease. Aleutian disease (AD) or mink plasmacytosis was first recognized in the mid-1950s in ranch-raised mink. Aleutian mink have a gun-metal gray-colored phase and tend to be more susceptible to infection and clinical disease with Aleutian disease virus (ADV) than other color variations of domesticated mink. AD tends to be a lethal disease in mink that progresses slowly after infection, often times taking up to a year before producing clinical symptoms. The disease is characterized by poor reproduction, gradual weight loss, oral and gastro-intestinal bleeding, renal failure, uremia, and frequently death. ADV infects mink, ferrets, and possibly other Mustelidae. AD causes significant economic loss to mink ranchers and now appears to be spreading to wild mink populations. It is also becoming a significant threat to pet ferrets.

Etiologic Agent

Physical, Chemical, and Antigenic Properties. ADV is the only known member of the genus *Amdovirus* in the family Parvoviridae and is similar to "true" parvoviruses in the genus *Parvovirus*. ADV-infected animals shed the virus in saliva, feces, and urine, and these secretions may be infectious for months or even years. ADV is a small, naked virus containing a single linear strand of DNA that is highly resistant to inactivation by pH solvents, extreme temperatures, and most disinfectants. Decontamination of infested pens is best achieved by steam cleaning followed by prolonged contact with a 5% bleach solution or a disinfectant that has been demonstrated to be efficacious against parvoviruses. The virus is genetically and antigenically distinct from the mink enteritis virus as well as other carnivore parvoviruses.

Infectivity for Other Species and Cell Systems. ADV infects mink of all types (domestic and wild), although disease is more severe in mink that have the Aleutian color phase. There is some serological evidence that ADV is spreading in wild mink populations in Canada. which may be associated with the decline of wild mink. Ferrets can be infected with ADV but do not always develop clinical disease, and the animals that do develop disease often show no apparent clinical signs until shortly before death. Some strains of the virus can be propagated in fetal mink kidney cell cultures or in feline cell lines.

Host–Virus Relationship

Distribution, Reservoir, and Transmission. AD of mink is present in many mink ranches around the world. Infected animals shed the virus in blood, saliva, feces, and urine, and the virus is transmitted by fecal–oral or possibly respiratory routes. The historical reservoir for ADV has been infected domestic mink with overt clinical signs or with undetected infections. In recent times, cross-transmission between ranch-raised mink and wild populations has been observed in Canada and Europe. AD in pet ferrets is receiving attention because asymptomatic animals are carriers of the virus and are capable of transmitting it at ferret shows and other gathering places. There has been a recent report of possible human disease associated with ADV. Two unrelated incidents of mink ranchers with vascular disease and microangiopathy were found to have ADV antibodies and viral nucleic acid.

Pathogenesis and Pathology. ADV replicates rapidly in experimentally infected mink, and virus titers are observed 10 days postinoculation. Most animals become persistently infected and harbor the virus in the viscera, serum, and urine for the remainder of their lives. Antibody response following infection reaches very high levels and binds with circulating ADV to form infectious immune complexes. Arterial and glomerular lesions that are classic of AD are caused by deposition of immune complexes and the subsequent inflammatory response. The disease process observed in natural infections is a slowly progressive one that can take up to a year to manifest and produce noticeable symptoms. During this time infected mink shed the virus in urine and feces and can infect naïve animals. Infected mink do not exhibit symptoms until several weeks or months after they are infected, at which time loss of appetite, decreased activity, weight loss, tarry diarrhea, and a rough coat are observed. Once the symptoms become obvious, death of the mink is certain. Gross lesions include splenomegaly, glomerulonephritis, and enlarged mesenteric lymph nodes. Histologic lesions are characterized by plasma cell infiltration in the kidneys, liver, spleen, lymph nodes, and bone marrow. Infection of young mink results in a more rapid onset and death is often due to acute interstitial pneumonia. In all cases the animals are immunocompromised and subject to secondary infections.

Infection in pet ferrets occasionally results in clinical presentation very similar to adult mink infection; however, most ferrets that become infected remain asymptomatic and clear the virus over time.

Host Responses to Infection. Following infection, immunoglobulin levels rise markedly and the antibody complexes with the circulating virus to form infectious immune complexes that are not cleared from circulation. Antibody response following infection can be detected in a number of assays including indirect fluorescent antibody detection and counterimmunoelectrophoresis.

Laboratory Diagnosis. Following infection, immunofluorescence, immunohistochemistry, and PCR assays may be used to detect the virus in body secretions and tissues. Serological methods for detection of antibodies following infection include indirect fluorescent antibody testing and counterimmunoelectrophoresis. Both assays are useful for identifying infected carrier animals that need to be culled or quarantined from naïve mink. Both assays are also useful for monitoring the infection status of pet ferrets that may be shedding the virus.

Treatment and Control. For both mink and ferrets, biosecurity is the only effective control mechanism for maintaining seronegative animals. Secure physical separation between domestic and wild mink populations should be in place to minimize transmission. All animals entering an established seronegative mink ranch need to be screened for the antibody prior to entry. If seropositive animals are found on a mink ranch, they should physically separated and maintained from seronegative animals and then culled at harvest. Seropositive ferrets should be isolated from seronegative animals in order to prevent horizontal transmission. Contaminated pens should be thoroughly cleaned, preferably with steam treatment followed by prolonged exposure to a 5% Clorox solution or a disinfectant that is labeled as parvocidal.

Circoviridae

The term "circovirus" originates from the covalently closed circular arrangement of the single-stranded genome characteristic of these viruses. Currently, two genera, *Circovirus* and *Gyrovirus*, are included in the Circoviridae family. The genus *Circovirus* contains 11 species, including *Porcine circovirus* types 1 (PCV1) and 2 (PCV2), *Canary circovirus, Duck circovirus, Finch circovirus, Goose circovirus, Gull circovirus, Pigeon circovirus, Starling circovirus, Swan circovirus*, and *Beak and feather disease virus* (BFDV). Additional circovirus species have been reported in chimpanzees, bats, bovine, fish, and canines; however, whether they play a significant role in disease manifestation is unknown. While chicken anemia virus is the only member of the *Gyrovirus* genus, additional *Gyrovirus* species have been reported in other avian species and humans. Recently, a new genus termed *Cyclovirus* has been proposed within the family Circoviridae. Cyclovirus sequences have been identified in chimpanzees, goats, sheep, camels, bats, chickens, and dragonflies. Furthermore, cyclovirus sequences have been found in beef products and human stool samples. Currently, knowledge of cycloviruses is based strictly on genomic sequence data.

The family Circoviridae encompasses some of the smallest known viruses with genomes ranging from 1 to 4 kb. The small genome size limits their capacity to only the most essential genes, including a viral replicase and capsid protein. Similar to parvoviruses, members of Circoviridae rely on host enzymes during their life cycle. Virus propagation within the host requires an actively replicating cell.

Characteristic Physical and Chemical Properties

Circoviridae are characterized as nonenveloped, single-stranded circular DNA viruses, with genomes ranging from 1 to 4 kb. Virions range in size from ~17 to 28 nm and are composed of 60 capsid protein subunits arranged in T = 1 icosahedral symmetry. Virions have a buoyant density of 1.37 g/ml in a CsCl gradient.

Resistance to Physical and Chemical Agents. Circoviruses are stable at a pH of 3.0 and at temperatures of 56 °C for 1 h, or 70 °C for up to 15 min. Disinfectants aimed at dissolving lipids such as those utilizing bases of alcohol, chlorhexidine, iodine, and phenol are ineffective. Virus inactivation requires alkaline disinfectants (sodium hydroxide), oxidizing agents (sodium hypochlorite), or quaternary ammonium compounds.

Beak and Feather Disease

Disease. While avian-specific medicine for poultry has significantly progressed over the years, only minimal information is available for psittacine birds. Viral infectious diseases such as beak and feather disease, also termed psittacine beak and feather disease (PBFD), are some of the most common problems with psittacine birds. PBFD was first observed in Australia in the early 1970s, and since then it has emerged in multiple countries. The onset and severity of disease is dependent on the age of the host. PBFD typically presents as necrotic or otherwise abnormal feathers such as feathers that are bent, contain hemorrhages, or are prematurely shed. Chronic infection may result in beak and nail deformities. Neonatal birds are particularly susceptible to severe acute disease characterized by pneumonia, enteritis, rapid weight loss, and death.

Etiologic Agent

Infectivity for Other Species and Culture Systems. The primary host for the causative agent of PBFD, the BFDV, is psittacine birds. There is currently no cell culture system available for virus propagation.

Host–Virus Relationship

Distribution, Reservoir, and Transmission. PBFD has been described among birds in many countries including Japan, Germany, Italy, New Zealand, South Africa, Taiwan, Thailand, the United States, and Australia. Movement of infected Australian psittacine birds is likely the cause of dissemination since BFDV is endemic in free-ranging populations of several psittacine species in Australia. BFDV has been identified in over 60 species of captive and free-ranging psittacine birds. Transmission of the virus occurs through both horizontal and vertical routes.

Pathogenesis and Pathology. Exposure to BFDV results in subclinical infection in the majority of free-ranging and captive birds. However, the outcome of infection is dependent on many factors, such as the age of the bird at initial exposure, the presence and levels of protection provided by the maternal antibody, and the route and titer of the infecting virus. The incubation time for BFDV may be prolonged with resulting clinical signs appearing long after the initial infection. Clinical signs in young birds may present as inappetance, lethargy, crop stasis, progressive feather abnormalities, and eventual death. In some cases, secondary infections stemming from immune suppression are the primary cause of death. Histologic lesions are dependent upon multiple factors including the duration and severity of the disease. However, characteristic intranuclear and intracytoplasmic inclusion bodies may be present in macrophages in the thymus, bursa, and other lymphoid tissues, as well as in epithelial cells lining the shaft of the feather.

Host Responses to Infection. Exposure to BFDV results in resistance to reinfection. Maternal antibodies likely provide passive protection of chicks against BFDV infection for several weeks after birth.

Laboratory Diagnosis. Diagnosis of PBFD is based on identification of the clinical signs and characteristic gross and histologic changes in the tissues of affected birds. Assays for the identification of BFDV infection include *in situ* hybridization, hemagglutination and HAI, electron microscopy, PCR, and real-time PCR.

Treatment and Control. The most effective method to control PBFD involves elimination or quarantine of carrier birds to prevent transmission of BFDV. Currently, there are no commercially available vaccines for BFDV, although experimental efforts involving recombinant BFDV capsid protein are underway.

Chicken Infectious Anemia Disease. Chicken infectious anemia (CIA) was first recognized in 1979 as a highly contagious disease of young chickens (2–4 weeks of age). Clinical disease resulting from infection with chicken anemia virus (CAV), the etiological agent of CIA, is rare due in large to the practice of widespread vaccination. However, the subclinical form of disease, which occurs at all stages of production, remains prevalent worldwide. Clinical signs in young birds include aplastic anemia, generalized lymphoid atrophy, and profound immune suppression often resulting in secondary viral, bacterial, and fungal infections. The subclinical form of disease, characterized by prolonged viremia and reduced growth performance, results in serious economic losses to the poultry industry. Within the Circoviridae family, CAV represents the most distinct virus, with a genetic organization that more closely resembles viruses classified within the Anelloviridae family. Genetically distinct strains of CAV have been identified, although strains are similar in terms of antigenicity and virulence.

Etiologic Agent

Infectivity for Other Species and Culture Systems. The primary host for CAV is the chicken. CAV can be propagated in chicken embryos, chicken primary blood mononuclear cells, and the MDCC-MSB-1 cell line *in vitro*.

Host–Virus Relationship

Distribution, Reservoir, and Transmission. CAV is ubiquitous in commercial and specific pathogen-free chicken stocks. While all ages of chickens are susceptible to infection, older chickens are more resistant to clinical disease. Transmission of the virus occurs through both the horizontal and vertical routes.

Pathogenesis and Pathology. In nonprotected chicks, CAV targets hemocytoblasts in the bone marrow and lymphocytes in the thymus, resulting in aplastic anemia, leukopenia, thrombocytopenia, and thymic atrophy. Clinical signs generally appear 7–14 days after infection, presenting as gangrenous lesions on the wings. Furthermore, immunosuppression often results in opportunistic infections from other viruses, bacteria, or fungi. Early investigations indicate that maternal antibodies play a significant role in the prevention of disease. However, older chickens become susceptible to CAV infection once maternal antibodies decay, which may result in the subclinical form of disease. In addition to reduced growth performance, immunosuppression has recently been identified as a disease manifestation in older chickens.

Host Responses to Infection. Maternal antibodies provide passive protection to CAV infection and disease for several weeks after birth. Upon decay of maternal antibodies, CAV exposure may result in a persistent infection, resulting in reduced growth performance and immunosuppression.

Laboratory Diagnosis. A clinical diagnosis of CIA is based on flock history, clinical signs, and pathological findings. Assays to confirm infection with CAV include virus isolation, PCR, real-time PCR, or immunohistochemical staining of tissues with CAV-specific antibodies. Serological assays for the detection of CAV infection include ELISA, indirect immunofluorescence (IFA), and virus neutralization assay.

Treatment and Control. The most effective practice for controlling CAV involves vaccination of breeding flocks with a modified live virus, which prevents vertical transmission of the virus and provides protective maternal antibodies. No specific treatment is available for chickens infected with CAV.

Porcine Circovirus-Associated Disease

Disease. Porcine circoviruses (PCV) were first discovered as a cell culture contaminant in the 1970s. At that time, the virus was considered nonpathogenic and ubiquitous within the swine population. In the early 1990s, a novel wasting syndrome was described in pigs. Subsequently, the etiological agent was identified as a PCV, which shared approximately 60% sequence identity with the previously identified virus. Since then, the viruses have been termed PCV1 and PCV2 to distinguish the nonpathogenic and pathogenic viruses, respectively. To date, PCV2 infection has been linked with a variety of syndromes, collectively termed porcine circovirus-associated disease (PCVAD).

PCVAD describes a group of complex multifactorial syndromes that occur during all stages of pork production. Manifestations of PCVAD can range from nonovert clinical signs to acute death. Clinical signs typically present as wasting, diarrhea, respiratory distress, dermatitis, or reproductive failure. PCVAD first appeared in the early 1990s, and continues to impact the world's pork industry. The primary factor for the onset of PCVAD involves infection with PCV2. PCV2 isolates are divided into two main genotypes, known as PCV2a and PCV2b. Recently, a new classification scheme has been proposed to describe PCVAD syndromes. Typical PCVAD syndromes include porcine multisystemic wasting syndromes (PMWS), PCV2-associated enteritis, PCV2-associated respiratory disease, proliferative and necrotizing pneumonia, PCV2-associated reproductive failure, porcine dermatitis and nephropathy syndrome, and acute pulmonary edema.

Etiologic Agent

Infectivity for Other Species and Culture Systems. Domestic and feral pigs are the primary hosts for PCV2. Porcine epithelial cells from kidney and testicle support PCV2 replication in cell culture systems. Experimental infections with PCV2 have been established in mice.

Host–Virus Relationship

Distribution, Reservoir, and Transmission. Historically, PCV2 isolates were classified based on similarities with isolates from North America (PCV2a) or Europe (PCV2b). However, both genotypes are considered endemic within the world pig population. PCV2 establishes a long-term infection and is shed in oronasal fluid, urine, blood, and feces in pigs for up to 28 weeks of age on PCVAD-affected farms. Transmission most often occurs pig to pig through the horizontal route. In addition, PCV2 is very stable within the environment, which likely plays a role in virus transmission.

Pathogenesis and Pathology. The clinical manifestation and severity of PCVAD are linked to a variety of cofactors, such as the disease potential of the PCV2 isolate, the presence of pathogenic or opportunistic infections, host genetics, and use of immunostimulating agents such as vaccines.

In general, clinical and pathological signs are syndrome specific. Clinical signs of PMWS, the most common PCVAD syndrome, include lethargy, diarrhea, lymphadenopathy, discoloring of the skin, jaundice, and wasting. Gross pathological signs include enlargement of the submandibular, inguinal, and bronchial lymph nodes, noncollapsed mottled lungs, occasional spleen infarcts, atrophic and discolored liver, and enteritis. Histopathological characteristics of PMWS may include lymphocyte depletion with granulomatous inflammation of lymphoid tissues, which may include intracytoplasmic inclusion bodies, granulomatous to lymphohistiocytic interstitial pneumonia, lymphohistiocytic hepatitis, interstitial nephritis, and granulomatous enteritis. An electron microscopic image of a

FIGURE 49.1. *Electron microscope image of swine testicle cells infected with PCV2.*

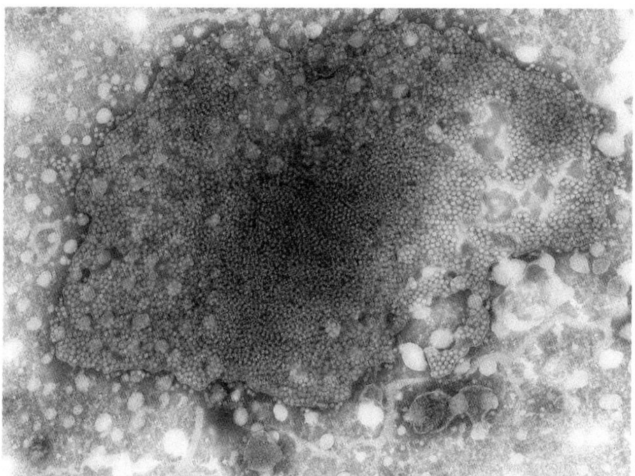

PCV2a-induced inclusion body following infection of swine testicle cells is shown in Figure 49.1.

Host Response to Infection. PCV2 infection results in a pronounced humoral and cell-mediated response that, in general, is incapable of clearing viral infection. Maternally derived antibodies resulting from natural infection typically provide minimal protection against PCV2 infection.

Laboratory Diagnosis. Clinical signs, history, and histopathological examinations are useful in a presumptive diagnosis of PCVAD. Laboratory procedures used to confirm PCV2 infection include the following:

1. Isolation of PCV2 from serum or tissues of infected animals on susceptible cell cultures, or by identification of PCV2 nucleic acid in infected tissues by PCR.
2. Detection of PCV2 antigens in histological sections of lung or lymphoid lesions by immunofluorescent or immunohistochemical staining with virus-specific antibodies.
3. Detection of PCV2-specific antibodies in serum using serologic tests such as IFA, virus neutralization assay, or ELISA. Figure 49.2 shows the typical PCV2 staining of an IFA-positive serum sample.

Treatment and Control. Before the advent of vaccines, multiple measures were incorporated with varying effects. These included proper housing, stress reduction, practicing an "all-in-all-out" policy, and the prevention of age mixing. Further methods that were used with minimal success included antibiotics to control secondary infections, serum therapy, and depopulation. The most effective method for controlling PCV2 today is vaccination. Field and experimental vaccine trials have demonstrated prevention of PCVAD, decreased viremia, and increased growth performance.

FIGURE 49.2. *Immunofluorescent staining of PCV2 antigens in swine testicle cells.*

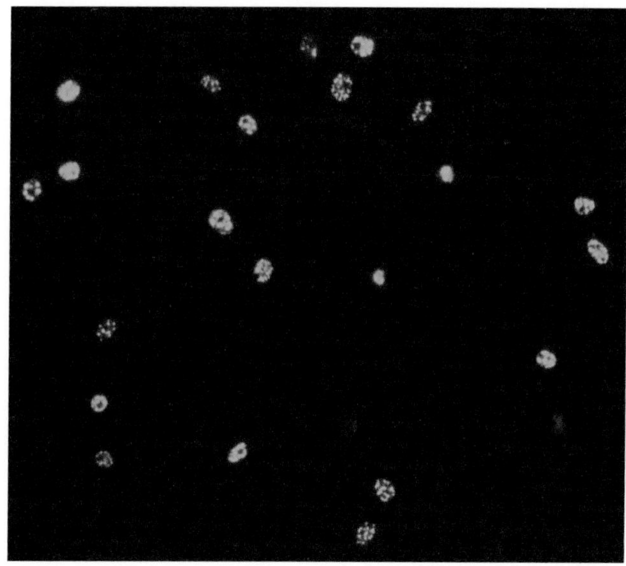

Currently, several commercial vaccines incorporate the PCV2a ORF2 antigen, which may be expressed in baculovirus, inactivated PCV2, or an inactivated PCV1/2 chimera. Of the five commercial vaccines currently available, four are recommended for use in piglets and only one for sows. Vaccine schedules for piglets are either one or two doses with the first dose administered at 3 weeks of age. In the case of the two-dose vaccine, the second dose is administered 3 weeks later. Sow vaccination is recommended at 2 and 5 weeks antepartum.

Further Reading

Allison AB, Harbison CE, Pagan I *et al.* (2012) Role of multiple hosts in the cross-species transmission and emergence of pandemic parvovirus. *J Virol*, **86**, 865–872.

American Ferret Association (2012) *Aleutian Mink Disease: A Hidden Danger to Your Ferret*, http://www.ferret.org/read/aleutianarticle.html (accessed January 11, 2013).

Bachmann PA, Sheffy BE, and Vaughan JT (1975) Experimental in utero infection of fetal pigs with a porcine parvovirus. *Infect Immun*, **12**, 455–460.

Balamurugan V and Kataria JM (2006) Economically important non-oncogenic immunosuppressive viral diseases of chicken—current status. *Vet Res Commun*, **30**, 541–566.

Battilani M, Balboni A, Ustulin M *et al.* (2011) Genetic complexity and multiple infections with more *Parvovirus* species in naturally infected cats. *Vet Res*, **42**, 43.

Bonne N, Shearer P, Sharp M *et al.* (2009) Assessment of recombinant beak and feather disease virus capsid protein as a vaccine for psittacine beak and feather disease. *J Gen Virol*, **90**, 640–647.

Cheng F, Chen AY, Best SM *et al.* (2010) The capsid proteins of Aleutian mink disease virus activate caspases and are specifically cleaved during infection. *J Virol*, **84**, 2687–2696.

Cutlip RC and Mengeling WL (1975) Pathogenesis of in utero infection of eight and ten-week-old porcine fetus with porcine parvovirus. *Am J Vet Res*, **36**, 1751–1754.

Ettinger SJ and Feldman EC (1995) *Textbook Vet. Internal Med*, W.B. Saunders Company.

Farid AH, Rupasinghe P, Mitchell JL, and Rouvinen-Watt K (2010) A survey of Aleutian mink disease virus infection of feral American mink in Nova Scotia. *Can Vet J*, **51**, 75–77.

Gillespie J, Opriessnig T, Meng XJ *et al.* (2009) Porcine circovirus type 2 and porcine circovirus-associated disease. *J Vet Intern Med*, **23**, 1151–1163.

Grau-Roma L, Fraile L, and Segalés J (2011) Recent advances in the epidemiology, diagnosis and control of diseases caused by porcine circovirus type 2. *Vet J*, **187**, 23–32.

Hoerr FJ (2010) Clinical aspects of immunosuppression in poultry. *Avian Dis*, **54**, 2–15.

Ikeda Y, Mochizuki M, Naito R *et al.* (2000) Predominance of canine parvovirus (CPV) in unvaccinated cat populations and emergence of new antigenic types of CPVs in cats. *Virol*, **278**, 9–13.

Jepsen JR, d'Amore F, Baandrup U *et al.* (2009) Aleutian mink disease virus and humans. *Emerg Infect Dis*, **15**, 2040–2042.

Johnson RH (1973) Isolation of swine parvovirus in Queensland. *Aust Vet J*, **49**, 257–259.

Johnson RH and Collings DF (1971) Transplacental infection of piglets with a porcine parvovirus. *Res Vet Sci*, **12**, 570–572.

Jones TC (1997) *Vet. Patho*, Blackwell Publishing Ltd.

Katoh H, Ogawa H, Ohya K, and Fukushi H (2010) A review of DNA viral infections in psittacine birds. *J Vet Med Sci*, **72**, 1099–1106.

Lobetti R (2003) Canine parvovirus and distemper. Proceedings 28th World Congress. World Small Animal Veterinary Association.

Mengeling WL and Cutlip RC (1975) Pathogenesis of in utero infection: Experimental infection of 5-week-old porcine fetuses with porcine parvovirus. *Am J Vet Res*, **36**, 1173–1177.

Mengeling WL, Cutlip RC, and Barnett D (1978) Porcine parvovirus: Pathogenesis, prevalence, and prophylaxis. *Proc Int Congr Pig Vet Soc*, **5**, 15.

Miller MM and Schat KA (2004) Chicken infectious anemia virus: an example of the ultimate host-parasite relationship. *Avian Dis*, **48**, 734–745.

Nituch LA, Bowman J, Beauclerc KB, and Schulte-Hostedde AI (2011) Mink farm predicts Aleutian disease exposure in wild American mink. *PLoS One*, **6**, 7.

Opriessnig T and Halbur PG (2012) Concurrent infections are important for expression of porcine circovirus associated disease. *Virus Res*, **164** (1–2), 20–32.

Redman DR, Bohl EH, and Ferguson LC (1974) Porcine parvovirus: Natural and experimental infections of the porcine fetus and prevalence in mature swine. *Infect Immun*, **10**, 718–723.

Segalés J (2012) Porcine circovirus type 2 (PCV2) infections: clinical signs, pathology and laboratory diagnosis. *Virus Res*, **164** (1–2) 10–19.

Segalés J, Allan GM, and Domingo M (2012) Porcine circoviruses, in *Diseases of Swine*, 10th edn, Blackwell Publishing Ltd, Ames, pp. 405–417.

Tapscott B (2010) *Aleutian Disease in Mink*, Ministry of Agriculture, Food and Rural Affairs, Ontario.

Trible BR and Rowland RRR (2012) Genetic variation of porcine circovirus type 2 (PCV2) and its relevance to vaccination, pathogenesis and diagnosis. *Virus Res*, **164** (1–2), 68–77.

Varsani A, Regnard GL, Bragg R *et al.* (2011) Global genetic diversity and geographical and host-species distribution of beak and feather disease virus isolates. *J Gen Virol*, **92**, 752–767.

50 Asfarviridae and Iridoviridae

MELISSA KENNEDY

Asfarviridae

The family Asfarviridae includes just one genus, the genus *Asfivirus*, of which *African swine fever virus* is the type species.

African Swine Fever Virus

African swine fever (ASF) is a highly contagious disease of domestic and some species of wild swine. Disease in ASF virus-infected pigs ranges from peracute to chronic and inapparent. The primary natural reservoirs of the virus are warthogs and arthropod vectors in sub-Saharan Africa. While present in its wildlife host for a long time, it was first noted in domestic swine in 1921 in Kenya. It was first noted outside of Africa occurring in Portugal in 1957. Since this time, the virus has been identified at various times in European countries and Caribbean islands. In recent years, outbreaks have occurred in Russia (reviewed in Costard *et al.* 2009). Incursions of the virus into populations of domestic and swine typically result in extensive outbreaks of acute ASF, and the subacute and chronic forms appear after the virus becomes established in the pig population. Whether endemic or newly introduced, ASF has a profound impact on economics and food security. Given that several species of wild and domestic pigs as well as tick vectors are susceptible, it continues to be a global threat.

Disease. Acute, severe ASF has a high mortality, often approaching 100%, and death may occur prior to development of clinical signs. The disease is characterized by high fever and leukopenia, often followed by the appearance of erythema (red areas on the skin), weakness, accelerated respiration and pulse, vomiting, bloody diarrhea, and nasal and conjunctival discharges. Subacute ASF is characterized by less dramatic clinical signs and death or recovery in 3–4 weeks. Affected pigs typically experience a high fever; abortion is common and may be the only sign of illness. Pigs with chronic ASF fail to thrive (stunting and emaciation), and exhibit swollen joints and lameness, skin ulcerations, and pneumonia.

Etiologic Agent

Physical, Chemical, and Antigenic Properties. The ASF virus is an enveloped DNA virus with a nucleoprotein core of 70–100 nm that is surrounded by lipid layers and an icosahedral capsid of 170–190 nm in diameter (Figure 50.1). The genome is a single large (170–190 kb) molecule of double-stranded DNA that includes approximately 150 open reading frames. Virions contain more than 50 different proteins, including a large number of enzymes and proteins required for replication. The viral genome also encodes proteins that appear to modulate the protective host antiviral response.

Several genetically distinct groups of ASF viruses have been identified by restriction endonuclease analysis of the genomes of ASF viruses isolated in different regions of the world. Strains of the ASF virus can vary markedly in their virulence in swine. The greatest genetic variation occurs in regions where the sylvatic cycle is present.

Resistance to Physical and Chemical Agents. The ASF virus is stable in tissues and excretions. It can withstand pH in a considerable range (pH 4–13). The virus is inactivated by heating to 60 °C for 20 min and by lipid solvents and some disinfectants (paraphenylphenolic disinfectants are very effective against the virus).

Infectivity for Other Species and Culture Systems. The ASF virus infects domestic and wild pigs (including European wild boars), warthogs, giant forest hogs, and bush pigs. Soft ticks of the genus *Ornithodoros* transmit the virus as biological vectors. Only domestic and wild pigs (feral pigs and European wild boars) express clinical disease, whereas African wild pigs do not.

The ASF virus replicates in pig macrophages, and can be propagated *in vitro* on cultures of swine bone marrow cells, monocytes, and alveolar macrophages. The virus can also be adapted to various established cell lines (pig kidney, VERO, and baby hamster kidney).

Veterinary Microbiology, Third Edition. Edited by D. Scott McVey, Melissa Kennedy and M.M. Chengappa.

FIGURE 50.1. ASF virus in thin section of infected tissue culture cells (58 000×). (Courtesy of I.C. Pang.)

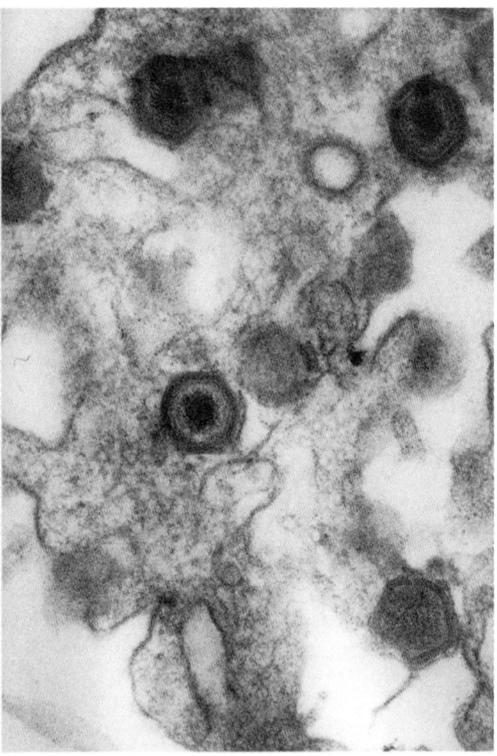

Host–Virus Relationship

Distribution, Reservoir, and Transmission. ASF was first described in European domestic pigs in Kenya in the early 1900s, and the disease regularly has emerged into other regions of the world since that time. The disease spread outside of Africa for the first time in 1957 when it appeared on the Iberian Peninsula, and subsequently has occurred in Mediterranean Europe (Spain, France, Italy, Malta, and Sardinia), northern Europe (Belgium and the Netherlands), the Caribbean (Cuba, the Dominican Republic, and Haiti), and South America (Brazil). ASF has been described throughout much of Africa.

The ASF virus exists in two distinct cycles of infection: first, a sylvatic cycle in ticks and wild pigs in Africa; and, second, epidemic and endemic cycles in domestic swine. The reservoirs of the sylvatic cycle of ASF virus infection in Africa are persistent or inapparent infections in African wild pigs (warthogs in particular) and the soft tick vector. Vertical transmission of the ASF virus in the tick vectors makes them an especially efficient reservoir of the virus. The virus spreads into domestic swine through the bites of infected ticks, or by ingestion of tissues from carrier swine. The virus is then readily transmitted to susceptible pigs by direct contact, including aerosols and fomites. The virus is easily transmitted over long distances because of its stability in infected tissues, including uncooked and some cured pork products. Importantly, soft ticks become infected with the virus after they feed on viremic swine, and thus they can become reservoirs of the virus after it incurs into previously noninfected regions. Pigs that survive infection with the ASF virus become carriers of the virus.

Pathogenesis and Pathology. Following oral or nasal exposure of domestic pigs to the ASF virus, virus replication initially occurs in the upper respiratory tract with subsequent dissemination to adjacent lymph nodes and then systemic spread via leukocytes, erythrocytes, or both in the lymph and blood; this occurs within 3 days postinfection and corresponds closely with the onset of pyrexia. The virus replicates in macrophages; thus, the highest titers of the virus occur in those tissues in which macrophages are most abundant.

Acute severe ASF is characterized by edema and hemorrhage within internal organs, particularly the lymph nodes and spleen, which can be very large and intensely hemorrhagic. Pulmonary edema and intestinal congestion and hemorrhage are also common. The lesions of subacute ASF are similar but less pronounced, whereas animals with chronic ASF may show fibrinous pericarditis and pleuritis, lobular consolidation of the lungs, swollen joints, and patchy necrosis of the skin. Lesions in aborted piglets are relatively nonspecific, but may include disseminated petechial hemorrhages.

Microscopic lesions are most pronounced in the lymphoid tissues, and include extensive necrosis of both lymphocytes and mononuclear phagocytic cells. Endothelial cell necrosis and thrombosis of the pulmonary vasculature is common in fulminant cases of acute ASF.

Host Responses to Infection. Pigs that survive infection with ASF virus develop a strong humoral immune (antibody) response; however, this response is largely ineffectual in neutralizing the virus. Why the antibody response of swine to ASF is largely ineffectual remains uncertain, but it is clearly a reflection of the inherent properties of the ASF virus itself. Nevertheless, efforts at developing an effective vaccine are complicated by the inability of swine to produce high titers of neutralizing antibodies to the virus. It appears that cell-mediated immunity is important in protection.

Laboratory Diagnosis. Laboratory tests are required to distinguish between hog cholera and ASF because the two diseases cause very similar signs and lesions in susceptible pigs, including fever, high mortality, and hemorrhages within internal organs. Tissues submitted should include spleen, liver, lymph nodes, and blood. Virus isolation can be used to identify the ASF virus, and then confirmed with hemadsorption. Immunofluorescent or immunoperoxidase staining of sections of tissue from affected pigs using ASF virus-specific antisera provides a rapid method of diagnosis. Techniques based on polymerase chain reaction can also be used to rapidly identify the presence of ASF virus genomic material.

Treatment and Control. There is no effective vaccine or treatment for ASF. Eradication of the disease is accomplished by slaughter and disposal of all exposed pigs after the virus incurs into new areas. These drastic measures, however, may not prevent the virus from spreading to the local populations of soft ticks and wild pigs. Premises that undergo eradication procedures not only must slaughter all pigs but also must be treated with insecticides and disinfectants containing O-phenylphenol with surfactants and must remain free of livestock for at least a month. Prior to restocking, susceptible sentinel animals should be placed on the premises to confirm eradication of the virus.

In endemic areas, contact between domestic and wild swine must be avoided. Early detection is critical in control of outbreaks in domestic swine. Localized disease eradication with the establishment of ASF-free zones is beneficial, and can enhance support of larger scale eradication programs.

Iridoviridae

The family Iridoviridae includes five genera (*Iridovirus*, *Chloriridovirus*, *Ranavirus*, *Lymphocystis virus*, and *Megalocytivirus*) that are serologically distinct. Viruses in the genera *Megalocytivirus* and *Lymphocystisvirus* cause important diseases of fish, while viruses in the genus *Ranavirus* are significant pathogens of reptiles and amphibians as well as fish. In particular, *Megalocytivirus* and *Ranavirus* have emerged as important economically, causing systemic disease in freshwater and marine environments (Whittington 2010).

Iridoviruses are enveloped viruses that have icosahedral symmetry with a virion diameter of 120–200 nm but occasionally up to 350 nm. The genome is a single molecule of double-stranded DNA of between 140 and 300 kb pairs. Iridoviruses, like asfarviruses, are structurally complex with large numbers of virus-specific proteins (at least 36) encoded by the genome. A single protein constitutes the majority of the outer capsid. The double-stranded DNA genome is circular and terminally redundant with many of the internal cytosine residues being highly methylated. Viral replication occurs in the nucleus and cytoplasm of infected cells. These viruses are resistant to drying, and can persist in water for months. Definitive diagnosis is best made by viral isolation and/or characterization of the genome by molecular biology techniques.

The lymphocystis virus infects a wide variety of fish and causes unsightly wart-like cutaneous lesions. These lesions consist of benign proliferations of hypertrophied, virus-infected cells (fibroblasts and osteoblasts) on the skin, peritoneum, and mesentery. The lesions typically resolve with minimal mortality. The virus spreads by direct contact through abrasions, especially when fish are crowded; thus, disease caused by the lymphocystis virus is especially important in fish raised in aquaria and in some commercial aquaculture operations. Two strains of lymphocystis disease virus (LCDV) have been described, with LCDV-1 being associated with flounder and LCDV-2 being associated with dabs.

FIGURE 50.2. *Cope's gray tree frog (*Hyla chrysoscelis*) larvae experimentally exposed to ranavirus. The body and legs are swollen and there is hemorrhage in the legs, consistent with ranaviral disease.*

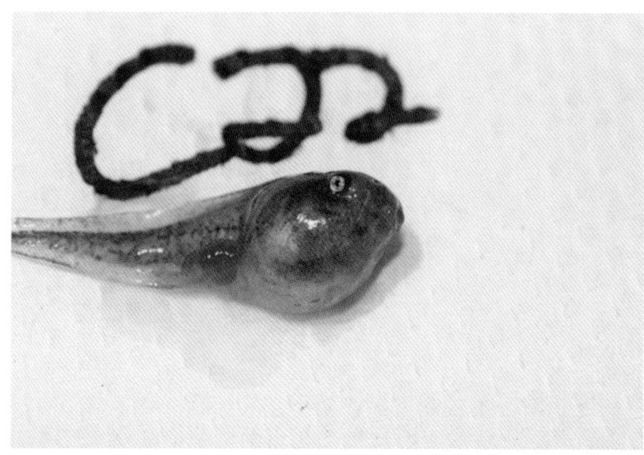

In contrast, the *Ranavirus* genus has been associated with high mortality in both farmed and free-ranging fish. These pathogenic iridoviruses causing fatal systemic disease are closely related to frog virus 3, the latter serving as the prototype ranavirus. Members of this genus have been reported to cause epizootic hematopoietic necrosis and systemic hemorrhagic disease in fish. Ranaviruses of amphibians are virulent for larval anurans, though susceptibility varies among different species. Recent widespread die-offs in amphibian populations may be the result of a combination of host immunity, natural and man-made stressors, and the emergence of novel strains (Figure 50.2). Megalocytiviruses affect a wide variety of tropical marine and freshwater fish leading to systemic infection with significant mortality. The commercial trade and movement of fish, amphibians, and reptiles may contribute to the emergence of new iridoviruses (Gray *et al.* 2009).

References

Costard S, Wieland B, de Glanville W *et al.* (2009) African swine fever: how can global spread be prevented? *Phil Trans R Soc B*, **364**, 2683–2696.

Gray MJ, Miller DL, and Hoverman JT (2009) Ecology and pathology of amphibian ranaviruses. *Dis Aquat Organ*, **87**, 243–266.

Whittington, RJ, Becker JA, and Dennis MM (2010) Iridovirus infections in finfish—critical review with emphasis on ranaviruses. *J Fish Dis*, **33**, 95–122.

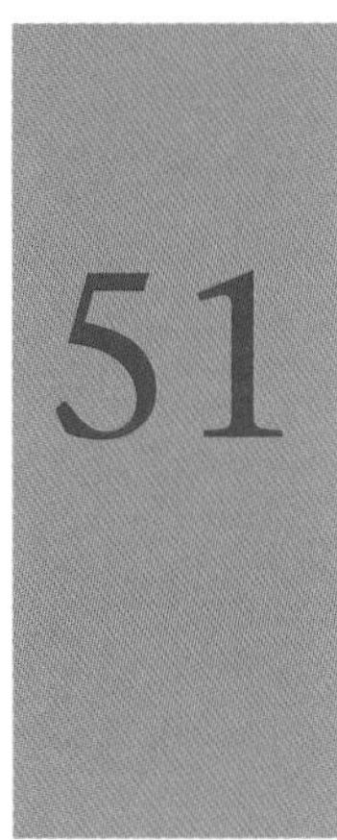

Papillomaviridae and Polyomaviridae

Melissa Kennedy

Papillomaviridae

Papillomaviruses are widespread among mammals, having been identified in cattle, sheep, goats, deer, elk, horses, rabbits, dogs, monkeys, pigs, opossums, mice, elephants, and several species of birds. *Cottontail rabbit papillomavirus* is the type species. Virus-induced papillomas (warts) are benign, hyperplastic epithelial proliferations of the skin or mucous membranes that may undergo malignant transformation in certain circumstances. Some papillomaviruses also cause proliferations of mesenchymal tissues in the skin, with or without associated epithelial pro-liferations. Those with exclusively epithelial proliferation are papillomas, whereas those with proliferation of both mesenchymal (fibrous tissue) and epithelial tissue are termed fibropapillomas. Papillomaviruses are highly species specific, and thus are generally contagious only to the animal species in which they naturally occur. Virus-induced cutaneous papillomas (warts) are common in horses and cattle and infrequent in dogs, sheep, and goats. In some cases, papillomaviruses may play a role in neoplastic development as occurs in humans.

Etiologic Agents

Papillomaviruses have naked icosahedral capsids approximately 55 nm in diameter (Figure 51.1). The viral genome is a single circular molecule of double-stranded DNA that encodes between 8 and 10 proteins; two are structural (L1 and L2) and the remainder are nonstructural proteins that are essential for virus replication.

Papilloma Types

Papillomaviruses are distinguished by their host specificity, tissue and cell tropism, and sequence relatedness. However, some papillomaviruses may abortively infect other species leading to neoplastic development, such as sarcoids in horses linked to bovine papillomavirus types 1 (BPV-1) and 2 (BPV-2).

Papillomaviruses are also distinguished on the basis of the lesions they induce, including skin papillomas (warts), proliferation of nonstratified squamous epithelium (polyps), and subcutaneous fibromas with or without associated cutaneous papillomas (fibropapillomas).

Bovine Papillomaviruses. At least six types of bovine papilloma virus are distinguished on the basis of their antigenic and nucleotide sequence homologies. They can be further distinguished on the basis of the nature of the lesions that they cause in cattle. This has led to the establishment of three genera of bovine papillomaviruses: *Xipapillomavirus*, which is epitheliotropic; *Deltapapillomavirus*, which causes fibropapillomas; and *Epsilonpapillomavirus*, which contains properties of both xipapillomaviruses and deltapapillomaviruses. However, most bovine papillomaviruses are referred to by type number, of which there are at least ten. Cutaneous fibropapillomas (warts) caused by papillomavirus types 1, 2, and 5 occur commonly in calves less than 2 years old. They appear most frequently on the head, especially in the skin around the eyes. They may also appear on the sides of the neck and less commonly on other parts of the body. They begin as small, nodular growths that then grow rapidly into dry, horny, whitish, cauliflower-like masses that eventually regress spontaneously. The histological appearance is a variable mixture of proliferating dermal fibrous tissue and overlying epithelium. Infectious papillomas (without a fibrous tissue component) that occur on the skin and teats of dairy cattle are also associated with infection by bovine papillomaviruses, as are some epithelial proliferations (polyps) that occur in the bladder and gastrointestinal tract, particularly those that affect the esophagus, forestomachs, and intestines.

Fibropapilloma is a papillomavirus-induced tumor that occurs on the penis of young bulls and the vagina and vulva of young heifers. These are fleshy, raised multinodular proliferations that consist of abundant fibrous tissue covered by epithelium of variable thickness.

Host immune responses eventually control papillomavirus infections because most warts persist for variable periods and usually regress spontaneously. The host is then immune to reinfection with the same virus, but not to other types of bovine papillomaviruses. Occasionally, they may evolve into cancers of epithelial or mesenchymal origin.

Veterinary Microbiology, Third Edition. Edited by D. Scott McVey, Melissa Kennedy and M.M. Chengappa.

FIGURE 51.1. *Negatively stained preparation of equine papillomaviruses (75 000×). (Reproduced with permission from Sundberg and O'Banion 1986.)*

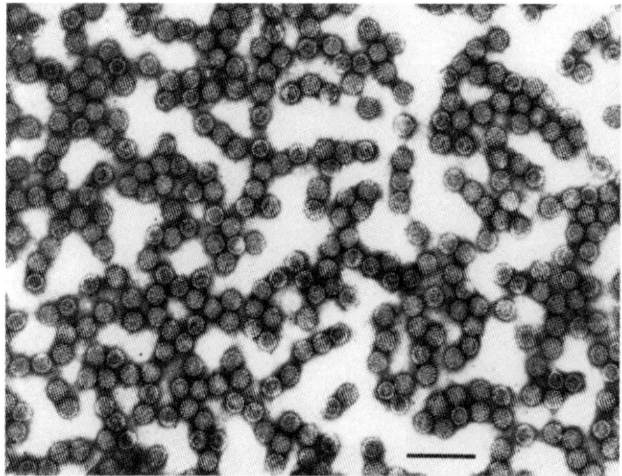

In cattle grazing on bracken ferns, BPV-2 and BPV-4 have been associated with urinary bladder and upper gastrointestinal tumors, respectively. Conversely, DNA of BPV has been identified in normal bovine skin, indicating that it can persist in a latent state causing no clinical signs. Treatment of bovine papillomatosis with finely ground wart tissue suspended in a 0.4% formalin solution has been used for many years to combat outbreaks of the disease, but it is difficult to evaluate the efficacy of this procedure since the disease is self-limiting and its duration varies between individual animals. A significant proportion of vaccinated animals apparently fail to reject their warts after vaccination with autologous tumor preparations. Cattle vaccinated with the L2 structural protein of BPV-4 did not develop alimentary papillomas when challenged with that virus type.

Equine Papillomavirus and Equine Sarcoids. Skin warts of horses are not as common as those affecting cattle. They develop most often on the nose and around the lips of young horses, appearing as small, elevated, papillary (horny) masses. They also occur in the inner aspects of ear (aural plaques). The causative virus is spread by direct contact of infectious material through wounds and cutaneous abrasions. The virus can be experimentally transmitted to horses by intradermal inoculation of a suspension of wart tissue, but not to other animal species. Equine papillomas are usually self-limiting and disappear spontaneously in 4–8 weeks, although they can progress to squamous cell carcinoma (SCC) in rare instances. Natural infection provides solid immunity.

Sarcoids are common skin tumors of horses that grossly and histologically resemble fibropapillomas of cattle. Interestingly, the genome of BPV-1 or BPV-2 is present within some of these tumors, whereas that of equine papillomavirus is not. Sarcoids have been reproduced by direct inoculation of bovine papillomavirus into susceptible horses. The tumors range from being largely epithelial in nature to intensely fibroblastic, and the histological diagnosis is dependent on demonstrating both epithelial and mesenchymal components to the tumor. Sarcoids are frequently multiple in affected horses, and they are commonly ulcerated. Recurrence after surgical removal is common, but metastasis has not been described; thus, they are not malignant tumors despite their locally aggressive behavior.

Canine Oral Papillomavirus. Canine papillomavirus induces warts in the mouths of dogs. The warts generally develop on the lips and spread to the buccal mucosa, tongue, palate, and pharynx. The warts are usually benign and disappear spontaneously after several months. Occasionally, the papillomas may interfere with eating, or may compromise breathing necessitating excision. Dogs recovered from the infection develop immunity to reinfection. The infection is highly contagious, often spreading through all the dogs in a kennel. Dogs that are immunosuppressed have been reported to be more susceptible to development of papillomatosis.

Warts have been experimentally transmitted by rubbing pieces of wart tissue on scarified mucous membranes of susceptible dogs. Under such conditions the incubation period was 4–6 weeks. Infectious venereal papillomas (warts) have also been described in dogs.

Azithromycin, a macrolide antibiotic, has been shown to be effective for treatment of human papillomatosis. Recent studies indicate that it may also be effective in treating canine papillomatosis. While the mechanism of this activity is unknown, it may aid resolution in chronic cases.

Feline Papillomavirus. Recently, DNA of a papillomavirus has been identified in feline viral plaques. These skin lesions are often of little clinical significance, but occasionally may progress to SCC. To date, at least two novel papillomaviruses, designated Felis domesticus papillomaviruses (FdPV) 1 and 2, have been associated with feline viral plaques. The identification of papillomavirus DNA has led to speculation that it may play a role in this neoplastic development in cats. However, as with other papillomaviruses, viral DNA has been found in normal feline skin. Additional research is needed to define the role, if any, of FdPV in viral plaques and SCC in cats.

Polyomaviridae

Polyomaviruses have not been associated with diseases of domestic animals with the notable exception of an avian polyomavirus that causes an acute generalized infection in fledgling budgerigars. Polyomaviruses are nonenveloped 40 nm in diameter, with an icosahedral capsid and a genome of a single molecule of circular double-stranded DNA. The genome encodes at least three structural and five nonstructural proteins.

The avian polyomavirus is the agent of budgerigar fledgling disease, a disease characterized by abdominal distention, feather abnormalities, and acute death. To date, at least four polyomaviruses of birds have been identified, with some occurring in species other than psittacines, including finches and crows. The virus is transmitted horizontally and vertically. It targets endothelial cells and macrophages, and may be found in any tissue. Nestling and juvenile birds are the most susceptible and asymptomatic adults are the major source. Diagnosis is made through clinical signs and polymerase chain reaction detection of the virus. There is no treatment.

Reference

Sundberg JP and O'Banion MK (1986) Cloning and characterization of an equine papillomavirus. *Virology*, **152**, 100.

Further Reading

Borzacchiello G and Roperto F (2008) *Bovine papillomaviruses*, papillomas and cancer in cattle. *Virus Res*, **39**, 45.

Hiroshi K, Ogawa H, Ohya K, and Fukushi H (2010) A review of DNA viral infections in psittacine birds. *J Vet Med Sci*, **72** (9), 1099–1106.

Potti J, Blanco G, Lemus JA, and Canal D (2007) Infectious offspring: how birds acquire and transmit an avian polyomavirus in the wild. *PLoS One*, **2**, e1276.

52 Adenoviridae

MELISSA KENNEDY AND D. SCOTT MCVEY

Adenoviruses have been isolated from many species of animals, but it is likely that additional animal adenoviruses exist that have not yet been identified. The host range of individual adenoviruses is frequently highly restricted. Although adenovirus infections of animals are often asymptomatic or subclinical, some adenoviruses are pathogenic and cause respiratory and/or systemic diseases. Table 52.1 lists the diseases of domestic animals caused by adenoviruses.

The family Adenoviridae is divided into four genera: *Mastadenovirus*, which includes many of the adenoviruses that infect mammals, and *Aviadenovirus*, which includes adenoviruses that infect birds. In recent years, some members of these genera have been reclassified into separate genera: *Atadenovirus*, which includes adenoviruses of reptiles as well as the agent of egg drop syndrome of fowl, and *Siadenovirus*, which includes the agent of hemorrhagic enteritis of turkeys and marble spleen disease of pheasants. Members of these genera do not share a common group antigen. Adenovirus virions are nonenveloped icosahedrons that are 70–90 nm in diameter and are composed of 252 capsomers. Extended fibers project from the virion surface and are used for attachment to target cells. The genome of adenoviruses is a large molecule (26–45 kb) of linear double-stranded DNA. Approximately 40 different proteins are encoded by the adenovirus genome. Adenoviruses replicate in the nucleus of infected cells. They affect cells in which they replicate profoundly, inhibiting protein and DNA synthesis and causing cell death.

Infectious Canine Hepatitis (Canine Adenovirus 1)

Disease

Infectious canine hepatitis (ICH) is a disease of dogs caused by canine adenovirus 1 (CAV-1). Although once an important disease of dogs, ICH is increasingly rare in much of the world, perhaps as a result of widespread vaccination. Outbreaks are still observed in regions where CAV vaccines are not routinely used. The majority of infections are asymptomatic, but the disease in susceptible dogs is characterized by fever, hepatic necrosis, and widespread hemorrhage as a consequence of vascular injury. Affected dogs may exhibit increased thirst, anorexia, tonsillitis, petechial hemorrhages on the mucous membranes, and diarrhea, and be reluctant to move. During the acute phase of illness, dogs may also develop conjunctivitis and photophobia. Severe ICH is most likely to occur in pups that are not immune to the disease.

Most dogs that survive acute ICH recover uneventfully, but transient corneal edema may occur in some convalescent animals after acute signs disappear. The CAV-1 also has been implicated as a cause of chronic progressive hepatitis and interstitial nephritis, but its role in spontaneous occurrence of these disorders in dogs is highly conjectural (CAV-1 is most unlikely to be a significant cause of either of these two common diseases of dogs).

Etiologic Agent

Physical, Chemical, and Antigenic Properties. CAV-1 is antigenically related but distinct from CAV-2. CAV-1 is morphologically similar to other adenoviruses, but antigenically distinct.

Resistance to Physical and Chemical Agents. CAV-1 is resistant to ether, alcohols, and chloroform. It is stable for at least 30 min at a wide range of pH (3–9), and is also stable in soiled material at room temperature for several days. Viral infectivity is lost after heating at 50–60 °C for 10 min. Steam cleaning and treatment with iodine, phenol, sodium hydroxide, or lysol are effective means of disinfection.

Infectivity for Other Species and Culture Systems. CAV-1 causes clinical disease in dogs and other canids (wolves, foxes, and coyotes). Skunks and bears also are susceptible. Antibodies to CAVs have been detected in marine mammals as well as other terrestrial carnivores. Infection in foxes can manifest as encephalitis. CAV-1 replicates well in canine kidney cells.

Although some strains of CAV-1 and CAV-2 are oncogenic in inoculated hamsters, these viruses have not been associated with neoplastic disease in dogs.

Host—Virus Relationship

Distribution, Reservoir, and Transmission. ICH has a worldwide distribution, although clinical disease is

Veterinary Microbiology, Third Edition. Edited by D. Scott McVey, Melissa Kennedy and M.M. Chengappa.

Table 52.1. Diseases of Domestic Animals Caused by Adenoviruses

Virus	Type of Disease
Mastadenovirus	
Bovine adenovirus, types 1–10	Conjunctivitis, pneumonia, diarrhea, polyarthritis
Canine adenovirus type 1 (CAV-1; infectious canine hepatitis)	Hemorrhagic and hepatic
Canine adenovirus type 2	Respiratory
Equine adenovirus types 1–2	Respiratory
Ovine adenoviruses types 1–6	Respiratory and enteric
Porcine adenoviruses types 1–4	Diarrhea or meningoencephalitis, or both
Deer adenovirus	Systemic vasculitis, with hemorrhage and pulmonary edema
Aviadenovirus	
Chicken adenoviruses types 1–12	Respiratory disease, enteric disease, egg-drop syndrome, aplastic anemia, atrophy of the bursa of Fabricius
Turkey adenoviruses types 1–4	Respiratory disease, enteritis, marble spleen disease

Deer adenovirus, egg-drop syndrome virus of poultry, bovine adenovirus 4, and duck adenovirus 1 are proposed to be members of a new genus *Atadenovirus*, similarly, hemorrhagic enteritis of turkeys virus and marble spleen disease of pheasants virus are proposed to be members of a new genus *Siadenovirus*.

increasingly rare. The infection is spread through the urine of infected dogs. Dogs may retain the virus in their kidneys and shed it in urine for months after infection.

Pathogenesis and Pathology. Following aerosol infection, the virus localizes in the tonsils and spreads to regional lymph nodes and then to the systemic circulation. Viremia results in rapid dissemination of the virus to all body tissues and secretions, including saliva, urine, and feces. The virus has a particular tropism for hepatocytes and endothelial cells, which produces the characteristic signs of the disease. Virus-induced injury to endothelial cells leads to consumptive coagulopathy (disseminated intravascular coagulation) and a generalized bleeding tendency (hemorrhagic diathesis) that is reflected by abnormal clotting parameters.

Dogs that die during the acute phase generally have edema and hemorrhage of superficial lymph nodes and cervical subcutaneous tissue. The abdominal cavity often contains fluid, which may vary in color from clear to bright red. Hemorrhages are present on all serosal surfaces. A fibrinous exudate may cover the liver, which can be swollen and congested. The gallbladder is characteristically edematous. Large characteristic intranuclear inclusion bodies may be present in hepatocytes, vascular endothelium, and macrophages.

The ocular lesions that develop in some dogs that recover from ICH are the result of deposition of immune complexes within the ciliary body of the eye. Interstitial nephritis may also occur as a consequence of immune complex deposition 1–3 weeks after recovery.

Host Response to Infections. Recovery from ICH, regardless of the severity of illness, results in long-lasting immunity that likely is lifelong. Recovered animals have high titers of neutralizing antibodies to CAV-1.

Laboratory Diagnosis

The diagnosis of ICH can be confirmed by serologic testing (complement fixation, hemagglutination inhibition, or enzyme-linked immunosorbent assay) to demonstrate rising titers of antibodies to CAV-1, polymerase chain reaction (PCR) detection of viral nucleic acid or virus isolation from affected tissues, or immunohistochemical staining of tissues with CAV-1-specific antibodies. Antemortem, ocular and oropharyngeal swabs, feces, and urine may be used for virus identification.

Treatment and Control

Therapy for dogs that develop ICH involves supportive and symptomatic treatment. Control is achieved by vaccination and strict sanitation of affected premises with quarantine of exposed dogs. Available vaccines include both inactivated and modified live virus varieties, including CAV-2 vaccines that induce heterologous protection against CAV-1. CAV-2 vaccines do not induce immune complex uveitis in dogs as do some other modified live virus vaccines. Care must be exercised to ensure that maternal antibodies do not interfere with active immunization of pups, because vaccination success is directly related to the level of neutralizing antibodies.

Canine Adenovirus Type 2

CAV-2 has been isolated from dogs with acute cough and is one of several infectious agents implicated in infectious tracheobronchitis (kennel cough). Experimental infection produces mild pharyngitis, tonsillitis, and tracheobronchitis, and the virus persists in the respiratory tract for up to 28 days. Unlike CAV-1, CAV-2 does not produce generalized disease, is not excreted in the urine, and does not produce renal and ocular lesions. CAV-2 is antigenically related to CAV-1, and CAV-2 vaccines have been developed as ICH vaccine since they do not produce postvaccinal ocular lesions.

Bovine Adenoviruses

Bovine adenoviruses (BAV) are currently classified into 10 serotypes (BAV-1–BAV-10), of which BAV-3 and BAV-5 appear to be more pathogenic than the other serotypes. Adenoviruses typically produce pneumonia or enteritis but only in very young or immunosuppressed cattle. Adenoviruses are frequently isolated from apparently normal cattle, and serologic surveys indicate that asymptomatic or subclinical BAV infection of cattle occurs worldwide. BAV-3 can produce mild pneumonia in susceptible calves, with necrosis of the epithelium lining terminal airways in the lungs, causing necrotizing bronchiolitis with characteristic intranuclear inclusion bodies in the affected epithelial cells.

Immunocompetent calves inoculated with BAV develop neutralizing antibodies in 10 to 14 days, and immunity after natural infection is long-lasting. Diagnosis requires viral isolation or serology. Bovine adenoviruses can be isolated from rectal, nasal, or conjunctival swabs. Most types do not produce characteristic cytopathogenic effects until after several blind passages.

Although no vaccines are licensed for use in the United States, there is limited use of vaccines against BAV-1, BAV-3, and BAV-4 in Europe.

Equine Adenovirus

Adenovirus infection rarely results in respiratory tract disease in healthy horses, and immunocompetent foals normally develop either subclinical or asymptomatic infections. However, Arabian foals with severe combined immunodeficiency (SCID) are highly susceptible to infection with equine adenovirus 1. The respiratory disease induced by equine adenovirus in SCID Arabian foals is protracted and characterized by coughing, dyspnea, and fever. These foals also develop generalized adenovirus infections, with involvement of a variety of organs and tissues.

There are two serotypes of equine adenovirus, as determined by serum neutralization. For laboratory diagnosis, the virus may be isolated from infective tissue and nasal and ocular swab material in equine fetal kidney or equine fetal dermis cell cultures. The virus can be identified by electron microscopy or by immunofluorescent (IF) or immunohistochemical staining of infected tissues. Adenovirus nucleic acid can also be detected by PCR assay. Viral neutralization and hemagglutination-inhibition test are used to detect the presence and rise of antibody titers for serological diagnosis of adenovirus infections.

There is no commercially available vaccine.

Ovine Adenoviruses

Adenoviruses have been isolated from the feces of apparently normal sheep and from lambs with respiratory disease. Six serotypes have been identified. The pathogenic role of most of the ovine adenoviruses is uncertain because they typically produce only mild or inapparent infection of the respiratory or gastrointestinal tracts. However, apparent outbreaks of adenovirus-induced pneumonia and enteritis have been described in lambs, as have sporadic cases of generalized (systemic) infections of very young lambs.

Deer Adenovirus

A unique adenovirus was recently identified as the cause of a fatal systemic hemorrhagic disease of mule deer (including black-tailed deer). The virus was originally identified as the cause of extensive outbreaks of fatal disease in mule deer in North America (California), both captive and free-ranging, but subsequently has been recognized to have a much wider distribution. A similar disease has also been identified in moose. The causative adenovirus is genetically unique and is serologically related to some adenoviruses of cattle (BAV) and goats. It is proposed that deer adenovirus be included in the genus *Atadenovirus*, along with BAV-4, duck adenovirus 1, and certain other adenoviruses. The virus causes either localized or systemic vascular injury as a consequence of infection of endothelial cells and subsequent thrombosis, leading to severe pulmonary edema, ulceration of the oral cavity and gastrointestinal tract, and widespread hemorrhages. Mortality can be high, especially among fawns. The virus can be propagated in primary deer respiratory epithelial cell cultures, but diagnosis is based on the characteristic gross and histologic lesions, immunohistochemical staining with antisera to BAV, and electron microscopy.

Avian Adenoviruses

Adenoviruses infect poultry and other bird species worldwide. Although adenoviruses are often isolated from apparently normal birds, specific diseases are also associated with adenovirus infections. These include egg drop syndrome, a disease of both wild and domestic birds that is characterized by production of eggs that lack shells or have abnormally soft shells, and hemorrhagic enteritis of turkeys and marble spleen disease of pheasants, which are similar diseases characterized by intestinal hemorrhage and enlargement of the spleen of affected birds and are classified as siadenoviruses. Aviadenoviruses are associated with inclusion body hepatitis, usually seen in 3- to 7-week-old broilers, and quail bronchitis, and may have significant mortality in young birds. A relatively new syndrome of broilers, hydropericardium or Angara disease, has been associated with fowl adenovirus 4, and has a mortality approaching 75% among 3- to 5-week-old chicks.

Among psittacines, adenoviruses have been associated with clinical depression and diarrhea with cloacal hemorrhage; birds may be found dead in their enclosures. Lesions affecting liver, spleen, kidneys, lungs, and gastrointestinal tract have been identified. Basophilic intranuclear inclusions are often seen associated with liver and splenic necrosis.

53 Herpesviridae

Rebecca P. Wilkes

Herpesviruses have been found in virtually every species that have been investigated and cause significant disease in each domestic animal species except sheep. Within this group of viruses, there is wide variation in biological properties including pathogenicity and oncogenic potential. Herpesviruses are morphologically similar, with a double-stranded DNA core and an icosahedral capsid consisting of 162 capsomeres, surrounded by a granular zone composed of globular proteins (tegument) and encompassed by a lipid envelope (Figure 53.1). The genome of herpesviruses is large, 125–290 kilobases (kb), and encodes many different proteins; functions of the proteins encoded by the viral genome include virus replication, virus structural proteins, and a variety of proteins that regulate cell growth and modulate the host's antiviral response.

Viral replication and encapsidation occur in the nucleus, and the envelope is obtained by budding through the inner layer of the nuclear envelope. Intranuclear inclusion bodies are a characteristic feature of infection (Figure 53.2). Infection with herpesviruses results in lifelong latent infection with subsequent recrudescence and intermittent or continuous shedding of virus.

Herpesviruses do not survive well outside of the host. Transmission usually requires close contact, but respiratory droplet spread is important in facilities with confined populations, such as cattle feedlots and animal shelters. The virus may survive longer in cool, moist environments, but latently infected animals serve as the reservoir for transmission.

Herpesviruses have been assigned to the order Herpesvirales, which contains three distinct families: Herpesviridae includes herpesviruses of birds, mammals, and reptiles; Alloherpesviridae includes herpesviruses of fish and frogs; and Malacoherpesviridae contains a single virus isolated from oysters (ostreid herpesvirus 1). The family Herpesviridae consists of three major subfamilies, alpha-, beta-, and gammaherpesvirinae, which were initially distinguished by host range, duration of replication, reproductive cycle, cytopathology, and latent infection characteristics. The alphaherpesvirinae are generally highly cytopathic in cell culture, have a relatively short replication cycle (24 h), and frequently cause latent viral infections in sensory ganglia. Most of these viruses are restricted in their host range, indicating that they evolved with their hosts over long periods of time. Betaherpesvirinae have a variable host range and a long replication cycle; infected cells often become enlarged (cytomegaly), thus their designation as cytomegaloviruses. Latency can be established in numerous tissues, including secretory glands and lymphoreticular tissues. Gammaherpesvirinae, with some exceptions, tend to be tropic for B or T lymphocytes (lymphotropic), replicate in lymphoblastoid cells, and may cause lytic infections in certain types of epithelial and fibroblastic cells. Infection is frequently arrested at a prelytic stage with persistent and minimum expression of viral genome in the cell. Latency is established frequently in lymphoid tissue. Host range is narrow with experimental hosts usually limited to the order of the natural host.

Equid Herpesviruses

Both alpha- and gammaherpesviruses have been identified in equids. The alphaherpesviruses isolated from domestic horses are equid herpesvirus 1 (EHV-1; equine abortion virus), EHV-3 (equine coital exanthema (ECE) virus), and EHV-4 (equine rhinopneumonitis virus). Alphaherpesviruses have also been isolated from donkeys, including EHV-6 (asinine herpesvirus 1) and EHV-8 (asinine herpesvirus 3). Asinine herpesvirus 1 produces a disease that resembles EHV-3 and asinine herpesvirus 3 is related to EHV-1. In addition to infecting donkeys, these viruses also infect zebra and asses. Another equid alphaherpesvirus is EHV-9, which genetically resembles EHV-1 and was first isolated from Thomson's gazelles. Infection causes little or no illness in equid species, and zebra are suggested to be the natural host and reservoir of EHV-9. EHV-9 produces neurotropic pathogenicity in nonequids and has been associated with encephalitis in giraffes and polar bears.

Equid gammaherpesviruses include EHV-2, EHV-5, and EHV-7 (asinine herpesvirus 2). Some additional gammaherpesviruses have been isolated from donkeys with neurologic disease or severe interstitial pneumonia, but these viruses have not been well characterized.

EHV-1 (Equine Abortion Virus)

Disease. EHV-1 causes abortion in mares, respiratory tract disease, and occasional neurologic disease. While abortion in mares may occur as early as 4 months of gestation, it

Veterinary Microbiology, Third Edition. Edited by D. Scott McVey, Melissa Kennedy and M.M. Chengappa.

FIGURE 53.1. *Negatively stained preparation of infectious bovine rhinotracheitis virus. n, nucleocapsid; ev, envelope; rv, enveloped virus; tn, twin nucleocapsids. 17 000×. Inset: Minute projections on the envelope of a matured virus. sp, virus spikes; cd, virus core; ve, virus envelope. 100 000×. (Reproduced with permission from Talens and Zee 1976.)*

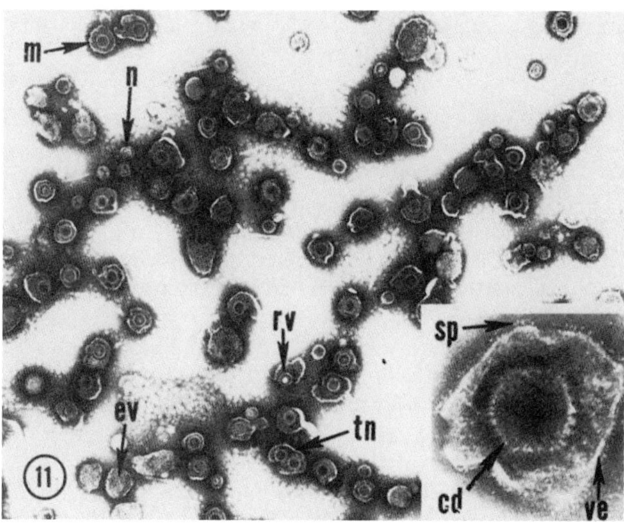

most frequently occurs between the seventh and eleventh months of gestation and usually without any premonitory signs. Foals infected in utero may be born alive but are usually weak and die within 2–3 days. Naturally occurring respiratory disease due to EHV-1 is characterized by fever, anorexia, nasal discharge of varying severity, and ocular discharge. Experimentally, EHV-1 causes a much more severe respiratory disease than that induced by equine herpesvirus 4 (equine rhinopneumonitis virus).

Equine herpesvirus myeloencephalopathy (EHM) with variable neurologic signs ranging from ataxia, urinary incontinence and limb paresis to paralysis and death has been associated with certain strains of EHV-1. EHM is a relatively uncommon manifestation of EHV-1 infection, but recently these outbreaks have been reported with increased frequency, and devastating losses can occur. A study has shown that EHV-1 strains with increased genetic propensity to cause neurologic disease are continuing to increase in prevalence within the latent reservoir of the virus, leading to greater risks for outbreaks of EHM.

FIGURE 53.2. *Photomicrograph of the liver (100×) stained with hematoxylin and eosin. Several nuclei with peripheralized chromatin and herpesviral eosinophilic intranuclear inclusion bodies are indicated by arrows. (Photo courtesy of Dr Robert Donnell, The University of Tennessee.)*

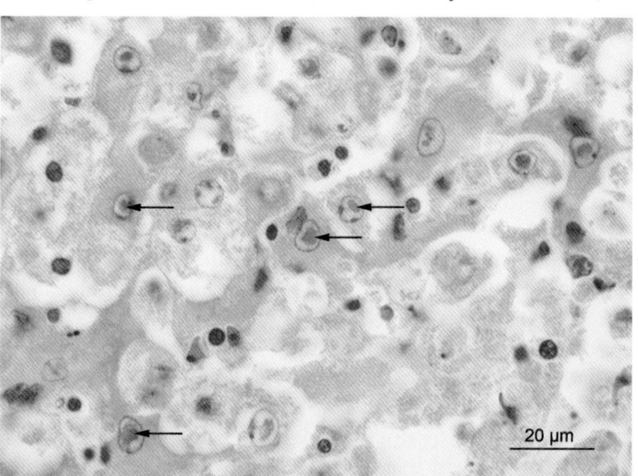

Etiologic Agent

Physical, Chemical, and Antigen Properties. The equine herpesviruses have typical morphology and cannot be distinguished from each other based on their morphology. They are, however, antigenically distinct and can be distinguished by serological assays.

Resistance to Physical and Chemical Agents. The equine herpesviruses are inactivated by ether, acid (pH 3), drying, exposure to heat of 56 °C for 30 min, and detergents and commonly used disinfectants.

Infectivity for Other Species and Culture Systems. EHV-1 usually infects only horses; however, ocular disease due to EHV-1 characterized by vitritis, retinitis, and optic neuritis leading to blindness has been described in new-world camelids (alpacas, llamas). EHV-1 also produces encephalitis and acute death in these species. Abortions due to EHV-1 have been described in cattle and zebras.

EHV-1 can be propagated in equine fetal kidney, rabbit kidney, and L (mouse fibroblast) cells, resulting in formation of cytopathic effect (CPE) and intranuclear inclusion bodies.

Host–Virus Relationship

Distribution, Reservoir, and Transmission. EHV-1 is prevalent in horses worldwide. The virus appears to be maintained in the horse, but it is possible that dogs, foxes, and carrion birds may carry infection with fragments of aborted fetuses from one farm to another. Transmission may occur by direct contact with virus-laden aborted fetuses or placentas. Aerosol transmission is considered less important than direct contact or spread of secretions on fomites between horses by handlers.

Pathogenesis and Pathology. Primary EHV-1 replication occurs in the upper respiratory tract epithelial cells and local lymph nodes resulting in leukocyte-associated viremia. This leukocyte-associated viremia in an acute infection has been shown to be a prerequisite for abortion and EHM by initiating replication of EHV-1 in endothelial cell lining of blood vessels in the pregnant uterus or central nervous system (CNS). A widespread infection of endometrial blood vessels results in severe vasculitis and multifocal thrombosis, which could result in an abortion of a virus negative fetus. Less extensive uterine vascular pathology may allow focal transfer of virus across the utero-placental barrier and abortion of a virus-infected fetus. A near term transplacental EHV-1 infection could result in the birth of live infected foals, which usually die a few days afterward—a condition known as neonatal foal disease. These differences in abortigenic potential may relate to differences in the level of viremia or endothelial cell infection induced by different virus strains.

Macroscopically, the most prominent lesions of the virus-infected fetus are jaundice, mucous membrane petechiation, subcutaneous and pleural edema, splenic enlargement with prominent lymphoid follicles, and focal hepatic necrosis. Histologically, there is bronchiolitis, pneumonitis, severe necrosis of the splenic white pulp, and focal hepatic necrosis, all accompanied by intranuclear inclusion bodies. The early fetus (<3 months) shows little or no response to the viral infection. However, the fetus in its last 4 months of gestation shows a marked ability to react in a specific manner to the presence of the virus. Lesions in the fetus less than 7 months of age differ from those in older fetuses, suggesting that the lesions represent a fetal response to the virus.

The neurological signs of EHM do not result from direct damage to neurons or glial cells by viral infection but instead result from diffuse, multifocal myeloencephalopathy secondary to vasculitis, hemorrhage, thrombosis, and ischemic neuronal injury due to viral replication in the endothelial cells lining the arterioles of the CNS. The lesions are focal and neurologic signs are associated with the sites and extent of CNS infection. Clinical signs initially reflect lower motor neuron defects, including an initial dysuria, constipation, perineal analgesia, protrusion of the penis, locomotor dysfunction varying from mild ataxia to severe paralysis, and possible tetraplegia. When the cortex or brainstem is involved, encephalitic signs, including convulsions, may occur.

Host Responses to Infection. Virus persists in circulating leukocytes for as long as 9 days following infection. Abortion in mares may occur as long as 90–120 days following infection. Both complement-fixing and virus-neutralizing antibodies appear in the sera of infected horses. In general, complement-fixing antibodies are demonstrable for 6 months after infection, with virus-neutralizing antibodies persisting longer. IgG antibodies against the viral envelope neutralize virus, while those against the nucleocapsid do not. Results from an experimental challenge study failed to reveal any significant relationship between preexposure virus neutralizing antibody titer and the magnitude of postinfection EHV-1 viremia. The intracellular location of EHV-1 during most of its infection cycle within horses may limit the effectiveness of virus neutralizing antibody in controlling cell-associated EHV-1 viremia. Experimentally, pregnant mares with antibody to EHV-1 may abort when challenged with EHV-1.

Also, the concentration of antibodies prior to virus inoculation does not correlate with protection against challenge with neuropathogenic EHV-1. Although the specific immune mechanisms required for control of EHV-1 neurologic disease are largely unknown, data suggest that presence of a high frequency of preexposure EHV-1 specific memory cytotoxic T lymphocytes is significantly correlated with protective immunity against development of EHM. A previous study also demonstrated an association between a high frequency of memory cytotoxic T lymphocytes and a resistance to abortion in ponies exposed to EHV-1. Neuropathogenic strains of EHV-1 are thought to replicate more efficiently than nonneuropathogenic strains, and the quantitative load of circulating virus that follows infection by EHV-1 was defined as a major risk factor for postexposure development of EHV-1 CNS disease, and cytotoxic T lymphocytes appear to have a role in maintaining immunologic control of EHV-1 viremia.

Laboratory Diagnosis. In cases of abortions, diagnosis is based on characteristic lesions with intranuclear inclusions present in the fetal liver, spleen, lung, and thymus. The same tissues provide a good source of virus, which can be demonstrated by immunofluorescence or immunohistochemical staining of tissue sections. Histopathological examination of the brain and spinal cord is essential in confirming EHV-1 infection in a horse with suspected EHM. Vasculitis and thrombosis of small blood vessels in the spinal cord or brain are consistent changes and virus detection in the CNS is achieved using immunohistochemistry, *in situ* hybridization, or polymerase chain reaction (PCR). Virus isolation can be used to confirm the diagnosis in abortion cases, but isolation from neural tissues in EHM cases is difficult.

PCR has become the diagnostic test of choice due to its high sensitivity and specificity, and PCR detection of EHV-1 is routinely performed on secretions from nasal or nasopharyngeal swabs or from uncoagulated blood samples. A variable region in the EHV-1 DNA polymerase gene (ORF 30) involved in initial viral replication within cells has been linked to EHM. PCR assays based on ORF 30 have been developed and used to differentiate between EHV-1 isolates from neurologically and nonneurologically affected horses (Allen 2007). However, the genotyping of field isolates needs to be interpreted carefully, because between approximately 14% and 24% of EHV-1 isolates from horses with EHM do not have this neuropathogenic marker (Nugent *et al.* 2006; Perkins *et al.* 2009). Strain characterization may be important; however, given that the odds of neurological disease when infected with the neurotropic EHV-1 genotype versus the nonneurotropic genotype are 162 times greater.

Serology that demonstrates a fourfold or greater increase in serum antibody titer, using serum neutralization tests, on acute and convalescent samples collected 7–21 days apart provides presumptive evidence of infection. The mares' sera may, but does not invariably, demonstrate a rise in titer. Also, many horses with EHM do not exhibit a fourfold rise in serum neutralization titer, because titers rise rapidly and may have peaked by the time neurological signs appear.

Treatment and Control. Both modified live and inactivated vaccines are commercially available and widely used; however, the vaccines do not block infection, the development of viremia, or the establishment of latency. Regular vaccination of mares has been shown to reduce the risk of EHV-1 induced abortion, but no vaccine currently offers protection against the development of EHM and it has been observed in horses regularly vaccinated against

EHV-1 at 3–5 monthly intervals with inactivated or modified-live vaccines. To achieve protective efficacy against EHV-1 myeloencephalopathy by vaccination, the vaccines must be able to stimulate the equine immune response toward the production of functional effector cytotoxic T lymphocytes. Horse owners must develop an understanding of the concept of boosting herd immunity to help protect individual horses rather than having an (as yet unattainable) expectation that the attending veterinarian can reliably protect an individual horse from developing potentially fatal EHM by administering one of the currently available vaccines.

Thus, disease control measures are important for preventing the spread of virus. Limiting traffic in and out of brood-mare bands and weanling fields, minimizing stress to pregnant mares, and separating pregnant mares from the remaining population have been suggested to help prevent abortion disease.

It is known that the nasal secretions of horses with EHM contain large amounts of replicating virus and these secretions in particular contribute to the spread of disease to other susceptible individuals. As a consequence, horses suspected of having EHM must be removed from the stable environment as quickly as possible and placed in strict isolation until they have been shown to be asymptomatic for 21 days. The treatment of EHM is challenging and the outcome is directly related to the severity of the neurological deficits in the affected horse. As no specific treatment is available, the management of affected animals is directed toward supportive nursing and nutritional care and in reducing CNS inflammation. Affected horses that remain standing have a good prognosis, and improvement is generally apparent within a few days, though some horses may be left with residual neurological deficits.

Equid Herpesvirus 2

Disease. EHV-2 is prevalent in horses worldwide and has been isolated from both clinically healthy and ill horses. It has been isolated from cases of superficial and chronic pharyngeal lymphoid follicular hyperplasia, mild respiratory disease, and horses with gastroesophageal ulcers, foals with pneumonia, and foals with keratoconjunctivitis. It has also been associated with granulomatous dermatitis and abortion. There is considerable skepticism by some concerning its role in disease. The relationship of EHV-2 to disease causality is uncertain because of the ubiquity of the virus in horse populations worldwide. The fact that gammaherpesviruses are optimally adapted to their natural hosts means that significant clinical expression of infection is rarely encountered.

Etiologic Agent

Physical, Chemical, and Antigen Properties. EHV-2 is a typical gammaherpesvirus.

Resistance to Physical and Chemical Agents. The virus is labile in the environment and infectivity is destroyed by heat, drying, detergents, and common disinfectants.

Culture Systems. Primary rabbit kidney and equine dermal cells as well as hamster embryos can be used for virus isolation.

Host–Virus Relationship

Distribution, Reservoir, and Transmission. EHV-2 has been isolated from horses worldwide. Ninety-seven percent of horses less than 1 year old have antibodies to EHV-2, and in one study, the virus could be isolated from the leukocytes of 88.7% of normal horses. Similarly, virus was isolated from 68 of 69 foals sampled once between 1 and 8 months of age. Both "healthy" and clinically ill horses act as a reservoir for the virus. In ponies experimentally inoculated with EHV-2, the virus was recovered up to 118 days postinoculation. The virus is latent in B lymphocytes and is frequently isolated from nasopharyngeal swabs following infection or viral recrudescence. Foals generally shed higher loads of EHV-2 in nasal secretions early in infection, and progressively less with age.

Pathogenesis and Pathology. Little is known about the pathogenesis of EHV-2. It is suggested that infection is initiated in tonsils, with replication in other sites based on an observed viremia and its cell-associated nature. Young foals are probably infected by their dams and can be infected despite the presence of maternal antibodies. The virus can then be spread horizontally to in-contact foals. Sequence heterogeneity exists among strains and horses may be infected with more than one strain at a time. One study suggests the heterogeneity may be due to positive selection, producing variation in a neutralization domain; however, strain variation and viral load were not correlated to any clinical manifestation of disease. A recent study suggests disease produced by EHV-2 may be immunologically mediated, similar to infectious mononucleosis caused by the related gammaherpesvirus, Epstein–Barr virus (human herpesvirus 4). Fever in individual foals was associated with an increase in EHV-2-specific responses of PBMC, though the results were not statistically significant. Several aspects of the immune response of the foals and EHV-2 infection status were unrelated to occurrence of clinical disease in the foals.

Laboratory Diagnosis. There are no specific diagnostic features associated with EHV-2 infection. The virus can be isolated from nasal and pharyngeal swabs and from blood buffy coats and identified by PCR assay. EHV-2 slowly induces CPE in culture and cannot be differentiated from other equid gammaherpesviruses such as EHV-5 solely on its growth characteristics. The CPE of EHV-2 are usually detected within 12–21 days.

Treatment and Control. Control methods have not been established, and a vaccine is not available for EHV-2.

EHV-3 (ECE Virus)

Disease. ECE, caused by EHV-3, is an acute, sexually transmitted disease characterized by the formation of papules, vesicles, pustules, and ulcers on the penis and prepuce of stallions and on the external genitalia and perineal skin of mares. The lesions usually heal after approximately 14 days. Lesions have occurred, infrequently, around the lips, external nares, nasal mucosa, and conjunctiva. The virus does not cause systemic disease, nor does it cause infertility or abortion. The negative impact of the virus results from potential serious economic consequences as a result of temporary disruption of mating activities in affected animals (specifically the thoroughbred breed) and the risk of iatrogenic EHV-3 dissemination and outbreaks of ECE in artificial insemination and embryo transfer facilities.

Etiologic Agent

Physical, Chemical, and Antigen Properties. EHV-3 is a typical alphaherpesvirus and is antigenically, genetically, and pathogenically distinct from the other equid herpesviruses.

Resistance to Physical and Chemical Agents. The virus is labile in the environment and infectivity is destroyed by heat, drying, detergents, and common disinfectants.

Infection for Other Species and Culture Systems. The only known reservoir for the virus is the horse, and EHV-3 only replicates in cell cultures of equine origin.

Distribution, Reservoir, and Transmission. EHV-3 was first isolated in 1968 concurrently in North America and Australia and is endemic in most horse breeding populations worldwide. The usual mode of transmission is venereal, but EHV-3 can be spread without coitus. EHV-3 can be potentially transmitted to the ejaculate through penile contact with an artificial vagina or sleeve and, consequently, by fresh or frozen semen. The infection may also spread via fomites, or insects may act as mechanical carriers. The vulva and vagina need not be damaged for infection to occur. It is suggested that in some infected stallions and mares, EHV-3 becomes latent in the nonbreeding season and is reactivated during the breeding season. The anatomical site that harbors latent EHV-3 is unknown, but it is hypothesized that the virus establishes a latent infection in sciatic and/or sacral ganglion cells.

Pathogenesis and Pathology. Viral replication is limited to the stratified epithelium of epidermal tissue present within the skin or at muco-cutaneous margins. The destruction of epithelium caused by the lytic virus infection elicits a vigorous, localized inflammatory response that gives rise to the formation of the characteristic cutaneous lesions of ECE. Microscopic examination of vulvar tissue demonstrates shallow erosions along with occasional typical intranuclear inclusions scattered in germinal epithelium or in nuclear remnants in necrotic areas.

Host Responses to Infection. Immunity to EHV-3 has not been studied in detail; the horse responds to infection by EHV-3 with the production of serum complement-fixing (CF) and virus-neutralizing (VN) antibodies that reach maximal levels 14–21 days after infection.

Laboratory Diagnosis. ECE genital lesions in both mares and stallions are usually characteristic enough for a clinical diagnosis to be made with reasonable certainty. A presumptive diagnosis can be confirmed in the laboratory by isolation of the virus. Detection of EHV-3 DNA by PCR or demonstration of either seroconversion or a fourfold or greater rise in antibody titer in paired serum samples can also confirm diagnosis. Reactivation from latency can be associated with low or decreasing neutralizing antibody titers.

Treatment and Control. At the present time, ECE vaccines are not commercially available, and vaccination to prevent the disease has not been investigated. Treatment includes daily cleansing of the affected areas with antiseptics, using anti-inflammatory agents to reduce inflammation, and preventing secondary bacterial infections with antimicrobials. Recovery from ECE is complete in a matter of 2–3 weeks and occurs without permanent sequelae. Prevention of ECE in stallions requires examination of mares before breeding; however, as reactivation of latent virus is not preventable, and subclinical virus excretion does occur, the basis for controlling ECE outbreaks in breeding establishments is containment of the spread of infection. Clinically affected animals should not be bred until lesions have healed and virus excretion has ceased. Mechanical transmission of the virus can be prevented by early recognition of new clinical cases and strict adherence to hygiene procedures.

EHV-4 (Equine Rhinopneumonitis Virus)

Clinical manifestations of EHV-4 are seen principally in foals and younger horses as protection from maternal antibody wanes. Though historically the clinical condition equine rhinopneumonitis was associated with EHV-1, this terminology is now assigned to EHV-4. Signs often include malaise and elevated temperature up to 105 °F, which may persist for 2–5 days; watery nasal discharge, which becomes mucopurulent in the later stages; congested conjunctiva; and, infrequently, enlarged submandibular nodes. Bacterial proliferation in nasal passages may be a contributory factor in the development of rhinopneumonitis. Sporadic cases of equine abortion have also been associated with this virus. In contrast to EHV-1, the pathogenesis of EHV-4 has not been well studied. Leukocyte-associated viremia is not a consistent feature of EHV-4 infection. The agent appears to have worldwide distribution; however, it is infrequently isolated. EHV-1 and -4 share many antigens, resulting in serologic cross-reactivity between these viruses, and protection against EHV-4 can be produced with use of EHV-1 vaccines. There are also vaccines available that contain both EHV-1 and -4. Both inactivated and modified live vaccines are used, but results are not uniformly favorable. With a specific enzyme-linked immunosorbent assay (ELISA) now available, it is possible to distinguish EHV-1 from EHV-4 serologically. PCR assays can also distinguish between EHV-1 and EHV-4 infection.

Equid Herpesvirus 5

In a study of multiple EHV-5 isolates, several were found to differ significantly genomically and in their protein composition. EHV-5 has been proposed for this group of viruses that were isolated from equine respiratory tracts. EHV-5 has been isolated from peripheral blood lymphocytes and nasal swabs of clinically normal adult horses in New Zealand, Australia, and the United States. EHV-5 can also be cultured from samples of horses with clinical respiratory disease and the virus has been associated with equine multinodular pulmonary fibrosis (EMPF), a novel pathological entity with characteristic gross and histopathological pulmonary lesions. Pulmonary interstitial fibrosis of alveolar parenchyma with intraluminal accumulation of neutrophils and macrophages within the alveoli and airways has been described. Eosinophilic intranuclear viral inclusion bodies are rarely seen in macrophages. The exact pathogenic role this virus plays in EMPF is unknown; EHV-5 may be an etiologic agent or cofactor in the development of EMPF. EHV-5 can be isolated on RK13, equine fetal kidney, equine dermal, and Vero cells. Slow development of CPE is described over three to four passages with evidence of ballooning, resulting in syncytia formation on equine dermal cells.

Ruminant Herpesviruses

Herpesviruses, representing alpha- and gammaherpesviruses, are responsible for a wide range of conditions in ruminants, including neurologic, genital, fetal, and respiratory diseases. Infections may range from unapparent to fatal. Several herpesviruses infect cattle (bovine herpesviruses (BHV)): infectious bovine rhinotracheitis (IBR) virus (BHV-1), bovine mammillitis virus (BHV-2), and bovine encephalitis virus (BHV-5) are alphaherpesviruses. BHV-1 causes both respiratory (IBR) and genital disease (infectious pustular vulvovaginitis (IPV)) in cattle. BHV-4 is a gammaherpesvirus, but its role in causing disease is uncertain. Another gammaherpesvirus, Alcelaphine herpesvirus 1 (AlHV-1), is the cause of African malignant catarrhal fever (MCF) associated with wildebeest and the sheep gammaherpesvirus ovine herpesvirus 2 (OvHV-2) is the cause of the sheep-associated form of MCF. Alphaherpesviruses have also been isolated from goats (CpHV-1) and deer (CerHV-1 and CerHV-2), and CpHV-1 is the cause of reproductive disease in goats.

Bovine Herpesviruses

Bovine Herpesvirus 1 (IBR and IPV Viruses)

Disease. BHV-1 infection in cattle may present as ocular, genital, and respiratory disease. Respiratory disease typically presents as rhinotracheitis (IBR), which may lead to severe and often fatal bronchopneumonia. Conjunctivitis is common. Occasionally, the cornea is involved and a panophthalmitis may occur. BHV-1 can infect genitalia, resulting balanoposthitis and vulvovaginitis (IPV). BHV-1 has been isolated from vesicular lesions on the udder and teats of a cow with mastitis. Previous reports of meningoencephalitis in young calves associated with BHV-1 are now being attributed to a different BHV-5. Rarely can BHV-1 reach the brain of infected cattle, but a few cases of BHV-1 associated encephalitis have been reported in cattle.

Etiologic Agent

Infectivity for Other Species and Culture Systems. Although cattle appear to be the major species affected by BHV-1, the virus has been incriminated in swine vaginitis and balanitis, and has been isolated from stillborn and newborn pigs. Approximately, 11% of swine tested in parts of North America (Iowa and Texas) had antibodies to IBR. The virus has been isolated from red deer with ocular disease, and could be reactivated in Malaysian buffalo by steroid administration. It does not appear that BHV-1 virus is a significant pathogen of goats. Only 3% of 1146 serum samples of captive ruminants in United States zoos had antibodies to IBR virus.

BHV-1 virus can be grown in a wide variety of cells, including bovine, canine, feline, equine, ovine, rabbit, monkey, and human, where it produces a characteristic CPE.

Host–Virus Relationship

Distribution, Reservoir, and Transmission. The disease occurs worldwide, though several countries in the European Union have eradicated the virus. It has been suggested that wildlife may play a role in disease transmission, but in light of demonstrated viral recrudescence, cattle must be considered the primary reservoir. Virus is transmitted by respiratory, genital, and conjunctival secretions of infected cattle.

Pathogenesis and Pathology. IBR is commonly diagnosed in cattle in feedlots as a result of close contact between cattle and respiratory droplet transmission. The virus induces injury to the respiratory mucosa, which becomes hyperemic and lesions within the nasal cavity progress from areas of focal epithelial necrosis to large areas of ulceration, covered by a pseudomembrane composed of fibrin and cellular debris that results from an intense inflammatory response to the virus. The injury predisposes the cattle to bacterial infection and subsequent bacterial bronchopneumonia (shipping fever complex). Virus can be recovered from nasal secretions for almost 2 weeks following infection. Although viremia is difficult to demonstrate, experimental infections have yielded virus from various organs, perhaps as a consequence of a leukocyte-associated viremia.

Conjunctivitis is common in BHV-1 infection. Typically, it presents with profuse lacrimation and occasionally extends into the cornea, resulting in a keratitis. In some cattle, a multifocal lymphoid hyperplasia may be seen in the palpebral conjunctiva.

Genital infections are most common in dairy cattle and most likely venereally transmitted, though mechanical transmission between bulls is possible in artificial insemination centers. Artificial insemination with infected semen may also produce genital infection. Lesions consisting of pustules and later fibronecrotic plaques are usually limited to the vulva and posterior vagina in the female. Similar lesions are seen on the prepuce of affected bulls. Lesions typically heal in 10–14 days, and many cases are subclinical. Respiratory disease has been produced with genital isolates, and genital lesions have been produced with respiratory isolates. Natural outbreaks of simultaneous respiratory and genital disease are rare. Abortion may be seen in pregnant cattle with IBR or occasionally following vaccination with modified live virus vaccine. The incubation period between infection of the dam and fetal death varies from 15 to 60 days. Since fetal death occurs several days before abortion, the fetus is often severely autolyzed. Fetal edema, especially of the fetal membranes, occurs along with extensive hemorrhagic edema in the perirenal tissue. Extensive hemorrhagic necrosis of the renal cortex is seen along with a focal necrosis in the liver and usually in the lymph nodes. Some necrosis may be observed in placentomes, which are usually good sources of virus for isolation attempts.

Sites of latency are the trigeminal and sciatic ganglia following respiratory and genital disease, respectively. Recrudescent shedding of virus has been observed naturally and in response to corticosteroid administration.

Host Response to Infection. The immune response to BHV-1 involves many factors in addition to the stimulation of neutralizing antibodies, most of which are directed toward surface glycoproteins. IgG and IgM antibodies appear 7 days following exposure.

Laboratory Diagnosis. The fibrinonecrotic plaques commonly present in the external nares and on the nasal septum of cattle with IBR are good sources of material for viral isolation. The conjunctival form can be tentatively diagnosed by the observation of multifocal white lesions in the palpebral conjunctiva. In their absence, viral isolation or PCR detection of viral DNA is needed. The virus can be readily isolated from the conjunctival swabs. Abortion may be difficult to diagnose as the fetus is often presented in an autolyzed condition. If placenta is available and relatively fresh, isolation attempts can be made from the placentomes. Immunohistochemical staining of aborted fetal tissues as well as PCR detection of viral DNA can be used for diagnosis. Diagnosis based on serology may be difficult because animals often have high titers at the time of abortion, regardless of cause, making it difficult to demonstrate rising titers. Detection of BHV-1 in semen is possible by PCR-based techniques.

Treatment and Control. Both modified-live and inactivated vaccines are available for BHV-1 and are used extensively in areas where BHV-1 is endemic. Experimental recombinant DNA vaccines have also been developed. Breeding animals should be vaccinated prior to coitus to prevent abortion, and vaccination prior to weaning or transport is also useful to maintain herd immunity during stressful situations. Vaccination does not prevent infection but does reduce the incidence and severity of disease.

Eradication. Several countries within the European Union (EU) have either successfully eradicated BHV-1 (Denmark, Finland, Sweden, Switzerland, Austria, province of Bolzano in Italy) or implemented an EU-approved compulsory program (Germany). Use of attenuated or whole-virus vaccines is prohibited in these areas and strict import restrictions are aimed at preventing the reintroduction of virus-positive animals and embryos or obtaining semen from positive bulls.

BHV-2 (Bovine Mammillitis Virus)

BHV-2 has been isolated from cattle with generalized skin disease (pseudolumpy skin disease), mammillitis, and stomatitis. BHV-2 will replicate in a wide range of cells, but bovine kidney cell culture is most widely used. Cattle appear to be primarily infected, with mild experimental disease produced in sheep, goats, and pigs.

BHV-2 has been isolated from cattle skin and mucosal infection in the United States, Africa, Europe, and Australia. Originally virus was isolated from South African cattle with generalized skin disease, subsequently termed pseudolumpy skin disease. Mammillitis due to BHV-2 was described in Africa and England, and subsequently in the United States. Stomatitis in bovine and buffalo calves has been described in association with calves nursing cows with mammillitis. Suggested modes of infection include transmission at milking, by insects, or activation of latent virus. Intravenous exposure produces generalized skin lesions, which are characterized by a severe intercellular edema in the epidermis along with syncytia with intranuclear inclusions. An epidermal mononuclear cell and neutrophil infiltrate is present along with mononuclear and lymphocytic dermal perivascular infiltration.

The diagnosis of pseudolumpy skin disease and mammillitis can be based on clinical signs and viral isolation in cell culture. Serology on paired samples will demonstrate an increase in antibody.

Bovine Herpesvirus 4

BHV-4 consists of a group of gammaherpesviruses that have been isolated from different clinical syndromes and normal cattle. Their importance as pathogens is unclear. Only strain DN-599 has been reported to produce conjunctivitis and respiratory disease. Viruses related to this group have been repeatedly isolated from cases of metritis in some North American cattle and are suspected of causing vaginitis in heifers. There is no proven etiologic association between the virus and these diseases and when experimentally inoculated into susceptible cattle, no disease is produced. The North American and European strains appear to be closely related. Latency has been suggested for this group as there appears to be reactivation in response to other inflammatory processes.

Bovine Herpesvirus 5

BHV-5 is an alphaherpesvirus responsible for nonsuppurative meningoencephalitis in young cattle and is closely antigenically and genetically related to BHV-1. Although a case of BHV-5 associated disease in Europe and some outbreaks in United States and Australia have been reported, the current geographical distribution of BHV-5 infection is mainly restricted to South America, especially Brazil and Argentina. However, since this virus is closely related to BHV-1 and currently available serological tests do not differentiate antibodies against each virus, the true prevalence of BHV-5 infection remains unknown. PCR-based methods can differentiate between the two viruses and monoclonal antibodies can also be used for serological differentiation.

Cattle are the natural hosts and latently infected cattle are reservoirs of BHV-5. Natural occurrence of BHV-5 antibodies has also been reported in sheep. Based on experimental evidence, sheep and goats may be potential reservoirs of the virus. There are scarce data regarding BHV-5 transmission. Viral DNA and infectious virus have been detected in semen of subclinically infected bulls. BHV-5 initially infects epithelial cells at the portal of entry. After initial replication, spread of virus probably occurs by three routes, as described previously for BHV-1: local dissemination, systemic spread by viremia, and neuronal spread. Systemic spread by viremia does not appear to be an important part of the pathogenesis of BHV-5, and BHV-5 infection induces either a subclinical infection or disease of moderate severity in adult cattle. However, it can induce lethal encephalitis in young animals (less than 6 months of age). Although BHV-5 and BHV-1 are related, they differ in their neuroinvasion and neurovirulence capacities. BHV-1 neuroinvasion usually does not go further than the first order neuron located in the trigeminal ganglion, where the latent infection is established, whereas BHV-5 is able to infect different regions of the brain. The main macroscopic lesions reported following BHV-5 infection consist of softening of the parenchymal tissue, focal meningeal hemorrhages in the frontal and/or ventral areas and hemorrhagic foci in the pons and left parietal lobe. Gross respiratory lesions, such as nasal congestion, petechial hemorrhages and congestion of the pharyngeal and laryngeal mucosa, as well as bronchopneumonia, have also been detected. BHV-5 can be reactivated and re-excreted without clinical signs or cattle may develop clinical manifestations of encephalitis similar to those observed during acute infection. Specific BHV-5 vaccines remain at an experimental stage of development. The use of BHV-1 vaccines is, therefore, considered to be the best option to protect against BHV-5; however, several studies show that full protection against BHV-5 infection is difficult to induce with a BHV-1 vaccine.

Alcephaline Herpesvirus 1 and Ovine Herpesvirus 2 (MCF)

MCF, an often fatal infection of many species of bovidae and cervidae, occurs as two epidemiologically distinct entities: wildebeest-associated and sheep-associated MCF. Alcephaline herpesvirus 1 (AlHV-1) is responsible for wildebeest-derived (or African) MCF, which occurs when cattle or other susceptible wild ruminants and wildebeest graze together. This form of the disease occurs in Africa and has occurred in zoos that house African ungulates. The sheep associated form of MCF has been described in cattle, bison, and deer outside of Africa and in zoos where animals have had contact with sheep. An etiologic agent for the sheep-associated form of MCF has not been isolated; however, MCF can be transmitted to cattle or bison by aerosolization of nasal secretions from sheep experiencing viral shedding of ovine herpesvirus 2 (OvHV-2), implicating OHV-2 as the cause of this form of MCF. The genome of OHV-2 has been completely sequenced and it is closely related genetically to AlHV-1. AlHV-1 and OvHV-2 are both gammaherpesviruses and are not recognized as significant causes of disease in their natural hosts, wildebeest and sheep, respectively.

AlHV-1 MCF is associated with mixing wildebeest and cattle during periods when the wildebeest are calving. Newborn wildebeest calves shed virus in nasal and ocular secretions up to 3 months of age. Viral shedding also occurs in adult wildebeest given corticosteroid. There is no evidence for congenital infection of sheep with OvHV-2; rather, lambs appear to become infected during the first year of life and typically do not shed virus until after 5 months of age. While sheep-associated MCF in cattle has been associated with lambing, it appears that the newborn lamb does not play the same role as the newborn wildebeest. It also appears that all domestic United States sheep carry OvHV-2. Cattle are considered dead-end hosts for OvHV-2 because cow-to-cow transmission has not been demonstrated.

Both AlHV-1 and OvHV-2 produce similar clinical disease syndromes in cattle. Affected animals present with mucopurulent nasal and ocular discharge and bilateral corneal opacity. Oral lesions may be present, consisting of multiple erosions preceded by a diffuse hyperemia and profuse salivation. Central nervous disturbances are frequent and diarrhea is common.

Histologic lesions are those of a lymphoproliferative disorder characterized by perivascular mononuclear infiltration, necrotizing vasculitis, and tissue lymphoid infiltration, resulting in enlarged, edematous and potentially hemorrhagic lymph nodes. Deposition of immunoglobulin and complement has been described in the glomeruli of affected cattle, suggesting an immune-mediated disease. Death usually occurs in 2–7 days following the onset of clinical signs. History, clinical signs, and histopathology suggest the diagnosis of MCF. Confirmation of the diagnosis of AlHV-1 can be made by isolation of the virus from peripheral blood leukocytes in calf thyroid cells or by PCR detection of the viral DNA. OvHV-2 has not been isolated in cell culture but viral DNA may be detected in the tissues of infected animals by PCR. There is currently no vaccine available for MCF and control is aimed at preventing contact between susceptible hosts and viral carriers.

OvHV-2 associated MCF has also been reported in swine. DNA was detected in the blood and semen of asymptomatic boars and from the brain of symptomatic sows and gilts with MCF that was probably transmitted by artificial insemination. Signs in symptomatic sows and gilts included depression, fever, anorexia, abortion, followed by neurologic signs including ataxia, tremors, convulsions, and aggressive behavior and death. Pigs that survived displayed forelimb paralysis. Pigs are terminal hosts and are not believed to spread the virus.

Caprine Herpesvirus 1

Caprine herpesvirus 1 (CpHV-1) is an alphaherpesvirus that is spread worldwide where goat husbandry is practiced. In the United States, neither the prevalence of seropositive goats nor the prevalence of disease associated with them is known. CpHV-1 is genetically and antigentically related to BHV-1 and though the virus can infect cattle, it has not been associated with disease in cattle.

CpHV-1 induces generalized, often lethal, infection in 1–2-week-old kids. Gross lesions are limited to the gastrointestinal tract with necrosis and ulceration in rumen, cecum, and colon. Intranuclear inclusions are present in epithelial cells near the necrotic areas. In adult goats, the infection is mild or subclinical, with affected animals showing very slight signs of respiratory distress, vaginitis, balanoposthitis, or occasionally, abortion.

CpHV-1 establishes latent infections, but, unlike other herpesviruses, its reactivation is extremely difficult to demonstrate under both natural and experimental conditions. In the natural infection, CpHV-1 reactivates during estrus, but only in animals with low neutralizing antibody titers. After a primary infection, neutralizing antibodies are detected in the serum 1–2 weeks after infection; they reach a peak in the following third or fourth week and decrease slowly about 6–10 months later. If the animals are stressed at this stage, CpHV-1 can reactivate and be shed, especially by the genital route. In response to the reactivation, humoral and cell-mediated immune responses are boosted. It should be noted that a residual sero-neutralizing activity persists even years after the primary CpHV-1 infection.

The disease can be diagnosed by viral isolation from nasal secretions and fecal material. CpHV-1 replicates in canine, rabbit, feline, equine, bovine, and lamb cells. PCR assays for DNA detection are also available. Serum neutralization is the gold standard for serological diagnosis and an ELISA has also been developed.

No CpHV-1 vaccine is presently available in the United States, and it is unlikely that such a vaccine will be developed because of the small market size. Antibodies directed against BHV-1 will react with CpHV-1; thus, it has been suggested that BHV-1 vaccines could be used in goats to protect against CpHV-1 infection. However, a challenge study found that vaccinating goats with an attenuated BHV-1 vaccine induced only partial protection against CpHV-1 infection. No studies have determined whether vaccination would protect against CpHV-1 abortion.

Suid herpesvirus 1 (Pseudorabies; Aujeszky's Disease Virus)

Disease. Pseudorabies in swine is a notifiable disease that causes substantial economic loses to the swine industry in countries where the virus is present in domestic pigs. The virus is most severe in younger animals. The virus commonly affects the nervous system and the mortality rate varies from 5% to 100%. Infection of sows during mid- to late pregnancy can result in abortion, fetal death, mummification, or stillbirths. In adult pigs, severe nervous disorders are rare, and pseudorabies usually presents as a rather vague illness of transient pyrexia, dullness, inappetence, incoordination, and ataxia. Respiratory disease can also be seen in pigs of various ages but is most common in grower and finishing pigs. Inapparent or mild disease may be missed or misdiagnosed in older swine. Pseudorabies also occurs in a number of other species, including cattle, sheep, dogs, cats, and raccoons, in which the clinical signs are usually neurologic and manifested by an intense pruritis.

Etiologic Agent

Physical, Chemical, and Antigenic Properties. The pseudorabies virus (PRV) is an alphaherpesvirus that is designated Suid herpesvirus 1 (SuHV-1). Only one serotype has been identified; however, strain variability has been shown by restriction endonuclease digestion of viruses from different geographic areas. Attenuated strains have been demonstrated to have a deletion in their genome, suggesting that specific regions are associated with virulence.

Sensitivity to Physical and Chemical Agents. The PRV is fairly sensitive to high temperatures and is stable in cell culture fluid between a pH of 6–8 at cooler temperatures. Virus has been observed to survive in nonchlorinated water for 7 days and for 2 days in an anaerobic lagoon. Chemicals that cleave chlorine appear to be the most effective disinfectants.

Infectivity for Other Species and Culture Systems. The disease occurs naturally in cattle, sheep, dogs, cats, and rats. In all but adult swine, the disease is almost always fatal; hence, other animals are essentially "dead-end" hosts. Although one report exists of human infection, PRV is not readily transmitted to humans.

The virus replicates readily in cell cultures from many species and tissues, including cat, dog, cattle, badger, coyote, deer, buzzard, chicken, and goose.

Host–Virus Relationship

Distribution, Reservoir, and Transmission. Pseudorabies has been eradicated from domestic pigs in several parts of Europe, Canada, New Zealand, and the United States. However, it is recognized as one of the most important diseases of domestic pigs, particularly in regions with dense pig populations, including some remaining regions in Europe and also in Latin America and Asia. The principal reservoir of PRV appears to be the pig and transmission is frequently pig to pig. The virus is transmitted by ingestion and inhalation, and during coitus the virus can be transmitted from boar to sow or vice versa. The virus is not shed in urine or feces. Transmission can occur in a contaminated environment under crowded conditions.

Feral swine can transmit the virus to domestic swine and endemic infections in wild swine populations in the United States and Europe represent a constant danger for reintroduction of PRV into free domestic pig herds and regions. The pig is the primary source of viral spread to other species. Cases in dogs have been linked to consumption of feral swine tissues. The cat appears to be more sensitive, and infection in cats was observed in 51% of PRV-infected farms where cats were present.

Pathogenesis and Pathology. The virus replicates primarily in the upper respiratory epithelium including the tonsillar tissue. Virus can be isolated from the brain 24 h following infection, which suggests that the route of infection is via the axoplasm. Viremia is difficult to demonstrate; however, viral shedding may persist in nasal secretions for up to 14 days. Lower airway infection often results, and cardiac and splanchnic ganglia become involved.

The virus produces a nonsuppurative meningoencephalomyelitis with extensive damage to neurons, widespread perivascular cuffing, and gliosis. The brain stem is particularly affected, but lesions also occur throughout the cerebral cortex and cerebellum. There may be intranuclear inclusion bodies in all types of cells. In the respiratory form of the disease, a necrotizing tracheitis and pneumonia occur that result in loss of epithelium in airways and necrosis of alveolar cells.

Microscopic lesions in aborted fetuses include necrosis of many organs, but primarily liver, spleen, visceral lymph nodes, and adrenal glands. Intranuclear inclusion bodies are often present in degenerating hepatocytes, cells of the adrenal cortex, and occasionally mononuclear phagocytic cells of the spleen and lymph nodes. Placental lesions are characterized by degeneration and necrosis of the trophoblasts and mesenchymal cells of the chorion.

Host Response to Infection. IgM antibodies are first detectable about the fifth day after infection followed by measurable IgG antibodies about the seventh day, reaching maximum levels by the twelfth to fourteenth day.

Laboratory Diagnosis. Because signs of the disease in swine vary widely with the age of the animal, the dose of virus received, the strain of virus, and the route of exposure, clinical diagnosis is often difficult.

In the laboratory, a definitive diagnosis of pseudorabies can be made by viral isolation or detection of viral DNA by PCR. Immunofluorescent staining of frozen tonsil or brain tissue can provide a rapid diagnosis. ELISA tests are used to differentiate antibody response to gene-deleted vaccines and field infection and have been used in eradication programs. In an acute outbreak, serology may not be helpful because of the time needed for antibodies to develop.

Prevention and Control. In PRV free areas, biosecurity should be maintained to prevent contact between infected wild swine populations and domestic pigs. Yearly serologic monitoring of domestic pigs is required for maintaining pseudorabies free status. In areas with endemic disease in domestic pigs, efforts should be taken to avoid the disease in a breeding herd. In infected herds, quarantine is the most urgent obligation and it is recommended that the movement of swine be limited for slaughter only. Attenuated live vaccines are available and have been successful in reducing death losses in endemic areas. These vaccines do not prevent reinfection with virulent field virus or the shedding of virulent virus for variable periods. Latently infected and vaccinated animals may shed the virus for indeterminate periods while asymptomatic.

Inactivated vaccines are commercially available. Their principle use has been in susceptible sows in endemic areas to provide antibodies to colostrum for protection of newborn pigs during the first few weeks of life. In certified pseudorabies free areas, vaccination is prohibited.

Canid Herpesvirus 1

Disease. Canid herpesvirus 1(CHV-1) causes a fatal systemic infection in newborn pups and relatively mild infections in older dogs. CHV has been isolated from dogs with respiratory diseases, and, with other viruses and bacteria may be involved in the "kennel cough" syndrome. CHV-1 may be associated with outbreaks of highly contagious ocular infection in susceptible adult dogs, in the absence of concurrent overt systemic disease. CHV-1 can induce genital lesions in male and female dogs. Affected animals appear healthy but often present with a history of infertility.

Etiologic Agent

Physical, Chemical, and Antigenic Properties. Canine herpesvirus is a typical alphaherpesvirus. There is no cross-neutralization between CHV-1 and the viruses of herpes simplex, PRV, or IBR. However, CHV-1 appears to be antigenically related to herpes simplex virus. Only one serotype of CHV-1 is recognized; however, restriction endonuclease analysis of CHV-1 isolates has detected genotypic differences between viruses. Currently, no correlation between different CHV-1 genomes and disease patterns has been demonstrated.

Infectivity for Other Species and Culture Systems. The host range for CHV-1 is restricted to domestic and wild canids. Limited growth occurs in human lung cells and calf, monkey, pig, rabbit, and hamster kidney cells.

Host–Virus Relationship

Distribution, Reservoir, and Transmission. CHV-1 has a worldwide distribution. CHV-1 seroprevalence is high in many domestic canine populations, and primary infection is generally believed to occur at a young age in most dogs. The only known reservoir of CHV-1 in all geographic areas is the dog, with the possible exception of coyotes in the United States. Pups born to seronegative bitches are infected oronasally either from the bitch or from other infected dogs from viral shedding in venereal, ocular, or nasal secretions.

Pathogenesis and Pathology. Clinical manifestations and disease severity during primary infection with many alphaherpesviruses, including CHV-1, are host age dependent. In pups less than 4 weeks of age, primary CHV-1 infection may result in severe generalized disease due to hematogenous spread of the virus. This produces a necrotizing vasculitis in many organs, and the disease is often fatal. Grossly, the kidneys may appear mottled and there may be pulmonary congestion and edema, splenomegaly, lymphadenitis, and nonsuppurative meningoencephalitis. Widespread foci of necrosis and hemorrhages characterize the histologic lesions in affected organs such as kidney, liver, lung, and the gastrointestinal tract. Intranuclear inclusions may be present in areas adjacent to necrotic lesions, specifically in the liver. Primary CHV-1 infection in older canids is frequently subclinical or results in localized respiratory tract, genital mucosa, or ocular disease. Ocular lesions associated with primary CHV-1 infection in adult dogs include conjunctivitis and less frequently, keratitis. Viremia is not typical of CHV-1 infection in immunocompetent adult dogs; however, generalized disease resulting from viremia has been reported in an immunocompromised adult dog.

Host Response to Infection. Neutralizing antibodies develop in dogs inoculated with CHV-1 and are detectable by day 7 postinoculation. Titers peak by day 21 and slowly decrease, persisting approximately 8 months postinoculation. Reactivation of CHV-1 in experimentally infected pups and dogs has been demonstrated with administration of corticosteroids. Latency is established in neurons of the sensory ganglia. During viral reactivation, CHV-1 neutralization titers become detectable and elevate in as few as 7 days, but rapidly decline in a matter of weeks following active infection resolution.

Laboratory Diagnosis. Clinical signs and histopathology can be useful in diagnosis. Definitive diagnosis is by viral isolation and more rapidly by immunofluorescent staining of affected tissues or by detection of genomic DNA by PCR.

Prevention and Control. Commercial CHV vaccines are not available in the United States; a killed virus vaccine is available in Europe. Hyperimmune globulin may be useful but difficult to obtain because the virus is poorly immunogenic. Removal or separation of infected animals should be considered. Optimal temperature for viral replication is approximately 33 °C. Due to the poor ability of puppies to control their body temperature until about 4 weeks of age, younger animals are susceptible to severe disease. Maintenance of normal body temperature in exposed puppies may have therapeutic value.

Felid Herpesvirus 1 (Feline Viral Rhinotracheitis Virus)

Disease. Felid herpesvirus 1 (FHV-1) is the cause of feline viral rhinotracheitis (FVR). Primary infection causes acute rhinitis and conjunctivitis, usually accompanied by fever, depression, and anorexia. Ulcerative keratitis is a frequent sequela to recurrent FHV-1 infection and should be considered the cause of corneal ulceration in cats unless proven otherwise. The virus has also been associated with ulcerative stomatitis, abortions, pneumonia, and facial dermatits.

Etiologic Agent

Physical, Chemical, and Antigenic Properties. FHV-1 is a typical alphaherpesvirus. Serologic comparisons suggest that FHV-1 from around the world belong to a single known serotype; however, differences in the clinical manifestations caused by various isolates have been observed. Viral DNA analysis suggests genetic differences between strains.

Sensitivity to Physical and Chemical Agents. The virus is inactivated by most commercially available detergents, disinfectants, and antiseptics. Virus in cell culture fluid loses 90% of its viability within 6 h at 37 °C, 6 days at 25 °C, and 1 month at 4 °C. The virus is most stable at pH 6, and complete activity is lost in 3 h at pH 3 and pH 9. FHV can be recovered for up to 18 h in a moist environment at 15 °C, but for less than 12 h in a dry room.

Infectivity for Other Species and Culture Systems. Natural infections with FHV-1 have been observed only in the cat family. FHV-1 *in vitro* growth is limited to cells of feline origin. The virus propagates to high titers with demonstrated CPE in primary cell cultures of feline testicle, lung, and renal cells.

Host–Virus Relationships

Distribution, Reservoir, and Transmission. Serological studies show that FHV-1 is widespread in the feline population worldwide, with reported exposure rates of up to 97%. Cats serve as reservoirs. Healthy cats that are latently infected with FHV-1 may shed virus when stressed and following corticosteroid administration, and viral transcripts have been detected in trigeminal ganglia of latently infected cats. The major avenue for spread of FHV-1 is by direct cat-to-cat contact through infectious discharges, particularly respiratory secretions. Overcrowded conditions and close housing greatly increase the likelihood of viral transmission as FHV-1 is short lived in the environment. Indirect or fomite transmission via a contaminated environment, personnel, or feeding and cleaning utensils appears important only in multi-cat situations such as catteries, shelters, and multi-cat households. Strict attention to hygiene should be sufficient to prevent this route of infection. Given that parturition and lactation have been shown to precipitate viral shedding, neonatal infection is highly probable, and the primary infection typically occurs in kittens. Transplacental infection has not been demonstrated in natural infections.

Pathogenesis and Pathology. FHV-1 has a tropism for the conjunctival, nasal and pharyngeal epithelium. The pathogenesis of the infection differs with the route of inoculation. As FHV-1 infection is often manifested in the upper respiratory tract; experimental studies have been done by nasal and ocular routes. When introduced intranasally, the virus produces rapid, cytolytic infection of epithelial cells of the nasal passages. The virus generally persists in the upper respiratory tract for 2 weeks. Damage to the nasal turbinates in acute disease predisposes some cats to chronic rhinitis. In cases of chronic rhinosinusitus, the virus does not replicate, suggesting the disease is perpetuated by immune-mediated mechanisms.

Although many cats develop conjunctivitis during the primary disease, very few develop corneal disease. Reactivation of FHV-1 latency is usually associated with conjunctivitis and may be accompanied by corneal epithelium invasion, which is associated with epithelial ulceration, initially of a pathognomonic dendritic form (Figure 53.3), but progressing rapidly to a larger irregular geographical form. Intranuclear inclusion bodies are numerous in the stratified squamous epithelium of the conjunctiva with conjunctival and corneal lesions. Histologically, corneal ulcers reveal disorientation and degeneration of the epithelial cells, some of which contain nuclear inclusions. Many of these ulcers are slow to heal, leading to a more chronic evolution than seen in primary disease. Chronic keratitis is an immune-mediated condition that results from persistence of virus antigen in the corneal stroma and leads to corneal vascularization and infiltration of inflammatory cells. Formation of corneal sequestra can occur secondarily to any chronic ulcerative keratitis, including FHV-1 ulceration.

FIGURE 53.3. *Dedritic corneal ulcer (arrow), pathognomonic for herpesviral infection. (Photo courtesy of Dr Diane Hendrix, The University of Tennessee.)*

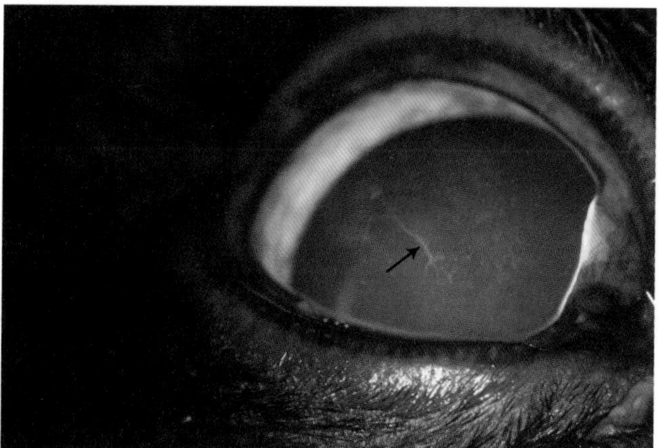

Host Response to Infection. In general, the immune response protects against disease, but not against infection, and mild clinical signs have been observed following reinfection only 150 days after primary infection. The primary immune response of cats to intranasal infection as measured by serum neutralizing antibodies is not impressive. Antibodies usually persist for 1–3 months, although titers have been observed to fluctuate in a cat over a 12-month period. Correlation between presence of antibodies and resistance to infection is not absolute. As with other alphaherpesviruses, cell-mediated immunity plays a very important role in protection, because vaccinated cats without detectable antibody are not necessarily susceptible to disease. By contrast, seroconversion has been shown to correlate with protection against virulent FHV challenge. In these cases, antibodies may serve as an indicator of cellular immune responses, because T lymphocytes are required for the maintenance of B lymphocyte function. Because FHV is a pathogen of the respiratory tract, mucosal cellular and humoral responses are important. Although a correlation exists between FHV antibodies and protection against clinical signs, there is no test available to predict protection in individual cats.

Laboratory Diagnosis. Immunofluorescent staining can demonstrate viral antigens in the tissues of infected cats. However, the test is not particularly sensitive and use of stains, such as fluorescein, may result in false positive results. PCR has become the mainstay for diagnosis of FHV-1 infections. Detection of virus may indicate either coincidental reactivation of latent infection, a consequential reactivation due to another disease process or the cause of the disease. Feline herpesvirus 1 may also be isolated from tissue samples and from swabs of the ocular, nasal, or oropharyngeal mucosa. The virus can be cultured for 14–21 days after infection, but most consistently during the first week. Virus isolation is more difficult in chronic cases. Virus-neutralizing antibodies can be detected in the serum of convalescent cats. Serology is complicated by vaccine virus and positive titers are independent of clinical signs. Titers may be low in both acute and chronic disease. Serology, therefore, is only of limited value in the diagnosis of FHV-1 infection.

Prevention and Control. Both modified-live and inactivated parenteral vaccines are available. Subunit FHV vaccines and modified-live intranasal vaccines are no longer available in Europe. Vaccination protects against disease, but not necessarily against infection. However, it can reduce virus excretion upon infection. Assessment of the duration of immunity is complicated: vaccination does not provide complete protection even shortly after vaccination and no protection against reactivation and shedding, and the degree of protection decreases with time. Even vaccinated cats remain at some risk because FHV-1 vaccines, both parenteral and intranasal, confer only partial immunity against clinical signs and no protection against reactivation/shedding. Maternally derived antibodies provide some degree of humoral protection in kittens up to the age of around 8 weeks, and therefore, primary vaccination should be instigated around 9 weeks of age, with a second vaccination 2–4 weeks later annual boosters are particularly important for cats in high-risk situations or environments. However, for cats in low-risk situations (e.g., indoor-only cats without contact with other cats), 3-yearly intervals are recommended. Care should be taken to avoid introducing cats with developing, subclinical, or latent infections to a colony.

Macacine Herpesvirus 1 (B-virus of macaques)

Herpesvirus B causes a natural infection in *Macaca*—a genus of Old World monkeys (rhesus and cynomolgus species). The infection in monkeys is characterized by oral vesicles similar to the cold sores in humans caused by herpes simplex virus. The disease is common in macaques, is not fatal and the virus may remain latent in the trigeminal and lumbosacral ganglia of infected animals. Direct contact is the most common means of viral spread in monkeys, because virus can be recovered from saliva and from the central nervous tissues of clinically asymptomatic, persistently infected animals.

The virus can cause fatal central nervous infection in humans and laboratory animals such as rabbits and unweaned mice. Most human infections are caused by a bite from a monkey secreting infectious virus, although handling virus-infected primary monkey kidney cell cultures can also lead to infection. The incubation period in humans is 10–20 days. Usually, there is local inflammation at the bite site followed by vesicle formation and necrosis of the area. Virus reaches the CNS by peripheral nerves, and in the majority of cases, death occurs due to acute encephalitis or encephalomyelitis.

Herpesvirus B is morphologically similar to other alphaherpesviruses. It is readily inactivated by detergents. The virus can be cultivated on the chorioallantoic membrane of embryonated chick eggs and in rabbit, monkey, and human cell cultures, producing intranuclear inclusion bodies and syncytia formation. Strong cross-reactivity exists between human herpes simplex viruses and herpesvirus B.

B virus infection can be diagnosed by isolating virus from the central nervous tissues of fatal human cases. A PCR-based assay has been developed for viral identification. Diagnostic detection of herpes B specific antibodies is difficult. An effective vaccine has not been developed. Rapid diagnosis and initiation of therapy, such as antiviral drugs like acyclovir can be of benefit and may prevent death or permanent disability in patients that survive. Caution and wearing of protective gear when handling monkeys remain the best ways to avoid infection.

Gallid Herpesvirus 1 (Infectious Laryngotracheitis Virus)

Disease. Infectious laryngotracheitis virus (ILTV) usually occurs as an acute disease in chickens and represents a serious problem in areas of intense poultry husbandry. The virus produces signs of respiratory distress and coughing that often produce a bloody discharge. Mild enzootic forms of ILTV infection may result in reduced egg production, conjunctivitis, and persistent nasal discharge with swollen nasal and infraorbital sinuses. The mild enzootic form is the most common form in modern poultry operations.

Etiologic Agent

Physical, Chemical, and Antigenic Properties. ILTV is a typical alphaherpesvirus that is also designated as gallid herpesvirus 1 (GaHV-1). There is one serotype of the virus, but genetic variation occurs among strains from different regions.

Sensitivity to Physical and Chemical Agents. ILTV is inactivated by 3% cresol, 1% sodium hydroxide, and 1% lye, 24 h exposure to ether, and 10–15 min at 55 °C. The virus can be stored for lengthy periods by lyophilization and freezing.

Infectivity for Other Species and Culture Systems. ILTV is primarily a disease of chickens and is most common in birds 4–18 months of age. The disease has also been reported in pheasants and peafowl. Young turkeys have been infected experimentally but natural infection rarely occurs in turkeys. Starlings, sparrows, crows, doves, ducks, pigeons, and guinea fowl have been found to be resistant to ILTV. There are no known wild bird reservoirs of this virus.

Chicken kidney monolayer cell cultures, embryonated chicken eggs, and chicken embryo (kidney, liver, and lung) cell cultures have been used to culture ILTV.

Host–Virus Relationship

Distribution, Reservoir, and Transmission. ILTV has been identified in almost every country in the world; it occurs primarily in areas with high concentrations of chickens. ILTV continues to cause disease problems, especially in the Americas and Australia. Chickens are assumed to be the primary reservoir and mode of transmission, which occurs by direct contact through droplet infection of the ocular and respiratory secretions. Mechanical transmission can occur via contaminated equipment and litter. Egg transmission of ILTV has not been demonstrated. A carrier state can develop in birds with sublethal disease, and ILTV has been isolated from chickens 2 years after infection. Unvaccinated birds are susceptible to infection from vaccinated birds, and vaccinated birds may become carriers. Acutely infected birds represent a greater source of virus than clinically recovered carrier birds.

Pathogenesis and Pathology. ILTV in natural conditions enters through the upper respiratory tract and ocular tract. In the natural disease, the greatest concentration of ILTV is found in the trachea, and the virus replicates only in the nasal cavity, trachea, and lower respiratory tract. Latent virus has been demonstrated in the trigeminal ganglion. Viremia has not been reported.

Lethal infections of ILTV can occur due to asphyxiation, resulting from extensive diphtheritic membrane formation that plugs the tracheal bifurcation. Histopathology demonstrates fibrinous laryngotracheitis, with detachment of the tracheal epithelium and large intranuclear inclusion bodies in detached cells that are the basis for a strong presumptive diagnosis.

Host Response to Infection. The first signs of ILTV infection usually appear 6–12 days following natural exposure. Resistance to disease following the infection or vaccination usually persists for approximately 1 year. Infected birds develop precipitating and serum-neutralizing antibodies; however, the cell-mediated response appears to be important in resistance. Full immunity can be demonstrated in bursectomized chickens in the absence of a humoral response.

Laboratory Diagnosis. Virus can be isolated from tracheal and lung tissue in embryonated chicken eggs, cell culture, and ILTV DNA can be demonstrated by PCR. Immunofluorescent staining of trachea can demonstrate presence of viral antigen up to 14 days postinfection. ELISA-based serology is widely used.

Prevention and Control. Use of live ILTV vaccine results in carriers, which can shed to nonvaccinated susceptible birds. Vaccine strains have been associated with outbreaks in some flocks following reversion of the strains to virulence. Because the virus can survive for 10 days at temperatures of 13 °C to 23 °C, the cleaning of infected premises is very important. Complete depopulation and disinfection of premises has been used to control the disease.

Use of attenuated vaccines is a common practice for breeding and egg production flocks, though vaccination does not protect against infection with virulent virus or development of latency. The development of genetically engineered vaccines holds promise for improved control strategies.

Gallid Herpesvirus 2 (Marek's Disease Virus)

Disease. Marek's disease (MD) is a lymphoproliferative disease, lymphoma being most common, of chickens that may involve numerous tissues. Most frequently peripheral nerves are affected. Prior to vaccine development, MD was responsible for heavy losses, and increased losses to MD in vaccinated flocks have suggested an evolution toward greater virulence.

Progressive paralysis of one or more extremities, incoordination, drooping wings, and lowered head position are the most common signs of MD. Mortality varies from 10% with mild MD to more than 50% in unvaccinated birds.

Etiologic Agent

Physical, Chemical, and Antigenic Properties. Gallid herpesvirus 2 (GaHV-2) is an alphaherpesvirus, and virulence varies greatly among strains.

Resistance to Physical and Chemical Agents. Cell-free virus is readily inactivated at temperatures greater than 37 °C and is only relatively stable at 25 °C (4 days) and 4 °C (2 weeks). MDV can be maintained for long periods at 27 °C. Virus is inactivated by pH 3 and pH 11. Infectivity of dried MDV-infected feathers is destroyed by chlorine, organic iodine, a quaternary ammonium compound, cresylic acid, synthetic phenol, and sodium hydroxide.

Infectivity for Other Species and Culture Systems. The chicken is the primary natural host for the MDV, and disease is rare in other species except for quail. MD virus has not been shown to affect any nonavian animals. No etiologic link has been demonstrated between MDV and human cancer. The virus is most often cultivated on chicken or duck embryo fibroblast cells. Chicken kidney cells have also been used.

Host–Virus Relationships

Distribution, Reservoir, and Transmission. MD is a major disease of domestic chicken flocks worldwide. The virus tends to remain highly cell associated but release of cell-free infectious virus is associated with productive infection of epithelial cells at the base of feather follicles and birds are usually infected through inhalation of this cell-free virus in feather dander. The virus can persist in litter and poultry house dust. The virus is not transmitted *in ovo*.

Pathogenesis and Pathology. The incidence of MD is variable, depending on the strain of the virus and the age of the chicken. It usually occurs in chickens between 2 and 5 months old and is commonly felt not to be seen in birds older than 22 weeks; however, disease has been observed in birds as young as 3–4 weeks and in 60-week-old laying hens. The virus primarily affects the nervous system although visceral organs and other tissues may also be involved. Lesions involve peripheral nerves and spinal roots. The principal infected nerve trunk shows gross lesions consisting of a grayish-white swelling, which histologically are characterized by extensive lymphocytic infiltrations. Nerve enlargement is frequently unilateral. Edema may be present and myelin degeneration of nerve sheaths may be apparent.

Ocular lymphomatosis is another possible outcome of MDV infection, with blindness resulting due to iris involvement. Histologically, a similar infiltration of lymphocytes is present, which can also occur in the optic nerve.

In the visceral form, lymphoid tumors of varying degrees of severity infiltrate the gonads, liver, lung, and skin. Affected chickens have enlarged visceral organs with white nodular or miliary foci. Occlusive atherosclerosis has been observed experimentally.

Host Response to Infection. The immune response to MDV is complex, in that both humoral and cell-mediated immunity (CMI) develop in normal birds. Bursectomized birds survive experimental infection, suggesting that CMI is important. In chicks, passively acquired antibody is thought to limit the extent of infection rather than prevent it or clear the virus. Viral-specific antibodies appear within 1–3 weeks following infection and neutralizing antibodies persist for the life of the bird. The genome of MD virus has incorporated *onc* genes, which result in transformation of infected T cells and production of T cell lymphomas following infiltration and proliferation of these transformed cells. Following infection, transient CMI suppression is common; it may persist in birds that develop neoplasms. Genetic resistance is correlated with birds that carry the B21 alloantigen of the B red blood cell group. The basis for this resistance has not been fully characterized.

Laboratory Diagnosis. On necropsy, gross lesions are common in peripheral nerves, root ganglia, and the spinal roots. Lymphomatous lesions are characteristically composed of small lymphocytes, lymphoblasts, and reticulum cells. Arterial lesions of atherosclerosis are often present. Confirmatory diagnosis is made by viral isolation or by antigen detection using fluorescent antibody or immunoperoxidase, or by detection of viral DNA by PCR. Antibodies can be detected by agar gel immunodiffusion, indirect immunofluorescence, and viral neutralization and ELISA assays.

Prevention and Control. Experimentally, MDV-free flocks can be maintained by strict isolation, constant surveillance, and frequent monitoring for virus and antibody, but these techniques have been of limited commercial use. Commercial vaccines are available and have been effective in reducing the incidence of MD. Vaccination does not prevent infection or shedding of virulent MDV, but it does prevent tumor formation, particularly in visceral organs. Peripheral nerve lesions continue to occur, but at reduced rates. Turkey herpesvirus strains (HVT; MDV serotype 3) are antigenically related viruses that have been routinely used for vaccination, but the emergence of more virulent strains of GaHV-2 has resulted in vaccine failures and increased use of avirulent gallid herpesvirus 3 (MDV serotype 2) viruses or strains of low-pathogenicity GaHV-2 for vaccination. Birds are vaccinated annually in the United States and the vast majority are vaccinated *in ovo*.

References

Allen GP (2007) Development of a real-time polymerase chain reaction assay for rapid diagnosis of neuropathogenic strains of equine herpesvirus-1. *J Vet Diag Invest*, **19**, 69–72.

Nugent J, Birch-Machin I, Smith KC *et al.* (2006) Analysis of equid herpesvirus 1 strain variation reveals a point mutation of the DNA polymerase strongly associated with neuropathogenic versus nonneuropathogenic disease outbreaks. *J Virol*, **80**(8), 4047–4060.

Perkins GA, Goodman LB, Tsujimura K *et al.* (2009) Investigation of the prevalence of neurologic equine herpes virus type 1 (EHV-1) in a 23-year retrospective analysis (1984–2007). *Veterinary Microbiology*, **139**(3–4), 375–378.

Talens LT and Zee YC (1976) Purification and buoyant density of infectious bovine rhinotracheitis virus. *Proc Exp Biol Med*, **151**, 132.

Further Reading

Allen GP (2008). Risk factors for development of neurologic disease after experimental exposure to equine herpesvirus-1 in horses. *Am J Vet Res*, **69** (12), 1595–1600.

Azevedo Costa E, de Marco Viott A, de Souza Machado G, *et al.* (2010) Transmission of ovine herpesvirus 2 from asymptomatic boars to sows. *Emerg Infect Dis*, **16** (12), 2011–2012.

Baigent SJ, Smith LP, Nair VK, and Currie RJW (2006) Vaccinal control of Marek's disease: Current challenges, and future strategies to maximize protection. *Vet Immunol Immunopathol*, **112**, 78–86.

Barrandeguy M and Thiry E (2012) Equine coital exanthema and its potential economic implications for the equine industry. *Vet J* **191** (1), 35–40.

Borchers K, Lieckfeldt D, Ludwig A *et al.* (2008) Detection of equid herpesvirus 9 DNA in the trigeminal ganglia of a Burchell's zebra from the Serengeti ecosystem. *J Vet Med Sci*, **70** (12), 1377–1381.

Brault SA, Blanchard MT, Gardner IA *et al.* (2010) The immune response of foals to natural infection with equid herpesvirus-2 and its association with febrile illness. *Vet Immunol Immunopathol*, **137**, 136–141.

Brault SA, Bird BH, Balasuriya UBR, and MacLachlan NJ (2011) Genetic heterogeneity and variation in viral load during equid herpesvirus-2 infection of foals. *Vet Microbiol*, **147**, 253–261.

Davison AJ (2010) Herpesvirus systematics. *Vet Microbiol*, **143** (1–2), 52–69.

Del Medico Zajac MP, Ladelfa MF, Kotsias F *et al.* (2010) Biology of bovine herpesvirus 5. *Vet J*, **184**, 138–145.

Donovan TA, Schrenzel MD, Tucker T *et al.* (2009) Meningoencephalitis in a polar bear caused by equine herpesvirus 9 (EHV-9). *Vet Pathol*, **46** (6), 1138–1143.

Fortier G, van Erck E, Pronost S *et al.* (2010) Equine gammaherpesviruses: pathogenesis, epidemiology and diagnosis. *Vet J*, **186**, 148–156.

Hartley C (2010). Aetiology of corneal ulcers assume FHV-1 unless proven otherwise. *J Feline Med Surg*, **12**, 24–35.

House JA, Gregg DA, Lubroth J *et al.* (1991) Experimental equine herpesvirus-l infection in llamas *(Lama glama)*. *J Vet Diag Invest*, **3**, 137–143.

Jones RC (2010) Viral respiratory diseases (ILT, aMPV infections, IB): are they ever under control? *Br Poult Sci*, **51** (1), 1–11.

Kasem S, Syamada S, Kipuel M *et al.* (2008) Equine herpesvirus type 9 in giraffe with encephalitis. *Emerg Infect Dis*, **14** (12), 1948–1949.

Kleiboeker SB, Schommer SK, Johnson PJ *et al.* (2002) Association of two newly recognized herpesviruses with interstitial pneumonia in donkeys (*Equus asinus*). *J Vet Diag Invest*, **14**, 273–280.

Ledbetter EC, Dubovi, EJ, Kim, SG *et al.* (2009) Experimental primary ocular canine herpesvirus-1 infection in adult dogs. *Am J Vet Res*, **70** (4), 513–521.

Ledbetter EC, Kim SG, Dubovi EJ. (2009) Outbreak of ocular disease associated with naturally-acquired canine herpesvirus-1 infection in a closed domestic dog colony. *Vet Ophthalmol*, **12** (4), 242–247.

Malone EK, Ledbetter EC, Rassnick KM *et al.* (2010) Disseminated canine herpesvirus-1 infection in an immunocompromised adult dog. *J Vet Inter Med*, **24**, 965–968.

Marinaro M, Bellacicco AL, Tarsitano E *et al.* (2010) Detection of caprine herpesvirus 1-specific antibodies in goat sera using an enzyme-linked immunosorbent assay and serum neutralization test. *J Vet Diag Invest*, **22** (2), 245–248.

McCoy MH, Montgomery DL, Bratanich AC *et al.* (2007) Serologic and reproductive findings after a herpesvirus-1 abortion storm in goats. *J Am Vet Med Assoc*, **231** (8), 1236–1239.

Muller T, Han EC, Tottewitz F *et al.* (2011) Pseudorabies virus in wild swine: a global perspective. *Arch Virol*, **156**, 1691–1705.

Nardelli S, Farina G, Lucchini R *et al.* (2008) Dynamics of infection and immunity in a dairy cattle population undergoing an eradication programme for Infectious Bovine Rhinotracheitis (IBR). *Prev Vet Med*, **85**, 68–80.

Patel JR, and Heldens J (2005) Equine herpesviruses 1 (EHV-1) and 4 (EHV-4)—epidemiology, disease and immunoprophylaxis: A brief review. *Vet J*, **170**, 14–23.

Pusterla N, Wilson W, David M *et al.* (2009) Equine herpesvirus-1 myeloencephalopathy: A review of recent developments. *Vet J*, **180**, 279–289.

Schrenzel MD, Tucker TA, Donovan, TA *et al.* (2008) New Hosts for Equine Herpesvirus 9. *Emerg Infect Dis*, **14** (10), 1616–1619.

Smith, KL, Allen, GP, Branscum, AJ *et al.* (2010) The increased prevalence of neuropathogenic strains of EHV-1 in equine abortions. *Vet Microbiol*, **141** (1–2), 5–11.

Thiry E, Addie D, Belak S *et al.* (2009) Feline herpesvirus infection ABCD guidelines and prevention and management. *J Feline Med Surg*, **11**, 547–555.

Vengust M, Wen X, and Bienzle D (2008) Herpesvirus-associated neurological disease in a donkey. *J Vet Diagn Invest*, **20**, 820–823.

Williams KJ, Maes R, Del Piero F *et al.* (2007) Equine multinodular pulmonary fibrosis: a newly recognized herpesvirus-associated fibrotic lung disease. *Vet Pathol*, **44** (6), 849–862.

Wong DM, Belgrave RL, Williams KJ *et al.* (2008) Multinodular pulmonary fibrosis in five horses. *J Am Vet Med Assoc*, **232** (6), 898–905.

54 Poxviridae

Gustavo A. Delhon

Viruses of the Poxviridae family are among the largest and more complex viruses infecting animals. The enveloped, pleomorphic, roughly brick-shaped poxvirus virions are 220–450 nm long and 140–260 nm wide, just at the limit of the resolution power of light microscopes, and consist of copies of approximately 80 different viral proteins. Characteristic tubular structures decorate the virion surface (Figure 54.1A). The size and morphology of poxvirus particles are so distinctive that many veterinary virology laboratories use negative-stain electron microscopic examination of lesion material for rapid preliminary diagnosis of poxviral infection.

The poxviral genome consists of a linear double-stranded DNA molecule with lengths ranging from 134 to 300 kilobase pairs and encodes for 130 to more than 300 genes. Genes with roles in virus structure and morphogenesis, transcription, and DNA replication are clustered into a large central genomic region and are conserved among poxvirus genera. Regions flanking the central genomic region are less conserved and contain genes with roles in immune evasion, host-range, and virulence. Many genes in the flanking regions of the viral genome exhibit homology to host genes that function in innate immunity, suggesting that poxviruses can manipulate host antiviral responses. It is believed that modulation of host antiviral responses is important for successful poxviral infection and disease. Exceptional for DNA viruses, poxviruses replicate in the cytoplasm of infected cells, implying that they can dispense with host nuclear functions. The presence of a relatively large number of replicative viral genes in poxviral genomes reflects independence of host nuclear enzymes and factors. Cytoplasmic replication of poxviruses occurs in virus infection-induced cytoplasmic compartments known as *viroplasm* or *virus factories*, where viral genome replication and virion assembly take place.

Viruses of the family Poxviridae are classified into two subfamilies, Chordopoxvirinae (poxviruses that infect vertebrates) and Entomopoxvirinae (poxviruses that infect insects). The current classification of chordopoxviruses is shown in Table 54.1. Some poxviruses are very host species specific, while others infect multiple species. Several poxviruses maintained in animals cause zoonotic infections in humans.

A common feature of chordopoxviruses is that, at some stage during infection of the host, they colonize, replicate, and induce pathology in the skin and, to a lesser extent, selected mucosae. Lesions in the skin may be localized or extend over a large surface. Frequently skin lesions adopt the form of exanthema, evolving through stages of erythema, papula, and scabs, with or without clear intermediate vesicular and pustular stages. Some poxviral diseases are characterized by nodular skin lesions, while others are prominently proliferative. For some diseases (e.g., swinepox), skin lesions may be the only manifestation of disease. For others, skin lesions are accompanied by fever and other manifestations of systemic disease such as lesions in internal organs (e.g., sheeppox and mousepox) and generalized lymphadenopathy.

In general, the main skin target cell for chordopoxviruses is the keratinocyte. Keratinocytes are found in different stages of differentiation in the epidermis and associated hair follicles, forming multiple strata from basal stem cells to apical corneocytes (i.e., keratin scales). Typical poxviral histopathology during the papular stage shows hyperplasia of the epidermis, ballooning degeneration of keratinocytes of the stratum spinosum, and aberrant keratinization (Figure 54.2A). Viral particles in different maturation stages are seen in infected keratinocytes with the electron microscope (Figure 54.1B).

A conspicuous feature of poxvirus-infected cells is the presence of cytoplasmic inclusion bodies. Two types of poxviral inclusion bodies are known. Most poxviruses induce formation of Guarnieri's or type B inclusion bodies, which are slightly basophilic and are composed of virus particles and protein aggregates (Figure 54.2A, inset). In addition, some poxviruses (e.g., cowpox virus and ectromelia virus) induce type A inclusion- or ATI bodies, which are acidophilic and consist largely of aggregates of one type of viral protein. The size and type of inclusion bodies as well as the time frame during infection in which they are detected vary broadly among poxviral diseases. Detection of inclusion bodies in tissue sections from lesions aids to the diagnosis of some poxviral diseases.

Poxvirus cannot infect intact skin. Contact of infectious material (e.g., scabs, secretions, and fomites) with broken or lacerated skin is a common route of poxvirus transmission. While some poxviruses have adapted for aerosol transmission (e.g., sheeppox virus), others are mechanically transmitted by biting arthropods (e.g., myxoma virus and avipoxviruses).

Veterinary Microbiology, Third Edition. Edited by D. Scott McVey, Melissa Kennedy and M.M. Chengappa.

FIGURE 54.1. *(A) Transmission electron micrograph of a contagious ecthyma virion. Note the ovoid shape of the particle and the cris-cross pattern of surface tubular structures. Negative stain; bar= 200 nm. (B) Transmission electron micrograph of a section of a capripoxvirus-infected keratinocyte. N, nucleus; C, cytoplasm; V, virus particles; T, tonofilaments; d, desomosomes; m, mitochondrium. Bar = 500 nm. Inset, enlargement of a mature viral particle. Bar = 100 nm.*

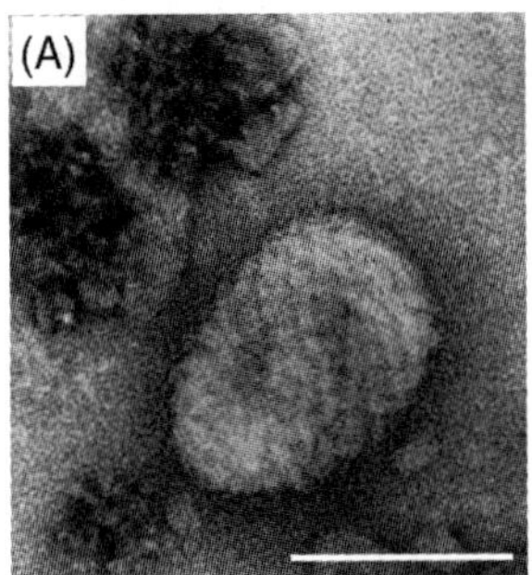

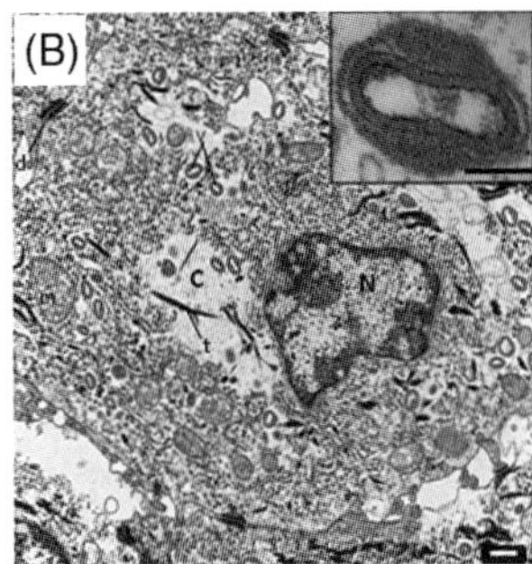

Orthopoxviruses

Members of the genus *Orthopoxvirus* are the best-known poxviruses. One reason for this is that variola virus, the human pathogen that causes *smallpox*, is an orthopoxvirus. Historically, smallpox was one of the most devastating human diseases until eradication in 1980. With mortality rates approaching 35%, and transmission by the respiratory route, smallpox caused massive epidemics that impacted human demographics worldwide. In its most frequent presentation (ordinary smallpox), the disease was characterized by fever, enanthema in the pharynx and oral cavity, and generalized exanthema. The most serious complication of the disease was bronchopneumonia, as a result of virus replication and/or secondary bacterial infection in the respiratory tract. Orthopoxviruses that cause disease in animals include cowpox virus, vaccinia virus, camelpox virus, and ectromelia virus.

Cowpox

Infections by cowpox virus are endemic in Europe and Western Asia. The virus is maintained in rodents, and naturally infects humans and multiple animal species. The name cowpox virus refers to its association with pustular lesions of the teats of milking cows, currently a rare condition. More recently cowpox virus infections have been associated with cats, dogs, mice, and a number of zoo animals, including elephants, large felids, foxes, anteaters, and rhinoceros.

Cowpox virus enters the host through broken skin. In most species, including humans, infection results in localized, self-limiting pustular, often erosive skin lesions that evolve to crust in a few days, and a swelling draining lymph node. In domestic cats, however, cowpox virus infection

Table 54.1. Poxviruses that Infect Vertebrate Species

Genus	Virus, Examples[a]	Reservoir Host	Other Infected Hosts	Geographic Distribution
Orthopoxvirus	Cowpox virus	Wild rodents	Cats, humans, cattle, zoo animals	Europe, Asia
	Monkeypox virus	Likely wild rodents	Monkeys, humans, zoo animals	Africa
	Variola virus	Humans	Nil	*Eradicated*
	Vaccinia virus	Unknown	Humans, cattle, water buffaloes	Worldwide
	Camelpox virus	Camels	Nil	Africa, Asia
	Horsepox virus	Unknown	Horses	Asia?
	Ectromelia virus	Unknown	Laboratory mice	Europe
Leporipoxvirus	*Myxoma virus*	Wild rabbits	European or common rabbit	Americas, Europe, Australia
	Rabbit fibroma virus	Wild rabbits	European or common rabbit	Europe
	Squirrel fibroma virus	Gray squirrel	Woodchuck	North America
Suipoxvirus	*Swinepox virus*	Swine	Nil	Worldwide
Capripoxvirus	*Sheeppox virus*	Sheep, goats	Nil	Africa, Asia
	Goatpox virus	Goats, sheep	Nil	Africa, Asia
	Lumpy skin disease virus	Unknown	Cattle	Africa
Cervidpoxvirus	*Deerpox virus*	Cervids	Unknown	North America
Yatapoxvirus	*Tanapox virus*	Monkeys	Humans, monkeys	Africa
	Yaba monkey tumor virus	Monkeys	Humans	Africa
Parapoxvirus	*orf virus*	Sheep, goats	Humans, camels, wild mammals	Worldwide
	Bovine papular stomatitis virus	Cattle	Humans	Worldwide
	Pseudocowpox virus	Cattle	Humans	Worldwide
	Parapoxvirus of red deer	Red deer	Unknown	New Zealand, Europe
Molluscipoxvirus	*Molluscum contagiosum virus*	Humans	Nil	Worldwide
Avipoxvirus	Canarypox virus	Canaries	Unknown	Worldwide
	Fowlpox virus	Chicken	Unknown	Worldwide
	Pigeonpox virus	Pigeons	Unknown	Worldwide
	Psittacinepox virus	Psittacidae	Unknown	Worldwide

[a] The prototype virus of the genus is indicated in italics.

FIGURE 54.2. *Histopathology of a skin lesion induced by poxvirus infection (contagious ecthyma). (A) Five days postinfection. The epidermis (e) exhibits hyperplasia of keratinocytes, most notably in the stratum spinosum, with the upper cells in the stratum undergoing ballooning degeneration. Pale cytoplasmic inclusion bodies are observed in a few keratinocytes (arrows). The dermis (d) is infiltrated with neutrophils and inflammatory mononuclear cells. H&E, X400. (B) Twenty days postinfection. The hyperplastic epidermis (e) grows inward forming epidermal pegs (p) that interdigitate with the infiltrated dermis (d); c= crust. H&E, X100.*

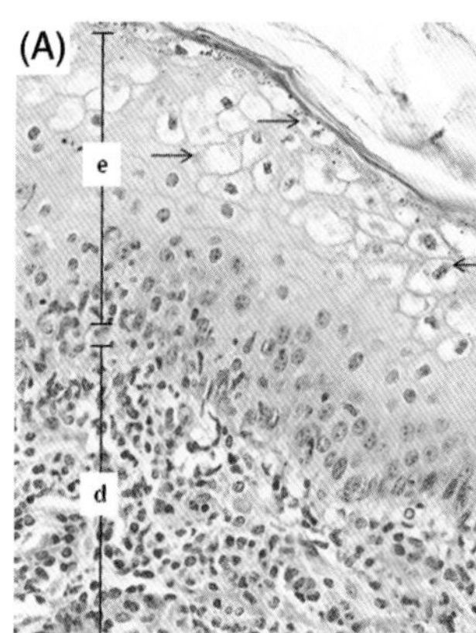

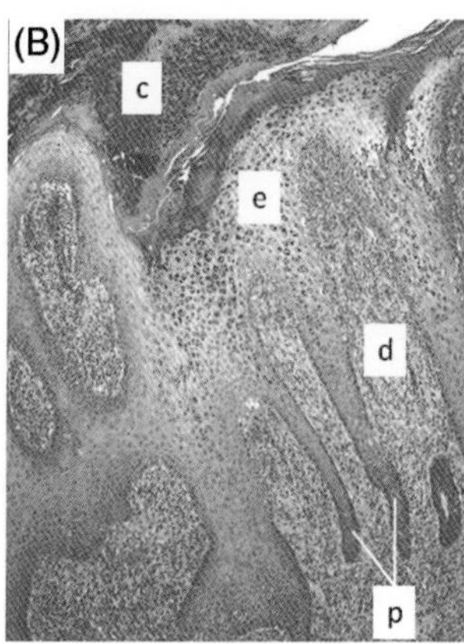

has a systemic character. A primary infection occurs at the site of virus entry followed by viremia. Seven to ten days later multiple lesions develop, primarily on the skin of the head, neck, and limbs and, occasionally, in the oral cavity. Some cats exhibit conjunctivitis and become pyretic. In rare cases, the infection is fatal, with lesions manifested in internal organs such as the liver and lungs. Most cowpox virus infections in cats occur in late summer and autumn due to a higher density of potentially infected rodents. Cat-to-cat transmission can occur but usually results in subclinical infection. Seroprevalence of cowpox virus in cats varies from 0% to 16%.

Zoonotic transmission of cowpox virus to humans occurs via contact with infected animals. Transmission to humans has been reported primarily from cats, especially in children, but also from cattle, mice, and zoo animals.

Vaccinia

Vaccinia virus, the prototype orthopoxvirus, is closely related immunologically to variola and cowpox viruses. Various vaccinia virus strains have been successfully used as vaccines during the worldwide smallpox eradication campaign by the World Health Organization. The name vaccinia derives from the Latin word *vacca* for cow, but there is no evidence that the virus is originated from cows. The natural host for vaccinia virus remains unknown.

Although smallpox vaccination has been suspended 30 years ago, infections by vaccinia virus have been sporadically reported in multiple species. For example, infections by various vaccinia virus strains have been reported in daily cattle and milkers in Brazil. Disease in cows, known as *bovine vaccinia*, is indistinguishable from cowpox, with papules, vesicles, and crust in the udders and teats. Unprotected milkers become infected by contact and may spread the disease in cattle. Vaccinia virus strains have been isolated from wild rodents in bovine vaccinia areas as well as Brazilian forests, providing a hypothesis for maintenance of the virus in Nature and outbreaks in cattle.

Similar to cowpox and bovine vaccinia viruses, buffalopox virus, a virus circulating in water buffalos in northern India and, to a lesser extent, in Pakistan, Egypt, and Indonesia, causes pustular lesions on the teats and udders of milking buffalos. Buffalopox can be enzootically transmitted to unprotected milkers, producing lesions on the hands and face. Buffalopox virus and rabbitpox virus (i.e., the causative agent of a highly lethal airborne disease of laboratory rabbits) are considered vaccinia virus strains that have adapted to buffalos and rabbits, respectively. Vaccine escape has been hypothesized to account for the origin of buffalopox and bovine vaccinia strains.

Camelpox

Camelpox is an economically significant disease in Middle East, and Asian and African countries with an indigenous camel population, in which the disease is endemic. New world camelids are also susceptible. DNA sequencing and analysis of virus genomes have shown that camelpox virus is most similar to variola virus. Indeed, in the past, camels have been successfully protected against camelpox with vaccinia virus-based vaccines.

Camelpox virus entry into the host is thought to occur via the respiratory route and by contact with skin abrasions. Arthropod vectors, including ticks and biting flies, may also play a role in virus transmission (reviewed in Bhanuprakash *et al.* 2010). Camelpox may adopt several clinical forms, ranging from local mild skin infections to moderate and severe systemic infections. The incubation time for systemic forms is 8–13 days, which is followed by fever and various degrees of exanthema and lymphadenopathy. Skin rash appears 1–3 days after the onset of fever, following the progression macula-papula-vesicle-pustule-scab. Lesions are first observed in the head, and then in the neck and limbs. In the most severe infections (generalized camelpox), skin lesions spread to the entire body surface and the mucosa of the oral cavity and respiratory and gastrointestinal tracts. In noncomplicated cases, lesions resolve in 4–6 weeks. Camels may exhibit lacrimation, salivation, and nasal discharge. In complicated cases, death occurs as a consequence of secondary bacterial infections. In epizootics involving young animals, the case-fatality rate may be as high as 25%. High rates of abortion have been described. Zoonotic transmission of camelpox to people in close contact with sick camels has been recently reported. Diagnosis of camelpox is based on clinical signs. Electron microscopic examination of lesion material and virus isolation confirms involvement of an orthopoxvirus. Mild forms of camelpox can be confounded with infections by Ausdyk virus, a poorly characterized parapoxvirus that cause localized skin lesions primarily in the face. Both inactivated and live attenuated virus-based vaccines can be used to protect camels from camelpox.

Mousepox

Mousepox is a rare fatal disease of laboratory mice caused by mousepox (ectromelia) virus. Although natural infection by mousepox virus in wild mice has been reported, the natural reservoir for the virus is unknown. Mousepox virus enters the body through skin breaks and causes an acute systemic disease, resulting is massive liver necrosis as well as necrosis of the spleen, lymph nodes, and Peyer's patches. If mice survive acute disease, they develop a generalized skin rash together with necrosis and ulceration of distal parts of the feet, snout, and tail. Conjunctivitis is often associated with mousepox, with large amount of virus being shed in ocular discharges.

Susceptibility to mousepox depends on virus strain, and mouse age, immune status, and genetic background (e.g., Balb/c and A/J mouse strains are highly susceptible, while AKR and C57BL6 mice resist severe disease). Highly susceptible mouse strains die rapidly after dissemination of infection without shedding significant amount of virus. Little virus is also shed by resistant strains that exhibit limited infection. Mice with intermediate susceptibility are, therefore, most important in spreading virus in a colony since they develop generalized disease and survive long enough to spread virus to other animals.

Mousepox outbreaks may significantly impact laboratory mouse colonies. Prevention and control are based on quarantine and regulation of mice traffic. Serological tests such as enzyme-linked immunosorbent assay (ELISA) are periodically performed on valuable mouse colonies.

Parapoxviruses

Viruses of the genus *Parapoxvirus* infect farm and wild animals worldwide. The genus includes contagious ecthyma virus, bovine papular stomatitis virus, pseudocowpox virus, and parapoxvirus of red deer in New Zealand. A distinct subclade of parapoxviruses infect seals and sea lions. Virus particles are ovoid, 260 nm long and 160 nm wide, and exhibit a regular array of superficial tubule-like structures arranged in a characteristic criss-cross pattern (Figure 54.1A). The size and morphology of virus particles allows for rapid diagnosis of parapoxvirus infection following electron microscopic examination of lesion material. In general, parapoxviruses cause self-limiting, nonsystemic, localized disease of the skin and oral mucosa, with a preference for mucocutaneous transitions. Many parapoxviruses zoonotically infect humans, with infections in immunocompetent persons being mild and self-limiting.

Contagious Ecthyma

Contagious ecthyma, orf, or contagious pustular dermatitis is a highly contagious ubiquitous disease of sheep and goats characterized by maculopapular and proliferative lesions affecting the skin around the mouth, nostrils, interdigital region, and teats, and the oral mucosa (Figure 54.3). Spread in a flock is rapid and occurs by contact with affected animals or shed crust. Contagious ecthyma primarily affects

FIGURE 54.3. *(A) Ecthyma contagiosum in a lamb. Thick crust surrounds the mouth and nostrils. The arrow indicates a proliferating mass originated from the inner side of the lower lip. (B) Papilomatous proliferative lesions in the mucosa lining the hard palate and upper lip. (Courtesy of Francisco A. Uzal.)*

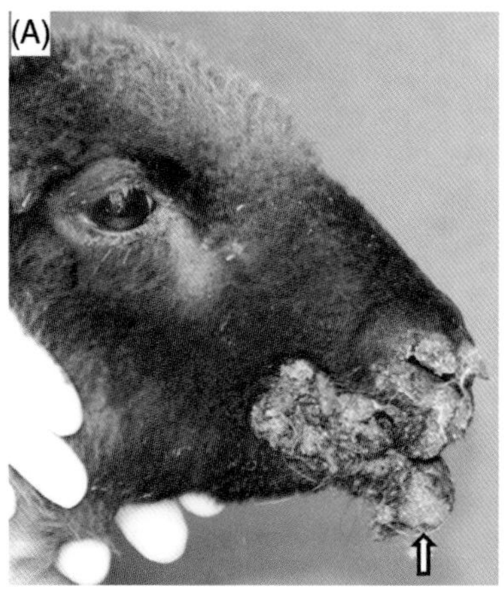

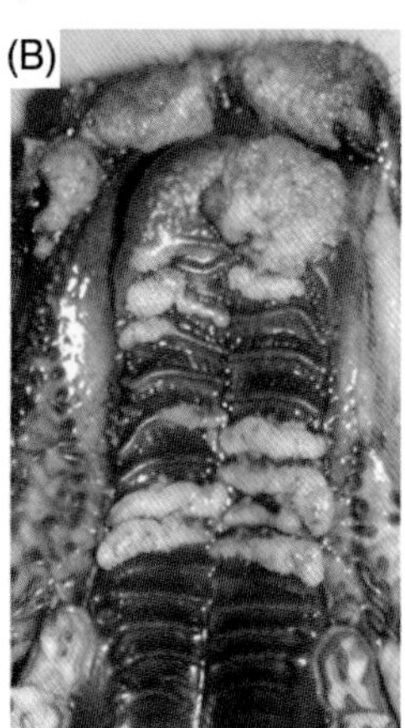

animals less than 1 year old, with morbidities in susceptible flocks that may reach 90%. Mortality is usually low; however, lesions in lips and udders may prevent affected lambs and kids from suckling, which can result in rapid emaciation. Lesions are largely confined to areas surrounding the virus entry sites, evolving through stages of erythema, papules, and crust. Histological examination shows classical poxviral lesions, including epidermal hyperplasia, ballooning degeneration of keratinocytes, hyperkeratosis, occasional inclusion bodies, infiltration of the dermis and epidermis with inflammatory cells, and deposition of scale-crust on the skin surface (Figure 54.2A). Intraepidermal microvesicles and micropustules rarely coalesce to form macroscopic vesicles and pustules. Evidence of angiogenesis is often seen in the infiltrated dermis. As the infection progresses, the epidermis grows deep into the dermis forming an intricate epithelial network (rete pegs) that persists beyond the macroscopic resolution of lesions Figure 54.2B). Advanced lesions, specially around the mouth, may progress to a more or less pronounced proliferative stage in the form of papillomatous growths (Figure 54.3B). In the absence of secondary infections, lesions are usually resolved in 6–8 weeks; however, persistent infections have been reported. Contagious ecthyma virus is a highly epitheliotropic virus and keratinocytes and their counterparts in the oral mucosa are the most important if not the only cell type to support virus replication. Viral antigen, most abundant in the second and third week postinfection, is seen in regenerating keratinocytes.

In spite of a vigorous and typical anti-viral T-helper type 1 (Th1) immune response, immunity elicited by contagious ecthyma virus is short-lived, and animals can be repeatedly infected, albeit lesions are smaller and resolve sooner than in primary infections. Contagious ecthyma is a zoonotic disease, affecting humans in close contact with infected animals. In general, lesions are solitary and nodular, usually in the hands. Evidence suggests that contagious ecthyma virus occasionally infects camels and wild mammals, including chamois, ibex, musk ox, and the Japanese serow.

Pregnant ewes can be vaccinated using nonattenuated virus derived from crust material collected from sick animals. The vaccines are applied to prescarified skin, which develops a localized lesion. While immunity achieved in this way is short lived, vaccinated animals and their offspring are less prone to develop ecthyma.

Bovine Papular Stomatitis

Bovine papular stomatitis is a mild disease of cattle characterized by the presence of papules, often mildly erosive, on the muzzle, lips, nares, dental pad, palate, tongue, and udder. Lesions can be occasionally seen in the esophagus and forestomach. Histologically, lesions are similar to but less extensive and proliferative than those in contagious ecthyma. The disease occurs worldwide with highest incidence in milking herds and animals less than 1 year old. Similar to contagious ecthyma, reinfection with bovine papular stomatitis virus is commonly observed, suggesting that virus infection does not confer significant immunity. Because its clinical resemblance to foot-and-mouth disease, the disease is reported to veterinary authorities for differential diagnosis. Like other parapoxvirus infections, bovine papular stomatitis is an occupational zoonotic disease.

Pseudocowpox

Pseudocowpox is a frequent enzootic infection of cattle worldwide caused by pseudocowpox virus. Infections by pseudocowpox virus are mild, affecting the teats and udder of milking cows, and occasionally the mucocutaneous transitions around the mouth and muzzle of nursing calves. Typical parapoxvirus lesions develop at these sites. Manual removal or natural falling of crust leaves exposed granulomatous tissue that heals centrifugally forming a characteristic scabby circular ring, a process that takes 1–2 weeks. Chronic infections have been reported. The infection spreads slowly in herds, likely by cross-suckling of calves and mechanical virus transmission by flies. Cattle may become reinfected in subsequent lactations. Electron microscopic examination of scab homogenates shows parapoxvirus particles, thus excluding cowpox and vaccinia virus infections and mechanical injuries. Pseudocowpox can spread from cattle to man by contact, leading to painful nodular lesions, usually in the hands, known as milker's nodules.

Capripoxviruses

The three recognized capripoxviruses, sheeppox virus, goatpox virus, and lumpy skin disease virus, are the causative agents of sheeppox, goatpox, and lumpy skin disease, respectively, arguably the most serious poxviral diseases of production animals. These are systemic diseases affecting domestic ruminants in regions of Asia and Africa. In addition to direct mortality, capripoxvirus diseases are associated with reduced milk production, increased abortion rates, decreased weight gain, and increased susceptibility to secondary bacterial infections. Capripoxvirus diseases can negatively impact on international animal trade, and are on the World Organization for Animal Health list of important animal diseases that need to be notified. Capripoxviruses are not present in the Americas, Southeast Asia, and Australasia. Although Europe has been free of capripoxviruses for decades, outbreaks of sheeppox have been recently reported in Greece.

Virus particles are ovoid, 300 nm × 270 nm in size, and morphologically indistinguishable between the three viruses (Figure 54.1B). Comparison of the genomic DNA sequences of sheeppox, goatpox, and lumpy skin disease viruses has shown that they are closely related viruses. A reflection of this is that infection with any virus induces cross-protection to heterologous capripoxviruses. While lumpy skin disease virus affects only cattle, some strains of sheeppox and goatpox viruses can infect both sheep and goats, with most virus strains causing more severe disease in the homologous host. Sheeppox and goatpox are clinically indistinguishable, and they are described as a single entity.

Sheeppox and Goatpox

Sheeppox and goatpox occur in Africa north of the Equator, southwest and central Asia, and Middle East. The diseases vary from inapparent to severe generalized disease. Factors influencing disease presentation are breed, age, and immune status of the animals, and virus strain. In the most frequent form, acute disease, the incubation time ranges from 6 to 12 days. Fever is the first clinical sign followed by skin rash 2–4 days later. Skin lesions start as erythema that develop into papules of 0.5–1.0 cm in diameter (Figure 54.4A). The skin lesions initially localize to wool-less areas such as the axilla, inner side of the tights, inguinal and perineal regions, and the face, and they tend to become confluent in a few days, especially in the lips, eyelids, and around the nose. Eventually, skin lesions may cover the entire body surface. Coincident with the appearance of papules, animals show excessive salivation, and nasal and conjuctival discharge. As the rectal temperature drops, the superficial lymph nodes become enlarged. If animals survive this stage, papules further develop into scabs, with or without intermediate vesicular and pustular stages. Scabs, which may persist for 6–8 weeks, remain infectious for months after detaching from the skin. Bronchopneumonia is a frequent complication in fatal cases, and is usually associated with a second peak in rectal temperature. Although the virus causes primary nodular lesions in the lungs, it is though that secondary bacterial infection is responsible for bronchopneumonia. Nodular lesions are also observed in the gastrointestinal tract, including the liver, and in the kidneys (Figure 54.4C). Lesions in the upper respiratory tract and oral cavity are short lived, and ulcerate, becoming a significant source of infectious virus (Figure 54.4B). Histologically sheeppox lesions frequently contain cells with a distinctly vacuolated nucleus and marginated chromatin known as sheeppox cells, which represent virus-infected epithelial and phagocytic cells, and perhaps other cell types (Figure 54.4D and E).

FIGURE 54.4. *Sheeppox lesions; lamb. (A) Papules in axillary skin. (B) Hemorrhagic ulcers in the tracheal mucosa. (C) Nodular lesions in the rumen wall. (D) Section of a papular lesion of the skin. Parakeratosis, and hyperplasia and ballooning degeneration of keratinocytes are shown. Keratinocytes with nuclei exhibiting chromatin margination are known as sheeppox cells, which are sites of virus replication (arrows), H&E, X380. (E) Macrophage with a sheeppox cell phenotype in the dermis (arrow) H&E, X400.*

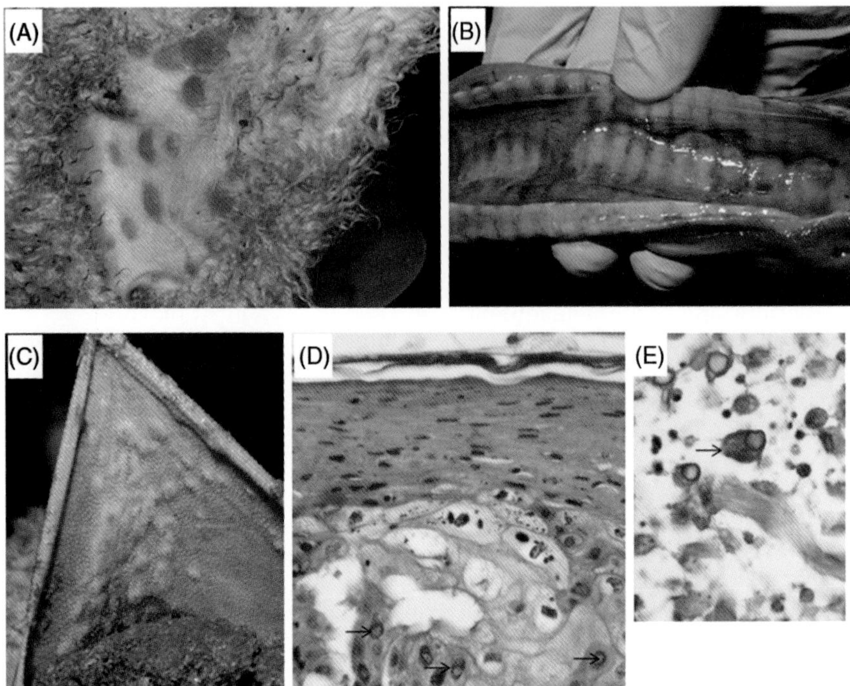

Mortality in young animals can be as high as 50–70%, and case-fatality rates may approach 100%. In adults mortality rates range between 1% and 10%. Sheeppox and goatpox viruses propagate mainly by aerosols, requiring close contact between animals. Experimental infections in sheep and goats suggest that extended excretion of virus in secretions may take place following clinical recovery. Mechanical transmission of virus by insect vectors has been suggested. Interestingly, high concentration of infectious virus in sick animals has been detected even in normal skin between lesions.

In endemic areas, clinical signs and necropsy findings are sufficient for the diagnosis. Several tests have been proposed for laboratory confirmation of sheeppox and goatpox, including ELISA and agar immunodiffusion tests to detect capripoxvirus antigen, polymerase chain reaction (PCR), and real-time PCR. Virus isolation in primary sheep cells (e.g., lamb testis or kidney cells) can be achieved using skin samples or nasal and oral secretions as source of virus. Virus neutralization is the most widely used assay for antibody detection.

Virus strains attenuated by serial passage in cell culture have been successfully used as vaccines, yet vaccine breakdown and short duration of protection have been reported.

Lumpy Skin Disease

Lumpy skin disease occurs in sub-Saharan Africa, although outbreaks have been reported in Egypt and Israel. It is essentially a cattle disease, with morbidity varying from 10% to 85%, and mortality of 1%, although mortality rates over 75% have been recorded. While virus neutralization activity has been occasionally detected in selected wildlife species, there is no decisive support for a role of these species as capripoxvirus reservoirs.

Lumpy skin disease is a subacute to acute generalized disease characterized by extensive cutaneous lesions. Following an incubation period of 4–14 days, fever of 40–41 °C develops, persisting for 1–2 weeks. At this time, animals show depression, salivation, nasal and ocular discharges, and enlarged superficial lymph nodes. Erythematous skin lesions appear in the first or second week after the onset of the disease, rapidly evolving to firm, well-circumscribed nodules of 0.5–5 cm in diameter. The nodules are first seen in the head, neck, and perineum, but they can eventually cover the entire body surface. Some nodules may persist for weeks or even months before becoming hard and dry. Nodules finally detach leaving ulcers that heal in a few weeks if not complicated with secondary bacterial infection.

Transmission of lumpy skin disease between cattle is inefficient. The disease is prevalent in wet seasons when insects are abundant, and wanes with the onset of the dry season. Experimental transmission of the disease to susceptible cattle by the mosquito *Aedes aegypti* has been reported. These observations suggest that biting insect-vectored transmission may be significant in epizootic outbreaks.

Live field strains of lumpy skin disease virus have been attenuated by serial passage in tissue culture or in the chorioallantoic membranes of embryonated hen's eggs and successfully used as vaccines.

Avipoxviruses

Avipoxviruses have been identified as the causative agents of disease in more than 200 bird species, including domestic, pet, and wild birds. They are classified on the basis of host species, disease characteristics, virus growth properties, and antigenicity. The genomes of fowlpox virus, the type member of the genus, and canarypox virus have been sequenced, revealing that avipoxviruses are the most complex poxviruses currently known. A distinctive feature of fowlpox virus is the presence in many field and vaccine strains of a near full-length reticuloendotheliosis provirus integrated into the viral genome (Hertig *et al.* 1997). Reiculoendotheliosis viruses are avian immunosuppressive retroviruses that cause lymphomas in chickens. While the selective advantage of this natural recombination for the viruses is unknown, some speculate that reticuloendotheliosis virus-induced immunosuppression might favor fowlpox virus infection of the host and subsequent transmission.

Fowlpox

Fowlpox is a serious slow-spreading, worldwide disease that affects chickens and turkeys. Transmission is by contact through abrasions in the skin and by biting insects. In its most frequent form, *cutaneous form* or dry fowlpox form, the disease is characterized by proliferative lesions primarily confined to the skin of unfeathered body parts such as eyelids, comb, wattle, legs, feet, and base of the beak. When lesions affect the eyelids, complete closure of the eyes is common (Figure 54.5). Lesions range from small nodules to wart-like masses that evolve to scars before healing. Histologically, the hyperplastic epidermis shows degenerate keratinocytes containing large cytoplasmic eosinophilic (H&E) inclusion bodies known as Bollinger's bodies. In noncomplicated cases, lesions heal in 3 weeks.

While mortality with fowlpox is low, the transient drop in egg production in laying hens and decreased growth rates in young birds may be economically significant. A less common, severe form of the disease known as *diphtheric fowlpox* or wetpox is characterized by caseous plaques or necrotic pseudomembranes firmly attached to the mucosa lining the upper respiratory tract and esophagus. Cutaneous and diphtheric forms may coexist in the same animal. Aerosols have been suggested to play a role in transmission of fowl diphtheria.

Diagnosis of fowlpox is based on clinical signs and histopathology (inclusion bodies). Virus can be isolated by inoculation of lesion material into avian cell cultures for appearance of cytopathic effect, or the chorioallantoic membrane of chicken embryos for development of pock lesions. While most strains induce pock lesions on the membrane by 3–5 days, not all isolates grow well in embryonated eggs. PCR allows for sensitive and specific detection of fowlpox virus DNA sequences as well as distinction between field and vaccine virus strains.

Insect control programs and sanitation of housing are important to reduce the likelihood of fowlpox outbreaks. Attenuated live fowlpox and pigeonpox virus strains are used to protect poultry from fowlpox. The vaccines are usually applied by wing web inoculation, a laborious method for large facilities. Highly attenuated vaccines obtained by serial passage *in vitro* or by recombinant DNA technology exist for inoculation *in ovo*.

FIGURE 54.5. *Fowlpox, cutaneous form. Shown are scab-stage lesions in unfeathered parts of the head, with those in the eyelids completely obliterating the eyes. (Courtesy of Francisco A. Uzal.)*

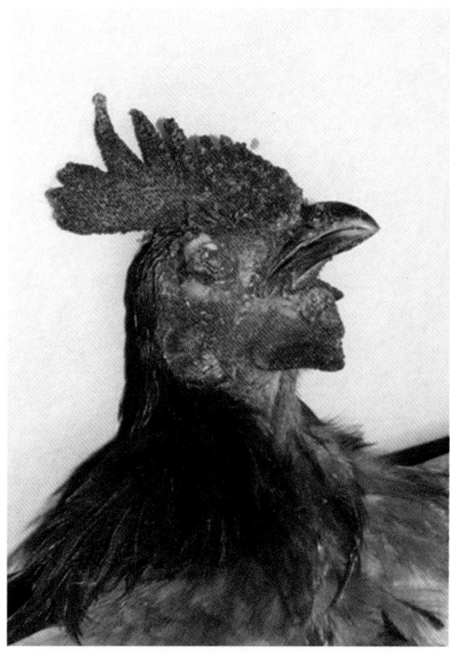

Poxviral Diseases in Other Bird Species

Avipoxviruses infect a variety of wild and caged birds, including penguins, ostriches, canaries, parrots, and sparrows. Disease ranges from cutaneous lesions in the head and feet to severe diphtheric forms. Disease in canaries is usually systemic, with hepatic necrosis and pulmonary nodules, and mortalities that may approach 90%. Vaccination is practiced by some canary breeders. With the exception of canarypox virus, little is known on the biology of causative viruses, strain variability, and their relationship to known avipoxviruses. Chickens are usually used to determine the pathogenicity of new isolates, but many viruses are not pathogenic or are marginally pathogenic in these species (e.g., pigeonpox virus), indicating host-specificity of isolates.

Avipoxviruses as Vaccine Vectors in Veterinary Medicine

As an alternative to conventional vaccines, poxviruses have been engineered to express heterologous genes and used as vaccine vectors. For this purpose, genes encoding immunogenic pathogen proteins are inserted into genomes of attenuated poxviruses and expressed upon infection of vaccine recipients. Avipoxviruses such as fowlpox virus are used as vaccine vectors for avian influenza, Newcastle disease, and infectious laryngotracheitis. The important observation that avipoxvirus can enter mammalian cells and undergo a nonproductive infection (i.e., progeny virus is not produced) led to development of safe avipoxvirus recombinant vaccines for mammals. Licensed canarypoxvirus-vectored vaccines exist for rabies, canine distemper, West Nile virus, feline leukemia virus, and equine influenza virus.

Swinepox

Swinepox, a mild acute disease of swine worldwide, is characterized by typical poxviral lesions of the skin. The disease is caused by swinepox virus, the sole member of the genus *Suipoxvirus* in the family Poxviridae. The virion is morphologically similar to vaccinia virus, exhibiting a brick-like structure approximately 320 × 240 nm in horizontal section.

Swinepox morbidity rates can be as high as 100%, but mortality is generally negligible (<5%). Young animals are the most susceptible, with adults usually developing a mild, self-limiting form of the disease. Multiple cutaneous lesions are commonly found on the flanks, belly, inner side of the legs, ears, and less frequently on the face of affected animals.

Swinepox is usually associated with poor sanitation conditions, which are rarely seen in modern production settings. Swinepox virus is mechanically transmitted by lice (*Haematopinus suis*), which affect the extent and distribution of cutaneous lesions that often occur in less keratinized abdominal and inguinal regions. However, swinepox without evidence of louse involvement has been described, suggesting the role for other insect vectors or the possibility of horizontal transmission. Vertical swinepox virus transmission is indicated by sporadic cases of congenital infection resulting in stillborn fetuses with generalized lesions.

Clinical signs and epidemiology are usually sufficient for swinepox diagnosis. Given that the disease is of relatively low economic impact, no vaccine has been developed. Good animal husbandry including ectoparasite control should be practiced.

Poxviral Infections of Horses

Although frequently reported in the nineteenth and early twentieth centuries, poxviral infections of horses are currently very rare. Several clinical forms of poxviral disease have been described in horses, but only in a few cases has the causative agent been characterized in any way. An orthopoxvirus recovered from Mongolian horses with severe pustular dermatitis and named horsepox was found to be very similar to but distinct from vaccinia virus. Vaccinia virus infections were relatively frequent in horses by the times of the smallpox eradication campaigns. Recently, an outbreak of orthopoxvirus-associated disease has been reported in horses in Brazil. Affected animals exhibited papular lesions around the muzzle and lips that progressed to vesicles and scabs before healing. A condition named *Uasin Gishu*, characterized by papillomatous skin lesions, affects horses in some regions of Africa, and is caused by a virus antigenically related to orthopoxviruses. Viruses morphologically similar to molluscum contagiosum, a poxvirus affecting humans (Table 54.1), have been demonstrated in small persistent lesions affecting the skin of horses.

References

Bhanuprakash V, Prabhu M, Venkatesan G *et al.* (2010) Camelpox: epidemiology, diagnosis and control measures. *Expert Rev Anti-Infective Ther*, **8**, 1187–1201.

Hertig C, Coupar BE, Gould AR, and Boyle DB (1997) Field and vaccine strains of fowlpox virus carry integrated sequences from the avian retrovirus, reticuloendotheliosis virus. *Virology*, **235**, 367–376.

Nollens HH, Gulland FMD, Jacobson ER *et al.* (2006) Parapoxviruses of seals and sea lions make up a distinct subclade within the genus Parapoxvirus. *Virology*, **349**, 316–324.

Further Reading

Babiuk S, Bowden TR, Boyle DB *et al.* (2008) Capripoxviruses: an emerging worldwide threat to sheep, goats, and cattle. *Transbound Emerg Dis*, **55**, 263–272.

Balinsky CA, Delhon G, Smoliga G *et al.* (2008) Rapid preclinical detection of sheeppox virus by a real-time PCR assay. *J Clin Microbiol*, **46**, 438–42

Baxby D and Bennett M (1997) Cowpox; a re-evaluation of the risk of human cowpox based on new epidemiological information. *Arch Virol*, **11**(Suppl), 1–12.

Bennett M, Gaskell CJ, Gaskell RJ *et al.* (1986) Poxvirus infections in the domestic cat: some clinical and epidemiological investigations. *Vet Rec*, **118**, 387–390.

Bennett M, Gaskell CJ, Gaskell RJ *et al.* (1989) Studies on poxvirus infections in cat. *Arch Virol*, **104**, 19–33.

Bera BC, Shanmugasundaram K, Barua S *et al.* (2011) Zoonotic cases of camelpox infection in India. *Vet Microbiol*, **152**, 29–38.

Bhanuprakash V, Indrani BK, Hosamani M, and Singh RH (2006) The current status of sheep pox disease. *Comp Immunol Microbiol Infect Dis*, **29**, 27–60.

Bowden TR, Babiuk SL, Parkyn GR *et al.* (2008) Capripoxvirus tissue tropism and shedding: a quantitative study in experimentally infected sheep and goats. *Virology*, **371**, 380–393.

Boyle DB (2007) Genus *Avipoxvirus*, in *Poxviruses* (eds AA Mercer, A Schmidt and O Weber), Birkhäuser Verlag, Basel-Boston-Berlin, pp. 217–251.

Brum MC, Anjos BL, Nogueira CE *et al.* (2010) An outbreak of orthopoxvirus-associated disease in horses in southern Brazil. *J Vet Diagn Invest*, **22**,143–147.

Carn VM and Kitching RP (1995a) The clinical response of cattle experimentally infected with lumpy skin disease (Neethling) virus. *Arch Virol*, **140**, 503–513.

Carn VM and Kitching RP (1995b) An investigation of possible routes of transmission of lumpy skin disease virus (Neethling). *Epidemiol Infect*, **114**, 219–226.

Chihota CM, Rennie LF, Kitching RP, and Mellor PS (2001) Mechanical transmission of lumpy skin disease virus by *Aedes aegypti* (Diptera: Culicidae). *Epidemiol Infect*, **126**, 317–321.

Davies FG (1991) Lumpy skin disease, an African capripox virus disease of cattle. *Br Vet J*, **147**, 489–503.

de Boer GF (1975) Swinepox, virus isolation, experimental infections and the differentiation from vaccinia infections. *Arch Virol* ,**49**, 141–150.

de la Concha-Bermejillo A, Guo J, Zhang Z, and Waldron D (2003) Severe persistent orf in young goats. *J Vet Diagn Invest*, **15**, 423–431.

Delhon GA, Tulman ER, Afonso CL, and Rock DL (2007) Genus *Suipoxvirus*, in *Poxviruses* (eds AA Mercer A Schmidt and O Weber), Birkhäuser Verlag, Basel-Boston-Berlin, pp. 203–215.

Diallo A and Viljoen GJ (2007) Genus *Capripoxvirus*, in *Poxviruses* (eds AA Mercer A Schmidt and O Weber), Birkhäuser Verlag, Basel-Boston-Berlin, pp. 167–181.

Essbauer S and Meyer H (2007) Genus *Orthopoxvirus*: Cowpox virus, in *Poxviruses* (eds AA Mercer A Schmidt and O Weber), Birkhäuser Verlag, Basel-Boston-Berlin, pp. 75–88.

Essbauer S, Pfeffer M, Meyer H. (2010) Zoonotic poxviruses. *Vet Microbiol*, **140**, 229–236.

Fenner, F (1981) Mousepox (infectious ectromelia): past, present, and future. *Lab Anim Sci*, **31**, 553–559.

Fleming SB and Mercer AA (2007) Genus *Parapoxvirus*, in *Poxviruses* (eds AA Mercer, A Schmidt and O Weber), Birkhäuser Verlag, Basel-Boston-Berlin, pp. 127–165.

Garner MG, Sawarkar SD, Brett EK *et al.* (2000) The extent and impact of sheep pox and goat pox in the state of Maharashtra, India. *Trop Anim Health Prod*, **32**, 205–223.

Griesemer RA and Cole CR (1961) Bovine papular stomatitis. II. The experimentally produced disease. *Am J Vet Res*, **22**, 473–481.

Haenssle HA, Kiessling J, Kempf VA *et al.* (2006) Orthopoxvirus infection transmitted by a domestic cat. *J Am Acad Dermatol*, **54**, S1–4.

Haig DM and Mercer AA (1998) Ovine diseases. Orf. *Vet Res*, **29**, 311–326.

Haig D M and McInnes CJ (2002) Immunity and counter-immunity during infection with the parapoxvirus orf virus. *Virus Res*, **88**, 3–16.

Heine HG Stevens, MP, Foord AJ, and Boyle DB (1999) A capripox virus detection PCR and antibody ELISA based on the major antigen P32, the homolog of the vaccinia virus H3L gene. *J Immunol Methods*, **227**, 187–196.

Hinrichs U, van de Poel PH, and van den Ingh TS (1999) Necrotizing pneumonia in a cat caused by an orthopox virus. *J Comp Pathol*, **121**, 191–196.

Jenkinson, DM, Mc Ewan PE, Moss VA *et al.* (1990) Location and spread of orf virus antigen in infected ovine skin. *Vet Dermatol*, **1**, 189–195.

Jubb TF, Ellis TM, Peet RL, and Parkinson J (1992) Swinepox in pigs in northern Western Australia. *Aust Vet J*, **69**, 99.

Kasza L, Griesemer RA (1962) Experimental swine pox. *Am J Vet Res*, **23**, 443–450.

Knowles DP (2011) Poxviridae, in *Fenner's Veterinary Virology*, 4th edn (eds NJ MacLachlan and EJ Dubovi), Academic Press, pp. 151–165.

Lange L, Marett S, Maree C, and Gerdes T (1991) Molluscum contagiosum in three horses. *J S Afr Vet Assoc*, **62**, 68–71.

Mazur C and Machado RD (1989) Detection of contagious pustular dermatitis virus of goats in a severe outbreak. *Vet Rec*, **125**, 419–420.

Moss B (2007) Poxviridae: the viruses and their replication, in *Fields Virology*, vol. **2**, 5th edn (eds DM Knipe and PM Howley), Williams & Wilkins, Lippincot, pp. 2905–2945.

Munz E and Dumbell K (1994) Horsepox, in *Infectious Diseases of Livestock—with Special Emphasis to Southern Africa*, vol. **1**, (eds JAW Coetzer, GR Thomson and RC Tustin), Oxford University Press, Oxford United Kingdom, pp. 631–632.

Paton DJ, Brown IH, Fitton J, and Wrathall AE (1990) Congenital pig pox: a case report. *Vet Rec*, **127**, 204.

Pfeffer M and Meyer H (2007) Poxvirus diagnosis, in *Poxviruses* (eds AA Mercer, A Schmidt and O Weber), Birkhäuser Verlag, Basel-Boston-Berlin, pp. 355–373.

Rao TVS, Negi BS, and Bansal MP (1997) Development and standardization of a rapid diagnosis test for sheep pox. *Indian J Comp Microbiol, Immunol Infec Dis*, **18**, 47–51.

Silva-Fernandes AT, Travassos CE, Ferreira JM *et al.* (2009) Natural human infections with vaccinia virus during bovine vaccinia outbreaks. *J Clin Virol*, **44**, 308–313.

Singh RK, Hosamani M, Balamurugan V *et al.* (2007) Buffalopox: an emerging and re-emerging zoonosis. *Anim Health Res Rev*, **8**, 105–114.

Tripathy DN (1993) Avipox viruses, in *Virus Infections of Birds* (eds JB McFerran and MS McNulty), Elsevier, London, pp. 5-15.

Tulman ER, Delhon G, Afonso CL *et al.* (2006) Genome of horsepox. *J Virol*, **80**, 9244–9258.

Vikøren T, Lillehaug A, Åkerstedt J *et al.* (2008) A severe outbreak of contagious ecthyma (orf) in a free-ranging musk ox (*Ovibos moschatus*) population in Norway. *Vet Microbiol*, **127**, 10–20.

Weli SC and Tryland M (2011) Avipoxviruses: infection biology and their use as vaccine vectors. *Virol J*, **8**, 49–63.

Picornaviridae

Luis L. Rodriguez and Peter W. Krug

Introduction

The family Picornaviridae comprises 12 genera, with most of them containing members of veterinary importance (Table 55.1). Common characteristics of the family include a genome consisting of single-stranded positive-sense RNA (ssRNA+) and a small nonenveloped icosahedral capsid. Although encompassing some of the smallest viruses, picornaviruses cause some of the largest animal health problems, such as foot-and-mouth disease (FMD), one of the most contagious and economically devastating diseases of livestock. Picornaviruses are characterized by their rapid replication cycle, remarkable stability in the environment, and swift transmission among susceptible hosts. These three general features are the main reasons why some animal picornaviruses are associated with high morbidity and extensive economic losses. This chapter discusses the picornaviruses of veterinary importance from the perspective of general virology, pathogenesis, diagnosis, and control.

Virion Structure, Genome Characteristics, and Replication

Electron micrographs of picornaviruses show icosahedral viral particles with sphere-like morphology and no projections (Figure 55.1). The viral capsid is composed of 60 identical units (protomers), each consisting of three surface proteins 1B, 1C, and 1D or VP3, VP2, and VP1, respectively, and an internal protein 1A or VP4.

Virion physicochemical properties vary among different genera with some members showing instability below pH 7 (e.g., aphthoviruses), and others highly resistant to pH changes (e.g., enteroviruses). All virions are insensitive to organic solvents such as ether and chloroform.

The genome consists of one molecule of ssRNA+, 7.0–8.8 kb in size with a single open reading frame (ORF). A poly(A) tail, of varying length located at the 3′-terminus and a small 2.2–3.9 kDa protein (3B or VPg), is linked covalently to the 5′-terminus. There is a highly structured 5′-untranslated region (UTR) containing signal sequences such as an internal ribosome entry site (IRES) to initiate translation of the viral polyprotein and a clover-leaf "S" fragment essential for viral replication.

Viral Replication

After entry into the cell via interaction of the viral capsid with receptors on the susceptible cell, the viral genome is released into the cytoplasm. The viral genome functions both as mRNA and as a template for genome replication. Protein synthesis initiates through recruitment of cellular ribosomal complexes by the viral IRES. Translation of the single ORF produces a 240–250 kDa polyprotein precursor that is cleaved by viral and host proteases into the viral structural proteins (SPs) derived from the P1 region and the nonstructural proteins (NSPs), derived from the P2 and P3 regions. Viral RNA replication in infected cells is carried out primarily by the viral RNA-dependent RNA polymerase (3Dpol), in conjunction with other viral or cellular proteins. The RNA is transcribed into a negative-strand RNA from which synthesis of the progeny plus-strand RNA is copied in a multistranded replicative intermediate complex. The negative-sense RNA serves as a template for the synthesis of multiple copies of genomic RNA, some of which are translated and others are packaged into viral particles. Due to the lack of proofreading activity of RNA-dependent RNA polymerase (3Dpol), errors are generated at a frequency of 1/10 000 bases incorporated during replication, resulting in every new genome containing at least one mutation. Therefore, the virus population consists of a collection of genetically diverse members (quasi-species) that provide the virus the ability to rapidly respond to selective pressure exerted by host factors (e.g. immune response).

Genus *Aphthovirus*

Foot-and-Mouth Disease Virus

Foot-and-mouth disease virus (FMDV), the type species of the *Aphthovirus* genus, is an antigenically variable virus with 7 serotypes: A, O, C, Asia-1, and South African Territories 1, 2, and 3. Infection with one serotype does not provide cross-protection against other serotypes and sometimes even among multiple subtypes within individual serotypes. Therefore, effective immunization requires a multiple serotype and subtype-specific vaccines. FMDV causes a highly contagious disease (FMD) in domestic and wild cloven-hoofed animals including cattle, buffalo,

Veterinary Microbiology, Third Edition. Edited by D. Scott McVey, Melissa Kennedy and M.M. Chengappa.

Table 55.1. Picornaviridae of Veterinary Significance

Genus	Species with Veterinary Relevance	Associated Major Disease
Aphthovirus	*Foot-and-mouth disease virus*	Vesicular disease, lameness
	Equine rhinitis virus A	Respiratory disease
	Bovine rhinitis virus	Respiratory disease
Erbovirus	*Equine rhinitis virus B*	Respiratory disease
Enterovirus	*Swine vesicular disease virus*	Vesicular disease, CNS disease
	Bovine enterovirus	Enteritis
Sapelovirus	*Porcine sapelovirus*	SMEDI, gastroenteritis, respiratory disease
	Avian sapelovirus	Growth inhibition
Kobuvirus	*Bovine kobuvirus*	Enteritis
Teschovirus	*Porcine teschovirus 1*	Encephalomyelitis, SMEDI
	Porcine teschovirus 2 to *Porcine teschovirus 11*	SMEDI, Talfan disease
Tremovirus	*Avian encephalomyelitis virus*	Encephalomyelitis
Avihepatovirus	*Duck hepatitis A virus*	CNS disease, hepatitis
	Duck hepatitis virus 1 and *Duck hepatitis virus 3*	CNS disease, hepatitis
	Turkey hepatopancreatitis virus	CNS disease, hepatitis
Cardiovirus	*Encephalomyocarditis virus*	Myocarditis
Senecavirus	*Seneca Valley virus*	Not known

CNS, central nervous system; SMEDI, stillbirth, mummification, embryonic death, and infertility.

swine, sheep, goats, and deer. The virus rapidly replicates in the host and readily spreads to susceptible animals by contact and aerosol. The disease is characterized by fever, lameness and vesicular lesions on the tongue, feet, snout, and teats resulting in high morbidity but low mortality in adult animals. However, mortality can be high in younger animals usually due to virus-induced pathology in the heart. FMD is considered the most contagious diseases of animals, and outbreaks require immediate notification by member countries to the World Animal Health Organization (OIE). Outbreaks result in trade bans and restrictions of susceptible animals and their products causing devastating economic consequences to the affected countries.

FMDV is enzootic in many countries and it has occurred in all continents except Antarctica. The disease was eradicated from Europe and North America. Large portions of South America control the disease through vaccination. However, disease outbreaks remain prevalent in endemic "pools" in South America, East, South East, and central Asia, southern Africa, northern Africa, and the Middle East. From these pools the virus makes incursions into FMDV-free countries, for example in Taiwan in 1997, in the United Kingdom in 2001, Japan in 2001 and 2010, and multiple outbreaks in the Republic of Korea in 2010–2011 including an outbreak in 2011 that was the largest in that country's history. Some of these outbreaks were controlled without

FIGURE 55.1. *FMDV purified from infected tissue-cultured cells and negatively stained with 2% phosphotungstic acid (magnification, 300 000×). (Courtesy of T.G. Burrage, Viral, Cellular and Molecular Imaging, Department of Homeland Security, Science and Technology Directorate, Plum Island Animal Disease Center.)*

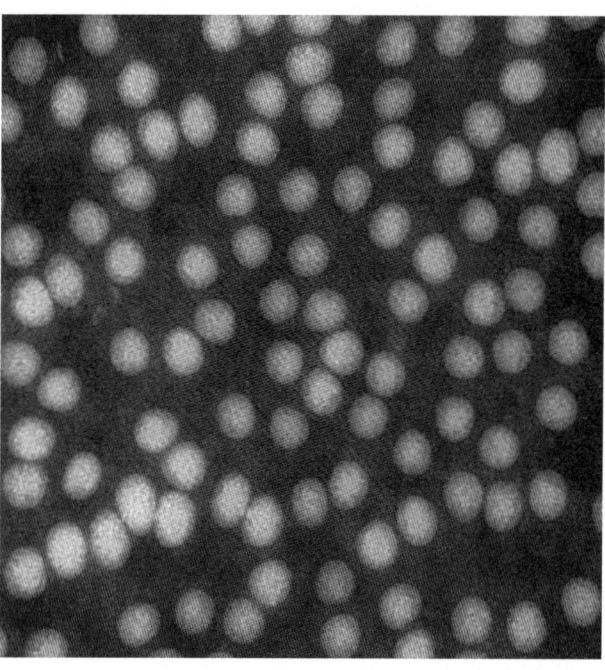

the use of vaccine resulting in the slaughter of millions of animals at a cost of billions of US dollars. Despite this effort, Republic of Korea had to implement general vaccination in order to control the disease.

Pathogenesis

FMDV can be transmitted by direct or indirect contact with infected animals, their secretions, or contaminated food products, and it has been documented that the virus can travel over extensive distances to cause incursions at previously virus-free premises. Natural infection of cattle and sheep with FMDV occurs primarily via the respiratory tract by aerosolized virus, whereas pigs are infected by consumption of virus-contaminated food or through abrasions on the skin or in the mucous membranes while in contact with infected animals or their secretions. Recent studies demonstrated that subsequent to exposure to infectious aerosols, the primary site of viral replication was in epithelial cells of the nasopharynx, followed by infection of pulmonary epithelium and onset of viremia. Viremia results in dissemination throughout the body; but high-titer viral replication only occurs at lesion predilection sites including the interdigital epithelia, coronary bands of the hooves, the oral cavity, and less frequently the myocardium. The specific factors determining tropism and high-titer replication at the lesion sites remain undetermined. Following the acute phase, up to 50% of FMDV-infected ruminants, whether vaccinated or naïve animals, become chronic, asymptomatic carriers of the virus. Carrier animals are those from which the live virus can be isolated 28 days postinfection. The role of carrier animals in the epidemiology, ecology, and long-term maintenance of FMDV in animal populations remains unclear. But in domestic cattle and African buffalo, the carrier state can last as long as 3.5–5.0 years, and there are some reports documenting transmission to cattle from African buffalo carriers.

Molecular Pathogenesis

FMDV enters cells via specific cellular receptors (integrins αvβ1, αvβ3, αvβ6, and αvβ8). *In vitro*, FMDV binds to cellular integrins via a highly conserved RGD (arginine, glycine, aspartic acid) sequence located on the G-H loop of capsid protein VP1. Studies in animals suggest that the integrin αvβ6 is the major viral receptor since it is expressed constitutively at high levels on the surface of epithelial cells in tissues susceptible to FMDV, and it is also expressed on the surface of FMDV-infected epithelial cells. Upon binding to cells, virus entry occurs by clathrin-dependent endocytosis followed by acidification of endosomes leading to capsid disruption and release of viral RNA.

Following uncoating and release of viral RNA into the cytoplasm, translation initiates internally in a cap-independent mechanism at the IRES located approximately 1500 bases downstream from the 5′ end of the genome. Two functional in-frame initiation codons (AUG), are present but translation, initiates mainly from the second AUG, resulting in a single polyprotein that is processed by viral-encoded proteinases L^{pro} and $3C^{pro}$ and protein 2A to yield SPs and NSPs. Four SPs form the capsid (Vp1–Vp4) and ten NSPs are necessary for viral replication and encapsidation. Once translated and processed, some NSPs interact with cellular factors to enhance viral replication. Viral proteins have diverse functions; for example, the RNA elongation polymerase activity is contained in 3D, 2C is an ATPase containing a nucleotide-binding sequence motif, and 2B is essential in the association to cellular membranes and formation of replication complexes. Protein VPg (3B in aphthoviruses) acts as a transcription primer after being uridylated to form VPgpUpUOH by a *cis*-acting replication element in the viral genome and the viral 3D polymerase.

Viral RNA replication in infected cells is carried out primarily by the viral RNA-dependent RNA polymerase (3Dpol), in conjunction with other viral or cellular proteins. Virus assembly starts with the formation of a virus particle containing three surface proteins, VP1–VP3, and an internal protein, VP4. The final steps in infectious virus formation are the maturation cleavage of VP4 and VP2 (from VP0) and the encapsidation of plus-strand viral RNA.

Viral Interference with the Host Immune Response

FMDV has evolved a variety of strategies to interfere with the host response (defense) to viral infection. The leader protein (L^{pro}), in addition to cleaving the viral polyprotein, also cleaves elongation factor eIF4G, which is involved in mRNA cap recognition by the ribosome to initiate protein translation. This cleavage effectively prevents cap-mediated translation of host mRNA. However, viral RNA translation continues mediated by the IRES signal in the viral 5′-UTR. In addition to this general mechanism of interfering with host protein translation, L^{pro} causes specific interference with the host innate response by translocating to the nucleus during viral infection and interfering with the signaling of the interferon response by the degradation of NF-κB, which regulates interferon-β transcription.

Infection of swine with FMDV results in a transient lymphopenia during the acute phase of infection, which correlates with viremia and T cell dysfunction but is resolved early after infection. Another effect on innate response by FMDV infection in swine is the decreased production of interferon-α by various types of dendritic cells during the acute phase. This viral-induced immunopathology results in a reduced and delayed innate response. There might be other effects on the porcine cellular immune responses including the decreased function of natural killer cells. Even though innate responses are inhibited, a solid antibody response develops quickly, within 4–6 days of infection, which is protective against reinfection by antigenically related strains of FMDV within the same serotype.

Another mechanism of interference with the host immune response used by FMDV is degradation of major histocompatibility complex class I molecules, thereby impairing the cytotoxic T cell response. In summary, FMDV infection has dramatic effects at the molecular, cellular, and host response levels, some of which as not yet fully understood. Understanding these viral mechanisms of pathogenesis will aid in the development of more effective vaccines and antiviral and biotherapeutic strategies against this devastating disease.

Control and Recovery

Approaches to control FMD vary dramatically from country to country, and depend primarily on the disease status (endemic vs. free), international commerce of animals and animal products, and political situation. The Food and Agriculture Organization has identified guidelines with stages for countries to follow in the progressive control program of FMD (for details visit http://www.fao.org/ag/againfo/commissions/en/eufmd/pcp.html, accessed January 25, 2013). Stage 0 countries do not monitor or control FMD, and countries at stages 1–3 include various levels of monitoring and control strategies including vaccination that result in no circulation of virus (stage 4), while countries at stage 5 maintain no disease circulation in the absence of vaccination (i.e., free without vaccination). Outbreak response in countries in stages 2–3 might involve some level of animal movement control and targeted vaccination and in some cases slaughter of animals in affected premises. Outbreak response in countries free with vaccination might involve some animal slaughter and revaccination of at-risk animal populations. In FMD-free countries without vaccination, the main response is usually stamping-out with minimal use of vaccination. This has had devastating consequences with millions of animals destroyed at a very high cost not only economically but also socially and morally as far as animal welfare is concerned. In some cases, stamping-out efforts have not been successful and countries have had to establish long-term mass vaccination campaigns in order to control the disease (e.g., Argentina and Uruguay in 2001 and Republic of Korea in 2011).

Vaccination

FMD vaccines have been available for decades and represent the largest share of the veterinary vaccine market worldwide in terms of sales. Commercial vaccines consist of killed whole-virus antigen preparations. Due to the high variability of FMDV serotypes and subtypes, the antigen composition of FMD vaccines is tailored for specific world regions and in many cases to specific countries or regions within. The use of vaccine in FMD-endemic regions requires an in-depth investigation of the epidemiology of disease, vaccine matching studies to determine whether the selected vaccine will be effective against the strain(s) circulating in the target area. Some FMD-free countries have established vaccine antigen banks to strategically store a number of viral serotypes and strains that would be used to control an outbreak at least during the early stages. Strain selection for these vaccine banks is based on risk analysis and must be regularly updated to ensure that emerging FMDV strains are well covered.

Commercial inactivated FMD vaccines are usually formulated as either regular potency for routine control in endemic settings or high-potency vaccines containing higher antigen payload for emergency use in nonendemic regions. These vaccines are effective in preventing clinical signs of disease and viral shedding and have been effectively used in eradication programs in various parts of the world. However, they have some shortcomings, such as the fact that manufacturing requires the use of live virus, which poses a risk of escape from manufacturing facilities. Another problem is duration of immunity, requiring multiple semiannual vaccinations in order to maintain protective immunity levels. Additional issues include the narrow antigenic coverage and the instability of the finished vaccines particularly those of the O serotypes. Potency is a major concern with FMD vaccines. The latest revision of OIE's *Manual of Diagnostic Tests and Vaccines for Terrestrial Animals* states that six protective doses (PD_{50}) for cattle are preferred. In FMD-free countries where specific vaccines to the outbreak-causing strain are not always available, higher potency vaccines are preferred since they confer greater protection against heterologous strains, quicker onset of immunity, and increased protection from viral shedding and transmission.

One of the important features of FMDV vaccines is the ability to differentiate infected from vaccinated animals (DIVA). For this purpose, it is very important that during vaccine manufacturing all nonstructural viral proteins (NSP) are removed from the vaccine, thus allowing testing for antibodies for these proteins that would be present only in infected and not in vaccinated animals. Only high-quality FMD vaccines devoid of NSP enable the differentiation of infected animals from vaccinated animals.

On-farm Control and Disinfection

In the recovery phase after an FMD outbreak it is necessary to disinfect the affected premises. FMDV is an acid-labile virus and begins to dissociate into pentamers at pH below 6.5 or over 7.5. This allows the use of acidic and basic disinfectants such as citric acid and sodium hypochlorite (bleach). Recent studies have shown that FMDV is readily inactivated by sodium hypochlorite (1000 ppm), citric acid (1%), and sodium carbonate (4%) when dried on non-porous surfaces. However, when disinfection was tested on a porous surface (wood), citric acid (2%) was more effective in virus inactivation than sodium hypochlorite even when tested at 2500 ppm. Based on these studies, chemicals containing very low pH are preferred for FMDV disinfection.

Other Members of Genus *Aphthovirus*

The dissolution of the *Rhinovirus* genus was the result of sequence analysis comparing human rhinoviruses with viruses causing bovine and equine rhinitis. These viruses—bovine rhinitis virus A-1, bovine rhinitis virus A-2, bovine rhinitis virus B, and equine rhinitis virus A (formally bovine rhinovirus types 1, 3, and 2 and equine rhinovirus type 1, respectively)—have been added to the *Aphthovirus* genus based on genomic organization and sequence similarity to FMDV. Specifically, the molecular evidence includes both genetic structural motif commonalities, substantial amino acid identity as well as the presence of a functional L^{pro} (only found in aphthoviruses and erboviruses). Bovine rhinitis viruses are thought to cause only minor respiratory disease since they have been isolated from both healthy and symptomatic cattle. Experimental infection with these agents results in mild disease or asymptomatic infection in the natural host. The detection of widespread preexisting antibodies in cattle populations suggests that these viruses often move unnoticed among susceptible hosts. The lack of serious disease associated with the rhinitis-causing aphthoviruses in cattle has limited the need for any control measures. Conversely, the equine rhinitis virus A (ERVA) has been associated with severe respiratory disease outbreaks in horses, with high fever and viremia. The virus can be isolated from feces. In addition, there is serological evidence for human infection by ERVA among workers with close contact to horses.

Genus *Erbovirus*

The genus *Erbovirus* includes equine rhinitis virus B (ERVB) types 1 and 2. These viruses were previously classified under the genus *Rhinovirus*. Erboviruses are distinct from other rhinitis viruses for their acid stability. ERVB types 1 and 2, formerly designated equine rhinitis virus types 2 and 3, respectively, are associated with upper respiratory disease and fever in horses similar to ERVA. The virus is shed from nasopharyngeal tissues, in some cases for a month after symptoms have resolved. It is thought there may be significant subclinical infection with ERVB and even in clinical infections the virus does not establish viremia in infected horses.

Genus *Enterovirus*

The enteroviruses are a large group of acid-resistant picornaviruses that mainly cause mild gastrointestinal disease or can be asymptomatic. They are transmitted via fomites, contaminated food products, fecal-oral routes, or direct contact and have wide distribution among cattle and swine populations. Because there tend to be multiple serotypes of each virus, there is little attempt to control these viruses in a veterinary setting.

A notable exception to this is swine vesicular disease virus (SVDV). This virus, once epidemic worldwide, is mostly limited to occasional outbreaks in Europe. Genetic evidence suggests that SVDV may be a porcine variant of human coxsackievirus B5. It is transmitted via fecal–oral and respiratory routes and may have a carrier state. The most important feature of infection with this virus is that its clinical features in swine resemble FMDV, vesicular stomatitis virus (VSV), and viral exanthema of swine virus (VESV). The vesicles on the feet and mouth are indistinguishable between those caused by these other viruses. Besides vesicles, other symptoms include fever, lameness, and loss of appetite. While mortality is low, there are severe symptoms in young animals associated with high morbidity. In these cases, there are signs of neurological involvement such as ataxia and chorea. A rapid differential diagnosis to FMDV, VSV, and VESV is required because these agents are reportable. SVDV diagnosis is done by virus isolation, antigen enzyme-linked immunosorbent assay (ELISA), or real-time polymerase chain reaction (RT-PCR). Serological tests are only useful for surveillance and are performed by virus neutralization or ELISA.

Genus Sapelovirus

The genus *Sapelovirus* (simian, avian, porcine entero-like viruses) consists of new and reassigned viruses with genetic similarity outside the clades of other picornavirus genera. Reassigned viruses include duck picornavirus, now avian sapelovirus, and porcine enterovirus A, now porcine sapelovirus. Newly discovered viruses are classified as new sapeloviruses by sequence similarity, for example, sea lion sapelovirus types 1 and 2. Porcine sapelovirus has been isolated from swine with respiratory disease and gastroenteritis, and it causes the same symptoms in experimentally infected naïve pigs. Porcine sapelovirus has been isolated from postmortem respiratory tissue of fetal piglets in utero with the syndrome known as stillbirth, mummification, embryonic death, and infertility (SMEDI). The symptoms are comparable to those caused by porcine parvovirus, the most common cause of SMEDI. Porcine sapelovirus has also been associated with cases of idiopathic vesicular disease, which is a differential diagnosis for FMD in swine.

Genus *Kobuvirus*

Kobuvirus is another genus organized by genomic similarity, members of which are found in human, bovine, and porcine hosts. These viruses are associated with gastroenteritis and have been shown to cause viremia in pigs. Bovine kobuvirus exhibits widespread prevalence in cattle feces. Transmission is thought to be fecal–oral based on studies on Aichi virus of humans. High levels of specific antibodies are found in the serum of unaffected animals. Isolates of putative kobu-like viruses have been detected in bat and sheep feces based on the phylogenetic analysis of partial genomes.

Genus *Teschovirus*

Porcine teschovirus (PTV) infection is limited to swine hosts. There are 11 serotypes but only serotype 1 (PTV-1) causes severe disease in adult pigs, known as Teschen disease or teschovirus encephalomyelitis. The virus has worldwide distribution, as encephalomyelitis has been reported in Eastern Europe and Africa over the last two decades, with a recent outbreak in Haiti (discussed later). Like all picornaviruses, PTV is very stable in the environment; it is often introduced into swine populations through incompletely heat-treated swill or other food products. The virus enters the host by ingestion, replicates in the gastrointestinal tract, and is shed in the feces. Most infections with serotypes other than PTV-1 result in subclinical disease except in very young piglets of naïve sows, which can sometimes display signs of neurological disease, but little mortality. Usually virus access to the central nervous system (CNS) is limited by circulating maternal antibodies, and the young pigs generate specific immunity subsequent to weaning. Mild pathogenesis is often referred to as Talfan disease. PTV serotype 1, 3, and 6 infections have been associated with SMEDI.

On the other hand, teschovirus encephalomyelitis affects swine of all ages and has up to a 90% mortality rate. Symptoms include fever, anorexia, depression, muscle tremors, encephalitis, and limb paralysis. Death can occur due to paralysis of the respiratory muscles as soon as 1 week after the onset of symptoms. As the virus invades the CNS, histopathological lesions are found in the brain, spinal ganglia, and cranial nerves. Because of the CNS involvement, differential diagnoses include pseudorabies virus, Japanese encephalitis virus, rabies virus, and porcine respiratory and reproductive syndrome virus. PTV is confirmed by virus isolation and the serotype determined by serological analysis, but since the antibody is widespread, cases of encephalomyelitis must be confirmed by virus isolation or histopathology of brain and spinal cord. There is no treatment for affected animals; in the past PTV vaccines have been available; however, they are no longer in use. Control is mediated by quarantine and disinfection.

A rapidly spreading outbreak of PTV-1 was reported in 2009 in Haiti, causing severe disease and devastating the pork economy already reeling from endemic classical swine fever. By 2010 the virus was found in almost all areas of the country and new cases were still developing in early 2011. Up to one-third of all swine in the country were affected and 25% mortality was observed in infected animals. Haiti's long eastern border with the Dominican Republic puts that country's swine population at high transmission risk.

In another recent report, a retrospective analysis of samples from 2002 suggested that PTV-1 caused swine polioencephalomyelitis on many farms in western Canada. While less than 1% of swine were affected on each farm, most animals exhibiting symptoms were euthanized prior to death. Infected survivors had lingering neurological impairments. The significance of this report is difficult to assess since there was no mention of possible sources of the virus and there was no evidence of spread beyond the initially affected sites.

Genus *Tremovirus*

The genus *Tremovirus*, whose sole member is avian encephalomyelitis virus (AEV), is the etiological agent of epidemic tremor disease in chickens. This virus can also affect a wide range of other avian hosts, including partridge, turkey, quail, guinea fowl, and pheasants. Originally detected in the New England region of the United States in the 1930s, AEV has a worldwide distribution, causing a range of symptoms from decreased egg production to neurological disease in young chicks less than 3 weeks of age. Neurological signs include tremors, ataxia, weakness, wing drooping, and paralysis. Mortality can be as high as 25% with extensive morbidity. Chicks will sit and fall over due to paralysis, and the survivors often recover with associated blindness. Hens have a 2-week temporary reduction in egg production. The virus is spread by the fecal–oral route. The virus replicates in epithelial cells of the digestive tract and is shed in feces 3 days after infection and can shed for up to 2 weeks. In young chicks, the virus establishes a viremia, spreading to the CNS and other organs. Diagnosis is made by histopathology of brain lesions or by virus isolation on embryonated eggs; antibodies only indicate prior exposure to disease. While there is no treatment for animals infected with AEV, there is a live attenuated vaccine that can be given as an eye drop or added to the drinking water.

Genus *Avihepatovirus*

Another genus born of consolidation is *Avihepatovirus*, consisting of the duck hepatitis A virus (DHAV), previously classified as an enterovirus. DHAV has worldwide distribution, a significant cause of high mortality in ducklings. DHAV has almost 100% mortality rate in ducklings aged less than 1 week; the mortality drops to less than 50% by 3 weeks of age. The clinical signs include paralysis, opisthotonus, paresis, enophthalmos, and sudden death. Clinical specimens show enlarged kidney, spleen, and liver, with the latter having massive hemorrhage and necrosis and a green color. The virus is diagnosed by inoculating embryonated duck and chicken eggs with liver homogenates or immunofluorescence of tissue sections. There is no treatment for this disease; while there is a vaccine available to help prevent spread, the best course of control for DHAV is to restrict contact of ducklings with adults until after the fourth week of life.

Related to the duck hepatitis A virus is the as-of-yet unclassified turkey hepatopancreatitis virus, the cause of turkey viral hepatitis. It is found mostly in North America and Europe, affecting young turkeys under the age of 6 weeks. It is transmitted via the fecal–oral route. Clinical signs include weight loss, anorexia, and sudden death, with neurological signs seen in some cases. Adults are mostly asymptomatic with a temporary drop in egg production. The virus can be isolated by inoculating embryonated chicken eggs with tissue homogenates of liver, pancreas, spleen, or kidney. Histopathological observations include multifocal necrosis manifested as depressed gray lesions on the pancreas and liver. Fatal cases demonstrate massive hemorrhage in both liver and pancreas with vacuolation and monocyte infiltration, as well as pooled blood in the organs.

Genus *Cardiovirus*

Encephalomyocarditis virus (EMCV), the type species for the cardioviruses, is a virus of rodents that is transmissible to farm animals as well as humans. Outbreaks of EMCV have also caused mortality in baboon colonies associated to wild rodent infestation of their cages. It is primarily a disease associated with unsanitary conditions as infection of animals, especially swine, is derived from contact with rodent feces. The virus replicates in the alimentary tract and establishes a viremia, providing access to the target organ, the heart. This disease manifests mostly as morbidity and mortality seen in young animals, but transplacental transmission can also occur, causing stillbirths. Young piglets die suddenly after primary symptoms of high fever, difficulty breathing, and a hallmark blue skin discoloration. Histopathological observations include edema in the lungs and abdomen as well as an enlarged liver. The heart becomes soft and pale with evident necrosis. Animals that survive infection have fibrosis. There is no treatment for infected animals; control is based on seclusion and disinfection of premises. An inactivated antigen vaccine is commercially available. Also, experimental inoculation with live Mengo virus (another cardiovirus of no veterinary relevance) can protect baboons, macaques, and swine against challenge with a lethal strain of EMCV.

Genus *Senecavirus*

Seneca Valley virus is the sole member of the newly created *Senecavirus* genus. The origin of this virus is unclear as it was originally discovered as a contaminant in cell culture. Virtually identical viruses were isolated during a retrospective analysis of swine clinical samples, and serological evidence suggests infection of swine, cattle, and wild mice. The lack of a disease association makes its relevance to veterinary virology unknown. However, there have been multiple cases of swine vesicular disease in the United States in which the only agent detected was SVV, confounding the diagnosis with other vesicular diseases such as FMD. Experimental infection of pigs with an SVV strain resulted in replication and spread to uninfected animals, with no associated signs of disease on the inoculated or contact-exposed animals. Interestingly, SVV is purported for use as an oncolytic therapeutic since the virus seems to be selective for replication in human cancer cells.

Further Reading

Diaz-Mendez AL, Viel J, Hewson P *et al.* (2010) Surveillance of equine respiratory viruses in Ontario. *Can J Vet Res*, **74**, 271–278.

Dynon KWD, Ficorilli BN, Hartley CA, and Studdert MJ (2007) Detection of viruses in nasal swab samples from horses with acute, febrile, respiratory disease using virus isolation, polymerase chain reaction and serology. *Aust Vet J*, **85**, 46–50.

Grubman MJ and Baxt B (2004) Foot-and-mouth disease. *Clin Microbiol Rev*, **17**, 465–493.

Honkavuori KS, Shivaprasad HL, Briese T *et al.* (2011) Novel picornavirus in Turkey poults with hepatitis, California, USA. *Emerg Infect Dis*, **17**, 480–487.

Lin F and Kitching RP (2000) Swine vesicular disease: an overview. *Vet J*, **160**, 192–201.

Lin JY, Chen TC, Weng KF *et al.* (2009) Viral and host proteins involved in the picornavirus life cycle. *J Biomed Sci*, **16**, 103.

Pogranichniy RM, Janke BH, Gillespie TG, and Yoon KJ (2003) A prolonged outbreak of polioencephalomyelitis due to infection with a group I porcine enterovirus. *J Vet Diagn Invest*, **15**, 191–194.

Reuter G, Boros A, and Pankovics P (2011) Kobuviruses—a comprehensive review. *Rev Med Virol*, **21**, 32–41.

Rodriguez LL and Gay CG (2011) Development of vaccines toward the global control and eradication of foot-and-mouth disease. *Expert Rev Vaccines*, **10**, 377–387.

Shan T, Li L, Simmonds P *et al.* (2011) The fecal virome of pigs on a high-density farm. *J Virol*, **85**, 11697–11708.

Tannock GA and Shafren DR (1994) Avian encephalomyelitis: a review. *Avian Pathol*, **23**, 603–620.

Tseng CH and Tsai HJ (2007) Sequence analysis of a duck picornavirus isolate indicates that it together with porcine enterovirus type 8 and simian picornavirus type 2 should be assigned to a new picornavirus genus. *Virus Res*, **129**, 104–114.

Yamada M, Kozakura R, Nakamura K *et al.* (2009) Pathological changes in pigs experimentally infected with porcine teschovirus. *J Comp Pathol*, **141**, 223–228.

Caliciviridae

Melissa Kennedy

Caliciviruses are small (27–40 nm in diameter), nonenveloped, icosahedral viruses with a genome of single-stranded, positive-sense RNA. The viral RNA serves as mRNA and is infectious. The name calicivirus is derived from the chalice-shaped spheres on the surface of negatively stained viral particles. There are four distinct groups in the family: *Lagovirus*, Norwalk-like virus, Sapporo-like virus, and *Vesivirus*. Hepatitis E virus, which had initially been classified in the family Caliciviridae, has been reclassified as a *Hepevirus* in the family Hepeviridae. Several members of Caliciviridae—specifically vesicular exanthema of swine virus, San Miguel sea lion virus, feline calicivirus (FCV), European brown hare syndrome, and rabbit hemorrhagic disease viruses—are important animal pathogens.

General Properties

The genome of caliciviruses has only two or three open reading frames. Virions are comprised of a single major capsid protein. The nonstructural proteins of caliciviruses share features with those of picornaviruses. Replication of caliciviruses occurs in the cytoplasm, although both cytoplasmic and intranuclear inclusions occur in infected cells.

Vesiviruses

Vesicular exanthema virus and FCV are classified together in the genus *Vesivirus*. Viruses within this genus are readily propagated in cell culture, in distinct contrast to caliciviruses in the other genera.

Vesicular Exanthema of Swine

Disease

Vesicular exanthema of swine (VES) is an acute viral disease characterized by the formation of vesicles in the oral cavity, interdigital spaces, and coronary band of the foot. VES is clinically indistinguishable from foot-and-mouth disease (FMD), swine vesicular disease, and vesicular stomatitis. The incubation period of the disease is approximately 24–72 h and the course is about 1–2 weeks. The disease has a high morbidity but a low mortality. It is of some economic importance as a disease in pigs; however, its main impact is that it mimics FMD, from which it must be distinguished. The last occurrence of this disease occurred in the United States in 1956. Subsequently, the US Department of Agriculture in 1959 declared VES an exotic disease; however, viruses capable of causing VES are endemic in marine mammals, where they also cause vesicular diseases and reproductive failure. A wide variety of seals, sea lions, walrus, and dolphins are infected with these viruses. Outbreaks of VES occur when these marine mammal caliciviruses spread to swine, likely as a result of feeding of dead marine mammals to swine.

Etiologic Agent

Physical, Chemical, and Antigenic Properties. Vesicular exanthema of swine virus (VESV) is a typical calicivirus, and viral particles are associated with cytoplasmic cisternae in infected swine cells (Figure 56.1) and in crystalline arrays in the cytoplasm (Figure 56.2). VESV is stable at low pH (pH 5). A large number of antigenically distinct types of VESV have been identified (at least 13), and a number of antigenically distinct viruses that originally were isolated from species other than swine are capable of causing VES and so are classified as VESV, including bovine calicivirus, cetacean calicivirus, primate calicivirus, and a number of so-called San Miguel sea lion viruses (17 types). Similar viruses have been isolated from fish, birds, reptiles, and other mammals, including skunks. These viruses are distinguished by serological tests, usually serum neutralization, and the virulence of these viruses to pigs varies significantly.

Resistance to Physical and Chemical Agents. VESV can persist in the environment and in contaminated meat products for very long periods. The virus is completely inactivated by 2% sodium hydroxide or 0.1% sodium hypochlorite.

Infectivity for Other Species or Culture Systems. Naturally occurring VES disease is confined only to swine of all ages and breeds. Experimentally, VESV causes vesicles at inoculated sites in seals. Vesicles are also produced at

Veterinary Microbiology, Third Edition. Edited by D. Scott McVey, Melissa Kennedy and M.M. Chengappa.

FIGURE 56.1. *Parallel rows of VESV particles in cytoplasmic cisternae (72 000×). (Reproduced with permission from Zee* et al. *1968.)*

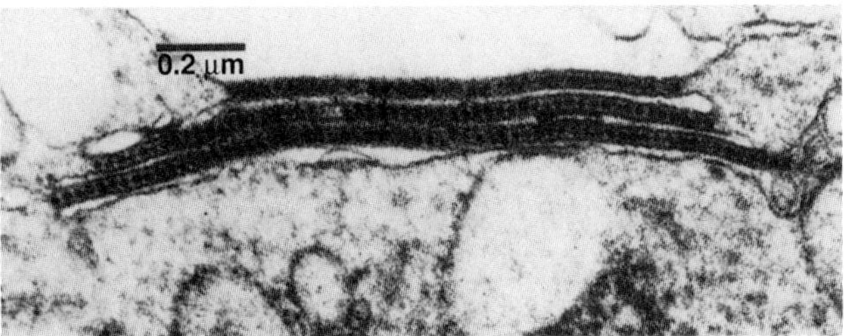

the sites of inoculation in horses and hamsters. The virus is isolated in low titers from some sites of inoculation and draining lymph nodes. VESV can be propagated in cell lines of swine kidney or Vero monkey kidney.

Host–Virus Relationship

Distribution, Reservoir, and Transmission. VES was first described in North America (California) in 1932, and outbreaks were reported every year in California between 1932 and 1951 (with the exception of 1937–1938). The disease first appeared outside of California in 1951, and from 1952 to 1953 it spread to a total of 42 states in the United States. The disease had never been reported elsewhere in the world except Iceland and Hawaii, and these two incidents resulted from shipping contaminated pork products from California.

FIGURE 56.2. *Section of a viral crystal in VESV-infected cells (64 000×). (Reproduced with permission from Zee* et al. *1968.)*

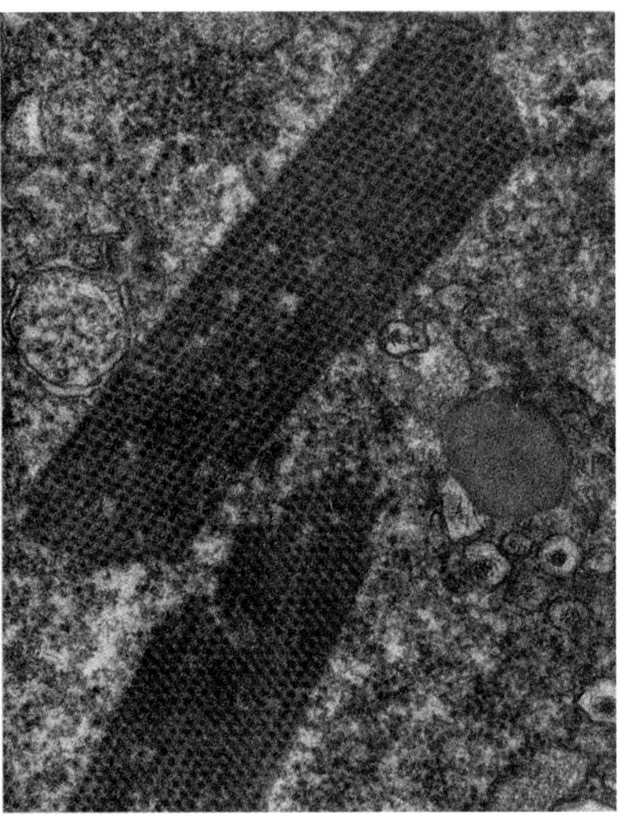

Marine mammals serve as reservoirs for VESV infection. A calicivirus was first isolated in 1972 from sea lions on San Miguel Island off the coast of southern California. This calicivirus was named San Miguel sea lion virus (SMSV), which was indistinguishable from VESV by morphological, biophysical, and biochemical criteria. Experimental SMSV infection of swine produces a disease indistinguishable from VES. SMSV has also been isolated from asymptomatic domestic swine. Serum-neutralizing antibodies to several serotypes of SMSV and VESV have been demonstrated in marine mammals and both wild and domestic swine in California. Earlier epidemiologic studies during the outbreaks of VES confirmed the relationship between feeding of raw garbage and outbreaks of the disease, and dead sea lions are known to have been utilized as a food source for swine.

Although outbreaks of VES likely originated from feeding SMSV-infected marine animal parts to swine, the infection subsequently spread rapidly within affected herds by direct contact.

Pathogenesis and Pathology. VES is characterized by the appearance of fluid-filled vesicles on the snout, coronary band, and tongue of infected swine. These same lesions develop in swine that are inoculated intradermally with either VESV or SMSV. Infected animals are febrile, and the virus is present in blood and nasal–oral secretions for several days after infection. Vesicles appear on the coronary band and interdigital space of the feet at 3–4 days after infection. The vesicles rapidly rupture and healing takes place unless complicated by secondary bacterial infection. High titers of viruses are present within the fluid in vesicles, which may also contaminate the environment. Mild encephalitis occurs in some swine infected with VESV, and the virus may also be recovered from brain tissue of swine infected with SMSV.

Host Response to Infection. Neutralizing antibodies to VESV and SMSV appear in the sera of animals infected with viruses soon after inoculation and titers peak within 7–10 days after infection.

Laboratory Diagnosis

VES must rapidly be differentiated from other vesicular diseases of swine, such as FMD, swine vesicular disease, and vesicular stomatitis. Laboratory diagnosis is accomplished by virus isolation in cell cultures, direct electron microscopic examination of vesicle fluid, or polymerase chain reaction (PCR). Although the vesicular diseases all produce similar signs in swine, there are major differences: whereas VES and swine vesicular disease are almost exclusively diseases of swine, vesicular stomatitis frequently affects horses as well as ruminants, and FMD also affects ruminants (Table 56.1).

Table 56.1. Susceptibility of Domestic Animals to Four Viruses That Cause Vesicles in Swine

Animal Species	SVD	VES	FMD	VSV
Cattle	–	–	++	++
Swine	++	++	++	+
Sheep	–	–	+	–[a]
Horse	–	–[a]	–	++
Guinea pig	–	–[a]	+	+
Suckling mice	+	–	+	+
Humans	+	–	–[a]	+

[a]Occasional lesions produced by specific virus strains; SVD, Swine vesicular disease; VES, Vesicular exanthema of swine; FMD, Foot-and-mouth disease; VS, Vesicular stomatitis.

Treatment and Control

There is no treatment for VES and there are no vaccines for control of the disease. It is now considered to be eradicated in the United States. Enforcement of laws requiring cooking of garbage before feeding it to swine was the most important factor in eliminating the disease.

Feline Calicivirus

Disease

FCV infects the oral cavity and upper respiratory tracts of cats to produce fever, sneezing, and nasal and ocular discharges. Clinical signs include rhinitis, conjunctivitis, oral ulcerations, and, in severe cases, pneumonia. Joint or muscle soreness, hyperesthesia, and chronic oral ulceration have also been attributed to FCV infection, and a disseminated highly virulent and fatal systemic disease associated with specific strains of FCV has recently been described. The incubation period of the disease is 2–3 days and infected cats usually recover in 7–10 days in the absence of secondary bacterial infections. Virulent systemic FCV infection is characterized by alopecia, cutaneous ulcers, subcutaneous edema, and high mortality.

Etiologic Agent

Physical, Chemical, and Antigenic Properties. FCV is classified into a single serotype, but there are multiple strains of FCV that vary in antigenicity, which impacts vaccine efficacy. The virulence of individual strains varies substantially as well, and is independent of antigenicity; that is, viruses that cause similar clinical syndromes are not necessarily as similar in antigenicity.

Resistance to Physical and Chemical Agents. FCV is resistant to many common disinfectants. It is readily inactivated by a 0.175% sodium hypochlorite solution (Clorox), which is the disinfectant of choice. Quaternary ammonium compounds are generally ineffective against FCV. The virus is stable at a pH of 4–5 and is inactivated at 50 °C within 30 min.

Infectivity for Other Species and Culture Systems. FCV is a ubiquitous pathogen that has been isolated from cats all over the world. There is no evidence that FCV produces disease in laboratory animals. The virus can readily be propagated in feline cell lines. Some strains have been grown in Vero monkey kidney and dolphin kidney cells.

Host–Virus Relationship

Distribution, Reservoir, and Transmission. The disease occurs worldwide, and all species of cats are likely susceptible. Infection and disease are most common in young cats, and older cats are usually immune. Infected cats recovered from the disease may carry the virus in their oropharynx for long periods of time and serve as reservoirs of infection. The virus is transmitted by horizontal aerosol infection and by contaminated fomites. The latter mode is of major importance because of the hardiness of the virus in the environment.

Pathogenesis and Pathology. Cats acquire FCV infection via the respiratory route, either by aerosol or from fomites. The primary sites of viral replication are epithelial cells of the oral cavity and respiratory tract and in the tonsils. Viremia occurs during acute infection.

The characteristic lesions in typical cases of FCV infection in susceptible kittens and young cats are vesicles within the oral cavity (tongue and hard palate) and on the nares. The vesicles rapidly rupture, leaving erosions and ulcers. Highly virulent strains can cause pneumonia in kittens. Regeneration of the oral mucosa occurs rapidly in uncomplicated cases. FCV has also been associated with a limping syndrome characterized by synovitis and increased synovial fluid. The mechanism of lameness is unknown, but may have an immune component.

Virulent systemic strains of FCV (VS FCV) cause epidemics of fatal disease in susceptible cats. VS FCV is characterized by vasculitis and multiorgan involvement. Affected animals may exhibit severe oral ulceration, extensive subcutaneous edema especially of head and limbs, and variable ulceration of the pinnae, paw pads, nares, and skin. Some affected cats also have pneumonia as well as liver and splenic necrosis. FCV antigen is detected by immunohistochemical staining in both epithelial and endothelial cells. Mortality is high and disease has occurred in vaccinated cats. Most commonly, VS FCV arises in rescue facilities or other multicat settings where FCV is circulating.

Host Response to Infection. Cats infected with FCV or vaccinated with inactivated or live modified FCV vaccines develop serum-neutralizing antibodies. Kittens born to cats that are immune to FCV acquire maternal serum-neutralizing antibodies to FCV via colostrum.

Laboratory Diagnosis

Laboratory tests are required to distinguish FCV infection from other agents that produce similar respiratory signs in cats, particularly feline viral rhinotracheitis (herpesvirus). These include the isolation of FCV in feline cell cultures from nasal secretions, throat swabs, or conjunctival scrapings and the identification of FCV antigens in conjunctival scrapings of tonsillar biopsies by immunohistochemical staining. Genetic detection by reverse transcription/PCR may also be used. However, positive results must be interpreted carefully, as asymptomatic carriers occur. In addition, false-negative results can occur due to the genetic variability of the virus. The characteristic appearance of the virus by electron microscopy can also be used for rapid diagnosis. VS FCV cannot be distinguished from classical FCV except by clinical manifestations.

Treatment and Control

Treatment for FCV infection in cats is mainly supportive and symptomatic. Broad-spectrum antibiotics help prevent secondary bacterial infections, and fluid therapy is useful in the event of dehydration. All strains of FCV are considered variants of a single serotype because there is considerable serologic cross-reactivity among viruses. Furthermore, cats immunized with one variant of FCV are protected against other strains, though protection can be incomplete. The use of viral neutralization assays in vaccine development is the best method for evaluating cross-protectivity of vaccines. Both inactivated and modified live FCV vaccines are commercially available and afford reasonable protection against FCV infection. The FCV vaccines are usually combined with feline rhinotracheitis (a herpesvirus) and feline panleukopenia (a parvovirus) and administered either intranasally or intramuscularly.

FCV infection is controlled primarily by isolating cats that show respiratory signs and disinfecting cages and premises with Clorox before susceptible animals are introduced.

Lagoviruses

Disease (Rabbit Hemorrhagic Disease and European Brown Hare Syndrome)

Rabbit hemorrhagic disease (RHD) and European brown hare syndrome (EBHS) are similar diseases that are caused by related but antigenically distinct caliciviruses. RHD is an acute infectious disease of the European rabbit, *Oryctolagus cuniculus*, and frequently has a very high mortality rate in susceptible rabbit populations. A novel feature of RHD is that the disease is only fatal to rabbits over 2 months of age. The disease is characterized by a short incubation period, followed by fever, disseminated hemorrhage in all body tissues, and rapid death. The disease was first described in China in 1984, and it then rapidly spread throughout much of the rest of the world. EBHS occurs in the European hare, *Lepus europaeus*.

Etiologic Agent

Physical, Chemical, and Antigenic Properties. Various strains of RHD and EBHS viruses are recognized and distinguished serologically.

Infectivity for Other Species and Culture Systems. Neither RHD nor EBHS viruses are readily propagated in cell culture, which means that the viruses have been largely characterized using homogenates of the livers of affected animals. The viruses appear to be highly species specific.

Host–Virus Relationship

Distribution, Reservoir, and Transmission. Although RHD was first reported in China, EBHS had been recognized earlier in Europe. It is possible that a mutation of the EBHS calicivirus led to the emergence of rabbit hemorrhagic disease virus (RHDV), causing the lethal pandemic of rabbits. The disease is transmitted by the oral–fecal route. Morbidity and mortality of RHD in European rabbits may approach 90–100%, and can have significant economic impact on affected farms.

Pathogenesis and Pathology. Rabbits with RHD have an enlarged spleen, swollen liver, and disseminated hemorrhages. Extensive liver necrosis is highly characteristic and potentially explains the disseminated intravascular coagulation (DIC) that occurs in affected animals. Lesions may also be found in other organs such as the kidneys, lungs, and heart. The DIC induced by RHDV is not characteristic of other calicivirus infections, but does occur in such flavivirus-induced diseases as yellow fever and dengue in humans.

Laboratory Diagnosis

Immunofluorescence and enzyme-linked immunosorbent assay tests have been developed for the rapid diagnosis of RHD. The genome of RHDV has been completely sequenced, so PCR readily can be developed and used for rapid diagnosis of the infection. The liver is the tissue of choice for viral detection.

Treatment and Control

There is no treatment for the acute disease. A formalin-inactivated vaccine that incorporates infected rabbit tissue provides effective immunization against the disease. Control can also be achieved through strict quarantine and isolation to prevent transportation of RHDV-contaminated materials into commercial rabbitries. Contaminated pelts and meat can serve as sources of the virus in nonendemic areas. It is interesting to note that, although most countries have focused on the control and prevention of RHD, RHDV has been used as a biologic weapon to control rabbit numbers in other countries.

Noroviruses

The first norovirus was identified in a human outbreak of gastroenteritis in Norwalk, Ohio, in 1968. Noroviruses have since been recognized in many species of animals, including mice, cattle, swine, sheep, and a lion cub where they have been associated with diarrhea in young animals. Several genotypes of noroviruses have been identified, most of which cannot be grown *in vitro*.

Transmission is fecal–oral, and the virus is stable in the environment after shedding. The virus appears to target enterocytes; disease is generally mild and self-limiting. Diagnosis can be done by electron microscopy or RT-PCR. The zoonotic potential for animal noroviruses is unknown though human and animal isolates are closely related.

Unassigned Caliciviruses

Enteric caliciviruses have been described in cattle, dogs, chickens, and pigs, among others. At least some of these appear to cause clinical signs of intestinal disease analogous to that caused by the Norwalk-like viruses in humans.

Reference

Zee YC, Hackett AJ, and Talens LT (1968) Electron microscopic studies on the vesicular exanthema of swine virus. II. Morphogenesis of VESV Type H54 in pig kidney cells. *Virology*, **34**, 596.

Further Reading

Chassey D (1997) Rabbit haemorrhagic disease: the new scourge of *Oryctolagus cuniculus*. *Lab Anim*, **31**, 33–44.

Scipioni A, Mauroy A, Vinje J, and Thiry E (2008) Animal noroviruses. *Vet J*, **178**, 32–45.

Togaviridae and Flaviviridae

Christopher C.L. Chase

Introduction

Togaviridae and Flaviviridae are two similar positive-sense single-stranded enveloped RNA virus families that are characterized by a single mRNA that results in a polyprotein that is posttranslationally modified. Both families contain several arboviruses. Originally, the genera *Flavivirus* and *Pestivirus* were included in the family Togaviridae, but based on differences in genomic organization and glycoproteins, a new family, Flaviviridae, was established in 1984 that included viruses in the genera *Flavivirus* and *Pestivirus*.

Togaviridae

The family Togaviridae derives its name from "toga," the Latin word for gown or cloak, which refers to the envelope possessed by all members of the family. The family includes two genera, *Alphavirus* and *Rubivirus*, which has a single member rubella virus the cause of human rubella (German measles). Viruses in the *Alphavirus* genus are predominately arboviruses that are transmitted by mosquitoes; thus, they have the capacity to replicate in insects and vertebrates. There are also four nonencephalitic alphaviruses that will be discussed: three recently discovered fish alphaviruses and an elephant seal virus (Table 57.1).

Alphavirus

Sindbis virus is the prototype of the genus *Alphavirus*. Alphaviruses of veterinary significance include eastern equine encephalitis (EEE), western equine encephalitis (WEE), and Venezuelan equine encephalitis (VEE, including subtype II Everglades) viruses, along with several other viruses (Fort Morgan, Highlands J, and Semliki Forest). The three equine encephalitis viruses (EEV) are also zoonoses. The three closely related salmonid alphaviruses (SAVs) are salmon pancreas disease virus (SPDV), sleeping disease virus (SDV), and Norwegian salmonid alphavirus. Another alphavirus, southern elephant seal virus (SESV), has been identified, but its role in disease is unknown.

Original chapter written by Drs. MacLachlan and Stott.

Physical, Chemical, and Antigenic Properties. Alphavirus virions are spherical, enveloped, and approximately 70 nm in diameter ($T = 4$) (Figure 57.1A). Alphaviruses are sensitive to lipid solvents, chlorine, phenol, acid pH, and heating to 60 °C for 30 min.

The envelope is derived from the plasma membranes of host cells through which virions bud as they mature. The envelope encloses an icosahedral nucleocapsid ($T = 4$) (Figure 57.1C) that is approximately 40 nm in diameter and consists of a single-capsid protein as well as the genome of linear single-stranded positive-sense RNA (Figures 57.1B–D). The envelope contains a heterodimer of two viral glycoproteins (E1 and E2) (Figures 57.1A and B) and some alphaviruses (Semliki Forest virus) have a third glycoprotein (E3). At least four different nonstructural viral proteins are produced in infected cells (Figure 57.1D). The alphaviruses are all antigentically related as determined by serological assays, and are grouped into distinct antigenic complexes with numerous subtypes or strains within each. The extensive genetic and antigenic variation that occurs within the various subtypes and variants of each antigenic complex is reflected by differences in their virulence, biochemical characteristics such as electrophoresis mobility of protein and RNA digests, physicochemical characteristics, host range, geographic distribution, and vector/host tropism. WEE virus is the result of recombination between EEE virus and a Sindbis-like virus in an event that has been estimated to have occurred thousands of years ago (Figure 57.2)

Infectivity for Other Species and Culture Systems. The EEV can infect a wide host range, including humans, horses, rodents, reptiles, amphibians, monkeys, dogs, cats, foxes, skunks, cattle, pigs, birds, and mosquitoes. Alphaviruses can be propagated in a variety of cell cultures, including chick and duck fibroblasts, Vero, L cells, and mosquito cells; cytopathology is often absent in the latter. A variety of laboratory animals can be experimentally infected, with suckling mice being the most common.

Veterinary Microbiology, Third Edition. Edited by D. Scott McVey, Melissa Kennedy and M.M. Chengappa.

Table 57.1. Viruses of Veterinary Importance in the Togaviridae Family

Genus	Serogroup/Agent	Vector	Affected Species	Distribution
Alphavirus	Family Alphavirus			
	Equine encephalitis group			
	Eastern equine encephalitis virus	Mosquitoes—*Culex Melanoconion* and *Cs. Melanura*	Horses, humans, pheasants, turkeys, emus, pigs, deer, dogs, sheep, penguins, cranes	Eastern North America, Caribbean Basin, Central America, South America
	Venezuelan equine encephalitis virus	Mosquitoes-enzootic *Culex melanoconion*-epizootic *Ades* and *Psophora* spp.	Horses, humans	Central America, South America
	Western equine encephalitis virus	Mosquitoes—*Culex tarsalis*	Horses, humans, emus	Western North America, South America
	Salmonid alphavirus group			
	Salmonid alphavirus 1 & 3 (pancreatic disease virus)	None	Salmon	Northern Europe
	Salmonid alphavirus 2 (sleeping disease virus)	None	Rainbow trout	Western Europe
	Getah virus (Sagiyama virus)	Mosquitoes—*Culex* spp.	Horse, pigs	Southeast Asia (India and Japan)
	Southern elephant seal virus	Lice—*Lepidophthirus macrorhini*	Elephant seal	Australasia

FIGURE 57.1. *Virion structure and genomic organization of Alphavirus: (A) Surface-shaded view of Sindbis virus, the prototype Togavirus. The flower-like trimeric spikes of E1-E2 heterodimers are seen in blue and turquoise, and small portions of the lipid bilayer are seen in green. (B) A central cross-section of the virus particle showing the organization of the particle with the E2 glycoprotein (blue), the E1 glycoprotein (turquoise), the lipid bilayer (green) penetrated by the transmembrane helices of glycoproteins, protease domain of the capsid protein (yellow), protein–RNA region (orange), and RNA region (red). (C) The nucleocapsid core showing the pentmeric and hexameric capsomeres viewed at the icosahedral twofold axis. (D) The genome of Venezuelan equine encephalitis virus (VEEV). The single positive-strand RNA genome encodes four nonstructural proteins (nsPs) and three main structural proteins. During infection, two mRNAs are synthesized—a full-length mRNA that forms the viral genome and a smaller mRNA that is used to produce virion proteins. The three structural proteins are translated from a subgenomic 26S message and combine with the genomic RNA to form virions. (Panels A, B, and C adapted from Jose et al. 2009 and Panel D from Weaver and Barrett 2004.)*

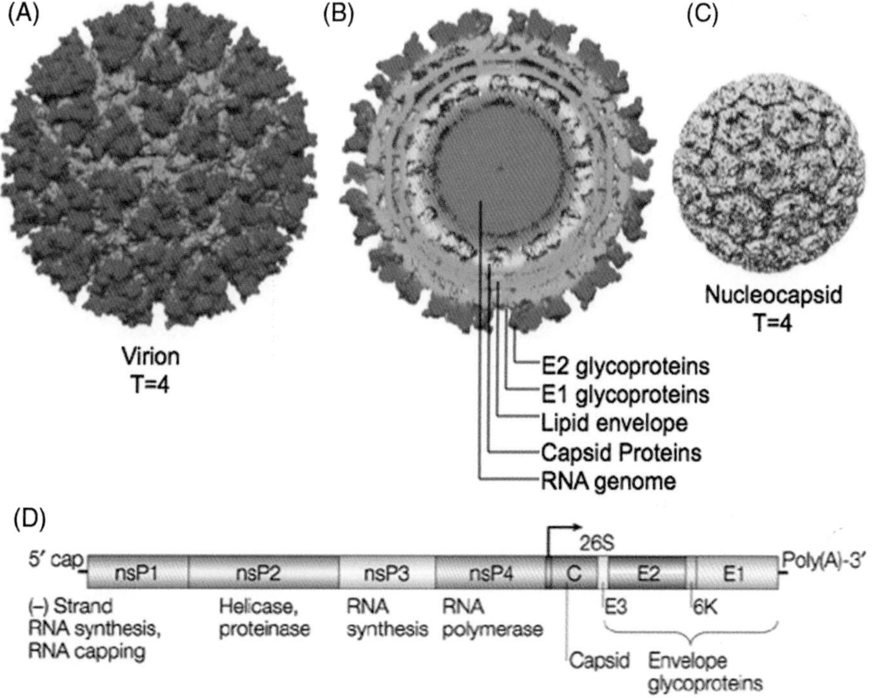

FIGURE 57.2. *Diagram of the Recombination Event That Led to WEE. (Adapted from Strauss and Strauss 1997.)*

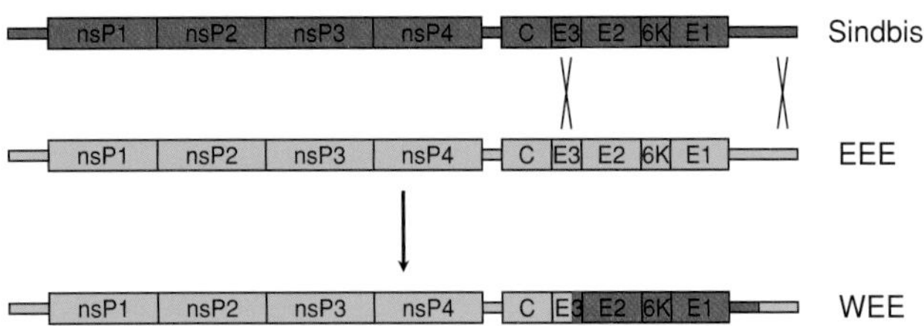

Embryonated chicken eggs and young chicks may also be susceptible to infection.

Veterinary and Zoonotic Alphaviruses

Equine Encephalitis Viruses

Disease. EEE, WEE, and VEE all cause encephalitis in horses, but the signs can vary from inapparent to fatal disease. Mild and/or inapparent infections are more common with WEE, whereas EEE and VEE are typically more virulent. Death from VEE may occur in the absence of neurologic signs. Central nervous system (CNS) involvement of horses following encephalitis virus infection is characterized by aimless walking, followed by severe depression and behavioral changes (dummy), central blindness, paralysis, and death soon after the onset of clinical signs. Mortality can be very high (up to 90%) with VEE and EEE. Young horses are more susceptible to severe disease. Other members EEE and WEE may also cause significant disease in domestic birds; EEE is more common and mortality can be very high.

Clinical disease is especially common in pheasants and ratites (emus, etc.). EEE also occurs in swine and cattle. EEE disease in birds is characterized by encephalitis with leg paralysis, torticollis, and tremors. Wild birds may also be infected but rarely experience disease, and they serve as vertebrate reservoirs of virus.

Epidemiology. The EEV occur in the Western Hemisphere, although related viruses occur elsewhere in the world (Figures 57.3A–C). EEE occurs in eastern North America (predominantly east of the Mississippi River and the Atlantic Seaboard region in particular), the Caribbean Basin, and Central and South America (Figure 57.3A). EEE is the most common EEV with an average of 254 cases per year (range from 65 to 712 cases per year) from 2003 to 2011 (Table 57.2). Often there are localized outbreaks in the United States. VEE is confined to South and Central America (Figure 57.3B), although incursions into North America have occurred periodically with last outbreak in the United States being in 1971. The United States considers VEE to be a foreign animal disease; however, an avirulent VEE virus (type II, Everglades) is endemic in portions of Florida. WEE occurs throughout much of North America, particularly in areas west of the Mississippi River, and South America (Figure 57.3C). Unlike EEE, WEE infection rates have declined dramatically with only a total of four cases diagnosed in the United States from 2003 to 2011 (Table 57.2). Other

FIGURE 57.3. *Range of EEE, WEE, and VEE. Map showing the distribution of the encephalitic alphaviruses: (A) EEEV, (B) VEEV, and (C) WEEV. (Adapted from Scott and Slobodan 2009.)*

(A)

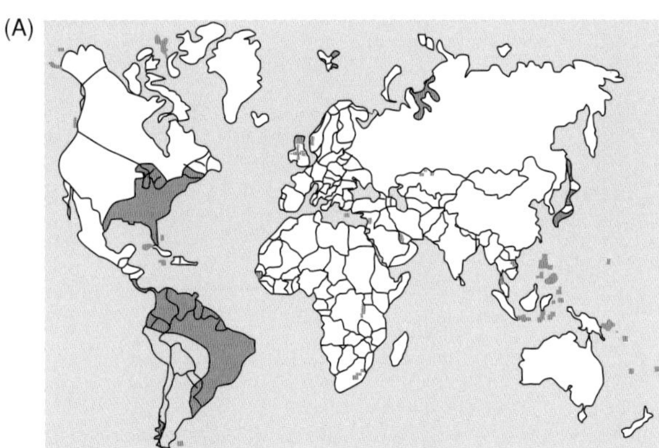

(B)

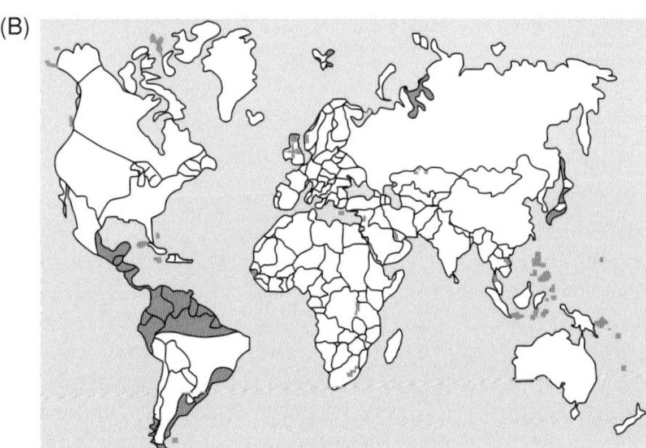

(C)

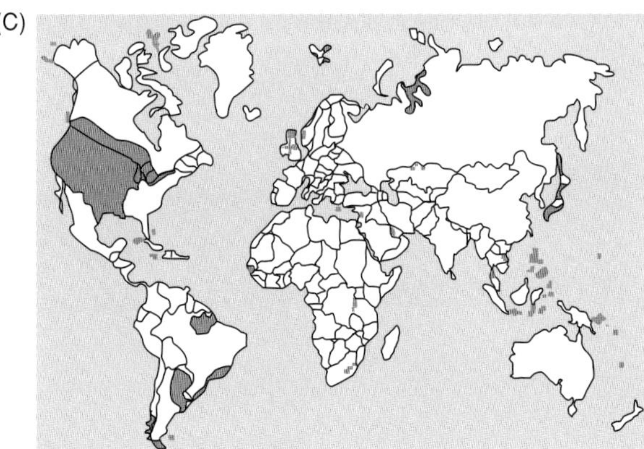

encephalitic alphaviruses sporadically occur in the United States but a much lower rates with the most prominent being Highland J virus that causes encephalitis in horses especially in Florida and is also pathogenic to turkeys and partridges.

Mosquitoes transmit the EEV, and despite their names, horses and humans are dead-end hosts that are unimportant to the natural cycle of EEE and WEE virus infections (Figure 57.4). These viruses were the first described arthropod-borne viruses (arboviruses). The viruses all persist in similar but distinct natural cycles of infection that include mosquitoes and birds or rodents that function as the vertebrate reservoirs of each virus. Except in tropical

Table 57.2. Number of Positive EEE and WEE in Horses in the US 2003–2011

Year	EEE[a,b]	WEE[b]
2003	712	1
2004	133	2
2005	330	0
2006	111	0
2007	206	0
2008	185	0
2009	301	0
2010	247	0
2011	65	1

[a]Data from USDA—Aphis Animal Health and Monitoring and Surveillance site 12/29/2011 http://www.aphis.usda.gov/vs/nahss/equine/ee/eee_distribution_maps.htm (accessed February 8, 2013).
[b]Data from USGS Disease Maps site 12/29/2011 EEE (http://diseasemaps.usgs.gov/eee_us_veterinary.html, accessed February 8, 2013) and WEE (http://diseasemaps.usgs.gov/wee_us_veterinary.html, accessed February 8, 2013).

areas where infection occurs year-round, the peak incidence of these diseases typically is in late summer and declines when climatic conditions are less favorable for the mosquito vectors. Mosquitoes are biological vectors of these viruses, which requires that the mosquito actually become infected with the virus rather than simply transmitting it mechanically. For a biological vector to become infected, it must obtain a blood meal from a viremic vertebrate host (Figure 57.5). The level of viremia required to infect the vector is dictated by viral strain and/or species of mosquito vector. Upon ingestion, the virus infects the insect gut and then spreads to the salivary glands, where replication provides a ready source of virus to infect additional vertebrate hosts during insect feeding. The time required for this process is the extrinsic incubation period (EIP) that varies with type of virus and species of mosquito. The EIP for EEE virus is quite short at 2–3 days (Figure 57.5). Once infected, the vector remains infected for life.

EEE virus exists in two distinct ecosystems: (1) North American (eastern United States and Canada) and the Caribbean and (2) Central and South America. *Culiseta melanura* mosquitoes transmit the North American strains of the virus. The virus is maintained in an enzootic cycle of infection that includes these ornithophilic (bird-feeding) mosquitoes and the passerine and wading birds that serve as vertebrate virus reservoirs in coastal and inland swamp environments (Figure 57.4). Periodic spillover of the virus occurs in adjacent horses, humans, birds, and other animals (Figure 57.4). A variety of mosquito species can transmit the virus during epidemics, and direct horizontal spread occurs among birds when they peck viremic birds. Another mosquito (*Culex melanoconion*) is responsible for transmission of EEE in Central and South America, where small mammals and birds serve as the vertebrate reservoirs of the virus.

The host–virus relationship of WEE is similar to that of EEE, with the virus being maintained in a transmission cycle between mosquitoes (*Culex tarsalis*) and domestic and passerine birds, with periodic spillover into humans, horses, and domestic birds. Other species of mosquitoes can transmit the virus during outbreaks.

The lifecycle of VEE is more complex. There are several distinct clusters of VEE viruses (types I–VI), most of which do not cause disease in horses (type 1, varieties D through F, types II–VI). These viruses are endemic throughout tropical and subtropical regions of the Americas (including Florida, where VEE type II [Everglades] occurs). These endemic VEE viruses are maintained in a natural cycle of infection

FIGURE 57.4. *The endemic and epidemic transmission cycles of eastern (EEEV), western (WEEV), and Venezuelan equine encephalitis viruses (VEEV). (From Pfeffer and Dobler 2010.)*

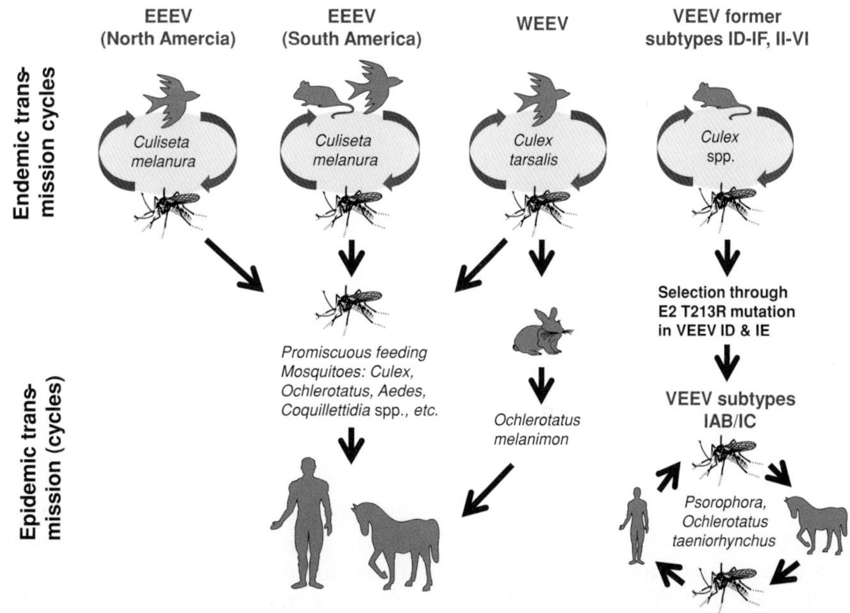

FIGURE 57.5. *Arbovirus replication in female mosquito following blood meal: (1) ingests infected blood; (2) virus infects and multiples in mesenteronal epithelial cells; (3) virus is released across the basal membrane of the epithelial cells and replicates in other tissues; (4) virus infects salivary glands; and (5) virus is released from cells of salivary glands and transmitted in saliva. The Extrinsic incubation period for EEE, JEV, and WNV is listed.*

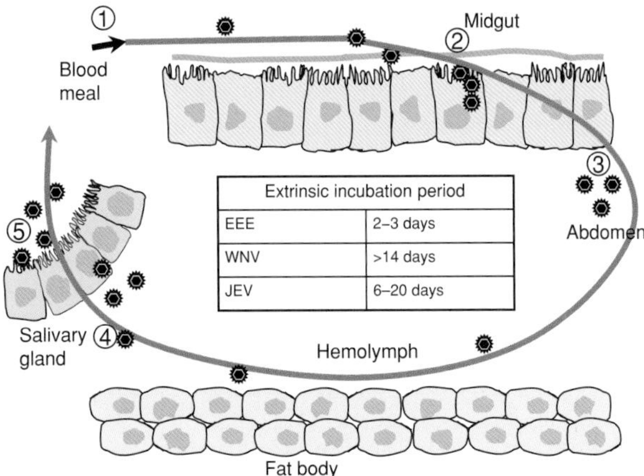

between *Culex* mosquitoes and small rodents in tropical swamps. Only VEE types 1AB and 1C are virulent to horses, and these are only isolated during the epidemics of VEE that regularly occur in northern South America. It is believed that these epidemic strains emerge after mutation of the E2 envelope glycoprotein of endemic type 1D strains of VEE that constantly are circulating in endemic areas but are not pathogenic to horses (Figure 57.4). Once strains of VEE emerge that are virulent to horses and humans, infected horses are a major source of virus because, unlike EEE and WEE, VEE replicates to high titers in horses. Thus, the endemic and epidemic (epizootic) VEE viruses have very different cycles of infection (Figure 57.4).

Pathogenesis and Pathology. Equine encephalitis alphavirus infections can range from inapparent to severe, fatal disease. Infection follows the bite of an infected mosquito. Primary viral replication occurs in regional lymph nodes adjacent to the site of the bite and is followed by generalized infection and viremia in which the virus replicates in the lymphoid tissues throughout the body, bone marrow, and certain other tissues. The encephalitis viruses likely gain entry into the CNS after replication in the endothelial cells lining blood vessels in the brain, and passage of virus to the brain occurs after the acute phase of infection and viremia. Lesions occur throughout the gray matter of the brain and include perivascular cuffing with inflammatory cells, infiltration of neutrophils into the gray matter with neuronal and parenchymal necrosis, and vasculitis, thrombosis, and hemorrhage. Neutrophils are especially characteristic of the early cerebral lesions of EEE and VEE.

Host Response to Infection. The development of neutralizing antibody to EEV appears to be important in limiting viral replication and spread and is clearly important in preventing reinfection. Antibodies develop to all viral proteins, and peak titers of neutralizing antibody typically develop within 2 weeks of infection in animals that survive. This antibody may be effective in neutralizing virus, enhancing viral clearance, and lysing infected cells via complement or natural killer cells. Cell-mediated immunity also appears to contribute to viral clearance and protective immunity. Cytotoxic T lymphocytes can be identified as early as 3–4 days postinfection.

Laboratory Diagnosis. Equine encephalitis alphavirus infection may be suspected based on the occurrence of neurologic disease among susceptible animal species in endemic areas, thus prior history and seasonal occurrence can be important. Definitive diagnosis requires laboratory confirmation, which usually is done by serology with an IgM-capture enzyme-linked immunosorbent assay (ELISA) to detect virus-specific antibodies in the serum of acutely affected animals. The diagnosis is unequivocally confirmed by virus isolation from blood or CNS tissue, the latter being preferable due to the variable occurrence of viremia by the time signs of encephalitis are manifest in infected animals. Antigen capture ELISA for EEE may be used to help identify the virus in CNS tissue. Immunohistochemistry and polymerase chain reaction (PCR) may also be used to identify virus in neurologic tissue. Virus may be isolated in a variety of systems, including cell cultures, chick embryos, and suckling mice.

Treatment and Control. There is no treatment for clinically ill animals. Control of equine encephalitis virus infections can be achieved through vaccination and pest management programs. Vector control can be approached through eliminating mosquito-breeding sites by water control or spraying programs. In the case of domestic bird farms, the use of tightly screened (insect-proof) rearing pens and locating such pens away from freshwater swamps is also a possibility. Effective inactivated (EEE, WEE, VEE) and attenuated (VEE) vaccines have been developed for the EEV. Regular annual vaccination of susceptible animals is required to maintain immunity if inactivated vaccines are used.

Salmonid alphaviruses

Disease. SAVs are recognized as serious pathogens of farmed Atlantic salmon, *Salmo salar* L., and rainbow trout, *Oncorhynchus mykiss*, in Europe. There are three alphavirus salmonid viral diseases. Salmon pancreas disease virus (SPDV or SAV subtype 1 (SAV 1) or subtype 3 (SAV 3)) is the causative agent of pancreas disease (PD). The disease occurs in farmed Atlantic salmon smolts during their first year at sea, with peak prevalence occurring from late July to early September but outbreaks have occurred at all stages of Atlantic salmon production. Clinical signs associated with PD in order of their appearance may be sudden inappetence, lethargy and an increased number of fecal casts in the cages, increased mortality and ill-thrift. Affected fish may appear to be unable to maintain their position in the water column/currents within the cages due to muscle damage, predisposing them to erosion and ulceration of the skin and fins. Apparently healthy fish may also die suddenly due to cardiac and skeletal muscle damage and exhaustion. Fish with normal or good-condition factor may sometimes be seen swimming in a spiraling or circular motion or appear dead at the bottom of the cage (similar to SD signs), but swim away if handled. Mortality rates in PD outbreaks have ranged from 1% to 48%. High mortality tends to occur in higher energy density feeding sites and when the fish are returning to feeding after a period of inappetence. Up to 15% of survivors fail to grow and become runts.

Sleeping disease (SD) is an infectious disease of rainbow trout reared in freshwater and it was confirmed by the isolation of SDV in France and is now SDV (SAV 2). SDV affects rainbow trout at all stages of production. The characteristic clinical presentation is of affected fish lying on their side on the bottom of the tank, hence the name "sleeping disease". These clinical signs are primarily due to extensive necrosis of skeletal red muscle. Reported mortality levels have been variable, from negligible to more than 22% in affected populations.

Epidemiology. The SAV have been found almost exclusively in farmed Atlantic salmon and rainbow trout in Europe. SPDV or SAV 1 found in farmed Atlantic salmon in Ireland and Scotland. SDV (SAV subtype 2 (SAV 2)) was first confirmed in France and is now SAV 2 has been isolated from diseased rainbow trout in England, Scotland, Italy, and Spain. SPDV (SAV 1) and SDV (SAV 2) are closely related subtypes of the same virus species with the proposed name salmonid alphavirus. Norwegian salmonid alphavirus (NSAV; (SAV 3) was isolated from farmed Atlantic salmon with pancreatic disease (PD) and has been detected only in Norway. The genomic organization of SAV 3 is identical to that of SAV 1 and SAV 2, and the nucleotide sequence similarity to the other two alphaviruses is 91.6% and 92.9%, respectively. PD was described only once in North America, in 1987, but no virus was detected and this remains the only report of a PD-like condition outside Europe. A dual infection of infectious salmon anemia virus (a member of the Orthomyxoviridae) and a toga-like virus was described in New Brunswick, Canada, in 2000.

Pathogenesis and Pathology. The principal gross findings at necropsy in the early stages of a PD outbreak are the absence of food in the gut and the presence of fecal casts. The significant lesions in naturally occurring PD occur sequentially in the pancreas, heart, and skeletal muscle of affected fish. Pancreatic necrosis, cardiomyopathy and skeletal myopathy, including esophageal muscle lesions, are the most significant PD lesions. Approximately, three out of four cases of PD have cardiac and/or skeletal myopathies. These myopathies are significant in the pathogenesis of PD outbreaks. Relatively small numbers of myopathies have acute pancreatic lesions (<2% of fish)

The acute infection phase of PD is relatively short-lived with rapid destruction of the majority of pancreatic acinar tissue and a variable inflammatory response. As skeletal muscle lesions tend to first appear 3–4 weeks after the appearance of pancreatic and heart lesions, fish sampled in late phase disease may only have skeletal muscle lesions.

SD has the same sequential histological lesions: exocrine pancreas, heart, and skeletal muscle as those described for PD. The major histological lesion sign is extensive necrosis of skeletal red muscle.

Host Response to Infection. Very few studies have been carried out on the specific immune responses to SAV infections in fish. There is cross-protection between SAV 1(SPD) and SAV 2 (SD) in both Atlantic salmon and rainbow trout. The specific VN antibody response occurred in 60% of fish by 14–16 dpi with all the fish seroconverting by 21 dpi. There have been no reported cases of recurrence of PD or SD in previously infected populations indicating that protection following natural infection is adequate for a complete production cycle.

Laboratory Diagnosis. Diagnosis of early acute SAV infections can be diagnosed using histology (pancreas, heart, and muscle) and immunohistochemistry (IHC-pancreas), detecting viremia and virus RNA in serum and heart tissue (real-time PCR). Chronic-stage SAV infections could be diagnosed by histology, serology (virus neutralization (VN) antibody detection), and virus RNA detection.

Treatment and Control. Vaccines have been developed for SAV 1 and SAV 2. A commercial PD vaccine is available. While it has proved to be very effective in some field trials there are concerns about the duration of immunity. Sea vaccination or revaccination is being currently investigated for sites where PD occurs in Atlantic salmon in the second year at sea. A recombinant SAV 2 live vaccine protected rainbow trout from wild type SAV 2 infection for 5 months.

SAV 1 can survive for more than 2 months in sterile seawater at low temperatures so endemic SAV 1 impact must be minimized by reducing stress through careful management and good hygiene methods. Some risk factors that have been identified include sea-site-to-sea-site movements and sea-site to harvest movements by well boat. Biosecure slaughter methods and safe disposal of offal and effluent are also important to minimizing the risk from these processes. Good sea lice control is desirable, not only for the health and welfare of the fish, but because sea lice may act as reservoirs or vectors of infection. Since most of the alphaviruses are arboviruses, the possibility of a biological transmission cycle between susceptible vertebrate hosts and blood-feeding arthropods is possible. While SAV infections can be transmitted without an insect vector, the potential role of sea and freshwater lice in SAV infections needs to be investigated. There is some evidence that SAV 2 can be transmitted vertically from brood stock to eggs and fry, but further work is required to confirm vertical transmission.

Other Medically Important Alphaviruses. A number of other alphaviruses can infect animals, including Sindbis, Semliki Forest, Highlands J, and Getah viruses. Highlands

J virus has a similar distribution in North America as EEE virus, but it rarely causes encephalitis in horses. It is, however, an important pathogen of turkeys, pheasants, chukar partridges, ducks, emus, and whooping cranes. Getah virus infects horses and swine in Asia and Southeast Asia. Infection in horses is sometimes characterized by fever, rash, and limb edema (but not encephalitis), and Getah virus also can cause abortion in pregnant swine. Getah virus is included within the Semliki Forest virus complex of alphaviruses, and Semliki Forest virus also can cause a febrile disease of horses in Africa. The SESV, an alphavirus, was isolated from the elephant seal louse, *Lepidophthirus macrorhini*, on Macquarie Island in Australasia, and given the high SES virus seroprevalence in the seal population suggest that the SESV is transmitted by the lice. Southern elephant seal population has decreased by 50% in the last 50 years, but there has been no causal effect of SESV on the seal population.

Flaviviridae

The family Flaviviridae contains a large number of viruses within three antigentically distinct genera (Table 57.3): *Flavivirus*, *Pestivirus*, and *Hepacivirus* (human hepatitis C virus). The family Flaviviridae includes a number of important human pathogens.

Flavivirus

Members of the genus *Flavivirus* include arboviruses that are transmitted by either mosquitoes or ticks. Those that are mosquito-transmitted include the Japanese encephalitis virus (JEV) group (including Japanese encephalitis, Murray Vallcy encephalitis, St. Louis encephalitis, and West Nile and Kunjin viruses), the Yellow Fever (YF) virus group (including YF and Wesselsbron viruses) and Dengue virus (DV) group (the cause of human Dengue hemorrhagic fever). The tick-borne flaviviruses include tick-borne encephalitis (TBE; European, Far Eastern, and Siberian), Powassan, and Louping ill viruses. These viruses cause either encephalitis or systemic hemorrhagic-septicemia in animals and/or humans.

Physical, Chemical, and Antigenic Properties. The name *Flavivirus* is derived from the Latin word "flavus," which means yellow, since YF virus is the family prototype. Members of the genus consist of spherical (50 nm in diameter) enveloped particles with small surface projection (peplomers) (Figure 57.6). Virions are stable at a pH of 7–9, but are inactivated by acid pH, temperatures above 40 °C, lipid solvents, ultraviolet light, ionic and nonionic detergents, and trypsin. A single nucleocapsid protein encapsulates the genome, and the envelope contains two viral membrane proteins (E and M). Several nonstructural viral proteins are also produced in virus-infected cells (NS1-5). The viral genome is a single linear strand of positive-sense RNA. The genomic RNA is infectious and encodes a single large polyprotein that is co- and posttranslationally cleaved into the various viral structural and nonstructural proteins. The flaviviruses are all serologically related as determined by group-specific assays such as ELISA and hemagglutination inhibition. They are distinguished by neutralization assays, although there is considerable cross-reactivity among viruses within the same serogroup (sero complex). The envelope E protein contains the major determinants of VN.

Veterinary and Zoonotic Flaviviruses

Japanese Encephalitis Group. JEV is the prototype of the JE antigenic complex within the *Flavivirus* genus. They are all mosquito-transmitted flaviviruses that cause encephalitis. The JE complex includes St. Louis encephalitis virus, Murray Valley encephalitis virus, and West Nile virus (WNV) (and related Kunjin virus), in addition to JEV itself. These are all human pathogens, but JEV and WNV are important veterinary pathogens as well.

Japanese Encephalitis Virus

Disease. JEV infection is typically inapparent but can cause clinical disease in humans, horses, and swine.

Table 57.3. Viruses of Veterinary Importance in the Flaviviridae Family

Genus	Serogroup/Agent	Vector	Affected Species	Distribution
Flavivirus				
	Japanese Encephalitis Group			
	Japanese encephalitis virus	Mosquitoes—*Culex* spp.	Horses, humans, swine, poultry	Southeastern Asia
	West Nile virus	Mosquitoes—*Culex* and *Aedes* spp.	Horses, humans, geese, raptors, corvids	Worldwide
	Yellow fever group			
	Wesselsbron virus	Mosquitoes—*Aedes* spp.	Sheep	Sub-Saharan Africa
	Tick-borne encephalitis Louping Ill virus	Tick-*Ixodes rincinus*	Sheep	British Isles, Southern Europe
Pestivirus				
	Bovine viral diarrhea virus	None	Cattle, sheep, wild ruminants	Worldwide
	Border Disease Virus	None	Sheep	Worldwide
	Classic swine fever virus	None	Swine	Asia, Africa, Europe, and South and Central America

FIGURE 57.6. *Virion structure and genomic organization of Flavivirus. (A) Flavivirus: Enveloped, spherical, about 50 nm in diameter. The surface proteins are arranged in an icosahedral-like symmetry. (B) Monopartite, linear, ssRNA(+) genome of about 9.7–12 kb. The genome 3′ terminus is not polyadenylated but forms a loop structure. The 5′ end has a methylated nucleotide cap (allows for translation) or a genome-linked protein (VPg). (From viralzone.expasy.org, SIB Swiss Institute of Bioinformatics. http://viralzone.expasy.org/all_by_species/43.html; accessed January 25, 2013.)*

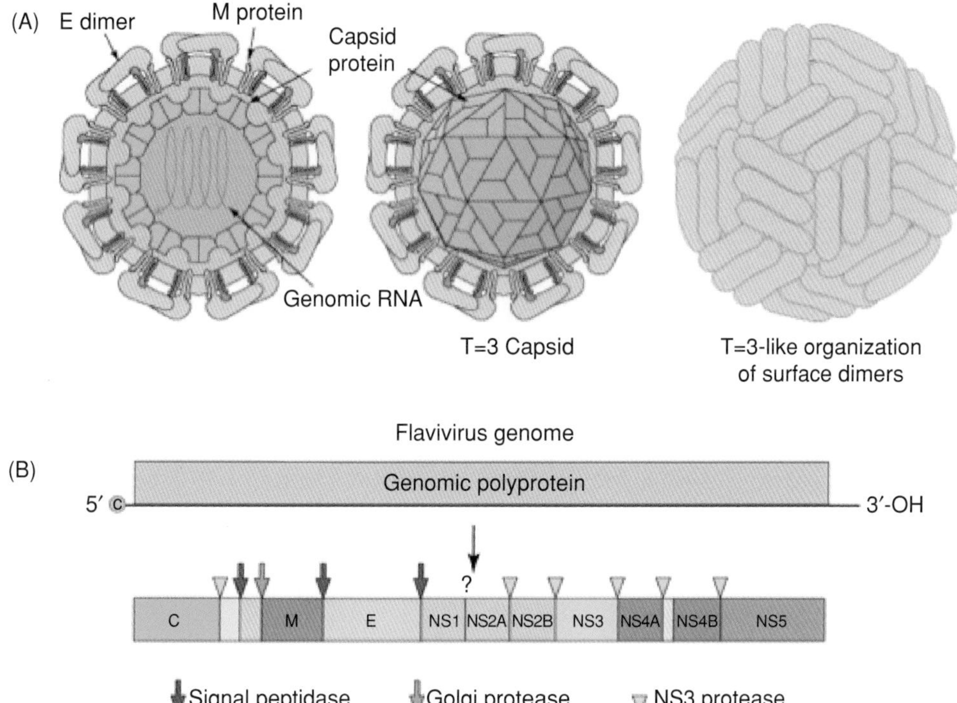

Infection of dogs and domestic poultry also occurs. JEV infection of swine is generally inapparent in swine but results in abortions and stillborns of naive pregnant sows. Infected horses can develop severe neurologic disease that resembles EEE, but mortality is lower.

Epidemiology. JEV infection currently is confined to temperate and tropical areas of Asia, where serological surveys indicate that infection of horses, cattle, and swine is widespread. The virus occurs throughout much of Asia, from the Indian Subcontinent to the west to the Pacific Islands in the east (Figure 57.7). Most infections are inapparent or mild. Horses and humans are unimportant to the epidemiology of JEV infection because viremias are very low titered in these species, insufficient to serve as a virus reservoir for susceptible mosquito vectors (Figure 57.8). In contrast, infected swine and birds serve as amplifying hosts for the virus because they have high-titered viremias (Figure 57.8). *Culex* spp. mosquitoes are the principal vectors of JEV and the EIP is moderate at 6–20 days (Figure 57.5). In swine, virus may also be transmitted from the infected dam to the fetus and from boar to sow via insemination of viral-contaminated semen. The virus is maintained in tropical regions probably by continual transmission between mosquitoes, birds, and swine.

Pathogenesis and Pathology. The pathogenesis and lesion of the disease in horses are similar to that described earlier for the EEV.

Host Response to Infection. Both humoral and cell-mediated immune responses develop in animals following JEV infection. Antibodies (HI and viral-neutralizing) develop within a few days after infection. Neutralizing antibodies largely are directed at the E envelope protein, whereas cytotoxic T lymphocyte responses are directed at the nonstructural viral proteins. Humoral responses appear to play an important role in both recovery and long-term protection against reinfection. Cell-mediated immune responses (cytotoxic T lymphocytes) likely contribute to viral clearance. Immunity is lifelong after natural infection.

Laboratory Diagnosis. Diagnosis of JEV is accomplished by isolating virus from the tissues or blood of affected animals using cell cultures (vertebrate or insect) or suckling mice. Viral RNA can be identified by PCR from any sample. Viral antigen may also be demonstrated directly in brain tissue sections by immunohistochemical staining. A variety of serological assays also are available, but demonstration of virus-specific IgM (indicative of recent infection) is generally required as IgG assays often detect antibodies to related flaviviruses, which complicates interpretation.

Treatment and Control. Vaccination is used for control of JEV infection in endemic areas, and both attenuated and killed vaccines are available. Vector control measures are also an important approach to control.

FIGURE 57.7. *Geographical distribution of Japanese encephalitis virus based on current and historical data. (From van den Hurk et al. 2009.)*

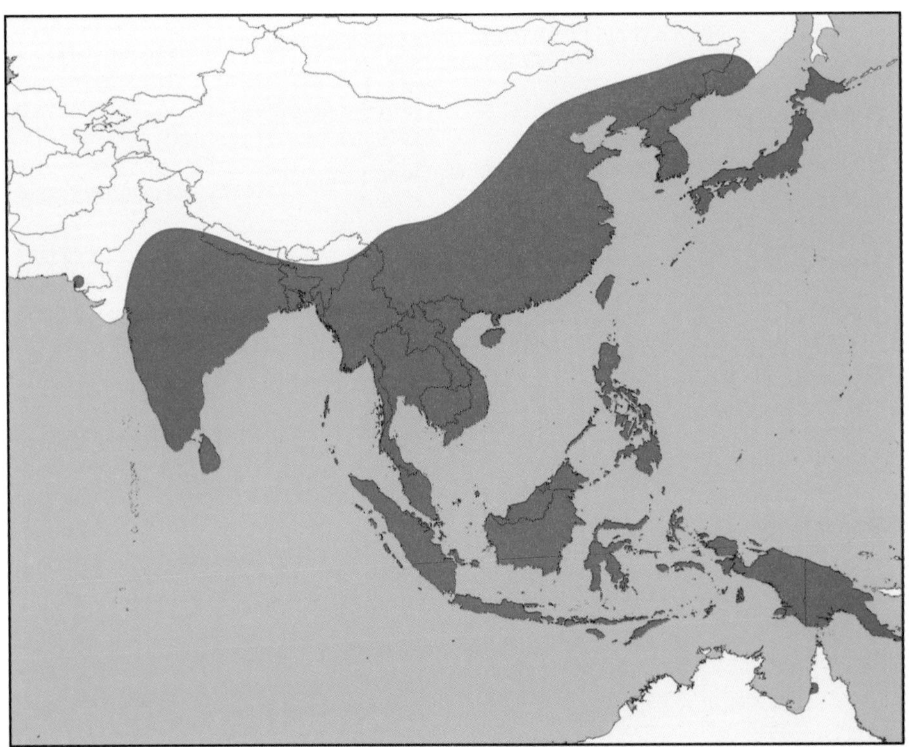

FIGURE 57.8. *Transmission cycles for Japanese encephalitis virus. (From Pfeffer and Dobler 2010.)*

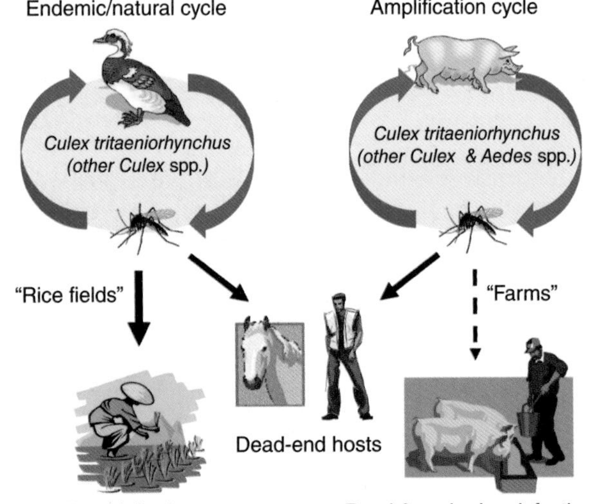

West Nile and Kunjin Viruses

Disease. WNV, a member of the JEV antigenic complex, recently emerged in the Western Hemisphere, precipitating a massive epidemic of disease in humans, horses, birds and an variety of other animals (alligators, squirrels, mountain goats, llamas, sheep, cats, dogs, etc.). Although most horses are asymptomatic (>90%), the neurological disease that occurs in WNV-infected horses is characterized by ataxia, weakness, recumbency, muscle fasiculations, and high fatality rates. Some species of birds suffer high mortality similar to horses including geese (particularly goslings, raptors, and corvids (crows)).

Epidemiology. Prior to 1999, WNV occurred throughout Africa as well as portions of Europe, the Middle East, Asia, and Australia (where it is called Kunjin virus). However in 1999, the virus was introduced into the New York City and the northeast United States and swept across two-third of the United States by 2002 and reached the West Coast of the United States by 2003 (Figure 57.9). Horse cases peaked in 2002 and have declined since the introduction of an inactivated WNV in 2003 (Table 57.4). Human cases peaked in 2004, but WNV is the leading cause of arbovirus infections in the United States (Table 57.4). The virus is maintained in a mosquito-bird cycle of infection, and humans and horses are "dead-end" hosts because viremia is not sufficient to infect susceptible mosquitoes that feed on infected individuals (Figure 57.10). There are two distinct genetic lineages of WNV, so-called lineage 1 and lineage 2. Lineage 2 viruses are endemic south of the equator in Africa, where they cause little if any disease in horses. In distinct contrast, lineage 1 strains of WNV have been associated with outbreaks of disease in Mediterranean and Eastern Europe, North Africa, Asia, and North America. Many bird species undergo subclinical or asymptomatic infection and have viremias of sufficient magnitude to serve as amplifying reservoir hosts of the virus. Specific species of mosquitoes transmit WNV in endemic areas, whereas a wide variety of mosquito species have been incriminated in

FIGURE 57.9. *Year of first reported human West Nile virus disease case, by state—United States 1999–2008. (From Lindsey* et al. *2010.)*

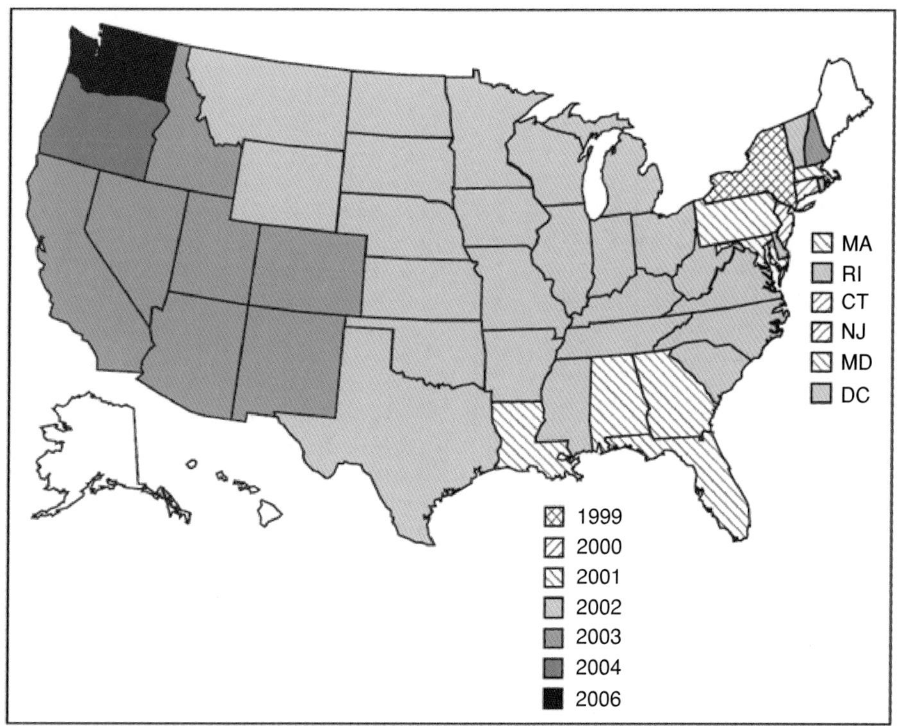

Table 57.4. Number of Positive WNV Cases in Humans and Horses in the US 1999–2011

Year	Human[a]	Horse[a,b]
1999	62	25
2000	21	60
2001	66	738
2002	4 156	15 257
2003	9 862	5 181
2004	2 539	1 406
2005	3 000	1 008
2006	4 268	1 121
2007	3 630	507
2008	1 356	224
2009	720	298
2010	1 021	157
2011	667	115

[a]Data from USGS Disease Maps site 1/2/2012 WNV (http://diseasemaps.usgs.gov/wnv_us_veterinary.html, accessed February 8, 2013; http://diseasemaps.usgs.gov/wnv_us_human.html, accessed February 8, 2013).
[b]http://www.aphis.usda.gov/vs/nahss/equine/wnv/wnv_distribution_maps.htm (accessed February 8, 2013).

the transmission of WNV infection in North America (Figure 57.10). The EIP for WNV is quite long (>14 days) compared to the other encephalitic arboviruses (Figure 57.5).

Pathogenesis and Pathology. The pathogenesis and lesion of the disease in horses are similar to that described earlier for the EEV.

FIGURE 57.10. *Transmission cycles for West Niles virus. (From Pfeffer and Dobler 2010.)*

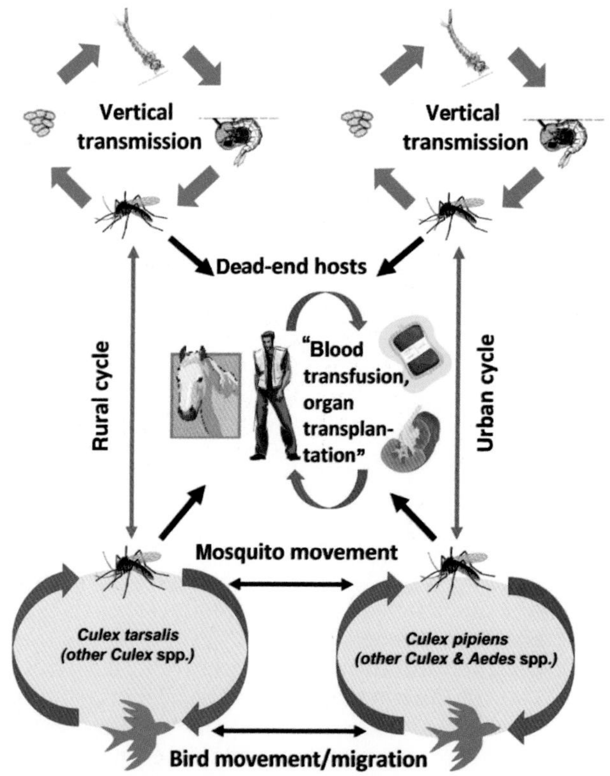

Host Response to Infection. The host immune response is similar to that described above for JEV.

Laboratory Diagnosis. Diagnosis of WNV is best done by PCR. Virus isolation in appropriate cell cultures is also possible. WNV-specific IgM capture ELISA is very useful for the serological identification of animals that are acutely infected with WNV.

Treatment and Control. There are four different WNV vaccines available for horses: an inactivated WNV vaccine, a canarypox recombinant WNV vaccine, a YF virus-WNV chimera vaccine, and a WNV DNA vaccine. Annual revaccination is highly recommended. Vector control measures are also an important approach to control.

Other Medically Important Members of the Flavivirus—Japanese Encephalitis Group. Murray Valley encephalitis virus, another member of the JE mosquito-borne encephalitis complex, is enzootic in New Guinea and Australia and causes sporadic encephalitis in humans. St. Louis encephalitis virus, another member of the JE complex is enzootic in North, Central and South America and also causes sporadic encephalitis in humans.

YF virus group. YF virus group are a small group of mosquito-borne flaviviruses that cause hemorrhagic fevers. YF virus is the prototype virus and this group includes Wesselsbron virus.

Wesselsbron Virus

Disease and Epidemiology. Wesselsbron virus causes disease of sheep in sub-Saharan Africa. Subclinical infection of cattle, horses, and swine also occur, and the virus is a zoonotic pathogen causing febrile disease in humans with headache, myalgia, and arthraglia. The virus causes extensive liver necrosis, jaundice, subcutaneous edema, gastrointestinal hemorrhage, and fever in infected sheep; mortality in lambs can be high, and abortion is common in pregnant ewes. *Aedes* mosquitoes transmit Wesselsbron virus.

Pathogenesis and Pathology. The virus infects and causes necrosis of the liver resulting in hemorrhage and systemic organ failure.

Host Response to Infection. All immune cells are depleted following infection.

Laboratory Diagnosis. Diagnosis may be based upon viral isolation using a variety of cell cultures (baby hamster kidney and lamb kidney), chick embryos, or suckling mice. Viral RNA can be identified by PCR from any sample. Vaccination and/or prior exposure to other flaviviruses complicate the interpretation of serological assays.

Treatment and Control. Attenuated virus vaccines are used to prevent the disease in endemic areas. Vector control measures are also an important approach to control.

Other Medically Important Mosquito-Borne Flaviviruses. YF virus is one of the most severe hemorrhagic viral fevers of humans. It occurs predominately in areas with jungle canopies in Central and South America and Africa. It involves an interaction between canopy mosquitoes, monkeys, and vector mosquitoes. *Aedes aegypti* is the predominant vector in the Western Hemisphere. YF occurred in the southern United States until the 1890s when vector control measures eliminated *A. aegypti*. There is an effective YF vaccine. DV is responsible for Dengue hemorrhagic fever, one of the greatest human arbovirus threats. DV occurs in a wide belt across Central and South America, Africa and Southeast Asia and has occurred in the Caribbean and the extreme southern United States. *A. aegypti* is also predominant vector of DV. Reinfection with DV results in immune-mediated enhancement that causes the subsequent DV infection to infect macrophages and cause severe disseminated intravascular coagulation and hemorrhagic fever. DV has four different serotypes that do not cross protect and there is no vaccine.

Tick-Borne Encephalitis group. This group of viruses includes a number of human pathogens including prototype virus, TBE virus with its three geographical subtypes (European (Western), Siberian, Far Eastern (Russian spring summer encephalitis virus)), Kyasanur forest disease virus, Omsk hemorrhagic fever virus, Powassan virus and the important veterinary pathogen, louping ill virus. This group is all transmitted by ticks making their epidemiology more complex, as the ticks serve as both a reservoir and a virus vector. Unlike mosquitoes, ticks can live for several years making them an effective reservoir. In addition, these tick-borne viruses are transmitted from one developmental stage to another (transstadial transmission) and vertically from one generation to another (transovarial transmission). The tick larvae and nymphs feed on birds or small rodents, while the adult ticks prefer larger animals (Figure 57.11).

Louping Ill Virus

Disease. Louping ill virus is a tick-transmitted *Flavivirus* that naturally infects many animal species, including humans, sheep, horses, deer, and birds. The virus causes encephalomyelitis in sheep, and high mortality may result when susceptible sheep are introduced into an endemic area. Louping ill is characterized by neurologic signs such as hyperexcitability, cerebellar ataxia, and progressive paralysis. The disease derives its name from the leaping gait sometimes observed in ataxic animals. Louping ill is a zoonotic disease causing influenza-like syndromes followed by meningoencephalitis in humans that resolves in 4–10 days. The disease also sometimes occurs in cattle, horses, and goats.

Epidemiology. Louping ill is confined to the British Isles and portions of continental Europe (Spain, Greece, and Turkey). *Ixodes rincinus* ticks are the principal vector.

Laboratory Diagnosis. Diagnosis of louping ill virus is done by viral isolation, immunohistochemical staining of CNS tissue sections from affected animals, or serology. Viral

FIGURE 57.11. *Transmission cycle of tick-borne encephalitis virus. (From Pfeffer and Dobler 2010.)*

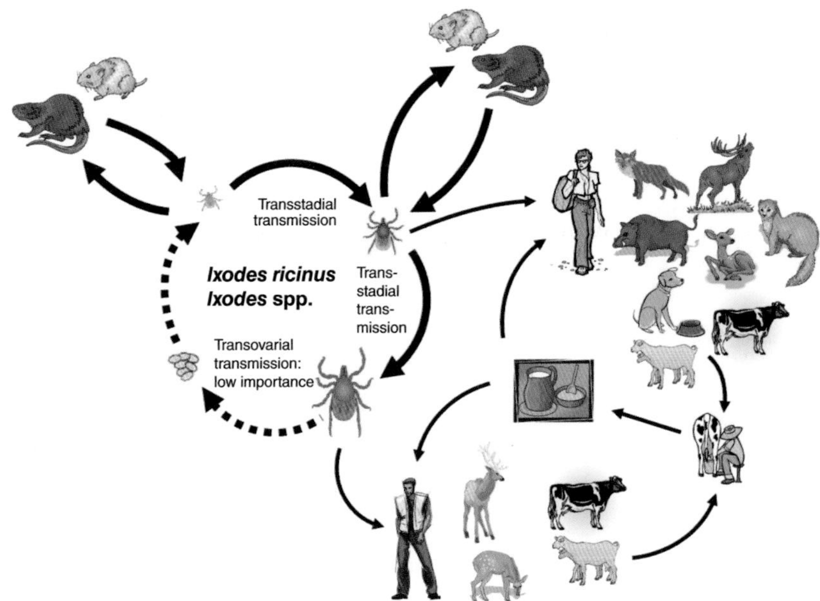

RNA can be identified by PCR from any sample. Virus can be isolated using vertebrate or insect cell cultures and intracerebral inoculation of suckling mice. Propagated virus can be definitively identified by viral neutralization.

Treatment and Control. Louping ill can be controlled through tick control by dipping and spraying of sheep. A formalin-inactivated cell culture-origin vaccine is available and effective. Lambs born to immune dams are protected by colostral antibody for approximately 4 months.

Other Medically Important Tick-Borne Encephalitides. Powassan virus is the cause of a tick-transmitted encephalitis of humans and horses in North America. The virus infects a wide variety of animal species, both wild and domestic, as well as several species of ticks. It causes encephalomyelitis in horses that mimics that caused by other flaviviruses like WNV, from which it must be distinguished by either PCR assay or by virus isolation. Similar tick-borne encephalidities of humans are caused by related viruses in Europe and Asia, including Omsk hemorrhagic fever virus, TBE viruses (European, Far Eastern, and Siberian), and Kyasanur Forest disease virus. The TBE encephalitis results in a high proportion (up to 50%) of the patients having permanent neurological disorders. These TBE viruses are maintained in a cycle of infection that includes ticks and vertebrates (livestock and dogs) that serve as amplifying hosts of the virus. The virus can be transmitted to humans in the milk or dairy products of TBE-infected cattle sheep and/or goats (Figure 57.11). Encephalitis occurs sporadically among animals in areas where these viruses are endemic.

Pestivirus

The genus *Pestivirus* includes bovine viral diarrhea virus (BVDV; types 1 and 2), border disease virus (BDV), and classical swine fever virus (CSFV; previously referred to as hog cholera virus), all of which are important pathogens of livestock. In contrast to the genus *Flavivirus*, members of the genus *Pestivirus* are not arthropod-borne.

Physical, Chemical, Biotype and Antigenic Properties. Pestiviruses are readily inactivated by low pH, heat, organic solvents, and detergents. Virions are spherical to pleomorphic (40–60 nm in diameter) and enveloped with small surface projections (spikes) emanating from the viral envelope. The virions consist of an envelope and nucleocapsid and include four structural proteins—a nucleocapsid protein (C) and three envelope glycoproteins (Erns, E1, and E2) (Figure 57.12). Some seven or eight viral nonstructural proteins are also produced in infected cells. The genome is a single molecule of positive-sense, single-stranded RNA that contains a single, large open reading frame that encodes a large polyprotein that is co- and posttranslationally cleaved into the various structural and nonstructural viral proteins (Figure 57.12).

Pestivirus infection of cell culture can results in one of two different phenotypes: cytopathic (CP) where the cells die or noncytopathic (NCP) where the cells appear normal. Although both BDV and CSFV CP isolates have been identified, BVDV is most frequently associated with CP viruses. NCP viruses are the predominate biotype in nature. All CP viruses arise from mutations to NCP usually from recombination events that include point single nucleotide, cellular genes or viral gene insertions or in deletions (Figure 57.13) in or near the NS2-3 gene resulting in the production of the NS3 gene product in CP viruses. These cell culture phenotypic differences do not reflect pathogenesis or severity of disease as the most pathogenic viruses are NCP.

The pestiviruses are very closely related and can only be distinguished by application of monoclonal antibodies and/or molecular biology techniques; however, they tend to be host specific. The pestiviruses are all antigentically

FIGURE 57.12. *Virion structure and genomic organization of Pestivirus. (A) BVDV virion: enveloped, spherical, about 50 nm in diameter; mature virions contain three virus-encoded membrane proteins (Erns, E1 and E2) in addition to the capsid protein. (B) BVDV genome: monopartite, linear, ssRNA(+) genome of about 12 kb; the genome 3′ terminus is not polyadenylated, but terminates with a short poly-(C) tract; there is an IRES at the 5′ end that mediates translation initiation; duplications, deletions, and other rearrangements are found in most cytopathic (CP) pestiviruses isolates. (From viralzone.expasy.org, SIB Swiss Institute of Bioinformatics. http://viralzone.expasy.org/all_by_species/43.html; accessed January 25, 2013.)*

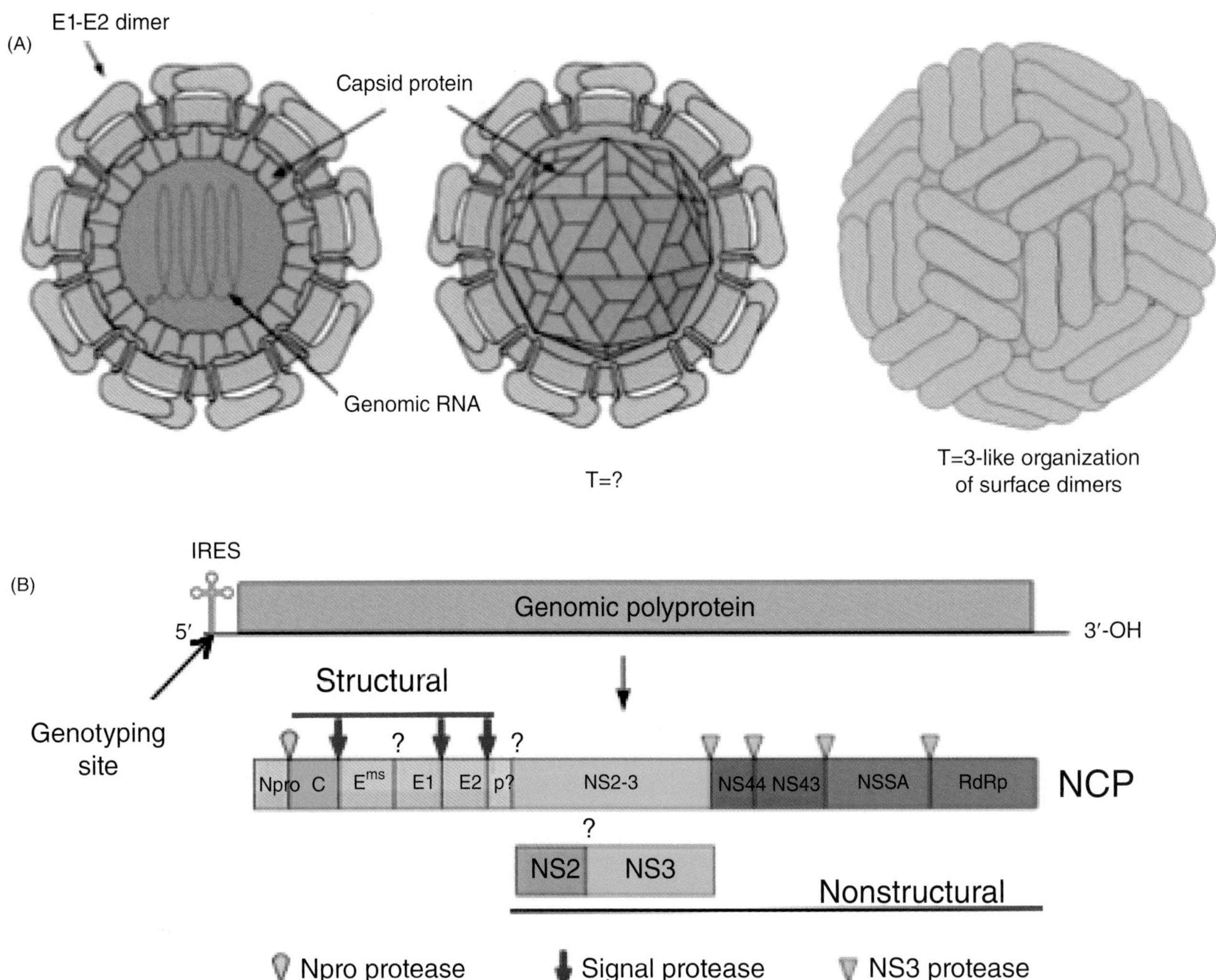

related and include cross-reactive epitopes. Several other pestiviruses have been isolated that are genetically distinct from BVDV (types 1 and 2), BDV, and CSFV, and it is proposed that pestiviruses isolated from a giraffe, for example, be identified as new species. Typing of pestiviruses is based on genetic sequence analysis of 5′ untranslated region (Figure 53.12). Neutralizing antibodies are directed against the Erns and E2 envelope glycoproteins. Animals infected with CP BVDV also mount a strong immune response against the NS3 protein, whereas the antibody response to other viral proteins is generally weak.

Infectivity for Other Species and Culture Systems. BVDV infect cattle, sheep, goats, pigs, and wild ruminants, but BVDV principally is an infectious pathogen of cattle and sometimes sheep. Isolates of BVDV, whether CP or NCP, can be grown in cell culture systems, including various bovine embryonic cell cultures. Immunofluorescence or other immunohistochemical staining methods are used to detect NCP strains of BVDV, which contaminate many commonly used cell lines. CP strains produce plaques and can be used for accurate viral titrations.

Infectivity for Host Species and Culture Systems. While BDV is classically associated with infection of sheep, it can also infect cattle and goats, and pregnant sows that were experimentally infected with BDV gave birth to piglets with cerebellar hypoplasia. The virus can be propagated in primary and secondary cell cultures of bovine and ovine origin and in established cell lines, including pig kidney, fetal lamb muscle, and bovine turbinate.

CFSV only infects domestic swine and wild hogs. CFSV replicates in cultures of porcine cells such as spleen, kidney, testicle, and peripheral blood leukocytes. Most strains

FIGURE 57.13. *Recombinations that generated four CP BVDV strains: (1) insertions of cellular sequences coding for ubiquitin; (2) duplications and rearrangement of viral sequences including the NS3 gene (>2 kb); (3) deletions that led to generation of cp defective interfering particles (DIs); and (4) a small duplication of a viral sequence (27 nucleotides); the insertion is identical with a sequence located about 300 nucleotides upstream. (From Kummerer* et al. *2010.)*

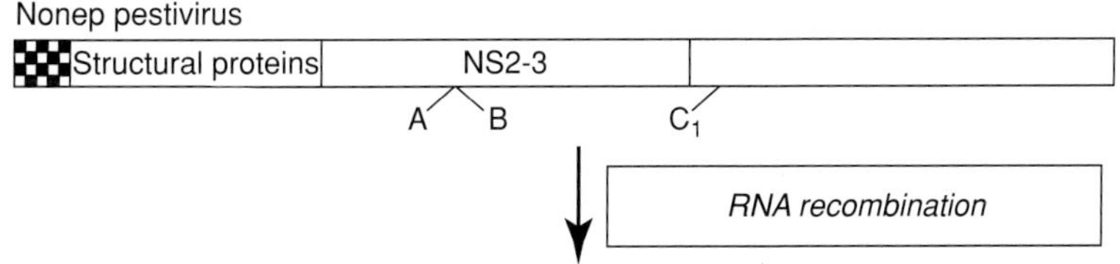

Insertion of cellular sequence

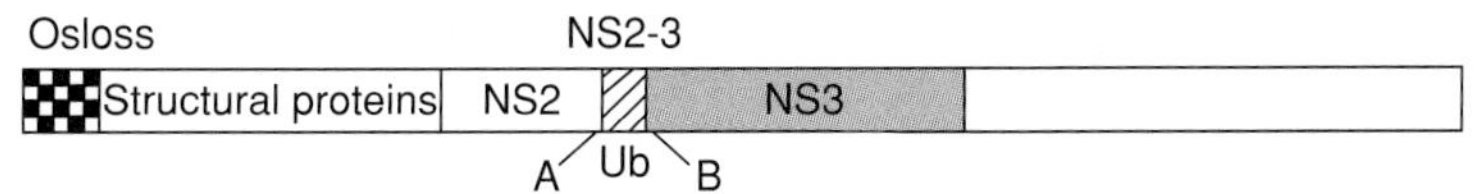

Duplication and rearrangement of viral sequences

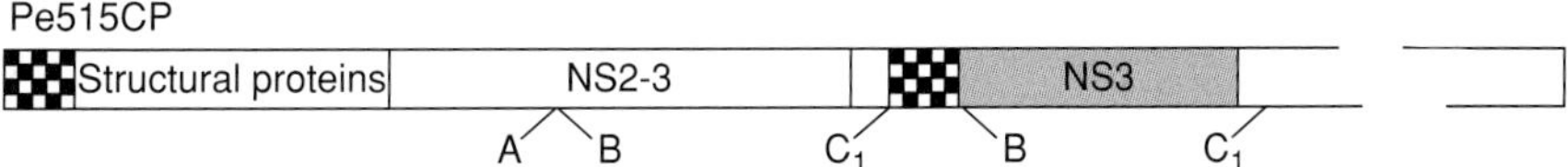

Deletion of viral sequences

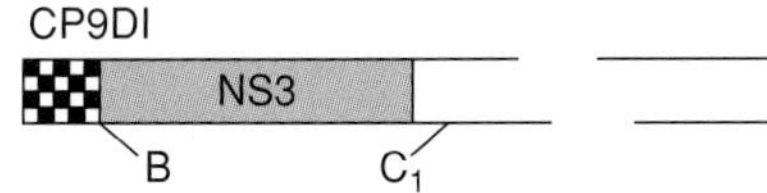

Small duplication of viral sequences

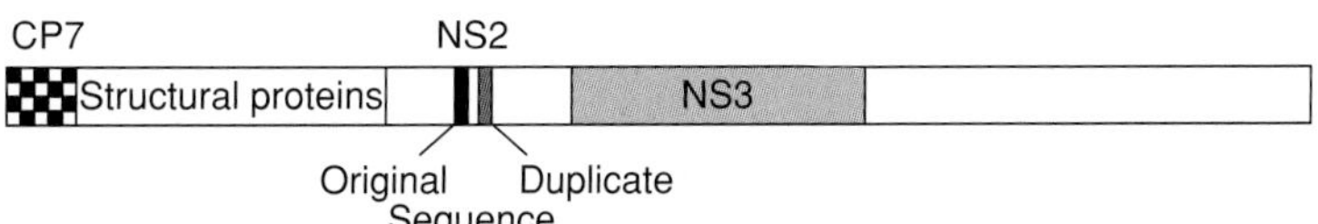

of the virus are noncytopathogenic and may persist in culture for many cell passages. The presence of HCV in infected cell cultures is readily demonstrated by immunofluorescent or immunohistochemical staining techniques. Some cytopathogenic strains have been reported.

Bovine Viral Diarrhea Virus

Disease. BVDV is responsible for a variety of respiratory, digestive tract, and reproductive syndromes. This disease complex actually includes three distinct disease syndromes:

1. The consequences of infection of cattle with BVDV vary from an inapparent infection to severe fatal disease. Acute BVDV infection is a usually mild disease of young calves characterized by leukopenia, fever, and erosions and ulcers of the upper gastrointestinal tract (particularly the hard palate and gums). The infection is typically characterized by high morbidity and low mortality if uncomplicated. Frequently BVDV infection is the viral component of the bovine respiratory disease complex, a disease complex that predisposes cattle to secondary bacterial and/or mycoplasma respiratory infections that result in severe bronchopneumonia, resulting in high morbidity and mortality. Occasionally acute BVDV infection can caused severe, fatal disease with high mortality in both calves and adult animals often accompanied by widespread hemorrhages as a consequence of thrombocytopenia. When this disease syndrome first arose in the 1990s, type II strains of BVDV are now increasingly associated with mild disease in calves, similar to that produced by most type I strains.
2. Reproductive BVDV infection results in a variety of syndromes depending on the stage of development of the fetal calf. Infections prior to 40 days of gestation will result in fetal death. BVDV infection of bovine fetuses with a NCP BVD virus prior to

FIGURE 57.14. *The generation of BVDV persistent infection. (From RL Larson, Kansas State University and D Connor, University of Missouri.)*

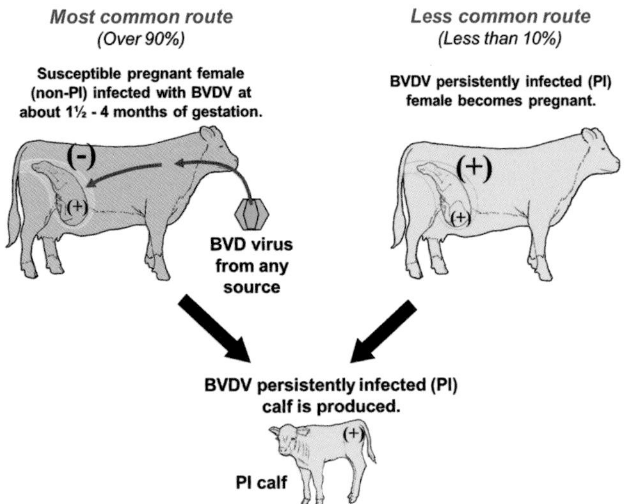

FIGURE 57.15. *The threat of BVDV persistent infection to a herd. (From Rodning and Givens 2010.)*

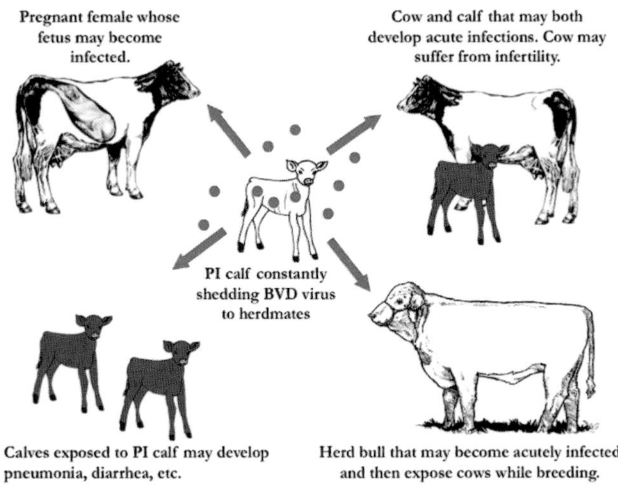

mid-gestation (40–150 days of gestation) often leads to the birth of calves that are persistently infected (PI) with BVDV (Figure 57.14). Usually other animals are the source but a PI cow will always produce a PI calf (Figure 57.14) These animals subsequently serve as a reservoir of virus in the herd, which they transmit both horizontally and vertically (to their own progeny)(Figure 57.15); furthermore, they develop weak or no obvious humoral immune response to the virus with which they are PI. PI animals have a high mortality rate in the first year of life. Calves infected with NCP BVDV after 150 days of gestation (after the immune response develops) are congenitally infected. Although they clear the BVDV infection, lifelong damage can occur to their immune and reproductive systems. Both PI and congenitally infected calves can exhibit "weak calf syndrome" where the calves fail to thrive following birth. Congenital abnormalities can also occur. BVDV can also cause abortion throughout pregnancy and is the most frequent diagnosed viral pathogen from abortions.

3. Mucosal disease (MD) is characterized by low morbidity but high mortality in cattle of several months to several years of age. It is characterized by severe, fatal disease with extensive ulceration of the upper gastrointestinal tract, diarrhea, and lymphopenia. MD occurs only in PI animals.

Epidemiology. BVDV has a worldwide distribution, and infection of cattle is very common with high seroprevalence in most countries of the world. Transmission is by contact and horizontal transfer of virus, particularly from PI carriers of the virus that shed high titers of virus in all of their body secretions and excretions for horizontal spread, and transmits the virus vertically to their progeny (Figure 57.15).

Pathogenesis and Pathology. The pathogenesis and consequences of BVDV infection of cattle are dependent on the age and immune status of cattle at infection, as well as the biological properties of the infecting virus strain. BVDV infection in calves results in systemic infection of variable severity. Lesions in affected calves range from mild erosion and ulceration of the upper gastrointestinal tract to severe ulceration throughout the gastrointestinal tract and disseminated hemorrhages. Highly virulent strains of BVDV can produce severe lesions in susceptible calves that mimic MD.

The lesions associated with congenital BVDV infection include ocular lesions (retinal degeneration and hypoplasia, optic neuritis) and cerebellar atrophy/hypoplasia. PI animals have BVDV virus in all tissues but the hair follicles have high levels of BVDV virus and can be used for diagnostic samples.

MD manifests when a CP strain of BVD virus emerges in the PI animal. The CP strain usually is a mutant of the NCP PI strain and these mutations arise as described earlier. These NCP and CP viruses in MD are referred to as a pair. MD is characterized by the presence of erosions and ulcers on the muzzle, throughout the oral cavity, esophagus, and small intestine (ulcers over Peyers patches are characteristic). There also is widespread necrosis of lymphocytes. The mechanism of tissue destruction in MD currently is uncharacterized but might involve apoptosis of cells.

Host Responses to Infection. BVDV infection of cattle usually results in the production of high titers of neutralizing antibodies in serum, and cattle that recover from infection have long-lasting immunity. BVDV infection of animals in utero prior to 150 days of gestation can result in immunotolerance to BVDV, resulting in persistent postnatal infection and no or very low titers of virus-specific antibodies.

Laboratory Diagnosis. Clinical diagnosis may be difficult. MD must be differentiated from other diseases that cause ulceration of the gastrointestinal tract, including malignant catarrhal fever and rinderpest. Rapid diagnosis is best accomplished by antigen capture ELISA or immunohistochemical staining of the tissues of affected animals with BVDV-specific antibodies. PCR can be used to detect viral nucleic acid from any sample. An ear biopsy has been shown to be an effective sample to use to identify PI animals. Virus isolation also can be used. The widespread use of vaccines complicates serological diagnosis of BVDV infection, as does the low or no obvious titers to BVDV in PI animals.

Treatment and Control. Control of BVDV infection of cattle involves good biosecurity that includes quarantine and testing of new introductions to the herd for PI. Purchased bred animals are a high risk to bring BVDV into the herd. Within the herd, all PI carriers need to be identified and removed. Vaccines are only an adjunct to control and will fail if PI animals are in the herd. Both attenuated (live) or killed BVDV vaccines are used. Concerns have been raised about the use of live attenuated BVDV vaccines, including their potential reversion to virulence, dissemination in cattle populations, and potential to cause immunosuppression as well as fetal infections. In the past, inadvertent contamination of bovine cell cultures used for vaccine production with virulent, but NCP BVDV strains have also occurred. Vaccination of PI cattle with attenuated vaccines can sometimes produce MD. Vaccination prior to 4 months of age in calves may not be effective due to maternal antibody interference and repeated revaccination may be necessary.

Border Disease Virus

Disease. Border disease is a congenital pestivirus disease of sheep characterized by the birth of lambs with abnormal ("hairy") wool and tremors that reflect abnormal myelination in the central nervous system (so-called hairy-shaker lambs). Expression of disease varies depending on gestational age of the lamb at infection as well as the infecting viral strain. Infection of the developing fetus may result in fetal death, mummification, abortion, stillbirth, or birth of abnormal lambs, whereas infection of adult sheep is subclinical.

Epidemiology. BDV was initially described in the late 1940s as a congenital disease of sheep in England and Wales. The disease has since been recognized in many European countries, Australia, New Zealand, Canada, and the United States. The virus persists in sheep, likely in a manner similar to that of BVDV in cattle, and extensive outbreaks of BDV can occur when the virus is introduced into immunologically naive flocks. Transmission of BDV is probably most common by the oral and intranasal routes, from infected animals or infected fetuses.

Pathogenesis and Pathology. BDV infection of immunologically naive sheep results in viremia, with subsequent spread of the virus to the fetus in pregnant animals. Generalized infection of the fetus can lead to fetal death, with or without expulsion, or teratogenesis. The consequences of fetal infection are inversely related to fetal age, thus infection during the first trimester is relatively more severe than infection later in gestation. Infection after 80 days' gestation often results in viral clearance without disease. The teratogenic effect of BDV infection is also dependent on fetal age. Infection of the developing central nervous system leads to reduced or altered myelination and demyelinization, resulting in the characteristic congenital tremors of the affected newborn lambs. Necrosis of the developing brain can cause more serious developmental injury, resulting in hydranencephaly, porencephaly, and/or cerebellar dysplasia.

Host Response to Infection. BDV infection of adult sheep usually results in a prompt humoral immune response characterized by the appearance of long-lived neutralizing antibody in serum. The fetal immune response reflects its gestational age at the time of infection. Infection during the first half of gestation usually leads to persistent postnatal infection and a minimal, inadequate immune response. Such animals may remain persistently infected and seronegative to BDV for the remainder of their lives. Infection during the second half of gestation, at a time when the fetus is gaining immunologic competence, usually results in immune responses that resolve the infection.

Laboratory Diagnosis. Detailed necropsy and histologic evaluation is often diagnostic, especially when immunohistochemical staining is used to identify viral antigens in the tissues of affected lambs. PCR can be used to detect viral nucleic acid from any sample.

Treatment and Control. Control of BDV is difficult. Losses can be high during initial infection of naive animals, whereas losses are relatively minimal when the virus is endemic on a farm. BVDV vaccines are sometimes used.

Classic Swine Fever Virus

Disease. CSFV is an important disease of swine worldwide; although it has been eliminated in many intensive swine-producing countries but often reemerges to cause serious, economically devastating outbreaks. CSFV is characterized by fever (104 °F or higher), leukopenia, and loss of appetite. Affected animals may appear dull and drowsy and crowd together as if chilled. Vomiting and diarrhea are common, as is conjunctivitis, erythema of the skin, and neurologic signs such as paralysis and locomotory disturbances. Infection of pregnant sows can result in small litters, fetal death, premature births, stillbirths, and the birth of piglets with cerebellar ataxia or congenital tremors. Morbidity and mortality are both high during epidemics caused by virulent strains of the virus in fully susceptible swine, whereas disease is less apparent when the virus is endemic, making detection and eradication more difficult.

Epidemiology. CSFV occurs worldwide, but it has been eradicated from North America, Great Britain and Ireland, Scandinavia, Australia and New Zealand, and portions of Europe. It is endemic in extensive areas of Asia, Africa, Europe, and South and Central America. Domestic swine and wild hogs serve as reservoir hosts, often as inapparent carriers. Pigs infected in utero may become persistently infected carriers of the virus, analogous to the reservoirs of other pestiviruses like BVDV and BDV. Transmission is by droplet, fomites, and ingestion of infected materials, particularly uncooked garbage.

Pathogenesis and Pathology. CFSV is an acute, highly contagious disease that is characterized by disseminated intravascular coagulation leading to hemorrhage and infarction in many tissues. The incubation period is short (3–8 days), and the virus first replicates in the lymphoid tissues of the upper respiratory tract or tonsils. The virus then spreads widely and replicates in endothelial cells and mononuclear inflammatory cells throughout the body. The characteristic lesions are petechial hemorrhages on all serous surfaces, lymph nodes (hemorrhagic lymphadenitis), and kidney, and the presence of infarcts in the spleen. More chronic forms of CSFV occur in some endemic areas. Affected pigs may exhibit growth retardation (stunting), chronic diarrhea, and secondary bacterial pneumonia.

Host Response to Infection. Animals that recover from hog cholera have a long-lasting immunity. Neutralizing antibody titers correlate with protection against CFSV infection. Suckling pigs acquire colostral antibodies from the immune dam. Pigs infected in utero with the virus are often persistently infected carriers, whether or not they are healthy at birth.

Laboratory Diagnosis. Diagnosis of CFSV can be suspected in free areas by explosive outbreaks of severe disease in pigs, but the diagnosis always requires laboratory confirmation to distinguish it from other septicemias. The virus is identified in the tissues of affected pigs by immunohistochemical staining or by virus isolation from the spleen, tonsils, lymph nodes, and blood. Since many strains are noncytopathogenic in cell culture, the fluorescent antibody method is required for the detection of CFSV. PCR can be used to detect viral nucleic acid from any sample. The diagnosis of chronic forms of CFSV is more difficult and requires careful laboratory investigation.

Treatment and Control. Control of CFSV depends on whether the virus is endemic in a particular country or region. In free areas, exclusion of the virus is accomplished by regulating the movement (importation) of swine from endemic areas and by prohibiting the feeding of garbage and/or food scraps containing pork products to swine. In endemic areas, vaccination and/or eradication are used. Vaccines for CFSV are attenuated and effective in preventing disease. The use of vaccines prevents serological diagnosis of CFSV infection, complicating efforts to eradicate CFSV from a region or country.

References

Jose J, Snyder JE, and Kuhn RJ (2009). A structural and functional perspective of alphavirus replication and assembly. *Future Microbiol*, **4**, 837–856.

Kummerer BM, Tautz N, Becher P, Theil H-J, and Meyers G (2000). The genetic basis for cytopathogenicity of pestiviruses. *Vet Microbiol*, **77**, 117–128.

Lindsey NP, Staples JE, Lehman JA, and Fischer M (2010) Surveillance for human west Nile Virus Disease—United States, 1999–2008. *MMWR*, **59**(SS02), 1–17, http://www.cdc.gov/mmwr/preview/mmwrhtml/ss5902a1.htm (accessed January 25, 2013)

Pfeffer M and Dobler G (2010) Emergence of zoonotic arboviruses by animal trade and migration. *Parasites & Vectors*, **3**, 35, http://www.parasitesandvectors.com/ content/3/1/35 (accessed January 25, 2013).

Rodning SP and Givens MD (2010) Bovine viral diarrhea virus. Alabama Cooperative Extension System ANR-1367, http://www.aces.edu/pubs/docs/A/ANR-1367/ index2.tmpl (accessed January 25, 2013).

Scott CW and Slobodan P (2009) Alphaviral encephalitides (Chapter 21), in *Vaccines for Biodefense and Emerging and Neglected Diseases* (eds DT Alan Barrettand LR Stanberry). Elsevier.

Strauss JH and Strauss EG (1997) Recombination in Alphaviruses. *Sem Virol*, **8**, 85–94.

van den Hurk AF, Ritchie SA, and Mackenzie JS (2009) Ecology and geographical expansion of Japanese encephalitis virus. *Ann Rev Entomol*, **54**, 17–35.

Weaver SC and Barrett ADT (2004). Transmission cycles, host range, evolution and emergence of arboviral disease. *Nature Rev Micro*, **2**, 789–801.

Further Reading

McLoughlin MF and Graham DA (2007) Alphavirus infections in salmonids—a review. *J Fish Dis*, **30**, 511–531.

OIE Technical Disease Cards: Japanese Encephalitis Virus, Classic Swine Fever Virus, Venezuelan equine encephalitis virus, http://www.oie.int/animal-health-in-the-world/ technical-disease-cards/ (accessed February 9, 2013)

Pfeffer M and Dobler G (2011) Emergence of zoonotic arboviruses by animal tread and migration. *Parasites & Vectors*, http://www.parasitesandvectors.com/content/3/1/35 (accessed January 25, 2013).

Thiel H-J, Collett, MS, Gould EA *et al.* (2005) Family flaviviridae: positive sense single stranded RNA viruses, in *Virus Taxonomy*, pp. 991–998, Academic Press/Elsevier.

Weaver, SC, Frey TK, Huang HV *et al.* (2005) Family togaviridae: positive sense single stranded RNA viruses, in *Virus Taxonomy*, pp. 999–1008, Academic Press/Elsevier.

58 Orthomyxoviridae

Wenjun Ma

The Orthomyxoviridae is a family of RNA viruses, which includes five genera: *Influenzavirus A*, *Influenzavirus B*, *Influenzavirus C*, *Isavirus*, and *Thogotovirus*. A novel genus of this family has been recently identified, which includes Quaranfil, Johnston Atoll, and Lake Chad viruses. Viruses in the first three genera, which are identified by antigenic differences in their nucleoprotein (NP) and matrix (M) proteins, cause influenza disease in vertebrates, including birds, humans, and other mammalian species. Isaviruses infect salmon; thogotoviruses infect both vertebrates and invertebrates, such as mosquitoes and sea lice.

Influenza

Influenza viruses are classified as members of the genus *Orthomyxovirus* in the family Orthomyxoviridae, and are named according to their type, species where isolated (except humans), location where isolated, the successive isolate number from that location, and year of isolation. Influenza viruses are divided into three types, including influenza A, B, and C viruses, based on antigenic differences in their NP and M proteins. All pandemics in human history were caused by the influenza A virus (1918–1919, 1957–1958, 1968–1969, 1977, and 2009) due to the emergence of new subtypes of this virus; the Spanish influenza pandemic in 1918–1919 is the most devastating one, resulting in the deaths of up to 50 million people worldwide.

Classification

Influenza A viruses are further divided into different subtypes based on the antigenic nature of the surface hemagglutinin (HA) and neuraminidase (NA). To date, there are 17 HA and 10 NA subtypes of influenza A virus, all of which except H17 and N10 have been isolated from wild aquatic birds, including waterfowl and shore birds that are the natural reservoir of influenza A viruses. Influenza A viruses are also able to infect a large variety of mammalian species including human, horse, swine, dog, cat, bat, and marine mammals. Influenza B and C viruses infect humans, and the influenza C virus also infects pigs and dogs. A key difference between them is their host range. Whereas influenza B and C viruses are predominantly human pathogens that have sporadically been isolated from seals and pigs, respectively, only influenza A and B viruses cause major outbreaks and severe disease in humans; influenza C is associated with common cold-like illness, principally in children. The nomenclature system for different subtypes of influenza A viruses includes the host of origin, geographic origin, strain number, and year of isolation. A description of the two major surface antigens, the HA and the NA, is given in parentheses, for example, A/swine/Kansas/8/2007 (H1N1). By convention, the host of origin for human strains is now omitted.

These antigenic subtypes are distinguished by double immunodiffusion assays (hemagglutination inhibition and neuraminidase inhibition) with hyperimmune animal sera because such tests revealed antigenic relationships among influenza A virus isolates that were not apparent with other methods.

Morphology

Influenza virus particles are pleomorphic; its envelope can be in spherical and filamentous forms, and the virion envelope is derived from the membranes of host cells. Normally, the virion morphology is irregularly shaped spherical particles 80–120 nm in diameter (Figure 58.1) or filamentous virions 20 nm in diameter and 200–300 nm long (Figure 58.1). There are two distinct types of surface spikes (peplomers): one is the HA with a rod-shaped form and the other is the NA with a mushroom-shaped form and possessing neuraminidase activity. Both the HA and the NA are viral glycoproteins that attach to the viral envelope by short sequences of hydrophobic amino acids (see Figure 58.2 for a representation of the influenza virus). The glycoprotein HA is interposed irregularly by clusters of NA over the virion surface, with a ratio of HA to NA of about 4–5 to 1. The viral envelope surrounds an M protein shell, which in turn surrounds the genome of eight (seven in type C influenza viruses) individual molecules of single-stranded RNA, along with the NP and three large proteins—polymerase basic 1 (PB1), polymerase basic 2 (PB2), and polymerase acidic (PA)—forming the ribonucleoprotein (RNP) complex that is responsible for RNA replication and transcription. Each of the eight genomic RNA segments encodes for one or two proteins. The segmented nature of the influenza virus genome results in the phenomena

Veterinary Microbiology, Third Edition. Edited by D. Scott McVey, Melissa Kennedy and M.M. Chengappa.

FIGURE 58.1. *Electron micrograph demonstrating irregularly shaped spherical particles (80–120 nm in diameter) of an avian influenza virus. (Courtesy of Dr David Swayne, Southeast Poultry Research Laboratory, USDA/Agricultural Research Service, Athens, Georgia.)*

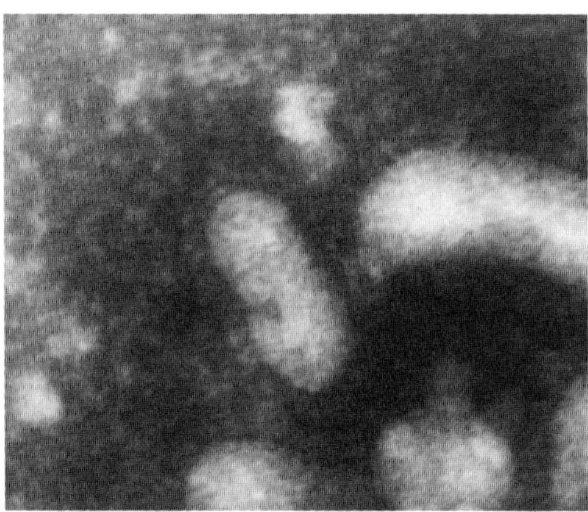

of high-frequency reassortment; when cells are infected with two or more different influenza A viruses, exchange of RNA segments from parental viruses allows the generation of progeny viruses containing a novel combination of genes.

Viral Genome

The genome of influenza A virus contains eight segments of negative-sense RNA, varying in length between 890 and 2341 nucleotides, which encode 10 or 11 proteins. The segments 1 and 3 encode RNA-dependent PB2 and PA proteins. The segment 2 encodes the PB1 and in some virus strains also encodes a second short protein PB1-F2 using an additional open reading. The segments 4 and 6 encode the surface glycoprotein HA and NA, respectively. The segment 5 encodes the NP that binds around the viral RNA (vRNA). The segments 7 and 8 encode two proteins (M1/M2 and NS1/NS2) due to differentially spliced transcripts. The function of each protein is described in the next paragraph. Influenza viral variation is frequent and occurs based on two major mechanisms: antigenic drift and shift. Antigenic drift is the accumulation of random mutations in viral genes because of low fidelity of the vRNA polymerase. Antigenic drift is responsible for the variability of the human seasonal influenza viruses. The segmented nature of the influenza genome contributes to antigenic shift or reassortment that occurs when a cell is infected with different influenza viruses, resulting in exchange of vRNA segments and generation of new viruses with a novel combination of genes. The 1957 Asian flu pandemic and the 1968 Hong Kong flu pandemic as well as the 2009 pandemic are a result of antigenic shift.

FIGURE 58.2. *Diagram of an avian influenza virus particle. Note the HA and NA surface proteins and the eight RNA segments of the viral genome. (Used by permission, Swayne and King .)*

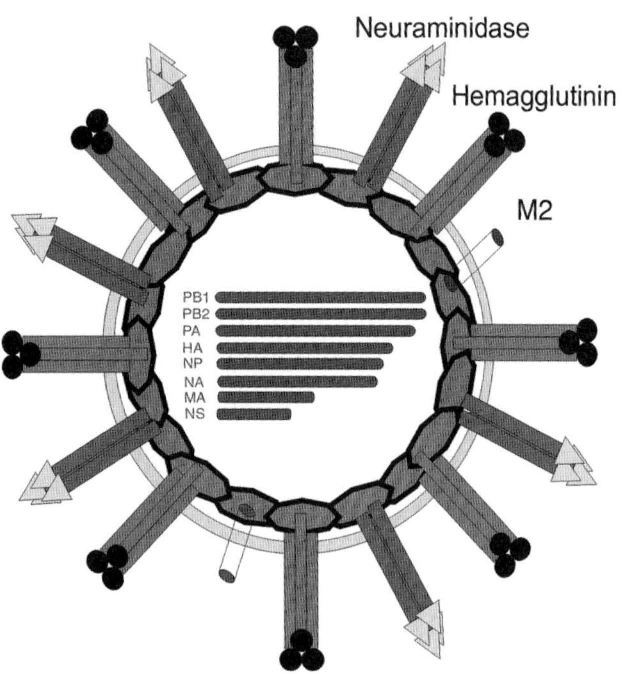

Viral Proteins

Hemagglutinin. Influenza A and B viruses have two major surface glycoprotein antigens: hemagglutinin (HA or H) and neuraminidase (NA or N). For influenza A virus, 17 antigenically distinct HAs have been recognized, all of which except the H17 can be found circulating in aquatic birds, where they are generally carried asymptomatically. The HA protein of influenza A virus is a type I transmembrane glycoprotein, which is initially synthesized as a single polypeptide precursor (HA0) with a molecular weight of approximately 76 kDa. The mature HA forms homotrimers, and each monomer is generated by cleavage of HA0 into HA1 and HA2 subunits by trypsin-like or furin-like proteases. The HA of influenza A virus has two functions during early steps of the replication of the virus in host cells: receptor binding and membrane fusion. First, it attaches the virus to the cell surface by binding to the cellular receptors that are sialic acids of cell surface glycoproteins and glycolipids. Second, once bound it promotes viral penetration by mediating fusion of the endosomal and viral membranes to release the viral genome into the cell cytoplasm of target cells. The conserved sialic acid receptor-binding pocket is located on the HA1 subunit at the distal end of the molecule. There are five major antigenic epitopes A–E on the HA1 subunits of the influenza HA. All strains of influenza viruses are capable of agglutinating erythrocytes from humans, guinea pigs, and chickens as well as many other species. Antibodies to the HA prevent infection of host cells via neutralizing the virus and are important to host immunity. In fact, it is the variation of this molecule that is primarily responsible for emergence of new strains of the virus leading to new outbreaks of influenza, and the failure to control them by vaccination.

Neuraminidase. The NA is a type II membrane glycoprotein that is located on the surface of the virus. The shape of NA protein is mushroom-shaped tetramers with an average molecular weight of approximately 220 kDa, which is composed of four identical monomers. The ectodomain of NA consists of a stalk and a globular head. The stalk and the transmembrane domain sequences are highly variable among the ten recognized NA subtypes. The NA stalk separates the head region with the enzymatic center from the transmembrane and cytoplasmic domains. The NA is responsible for the cleavage of the sialic acid residues from the virus and the infected cells during both entry and release from the cells. In addition, it seems that NA helps the virus to penetrate through the mucin layer in the respiratory tract to reach the epithelial cells, which are the target cells of the virus. The enzyme activity of the NA prevents self-aggregation and promotes release of the newly made virus from the infected cells. The antibody against the NA does not protect against infection but does confer protection against disease and reduces transmissibility.

Nucleoprotein. The NP was originally designated the soluble, or "S," antigen and is a structural protein with a molecular weight of approximately 56 kDa. NP encapsidates vRNA and interacts with PB1, PB2, and PA subunits in the vRNA polymerase forming the RNP, which is involved in viral genome transcription and replication. NP also forms homooligomers to maintain the structure of RNP. It is also thought to be the major switching factor that determines whether genomic vRNA is transcribed into mRNA or used as template to synthesize complementary RNA (cRNA) for genome replication.

The NP is one of the type-specific antigens used to distinguish genera of influenza virus, and can be identified by enzyme-linked immunosorbent assay (ELISA), double immunodiffusion, complement fixation, single radial diffusion, and agar gel precipitation. Antibodies to the NP do not provide passive protection. However, the NP of influenza A viruses is a major protein recognized by cytotoxic lymphocytes (CTLs).

Matrix Protein. RNA segment 7 of influenza A viruses encodes two proteins M1 and M2 by RNA transcript splicing, and both matrix proteins are nonglycosylated and type-specific antigens. The matrix protein (M1), the most abundant protein in virus particles, which lies inside the lipid envelope, is associated with both the RNP and the viral envelope. The M1 protein is thought to play a fundamental role in virus assembly budding processes. The functions of the M1 include (i) interaction with vRNP and nuclear export protein (NEP) and regulation of vRNP transport between the cytoplasm and the nucleus; (ii) regulation of vRNP transcription and replication; (iii) interaction with viral envelope proteins including HA, NA, and M2; (iv) recruitment of viral components at the assembly site and initiation of budding; and (v) recruitment of host components for bud completion and virus release.

The M2 protein acts as an ion channel and plays a role in triggering the viral uncoating in the endosome. It has been well studied because virus ion channel is an ideal antiviral drug target. Amantadine and rimantadine have been developed and used clinically as an anti-influenza drug. However, amantadine-resistant strains have been detected widely and contain mutations in the transmembrane domain of the M2 protein. Antibodies against M1 protein provide little, if any, protection against infection. The M2 protein is one of important proteins of influenza A viruses recognized by CTLs.

Nonstructural Proteins. RNA segment 8 of influenza A viruses encodes two proteins by mRNA splicing: nonstructural protein 1 (NS1) and nuclear export protein (NEP), formerly referred to as the NS2 protein. The NS1 protein of influenza A viruses is not a structural component of the virion, but is expressed at very high levels in infected cells. The NS1 protein is a multifunctional protein with a molecular weight of 26 kDa, and is an antagonist of innate host type I interferon-mediated antiviral response and the antiviral effects of interferon-induced proteins, such as dsRNA-dependent protein kinase R and 2′-5′-oligoadenylate synthetase/RNase L. NS1 also acts directly to modulate other important aspects of the virus replication cycle including (i) temporal regulation of vRNA synthesis; (ii) enhancement of viral mRNA translation; (iii) regulation of virus particle morphogenesis; (iv) suppression of host immune/apoptotic responses; and (v) activation of phosphoinositide 3-kinase pathway.

The NEP was thought to be a nonstructural protein, but is present in small amounts in the virions in association with the RNP through interaction with the M1 protein. The NEP functions to mediate the export of newly synthesized RNPs from the nucleus.

Polymerase Proteins. The three largest vRNAs encode the three subunits of the RNA-dependent RNA polymerase: PA and PB1 and PB2. The polymerase subunits PB2, PB1, and PA together with the NP and vRNAs form the RNP complex, which is responsible for viral transcription and replication. In the nucleus, influenza polymerase employs a "cap-snatching" mechanism to initiate vRNA replication. The PB2 binds cap-containing cellular mRNA in order to produce primers for RNA synthesis. An endonuclease from the PA subunit cuts the capped oligonucleotide pre-mRNA as primers for viral mRNA synthesis. The polymerase then transcribes vRNA by elongation, leading to the formation of viral mRNA. The PB1 subunit is thought to be involved in the catalytic activity of nucleotide elongation. During the viral genome replication, the vRNAs are used as templates to synthesize cRNAs that are positive-sense antigenomic RNAs, and then the cRNAs are transcribed into vRNAs that are incorporated into progeny viruses. The influenza polymerase has no proofreading activity, resulting in a high gene mutation rate of approximately one error per replicated genome.

PB1-F2, a short polypeptide expressed from an alternative -1 open reading frame of the PB1 in some influenza A stains, is believed to be an important determinant of influenza virus virulence. However, the PB1 segment of many influenza A viruses encodes a truncated PB1-F2.

Equine Influenza

Disease

Influenza is an acute respiratory disease of horses. While horses of all ages are affected, those between 2 and 6 months of age are at greatest risk. The mortality rate of equine influenza is low, whereas the morbidity rate can approach 100%. The incubation period lasts 1–5 days. Disease is manifested by a high fever, up to 106 °F, which lasts about 3 days. Other clinical signs include a frequent, strong, dry cough lasting 1–3 weeks, a nasal discharge that is initially serous in character but that later becomes mucoid, anorexia, depression, photophobia, lacrimation with a mucopurulent ocular discharge, and corneal opacity (sometimes with loss of sight). Limb edema and muscle soreness can occur and, in some severe outbreaks, acute deaths due to fulminant pneumonia have occurred. Enteritis was described in a 1989 outbreak in northern China due to a new equine influenza virus, A/equine/2/Jilin; this virus is considered to have emerged from birds into horses.

Equine influenza is caused by two subtypes of influenza A viruses: A/equine/1 (H7N7) and A/equine/2 (H3N8), based on antigenic differences in their HA and NA. There is no immunological cross-reaction between these two subtypes. A/equine/1 has one prototype, A/equine/1/Prague, which was first isolated in 1956. Antigenic drift has occurred among A/equine/1 viruses with the subsequent designation of two subgroups that do not appear to differ significantly in terms of their immunity after vaccination. In recent years, the H7N7 subtype has not been isolated from horses and is believed to be extinct or to be persisting at a very low level in some regions. Strains of A/equine/2 virus have been responsible for all known outbreaks of the disease since 1980. Significant drift has occurred among A/equine/2 viruses from the original prototype A/equine/2/Miami/63 that was first isolated from a severe outbreak in Florida horses in 1963, resulting in the evolution of two distinct lineages that have been designated the “American-like” and “European-like” lineages based on the initial geographical distribution of the viruses. In August 2007, an outbreak of equine influenza occurred in Australia, which is one of previously equine influenza virus-free countries, and was caused by the American-like lineage. Emergence of variant strains has shown that considerable antigenic drift occurs in the A/equine/2 viruses, which may have implications for efficacious vaccination. Influenza occurs in horses worldwide, and is a common and troublesome problem when horses are congregated at shows, sales, stables, and racetracks.

Etiologic Agent

Resistance to Physical and Chemical Agents. Equine influenza virus is usually inactivated at 56°C in 30 min. Like type A influenza viruses, the virus is inactivated by phenol, lipid solvents, detergent, formalin, and oxidizing agents such as ozone.

Infectivity for Other Species and Culture Systems. Equine influenza virus normally infects horses, asses, and mules, and also is able to cross the species barrier to infect dogs. The first cross-species transmission of the equine influenza H3N8 virus to racing greyhounds was reported in the United States in 2004, resulting in respiratory disease and death of infected dogs. Retrospective studies in the United Kingdom have shown that the equine influenza H3N8 virus is responsible for severe outbreaks of respiratory disease in dogs. Equine influenza virus can be experimentally adapted to infect mice when introduced intranasally. All orthomyxoviruses, including equine influenza virus, can be propagated in the allantoic cavity of embryonated chicken eggs. Equine influenza virus can also be grown in chick embryo kidney, bovine kidney, rhesus monkey kidney, and human embryo kidney cells.

Host–Virus Relationship

Pathogenesis and Pathology. Equine influenza virus infects both the upper and lower respiratory tracts. Virus antigen has been detected in samples collected from the nasopharynx, trachea, bronchus, and alveoli by bronchoalveolar lavage. There is an early lymphopenia with accompanying enlargement of the lymph nodes of the head. Initially there may only be a slight serous nasal discharge, which later becomes mucoid. Fatal pneumonia can occur in foals and on occasion in older animals. Occasionally there is ventral edema of the trunk and lower limbs. A/equine/2 has been known to cause a postinfection encephalopathy in foals. Catarrhal and even hemorrhagic enteritis may occur. Necrotizing bronchiolitis in which the bronchioles are progressively obstructed is characteristic of equine influenza. Severe necrotizing myositis with elevated serum enzyme levels has been observed with A2 infections. Most animals recover within 2–3 weeks; those that do not may develop chronic obstructive pulmonary disease. Prolonged recovery and severity of disease appear to be related to the level of stress that an affected horse undergoes, thus adequate rest is important for recovery.

Equine influenza virus is most commonly transmitted via aerosol and can spread extremely rapidly due to the frequent, violent cough of infected horses. Infected animals continue to shed the virus for about 5 days after the first signs appear. The virus can also be spread by fomites, for example, the contaminated vehicles.

Laboratory Diagnosis

A tentative clinical diagnosis of equine influenza can be made from the characteristic rapid spread of the disease, especially among stabled horses, and the frequent dry cough of affected horses. A definitive diagnosis requires isolation of the virus, demonstration of viral antigen, or demonstration of rising antibody titers between acute and convalescent sera by complement fixation and hemagglutination inhibition tests. During outbreaks it is important to isolate and type the causative strains of the influenza virus for the success of future vaccination programs.

The clinical samples are taken by nasal or nasopharyngeal swabs or by nasal or tracheal washings. The washings are usually taken by endoscopy. The virus can be isolated in embryonated chicken eggs or cell cultures, and it can take 5–10 days to complete. Once isolated, the virus can be sequenced to determine its phylogeny. There are three tests for detecting the presence of antibodies to equine influenza viruses in the horse blood: the hemagglutination inhibition, the single radial hemolysis, and the competitive ELISA. Other assays have been developed that rely on detecting vRNA (real-time polymerase chain reaction test, qPCR), viral proteins (antigen-capture ELISA test) or various commercially available rapid assay kits (such as Directigen Flu A, Directigen Flu EZ, and A+B tests).

Treatment and Control

Vaccination is somewhat an effective method in preventing influenza in horses. Protection, however, is dependent on the manner of vaccination and the quality of the vaccine, with particular emphasis placed on proper selection of vaccine strains. Available vaccines contain the inactivated virus of both A/equine/1 and A/equine/2 subtypes. Classically, A/equine/Prague/56 (H7N7) and A/equine/Miami/63 (H3N8) have been used as the prototype A/equine/1 and A/equine/2 strains, respectively. There is increasing evidence of antigenic diversity among contemporary equine influenza viruses that circulate in nature, suggesting that the effectiveness of the conventional vaccine strains in providing protection will become limited with time. For this reason, current vaccines include some of the newer variant A/equine/2 viruses. However, the level of protection has varied as a result of the higher rate of antigenic drift of H3N8 strains. The various inactivated vaccines available are incorporated with adjuvants that have proved to significantly augment their immunogenic potential. Initial immunization requires two doses of vaccines 2–4 weeks apart. These should be followed by a single booster when the horse is 1 year of age and then repeated every 6 months until the horse is about 3 years of age, at which time the booster interval may be increased to not more than 1 year. More recently, live attenuated vaccines have become available in some countries.

In horses, a relationship has been shown between titers of the nasal antibody to the influenza virus and resistance to infection. The presence of prechallenge serum antibody has also been shown to shorten the duration of viral excretion and febrile response.

In addition to vaccination, isolation and quarantine measures are advised during outbreaks to reduce the spread of disease, and disinfection of affected premises, equipment, and clothing is essential to prevent mechanical transmission of the virus.

Swine Influenza

Disease

Swine influenza is an important respiratory disease of pigs. The natural disease commonly affects large numbers of animals in the herd with high morbidity (approaching 100%) and generally low mortality (<1%) rates. Swine influenza occurs more frequently during colder months. Disease caused by swine influenza alone is usually mild; however, disease may be severe when secondary infections occur. The incubation period is short, between 1 and 3 days, with rapid recovery beginning 4–7 days after onset. Disease symptoms include fever, anorexia, weakness, dyspnea, sneezing, coughing, and nasal discharge. Some animals develop conjunctivitis, pulmonary edema, or bronchopneumonia.

Swine influenza was first recognized during the massive human influenza pandemic in 1918, and subsequent studies confirm that a similar H1N1 virus caused disease in both humans and swine. Swine influenza virus can spread from pigs to humans causing illness, and there is concern that swine may serve as a reservoir from which influenza virus can emerge to precipitate human epidemics and pandemics. Although 16 HA and 9 NA subtypes have been isolated from birds, only the H1N1, H3N2, and H1N2 subtypes have established in swine and are most commonly responsible for disease outbreaks in pigs worldwide. Genetic and antigenic differences among strains of swine influenza viruses have been observed; for example, Eurasian avian-like H1, human-like H1, and classical H1 swine influenza viruses exist in pigs worldwide, and at least five clusters of H3N2 swine influenza viruses have been found in swine herds in North America.

Host–Virus Relationship

Pathogenesis and Pathology. On postmortem examination of swine with influenza, the mucosa of the upper respiratory tract is congested and the bronchial and mediastinal lymph nodes are enlarged and edematous. Affected lungs display a purple-red, multifocal to coalescing consolidation of predominantly cranioventral portions of the lung. Microscopic lesions usually consist of airways filled with exudate, widespread alveolar atelectasis, interstitial pneumonia, and emphysema. Peribronchial and perivascular cellular infiltration is also seen.

Swine influenza virus can be transmitted by droplet and aerosol infection, and also direct contact between infected and uninfected animals. Infection with aerosols and droplets produced by pigs coughing and sneezing is an important way of transmission of swine influenza. The virus can be spread rapidly through a herd, resulting in infection of all the pigs in a few days. The direct contact is the main route of transmission of swine influenza by pig touching noses. The virus is shed by nasal secretions, which are laden with viruses during the acute febrile stage. If the pigs are raised in the concentrated feeding operations, it will increase the risk of transmission of swine influenza virus. Transmission can also happen through humans and wild animals, which can spread disease to uninfected farms from infected farms.

Laboratory Diagnosis

Swine influenza is suspected whenever there is an "explosive" appearance of respiratory disease involving many pigs, particularly during the fall or winter months. A definitive diagnosis requires either viral isolation from nasal secretions or the lung of dead pigs or demonstration of a rising titer between acute and convalescent sera or vRNA and antigen detection. Swine influenza virus can be cultivated in 10- to 12-day-old embryonated chicken eggs and various tissue culture monolayer systems involving primary or stable cell cultures, such as Madin–Darby canine kidney, PK15 (porcine kidney), and Swine testicular cells.

Treatment and Control

Swine that have recovered from influenza develop the neutralizing antibodies, which normally can protect animals with infection of homologous viruses. Therefore, vaccination is one of efficient measures to control swine influenza. Swine flu vaccines have been developed and commercially available and widely used in European countries and the United States. Commercial swine influenza-inactivated vaccines contain H1N1 and H3N2 subtypes of circulating viruses and are effective when the virus strains used in vaccines match the epidemic viruses. Prevention and control of swine influenza by vaccination has become very difficult in recent years because the rapid evolution of the virus and emergence of the novel virus resulted in evading immune responses to the traditional vaccines. Since much of the illness and death associated with swine flu involves secondary infection by other pathogens, control strategies that rely on vaccination may be insufficient. The best way to deal with swine influenza is to prevent the occurrence and spread of the disease. Therefore, facility and herd management is also essential to control swine influenza. Facility management includes using standard sanitary measures to control viruses in the environment. Influenza A viruses are easily inactivated by disinfectants, heat, and formalin. Be sure to clean and disinfect trucks, trailers, and any equipment that may be contaminated. If a group of finishing pigs had swine influenza, it is necessary to clean and disinfect the house completely before the next group enters. Pigs carrying or exposed to influenza virus are normally responsible for the introduction of viruses to uninfected herds; therefore, new animals should be quarantined before they are added into herds. Treatment entails supportive measures including a draft-free environment with clean, dry, dust-free bedding; fresh clean water; and a good source of feed. Antibiotics given on a herd basis may help prevent secondary bacterial infection.

Avian Influenza

Disease

The first description of avian influenza, a contagious disease of poultry associated with high mortality, was reported in northern Italy in 1878 and was termed "fowl plague" initially. Influenza A virus was found to be the pathogeny of "fowl plaque" until 1955. The term "fowl plaque" was replaced by "highly pathogenic avian influenza (HPAI)" at the First International Symposium on Avian Influenza in 1981. To date, 16 different HA and 9 different NA subtypes of influenza A viruses have been isolated from waterfowl and shorebirds. There are 144 theoretical combinations (e.g., H5N1, H9N2, and H6N1) between 16 HA and 9 NA that make up different subtypes of avian influenza viruses. Avian influenza is further classified as HPAI and low pathogenic avian influenza (LPAI) on the basis of specific molecular genetics and pathogenesis criteria. The HPAI is an extremely contagious, multiorgan systemic disease of poultry resulting in high mortality. Up to now, all HPAI outbreaks have been caused by the H5 or H7 subtype of viruses in which their HA proteins possess multiple basic amino acids at the cleavage site. Most of avian influenza viruses are the LPAI viruses, which are usually associated with mild disease in poultry, and they only replicate in respiratory and intestinal tracts. The HAs of LPAI viruses normally have a single basic amino acid at the cleavage site.

Infection of the domestic poultry with avian influenza viruses including the LPAI or HPAI virus has caused significant losses for the industry worldwide. Waterfowl and shorebirds, the natural reservoir of influenza A viruses, normally do not show any clinical signs with infection of different subtypes of viruses. In wild ducks, influenza virus replicates in intestinal mucosal cells and is excreted in high concentrations. The virus has been isolated from lake and pond water, and surveys have demonstrated that as many as 60% of juvenile birds may be infected as they congregate prior to migration. In 2005, over 6000 wild migratory birds died from HPAI H5N1 infection in Qinghai Lake in China. From then on, the HPAI H5N1 virus has been spread to Europe, the Middle East, and Africa, most likely through the migratory birds.

Host–Virus Relationship

Geographic Distribution, Reservoir, and Mode of Transmission. Although LPAI viruses exist in wild birds and poultry worldwide, HPAI is a major threat to the world's poultry industry. Before 2002, only few HPAI outbreaks in poultry were documented. Large-scale outbreaks of HPAI H5N1 started in domestic poultry in several countries in Southeast Asia from 2003, including China, Indonesia, Thailand, and Vietnam. Subsequently, the HPAI H5N1 spread to Europe, the Middle East, and Africa after wild birds were killed by the H5N1 virus at Qinghai Lake in China in 2005, resulting in HPAI outbreaks worldwide. This phenomenon caused influenza experts to believe that the H5N1 virus would cause the next pandemic. Luckily, the field H5N1 isolates still have not gained the ability of human-to-human transmission.

The disease is transmitted through poultry flocks mainly through ingestion of the virus, but it may also be transmitted by inhalation and by mechanical means involving movement of personnel throughout flocks or between premises. In birds, avian influenza viruses are shed in the feces as well as in saliva and nasal secretions. The feces contain large amounts of virus, and the fecal–water–oral transmission is a major route in waterfowl, but fecal–water–cloacal route of transmission is also possible. Furthermore, avian influenza may be transmitted on such objects as shoes, clothing, and crates that come in contact with infected birds or premises. While the possibility of vertical transmission of avian influenza through infected eggs exists, no evidence demonstrates its spread by this means. The transmission mode of HPAI H5N1 viruses is intensely debated; migratory birds and poultry trades have been discussed as potential factors.

Waterfowl have been implicated as the major natural reservoir for influenza. Infected ducks can shed the virus for prolonged periods without showing clinical signs or producing a detectable antibody response. There is evidence that influenza can persist in some birds for several months after infection. Various factors affect the viral life cycle, including cell surface receptors, host body temperature, immune responses, thus different species-specific virus lineage formed after adaptation in different animal species. Avian influenza viruses have been found to be capable of infecting a wide range of mammalian species in addition to birds, including humans, pigs, horses, dogs, cats, and terrestrial birds, exhibiting their interspecies transmissibility.

Pathogenesis and Pathology. The pathogenesis of avian influenza varies widely depending on strains of the virus, age, and species infected, concurrent infections, and husbandry. It appears that the HA gene is important in pathogenicity. The HAs of highly pathogenic H5 and H7 viruses contain multiple basic amino acids at the cleavage site that are recognized by ubiquitous proteases, such as furin and PC6, resulting in a systemic infection. By contrast, the HAs of LPAI viruses lack this series of basic residues at the cleavage site and thus are cleaved by proteases in a limited number of organs, restricting viral replication to the respiratory system. In addition to the HA gene, other genes such as PB2 and NS1 have also been identified to affect viral pathogenicity.

Sudden deaths without any clinical signs may occur in poultry infected with an HPAI virus; at necropsy, no obvious lesion exists in the dead avian body. Chickens without immediate death may exhibit listless, edema, and cyanosis of the comb, wattles, and legs. At necropsy, lesions include foci of necrosis of various sites including the skin, comb, wattles, spleen, liver, lung, kidney, intestine, and pancreas. There may be fibrinous exudates in the air sacs, oviduct, pericardial sac, or peritoneum. Other lesions include petechiation of the heart muscle, abdominal fat, and the mucosa of the proventriculus, nonsuppurative encephalitis, and serofibrinous pericarditis. Studies showed that chickens infected by the LPAI virus had histologic lesions limited to the respiratory system or lacked histologic lesions. The other poultry species, such as ducks, geese, ratites, and pigeons, is less vulnerable to avian influenza; however, infection with HPAI viruses may cause nervous symptoms including ataxia, torticollis, and seizures.

Laboratory Diagnosis

Avian influenza viruses can be identified by reverse transcription polymerase chain reaction (RT-PCR) assays, antigen detection, and virus isolation. Influenza A subtype-specific RT-PCR or real-time RT-PCR tests have been developed and utilized widely; these kinds of assays are usually used for the primary and rapid detection of avian influenza with high sensitivity. However, these assays need to be targeted at genes that are highly conserved among different subtypes to avoid false negative. Antigen-capture ELISA tests have been used for rapid viral detection. However, the main limitation of antigen-capture tests is the low sensitivity, which makes this assay unsuitable for monitoring and early detection of avian influenza. Virus isolation is a traditional method for the detection and identification of avian influenza viruses. Avian influenza viruses can be cultivated in chick embryos; duckling, calf, and monkey kidney cell cultures, so viruses could be isolated from samples of trachea, lung, air sac, sinus exudate, or cloacal swabs. The presence of influenza A virus in allantoic fluids or cell culture can be confirmed by HA assay, antigen-capture ELISA, or sequencing. For further subtyping of the virus, hemagglutination and neuraminidase inhibition tests should be conducted by using a battery of antisera against each of the 16 hemagglutinin (H1–H16) and 9 neuraminidase (N1–N9) subtypes.

Treatment and Control

Recovered birds remain immune to subsequent challenge by a homologous strain for at least several months. It has been demonstrated that the anti-HA antibody is important for protection against infection while the anti-NA antibody protects against disease and reduces virus shedding but does not prevent infection. Different avian influenza vaccines, such as inactivated whole virus vaccine, Newcastle disease virus vectored, or fowlpox virus vectored vaccine expressing the HA from avian influenza viruses, have been developed and commercially available and used to control avian influenza. Normally, they have been shown effective in protection against infection of viruses. However, there are a lot of challenges for the control of avian influenza owing to great genetic and antigenic diversity among avian viruses and rapid evolution of influenza A virus. Therefore, only relying on vaccination is not enough to control avian influenza. Careful husbandry and strict biosecurity is necessary for the control and prevention of avian influenza. Careful husbandry to prevent the introduction of the virus into the flock is important. New birds should not be introduced into a started flock, and careful precautions should be taken to prevent either direct or indirect contact with wild, migratory, or exotic birds. Since turkeys have been found also to be susceptible to a swine influenza virus, it is a good management practice not to have pigs on the same farm as turkeys. Eggs for hatching should come from flocks demonstrated to be free of the virus. The virus has been demonstrated to persist for 105 days in liquid manure following depopulation. Strict measures should be employed to eliminate movement of personnel and equipment, potentially contaminated by manure, between flocks and premises. During an outbreak, isolation of a flock along with orderly marketing of the flock should be considered. Treatment of infected flocks with broad-spectrum antibiotics is useful in controlling secondary bacterial infections, and proper nutrition and husbandry may help reduce mortality.

Zoonotic Significance of Animal Influenzas

A growing body of evidence suggests that pandemic strains of human influenza arise as a result of reassortment between different (human and animal or animal and animal) strains of influenza A virus. For example, both 1957 H2N2 Asian flu and 1968 H3N2 Hong Kong flu viruses are reassortants between human and avian influenza viruses, and 2009 pandemic H1N1 virus is generated by reassortment between North American and Eurasian swine influenza viruses. Waterfowl appear to be of particular significance in the origin of new human isolates. Ducks appear to act as a "melting pot" where various strains of influenza can come together and undergo genetic reassortment, resulting in the generation of new strains of influenza. Although little is known whether the past pandemic viruses are produced in pigs, swine have been considered as the "mixing vessels" of "avian-like" and "human-like" influenza viruses. The supportive evidences include that pigs have receptors for both avian and human influenza viruses; and that triple-reassortant swine influenza viruses carrying the gene from swine, avian, and human influenza viruses have been circulating in swine herds in North America for more than 12 years and sporadically transmitted to and infected humans. Since the internal and HA genes are critical for host range, and the HA and NA are important to host immunity, reassortment events in an intermediate host, such as swine or quail, can result in the formation of new virus strains. They contain the same or similar internal genes but possess very different HA and NA proteins and this HA is able to bind the mammalian receptors. The novel viruses generated in this manner might still be infective to humans but possess surface antigens that are very different than those to which the human population previously was exposed (and immune). The result could be a substantial influenza pandemic as the new strain rapidly spreads through a susceptible population.

Normally avian influenza viruses do not cross the species barrier to infect humans and other mammalian hosts directly. However, the accumulated evidences demonstrate that avian influenza viruses can directly infect human beings. The first outbreak of H5N1 avian influenza in Hong Kong in 1997 caused death of 6–18 infected people. Since 2005 the H5N1 HPAIV has caused an outbreak in wild birds in Qinghai Lake in China, and the H5N1 HPAIV has been spread to Europe, the Middle East, and Africa from southeast countries. Currently, the H5N1 HPAI is endemic in poultry in several countries, for example, Egypt and Vietnam, and human infection with this virus continues to be reported. As of February 24, 2012, 586 of confirmed human cases for H5N1 HPAIV have been reported to World Health Organization and 346 of them died. The H5N1 HPAIV has been considered to be the candidate to cause the next pandemic. Furthermore, other subtypes of avian influenza viruses, such as H9N2 and H7N7, have also been found to infect humans directly. Fortunately, all of these avian influenza viruses including H5N1 and H9N2 do not have the ability of human-to-human transmission. Obviously, avian influenza is an important zoonotic disease for humans.

Swine are susceptible to infection with human, avian, and swine influenza viruses, suggesting that the novel virus might be generated by reassortment in this host to cause epidemic and pandemic due to no immunity against this virus in humans. Especially, the H5N1 and H9N2 avian influenza viruses have been isolated from pigs in Southeast Asian countries. Southeast Asia has been considered as "influenza hotbeds" because of the proximity of human habitations to the farms, and in close association with swine, poultry, and humans in family farms. It has been implicated as an ideal situation for establishing new antigenic strains and introducing these viruses to the human population. The fact emphasizes importance of surveillance for animal and human influenza viruses in this area in order to prevent next pandemic. However, the H1N1 virus caused the 2009 pandemic in the twenty-first century, which first occurred in Mexico. Lessons we learnt from the 2009 pandemic are that the pandemic virus could also be generated in other locations including the highly industrialized countries in North America or Western Europe with the modern swine and poultry facilities except the Southeast Asia.

Further Reading

Wright PF and Webster RG (2001) Orthomyxoviruses, in *Fields Virology*, 4th edn (eds DM Knipe and PM Howley), Lippincott, Philadelphia, pp. 1533–1579.

Landolt GA, Townsend HG, and Lunn DP (2007) Equine influenza infection, in *Equine Infectious Diseases*, 2nd edn (eds DC Sellon and MT Long), St. Louis, MO, pp. 124–133.

Vincent AL, Ma W, Lager KM *et al.* (2008) Swine Influenza Viruses: A North American Perspective, in *Advances in Virus Research*, (eds K Maramorosch, AJ Shatkin, and FA Murphy), Academic Press, Burlington, pp. 127–154.

Swayne DE (2009) Avian Influenza, John Wiley & Sons/Wiley-Blackwell.

Werner O and Harder T (2006) Avian influenza, in *Influenza Report*, (eds BS Kamps, C Hoffmann, and W Preiser), Flying Publisher, Paris, Cagliari, Wuppertal, Sevilla, pp. 48–86.

59 Bunyaviridae

D. Scott McVey, Barbara Drolet, and William Wilson

Introduction

The family Bunyaviridae is the largest family of viruses and includes the genera *Orthobunyavirus*, *Hantavirus*, *Nairovirus*, *Phlebovirus*, and *Tospovirus*. There are several hundred bunyaviruses, and viruses of veterinary significance are classified within the genera *Bunyavirus*—California encephalitis serogroup viruses and Akabane virus (as well as Aino and Cache Valley viruses); *Phlebovirus*—Rift Valley fever virus (RVFV); *Nairovirus*—Nairobi sheep disease virus; and *Hantavirus*. Many of the bunyaviruses are arboviruses that are transmitted by arthropods such as mosquitoes, ticks, and biting flies, and thus have the capacity to alternately replicate in vertebrate animals and insects. A description of significant bunyavirus veterinary pathogens is in Table 59.1.

Several bunyaviruses are important zoonotic pathogens, including hantaviruses (the cause of hantavirus pulmonary syndrome and hemorrhagic fever with renal syndrome in people); RVFV; Crimean–Congo hemorrhagic fever virus; and Nairobi sheep disease virus.

General Family Properties

Bunyaviruses are enveloped, pleomorphic viruses that are 80–120 nm in diameter with surface projections (spikes) emanating from the envelope surface of mature virions (Figure 59.1). The virions consist of four structural proteins, including two external glycoproteins in the envelope, a nucleocapsid protein that encapsidates the genome, and a transcriptase protein (L). The envelope glycoproteins are responsible for neutralization and hemagglutination. A variety of nonstructural proteins are also encoded by the viral genome. The nucleic acid is helical and included in three distinct segments—large (L), medium (M), and small (S)—each comprised of single-stranded, negative-sense, or ambisense RNA. The organization and structure of the genomes determine the genera of these viruses. In addition, serological methods are used to provide further classification. However, many epitopes on envelope and capsid proteins are highly conserved. This creates unique challenges for taxonomic efforts. There is considerable genetic diversity and serological cross-reactivity among viruses within the various genera of the Bunyaviridae. Genetic reassortment may occur when cell cultures or insects are simultaneously infected with multiple, but closely related, bunyaviruses. Within established geographic ranges, the bunyaviruses undergo genetic drift and selection, especially in arthropod hosts. Nevertheless, it is unusual for new, serologically distinct strains to emerge.

The bunyaviruses are generally susceptible to drying, heat, acids, bleaches, detergents, and most common disinfectants.

Genus *Orthobunyavirus*—Akabane, Aino, and Cache Valley Viruses

Akabane virus is the cause of periodic outbreaks of fetal malformation in ruminants, especially cattle, in Asia, Australia, the Middle East, and Africa. The virus is transmitted by mosquitoes and *Culicoides* midges and causes distinctive teratogenic defects of the musculoskeletal and nervous systems (arthrogryposis–hydranencephaly) in fetuses from dams infected during pregnancy. The gestational age of the fetus at the time of infection determines the type of lesions that will be present at birth; fetuses infected prior to midgestation are typically born with their limbs held in rigid flexion (arthrogryposis), with variable deviation of their vertebral columns. The brains of affected fetuses may lack cerebral hemispheres or these may be represented only as fluid-filled sacs as a consequence of virus-mediated destruction of the developing cerebrum during gestation (hydranencephaly). An inactivated vaccine is used to protectively immunize ruminants prior to breeding.

Aino virus causes a similar disease as Akabane virus and has much the same global distribution. Cache Valley virus has been documented as the cause of outbreaks of arthrogryposis–hydranencephaly of sheep in the western and southwestern United States. A similar virus isolated from sheep in the Netherlands, Germany, and the United Kingdom in 2011 and 2012 causes similar teratogenic effects in sheep. This Schmallenberg virus is thought

Veterinary Microbiology, Third Edition. Edited by D. Scott McVey, Melissa Kennedy and M.M. Chengappa.

Table 59.1. Genera of Bunyaviridae, Diseases, Hosts, Principal Vectors, and Zoonotic Status

Virus	Distribution	Arthropod Vector	Target Species	Disease in Animals	Zoonotic?
Bunyavirus					
Akabane virus	Australia, Asia, Africa, the Middle East	Mosquitoes, *Culicoides*	Cattle, sheep	Abortion, congenital defects	No
Cache Valley virus	The United States	Mosquitoes	Sheep, cattle	Congenital defects	Rarely, fetal infection
La Crosse virus, California encephalitis group	North America	Mosquitoes	Rodents, humans	None in animals	Yes, encephalitis
Schmallenberg virus	The Netherlands, France, Germany	*Culicoides*	Sheep, cattle	Abortion, congenital defects	No
Phlebovirus					
RVFV	Africa	Mosquitoes	Sheep, cattle, wild ruminants, camels, humans	Systemic disease, hepatitis, encephalitis, abortions	Yes, hepatitis, encephalitis, hemorrhagic disease
Nairovirus					
Crimean–Congo hemorrhagic fever virus	Africa, Asia, Europe	Ticks	Sheep, cattle, goats, humans	Few clinical signs	Yes, hemorrhagic fever, hepatitis
Nairobi sheep disease virus	Eastern Africa	Ticks	Sheep, goats	Hemorrhagic enteritis	Mild febrile illness
Hantavirus					
Hantaan virus	China, Russia, Korea	None	Striped field mouse	None documented	Hemorrhagic fever and renal failure
New World hantavirus	Western hemisphere	None	Multiple rodent species	None documented	Pulmonary syndrome

to be an orthobunyavirus of the Simbu serogroup and is likely a Shamonda/Sathuperi virus reassortant.

California Encephalitis Serogroup Viruses

California encephalitis serogroup viruses are serologically cross-reactive, mosquito-transmitted viruses of the genus *Bunyavirus* and include La Crosse, snowshoe hare, and Jamestown Canyon viruses. These viruses occur in endemic cycles of infection in different regions of North America and, although infection occurs in a variety of mammalian species, encephalitis is rarely documented even in humans.

Other members of the genus *Bunyavirus* have been sporadically incriminated as the cause of encephalitis in animals—Main Drain virus in horses, for example.

FIGURE 59.1. *Representations of bunyavirus structure and genomic organization including the structure of the surface glycoproteins, G_C and G_N. (A) The two glycoproteins G_N and G_C are incorporated into the lipid bilayer during the budding process. The three encapsidated genome segments (associated with the nucleoprotein N and the polymerase L) are incorporated into the virion. (B) Schematic representation of the three RVFV RNA genome segments and coding strategy. The arrow indicates the open reading frames in each segment, which are flanked by noncoding regions. (Courtesy of Mandell and Flick 2011.)*

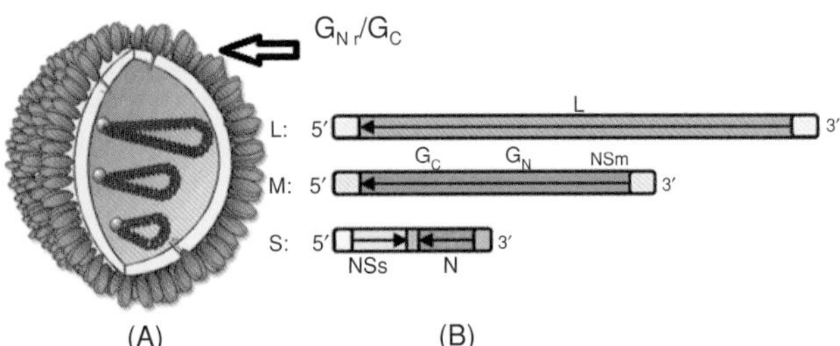

Genus *Phlebovirus*—Rift Valley Fever

Rift Valley fever virus (RVFV) is a zoonotic, mosquito-transmitted virus that causes epidemics of severe, frequently fatal systemic disease of ruminants, especially sheep and goats. Mortality is highest in young animals, and pregnant ruminants often abort following infection. RVFV causes extensive liver necrosis in affected sheep and goats and widespread hemorrhages are common. Encephalitis with neuronal necrosis also occurs in some affected animals.

Rift Valley fever (RVF) is endemic in sub-Saharan Africa and periodically incurs into adjacent northern regions such as Egypt, Saudi Arabia, and Yemen (Table 59.2). Climatic conditions influence the occurrence of epidemics, particularly high rainfall that results in rapid expansion of the populations of *Aedes* mosquitoes that harbor the virus. RVF is a zoonotic. The overall human mortality rate is

Table 59.2. Distribution of Recent RVF Disease in Africa and Asia (as of February 2012)

Countries with endemic RVF	Gambia, Senegal, Mauritania, Namibia, South Africa, Mozambique, Zimbabwe, Zambia, Kenya, Sudan, Egypt, Madagascar, Saudi Arabia, Yemen
Countries with some cases or serological evidence of infection	Botswana, Angola, Democratic Republic of the Congo, Congo, Gabon, Cameroon, Nigeria, Central African Republic, Chad, Niger, Burkina Faso, Mali, Guinea, Tanzania, Malawi, Uganda, Ethiopia, Somalia

approximately 1%, but has been reported as high as high as 30% in recent outbreaks.

RVFV is widely feared because of its virulence to humans and multiple species of animals, as well as its capacity for rapid spread by a variety of species of mosquitoes during epidemics. Thus, rapid diagnosis is imperative, usually by virus isolation or serology. An inactivated investigational vaccine is available for select at-risk veterinarians and laboratory staff working with RVFV-infected animals and materials.

Physical, Chemical, and Antigenic Properties and Virus Structure

RVFV is a spherical, enveloped virus of 80–90 nm diameter. The viruses have glycoprotein spikes (G_N/G_C) but do not have a matrix protein. The genome is composed of three RNA segments: (i) an ambisense S segment that encodes N and NSs nonstructural proteins, (ii) a negative-sense M segment that encodes the G_N and G_C spike proteins, and (iii) a negative-sense L segment that encodes the transcriptase. After the RVFV attaches to target cells through multiple receptors by endocytosis, replication occurs in cellular cytoplasm. The virus is uncoated and the RNA-dependent polymerase (transcriptase) begins initial transcription of nonstructural proteins critical for viral replication. Subsequent rounds of replication result in synthesis of the structural proteins essential for virus assembly and release by budding from intracytoplasmic vesicles from the Golgi apparatus. Virus particles are then released by exocytosis from apical or basolateral plasma membranes.

Distribution, Reservoirs, and Transmission. RVFV survives in multiple enzootic regions of Africa, primarily Kenya and South Africa (Table 59.2). It is not completely understood how the virus survives the interepizootic periods, but mosquito and wild ruminant cycles are thought to be important. During periods of disease emergence, which are associated with heavy rainfall, infected mosquitoes spread the virus to wild and domestic ruminants. From this point, expansion and spread occur through multiple species of *Aedes*, *Culex*, and *Anopheles* and other species of mosquitoes. The virus may also be contracted by direct contact with infected tissue and milk or by aerosols from these sources.

Pathogenesis. Incubation periods for this disease are relatively short at 3–5 days. Sheep, cattle, humans, and camels are frequently affected. Clinical signs include fever, loss of appetite, purulent nasal discharge, and diarrhea. Almost all pregnant ewes will abort. Mortality may approach 100% in lambs and up to 60% in adults. In cattle, the disease is usually less severe with mortality rates under 30%; however, abortion in pregnant animals may approach 100%. Horses, camels, cats, and dogs may also be infected during epizootic periods, but only very young animals will develop clinically significant disease. The disease is an influenza-like illness in humans. Most cases are usually relatively mild with a less than 2% mortality rate. However, up to 10% of cases may be associated with hepatitis or neurologic complications (blindness and encephalitis)(Figure 59.2).

FIGURE 59.2. *Immunohistochemical demonstration of virus antigen associated with a focal necrotic lesion in the liver of an RVFV-infected lamb. (Reproduced with permission from Drolet et al. 2012.)*

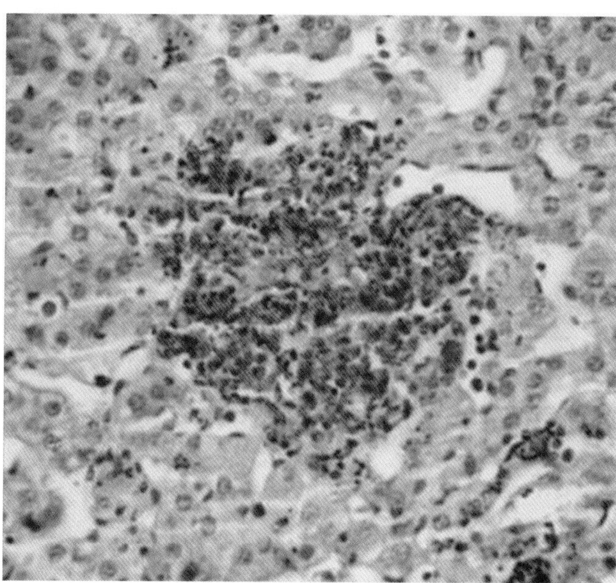

Host Response. As the virus spreads rapidly to hepatic and primary lymphoid tissues, liver necrosis, splenomegaly, and subserosal hemorrhages are observed (Figure59.3). Fever, as well as local and systemic inflammation, is associated with the tissue necrosis. These tissue changes are seen within 3–5 days. In the more severe cases, liver and kidney failure, hemorrhagic fever syndrome, and encephalitis all may occur. Animals usually respond by producing detectable IgM antibodies by day 5 and IgG antibodies by days 10–14. This immune response is associated with recovery and immunity is generally long lasting.

Diagnosis. Multiple polymerase chain reaction (PCR) assays are available to detect the presence of virus in blood or other tissues. These assays are very specific and sensitive. Virus isolation in cell culture may also be used as a gold standard test. However, this requires direct laboratory exposure of technicians to a virulent, zoonotic virus. Also, IgM-capture assays, direct antigen detection dip-sticks, and immunohistochemical assays are under development and/or are available for detecting recent RVFV infection or virus antigen detection. These assays can be performed using recombinant protein antigen and are therefore also be used safely to detect viral antigens in infected tissue specimens submitted to diagnostic laboratories (Figure 59.2).

Control. Vaccination of susceptible livestock in endemic regions is a primary method of control. Both inactivated virus and attenuated virus vaccines have been used with reasonable success. Vaccines made from attenuated strains of virus (MP-12 and Clone-13) are efficacious in cattle and sheep and licensed in some countries in Africa. These vaccines are undergoing registration and development in other regions. Further development of these and other

FIGURE 59.3. *Hepatitis in a lamb infected with RVFV: (A) gross lesions and (B) necrosis and inflammation in the liver. (Reproduced with permission from Drolet et al. 2012.)*

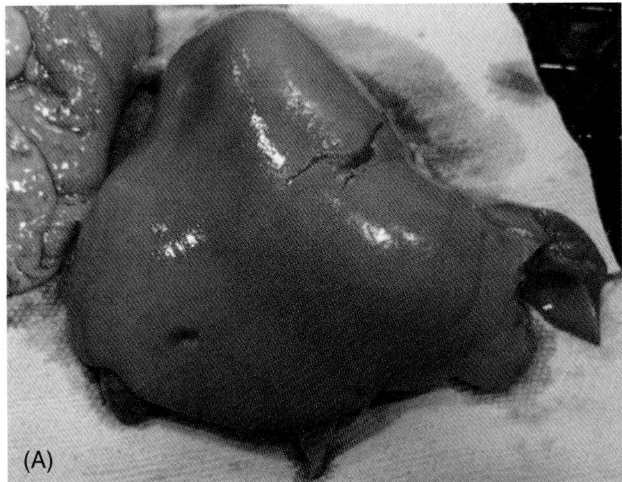

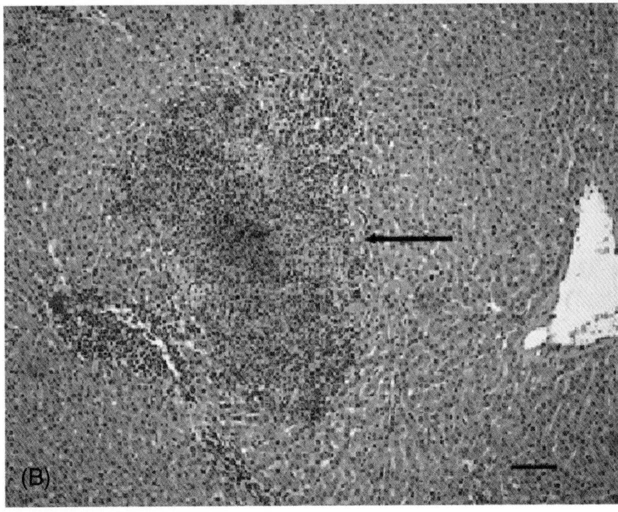

vaccines may provide the ability to distinguish vaccinated from infected animals.

Control of vectors in endemic zones, as well as restricting animal movement and subsequent human exposure, is also moderately effective methods of control.

Genus *Nairovirus*—Nairobi Sheep Disease

Nairobi sheep disease (NSD) and related viruses cause severe disease of sheep and goats in Africa and Asia. The virus is transmitted by the brown ear tick. NSD is characterized by high fever, intestinal hemorrhage, and death of susceptible ruminants. Pregnant animals typically abort. NSD is also an occasional zoonotic pathogen causing disease in veterinarians and laboratory staff exposed to infected animals or materials.

Other members of the genus *Nairovirus* that are of potential veterinary significance include Crimean–Congo hemorrhagic fever, a zoonotic disease that occurs throughout Africa, eastern Europe, the Middle East, and Asia. The virus is transmitted by Ixodidae (hard ticks). Although both wild and domestic animals can serve as reservoirs of the virus, clinical disease is typically only seen in humans and can include severe flu-like illness, jaundice, and hemorrhage. Transmission can also occur from contact with infected animal blood, and person-to-person transmission is possible through contact with infected blood or other tissue fluids.

Genus *Hantavirus*

There are at least 20 members of the genus *Hantavirus*. These viruses are not maintained through chronic infections of arthropod vectors, but rather in rodents. The Old World hantaviruses usually cause a hemorrhagic fever and renal syndrome disease, while the New World hantaviruses cause pulmonary disease. One major feature associated with hantaviruses is that they are difficult to isolate and maintain in cell culture. Thus, PCR assays are critically important for diagnosis.

The vast majority of hantavirus infections occur in Korea, China, eastern Russia, and the Balkans. Human disease usually occurs after direct contact with rodent feces. Viremia is transient and is suppressed by the appearance of neutralizing antibodies. However, the virus persists in kidneys and lungs, where the presence of necrosis and inflammation causes disease. Diagnosis is usually made by demonstration of the virus in tissue by immunologic or molecular (PCR) methods. Inactivated vaccines have been used in Korea and China, but the most effective means of control is through rodent control and personal hygiene.

References

Drolet BS, Weingartl HM, Jiang J *et al.* (2012) Development and evaluation of one-step rRT-PCR and immunohistochemical methods for detection of Rift Valley fever virus in biosafety level 2 diagnostic laboratories. *J Virol Methods*, **179** (2), 373–382.

Mandell RB and Flick R (2011) Virus-like particle-based vaccines for Rift Valley fever virus. *J Bioterr Biodef*, **S1,** 008. doi:10.4172/2157-2526.S1-008.

Further Reading

Bird BH, Ksiazek TG, Nichol ST, and Maclachlan NJ.(2009) Rift Valley fever virus. *J Am Vet Med Assoc*, **234** (7), 883–893.

Boshra H, Lorenzo G, Busquets N, and Brun A (2011) Rift valley fever: recent insights into pathogenesis and prevention. *J Virol*, **85** (13), 6098–6105. Epub March 30, 2011.

Goris N, Vandenbussche F, and De Clercq K.(2008) Potential of antiviral therapy and prophylaxis for controlling RNA viral infections of livestock. *Antivir Res*, **78** (1), 170–178. Epub November 5, 2007.

Gould EA and Higgs S.(2009) Impact of climate change and other factors on emerging arbovirus diseases. *Trans R Soc Trop Med Hyg*, **103** (2), 109–121. Epub September 16, 2008.

Haller O and Weber F (2009) The interferon response circuit in antiviral host defense. *Verh K Acad Geneeskd Belg*, **71** (1–2), 73–86.

Hollidge BS, González-Scarano F, and Soldan SS (2010) Arboviral encephalitides: transmission, emergence, and pathogenesis. *J Neuroimmune Pharmacol*, **5** (3), 428–442. Epub July 22, 2010.

LaBeaud AD, Kazura JW, and King CH (2010) Advances in Rift Valley fever research: insights for disease prevention *Curr Opin Infect Dis*, **23** (5), 403–408.

Linthicum K, Anyamba A, Britch SC *et al.* (2007) A rift valley fever risk surveillance system for Africa using remotely sensed data: potential for use on other continents. *Vet Ital*, **43**, 663–674.

Métras R, Collins LM, White RG *et al.* (2011) Rift Valley fever epidemiology, surveillance, and control: what have models contributed. *Vector Borne Zoonotic Dis*, **11** (6), 761–771. Epub May 6, 2011.

Walter CT and Barr JN (2011) Recent advances in the molecular and cellular biology of bunyaviruses. *J Gen Virol*, **92** (11), 2467–2484. Epub August 24, 2011.

Weaver SC and Reisen WK (2010) Present and future arboviral threats. *Antivir Res*, **85** (2), 328–345. Epub October 24, 2009.

Wilson WC, Weingartl H, Drolet BS *et al.* (2013) Diagnostic approaches for rift valley fever. In vaccine and diagnostics for transboundary and zoonotic diseases. *Devel Biol (Basel)*, **135**, 73–78.

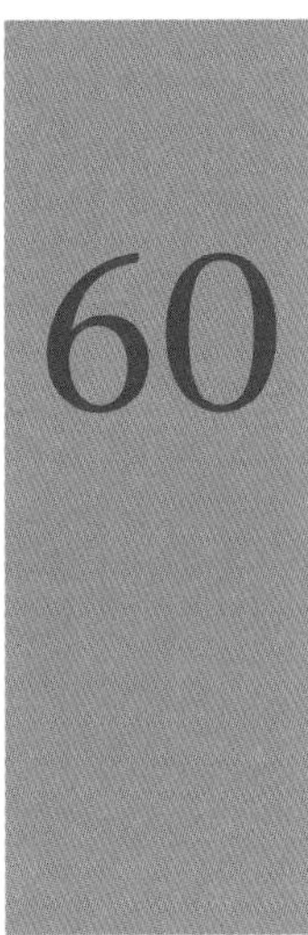

60 Paramyxoviridae, Filoviridae, and Bornaviridae

STEFAN NIEWIESK AND MICHAEL OGLESBEE

The order Mononegavirales includes viruses within the families Paramyxoviridae, Filoviridae, Bornaviridae, and Rhabdoviridae (Chapter 61). These viruses are ancestrally related as reflected by their common characteristics such as a single-stranded genome of negative-sense RNA, similar replication strategy and gene order, and virion morphology that includes an envelope.

Resistance to Physical and Chemical Agents

Mononegavirales can be inactivated by standard physical measures and chemical agents effective against enveloped viruses. These measures include treatment with heat, ultraviolet light, acidic or alkaline solutions, or chemical agents such as lipid solvents, lysol, phenol, quaternary ammonium compounds, and butylated hydroxytoluene. Disinfection is most effective after thorough cleaning of materials. The rate of viral inactivation varies with the strain of virus, quantity of virus initially exposed, time of exposure, and presence of organic matter in the environment. Infectious virus can survive for long periods in organic and frozen matter.

Paramyxoviridae

The Paramyxoviridae family is divided into two subfamilies: the Paramyxovirinae and the Pneumovirinae that are further subdivided into five (*Avulavirus*, *Henipahvirus*, *Morbillivirus*, *Respirovirus*, and *Rubulavirus*) and two genera (*Metapneumovirus* and *Pneumovirus*), respectively (Table 60.1). Viruses in this family cause a number of serious respiratory and/or systemic diseases of humans, animals, and birds.

Paramyxoviruses are characterized by virions that are enveloped, pleomorphic (filamentous or spherical; approximately 150 nm or more in diameter), and contain a genome of linear, negative-sense, single-stranded RNA. The viral nucleocapsid has helical symmetry and is approximately 13–18 nm in diameter (Figure 60.1). At least three proteins are associated with the nucleocapsid, including an RNA-binding protein (N or NP), a phosphoprotein (P) that enables transcription, and the viral polymerase (L = large protein). The nucleocapsid is enclosed by a lipoprotein envelope derived from the host cell plasma membrane, and contains two or three transmembrane viral glycoproteins that form spikes (8–12 nm) projecting from the surface. The spikes are formed by the receptor-binding attachment protein (hemagglutinin (H) or hemagglutinin-neuraminidase (HN) in the Paramyxovirinae; G protein in the Pneumovirinae) and the fusion protein (F) that is essential for virus infectivity and for cell-to-cell spread. Another protein, the matrix (M) protein, lines the inner surface of the envelope. Various nonstructural viral proteins are also formed in infected cells that usually regulate virus replication. Paramyxoviridae are monotypic; for example, antibodies against one virus strain can neutralize all strains of the same species.

Vaccination

All vaccines developed against infection with paramyxoviruses are based on live tissue culture attenuated viruses that do not cause disease but induce a protective immune response. In same cases, inactivated virus vaccines are being used which in general are not as efficient as the live virus vaccine. For canine distemper (CD) virus, an additional vaccine has been developed based on a canarypox virus vector.

Paramyxovirinae

Avulaviruses

Newcastle Disease

Disease. Newcastle disease (ND) is a highly contagious disease of chickens that is characterized by respiratory

Veterinary Microbiology, Third Edition. Edited by D. Scott McVey, Melissa Kennedy and M.M. Chengappa.

Table 60.1. Order: Mononegavirales

Family	Genus	Species
Bornaviridae	*Bornavirus*	Borna disease virus
Filoviridae	*Ebolavirus*	Zaire ebolavirus
	Marburgvirus	Lake Victoria marburgvirus
Paramyxoviridae		
Paramyxovirinae	*Avulavirus*	Newcastle disease virus
	Henipavirus	Hendra virus
		Nipah virus
	Morbillivirus	Canine distemper virus
		Peste-des-petits-ruminants virus
		Phocine distemper virus
		Rinderpest virus
	Respirovirus	Bovine parainfluenza virus 3
		Human parainfluenza virus 3
	Rubulavirus	Mumps virus
		Parainfluenza virus 5 (Canine)
Pneumovirinae	*Metapneumovirus*	Avian metapneumovirus
		Human metapneumovirus
	Pneumovirus	Bovine respiratory syncytial virus
		Human respiratory syncytial virus
		Murine pneumonia virus

distress, diarrhea, and neurological signs. The severity of the disease is dependent upon the age and immune status of the birds, and on the virulence of the strain of ND virus that is responsible for the infection. The most virulent strains are designated as velogenic and produce mortality rates in affected birds as high as 90% or more. The disease caused by mesogenic strains is less severe and the mortality rate is often less than 25%. The lentogenic strains are relatively avirulent and are often used as vaccines.

Host–Virus Relationship

Geographic Distribution and Transmission. Newcastle disease virus (NDV) infects chickens, guinea fowls, turkeys, and a large number of species of domestic and wild birds. Sea birds are less susceptible but may act as carriers. Humans accidentally infected with NDV when exposed to infected birds or live viral vaccines may develop a self-limiting conjunctivitis.

ND occurs worldwide and domestic birds are the major reservoir for NDV. Although NDV has been isolated from a large number of wild birds such as sparrows, crows, ducks, and geese, they appear to play a minimal role in transmitting this disease. The epizootic outbreak of the exotic velogenic strain of NDV in North America (California) in 1971 has been attributed to the introduction of caged birds.

Aerosol respiratory infection is the most common route for transmission of NDV. Infected birds begin to shed virus 2–3 days after exposure from their respiratory tracts and continue to shed virus for several weeks. The virus is also readily spread by fomites.

Pathogenesis and Pathology. Initial replication of NDV occurs in the mucosa of the upper respiratory tract following aerosol infection. Viremia then disseminates the virus throughout the body, and widespread multiplication of virus in cells of parenchymal organs leads to a secondary viremia, which in some instances leads to the infection of the cells of the CNS. Disease takes several different forms in chickens, depending on the virulence of the strain involved. Differences in the virulence of individual strains of NDV are due to differences in the proteases used to cleave the fusion protein. Less virulent strains use typsin-like proteases that are present in the respiratory and gastrointestinal tract, only, whereas more virulent strains use the more ubiquitously expressed furin-like proteases. The very virulent (velogenic) strains cause very rapidly fatal

FIGURE 60.1. *CDV infection of dog lung. (A) The initial infection of airway epithelium is noncytopathic and results in extensive viral shedding into the airway lumens. Numerous eosinophilic (pink) cytoplasmic inclusions are present within the infected cells. (B) Cytopathic effects are observed as the infection progresses, resulting in loss of cell differentiation, rounding, and sloughing, resulting in a denuded mucosal surface. (C) Secondary bacterial bronchopneumonia is a sequel to the mucosal injury and virus-induced immune suppression. Airway lumens (top) are filled with sloughed epithelial cells and neutrophils, and alveolar spaces (bottom) in the vicinity of these airways are filled with neutrophils and alveolar macrophages. Hematoxylin and eosin-stained tissue sections.*

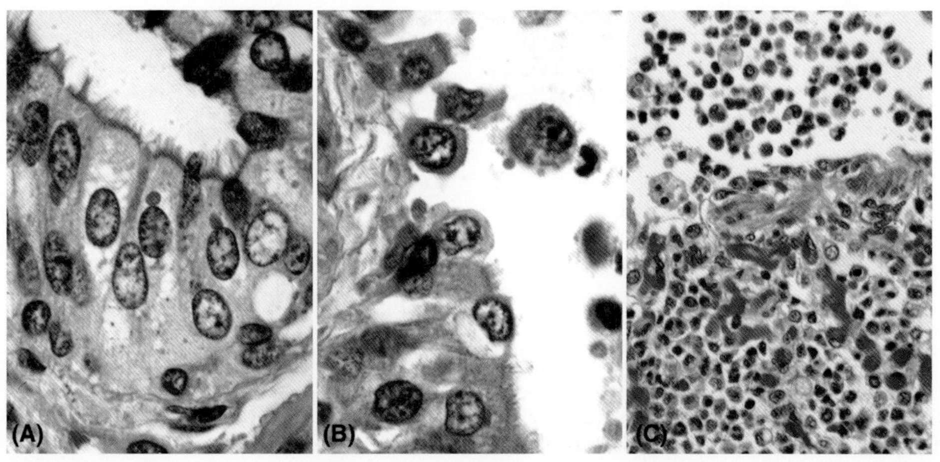

infections involving the visceral organs or the CNS. Mesogenic strains of NDV cause respiratory and, occasionally, neurologic disease in infected chickens with low mortality, while lentogenic strains produce a mild or often inapparent disease.

Lesions in ND vary greatly. Inapparent infections cause few, if any, lesions whereas hemorrhagic necrosis that affects the intestinal tract, respiratory tract, and visceral organs is characteristic of more severe forms. In chickens with CNS involvement, necrosis of the glial cells, neuronal degeneration, perivascular cuffing, and hypertrophy of endothelial cells are often present.

Host Response to Infection. Chickens infected with NDV produce antibodies 6–10 days after infection. Antibodies to the envelope glycoprotein, HN, exhibit viral neutralizing and hemagglutination inhibition activities and are responsible for host immunity to the disease.

Laboratory Diagnosis. As the clinical signs and pathologic lesions of ND are variable and nonspecific, definitive diagnosis of the disease must depend on laboratory methods to identify NDV. This now is best accomplished using PCR, and sequence and/or nucleic acid hybridization analysis to distinguish whether the virus is a velogenic field strain or a live vaccine strain. Alternatively, NDV can be isolated by inoculating embryonated eggs or cell cultures with respiratory exudate or tissue suspensions (spleen, lung, or brain), and NDV antigen in affected tissues or cell cultures can be identified by immunofluorescence or immunohistochemical staining. Serological diagnosis requires demonstration of rising NDV antibody titers by the hemagglutination inhibition or neutralization assay, or enzyme-linked immunosorbent assay (ELISA).

Control and Prevention. Sanitary management to prevent exposure of susceptible chickens to NDV is an important aspect of control against the disease. Since there is only one serotype of NDV, vaccination with either inactivated or live virus vaccines is also used to prevent ND. The majority of live vaccines incorporate lentogenic strains of NDV administered in drinking water or applied as aerosols.

Henipaviruses

Hendra Virus. Hendra virus disease is unique to Australia, where it was first recognized in 1994 as the cause of an outbreak of severe disease with respiratory and neurological symptoms that killed a number of horses and their trainer. The virus was named after the suburb of Brisbaine in which the disease was first described. Affected horses develop severe interstitial pneumonia and pulmonary edema as well as neurological symptoms that rapidly are fatal. The virus is harbored asymptomatically by several species of fruit bat (flying foxes). Although fruit bats are the reservoir of Hendra virus, the virus is contagious between horses and to humans by direct contact with nasal secretions or fomites that contain the virus.

Nipah Virus. Nipah viruses are closely related to Hendra virus. It has been found in several outbreaks in Malaysia, Singapore, Bangladesh, and India since 1998. The virus reservoirs are bats of (mostly) the Pteropus species that are subclinically infected and excrete virus through urine. When pigs become infected (presumably through infected feed) the illness presents with pneumonia and encephalitis. Close contact with infected pigs and food-borne (contaminated palm sap) transmission have been shown to lead to human illnesses with the same clinical symptoms observed in infected pigs. The case fatality rate in humans is high due to encephalitis. In humans, ribavirin treatment has been demonstrated to reduce fatalities.

Morbilliviruses

Although the various morbilliviruses are all closely related as evidenced by extensive serological cross-reactivity between them, they are distinguished on the basis of their individual host range, genome sequence, and antigenic differences. These viruses all have a hemagglutin (H) surface protein, but only rinderpest virus has a neuraminidase (HN). The receptor for wild-type morbilliviruses is the CD150 molecule of the respective species (Figure 60.1).

Canine Distemper Virus

Disease. CD is an important viral disease of dogs (Figures 60.2, 60.3, and 60.4). Acute CD is characterized by any combination of diphasic fever, ocular and nasal discharges, anorexia, depression, vomiting, diarrhea, dehydration, leukopenia, pneumonia, and neurologic signs. The severity of clinical signs exhibited by individual animals can vary markedly. The disease has an incubation period of 3–5 days. The mortality rate depends largely on the immune status of the infected dog and is highest among puppies. Animals that survive the acute disease may develop other signs, including hyperkeratosis of the footpads (hard pad disease) and neurologic disease that is characterized by any combination of convulsions, tremor, myoclonus, locomotor disturbances, paralysis, and blindness. The onset of neurologic signs frequently is delayed until several weeks after the systemic signs of acute CD are manifest. Old dog encephalitis is a rare form of chronic neurologic disease caused by defective CD virus.

Host–Virus Relationship

Host Range, Geographic Distribution and Transmission. CD viruses infect a wide range of animals. In addition to dogs, other members of the Canidae (e.g., fox, coyote, wolf, and wild dogs), Ailuridae (red panda), Hyaenidae (hyena), Mustelidae (e.g., ferret, mink, skunk, and badger), Tayassuidae (javelinas (collared peccaries)), Ursidae (bears), Viverridae (civet, mongoose), and Procyonidae (e.g., raccoon and panda) are susceptible. Some members of the Felidae (lion, tiger, and leopard) also are susceptible, and devastating outbreaks of distemper have occurred among lions in Africa.

CD occurs worldwide and remains endemic in many areas despite the widespread use of vaccines that are highly effective in preventing the disease. Infected dogs secrete virus in their nasal and ocular secretions, and CDV

FIGURE 60.2. *CDV cytoplasmic inclusions are the result of accumulations of virus core particles (nucleocapsids) during replication. (A) Nuclecapsids are formed by a helical arrangement of N protein (inset, blue) that packages the virus' single-stranded genomic RNA (inset, red). Negative stain transmission electron microscopy illustrates the length of these particles, and the superimposition of N proteins on the sides of the nucleocapsids creates a herringbone pattern that is typical of paramyxoviruses. (B) Transmission electron microscopy of an infected cell cytoplasm shows that nucleocapsids tend to form large aggregates that are the basis for the light microscopic inclusions. Osmium tetroxide-stained section.*

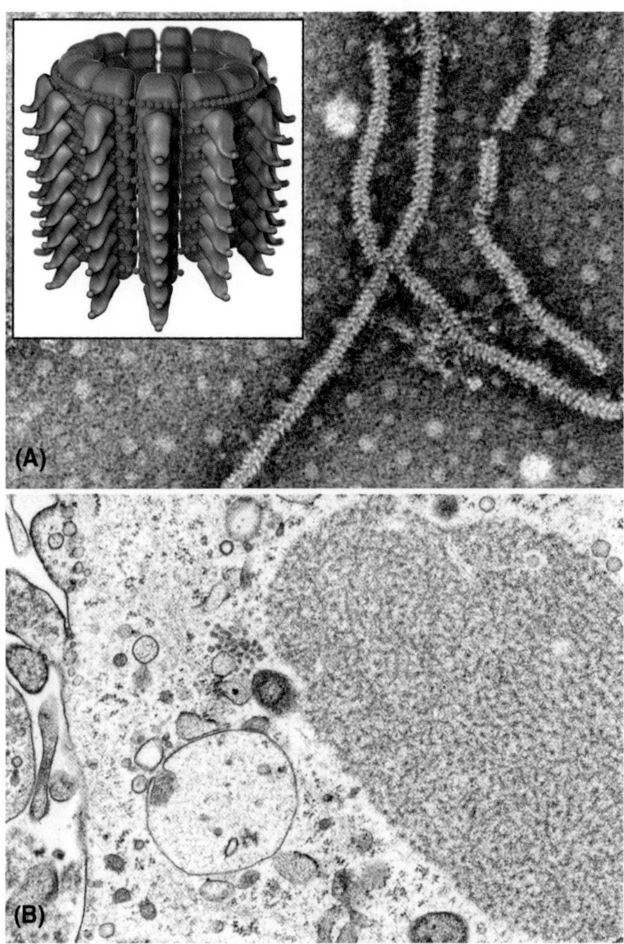

is present in the urine of experimentally infected dogs 6–22 days after infection. Feces of infected dogs may also contain CDV. Infection usually is transmitted by aerosol or by direct contact, leading to respiratory infection of susceptible animals.

Pathogenesis and Pathology. CDV is pantropic and has an especially strong tropism for epithelium and lymphoid tissues. The lungs are also central to the pathogenesis of CDV infection. Initial replication of CDV occurs in macrophages in the bronchial lymph nodes and tonsils immediately following respiratory infection. The virus then is spread to other lymphoid tissues (lymph nodes, spleen, thymus, and bone marrow) where further replication occurs prior to

FIGURE 60.3. *CDV forms both intranuclear and cytoplasmic inclusion bodies, a feature unique to morbilliviruses. (A) Eosinophilic (pink) intranuclear and intracytoplasmic inclusions are present in an astrocyte of an infected raccoon brain (H&E stain). The intranuclear inclusion is contrasted with the basophilic (blue) nucleolus. Cytoplasmic inclusions are aggregates of viral nucleocapsid, often referred to as a viral "factories." (B) Intranuclear inclusions are a unique cell structure known as complex nuclear bodies, shown here by transmission electron microscopy (osmium tetroxide stain). The nuclear bodies contain coarse filaments surrounded by a fine fibrillar capsule (top) and are readily distinguished from the compact reticulate nucleolus (bottom). The structures are induced by intranuclear trafficking of the viral N protein, contain abundant amounts of N protein, and are though to influence cellular RNA metabolism in a manner that supports viral replication.*

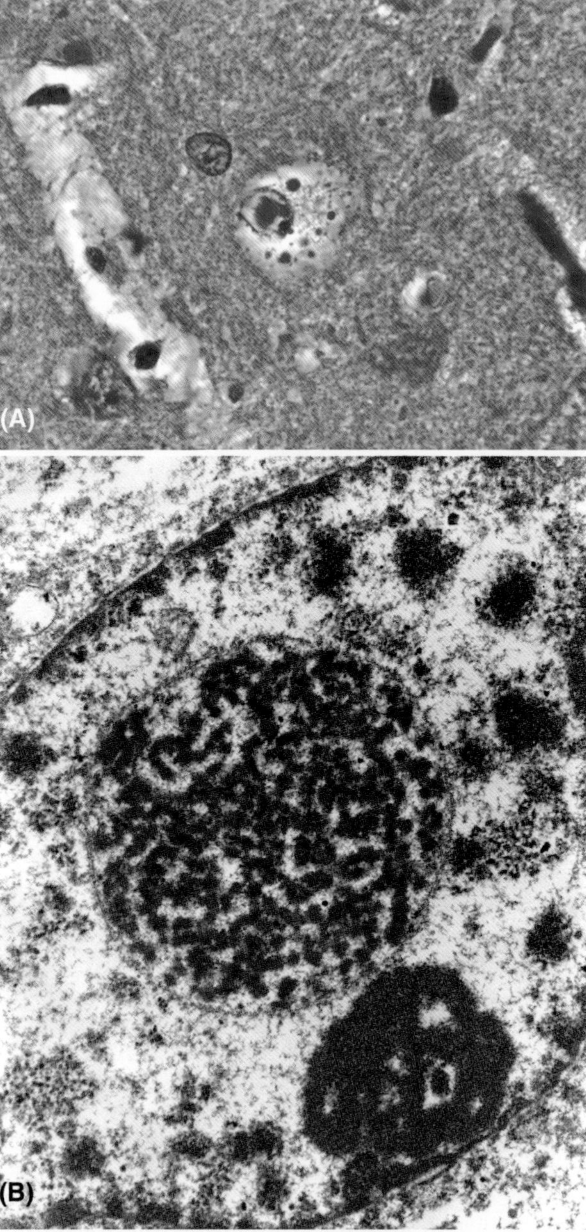

FIGURE 60.4. *BPIV3 infection of a seronegative calf, 7 days postchallenge. (A) Immunoperoxidase staining of viral antigen in lung (brown) shows extensive infection of epithelium in an airway (center). Discrete aggregates of viral antigen in the cytoplasm are the basis for eosinophilic (pink) inclusion bodies that are readily identified by routine hematoxylin and eosin staining, and represent aggregates of virus core particles. Viral envelop proteins mediate fusion of infected epithelial cells to form syncytia (white arrows). Viral antigen positive pulmonary alveolar macrophages are also observed (black arrow). (B) Virus-infection precipitates a secondary bacterial bronchopneumonia, and also collapse of lobules associated with airway obstruction by inflammatory cells (atelectasis), illustrated by the brown discoloration of lobules in the cranial and ventral aspects of the lung lobe. (Illustrations courtesy of John Ellis, University of Saskatchewan.)*

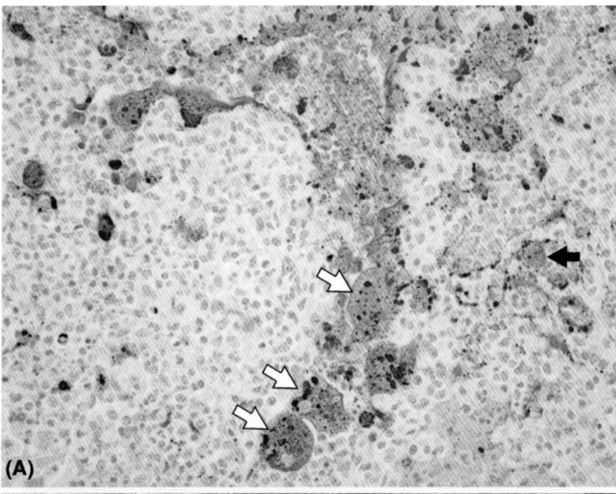

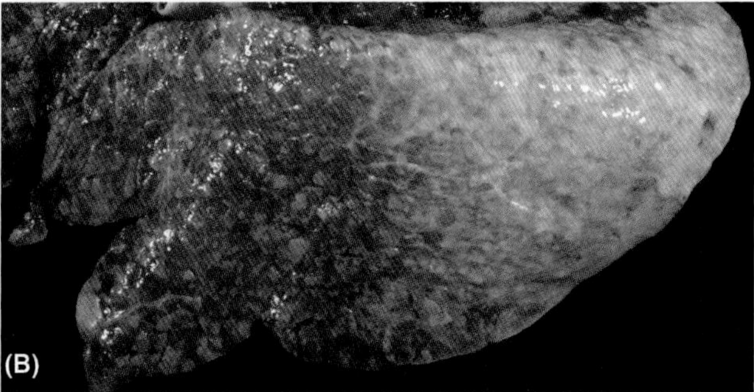

viremia that disseminates CDV to virtually all organs of the body, including the central nervous system (CNS) and eyes. The generalized dissemination of CDV results in infection of the epithelium of the alimentary, respiratory, and urogenital tracts; the skin and mucous membranes; endocrine glands and the CNS, the latter occurring approximately 8 or 9 days after infection and only in dogs that fail to develop sufficient titers of neutralizing antibodies to CDV by that time.

The lesions of CD occur in the organs in which the virus replicates, and the respiratory and alimentary tracts are especially affected, these being the organs primarily involved in viral shedding and transmission. The lungs of dogs with acute CD have diffuse bronchointerstitial pneumonia, reflecting viral replication in airway epithelium. Secondary bacterial bronchopneumonias are common in dogs as a consequence of virus-induced mucosal damage and immune suppression. Characteristic eosinophilic intranuclear and intracytoplasmic inclusion bodies are often present within respiratory epithelium and in the epithelium lining the stomach, urinary bladder, and renal pelvis. Extensive necrosis of lymphocytes is characteristic of acute CD, leading to lymphoid depletion that is one basis for immune suppression. Immune suppression may assist the virus in gaining access to the nervous system.

Dogs that survive acute CD may subsequently develop neurologic signs that are associated with virus-induced demyelination. The lesions within the central nervous system of these dogs begin as focal areas of demyelination that are accompanied by lymphocytic inflammation and accumulation of macrophages. Lesions occur within the cerebellum, brain stem, and cerebrum, and CDV inclusion bodies may occur in astrocytes and neurons. Although CDV predominately replicates in astrocytes and microglial cells within the brains of infected dogs, virus-mediated injury to oligodendrocytes is proposed to be responsible for much of the initial virus-induced demyelination.

Old dog encephalitis is a rare disease of mature dogs that results from very long-term persistent CDV infection of the central nervous system, leading to dementia. The disease is characterized by severe lymphocytic encephalitis with neuronal degeneration and, often, the presence of CDV inclusion bodies. Demyelination is not a typical feature of this disease.

Host Response to Infection. CD virus infection induces long-lasting immunity in dogs that recover from natural infection. Protective neutralizing antibodies first appear in serum of infected dogs 8–9 days after infection and persist for years thereafter. Cell-mediated immune responses are also generated by dogs infected with CDV. Virus-induced immune suppression contributes to the pathogenesis of CDV infection by predisposing affected dogs to secondary bacterial infections and by facilitating spread of the virus to the CNS.

Laboratory Diagnosis. Since the clinical signs of CD are variable and sometimes nonspecific, definitive diagnosis requires identification of CDV by virus isolation or the staining of CDV antigen in the cells or tissues of affected dogs using CDV-specific antibodies and immunohistochemical or immunocytochemical staining. Routine histological evaluation of postmortem cases allows a presumptive diagnosis based upon distribution of lesions and the occurrence of cytopathic effects that include formation of intranuclear and intracytoplasmic inclusion bodies and formation of virus-induced syncytia. Alternatively, serological diagnosis can be done by demonstration of rising IgG titers in paired sera by ELISA.

Control and Prevention. Treatment for CD is supportive, such as the use of antibiotics to control secondary bacterial infections and electrolyte solutions to restore fluids and electrolytes. Vaccination against CD is the best means of preventing the disease. Both modified live and inactivated

CD viral vaccines are available, and vaccination has greatly reduced the incidence of this disease in dogs. Maternally derived antibody to CDV can interfere with the successful vaccination of puppies against CDV. Puppies should be vaccinated for CD at an age when maternally derived antibody has been metabolized. Although both inactivated and modified live virus CDV vaccines safely have been used to immunize a variety of wild animal species, including foxes, ferrets, mink, bush dogs, and maned wolves, there have been reports of vaccine-induced CD in a variety of species, including mink, kinkajous, and lesser pandas after immunization with modified live CDV vaccine. For this reason, killed vaccines should always be used in species for which vaccine safety has not been established. Similarly, instances of vaccine-induced CD have been described in dogs. In order to provide a safer vaccine, a canarypox virus vector vaccine has been developed that expresses both the hemagglutinin and the fusion protein of CDV.

Morbilliviruses of Aquatic Mammals (Phocine Distemper and Cetacean Morbilliviruses)

A number of epidemics in pinnipeds and cetaceans have been determined to be due to morbillivirus infections. Phocine distemper is an infectious disease of seals that resembles CD. The disease first was recognized in the late 1980s when massive die-offs of seals occurred in the Baltic and North seas. The lesions and clinical signs in affected seals were remarkably similar to those of CD, and the disease of seals subsequently was shown to be caused by phocine distemper virus (PDV), a *Morbillivirus* that is closely related to CD virus. A similar disease caused by dolphin distemper virus caused extensive mortality among dolphins on the Atlantic coast of North America in the early 1990s, and porpoise morbillivirus was found to be responsible for the infection of porpoises. The dolphin, porpoise and phocine distemper viruses are closely related. In addition, infection with CD virus was detected in seals leading to the speculation that morbilliviruses infecting aquatic mammals might be derived from CDV. Like CD in dogs, infection with morbilliviruses in aquatic mammals leads to pneumonia and sometimes manifestation in the CNS.

Rinderpest

Rinderpest virus has been declared eradicated on May 25, 2011. After human poxvirus (declared eradicated in 1979), Rinderpest virus is the second virus to have ever been eradicated worldwide and the first virus of veterinary importance.

Disease. Rinderpest (also known as cattle plague) was a devastating pandemic viral disease of domestic cattle, buffalo, and some wild ruminant species. Rinderpest virus infects a number of species of the order Artiodactyla, which includes cattle, water buffalo, pigs, warthogs, and many species of African antelope. The reported infection of sheep and goat is now thought to be due to peste de petits ruminants virus. Rinderpest is characterized by fever, lymphopenia, nasal and lacrimal discharges, diarrhea, and erosions and ulcers throughout the oral cavity (ulcerative stomatitis). The disease has an incubation period of 3–8 days and the virus is extremely contagious, so morbidity rates are very high. The mortality rate also can be high (up to 100%) in cattle that have no immunity, but varies depending on the virulence of the infecting virus strain.

Host–Virus Relationship

Geographic Distribution and Transmission. Rinderpest historically occurred throughout Europe, Africa, and Asia but never became established in either the Americas or in Australasia. Until recently, the virus was enzootic in certain regions of Asia, the Middle East, and Africa.

Rinderpest virus is present in high titers in the nasal discharges, saliva, ocular secretions, and excretions of infected animals, and transmission requires direct contact of susceptible animals with secretions and excretions of infected animals.

Pathogenesis and Pathology. Rinderpest virus infection normally occurs through the upper respiratory tract, although cattle can be experimentally infected by any parenteral route of inoculation. The virus first replicates in the tonsils and regional lymph nodes, and a predominantly lymphocyte-associated viremia then disseminates the virus throughout the body. The virus replicates in lymphoid tissues (spleen, bone marrow, lymph nodes), and the mucosa of the alimentary and upper respiratory tracts. Nasal and ocular secretions contain high titers of virus at this time. Fever (up to 107 °F) and leukopenia occur prior to the appearance of oral ulcers and onset of diarrhea that may contain blood (dysentery). Titers of virus in the tissues and secretions of infected cattle decline after the appearance of neutralizing antibodies in serum. The convalescent phase begins with the healing of mouth lesions, and complete recovery from the disease may take 4–5 weeks.

Lesions of rinderpest occur in the tissues in which the virus replicates. Oral ulcers are characteristic of severe cases of rinderpest in cattle, and these begin as areas of necrosis with the basal cell layer of the epithelium. Necrosis also occurs in the mucosa of the abomasum and small intestine. The presence of syncytial cells within the affected epithelium is highly characteristic of rinderpest, but not other ulcerative diseases like malignant catarrhal fever or bovine viral diarrhea. There also is extensive necrosis of gut-associated lymphoid tissues as a result of virus-mediated destruction of lymphocytes, and similar lympholysis occurs in other lymphoid tissues (lymph nodes, spleen, bone marrow).

Eradication. The concerted efforts of a number of international organizations led to the eradication of Rinderpest that over the last few years resided in pockets in east Africa. The following aspects of the eradication program were seen as essential for eradication: a short infectious period of infected animals, no persistent infection and no viral reservoirs, transmission only by close contacts, a safe and reliable vaccine protecting against all viral strains, easy and reliable diagnosis, and an economic incentive to comply with the program.

Peste des Petits Ruminants

Disease. Peste des petits ruminants (PPR) viruses infect goats and sheep. Clinical symptoms are similar to Rinderpest in cattle although both viruses are clearly distinct. Cattle and pigs can be infected and develop antibodies but no clinical symptoms. The infection leads to high fever in goats and sheep after an incubation period of 3–9 days with subsequent pneumonia and diarrhea. The severity of symptoms depends on species, breed, age and the presence of secondary infectious agents.

Host–Virus Relationship.

Geographic Distribution and Transmission. The PPR virus is found in both Africa and Asia and is one of the fastest spreading infections of veterinary importance. It has recently been found in China and African countries bordering Europe. Its economic impact is particularly important in lower economic layers of society that depend on small ruminants for their livelihoods. The virus induces an acute infection so that there is not persistently infected animal reservoir. It is passed through direct contact between animals or contact with respiratory secretions or feces of infected animals.

Pathogenesis and Pathology. Pest des petits ruminants virus infection occurs through the upper respiratory tract. The virus first replicates in the tonsils and regional lymph nodes, and a predominantly lymphocyte-associated viremia then disseminates the virus throughout the body. With the onset of fever, respiratory symptoms such as congestion of the mucous membranes of the eyes, nose and mouth, and ocular and nasal discharge are seen. Many animals show labored breathing, and a productive cough. Necrotic lesions begin to appear as white/gray spots that spread throughout the mucosa of the mouth, eventually turn yellow and become encrusted with exudate. Animals drink a lot but stop eating. Some animals develop diarrhea 1–3 days later due to infection of the gastrointestinal mucosa. In fatal cases, animals will die 8–12 days after the onset of disease. During infection and recovery, animals are immunosuppressed that is indicated by low white blood cell counts and susceptibility to secondary infections. At postmortem examination, congestion of lung tissue is seen with marked infiltration of macrophages and proliferation of pneumocytes. In contrast to RPV infection, syncytia are seen in lung epithelium.

Laboratory Diagnosis. PPR virus infection can often not easily be distinguished from other infectious diseases of goats and sheep due to similarities of clinical symptoms. The laboratory diagnosis of acute infection is based on the presence of virus as detected by PCR or capture ELISA, an overcome infection is diagnosed based on antibody by ELISA.

Control and Prevention. The best prevention of PPR virus infection is the separation of infected and not infected animals. In consequence, the movement of livestock from endemic areas should be banned. If that is not feasible, movement has to be controlled by quarantine and surveillance. As another preventive measure, vaccination with a live-modified virus should be performed. Vaccination induces immunity for at least three years and has been used to control outbreaks.

Pneumovirinae

Viruses in the subfamily Pneumovirinae differ antigenetically and in their replication strategy from those in the subfamily Paramyxovirinae. Most viruses utilize a G protein as receptor-binding protein and lack a hemagglutinin and neuraminidase.

Respiroviruses

Bovine Parainfluenza Virus Type 3

Disease. Clinical disease due to infection with bovine parainfluenza virus (BPIV) type 3 is most common in calves with poor passive transfer of or decayed maternal antibodies (Figure 60.2). It is usually a mild disease with fever, nasal discharge, and dry cough. Disease can be more severe in seronegative calves with high fever for up to 7 days and clinical signs ranging from tracheitis to pneumonia. BPIV type 3 infection is often part of the bovine respiratory disease complex (see Section "Bovine respiratory syncytial virus").

Host–Virus Relationship.

Geographic Distribution and Transmission. BPIV3 was first isolated in the United States but has been found to be endemic in cattle populations worldwide. It is transmitted through the respiratory route via nasal mucus and ocular secretions. The severity of disease is promoted by poor ventilation, close contact due to overcrowding and stressed feedlots. Although antibodies reactive with BPIV3 have been found in a number of species (mostly ungulate), the importance of cross-species transmission is not resolved.

Pathogenesis and Pathology. After gaining access to the respiratory system, BPIV3 infects epithelia cells. This leads to loss of ciliary function of epithelia cells. In addition, the virus infects pulmonary macrophages leading to a weakened immune response. The inhibitory effect on the clearance function of the mucociliary apparatus, and on the local and systemic immune responses contribute to the establishment of secondary bacterial infections that are commonly associated with the bovine respiratory disease complex. The histological hallmark of BPIV3 infection are bronchitis/bronchiolitis and alveolitis. During acute infection, typical eosinophilic inclusion bodies are seen in epithelium. During the repair phase beginning 14 days after infection, hyperplasia of airways and alveolar epithelium are seen.

Laboratory Diagnosis. During the acute infection virus can be cultivated from nasal secretions or be detected by PCR. To detect antibodies, the hemagglutination inhibition assay, the neutralization and (less often) ELISA are used. Antibody diagnosis may be complicated by the presence of maternal antibodies or antibodies due to the endemic nature of the virus. To demonstrate acute infection, an increase in antibody has to be observed in paired serum samples from acutely infected and convalescent animals.

Control and Prevention. Good husbandry practices that avoid overcrowding, stress and poor ventilation help to control the transmission and severity of disease. Inactivated and modified live PI-3 viral vaccines are available, usually combined with other viral or bacterial vaccines.

Rubulaviruses

Parainfluenza Virus type 5 (Canine Parainfluenza Virus)

Canine parainfluenza virus type 5 has been implicated as a cause of infectious tracheobronchitis (kennel cough) in dogs, along with canine adenovirus and Bordetella bronchiseptica. The disease is characterized by sudden onset, mild fever, slight to copious nasal discharge, and a harsh, nonproductive cough. Canine parainfluenza virus is antigenically related to the Simian virus-5 virus of monkeys, and it appears that the same or very similar viruses infect a wide variety of animal species. Live modified viral vaccines are available, usually combined with other canine viral vaccines such as CD and canine hepatitis or with a Bordetella bronchiseptica vaccine.

Pneumovirinae

Metapneumoviruses

Metapneumoviruses are distinguished from pneumoviruses on the basis of their gene order and virion protein composition. Avian and human metapneumoviruses are assigned to this group.

Four subtypes of avian metapneumovirus exist (A–D) with differences in host species and geographic distribution. Subtype C is found in the United States and causes rhinotracheitis in turkeys. Subtypes A, B, and D are found in other parts of the world. In addition to turkeys, they infect the respiratory tract and the oviduct of chicken resulting in rhinotracheitis and the loss of egg production. There are also case reports of ducks and pheasants infected with avian metapneumovirus. To prevent infection, killed and live-attenuated vaccines exist.

Pneumoviruses

Viruses within the genus *Pneumovirus* include respiratory syncytial viruses that infect humans, cattle, and mice, as well as those that infect sheep and goats, which are closely related to bovine respiratory syncytial virus. The viruses within this genus are distinguished on the basis of their host range and lack of cross-neutralization. The members of this group lack neuraminidase and the nucleocapsid has a diameter of 13–14 nm, which is smaller than the nucleocapsid of the paramyxoviruses (18 nm). All members of the genus Pneumovirus are antigenically related but are antigenically distinct from other paramyxoviruses. Their hemagglutin protein is designated as G, as compared to H or HN in members of the subfamily Paramyxovirinae.

Bovine Respiratory Syncytial Virus

Disease. The bovine respiratory syncytial virus (BRSV) is a major cause of respiratory disease in cattle (Figure 60.5). It causes an acute pneumonia in calves, which show such clinical signs such as coughing, fever, anorexia, nasal discharge, and respiratory distress. Infection of cattle with BRSV leads to major economic losses.

In addition, BRSV is a major contributor to the bovine respiratory disease complex that is characterized by coinfections with BPIV, Mannheimia hemolytica and/or

FIGURE 60.5. *BRSV infection of a seronegative calf, 8 days postchallenge. (A) Immunoperoxidase staining of viral antigen in lung (brown) shows extensive infection of airway epithelium. Expression of viral membrane proteins causes extensive fusion of epithelial cells to form large syncytia (white arrow), and syncytia are widespread in an airway present in the lower portion of this field (black arrow). The more linear pattern of immunoperoxidase staining reflects viral infection of alveolar epithelium. Cytoplasmic viral inclusion bodies are not conspicuous. (B) Virus-infection precipitates a secondary bacterial bronchopneumonia, and also collapse of lobules associated with airway obstruction by inflammatory cells (atelectasis), illustrated by the brown discoloration of lobules in the cranial and ventral aspects of the lung lobe. Airway obstruction leads to rupture of air spaces during labored breathing, giving rise to emphysematous change (large pockets of trapped air, white arrows). (Illustrations courtesy of John Ellis, University of Saskatchewan.)*

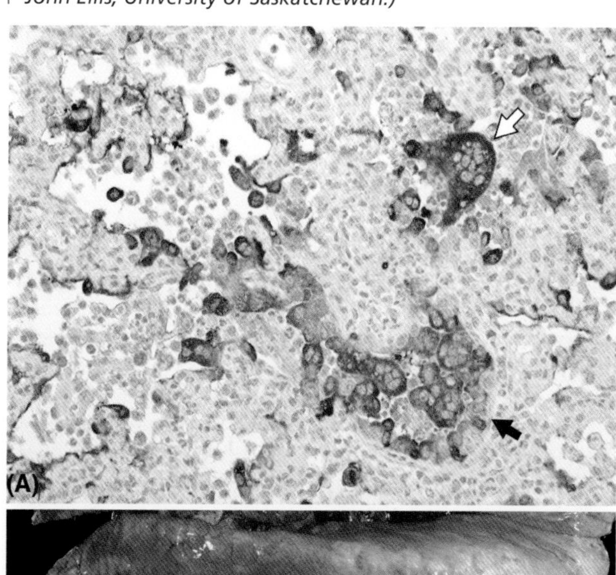

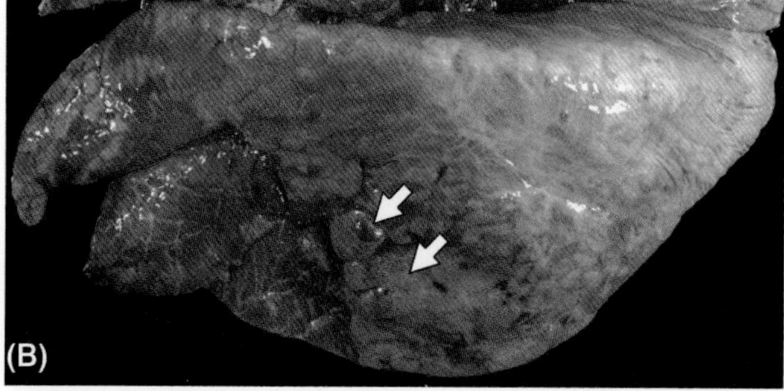

Mycoplasma species. The resulting clinical syndrome has been labeled bovine respiratory disease complex or "shipping fever." The disease is characterized by high fever, conjunctivitis, respiratory distress, mucopurulent rhinitis, and pneumonia, and occurs after cattle are congregated on feedlots. The disease is widespread in the United States and remains one of the major causes of economic losses in the cattle industry.

Host–Virus Relationship

Geographic Distribution and Transmission. BRSV was first identified in Europe in 1970 but has since been show to be present worldwide in cattle population causing respiratory diseases. The virus is transmitted through nasal secretions and close contact.

Pathogenesis and Pathology. After infection with the virus through the respiratory route, epithelial cells of the respiratory tract are infected. Animals develop fever, coughing, no or low nasal discharge and tachypnea between 3 and 9 days after infection. By gross pathology, lungs are red, depressed and firm after uncomplicated BRSV infection. Histologically, bronchial and bronchiolar epithelial necrosis and multinucleated syncytial cells are found. Sometimes intraepithelial inclusion bodies are detected in airways, although their formation is less conspicuous compared to that associated with bovine parainfluenza virus type 3. Younger animals are more severely infected than older ones, and the complication by secondary infections (see BRD complex) leads to more severe disease and economic losses.

Laboratory Diagnosis. The detection of BRSV in nasal secretion by immunofluorescence and quantitative RT-PCR assays are being used to diagnose BRSV. Paired serum samples (with a 10–14 days interval) can be used to determine infection through the increase in antibody titers by neutralization assay.

Control and Prevention. Given the high prevalence of BRSV worldwide, control of the virus has to be attempted by vaccination. Experimental vaccination using formalin-inactivated virus did not result in protection against infection but lead to an enhanced disease after infection with wild-type virus. This is very similar to findings with formalin-inactivated vaccine against human RSV in people. Currently, inactivated and modified live vaccines are being used, usually as combination with other viral and bacterial vaccines.

Filoviridae

Viruses within this family are characterized by enveloped, pleomorphic (filamentous) virions and a genome of single-stranded molecule of negative-sense RNA. There are two major groups of filoviruses: Ebola and related viruses, and Marburg and related viruses. Viruses within these groups cause severe, fatal diseases of humans that are characterized as "hemorrhagic fevers" because of the spectacular diseases they cause in affected humans. These viruses infect primates and can be adapted to laboratory animals. Outbreaks in human populations are rare and geographically restricted to certain parts of Africa. It is hypothesized that contact between humans and a rodent virus reservoir is the cause of these outbreaks.

Bornaviridae

Viruses within this family are characterized by enveloped spherical virions of 80–140 nm in diameter, and a genome of single-stranded, negative-sense RNA. In contrast to other viruses of the Mononegavirales family, bornaviridae use the nucleus of host cells for transcription and replication. Avian Bornavirus (ABV) and Borna disease virus (BDV) are members of this family.

Avian Bornavirus

An ABV is the causative agent of proventricular dilatation disease (PDD) in psittacine birds. The disease is also known as macaw wasting syndrome, proventricular dilatation syndrome, neuropathic gastric dilatation of psittaciforms or myenteric ganglioneuritis. Birds affected by PDD frequently show weight loss with reduced appetite and various degrees of gastrointestinal dysfunction. In a number of cases, central nervous disease symptoms like seizures, ataxia, and motor deficits can be observed. ABV infection in psittacine birds has been documented worldwide. In addition, case reports of ABV infection in other species of bird suggest that the host spectrum of this virus is larger than currently defined, and that persistent infection without clinical symptoms occurs often.

Borna Disease Virus

Originally, Borna disease was described as a neurological disease of horses in Germany, but since then, BDV infections have been discovered worldwide. The precise significance of BDV as a veterinary pathogen remains to be adequately defined. Natural infections with BDV are most frequently seen in sheep and horses. The natural reservoir for BDV is suspected to be insectivores. BDV is neutrotropic and persistently infects neurons in the brain that may or may not result in result in clinical symptoms. Experimentally cattle, rabbits, goats, dogs, cats, and rodents can be infected with BDV. Whether BDV is the cause of neuropsychiatric disorders in humans is fiercely debated.

Diagnosis, Control and Prevention. BDV infection can be determined by the presence of antibodies. ABV infection is currently diagnosed by PCR. No vaccine is available to prevent infection with either virus. To prevent infection, infected animals have to be kept separated from not infected animals. Bornaviruses are susceptible to common disinfectants against enveloped viruses.

Further Reading

Brodersen BW (2010) Bovine respiratory syncytial virus. *Vet Clin North Am Food Anim Pract*, **26**, 323–333.

Chatziandreou N, Stock N, Young D *et al.* (2004) Relationships and host range of human, canine, simian and porcine isolates of simian virus 5 (parainfluenza virus 5). *J Gen Virol* **85**, 3007–3016.

Di Guardo G, Marruchella G, Agrimi U, and Kennedy S (2005) Morbillivirus infections in aquatic mammals: a brief overview. *J Vet Med A Physiol Pathol Clin Med*, **52**, 88–93.

Dortmans JC, Koch G, Rottier PJ, and Peeters BP (2011) Virulence of newcastle disease virus: what is known so far? *Vet Res*, **42**, 122.

Ellis JA (2010) Bovine parainfluenza-3 virus. *Vet Clin North Am Food Anim Pract*, **26**, 575–593.

Lo MK, PA (2008) The emergence of Nipah virus, a highly pathogenic paramyxovirus. *J Clin Virol*, **43**, 396–400.

Martella V, Elia G, and Buonavoglia C (2008) Canine distemper virus. *Vet Clin North Am Small Anim Pract*, **38**, 787–797.

Morens DM, Holmes EC, Davis AS, and Taubenberger JK (2011) Global rinderpest eradication: lessons learned and why humans should celebrate too. *J Infect Dis*, **204**, 502–505.

Raghav R, Taylor M, DeLay J *et al.* (2010) Avian Bornavirus is present inmany tissues of psittacine birds with histopathologic evidence of proventricular dilatation disease. *J Vet Diagn Invest*, **22**, 495–508.

Staeheli P, Rinder M, and Kaspers B (2010) Avian Bornavirus Associated with Fatal Disease in Psittacine Birds. *J Virology*, **84** (13), 6269–6275.

61 Rhabdoviridae

DEBORAH J. BRIGGS

Rhabdoviruses are bullet-shaped, nonsegmented, single-stranded RNA that infect a wide variety of hosts including vertebrates, invertebrates, and plants. Viruses in the family Rhabdoviridae are grouped into six assigned and one unassigned genera (Table 61.1). Many of these viruses are of public health and economic importance causing severe infection and even death in both mammals and plants. For example, rabies virus is almost invariably fatal in both humans and animals once clinical signs are evident. Vesicular stomatitis virus causes a disease similar to foot-and-mouth disease (FMD), bovine ephemeral fever virus causes a disabling disease in cattle and water buffalo, and spring viremia of carp virus causes a severe hemorrhagic disease of cyprinids. Infectious hematopoietic necrosis virus causes a serious disease in salmonid fish. Plant rhabdoviruses can cause plant diseases that are economically devastating to food crops including maize mosaic, rice transitory yellowing, and potato yellow dwarf disease. The best-studied viruses in the Rhabdoviridae family are rabies virus and vesicular stomatitis virus. Most rhabdoviruses contain five structural genes coding for the nucleoprotein (N), phosphoprotein (P), matrix protein (M), glycoprotein (G), and large subunit protein (L). Some low-level serological cross-reactivity has been reported to occur between specific rhabdoviruses.

Rabies

Disease

Rabies is a progressive encephalitic disease that almost always results in the death of the victim although rare cases of prolonged life and the survival of one human without the administration of vaccine has been reported using the Milwaukee protocol. In humans, early symptoms of rabies are indeterminate, flu-like and may include general malaise, headache, fever, and weakness or discomfort. These signs progress into more specific symptoms and may include insomnia, anxiety, confusion, partial paralysis, hypersalivation, hydrophobia, hallucination, and painful spasms of the pharyngeal muscles. Pain or itching at the site of the initial exposure wound (paresthesia) may also occur. Without intensive medical support, death usually occurs within a few days of the onset of these symptoms. In animals, as in humans, the first signs of illness may be nonspecific and even overlooked. Early signs of rabies may include one or more of the following: lethargy, fever, vomiting, and anorexia. These signs progress rapidly to cerebral dysfunction, ataxia, weakness, paralysis, seizures, difficulty breathing and/or swallowing, hypersalivation, abnormal behavior, aggression, and/or self-mutilation. In dogs, rabies has a relatively short course and they may exhibit one or more of the following signs: drooping jaw and/or tongue, abnormal barking, vomiting, biting and eating unusual objects, aggression, biting without provocation, restlessness, or stiff gate. In cats, rabies also causes dramatic changes in behavior. Cats can become very aggressive and exhibit one or more of the following conditions: poor body condition, ruffled and dirty coat, high fever, restlessness, and pupil dilation. Approximately 90% of rabid cats exhibit aggressive behavior. Unexpected aggressive or abnormal behavior should be considered suspicious in cats that may have experienced an exposure to a potentially rabid animal. In horses, clinical signs of rabies include behavior changes ranging from aggression, ataxia, paresis, hyperesthesia, fever, colic, lameness, and recumbency. The disease generally results in death in 4–5 days once clinical signs are evident. In cattle, initial clinical signs may include depression, lack of eating, and seeking isolation. As the disease progresses, cattle exhibit weakness in legs, straining, and bellowing and may be unable to swallow, resulting in excessive salivation.

Etiologic Agent

Physical, Chemical, and Antigenic Properties. The rabies virion, approximately 180 nm in length by 80 nm in width, contains a single-stranded negative-sense genome RNA that is encapsidated with the nucleocapsid (N) protein, the RNA polymerase (L), and polymerase cofactor phosphoprotein (P). This ribonucleoprotein (RNP) core, along with the matrix protein (M), is condensed into the typical bullet-shaped particle characteristic of rhabdoviruses. Glycoprotein (G) spikes are anchored into the RNP-M structure and protrude through the virus envelope. Antibodies produced against the G protein after vaccination with cell culture rabies vaccines induce the production of protective antibodies and function to neutralize the virus.

Veterinary Microbiology, Third Edition. Edited by D. Scott McVey, Melissa Kennedy and M.M. Chengappa.

Table 61.1. Genus and Species of Family Rhabdoviridae

Genus	Species (Type Species in Bold)
Cytorhabdovirus	*Barley yellow striate mosaic virus* *Broccoli necrotic yellows virus* *Festuca leaf streak virus* *Lettuce necrotic yellows virus* *Northern cereal mosaic virus* *Sonchus virus* *Strawberry crinkle virus* *Wheat American striate mosaic virus*
Ephemerovirus	*Adelaide River virus* *Berrimah virus* *Bovine ephemeral fever virus*
Lyssavirus	*Aravan virus* *Australian bat lyssavirus* *Duvenhage virus* *European bat lyssavirus 1* *European bat lyssavirus 2* *Irkut virus* *Khujand virus* *Lagos bat virus* *Mokola virus* *Rabies virus* *Western Caucasian bat virus*
Novirhabdovirus	*Hirame rhabdovirus* *Infectious hematopoietic necrotic virus* *Snakehead virus* *Viral hemorrhagic septicemia virus*
Nucleorhabdovirus	*Datura yellow vein virus* *Eggplant mottled dwarf virus* *Maize fine streak virus* *Maize mosaic virus* *Potato yellow dwarf virus* *Rice yellow stunt virus* *Sonchus yellow net virus* *Sowthistle yellow vein virus* *Taro vein chlorosis virus*
Unassigned	*Flanders virus* *Ngaingan virus* *Sigma virus* *Tupaia virus* *Wongabel virus*
Vesiculovirus	*Carajas virus* *Chandipura virus* *Cocal virus* *Isfahan virus* *Maraba virus* *Piry virus* *Spring viremia of carp virus* *Vesicular stomatitis Alagoas virus* *Vesicular stomatitis Indiana virus* *Vesicular stomatitis New Jersey virus*

The N protein is the most highly conserved of all of the viral proteins but actually has a high degree of diversity within short segments. As a result, molecular analyses of the N protein have provided information on identifying rabies virus genotypes that can be used as a molecular epidemiological surveillance tool to explain the evolution of rabies viruses and to track movement of rabies over time. For instance, when rabies is detected in animals in a previously rabies-free zone, the virus can often be traced back to the point of origination.

Resistance to Physical and Chemical Agents. Rabies virus is readily destroyed through exposure to soap and other disinfectants, desiccants, and sunlight. The virus is inactivated by heating to 56 °C for 30 min or by various diluted chemicals and disinfectants including a 0.1% bleach solution and a 1% formalin solution. Saliva from a rabid animal is no longer considered infective in the environment or on intact skin after it has dried. In the case of human exposure, all wounds should be washed vigorously with soap and water for at least 15 min in order to inactivate the virus.

Infectivity to Other Species or Culture Systems. Rabies virus can theoretically infect all mammals, but each rabies virus variant tends to circulate in specific species of animals in each region with occasional spillover into animal species that coinhabit the same region. Over 98% of all human rabies deaths occur in Africa and Asia and are caused by exposure to an infected dog. In the Americas, most human deaths are caused by exposure to bat rabies virus variants although there are additional rabies virus variants circulating in other species of wildlife including raccoons, skunks, and foxes. Rabies virus can be propagated in many different mammalian and plant cell lines for research, diagnostic testing, and vaccine production purposes. Virus strains specifically used for diagnostic testing and vaccine production have been stabilized or "fixed" to have a predictable incubation period as opposed to "street" virus strains isolated directly from infected animals that may have varying incubation periods. There are several cell lines that are commonly used for diagnostic purposes including neuroblastoma cells (CCL-131) and baby hamster kidney cells (BHK-21). Several cell lines have been used to produce human and animal vaccines. The most commonly used types include embryonated egg cells, Vero cells, human diploid cells, and baby hamster kidney cells.

Host–Virus Relationship

Distribution, Reservoir, and Transmission. Rabies is an underreported disease that is present on every continent except Antarctica. Human rabies, especially paralytic rabies, may represent as much as 30% of total clinical rabies presentations and is often misdiagnosed as other encephalitic diseases such as malaria or Guillain–Barré syndrome, thus masking the true global burden of the disease. Although all mammals are susceptible to rabies, the primary reservoirs of the disease belong to the orders Carnivora and Chiroptera (dogs, foxes, jackals, coyotes, raccoon dogs, skunks, raccoons, mongoose, and bats). Maintaining rabies in a susceptible animal population is dependent upon several factors including the population and ecological characteristics of the host as well as susceptibility to infection and contact rate. Transmission of rabies from one mammal to another generally occurs through the contamination of tissue with virus-laden saliva inflicted during a bite wound. Transmission can also occur when virus-infected saliva or other body fluids enter a mucous membrane. Rabies virus cannot penetrate intact skin and therefore, even if infected saliva or body tissues come in contact with intact skin, it should not be considered an exposure. Aerosol transmission has been reported but it is extremely rare.

Pathogenesis and Pathology. Rabies virus infection begins with an exposure after which the virus attaches to the cell surface and penetration occurs. A specific rabies virus receptor site has not been reported, but various lipids, gangliosides, carbohydrates, and proteins have been implicated. After entering the peripheral nerves, rabies virus travels within motor and perhaps sensory axons centripetally to the central nervous system (CNS). Evidence indicates that the virus can travel at a rate of 50–100 mm/day. The virus crosses the synapse of one dendritic process to another eventually reaching the CNS and continually moving toward the brain. Once the virus reaches the brain, it moves centrifugally back through the peripheral nerves to various body organs including the salivary glands. In spite of the severe clinical neurological signs, the neuropathological findings in rabies-infected humans and animals are relatively mild, suggesting that neuronal dysfunction occurs in rabies without detectable morphologic changes. There may be some congestion of leptomeningeal and parenchymal blood vessels, perivascular cuffing, microglial activation with formation of "Babes' nodules," and neuronophagia, but subarachnoid or parenchymal hemorrhage is not a reported feature of rabies. Negri bodies, identified as neuronal intracytoplasmic bodies, may be found in brain tissue from animals or humans infected with "street" rabies virus strains as opposed to "fixed" viruses. However, Negri bodies are infrequently seen with "fixed" virus strains. Negri bodies are identified as dense, well-defined, oval or round, eosinophilic cytoplasmic inclusions that are typically 2–10 μm in diameter.

Host Response to Infection. Rabies virus synchronously infects the limbic system causing organically induced fury while the virus is being secreted into the saliva for transmission to the next victim through an inflicted bite. Human rabies patients experience episodes of arousal or hyperexcitability, aggression, confusion, and hallucinations interrupted by periods of lucidity when they are able to understand their condition. After an exposure occurs, the highly neurotropic virus initially replicates at the entry site, enters and moves along the peripheral nervous system to the spinal cord eventually reaching the brain. Once rabies virus reaches the brain, the virus continues to replicate and is disseminated centrifugally through the nerves to the body organs including the salivary glands where it is emitted into the saliva and is passed on to the next victim.

Hydrophobia, or "fear of water," is present only in humans. As with humans, initial signs of rabies in animals are nonspecific and may include anorexia, lethargy, fever, dysphagia, vomiting, stranguria, straining to defecate, and diarrhea. As the disease progresses, the behavior of animals changes and normally friendly animals may become more aggressive and vice versa. Wildlife may lose their fear of humans and normally nocturnal animals may be active in the daytime. Pressing or "head butting" may be observed. Clinical rabies in humans may include paresthesias, and a similar clinical sign may be observed in animals as they bite or scratch at the wound site where virus entered. Infected animals may also attack inanimate objects for no reason. The clinical representation of rabies is often categorized as being either "furious" or "dumb" rabies, but it is more likely that clinical signs such as these are likely to be a continuum of expressive behavior as the disease progresses to coma and death. Recovery from rabies is extremely rare although at least one human has been confirmed to have survived rabies without postexposure prophylaxis reported after administration of the Milwaukee protocol.

Laboratory Diagnosis

Bites or other exposures from suspected rabid animals and the disposition and testing of the animals in question should involve contacting and working with the appropriate public health departments. The decision whether animals that are exposed to humans or other animals should be isolated and observed, or humanely euthanized and submitted for testing, is ultimately the decision of professionals in the health department. If an animal is submitted for testing, it should be humanely euthanized and the head removed without damage. Tissue should be kept refrigerated to retard decomposition and provide reliable results because autolyzed samples can reduce the sensitivity and specificity of the test. Multiple regions of the brain are examined to ensure that if the virus is present, it will be detected. The fluorescent antibody test (FAT) is the "gold standard" assay, which confirms the presence of rabies virus in animal tissues. The FAT detects the virus in tissues through the binding of rabies virus-specific antibodies labeled with a fluorescent dye to rabies virus. Confirmatory testing on negative tissue samples often includes the use of the mouse inoculation test or the rabies tissue culture infection test. The use of the direct rapid immunohistochemical test (dRIT) has been extensively evaluated in the United States and abroad and is currently being expanded throughout the world. The dRIT is less expensive to use than the FAT and can be used in field conditions. Increased usage of the dRIT in resource-poor countries is a valuable tool to help increase surveillance and better evaluate the global epidemiology of rabies. Real-time polymerase chain reaction (RT-PCR) assays can assist in the detection and identification of specific lyssaviruses and are also useful tools to elucidate the global epidemiology of specific virus variants, but presently these tests require expensive equipment and well-equipped laboratories and are not cost-effective for routine diagnoses of animal tissues. Implementation of rapid laboratory diagnoses by a reliable laboratory after a bite incident from a suspected rabid animal can aid in significantly reducing the cost of post-exposure prophylaxis (PEP) for humans. PEP, consisting of washing the wound inflicted from a rabid animal and administration of rabies immunoglobulin and an injection series of rabies vaccine, is costly but must be administered to prevent rabies after an exposure has occurred. If the suspected animal is confirmed to be uninfected with rabies, PEP can be avoided or halted if it has already been initiated.

Treatment and Control

Rabies is virtually 100% fatal, and there are no treatment protocols for animals once clinical signs are evident. However, rabies can be prevented in domestic animals through effective vaccination. Animal rabies vaccines that are currently available include inactivated and recombinant vaccines. Inactivated rabies vaccines that are produced according to the OIE requirements protect against all strains of rabies genotype 1 isolated to date and are administered parenterally initially at 3 months of age, and then according to the recommendations of the manufacturer. Local and state ordinances may also regulate the timing of rabies vaccination. Modified live vaccines are not licensed for use in the United States, but may be produced and utilized in other countries. Recombinant vaccines are built on the backbone of another vector virus, for example, vaccinia or canarypox viruses, by incorporating the glycoprotein of the rabies virus into the carrier virus. The recombinant rabies vaccine produced from the canarypox vector is currently licensed for cats in the United States and is administered parenterally. The concept of developing oral rabies vaccines (ORV) to vaccinate wildlife to overcome the need of catching and vaccinating individual animals involved years of research. ORV was initially utilized in 1969 as a strategy in Switzerland to successfully eliminate rabies in red foxes and was a modified live vaccine (SAD Berne strain) imbedded in chicken heads and distributed throughout fox habitat. Newer, and safer, ORVs are manufactured as recombinant vaccines that have incorporated the rabies glycoprotein into the vaccinia virus vector. These ORVs have successfully eliminated rabies in foxes in Western Europe and in coyotes in the southern United States and continue to be an important component of the national strategy in both Europe and the United States.

Vesicular Stomatitis

Disease

Infection of vesicular stomatitis virus (VSV) causes an acute febrile disease of horses, cattle, and swine that is currently limited to the Americas. In cattle, vesicular stomatitis (VS) closely resembles FMD causing vesicles in the mucosal lining of the mouth and tongue. Vesicles can also be found on the teats, sink of the coronary band, and in the interdigital spaces of the hoof. In swine, the disease is similar to vesicular exanthema (VES) or swine vesicular disease (SVD). Neither VES nor SVD occurs in horses. Therefore, horses can serve as a sentinel species for VS when there is an outbreak of disease. Confirmation of VS is critical in order to prevent the potential spread of one of the three exotic diseases mentioned earlier and to limit spread within the Americas. VS is a self-limiting disease with infected animals generally recovering without residual disease impact. During outbreaks, milk production can be reduced in dairy cattle and the painful lesions can cause infected animals to reduce feed uptake or stop eating altogether thus impacting production.

FIGURE 61.1. *This negatively stained transmission electron micrograph revealed the presence of numerous negative-sense, single-stranded RNA VSV virions. (Courtesy of Dr Fred Murphy, Centers for Disease Control and Prevention; located in public health image library domain, http://phil.cdc.gov, accessed January 30, 2013; photo ID # 5611.)*

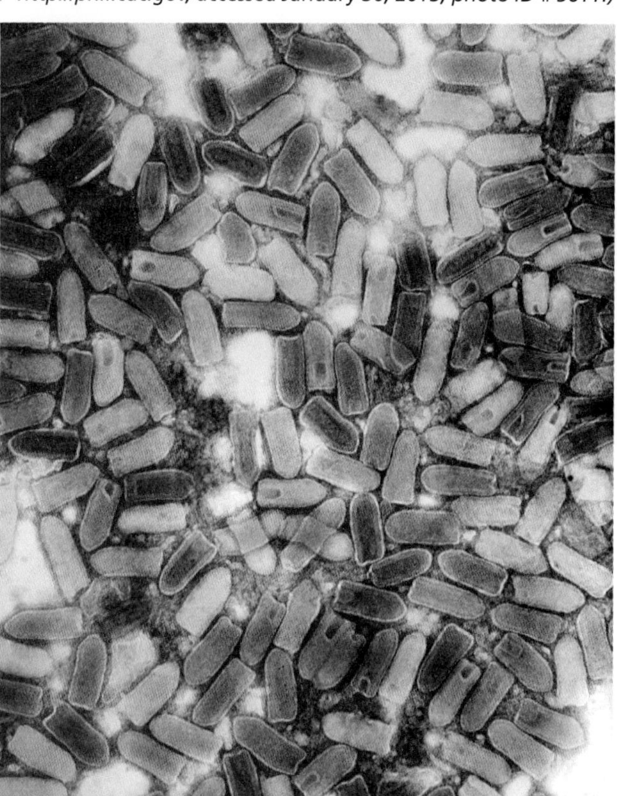

In humans, VS causes flu-like symptoms and can cause severe conjunctivitis when VSV is directly deposited into the mucous membrane of the eye.

Etiologic Agent

Physical, Chemical, and Antigenic Properties. VSV closely resembles rabies virus in morphology, genome, and protein structure (Figure 61.1). There are two distinct immunological classes of VSV currently identified including New Jersey (NJ) and Indiana (IND). In addition, the IND serogroup is divided into three subtypes including IND-1 (classical IND), IND-2 (Cocal virus), and IND-3 (Alagoas virus) (ICTV2012).

Resistance to Physical and Chemical Agents. VSV can be inactivated using an effective disinfectant including formaldehyde, ether and other organic solvents, chlorine dioxide, 1% formalin, 1% sodium hypochlorite, 70% ethanol, 2% glutaraldehyde, 2% sodium carbonate, 4% sodium hydroxide, and 2% iodophor disinfectants. Although the virus can survive for long periods at low temperatures, it is readily inactivated by direct sunlight or heating to 58 °C for 30 min. VSV can remain stable between pH

4 and 10 and is resistant to lye (2–3% NaOH will not fully inactivate VSV).

Infectivity to Other Species or Culture Systems. VSV can infect domestic animals including cattle, swine, horses, donkeys, and mules. Natural infection in sheep and goats is rarely reported, but both species can be infected experimentally. Wild animal hosts include white-tailed deer and many species of small mammals. Humans can be infected from handling infected livestock. In the laboratory, experimental infection has been confirmed in mice, rats, guinea pigs, deer, raccoons, bobcats, and monkeys. VSV is used as a laboratory model for studies in viral morphology, replication, and genetics.

Host–Virus Relationship

Distribution, Reservoir, and Transmission. Although VSV was historically described in France in 1915 and in South Africa in the late 1800s, its current distribution appears to be limited to the Americas. The NJ and subtype IND-1 are endemic causing more than 80% of all infections in regions of southern Mexico, Central America, Venezuela, Colombia, Ecuador, and Peru. Sporadic outbreaks of NJ and IND-1 VSV have been reported in northern Mexico and the western United States. IND-2 is currently only reported in horses in Argentina and Brazil. IND-3 subtype has also been identified sporadically in Brazil mostly in horses but to a lesser degree in cattle. Virus transmission is not fully understood, but VSV has been isolated from sandflies, mosquitoes, and other insects indicating that they may be involved in virus transmission although disease transmission through direct contact has also been confirmed.

Pathogenesis and Pathology. The pathogenesis of VS is not entirely clear, but clinically, it is indistinguishable from FMD, SVD, and VES. Other diseases to be considered in the differential diagnosis include infectious bovine rhinotracheitis, bovine viral diarrhea, malignant catarrhal fever, bovine popular stomatitis, rinderpest (eradicated in 2011), bluetongue, epizootic hemorrhagic disease, foot rot, and chemical or thermal burns.

The incubation period for VS is 2–8 days after exposure with the first sign usually presenting as fever and excessive salivation followed by blisters and eruption of vesicles, ulcerous erosions, and crusting of muzzle and lips. The disease is limited to the epithelial tissues of the mouth, nostrils, teats, and feet. The size of the vesicles is highly variable and can be as small as the size of a pea or large enough to cover the entire surface area of the tongue. In cattle, vesicles are usually found on the hard palate, lips, and gums and may extend to the nostrils and muzzle, whereas in horses, the first vesicles may go unnoticed until crusting scabs appear on the muzzle, lips, or ventral abdomen. In pigs, vesicles generally appear on the feet and frequently on the muzzle. Vesicles on the feet often cause lameness.

Dairy cattle with lesions on the teats may develop mastitis from secondary infection. VS occurs throughout the year in Latin America but is particularly common at the end of the rainy season. In the Southwestern United States, outbreaks of VS are common in the warmer months and are identified along rivers and in valleys.

Host Response to Infection. It has been reported that humoral-specific antibodies do not always prevent infection. Morbidity rate is 5–90% with deaths being rare in cattle and horses, but higher mortality rates are reported in some pigs infected with the NJ strain. Sick animals recover in approximately 2 weeks, and the most common complications during infection are mastitis and loss of production in dairy cattle. Disease incidence varies according to the serotype and species involved. Usually 10–15% of the adult animals in infected herds present with clinical signs. Cattle and horses less than 1 year of age are rarely reported affected and mortality is close to 0% in horses and cattle.

Laboratory Diagnosis

If VS infection is suspected, the proper authorities should be immediately notified. Sample collection should also comply with the required samples for FMD, VES, and SVD in order to facilitate ruleout of these diseases. To prevent spreading of VSV, all samples should be collected and sent under secured conditions to an authorized laboratory. Due to the painful nature of the vesicles and animal welfare concerns, sedation of the animal is highly recommended. Samples to be submitted should include vesicular fluid, the epithelium covering of unruptured vesicles or the epithelial flaps of ruptured vesicles from mouth, feet, and other sites of vesicle eruption. If epithelial tissue is not available, samples of esophageal/pharyngeal liquid should be collected. Samples from pigs should include throat swabs. All samples should be sent under refrigeration or frozen if the transport takes longer than 2 days. Paired serum samples taken 2 weeks apart may also be collected. In the United States, paired serum samples are only required for the index case. Once an outbreak has been confirmed, a single serum sample is all that is required to confirm infection. Assays to detect antigens include virus isolation, enzyme-linked immunoadsorbent assay (ELISA), complement fixation, and PCR. The indirect ELISA is the diagnostic method of choice to identify viral serotypes. Serological tests to confirm antibodies to VSV for international trade concerns include liquid-phase blocking ELISA or competitive ELISA, virus neutralization, and complement fixation for detection of IgM.

Treatment and Control

There is no treatment for VS, but antibiotics may prevent secondary bacterial infection in abraded tissues. Suspicion of VS includes quarantine of infected herds pending confirmatory testing. Vehicles and fomites should be disinfected, and subclinically infected animals should be kept indoors in isolation. Humans should use precautions when handling infected or suspected infected animals including gloves to prevent contamination and spreading of the disease. Cattle should not be moved from infected areas before 21 days after all lesions are healed with the exception of animals sent to slaughter. Insect control may help to prevent disease spread, and all breeding areas should be eliminated.

VSV-killed vaccines are currently sold in Venezuela and Columbia.

Bovine Ephemeral Fever

Disease

Bovine ephemeral fever (BEF) is a noncontagious epizootic arthropod-borne disease of cattle and water buffaloes commonly known as "3-day sickness," "3-day stiff sickness," or "dragon boat disease." It is an economically important disease in cattle due to the impact that it has on milk production, abortion, temporary infertility in bulls, and prolonged recovery in some animals. Mortality rates are low in cattle in good condition but can be more severe, with rates as high as 30%, in fat cattle. Ruleout diseases include Rift Valley fever, heartwater, bluetongue, botulism, babesiosis, and blackleg. Excess salivation may resemble FMD, but no vesicles are observed.

Etiologic Agent

Physical, Chemical, and Antigenic Properties. BEF is caused by bovine ephemeral fever virus (BEFV), a rhabdovirus that is antigenically related to several other nonpathogenic viruses, for example Adelaide River virus, as well as rhabdoviruses that cause similar diseases to BEF including Kotonkan and Puchong viruses.

Resistance to Physical and Chemical Agents. BEFV is destroyed by disinfectants like sodium hypochlorite.

Infectivity to Other Species or Culture Systems. BEFV is not spread by casual contact but is spread intravenously generally through the bite of an infected insect vector. Symptomatic infections have been reported in hartebeest, waterbuck, wildebeest, and goats. Additionally antibodies to BEFV have been detected in Cape buffalo, deer, and antelope in Africa and deer in Australia. BEF impacts trade in live animals and semen to disease-free zones.

Host–Virus Relationship

Distribution, Reservoir, and Transmission. BEF is endemic in tropical and subtropical zones in Africa, Asia, and Australia. Geographically, this includes all countries south of a line that also includes Israel, Iraq, Iran, Syria, India, Pakistan, Bangladesh, southern and central China, and southern Japan that extends through Southeast Asia to Australia. In Australia, the estimated economic impact of BEF is estimated to exceed US$100 million. The disease is spread by arthropods and has been isolated from the mosquito species of *Culex* and *Anopheles* and from *Culicoides* biting midges in Africa and Australia. The disease can also be spread through intravenous inoculation of blood from an infected animal. BEFV is not spread by close contact, body secretions including semen, or aerosol droplets. It is rapidly inactivated in meat and does not appear to be spread by consumption.

Pathogenesis and Pathology. Experimentally, the average incubation period is 2–4 days although as much as 9 days has been reported. Clinical signs of BEFV infection occur as a result of a vascular inflammatory response. The onset of fever and other clinical signs is accompanied by a marked leucopoenia, relative neutrophilia, elevated plasma fibrinogen, biochemical imbalance including hypocalcemia and elevated levels of cytokines. There have been reports of prolonged paralysis or ataxia in animals recovering from acute infection. Lesions include a small amount of fibrin-rich fluid in the pleural, peritoneal, and pericardial cavities. Fluid may also be found in the joint capsules. Serofibrinous polysynovitis, polyarthritis, polytendovaginitis, and cellulitis have also been reported. Patchy edema may be seen in the lungs and lymphadenitis is often observed. Petechial hemorrhages or edema occurs in the lymph nodes. Areas of focal necrosis are seen in the major muscle groups.

Host Response to Infection. Clinical signs of BEF are short lived but severe with infected cattle exhibiting a biphasic or triphasic fever. Morbidity rates range from 1 to 100% depending upon the epidemiological factors with mortality rates rarely reaching higher than 1%. Temperature peaks are approximately 12–18 h apart. The first indication of disease may be fever accompanied by a dramatic reduction in milk production that may not return to normal until the next lactation. Clinical signs are more severe during the second fever with animals exhibiting increased heart rate, tachypnea, depression, anorexia, ruminal atony, serous or mucoid discharge from nose and eyes, salivation, muscle twitching, shivering, joint pain, stiffness, and shifting lameness. Additionally, there may be submandibular edema or patchy edema on the head. Animals may become recumbent for 8 h to days with temporary loss of reflexes. Some animals will not be able to rise. Within a day or two, animals begin to recover. Complications are rare but may include temporary paralysis, gait impairment, aspiration pneumonia, emphysema, and the subcutaneous accumulation of air along the back.

Laboratory Diagnosis

If BEF is suspected, notification of the responsible authorities should be the first step. All samples collected for laboratory examination need to be sent securely to prevent spread of the disease. BEF is confirmed by serological testing, and submitted samples should include approximately 20 ml of clotted blood and 5 ml of uncoagulated blood using an anticoagulant other than EDTA (ethylenediaminetetraacetic acid). Paired serum samples, to demonstrate a rising titer, are tested by virus neutralization tests or ELISA. Cross-reactivity to related rhabdoviruses may occur. Virus isolation from blood samples is difficult. BEF has been confirmed by inoculating susceptible cattle or weaned mice with uncoagulated whole blood.

Treatment and Control

Sodium hypochlorite and other disinfectants will destroy BEFV, but generally disinfection is unimportant since the virus is transmitted through mosquitoes or midges rather than by direct contact. Anti-inflammatory drugs and calcium borogluconate injections are recommended in some cases to treat fever, anorexia, muscle stiffness, ocular and nasal discharge, ruminal stasis, and sternal recumbency. Immunity after infection has been reported and vaccination has an important role in the management of BEF. There are killed and live vaccines currently being sold in Asia and Africa.

Diseases of Fish Caused by Rhabdoviruses

Several rhabdoviruses in the genus *Vesiculovirus* and *Novirhabdovirus* cause serious diseases and economic losses in wild and farmed fish. Two specific viruses that have a high economic impact on farmed and wild fish are mentioned here: spring viremia of carp virus (SVCV), classified within the genus *Vesiculovirus*, and infectious hematopoietic necrosis virus (IHNV), classified within the genus *Novirhabdovirus*.

Spring Viremia of Carp

SVCV causes a fatal disease in cyprinid fish. Common carp, including the variety called koi carp, are the main species infected by SVCV although many species of fish in the minnow family are also susceptible to the disease. The disease has been reported in Europe, the Middle East, Asia, and North and South America. First signs of the disease include a change in behavior, and fish may begin to congregate in slow-moving water or lie on the bottom of ponds and streams. As the disease progresses, fish lie on their sides, become sluggish, and their rate of respiration decreases. Externally, fish may exhibit physical signs of darkening of the skin, swollen abdomen, exophthalmia, skin or gill hemorrhages, and a protruding vent. Internally infected fish exhibit edema in body organs, hemorrhages in the swim bladder, and inflammation of the bladder. Most outbreaks occur in the spring in cooler temperatures. When water temperatures rise to 15–18 °C, the immune system of carp can develop neutralizing antibodies and suppress virus replication. Viral transmission of SVCV occurs horizontally through contact with virus-infected feces, urine, and gill mucous. Vertical transmission is also a possibility since SVCV has been identified in ovarian fluids, but the lack of confirmed outbreaks in fry and fingerlings indicates that it may not be an important route of infection. Diagnosis of SVCV is confirmed through virus isolation, FAT, or ELISA. Prevention of SVCV includes using a source of water that is free from disease, especially in an endemic region, disinfection of eggs by iodophor treatment, regular physical and chemical disinfection of ponds and equipment, and proper disposal of infected fish.

Infectious Hematopoietic Necrosis

IHNV infection results in a serious viral disease of salmonid fish. IHNV is present in North America, Europe, and some Asian countries. Clinical infections are most common in young fish. IHNV can cause major financial losses for infected farms that raise young trout or salmon. Epizootics have also been reported in wild salmon. Susceptible species to IHNV include members of the trout and salmon family. Experimental infections have also been reported in pike fry, sea bream, and turbot. Transmission occurs horizontally from clinically ill fish and asymptomatic carriers through infected feces, urine, sexual fluids, and external mucous either by direct contact or through the water. Vertical transmission has also been reported. The incubation period is between 5 and 45 days, and clinical signs include abdominal distension, exophthalmia, darkened skin, and pale gills. Infected fish are lethargic exhibiting bouts of hyperexcitability and frenzy. Petechial hemorrhages are commonly seen at the base of the pectoral fins, mouth, skin behind the lateral line, muscles near the anus, and the yolk sac in sac fry. Surviving fish often have scoliosis. Postmortem lesions include lack of food in the digestive tract, pale kidney spleen, and focal necrosis of the liver. Petechiae are often seen in the internal organs. Hemorrhages may occur in the kidney peritoneum and swim bladder. Clinical disease occurs when water temperatures are between 8 °C and 15 °C although outbreaks have been reported in warmer water. Young fish, less than 2 months old, are most susceptible to disease. Fish that survive usually develop good immunity to IHNV, but they may also become viral carriers. Diagnosis is confirmed through virus isolation, FAT, and PCR. Serological tests have not been validated for international trade. If IHNV is suspected, appropriate authorities should be contacted. Outbreaks are controlled by culling, disinfection, and quarantines. Eggs should be disinfected with an iodophor solution, and virus-free water should be used to incubate eggs and raise fry. IHNV is inactivated by most common disinfectants including iodophors. A plasmid-based vaccine against IHNV has been developed and is applied one time intramuscularly to fry at the hatchery.

Reference

ICTV (2012) *Virus Taxonomy*. International Committee on Taxonomy of Viruses, www.ictvdb.org (accessed January 15, 2012).

Further Reading

Frymus T, Addie D, and Belák S (2009) Feline rabies: ABCD guidelines on prevention and management. *J Fel Med Surg*, **11**, 585–593.

Guleria A, Kiranmayi M, and Sreejith R (2011) Reviewing host proteins of Rhabdodoviridae: Possible leads for lesser studied viruses. *J Biosci*, **36**, 929–937.

Hemachudha T, Laothamatas J, and Rupprecht CE (2002) Human rabies: a disease of complex neuropathogenetic mechanisms and diagnostic challenges. *Lancet Neurol*, **1**, 101–109.

Hudson LC, Weinstock D, Jordan T, and Bold-Fletcher NO (1996a) Clinical features of experimentally induced rabies in cattle and sheep. *Zentralbl Veterinarmed B*, **43**, 85–95.

Hudson LC, Weinstock D, Jordan T, and Bold-Fletcher NO (1996b) Clinical presentation of experimentally induced rabies in horses. *Zentralbl Veterinarmed B*, **43**, 277–285.

Jackson AC and Wunner W (2007) *Rabies*, 2nd edn, Elsevier.

Meat and Livestock Australia (2006) Assessing the economic cost of endemic disease on the profitability of Australian beef cattle and sheep producers, Final Report, pp. 1–119, Meat and Livestock Australia.

Nandi S and Negi BS (1999) Bovine ephemeral fever: a review. *Comp Immunol Microbiol*, **22**, 81–91.

National Association of State Public Health Veterinarians, Inc. (2011) Compendium of animal rabies prevention and control. *MMWR Recomm Rep*, **60** (RR-6), 1–17.

OIE (2008) *OIE Manual of Diagnostic Tests and Vaccines for Terrestrial Animals*, 6th edn, OIE.

OIE (2009) *Manual of Diagnostic Tests for Aquatic Animals*, OIE.

Rodriguez LL (2002) Emergence and re-emergence of vesicular stomatitis in the United States. *Virus Res*, **85**, 211–219.

Slate D, Algeo TP, Nelson KM *et al.* (2009) Oral rabies vaccination in North America: Opportunities, complexities and challenges. *PLoS NTD*, **3**, e549.

Spickler AR and Roth JA (2006) *Emerging and Exotic Diseases of Animals*, 4th edn, Iowa State University.

WHO Expert Consultation on Rabies (2004) 2005 WHO Tech Rep Series 931. First Report. pp. 1–121. *www.who.int/rabies/trs931_%2006_05.pdf* (accessed January 30, 2013).

Willoughby RE Jr, Tieves KS, Hoffman GM *et al.* (2005) Survival after treatment of rabies with induction of coma. *N Engl J Med*, **352**, 2508–2514.

Coronaviridae

Udeni B.R. Balasuriya

Introduction and Classification

The virus families Coronaviridae, Arteriviridae, and Roniviridae are included in the order Nidovirales (Figure 62.1). All members of the order Nidovirales are enveloped viruses with linear, positive-sense, single-stranded RNA (ssRNA) genomes. They share a strikingly similar genome organization and replication strategy, but differ considerably in their genetic complexity and virion architecture (Figure 62.2). "Nido" derives from the Latin word nidus for nest, which refers to the 3′ co-terminal nested subgenomic viral mRNA that is produced during replication of these viruses. This chapter focuses on viruses of the family Coronaviridae that is further divided into two subfamilies, Coronavirinae and Torovirinae (Figure 62.1). The subfamily Coronavirinae consists of three genera (*Alphacoronavirus, Betacoronavirus*, and *Gammacoronavirus*), whereas the subfamily Torovirinae consists of two genera (*Bafinivirus* and *Torovirus*). Coronaviruses cause acute and chronic infections in humans and a wide variety of animals, resulting in respiratory, enteric, hepatic, and neurologic disease of varying degrees of severity. The toroviruses infect humans and animals (horses, cattle, and pigs) and are predominantly associated with enteric disease. The viruses belonging to the families Arteriviridae and Roniviridae will be discussed in Chapter 63.

Coronaviruses are well-known agents of respiratory, enteric, and neurologic disease in humans and domestic animals and are the only nidovirus group that has been reported to cause disease in humans. In spring 2003, severe acute respiratory syndrome (SARS) emerged from China as a potentially fatal and untreatable human respiratory disease that was caused by a previously unknown coronavirus (CoV) strain. Discovery of severe acute respiratory syndrome coronavirus (SARS-CoV) triggered a search for the reservoir species. After extensive investigative studies over a number of years, certain species of bats were identified as reservoir hosts of the virus. In addition, these studies led to the discovery of many novel human, bat, and avian coronaviruses. In 2008, a highly divergent coronavirus was identified from a deceased captive beluga whale and grouped as a gammacoronavirus. Coronaviruses infect a wide range of mammals (including humans, bats, and a whale) and birds. They exhibit a marked tropism for epithelial cells of the respiratory and enteric tracts, as well as macrophages of some animals. Coronaviruses cause a remarkably diverse spectrum of different diseases in different hosts (Table 62.1). They typically have a restricted host range, infecting only their natural host and closely related animal species. However, they have the capacity to cross the species barrier (species jumping) and infect new hosts.

Avian infectious bronchitis virus (IBV) was the first coronavirus to be isolated from chicken embryos in 1937. This was followed by mouse hepatitis virus (MHV) in the 1940s and other mammalian coronaviruses in the 1970s. These include several animal coronaviruses (e.g., porcine transmissible gastroenteritis virus (TGEV), bovine coronavirus (BCoV), and feline coronavirus (FeCoV)), as well as human coronaviruses (HuCoV; e.g., HuCoV-OC43 and HuCoV-229E). Since the emergence of the human SARS-CoV that was responsible for the SARS in the spring of 2003, coronaviruses became more recognized and generated a significant interest among researchers. Following the SARS outbreak, the number of full-length genome sequences deposited in public databases has almost tripled. These include two human coronaviruses (HuCoV-NL63 and HuCoV-HKU1), 10 other mammalian coronaviruses (bat SARS coronavirus, bat coronavirus (bat-CoV)-HKU2, bat-CoV-HKU4, bat-CoV-HKU5, bat-CoV-HKU8, bat-CoV-HKU9, bat-CoV-512/2005, bat-CoV1A, equine coronavirus (ECoV), and beluga whale coronavirus (BWCoV)), and four avian coronaviruses (turkey coronavirus (TCoV), bulbul coronavirus-HKU11 (BuCoV-HKU11), thrush coronavirus-HKU12 (ThCoV-HKU12), and munia coronavirus-HKU13 (MunCoV-HKU13)). The genus *Coronavirus* is divided into three groups (1–3) based on their serologic cross-reactivity. Groups 1 and 2 are composed of mammalian coronaviruses and group 3 consists of avian coronaviruses. The application of molecular biology techniques has generated a large amount of sequence data for these coronaviruses. Phylogenetic analysis of these coronavirus sequences has grouped them along the same boundaries of the traditional antigenic classification (groups 1–3). However, these phylogenetic analyses have also identified two additional subgroups in both groups 2 (2a, 2b, 2c, and 2d) and 3 (3a, 3b, and 3c). Recently, the Coronavirus Study Group of the International Committee for Taxonomy of Viruses has assigned the three traditional groups 1, 2, and 3 of

Veterinary Microbiology, Third Edition. Edited by D. Scott McVey, Melissa Kennedy and M.M. Chengappa.

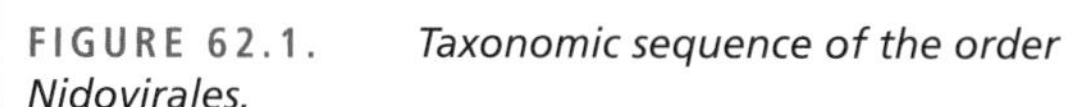

FIGURE 62.1. *Taxonomic sequence of the order Nidovirales.*

Order: Nidovirales

- **Family:** Arteriviridae → **Genus:** *Arterivirus*
- **Family:** Roniviridae → **Genus:** *Okavirus*
- **Family:** Coronaviridae
  - **Subfamily:** Coronavirinae → **Genera:** *Alphacoronavirus*, *Betacoronavirus (Subgroups A-D)*, *Gammacoronavirus*, *Deltacoronavirus**
  - **Subfamily:** Torovirinae → **Genera:** *Torovirus*, *Bafinivirus*

**Proposed new genus*

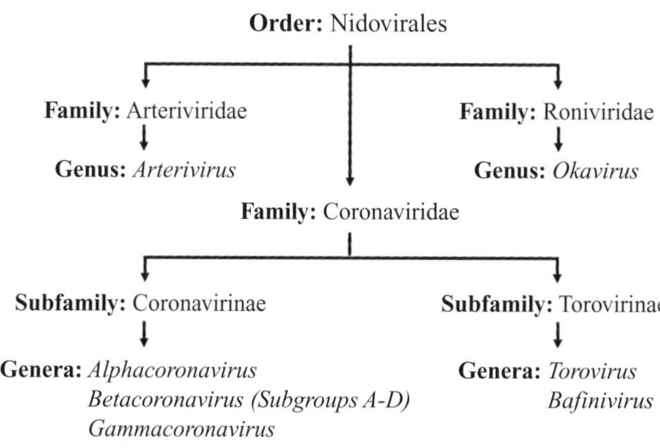

coronaviruses genera status and named them as *Alphacoronavirus, Betacoronavirus,* and *Gammacoronavirus,* respectively (Figure 62.1; http://www.ictvonline.org/virusTaxonomy.asp, accessed February 27, 2013). A fourth genus, *Deltacoronavirus,* to include newly identified bird coronaviruses, has been proposed. The genus *Alphacoronavirus* includes several human, feline, canine, porcine, ferret, rabbit, and bat coronaviruses. The genus *Betacoronavirus* includes human, bovine, porcine, equine, rat, mouse, and bat coronaviruses. Extensive homologous and heterologous recombination events have been documented in both human and animal coronaviruses in this genus, and this may have led to the generation of various subgroups and strains within the coronavirus species. This genus is further divided into four subgroups (A–D). All the animal coronaviruses in this genus are included in subgroup A, whereas SARS-CoV is included in subgroup B. The newly identified bat coronaviruses are included in groups C and D. The genus *Gammacoronavirus* includes old avian

FIGURE 62.2. *The members of order Nidovirales differ in their virion architecture. (Schematic diagrams and electron micrograph pictures were reproduced from Gorbalenya et al. 2006 (arterivirus, coronavirus, torovirus and okavirus), Schütze et al. 2006, and Enjuanes et al. 2008 (bafinivirus) with permission.)*

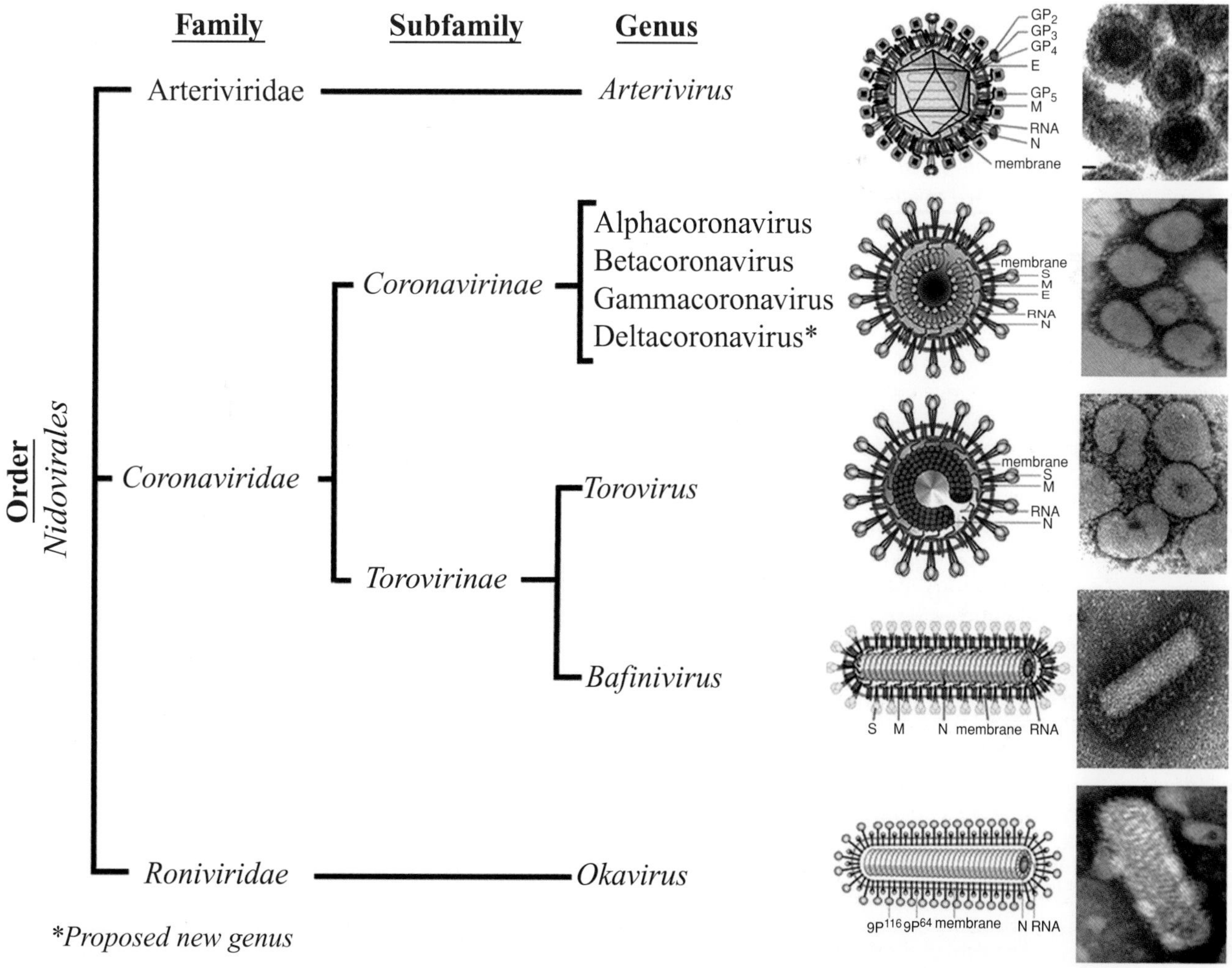

coronaviruses (IBV and TCoV) and the newly identified beluga whale coronavirus.

The human SARS outbreak followed by the discovery of bat-SARS-CoV marked the beginning of the hunt for coronaviruses in humans, bats, birds, and other animals. Since then, several new coronaviruses have been identified in humans, bats, beluga whale, Asian leopard cats, and birds (Table 62.1). Since most of the new viruses have been identified in bats and wild birds, it has been hypothesized that human and animal coronaviruses had evolved from a diverse population of coronaviruses present in bats and wild birds (Figure 62.3). The increased diversity of coronaviruses in bats and birds could be due to several reasons:

i. Bats and birds are highly diverse species. Bats represent 20% of the 5742 mammalian species and there are about 10 000 bird species around the world.
ii. Bats and birds can fly far distances. Bats have been found as high as 5000 meters, and some birds can fly for over 10 000 km during migration. This would allow bats and birds to exchange viruses with different species that come in close contact.
iii. Different environmental pressures (climate, food, shelter, and predators) would provide different selective pressures on establishment of different coronaviruses in different species of bats and birds.
iv. The habit of roosting (bats) and flocking (birds) in large numbers will facilitate exchange of viruses among individual bats and birds.

Recently, it has been proposed that the ancestor of the present coronavirus infected a bat and it jumped from a bat to a bird, or alternatively, it infected a bird and it jumped from a bird to a bat and evolved dichotomously. Consequently, the bat coronavirus jumped into other species of bats, giving rise to group 1 and group 2 coronaviruses (genera *Alphacoronavirus* and *Betacoronavirus* according to the new classification), and these evolved dichotomously. These bat coronaviruses in turn jumped to other bat species and other mammals, including humans, with each interspecies jump evolving dichotomously. On the other hand, bird coronaviruses jumped to other species of birds, and occasionally to some specific mammalian species, such as whale and Asian leopard cat. These coronaviruses have evolved dichotomously, giving rise to group 3 coronaviruses (*Gammacoronavirus*). Furthermore, the genetic diversity of the coronaviruses results from the high error rate in the viral RdRp enzyme (high mutation rates in the order of one per 1,000–10 000 nucleotides replicated), homologous and heterologous recombination mainly due to their large genome size that gives plasticity in accommodation and modification of genes. The evolutionary history of coronaviruses along with the identification of increasing numbers of more and more closely related coronaviruses from distantly related animal species clearly indicates their ability for interspecies jumping. Therefore, the coronaviruses have the potential to give rise to new veterinary and zoonotic pathogens that can pose a major threat to animal and public health.

The members of the subfamily Torovirinae (Genera *Bafinivirus* and *Toroviruses*) resemble coronaviruses in their genome organization and replication strategy but differ in virion morphology. Thus far, only four species have been recognized as members of the genus *Toroviruses* in the subfamily Torovirinae: equine torovirus (EToV), previously known as Bern virus; bovine torovirus (BToV), formerly known as Breda virus; porcine torovirus (PToV); and human torovirus (HuToV). Torovirus-like (TVL) particles have been detected by electron microscopy (EM) in feces from dogs, cats, and turkeys. HuToV has been identified as a potential pathogen inducing diarrhea in humans, specifically in young and/or immunocompromised individuals. Interestingly, close genetic and antigenic relationships between BToV and HuToV have been demonstrated. In addition, antibodies against toroviruses have been demonstrated in horses, sheep, goats, and pigs. Toroviruses are distributed throughout the world.

The recently isolated white bream virus (WBV) is the only member of the genus *Bafinivirus* in the subfamily Torovirinae. The virus was isolated from fish in Germany by inoculating tissue homogenate (heart, spleen, kidney, and swim-bladder) obtained from a white bream (*Blicca bjoerkna* L.; Teleostei, order Cypriniformes) into epithelioma papulosum cyprini (EPC) cell cultures. Until now, WBV has not been implicated in any fish disease and was first detected by EM and isolated in tissue culture during routine laboratory disease diagnostic investigation.

Virion Properties and Virus Replication

Coronaviruses

Coronaviruses have a unique morphologic appearance of a crown and the name "coronavirus" was derived from the Latin word *corona* (Greek κορωνα), *meaning crown*. They are spherical, enveloped virions with large club-shaped surface projections (peplomers) extending from the viral envelope (Figure 62.2). Virion size ranges from 100 nm to 160 nm in diameter. The coronavirus genome is a single-stranded, positive-sense RNA molecule that ranges in size from 26.4 to 31.7 kb and it is associated with the N phosphoprotein to form a long, flexible, helical nucleocapsid. However, in at least two coronaviruses (TGEV and MHV), the helical nucleocapsid is enclosed within an "internal core structure," 65 nm in diameter, that is spherical, or possibly icosahedral, in form. The virus core is surrounded by a lipoprotein envelope that is derived from the intracellular membranes during virus budding from the cell. The envelope is studded with 3–4 viral proteins depending on the coronavirus. These include the long spikes (20 nm), which consist of the S (spike) glycoprotein and the short spikes consisting of the hemagglutinin-esterase (HE) glycoprotein that are present in only some coronaviruses. The envelope also contains the glycoprotein M, a transmembrane protein that is more deeply embedded in the envelope. As indicated above, the M and N proteins form an internal core structure in at least two coronaviruses. The small envelope protein E is present in much smaller amounts than the other viral envelope proteins. The E

Table 62.1. Important Animal and Human Viruses in the Family Coronaviridae (subfamilies Coronavirinae and Torovirinae)

Family/Genus/Species	Abbreviation	Natural Host	Disease/Tissue Affected
Family: Coronaviridae			
Subfamily: Coronavirinae			
Genus: *Alphacoronavirus* (Group 1)			
Transmissible gastroenteritis virus	TGEV	Pig	Enteric infection
Porcine respiratory coronavirus	PRCoV	Pig	Respiratory infection
Porcine epidemic diarrhea virus	PEDV	Pig	Enteric infection
Canine coronavirus (Canine enteric coronavirus)	CCoV	Dog	Enteric and systemic infection
Feline infectious peritonitis virus	FIPV	Cat	Peritonitis, respiratory, enteric and neurologic infection
Feline coronavirus	FCoV	Cat	Enteric infection
Ferret enteric coronavirus	FRECV	Ferret	Enteric infection
Ferret systemic coronavirus	FRSCV	Ferret	Peritonitis and enteric infection
Rabbit coronavirus	RbCoV	Rabbit	Heart
Human coronavirus 229E	HCoV-229E	Humans	Respiratory infection
Human coronavirus NL63	HCoV-NL263	Humans	Respiratory infection
Scotophilus bat coronavirus 512	Sc-BatCoV-512	Lesser Asiatic yellow house bats	No clinical disease
Rhinolophus bat coronavirus HKU2	Rh-BatCoV-HKU2	Chinese horseshoe bats	No clinical disease
Miniopterus bat coronavirus HKU8	Mi-BatCoV-HKU8	Bent-winged bats	No clinical disease
Miniopterus bat coronavirus 1A	Mi-BatCoV-1A	Bent-winged bats	No clinical disease
Miniopterus bat coronavirus 1B	Mi-BatCoV-1B	Bent-winged bats	No clinical disease
Genus: *Betacoronavirus* (Group 2)			
Subgroup A			
Porcine hemagglutinating encephalomyelitis virus	PHEV	Pig	Enteric, respiratory and neurological infection
Bovine coronavirus	BCoV	Cattle	Enteric and respiratory infection
Enteric bovine coronavirus	EBCoV		
Respiratory bovine coronavirus	RBCoV		
Canine respiratory coronavirus	CRCoV	Dog	Respiratory infection
Equine coronavirus	ECoV	Horse	Enteric infection
Mouse hepatitis virus	MHV	Mouse	Hepatitis, enteric and neurological infection
Rat coronavirus	RCoV	Rat	Sialodacryadentis - salivary and
Sialodacryadentis virus	SDAV		lacrimal glands, and eyes
Parker's rat coronavirus	RCoV-P		Respiratory infection
Human coronavirus OC43	HCoV-OC43	Humans	Respiratory infection
Human coronavirus HKU1	HCoV-HKU1	Humans	Respiratory infection
Subgroup B			
SARS coronavirus	SARS-CoV	Humans	Respiratory infection
SARS-related Rhinolopus bat coronavirus	SARSr-Rh-Bat-CoV	Chinese horseshoe bats	No clinical disease
Subgroup C			
Tylonycteris bat coronavirus HKU4	Ty-BatCoV HKU4	Lesser bamboo bats	No clinical disease
Pipistrellus bat coronavirus HKU5	Pi-BatCoV HKU5	Japanese pipistrelle bats	No clinical disease
Subgroup D			
Rousettus bat coronavirus HKU9	Ro-BatCoV HKU9	Leschenault's rousette bats	No clinical disease
Genus: *Gammacoronavirus* (Group 3)			
Infectious bronchitis virus	IBV	Chicken	Respiratory, reproductive and kidney infection
Turkey coronavirus	TCoV	Turkey	Enteric infection
Beluga whale coronavirus SW1	BWCoV	Beluga whales	No clinical disease
Genus: *Deltacoronavirus*[a]			
Bulbul coronavirus-HKU11	BuCoV-HKU11	Chinese bulbuls	No clinical disease
Thrush coronavirus-HKU12	ThCoV-HKU12	Gray-backed thrushes	No clinical disease
Munia coronavirus-HKU13	MunCoV-HKU13	White-rumped munias	No clinical disease
Subfamily: Torovirinae			
Genus: *Torovirus*			
Equine torovirus	EToV	Horse	Enteric infection
Bovine torovirus	BToV	Cattle	Enteric infection
Porcine torovirus	PToV	Pig	Enteric infection
Human torovirus	HuToV	Humans	Enteric infection
Genus: *Bafinivirus*			
White bream virus	WBV	Fish	No clinical disease

[a]Proposed new genus.

FIGURE 62.3. *A proposed model of coronavirus evolution. Coronaviruses of bats and birds may have evolved from a common ancestor. Subsequently, coronaviruses from bats would have given rise to alphacoronavirus and betacoronaviruses (group 1 and 2), whereas coronaviruses from birds would have given rise to gammacoronaviruses (group 3).*

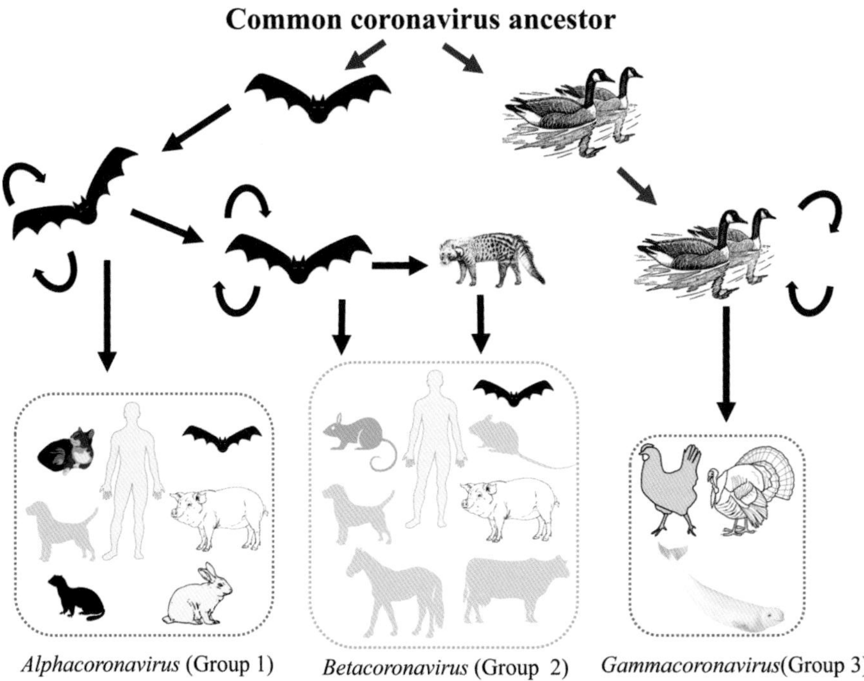

protein, together with the M protein, plays an essential role in coronavirus particle assembly. Coronaviruses have a buoyant density in sucrose of 1.15–1.20 g/cm^3. The buoyant density in CsCl is 1.23–1.24 g/cm^3 and the sedimentation coefficient (S20, w) is 300–500. Coronaviruses are sensitive to heat, lipid solvents, nonionic detergents, formaldehyde, oxidizing agents, and UV irradiation. Some coronaviruses are resistant to acid pH and/or desiccation.

The genome organization of the family Coronaviridae (subfamilies: Coronavirinae and Torovirinae) resembles the other members of the order Nidovirales (Figure 62.4). The coronavirus and torovirus genomic RNAs are 5′-capped, 3′-polyadenylated and can function as an mRNA. Thus, the purified genomic RNAs of these viruses are infectious. The coronavirus genomes consist of a 5′-leader sequence (65–98 nucleotides [nts]) followed by untranslated region (5′UTR; 200–400 nts). At the 3′-end of the viral genome there is another UTR of 200–500 nts (3′-UTR), followed by a poly A tail of variable length. The 5′ and 3′-UTRs flank an array of multiple genes (open-reading frames [ORFs]) whose number may vary among the members of the subfamily Coronavirinae. The coronaviruses have 9–14 ORFs that encode viral nonstructural and structural proteins. The 5′-proximal two-thirds (~20–22 kb) of the genome is occupied by the two largest ORFs (ORF1a and ORF1b) that encode for the nonstructural proteins (nsps). The ORF1a and ORF1b are connected by a -1 ribosomal frameshift site(RFS). The translation of genomic RNA starts at the start codon of ORF1a resulting in the production of a polyprotein, pp1a. In some cases, specific RNA signals promote ribosomal frameshifting at a -1 RFS or "slippery" sequence between ORF1a and ORF1b that results in the C-terminal extension of pp1a with the ORF1b-encoded polypeptide, pp1ab. The pp1a and pp1ab are co- and post-translationally processed by two virus-encoded proteases (papain-like protease (nsp3) and picornaviral 3C-like cysteine protease (nsp5) to produce 16 nsps. The nsp14 has the RNA-dependent RNA polymerase activity. These products of the large replicase protein, possibly with other viral and cellular proteins, assemble into a replication/transcription complex bound to modified intracellular membranes.

The structural proteins encoding ORFs are located in the 3′ one-third of the genome, for all coronaviruses, in the order 5′-S-E-M-N-3′. The ORFs encoding these proteins are interspersed with several ORFs encoding nsps (accessory proteins) and HE glycoprotein, which differ significantly among coronaviruses in number, nucleotide sequence, gene order, and method of expression (Figure 62.4). However, they are conserved within the same group of coronaviruses, thus they are called the group-specific proteins. When the HE protein is expressed, it is encoded 5′ to S protein. The structural and accessory proteins are expressed from a 3′ co-terminal nested set of subgenomic mRNAs (sgmRNAs). The coronavirus lifecycle (attachment, entry, replication of genome, transcription mRNAs, assembly, and release) is very similar to other members of the order Nidovirales (e.g., equine arteritis virus [EAV]). The genome replication, sgmRNA synthesis, and virus life cycle of EAV is depicted in Chapter 63. Briefly, replication of the genomic RNA involves synthesis of a full-length negative-stranded RNA that serves as template for full-length genomic RNA. The structural and accessory proteins are expressed from multiple overlapping 3′-co-terminal sgmRNAs. Each sgmRNA has a common leader sequence at its 5′-end that is

FIGURE 62.4. *Genome organization of selected members of genus Coronavirinae (HCoV-229E, TGEV, BCoV, SARS-CoV, and IBV) and Torovirinae (EToV and WBV).*

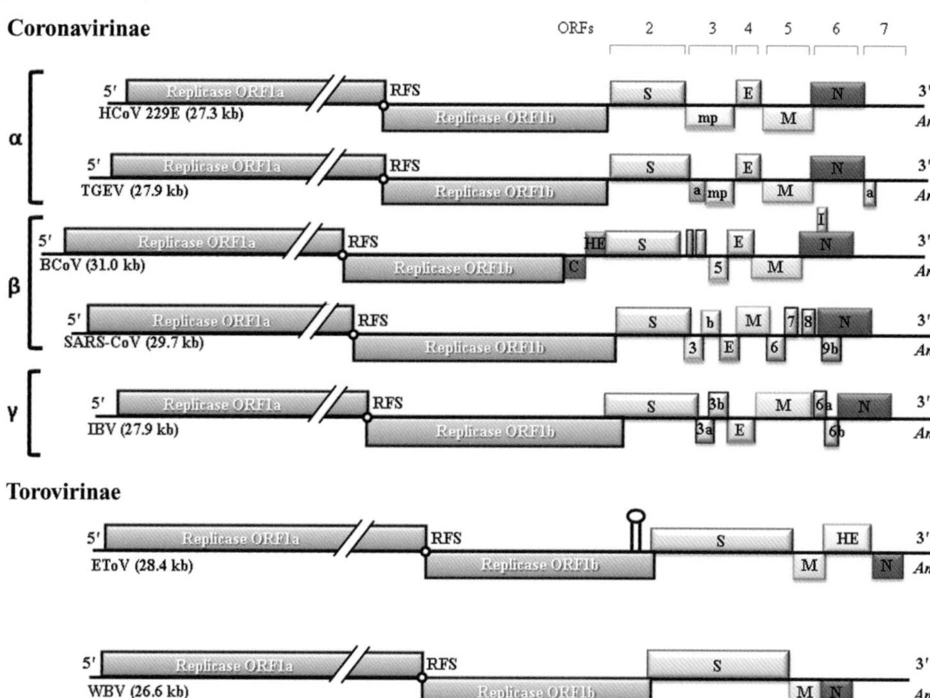

derived from the 5′-end of the genomic RNA. The sgmRNAs are synthesized from sg-negative-strand RNAs with the anti-leader sequences being added onto the 3′-ends of negative-stranded RNAs that then serve as templates for synthesis of sgmRNAs (discontinuous extension of minus-strand RNA synthesis; see Chapter 63). Most of the time, one viral structural protein is translated from individual sgmRNAs. However, in some cases, there may be two ORFs carried on and translated from one sgmRNA.

The S glycoprotein forms the large peplomers on the virion surface, giving the virus its corona or crown-like morphology when examined under the electron microscope. The S protein is a heavily glycosylated type I membrane glycoprotein that can be divided into three structural domains: a large N-terminal external domain further divided into two domains, S_1 and S_2; a transmembrane domain; and a short carboxyterminal cytoplasmic domain. The S_1 domain forms the globular portion of the spike and there is considerable sequence variation due to various deletions and substitutions within this region in different coronavirus strains. Thus, mutations in S_1 sequences have been associated with altered antigenicity, pathogenicity, and cellular tropism of the virus. In contrast, the S_2 domain is more conserved and constitutes the stalk of the spikes. There is evidence that mature S protein of some coronaviruses forms an oligomer, most probably assembled into a trimmer. In some coronaviruses (e.g., MHV and BCoV), the S protein gets cleaved by the cellular proteases during or after virus maturation and the S_1 and S_2 domains remain noncovalently associated in the viral spikes. The extent of S cleavage varies among coronaviruses and it also depends on host cell types. However, in some other coronaviruses (e.g., SARS-CoV), S protein cleavage occurs as part of the viral entry process. The S proteins of alphacoronaviruses (Group 1) are not cleaved, but they still could induce cell–cell fusion (e.g., feline infectious peritonitis virus (FIPV)). The S protein of coronaviruses has several biological properties that include binding to specific cellular receptor(s), inducing neutralizing antibodies, eliciting cell-mediated immune response, inducing fusion of the viral envelope with host cell membranes, inducing cell–cell fusion, and binding the Fc fragment of immunoglobulin (MHV and TGEV). The cellular receptors for many coronavirus S proteins have been identified.

The HE glycoprotein is found in all subgroup A betacoronaviruses and one member of the gammacoronaviruses (TCoV) as a disulfide-linked dimer that forms short spikes on the virion surface. The HE protein is not present on the virion of betacoronavirus members of subgroups B, C, and D. The absence of HE protein in some coronaviruses, and the frequent tendency of its structure to get mutated or completely deleted during serial cell culture passage suggest that this protein is not essential for viral replication. The HE gene of coronaviruses is believed to be acquired from influenza C virus by heterologous recombination. The HE protein of coronaviruses has several biological properties and these include hemagglutination, hemadsorption, the esterase activity that cleaves acetyl groups from 9-*O*-acetyl-neumeric acid, and may play a role in initial virus adsorption and entry or release from the infected cells.

The M protein of coronaviruses is glycosylated with a short aminoterminal domain that is exposed to the exterior surface, followed by a triple-membrane-spanning domain, an α-helical domain, and a large carboxyterminal domain inside the viral envelope. The glycosylation of the aminoterminal of the M protein either can be O-linked (MHV) or N-linked (IBV, TGEV, and SARS-CoV) and in some coronaviruses, the carboxyterminal of the M protein is exposed on the virion surface (TGEV). In MHV, monoclonal antibodies against M protein neutralize the virus. The M protein of coronaviruses interacts with both the N and S proteins and may play a key role in virus assembly. It may also play a major role in packaging viral RNA into nucleocapsids during virus assembly.

The E protein of coronaviruses acts synergistically with the M protein during virus budding from the infected cells. In addition to this, E protein also functions as an ion channel. The N protein interacts with the viral genomic RNA to form the viral nucleocapsid. The N protein has three relatively conserved structural domains and it interacts with M protein, leading to the incorporation of the nucleocapsid into the virus particle.

Toroviruses

Toroviruses are pleomorphic and measure 120–140 nm in diameter. Spherical, oval elongated, and kidney-shaped particles have been visualized under EM. Toroviruses are enveloped with a tubular nucleocapsid of helical symmetry. The nucleocapsid forms a doughnut-shaped structure and the envelope contains a large number of small spikes (15–20 nm) that resemble the peplomeres of coronaviruses. Torovirus particles consist of at least four structural proteins: nucleocapsid protein (N), unglycosylated membrane protein (M), spike glycoprotein (S), and HE protein. The torovirus genome consists of a polyadenylated, positive-sense, linear molecule of ssRNA, which is estimated to be 20-30 kb in length. Toroviruses have a buoyant density of 1.14–1.18 g/cm^3 in sucrose and an estimated sedimentation coefficient (S20, w) of 400–500. Virus infectivity is stable between pH 2.5 and 9.7 but rapidly inactivated by heat, organic solvents, and irradiation.

Bafinivirus

The WBV has a bacilliform shape (170–200 × 75–88 nm) with an envelope containing coronavirus-like spikes (20–25 nm). The virion consists of a rod-shaped nucleocapsid (120–150 × 19–22 nm) surrounded an envelope that consists of glycosylated S protein and integral membrane protein M. The virus replicates in various fish cell lines. The buoyant density of the virus in sucrose is 1.17–1.19 g/cm^3 and sensitive to lipid solvents.

Animal Diseases Caused by Members of the Genus *Alphacoronavirus*

Transmissible Gastroenteritis Virus and Porcine Respiratory Coronavirus

Disease. Transmissible gastroenteritis (TGE) is a highly contagious enteric disease of swine caused by TGEV. TGEV is antigenically related to coronaviruses of humans, dogs, and cats. Only one serotype of TGEV is recognized, but antibodies to TGEV can antigenically cross-react with porcine respiratory coronavirus (PRCoV). However, some antigenic sites of TGEV are absent from PRCoV because of a deletion in the amino terminus of the S protein in PRCoV. TGEV and PRCoV are inactivated by lipid solvents (ether and chloroform), sodium hypochlorite, quaternary ammonium compounds, iodines, heating at 56 °C for 45 min, and exposure to sunlight. Both viruses are stable when frozen but somewhat labile at room temperature. TGEV is stable for long periods when frozen at −80 °C, but when held at 37 °C for 4 days, there is total loss of infectivity. In liquid manure, infectious virus persists for more than 8 weeks at 5 °C, 2 weeks at 20 °C, and 24 h at 35 °C. TGEV resists inactivation by trypsin and acidic pH (pH of 3.0), and is relatively stable in pig bile. These properties allow the virus to survive in the stomach and small intestine.

TGEV is characterized by severe diarrhea, vomiting, dehydration, and high mortality in young piglets (less than 2 weeks of age). Mortality in older pigs (greater than 5 weeks) is usually low. Older growing and finishing pigs develop transient watery diarrhea but vomiting is uncommon. Most of the time TGEV infection of adult swine is asymptomatic, but sometimes infected sows exhibit anorexia, diarrhea, fever, vomiting, and agalactia.

More than 25 years ago, PRCoV was detected in swine herds with minor respiratory symptoms that are closely related to TGEV. A major difference between the two porcine coronaviruses is a large deletion in the spike protein S gene (deletion of nucleotides 621-681) of PRCoV. PRCoV is a natural deletion mutant of TGEV and has changed the tropism from porcine enteric epithelium to respiratory epithelium and alveolar macrophages. Because of this structural difference, TGEV but not PRCoV has a sialic acid binding activity that allows the attachment to mucins and mucin-type glycoproteins. The sialic acid binding activity may allow TGEV to overcome the mucus barrier in the gut and to get access to the intestinal epithelium for initiation of infection. As PRCoV shares some epitopes for neutralizing antibodies with TGEV, it acts like a nature-made vaccine against TGEV resulting in a drastic reduction of TGE outbreaks in Europe. Thus, PRCoV can infect pigs of all ages by aerosol or direct contact transmission. PRCoV infections are generally subclinical, but strains of the virus differ in the severity of the clinical signs they induce. Clinical signs include moderate to severe respiratory disease with interstitial pneumonia. In addition, PRCoV infection can be concurrently associated with other respiratory virus infections such as with porcine reproductive and respiratory syndrome virus (PRRSV), which can alter the severity of disease and associated clinical signs.

Host–Virus Relationship

Distribution, Reservoir, and Transmission. TGE has only been described in swine; however, TGEV has been isolated from the feces of experimentally infected cats, dogs, foxes, and starlings (*Sturnus vulgaris*) for up to 20 days. Serologic studies have also suggested natural infection of skunks, opossums, muskrats, and humans. Virus has also been demonstrated in house flies (*Musca domestica* Linneaus) following experimental and natural infection.

TGEV infection of swine occurs worldwide, and has been documented in North, Central and South America, Europe, and Asia. Epizootics of TGE are often seasonal in the United States, occurring in the winter months. The primary mode of TGEV transmission appears to be ingestion of feed contaminated with infected feces (fecal-oral). Persistence of TGEV in nature is likely via the fecal carrier/shedding state in recovered swine, thus the virus is maintained in endemically infected herds through ongoing fecal-oral infection of susceptible pigs. Infection of swine in endemically infected herds is often subclinical or mild, whereas the virus spreads rapidly in nonimmune herds and can cause devastating outbreaks of disease. In addition to movement by infected swine, TGEV is potentially transmitted between herds by fomites and other animals.

PRCoV has been isolated in North America and Europe. Infected pigs shed virus in their respiratory secretions, and PRCoV may persist in herds by continuous infection of newly weaned pigs. Although this is not an enteric pathogen, the virus has been demonstrated in feces by virus isolation and nested reverse transcription polymerase chain reaction (nRT-PCR) that may suggest the possibility of fecal-oral transmission.

Pathogenesis and Pathology. TGEV survives in the gastrointestinal tract after ingestion because of its resistance to low pH and trypsin, thus it passes through the stomach without inactivation. Six to twelve hours following intragastric inoculation, viral replication occurs in villus epithelial cells of the small intestine with highest titers of virus in the jejunum. TGEV infects and destroys the columnar epithelial cells lining the intestinal villi, resulting in atrophy of the villi. Villous blunting and increased crypt depth (as a consequence of replication of the progenitor cells in the crypts in an effort to repopulate the denuded villi) occurs 24–40 h postinfection and coincides with the occurrence of severe diarrhea. The loss of enterocytes lining the villi results in malabsorption and maldigestion, which in turn results in diarrhea and dehydration. Undigested lactose in the intestinal contents passes to the large bowel where it exerts an osmotic effect that further exacerbates the diarrhea in TGEV-infected swine. Affected piglets are dehydrated with fecal staining around the perineum. The typical lesions include thinning of the intestinal wall, villous atrophy, and gastrointestinal distension with yellow fluid containing curds of undigested milk.

The PRCoV is transmitted via respiratory aerosols and droplets to susceptible in-contact animals. The virus replicates in the tonsils, mucosal epithelium of the nasal passage and the airways of the lungs, and the type I and the type II pneumocytes in the alveolar lining. This cause inflammation and necrosis of terminal airways of the lungs leading to diffuse bronchointerstitial pneumonia. The severity of clinical signs and lesions may vary and subclinical infection can occur in herds.

Host Response to Infection. Neutralizing antibodies develop within approximately 7 days of TGEV infection of swine. The presence of secretory IgA plays a major role in protective immunity and viral clearance. Intramuscular immunization of pigs with TGEV results in development of a humoral IgG response but not protective immunity. Conversely, pigs immunized orally with TGEV develop protective virus-specific IgA in their intestinal mucosal secretions. Infection of sows with TGEV results in the secretion of protective IgA in colostrum (so-called lactogenic immunity), which is protective in suckling pigs. Cell-mediated immunity is also likely important in the immune response to TGEV infection, as passive transfer of mononuclear leukocytes from immune donor pigs to susceptible histocompatible piglets results in reduced disease expression. High levels of type I interferon are produced by infected intestinal cells, which also may play a role in controlling viral replication. Pigs infected with PRCoV develop neutralizing antibodies to the virus. Antibodies against PRCoV provide partial protection against TGEV, and therefore, the incidence and severity of TGE may decline in swine herds with endemic PRCoV infection.

Laboratory Diagnosis. TGEV infection of young pigs is usually diagnosed through the demonstration of viral antigen in mucosal scrapings or frozen sections of jejunum and ileum by immunohistochemical (IHC) or immunofluorescent (IF) staining with virus-specific antibodies. Definitive diagnosis of TGEV can be done by viral isolation through inoculation of animals (pigs 2–7 days old) or cell cultures (pig kidney, testis, or thyroid). EM or immuno-EM can also be used on fecal contents or intestine for diagnosis. Standard and real-time RT-PCR (rRT-PCR) assays for the detection and differentiation of TGEV and PRCoV have been described.

TGEV has been propagated in various cell culture systems, including pig kidney, testis, salivary gland, and thyroid; organ cultures of esophagus, intestine, and nasal epithelium; canine kidney cell cultures; and embryonated chicken eggs (amniotic cavity). Pig kidney (PK) and swine testicle (ST) cell lines have been the choice of cells for virus isolation from the feces or gut contents of infected pigs. Development of cytopathic effect may require multiple passages in cell culture. PRCoV replicates in PK and ST cells, as well as a cat fetus cell line.

Serologic diagnosis is appropriate when acute and convalescent sera are available. However, serologic diagnosis is complicated by the finding that both PRCoV and TGEV induce neutralizing antibodies that cross-neutralize each other. Therefore, TGEV strains are not distinguished from its nonenteropathogenic variant PRCoV by the virus neutralization test but can be distinguished by blocking enzyme-linked immunosorbent assay (ELISA).

Treatment and Control. Treatment of TGEV-infected pigs is usually unrewarding. Replacement of fluids and antibacterial drugs to reduce complications associated with enteropathogenic *Escherichia coli* may be of benefit. Inactivated and modified live attenuated virus vaccines are available for vaccination of pigs to prevent TGE. These can be used for vaccination of newborn piglets or immunization of sows, or both. Vaccination of pregnant sows provides lactogenic immunity that is passively transferred to piglets via colostrum. Vaccines have been variably successful in preventing TGE. Oral immunization provides optimal stimulation of local immunity (secretory IgA) in the intestine.

The practice of infecting sows with virulent TGEV at least 3 weeks prior to furrowing to induce an immune response by providing colostral immunity to piglets is complicated by the fact that this practice contaminates the environment with virulent TGEV that subsequently can spread infection to susceptible pigs.

Porcine Epidemic Diarrhea Virus

Coronavirus-like viruses have been isolated from swine with diarrhea, thus their designation as porcine epidemic diarrhea viruses (PEDV). These viruses are antigenically distinct from TGEV and porcine hemagglutinating encephalomyelitis virus (PHEV), and cause diarrhea, vomiting, and dehydration in inoculated swine. Pathogenesis studies indicate that PEDV replicates in both the small and large intestines, but lesions are confined to small intestines. Affected pigs have small intestines that are distended with yellow fluid; the lesions are similar to those of TGE.

PEDV particles can be demonstrated in the feces of infected pigs by direct EM, and the virus can be propagated in some African green monkey (Vero) cell lines but not in others. Viral growth depends on the presence of trypsin in the cell culture medium. Generally, field strains of PEDV need to be adapted to grow in cell culture before they can be used as a routine diagnostic assay. Virus can be adapted to grow in primary porcine cell culture or Vero cells (African green monkey cells). A direct immunofluorescence assay (IFA) and IHC technique applied on a section of small intestine are the most sensitive, rapid, and reliable methods of diagnosis of PEDV in pigs. A serologic diagnosis can be made by demonstration of PEDV antibodies by IF and ELISA. A multiplex rRT-PCR procedure developed for the simultaneous detection of PEDV and TGEV in preweaning pigs with diarrhea has been described.

Attenuated vaccines are available in some Asian countries for the prevention of PEDV infection in pigs. However, control of disease is dependent on management and husbandry practices.

Canine Enteric Coronavirus

Disease. Canine coronavirus (CCoV) infects domestic and wild canine species and the first CCoV was isolated from dogs with acute enteritis. CCoV infection of dogs is highly contagious and generally causes inapparent or mild gastroenteritis. CCoV is an important enteropathogen of dogs and is widespread in dog populations, mainly in kennels and animal shelters. Clinical signs include anorexia, lethargy, vomiting, fluid diarrhea, and dehydration. The virus is shed at high titers in the feces of infected dogs leading to typical fecal-oral route of transmission characterized by high morbidity and low mortality. Fatal infection usually occurs as a consequence of mixed infections with CCoV together with canine parvovirus type-2, canine adenovirus type-1, or canine distemper virus. CCoV is antigenically related to other coronaviruses, including TGEV, feline enteric coronavirus, and FIPV. Multiple antigenically and genetically distinct strains of CCoV have been recognized, including a novel respiratory coronavirus.

Based on genetic, antigenic and biological properties, the canine enteric coronaviruses can be broadly classified into two types: CCoV type I (CCoV-I) and CCoV type II (CCoV-II). The type I and type II CCoVs share up to 96% nucleotide identity. Recently, CCoV-II was divided into two subtypes, CCoV-IIa and CCoV-IIb, with the second of these arising as a result of a putative double recombination event between CCoV-II and TGEV (TGEV-like CCoV). In contrast to CCoV-I strains, the CCoV-IIa strains are highly virulent and cause systemic fatal disease in pups. CCoV-IIa strains include a pantropic variant causing systemic disease in pups that was identified in 2005 (CCoV CB/05). The virus was isolated from feces, as well as various paranchymatous organs of effected puppies. Subsequently, the disease was reproduced after experimental infection of dogs, with young puppies showing more severe clinical signs. Pantropic CCoV-IIa (e.g., CB/05 and NA/09 strains) cause severe systemic disease in dogs, characterized by fever, lethargy, anorexia, depression, vomiting, hemorrhagic diarrhea, severe leukopenia, and neurologic signs (seizures and ataxia) followed by death 48 h after the onset of symptoms.

In addition, various recombinants between CCoV-I and CCoV-II strains, as well as TGEV spike protein gene have been reported. Although TGEV-like CCoVs were detected in the internal organs of naturally infected dogs, experimental infection failed to cause systemic involvement or virus dissemination through the blood. CCoVs are inactivated by lipid solvents and are heat-labile. The viruses are acid-stable (pH of 3.0) and retain infectivity under cool conditions.

Host–Virus Relationship

Distribution, Reservoir, and Transmission. CCoV was first isolated in 1971 from an epidemic of diarrhea in dogs in Germany. The virus has since been recognized virtually worldwide, including North America, Europe, Australia, and Asia. Infected dogs excrete virus in their feces for 2 weeks or longer and fecal contamination of the environment is the primary source for its transmission via fecal-oral infection.

Pathogenesis and Pathology. Following an incubation period of 1–4 days, the virus causes infection of intestinal epithelial cells that progressively passes through the gastrointestinal tract. Diarrhea occurs 1–7 days postinfection, virus being present in feces within 1–2 days following the appearance of clinical signs. Viral replication in the intestinal epithelium results in desquamation and shortening of the villi. The diarrhea associated with CCoV infection occurs as a consequence of intestinal maldigestion and malabsorption. While CCoV infection is widespread, mortality is typically very low.

Host Response to Infection. Mucosal immunity appears to be protective as dogs orally infected with CCoV become immune while those immunized parenterally do not. It has been reported that immunity after natural exposure to enteric CCoV does not provide complete protection against infection with the new pantropic CCoV infections.

Laboratory Diagnosis. Virus or viral antigens can be visualized by EM or fluorescent antibody (FA) staining of feces or necropsy tissues. Antiserum specific for CCoV is commonly used to aggregate virus prior to negative staining for EM. Virus can be isolated from feces or intestinal tissue on cell culture. Several primary (kidney and thymus) and continuous canine lines of thymus, embryo, synovium, and kidney (line A-72) are susceptible to infection. The virus also infects feline kidney and embryo fibroblast cell lines. RT-PCR assays have been developed to detect CCoVs in feces. CCoV-I can be distinguished from CCoV-II by means of genotype specific conventional RT-PCR or rRT-PCR assays. Serum virus neutralization and ELISA tests for detection of CCoV antibodies have been developed. An ELISA based on recombinant spike protein S for the detection and differentiation of antibodies to TGEV-like CCoV from other CCoV-II strains has recently been described.

Treatment and Control. Treatment of CCoV-associated gastroenteritis is limited to relief of dehydration and electrolyte loss in severe cases. Inactivated and modified live virus (MLV) vaccines are available for parental administration for protection against CCoV infection. However, their use is questionable due to the apparent importance of local immunity at the level of the intestinal mucosa.

Feline Infectios Peritonitis and Feline Enteric Coronaviurus

Disease. Feline infectious peritonitis (FIP) is a contagious, progressive, and highly fatal disease of domestic and some wild feline species. The signs are highly variable and reflect the tissues affected by the disease, but persistent fever, weight loss, lethargy, dyspnea, and abdominal distension are all common clinical signs. The disease can occur in cats of all ages but is especially common in young and very old cats. Two distinct forms of FIP are recognized: (1) an effusive (wet) and (2) a noneffusive (dry) form. The effusive form, which is two to three times as common as the dry form, is characterized by accumulation of protein-rich fluid (exudate) in the peritoneal cavity. The noneffusive form is characterized by formation of granulomas in internal organs, central nervous system (CNS), and eyes. Mortality rates are high. FIP has an unusual and highly complex pathogenesis that involves the mutation of relatively apathogenic feline enteric coronavirus (FCoV) into FIPV that replicates in macrophages to produce an immune-mediated disease in affected cats. FCoV seems to be confined to the intestinal tract and causes mild, often unapparent enteritis especially in kittens. Comparative sequence analysis of FCoVs and FIPVs has shown that these viruses are genetically closely related but differ in their pathogenic potential (different pathotypes of the same virus). The FIPV efficiently infects macrophages and monocytes that escape from the intestine to cause lethal systemic disease with multiorgan involvement, in classical cases accompanied by accumulation of abdominal exudate (ascites). One of the hypotheses is that FIPV pathotype results from a mutation(s) in the FCoV genome. However, viral virulence determinants specifically associated with FIPV pathogenesis have not yet been identified. Some of the mutations in nonstructural protein 3c and spike appear to correlate with development of FIP.

Etiologic Agent

Physical, Chemical, and Antigenic Properties. Based on serological differences, FCoV strains have been separated into two types (more common FCoV type 1 and less common FCoV type 2), both being able to cause two forms of FIP (dry and wet form). The FCoV type 2 is genetically more closely related to canine coronavirus. FCoVs and FIPV are resistant to acid and trypsin but are readily inactivated by most disinfectants, including lipid solvents.

Infectivity for Other Species and Culture Systems. In addition to infecting domestic cats, FIPV has been associated with disease in wild *Felidae* such as lions, mountain lions, leopards, jaguar, lynx, caracal, sand cats, and pallas's cats. Young pigs can be experimentally infected with FIPV, resulting in development of lesions similar to those induced by TGEV. Suckling mice are susceptible to infection, with virus replicating in the brain. FIPV primarily replicates in macrophages, but virus can be propagated *in vitro* in feline organ cultures, cell lines, and mononuclear phagocytes.

Host–Virus Relationship

Distribution, Reservoir, and Transmission. FCoV and FIPV occur worldwide. FCoV spreads efficiently via the fecal-oral route but in contrast, FIPV is not well transmitted. FCoV may persist subclinically for up to a year or longer and these persistently infected cats serve as the virus reservoir that allows horizontal spread between cats.

Pathogenesis and Pathology. The pathogenesis of FIP is complex, and much remains to be resolved. Initial FCoV infection is rarely characterized by obvious disease, but results in persistent, low-level infection of macrophages in many tissues. The development of clinical FIP is associated with increased viral replication, usually secondary to some immunosuppressive event that suppresses cellular immunity. Increased virus replication results in the emergence of viral variants (FIPV) that replicate with increasing efficiency in macrophages where they persist, safe from immune clearance. Antibody exacerbates the disease, which suggests that FIP is at least in part an "immune mediated" disease. Virus-specific antibody actually facilitates uptake of FIPV by phagocytes in which pathogenic strains of the virus replicate.

Both "wet" and "dry" forms of FIP are characterized by the appearance of granulomas (or pyogranulomas) around blood vessels. It is proposed that deposition of complexes of FIPV and specific antibody (immune complexes) in the walls of blood vessels is responsible for the characteristic perivascular location of these lesions. These perivascular granulomas can occur in the bowel, kidneys, liver, lungs, CNS, eyes and lymph nodes of affected cats, and are especially common on the serosa of the abdominal viscera in cats with the wet form of FIP.

Host Response to Infection. The basis of immunity to FIPV is poorly understood. Cats develop humoral and cellular immune responses soon after FCoV infection, and these responses hold the infection in check until some stress or concurrent infection causes immune suppression. Antibodies to FCoV cross-react with FIPV and these cause disease expression rather than protection; this antibody facilitates viral uptake by phagocytic cells where the virus effectively replicates, and viral antigens complexed with specific antibodies (and complement) contribute to immune-mediated vasculitis.

Laboratory Diagnosis. FIP is a common disease of cats that often can be diagnosed based upon the characteristic clinical signs coupled with serology and hematology. Fluid accumulation in the peritoneal or pleural cavity, as determined by paracentesis, in association with a positive serum or fluid antibody titer, is indicative of effusive FIP. Noneffusive FIP is more difficult to diagnose and must be differentiated from other infectious, granulomatous, and neoplastic conditions. Histologic examination for pyogranulomatous or fibronecrotic inflammatory lesions and vasculitis, in association with serology, facilitates diagnosis. RT-PCR techniques have been developed for identification of FIPV sequences in clinical material, as has IHC staining for FIPV.

Serologic diagnosis may be determined by viral neutralization, ELISA, or indirect FA techniques. A serum titer of greater than 1 : 3200 supports the diagnosis of FIP although cats with FIP can have low titers of virus-specific antibody and, conversely, unaffected cats may have high titers of antibody to the virus.

Treatment and Control. No treatment for FIP has been described that consistently reverses the disease process. A temperature-sensitive mutant FIPV is available for vaccination of cats. Its use is not recommended in seropositive cats. Control of FIP is best realized by decontaminating (with quaternary ammonium compounds) infected premises, isolating serologically positive cats from those with no titer, and screening newly acquired cats for serum antibody.

Ferret Coronavirus

Recently a novel ferret enteric coronavirus (FRECV) was identified in domesticated ferrets (*Mustela putorius furo*) associated with epizootic catarrhal enteritis (ECE). ECE, a relatively new disease of domestic ferrets, was first described in the spring of 1993 on the east coast of the United States. Since then, FRECV has spread across the United States and to other countries. The disease is characterized by anorexia, lethargy, vomiting, and foul-smelling bright green diarrhea with high mucous content. The morbidity generally approaches 100% but the overall mortality rate is low (<5%), with juvenile ferrets often developing only mild or subclinical disease. Clinical signs are more severe in older ferrets and the mortality rate is often is higher. Phylogenetic analysis showed that FRECV is very closely related to the Alphacoronaviurses (Group 1). Another coronavirus has emerged in ferrets in the United States and Europe causing systemic disease (ferret systemic coronavirus (FRSCV) characterized by FIP-like clinical signs and lesions. Common clinical signs include anorexia, weight loss, diarrhea, and the presence of large palpable intra-abdominal masses. Gross lesions are characterized by the presence of widespread granulomas on serosal surfaces and within the parenchyma of the abdominal thoracic organs. Histopathologic examination shows a systemic pyogranulmatous inflammation involving the liver, kidney, spleen, pancreas, adrenal glands, mesenteric adipose tissue, lymph nodes, and lungs. Comparative nucleotide sequence analysis has demonstrated that FRECV and FRSCV differ significantly in their S genes (79.5% identity). Phylogenetically, FRSCV is more closely related to FRECV than to the other alphacoronaviruses.

Diagnosis of ferret coronaviruses can be achieved by demonstration of coronaviruses-like particles in clinical samples (e.g., feces and visceral organs) by EM or staining with anti-CoV monoclonal antibodies (e.g., FIPV3-70). Viral antigen can also be demonstrated in formalin fixed tissues by IHC. Microscopically, pyogranulomatous lesions can be observed in many visceral organs. The two ferret coronaviruses can be detected and distinguished by both conventional and rRT-PCR assays. Virus isolation in Madin–Darby canine kidney, Crandell feline kidney, Vero and rabbit kidney (RK-13b) cells has been unsuccessful.

Rabbit Coronavirus

Rabbit coronavirus (RbCoV) infection was first reported in 1961 by Scandinavian researchers who observed 50–75% mortality among laboratory rabbits. It was established that acute RbCoV infection targets the heart and results in virus-induced myocarditis and congestive heart failure in rabbits. RbCoV was demonstrated by EM examination of heart tissues of affected rabbits, and also by demonstrating complement fixing antibodies to the human coronaviruses 229E and 0C43 in surviving rabbits. Furthermore, immunofluorescence staining with anti-229E serum localized fluorescence in the interstitial tissue of the myocardium of affected rabbits. Antiserum to RbCoV cross-reacts with FIPV, CCoV, and TGEV by radioimmunoassay.

Animal Diseases Caused by Members of the Genus—*Betacoronavirus*

Porcine Hemagglutinating Encepahlitis Viurs

Disease. PHEV is the cause of vomiting and wasting disease (VWD) of young swine that is characterized by encephalomyelitis, vomiting and wasting. PHEV is antigenically related to BCoV. The virus hemagglutinates chicken, rat, mouse, hamster, and turkey erythrocytes. PHEV is sensitive to lipid solvents, including sodium deoxycholate; it is also heat labile and relatively stable when frozen. VWD occurs in pigs less than 3 weeks of age, although older swine may exhibit milder signs of the disease. VWD in young piglets is characterized by anorexia, lethargy, vomiting, constipation, and signs of CNS disturbance (hyperesthesia, muscle tremors, paddling of the legs). Mortality is high, up to 100%; pigs also may develop chronic infections and eventually die from starvation or secondary infections.

Host–Virus Relationship

Distribution, Reservoir, and Transmission. PHEV was first isolated and associated with VWD in Canadian swine in 1958. Subsequently, the virus has been identified in swine in many areas of the world. Pigs are the only known host of PHEV, and subclinical or inapparent carrier states likely exist. Nasal secretions contain virus and horizontal aerosol and direct animal contact are mechanisms of transmission.

Pathogenesis and Pathology. The pathogenesis of PHEV infection has been characterized by experimental inoculation of colostrum-deprived day-old pigs. Following oronasal inoculation, primary viral replication occurs in the epithelial cells of the nasal mucosa, tonsils, lungs, and small intestine. Virus subsequently spreads along peripheral nerves to the CNS. Prior to disease expression, viral antigen is present in the trigeminal, inferior vagal, and superior cervical ganglia, solar and dorsal root ganglia of the lower thoracic region, and the intestinal nerve plexuses. Infection in the brain stem is initiated in the trigeminal and vagal sensory nuclei and subsequently spreads to other nuclei and the rostral portion of the brain stem. Later stages of the infection may be characterized by viral replication in the cerebrum, cerebellum, and spinal cord; virus is typically found in the nervous plexuses of the stomach late in infection.

There are few characteristic gross lesions in natural PHEV infections; a mild catarrhal rhinitis is sometimes evident in encephalomyelitis cases, and gastroenteritis is sometimes observed in VWD. Lesions in the CNS are of a nonsuppurative encephalomyelitis characterized by perivascular cuffs of mononuclear cells, formation of glial nodes, neuronal degeneration, and meningitis. Respiratory tract lesions consist of focal or diffuse interstitial peribronchiolar pneumonia with cellular infiltrates composed of monocytes, lymphocytes, and neutrophils.

Host Response to Infection. Humoral immune responses may be quantitated by viral neutralization, hemagglutination inhibition (HI), and agar gel immunodiffusion (AGID). The clinical disease is self-limiting in pig populations due to the rapid development of maternal antibodies and transfer via colostrum.

Laboratory Diagnois. Diagnosis of PHEV encephalomyelitis or VWD in piglets requires IHC staining of viral antigens in the tissues of affected pigs, virus isolation on primary pig kidney (PK) or pig thyroid (PT) cells, or demonstration of a rising antibody titer. PHEV grows in primary PK or PT cells with formation of characteristic syncytia.

Treatment and Control. No effective treatment has been described for HEV-induced encephalomyelitis or VWD. Clinical outbreaks are self-limiting. No vaccines are available and good animal husbandry practices are essential for the prevention and control of the disease.

Bovine Coronavirus

Disease. BCoV is a pneumoenteric virus that infect upper and lower respiratory tracts, as well as the intestine of cattle and wild ruminants. In cattle, BCoV can cause three different disease syndromes: neonatal diarrhea in newborn calves (1–3 weeks, calf diarrhea (CD)) and winter dysentery (WD) in adult cattle with hemorrhagic diarrhea and respiratory infections in cattle of various ages. The respiratory infections in cattle include shipping fever or bovine respiratory disease complex (BRDC) in feedlot cattle.

The CD in newborn calves (1–3 weeks) is characterized by anorexia and a liquid, yellow diarrhea that persists for 4–5 days. WD is a sporadic acute disease in adult cattle that is characterized by explosive bloody diarrhea accompanied by decreased milk production, depression, and anorexia. The BCoV strains that are isolated from diarrheal fluid or intestinal fluid are now identified as enteropathogenic bovine coronaviruses (EBCoV). Other strains of BCoV have more recently been identified as respiratory pathogens in cattle; these strains of coronavirus have been isolated from the nasal secretions and lungs of cattle with severe shipping fever pneumonia, and are designated as respiratory bovine coronaviruses (RBCoV). Respiratory disease caused by RBCoV typically occurs in calves aged 6–9 months, and is characterized by fever, nasal discharge, and respiratory distress. The BRDC can be precipitated by RBCoV alone or in combination with several other respiratory viruses (e.g., bovine respiratory syncytial virus, parainfluenza-3 virus, bovine herpesvirus) and viruses capable of mediating immunosuppression (e.g., bovine viral diarrhea virus). Furthermore, there are other predisposing factors that allow commensal bacteria of the nasal cavity (e.g., *Mannheimia haemolytica, Pasteurella* sp., *Mycoplasma* sp.) to infect the lungs leading to a fatal fibrinous pneumonia associated with BRDC.

Etiologic Agent

Physical, Chemical, and Antigenic Properties. BCoV is acid stable (pH of 3.0), but is inactivated by lipid solvents, detergents, and high temperatures. Although there are significant phenotypic, antigenic and genetic differences between EBCoV and RBCoV strains, the precise relationship between enteric and respiratory strains of BCoV is uncertain. There is only one known serotype of BCoVs and as of now, no consistent antigenic or genetic markers have been identified to discriminate BCoV isolates from the three different clinical syndromes. BCoV is antigenically related to coronaviruses of other species. BCoV particles hemagglutinate erythrocytes from hamsters, mice, and rats.

Infectivity for Other Species and Culture Systems. The BCoV has been propagated in suckling mice, and following such passage will infect suckling rats and hamsters by both intracerebral and subcutaneous routes. EBCoV has been propagated in Madin–Darby bovine kidney, African green monkey kidney (Vero), bovine fetal thyroid, and bovine fetal brain cells. Trypsin treatment of the latter two fetal cell cultures enhances plaque formation and cell fusion. Certain isolates are difficult to propagate *in vitro* and may require passage in the natural host. In contrast, only a human rectal tumor cell line (HRT-18) is permissive for initial isolation of RBCoV.

Host–Virus Relationship

Distribution, Reservoir, and Transmission. The distribution of BCoV is worldwide, and transmission of EBCoV is likely fecal-oral by ingestion of virus from contaminated feed, teats, and fomites. RBCoV is shed in respiratory tract secretions of infected animals, and thus is spread horizontally by aerosol. However, RBCoV also can be found in feces leading to fecal-oral transmission of the virus. Bovine-like CoVs have also been identified in water buffalo calves and alpacas. Serological surveys using indirect IF tests have demonstrated circulation of CoVs antigenically closely related to BCoV circulating in captive and wild ruminants. Some of the CoVs from captive ruminants (sambar deer, white-tailed deer, elk, waterbuck, and giraffe) are biologically, genetically and antigenically (cross-neutralizing) very closely related to BCoVs. Sequencing of these closely related CoVs from captive ruminants have shown very close amino acid identity (93–99%) in some viral proteins to enteric and respiratory BCoV strains, further confirming their close genetic relationship. Thus, the possibility exists that wild and captive ruminants could transmit bovine-like CoVs to cattle or vice versa. Such interspecies transmission (species jumping) of BCoVs combined with their ability to recombine would lead to emergence of more genetically divergent CoVs. Sequence analysis has revealed that porcine HEV and HCoV-OC43 likely may have evolved from ancestral BCoV strains. Furthermore, genetic and antigenic similarity between canine respiratory coronavirus (CRCoV) and BCoV has been demonstrated.

Pathogenesis and Pathology. Diarrhea develops within 24–30 h following oral infection of calves with EBCoV. Four hours after onset of diarrhea, viral antigen is detectable in the epithelium of the small intestine and colonic crypts. Initiation of infection is facilitated by proteolytic enzymes in the intestinal tract since trypsin treatment of coronaviruses in cell culture results in enhanced viral growth. The virus also infects the adjacent mesenteric lymph nodes. Destruction of the mature enterocytes that line the intestinal villi leads to atrophy and fusion of affected villi, with subsequent intestinal maldigestion and malabsorption, rapid loss of fluids and electrolytes, and, in severe cases, dehydration, acidosis, shock and death.

RBCoV infection in calves causes interstitial pneumonia with congestion, hemorrhage and edema of the interlobular septa of the lung. Histologically, there is interstitial pneumonia with infiltration of mononuclear inflammatory cells and thickenings of alveolar septa.

Host Response to Infection. Both EBCoV and RBCoV infections in calves result in a humoral immune response that can readily be quantitated by viral neutralization, HI, hemadsorption inhibition (HAI), and ELISA tests. Local immune responses play an important role as circulating antibodies do not protect calves from infection. Neonatal ingestion of colostral IgA protects the intestinal lumen against EBCoV infection for a limited period of time.

Laboratory Diagnosis. BCoV infections can be diagnosed by detection of infectious virus, viral antigen, or viral RNA in clinical specimens (e.g., feces, respiratory secretions, tissues). Diagnosis of EBCoV-induced neonatal diarrhea requires identification of the virus in fecal samples or intestinal sections. This can be achieved by viral isolation, EM, or fluorescent antibody or IHC staining. Nasal swabs collected during the acute stage of upper respiratory tract disease are the specimens of choice for the diagnosis of RBCoV. Respiratory epithelial cells present in the nasal swabs are spotted onto slides for examination by direct fluorescent antibody test.

BCoV RNA in feces, nasal secretions or tissues can be detected by conventional RT-PCR, nRT-PCR, and rRT-PCR assays. Because of BCoV antibodies are widespread in cattle, it is important to test paired acute and convalescent serum samples for serologic diagnosis of BCoV infections.

Treatment and Control. Treatment is dictated by the severity and type of disease. Electrolyte solutions can be administered for dehydration in calves with diarrhea caused by EBCoV infections, and antibiotic therapy may be used to control secondary infections. All BCoV infections are best controlled by good management practices to minimize exposure to these viruses, such as avoiding introducing new (infected) animals into an intensive calving operation. It is difficult to control enteric disease by vaccination because very young calves are most affected before they have the opportunity to respond to vaccination. The alternative is to immunize the dam to increase antibody levels in colostrum. However, there are no BCoV-vaccines have been developed to prevent BCoV associated respiratory disease in young calves or BRDC of feedlot cattle.

Canine Respiratory Coronavirus

In 2003, a new coronavirus was identified in the respiratory tract of dogs housed in a rehoming kennel in the United Kingdom. This virus was referred to as CRCoV. Nucleotide sequence analysis of CRCoV spike protein gene demonstrated 97.3% and 96.9% identity to the betacoronaviruses (Group 2) BCoV and HCoV-OC43, respectively. It has been recently demonstrated that HCoV-OC43 has emerged after viral transmission from cattle to people. Interestingly, the genetic relationship of CRCoV to BCoV spike protein suggests that the virus was probably transmitted to dogs from cattle. The CRCoV shares only 21.2% amino acid identity to CCoV-I in the spike protein. CRCoV is responsible for mild respiratory disease in dogs. However, in most of the cases it contributes to the development of canine infectious respiratory disease (CIRD) together with other canine respiratory pathogens (e.g., *Bordetella bronchiseptica*, canine adenovirus type 1 and type 2, canine parainfleunza virus, canine herpesvirus, reoviruses, and influenza viruses).

Serological studies have shown antibodies to CRCoV in dog serum samples surveyed in the United Kingdom, Canada, Ireland, Italy, United States, and Japan. CRCoV infection associated with CIRD in kennels can occur throughout the year, but it can be more common in the winter months of the year. Isolation of CRCoV in canine cell lines is difficult, but it can be isolated in human rectal tumor cell line (HRT-18) and its clone HRT-18G. However, not all strains of CRCoV can be isolated in HRT-18 or HRT-18G cells. Hemagglutination assay using chicken RBCs at 4 °C can be used to detect CRCoV-infected cell cultures. CRCoV nucleic acids can be detected in clinical samples by standard RT-PCR or real-time RT-PCR. CRCoV can also be detected by immunohistochemistry on formalin-fixed tissues using anti-BCoV cross-reactive antibody. Several ELISAs either using BCoV antigen or CCRoV antigen have been developed. However, an ELISA assay using CRCoV antigen was found to have higher sensitivity and specificity compared with an assay based on BCoV. Antibodies to CRCoV can also be detected by using an IFA on CRCoV-infected HRT-18 cells. Antibodies to CRCoV do not cross-react with enteric CCoVs. There is no specific treatment for infections caused by CRCoV but dogs should be treated for other bacterial causes of CIRD. There are no vaccines against CRCoV and vaccines against CCoV are unlikely to protect against CRCoV because of low antigenic similarity in the spike protein of these viruses.

Equine Coronavirus

Coronavirus-like agents have been identified by EM examination of fecal samples from foals and adult horses having enteric disease and fever. First isolation and characterization of ECoV (NC99 strain) from feces of a diarrheic foal was described in 2000. Phylogenetic analysis has demonstrated that ECoV NC99 strain is most closely related to BCoV, HCoV-OC43, and PHEV. In 2011, isolation of ECoV (Tokachi09 strain) from adult horses with fever and enteric disease was described from Japan. Comparative nucleotide and amino acid analyses of nucleocapsid and spike protein genes showed that the Tokachi09 strain is very similar to the NC99 strain from North America (98.0% and 99.0% at the nucleotides, 97.3% and 99.0% at the amino acids, respectively). However, the Tokachi09 strain had a 185-nucleotide deletion from four bases after the stop codon of the spike gene, resulting in the absence of the open reading frame predicted to encode a 4.7-kDa nonstructural protein in strain NC99. Nevertheless, the pathogenicity of these equine coronaviruses, as well as their role in enteric disease, has not been examined in detail. ECoV has been implicated in an increasing number of enteric disease outbreaks in foals and adult horses in the United States in recent years. Further studies are needed to determine the prevalence of ECoV infection in healthy and sick horses, the occurrence of mixed infections with other enteric equine pathogens, and relative importance of ECoV as a cause of enteric disease in horses.

The diagnosis of ECoV can be achieved by demonstration of coronavirus particles in feces under electron microscopic examination. However, it may be difficult to find a sufficient number of ECoV particles in diagnostic fecal specimens and thus, it may be less rewarding. ECoV can be difficult to isolate and propagate in cell culture. Nevertheless, ECoV has been successfully isolated from feces by inoculating HRT-18 cells. Recently, conventional RT-PCR and rRT-PCR assays targeting the conserved nucleocapsid protein gene have been described. Antibodies to ECoV cross-react with the BcoV, and therefore, demonstration of rising neutralizing antibody titers (fourfold or more) to BCoV in paired serum samples indicates exposure to ECoV.

Mouse Hepatitis Virus

MHV is highly contagious and causes explosive outbreaks of disease in mouse colonies throughout the world. The severity of the clinical disease depends on several factors. These factors can be broadly classified into viral (strain, dose, and route of infection) and host factors (strain of mice, age, and immune status). There are many different strains of MHV, each with characteristic tissue tropism and associated clinical manifestations. Infection of mice with different virus strains can cause enteritis, hepatitis, nephritis, and demyelinating encephalomyelitis. For example the A59 strain of MHV induces moderate to severe hepatitis, whereas the MHV-4 strain does not. The enteropathogenic strains of MHV cause severe diarrhea in suckling mice with nearly 100% mortality. The intestines are distended and filled with yellowish fluid. Older mice develop jaundice, lose weight, and cease breeding. Characteristic histological lesions include blunted (club-shaped) intestinal villi with extensive syncytium formation. All mice develop acute hepatitis with focal hepatocellular necrosis and inflammatory cell infiltration. Other strains of MHV are the cause of respiratory and CNS disease in mouse colonies. A59 and JHM strains of MHV are the most commonly studied neurotropic strains of this virus. A59 causes moderate to severe hepatitis and in the brain, mild encephalitis and demyelination. A59 is a tissue culture adapted dualtropic strain that infects the liver as well as the brain. CNS infection with neurotropic strains of MHV causes paralysis due to demyelination (used as a model of chronic demyelinating diseases of humans like multiple sclerosis).

MHV infection in mouse colonies is diagnosed with the detection of characteristic gross and histological lesions in the intestines and liver, although some strains of MHV are highly attenuated and cause little pathology or disease. The diagnosis is confirmed by immunohistochemistry and serology using an enzyme immunoassay. Virus can be isolated using any of several mouse cell lines.

The virus persists following epidemics in persistently infected mice that continually infect susceptible mice that are introduced into the colony. Control is achieved by breaking this cycle of transmission through the use of strict quarantine measures.

Rat Coronavirus

Two prototype strains of rat coronavirus (RCoV) with different tissue tropism and disease associations have been described. The first, sialodacryadentis virus (SDAV) is the etiologic agent of sialodacryadenitis in laboratory rats. It is a severe, self-limiting inflammatory disease of the upper respiratory tract, salivary and lacrimal glands, and eyes of rats. SDAV has also been isolated from the lower respiratory tract and can cause mild interstitial pneumonia in young rats. The virus is highly contagious and causes high morbidity and low mortality in infected colonies. Clinical signs of infection include swelling of the face and neck, excessive lacrimation, blinking, squinting, and exophthalmia. Lesions in the lacrimal duct may lead to corneal drying. Lesions typically resolve within 2 weeks. The virus is transmitted by aerosol, direct contact, and fomites.

The second prototype, Parker's RCoV (RCoV-P) has only been isolated from the respiratory tract and causes fatal pneumonia in suckling rats. Following intranasal experimental infection, RCoV-P replicates in both upper and lower respiratory tract leading to interstitial pneumonia and focal edema in the alveoli, which resolves by day 8 after infection.

Animal Diseases Caused by Members of the Genus *Gammacoronavirus*

Avian Infectious Bronchitis Virus

Disease. Avian bronchitis virus (IBV) is one of the most significant causes of economic losses within the poultry industry, affecting the performance of both egg-laying and meat-style (broiler) birds. Avian IBV causes respiratory disease in chicks 10 days to 4 weeks of age; however, all ages, sexes, and breeds are susceptible to infection although mortality is low in birds greater than 6 weeks of age. The virus replicates not only in the upper and lower respiratory tract but also in the alimentary tract (e.g., esophagus, proventriculus, duodenum, jejunum, cecal tonsils, rectum, cloaca, and bursa of Fabricious) and other tissues such as reproductive tract (e.g., oviduct and testes) and kidneys. The respiratory disease is characterized by respiratory distress, rales, coughing, nasal discharge, and depression. The clinical course lasts 6–18 days. Morbidity is 100% and mortality may exceed 25%. Chicks with no maternal antibody may experience permanent oviduct damage and fail to lay eggs when mature. Infection of the alimentary tract tissues does not manifest clinically. However, nephritis is not uncommon among some of the IBV infected broilers. IBV-associated renal disease is dependent upon viral strain. Many viral strains with an affinity for the kidneys cause only mild or inapparent respiratory signs, but can cause substantial mortality in susceptible birds. Infection of laying flocks results in a drop of egg production and hatchability. Pullets in good condition return to normal production within a few weeks. Oviduct infection of is believed to contribute to diminished egg production.

Etiologic Agent

Physical, Chemical, and Antigenic Properties. IBV is antigenically distinct from other coronaviruses, and multiple distinct virus strains have been identified and grouped by serologic techniques, polypeptide patterns in polyacrylamide gel electrophoresis, oligonucleotide fingerprinting, and nucleotide sequencing. Strain-specific epitopes for viral neutralization and hemagglutination have been identified on the S1 protein (S protein is cleaved to generate two subunits, aminoterminal S1 and carboxyterminal S2) with monoclonal antibodies. However, serotyping based on the reaction between an IBV strain and chicken-induced IBV serotype-specific antibodies has become less practical due to the emergence of an increasing number of antigenic variants with new neutralization phenotypes. A small percentage of amino acid changes in the S1 protein can result in a change in virus neutralizing epitopes leading to emergence of new antigenic variants and serotypes. Thus, IBV variants may belong to over a hundred serotypes. Genotyping of IBV strains has been achieved primarily by RT-PCR implication and sequencing of the S1 subunit of the spike glycoprotein, which is the major inducer of protective immunity and expresses most of the virus-neutralizing epitopes, including the serotype specific epitopes. In general, the IBV strains with high level of homology in the S1 gene will provide a good level of cross-protection which is not seen with strains with a low homology in this region.

Resistance to Physical and Chemical Agents. Most strains of IBV are inactivated within 15 min at 56 °C. The virus is quite stable at cold temperatures. Stability at acidic pH is strain-variable; with some strains surviving at pH 3.0 for 3 h at 4 °C. Lipid solvents inactivate the virus.

Infectivity for Other Species and Culture Systems. The chicken is the only known natural host of IBV. However, quail and sea gulls have been experimentally infected. Suckling mice can be infected by intracerebral inoculation. The virus can be cultivated in developing avian embryos, cell cultures, and organ cultures. Turkey embryos have also been successfully infected with IBV, but less efficiently. IBV can be grown in chick embryo cells (kidney, lung, and liver), embryonic turkey kidney cells, and monkey kidney (Vero) cells. Organ cultures have been used to propagate IBV including tracheal and oviduct cultures.

Host–Virus Relationship

Distribution, Reservoir, and Transmission. A large number of IBV variants exist around the world. Interestingly, some of the IBV variants are unique to a particular area, whereas others have a more general distribution. The virus likely persists in persistently infected birds and/or continuous cycles of transmission. Virus has been recovered for up to 49 days from infected chickens held in isolation and for even longer periods in those held under natural conditions. Viral transmission occurs by inhalation, with the respiratory tract being the primary site of infection. Virus is shed in respiratory and fecal materials, with subsequent spread by contaminated fomites and aerosol.

Pathogenesis and Pathology. The incubation period of IBV infection is 18–36 h. Virus gains entry via the respiratory tract, and the respiratory form of IBV results in tracheitis and bronchitis. Mortality may be as high as 25% in young chicks. Strains exhibiting an affinity for the kidneys damage the renal tubules, resulting in renal failure. Chickens infected with nephrotropic viral strains develop renal tubular necrosis characterized by swollen and pale kidneys with accumulation of uric acid crystals causing distension of the tubules and ureters. Infection produces primarily a serous, catarrhal, or caseous exudate in the trachea, nasal passages, and sinuses. The air sacs may contain a caseous exudate, and small foci of bronchopneumonia may be apparent. Young chicks may experience a more severe infection, with lesions developing in the oviduct. Microscopic lesions of the respiratory tract include cellular infiltration, mucosal edema, vascular congestion, and hemorrhage.

Host Response to Infection. IBV elicits humoral and cellular immune responses. Humoral responses can be measured by ELISA, viral neutralization, and HI tests. Following infection with IBV, chickens first develop ELISA antibodies, followed by virus neutralizing, and HI antibodies. Titers of passively transferred maternal antibody decrease to negligible levels within 4 weeks of hatching. Chickens recovered from natural infection are resistant to homologous viral challenge. The duration of immunity is variable and difficult to determine due to the multiplicity of IBV strains. Passive transfer of maternal antibody does not confer total protection to the chick but reduces disease severity and mortality. Local tracheal immunity appears to play a major role in resistance to IBV. The relative importance of humoral versus cellular immunity is unclear. However, it has been demonstrated that cytotoxic T-cell responses to IBV infection in chickens correlated with initial decrease in infection and clinical signs. The observation that chickens may be protected in the absence of demonstrable antibody would suggest an important role for cell-mediated immunity.

Laboratory Diagnosis. Diagnosis of infectious bronchitis may be based upon direct visualization of viral antigen in tracheal smears using IHC or fluorescent antibody staining, viral isolation, or serology. Infectious bronchitis must be differentiated from other acute respiratory diseases of birds, such as Newcastle disease, laryngotracheitis, and infectious coryza.

Viral isolation is conducted by inoculation of tracheal or respiratory exudates into the chorioallantoic sac of 10- to 11-day-old embryonated chicken eggs (ECE). Serial passage in ECEs may be required before embryo dwarfing or mortality occurs. Recently, real-time RT-PCR assays for the detection of IBV nucleic acid have been described. Serologic diagnosis of IBV infection requires paired serum samples and the use of IBV-specific viral neutralization, HI, AGID, or ELISA assays.

Treatment and Control. No specific treatment for infectious bronchitis is available. Proper husbandry practices that reduce environmental stress are logical. Control of infectious bronchitis may be approached through management procedures and vaccination. Spread of the virus may be reduced by strict isolation of an affected flock and restocking with day-old chicks reared in isolation. Attenuated and inactivated vaccines have been developed for the control of IB. Inactivated vaccines induce neutralizing antibodies, but their efficacy has been questioned. MLV vaccines attenuated by serial passage in embryonated chicken eggs have not only reduced pathogenicity but also decreased immunogenicity. Vaccination with MLV vaccines produce short-lived protection and start to decline after 9 weeks. Consequently, commercial layers which are kept for a year or more should be vaccinated several times with MLV vaccines, perhaps with more than one serotype. Vaccines may be administered via aerosol or in drinking water. High passage vaccine viruses apparently have a reduced invasiveness and generally require aerosol administration.

The multiplicity of IBV strains and serotypes has made it difficult to develop efficacious vaccines. No single strain has been identified as capable of inducing more than limited protection to heterologous viruses. Multivalent vaccines are available, but in certain instances prolonged reactions to vaccination and some interference between vaccine strains have been reported. Vaccines have not been developed commercially with nephropathogenic strains of IBV. Inactivated and subunit vaccines have been developed against IBV but they do not provide good protection against infection.

Turkey Coronavirus

Disease. TCoV is the causative agent of coronavirus enteritis (CE) of turkeys. It is an acute and highly contagious disease of turkeys of all ages and is of major economic importance to the turkey industry. Synonyms of the disease include bluecomb disease, mud fever, transmissible enteritis, and infectious enteritis. The disease affects primarily the alimentary tract and is characterized by depression, subnormal body temperature, anorexia, inappetence, loss of body weight, and wet droppings. Darkening of the head and skin and tucking of the skin over the crop are characteristics of infected growing turkeys. A rapid drop in egg production with formation of chalky eggshells occurs in producing breeder hens. Morbidity is essentially 100%, and mortality varies with age and environmental conditions.

Etiologic Agent

Physical, Chemical, and Antigenic Properties. TCoV is inactivated by lipid solvents and detergents, but is resistant to acidic pH (pH of 3.0 at 20 °C for 30 min). The virus is resistant to 50 °C for 1 h. TCoV is apparently unrelated antigenically to other coronaviruses and is readily distinguished from IBV based on antigenic and biological differences. However, phylogenetic analysis based on the nucleocapsid gene has demonstrated that TCoV is more closely related to IBV than to other mammalian coronaviruses. TCoV agglutinates rabbit and guinea pig erythrocytes, but not those from cattle, horse, sheep, mouse, goose, monkey, rooster, or chickens.

Infectivity for Other Species and Culture Systems. TCoV infection is confined to turkeys and virus replication occurs exclusively in the intestinal epithelium and the epithelium of the bursa of Fabricious. Using IHC, TCoV antigens can be demonstrated in these tissues. Experimental infection of chickens, pheasants, sea gulls, and coturnix quail were shown to be refractory to infection. Laboratory propagation of the virus has been limited to turkey and chicken embryos, and attempts to grow TCoV in cell cultures have been unsuccessful.

Host–Virus Relationship

Distribution, Reservoir, and Transmission. CE has been described in North America and Australia. The virus persists in turkeys for life following recovery from the disease. It is stable in frozen feces and survives throughout the winter months in infected droppings, thus transmission of TCoV is principally fecal-oral from the infected feces of carrier birds. Introduction of virus onto a premise may occur via carrier turkeys, feces-contaminated fomites such as personnel and equipment, and possibly mechanical transmission by free-flying birds.

Pathogenesis and Pathology. The incubation period of CE varies from 1 to 5 days. Gross lesions are largely confined to the intestinal tract, with petechial hemorrhages sometimes apparent on the serosal surface. Lesions are most distinct in the jejunum but may also occur in the duodenum, ileum, and cecum. Gas and fluid typically distend the small intestine and ceca. The breast muscles are typically dehydrated and the carcass generally appears emaciated. Microscopic lesions include destruction of enterocytes lining the intestinal villi, leading to their shortening, loss of microvilli, and mononuclear cell infiltration of the lamina propria of the affected bowel.

Host Response to Infection. Turkeys respond to TCoV infection with a humoral and cellular immune response. Serum antibodies (IgM, IgA, and IgG) develop following infection, but only IgG is present by 21 days. Local IgA antibody appears in intestinal secretions and bile for at least 6 months. Passive transfer of maternal immunity has not been observed and administration of antiserum to young poults does not afford protection.

Laboratory Diagnosis. Definitive diagnosis of CE requires identification of viral antigen in intestinal tissue sections by IHC staining, viral isolation, or demonstration of serum antibody. Virus may be isolated by inoculation of embryonated turkey eggs or young poults and its presence confirmed by fluorescent antibody staining of infected tissues. Attempts to propagate TCoV in a variety of avian and mammalian cell cultures generally have been unsuccessful. Serologic diagnosis can be conducted on paired serum samples by viral neutralization or indirect FA tests.

Treatment and Control. No specific treatment is effective in reducing morbidity of CE, although various treatments may be used to prevent other intestinal infections. TCoV vaccines are not available, but prevention of infection is possible. The disease has been eliminated in some areas by depopulation and decontamination of affected premises. An alternative to viral elimination is exposing poults (5–6 weeks of age) to recovered carrier birds under ideal environmental conditions for the purpose of inducing protective immunity. Such a program is recommended only on farms with continued problems and when all other methods of control have failed.

Animal Diseases Caused by Members of the Genus *Torovirus*

Four species of toroviruses have recently been identified: BToV, PToV, EToV, and HuToV (Table 62.1). TVL particles have been observed in fecal samples of horses, cattle, pigs, cats, dogs, and humans. In addition, serological evidence for torovirus infections has been demonstrated in horses, cattle, sheep, goats, pigs, rabbits, rats, and two species of wild mice. It has been speculated that toroviruses are associated with enteric disease in many animal species, but as yet, only the BToV (also known as bovine enteric torovirus) has been definitely ascribed to be associated with gastroenteritis in animals.

Seroepidemiological studies indicate that BToV infection of cattle seems to be common throughout the world. Diarrhea due to BToV infections has been reported both in young and old cattle. The clinical manifestations of BToV infections include watery diarrhea with dehydration, weakness, and depression. Predominantly affected are 2–3-week-old calves and they tend to have only mild diarrhea by 3–4 months of age but continue to shed the virus. Diarrhea outbreaks associated with BToV in adult cattle have been described. Most of the affected cattle develop watery diarrhea, anorexia, and decreased milk production. BToV infections are usually limited to the intestine, but there is some evidence for respiratory tract involvement in adult cattle leading to pneumonia in older cattle. Recently, BToV nucleic acid has been detected by RT-PCR in nasal swabs collected from Japanese calves with respiratory symptoms, suggesting that this virus may be a predisposing factor and/or causative agent for bovine respiratory disease. Toroviruses infect the epithelial cells of the small and large intestine extending from mid-jejunum to colon. Transmission of BToV probably occurs via oral and respiratory routes. Following infection, cattle develop neutralizing antibodies to BToV and these antibodies can cross-react with toroviruses from other animal species. Diagnosis of BToV infection is achieved by demonstration of virus particles with a doughnut-shaped nucleocapsid surrounded by an envelope containing a large number of small spikes that resemble the peplomeres of coronaviruses. Although isolation of EToV from a rectal swab has been previously reported, attempts to isolate the other members of this genus have proved to be difficult. However recently, BToV from fecal samples of diarrheic cows in Japan has been isolated in HRT-18 cells. The diagnosis of BToV infection is mainly achieved by demonstration of antigen or demonstration of antibodies to the virus by immunological methods. Virus in fecal samples can be detected by indirect immunofluorescence using bovine anti-BToV antiserum. Antibodies to BToV can be demonstrated by neutralization assay or ELISA. Recently, standard and real-time RT-PCR assays have been described for the detection of both BToV and PToV nucleic acid in fecal samples.

PToV was originally isolated in 1998 from the feces of piglets that did not show any signs of enteritis or diarrhea, but it since has been isolated from pigs with diarrhea at the time of weaning. In recent years, PToV has been identified from piglets in many countries in the world but its potential to cause diarrhea in pigs remains unclear. EToV (Bern virus) was originally isolated from the rectal swab of a diarrheic horse. This is the only EToV isolate that has been reported to date. Limited seroepidemiological studies indicate that the virus is present in the United States and Europe. Much remains to be determined regarding the pathogenic importance of torovirus infections of animals.

References

Enjuanes L, Gorbalenya AE, de Groot RJ *et al.* (2008) Nidovirales, in *Encyclopedia of Virology* (eds BWJ Mahy and MHV Regenmortel), Elsevier, Oxford, pp. 419–430.

Gorbalenya AE, Enjuanes L, Ziebuhr J, and Snijder EJ (2006) Nidovirales: Evolving the largest RNA virus genome. *Virus Res*, **117**, 17–37.

Schütze H, Ulferts R, Schelle B *et al.* (2006) Characterization of *White Bream virus* reveals a novel genetic cluster of *Nidoviruses*. *J Virol*, **80** (23), 11598–11609.

Further Reading

Decaro N and Buonavoglia C (2008) An update on canine coronaviruses: Viral evolution and pathobiology. *Vet Microbiol*, **132**, 221–234.

de Groot RJ, Baker SC, Baric R *et al.* (2012) Order Nidovirales, in *Virus Taxonomy, Ninth Report of the International Committee on Taxonomy of Viruses* (eds AMQ King, MJ Adams, EB Carters, and EJ Lefkowitz), Elsevier Academic Press, London, Nidovirales, pp. 806–828.

de Groot RJ, Cowley JA, Enjuanes L *et al.* (2012) Order Nidovirales, in *Virus Taxonomy, Ninth Report of the International Committee on Taxonomy of Viruses* (eds AMQ King, MJ Adams, EB Carters, and EJ Lefkowitz), Elsevier Academic Press, London, Nidovirales, pp. 785–795.

Faaberg KS, Balasuriya UBR, and Brinton MA (2012) Family *Arteriviridae*, in *Virus Taxonomy, Ninth Report of the International Committee on Taxonomy of Viruses* (eds AMQ King, MJ Adams, EB Carters, and EJ Lefkowitz), Elsevier Academic Press, London, Nidovirales, pp. 796–805.

Lai MMC, Perlman S, and Anderson LJ (2007) *Coronaviridae*, in *Fields Virology*, 5th edn (eds DM Knipe and PM Howley), Lippincott Williams & Wilkins, Philadelphia, PA, pp. 1305–1335.

Perlman S, Gallagher T, and Snijder EJ (ed.) (2008) *Nidoviruses*, ASM Press, Washington DC.

Saif L (2010) Bovine respiratory coronaviruses. *Vet Clin Food Anim*, **26**, 349–364.

Siddell SG, Ziebuhr J, and Snijder EJ (2005) Coronaviruses, toroviruses and arteriviruses, in, *Topley & Wilson's Microbiology and Microbial Infections, Virology* (eds BWJ Mahy and V ter Meulen), Hodder Arnold. London, pp. 823–856.

Woo PCY, Lau SKP, Huang Y, and Yuen KY. (2009) Coronavirus diversity, phylogeny and interspecies jumping. *Exp Biol Med*, **234**, 1117–1127.

Woo PCY, Huang Y, Lau SKP, and Yuen KY. (2010). Coronavirus genomics and bioinformatics analysis. *Viruses*, **2**, 1804–1820.

Arteriviridae and Roniviridae

Udeni B.R. Balasuriya

Introduction and Classification

The virus families Arteriviridae and Roniviridae are included in the order Nidovirales along with Coronaviridae. The members of Arteriviridae and Roniviridae are enveloped viruses with linear, positive-sense, single-stranded RNA (ssRNA) genomes. The genome of arteriviruses and roniviruses contains a 5′-cap structure and a 3′-poly (A) tail and includes untranslated regions (UTR) at their 5′- and 3′-termini. They share a strikingly similar genome organization and replication strategy to that of coronaviruses, but differ considerably in their genetic complexity and virion architecture (Figures 63.1 and 63.2 and Tables 63.1, 63.2, and 63.3). The family Arteriviridae (genus *Arterivirus*) contains four species-specific viruses that infect as follows: (i) horses, donkeys, mules and zebras (members of the family Equidae), equine arteritis virus (EAV); (ii) pigs, porcine reproductive and respiratory syndrome virus (PRRSV); (iii) monkeys, simian hemorrhagic fever virus (SHFV); and (iv) mice, lactate dehydrogenase-elevating virus (LDV). The arteriviruses primarily target macrophages in their respective hosts, and the disease outcome is highly variable and includes persistent asymptomatic infections, respiratory disease, reproductive failure (abortion), and lethal hemorrhagic fever. All four members of the family Arteriviridae are capable of establishing asymptomatic, long-term infection or persistent infection in their respective natural hosts. The family Roniviridae (genus *Okavirus*) contains a number of closely related viruses that infect crustaceans (shrimp, prawns, and crabs). The name *Okavirus* is derived from the observation that these viruses have the ability to infect the shrimp lymphoid or "Oka" organ. Members of this genus include yellow-head virus (YHV) and gill-associated virus (GAV), both of which infect and cause high mortalities in farmed black tiger prawns (*Penaeus monodon*) in Asia and Australia, respectively.

Virion Properties and Virus Replication

Genus Arterivirus

Arterivirus virions are spherical, 45–60 nm in diameter, and consist of an isometric nucleocapsid of 25–39 nm in diameter, surrounded by a lipid envelope. The envelope includes 12–15 nm diameter ring-like surface projections. The large spikes that are typical of coronaviruses and roniviruses are absent from the arterivirus envelope. The buoyant density of arteriviruses ranges from 1.13 to 1.17 g/cm^3 in sucrose, whereas the sedimentation coefficient is 214–230S. The arterivirus genome is a linear, positive-sense, ssRNA molecule of 12.7–15.7 kb and includes 10–14 open reading frames (ORFs) (Table 63.2 and Figure 63.2). Arteriviruses are readily inactivated by lipid solvents (ether and chloroform) and by common disinfectants and detergents (e.g., 0.01% NP-40 or Titron X-100). Arteriviruses are also highly heat labile, and their half-life progressively decreases with increasing temperature. EAV survives 75 days at 4 °C, 2–3 days at 37 °C, and 20–30 min at 56 °C. Tissue culture fluid or organ samples containing EAV can be stored at −70 °C for years without significant loss of the infectivity. PRRSV infectivity is lost within 1 week at 4 °C, but is stable for a long time (months to years) when frozen (−70 or −20 °C). PRRSV is rapidly inactivated by low and high pH (<6 and >7.5). LDV is not stable at −20 °C and rapidly loses its infectivity.

The virions of EAV and PRRSV consist of a nucleocapsid protein (N) and seven envelope proteins (E, GP2, GP3, GP4, ORF5a protein, GP5, M; Figure 63.1A and Table 63.2). The GP5 (glycosylated) and M (unglycosylated) are the major envelope proteins of EAV and PRRSV, and they form a disulfide-linked heterodimer in the mature virus particles. In addition, the arterivirus envelope contains a heterotrimer of three minor membrane glycoproteins (GP2, GP3, and GP4) and two unglycosylated envelope proteins

Veterinary Microbiology, Third Edition. Edited by D. Scott McVey, Melissa Kennedy and M.M. Chengappa.

FIGURE 63.1. *Structure and morphology of arteriviruses and roniviruses. (A) Schematic representation of arteriviruses (e.g., EAV); (B) electron micrographs of arteriviruses: (a) EAV, (b) PRRSV, (c) SHFV, and (d) LDV; (C) schematic representation of ronivirus; and (D) electron micrograph of roniviruses: (a) GAV and (b) EsRNV. (Adapted from Snijder et al. 2005 (EAV and GAV), Spilman et al. 2009 (PRRSV), Gravell et al. 1980 (SHFV), Brinton-Darnell and Plagemann 1975 (LDV), and Zhang and Bonami 2007 (EsRNV) with permission.)*

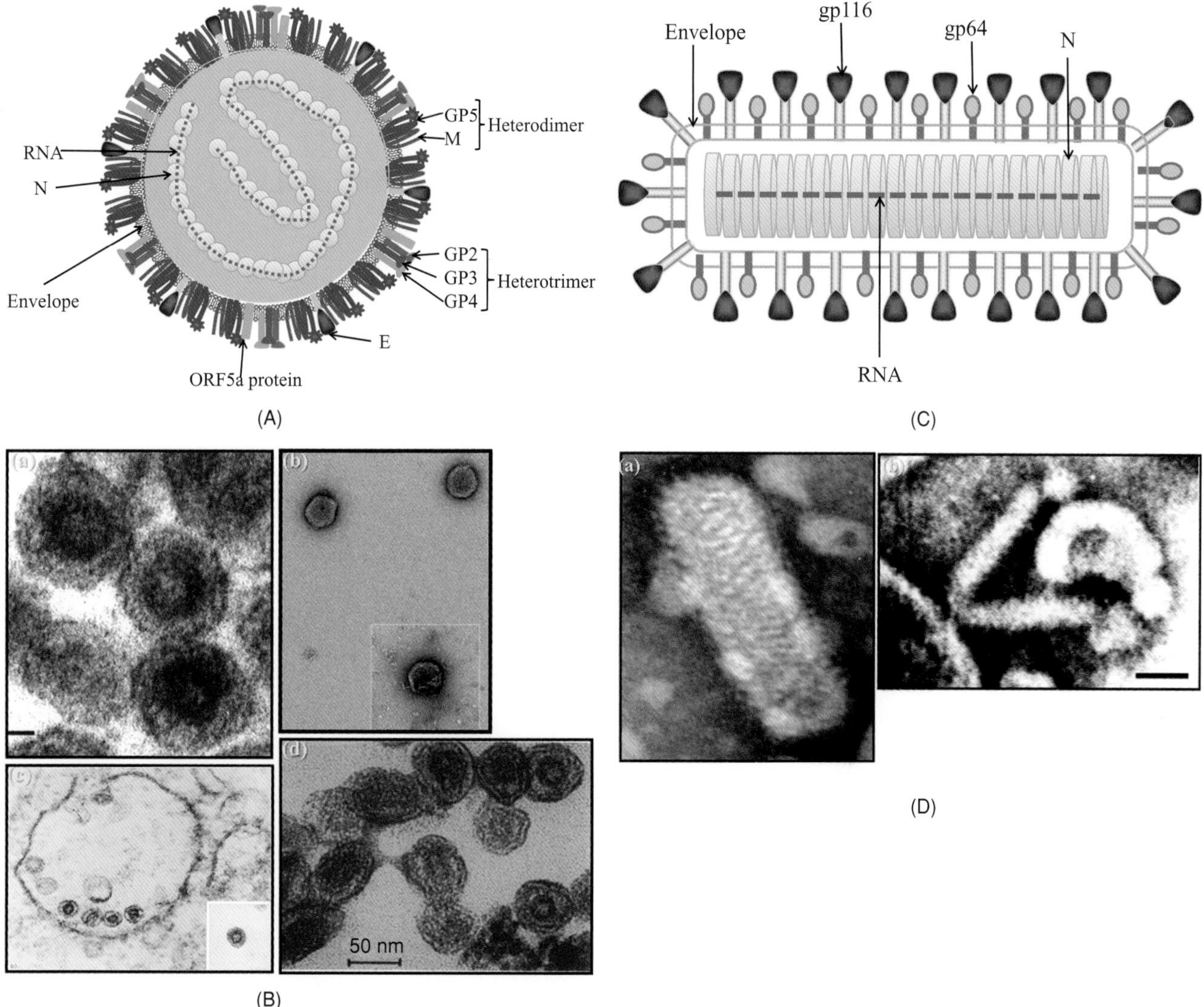

(E and ORF5a protein). It has been shown that all major structural proteins (N, GP5, and M) and four of the minor envelope proteins (E, GP2, GP3, and GP4) are essential for the production of infectious progeny virus. It has been shown by reverse genetics that the elimination of ORF5a protein expression will cripple the EAV virus, which leads to progeny virus with small plaque phenotype and significantly reduced virus titer. In LDV the proteins encoded by ORF2a, ORF2b, ORF3, ORF4, and ORF5a have not been confirmed as structural proteins of the virus. The cells infected with the North American PRRSV (type 2) and LDV have been shown to produce a non-virion-associated form of the GP3 that is released into the culture medium. The GP5 protein contains the known neutralization determinants of EAV, PRRSV, and LDV (Figure 63.3), and it has been clearly demonstrated that heterodimerization of GP5 and M proteins is critical for the authentic posttranslational modification (glycosylation) and conformational maturation of neutralization determinants in GP5 of both EAV and PRRSV. The M protein may act as an essential scaffold on which the GP5 protein folds from the epitopes that induce neutralizing antibodies in mice, horses, and pigs.

In addition, it has been shown that the GP4 of the European prototype PRRSV strain leylystad virus (LV) contains a highly immunogenic linear neutralizing epitope (amino acids 57–68). Monoclonal antibodies (Mabs) against this neutralizing epitope on GP4 of LV do not recognize or neutralize other European field isolates that differ in the corresponding region, indicating that porcine neutralizing antibodies might be responsible for the selection of neutralization-resistant variants with amino acid substitutions in the neutralization epitope in GP4. The GP2, GP3, and GP4 heterodimer is involved in virus attachment and receptor binding. Recently, it has been shown that GP2 and

FIGURE 63.2. *Schematic representation of genome organization of arteriviruses and roniviruses. The genomic RNA of representative viruses of the families Arteriviridae (EAV, PRRSV-NA, and SHFV) and Roniviridae (GAV) is shown to the same scale. The open reading frames (ORFs) encoding replicase proteins and viral structural proteins are depicted. The duplicated SHFV structural protein ORFs are indicated by boxes with broken lines. The 5′-cap structure, 5′-leader sequence (L), ribosomal frame shift (RFS) of the ORF1a/1b, and the 3′ poly A tail (A_n) are indicated. (Modified from Gorbalenya et al 2006.)*

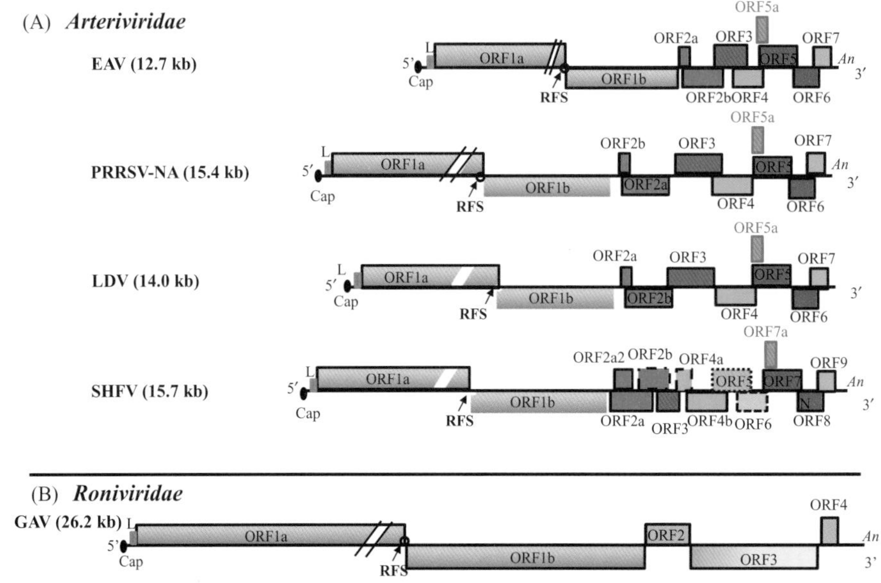

Table 63.1. Viruses in the Families Arteriviridae (Genus *Arterivirus*) and Roniviridae (Genus *Okavirus*)

Family/Genus/Species	Year of Isolation	Natural Host	Disease/Tissue Affected	Transmission
Family Arteriviridae, Genus *Arterivirus*				
Equine arteritis virus[a]	1953	Horse, donkey, and mule	Equine viral arteritis—respiratory disease (influenza-like disease), abortion, interstitial pneumonia in young foals	Aerosol, contact, fomites, venereal (breeding), embryo transfer, and congenital infection
Porcine reproductive and respiratory syndrome virus[b]	1990	Pig	Porcine reproductive and respiratory syndrome—respiratory distress, abortion, stillbirths, mummified fetuses	Aerosol, contact, fomites, venereal (breeding)
Lactate dehydrogenase-elevating virus[c]	1960	Mice	No clinical disease, but elevated lactate dehydrogenase-elevating enzyme in blood	Biting and coprophagy
Simian hemorrhagic fever virus[d]	1964	Monkeys	Systemic hemorrhagic disease	Aerosol, contact, fomites, biting, and iatrogenic
Family Roniviridae, Genus *Okavirus*				
Yellow-head virus[e]	1990	Shrimp and prawns	Yellowing of the hepatopancreas	Horizontal (water-borne), cannibalism, and vertical
Gill-associated virus[f]	1993	Shrimp and prawns	Gills and lymphoid organs	Horizontal (water-borne), cannibalism, and vertical
Eriocheir sinensis ronivirus (EsRNV)	1996	Crabs	Affect lymphoid organs, gills and hepatopancreas, and cause "sighs disease"	Horizontal (water-borne)

GenBank accession numbers for the full-length genome sequence of each of the *Arterivirus* species:
[a]EAV virulent Bucyrus strain (EAV-VBS)—DQ846750; cell culture-adapted Bucyrus strain—X53459 (=NC_001639).
[b]PRRSV type 1 (PRRSV-1 or PRRSV EU [Lelystad virus])—M96262; PRRSV type 2 (PRRSV-2 or PRRSV-NA [VR-2332])—U87392.
[c]LDV Plagemann (LDV-P)—U15146 (=NC_001639); LDV-C (L13298).
[d]SHFV—AF180391 (=NC_003092).
[e]YHV(YHV1992)—FJ848673.
[f]GAV—NC_010306.

Table 63.2. Molecular Properties of Arteriviruses

	Replicase Proteins			Structural Proteins		
Virus (Genome Size; bp)	ORFs	Nsp Name	Size (aa)	ORFs	Protein Name	Size (aa)
EAV	ORF1a	8/9	1727	2a	EGP2	67
(12 704–12 731)	ORF1ab	11	3175	2b	GP3	227
				3	GP4	163
				4	ORF5a	152
				5a	GP5	59
				5b	M	255
				6	N	162
				7		110
PRRSV-NA	ORF1a	9/10	2504	2a	GP2	256
(15 047–15 465)	ORF1ab	12	3962	2b	E	73
				3	GP3	2254
				4	GP4	178
				5a	ORF5a	51[a]
				5b	GP5	200
				6	M	174
				7	N	123
PRRSV-EU	ORF1a	9/10	2397	2a	GP2	249
(15 111)	ORF1ab	12	3854	2b	E	70
				3	GP3	265
				4	GP4	183
				5a	ORF5a	43
				5b	GP5	201
				6	M	173
				7	N	128
LDV	ORF1a	9	2206	2a	E	70
(14 104)	ORF1ab	12	3616	2b	GP2	227
				3	GP3	191
				4	GP4	175
				5a	ORF5a	47
				5b	GP5	199
				6	M	171
				7	N	115
SHFV	ORF1a	9/10	2105	2a	GP2a	281
(15 717)	ORF1ab	12/13	3594	2a2	E	94
				2b	GP2′	204
				3	GP3	205
				4a	E′	80
				4b	GP4	214
				5	GP3′	179
				6	GP4′	182
				7a	ORF7a	64
				7b	GP7	278
				8	M	162
				9	N	111

Molecular data are based on the following GenBank sequences: DQ846750 (EAV virulent Bucyrus strain), U87392 (PRRSV-NA [VR-2332]), M96262 (PRRSV-EU [Lelystad virus]), U15146 (LDV-P), and AF180391 (SHFV).
[a]Size varies between 46 and 51 amino acids among North American PRRSV strains.

GP4 proteins of North American PRRSV interact with all the other envelope GPs to form a multiprotein complex. The interaction between GP4 and GP5 is suggested to be much stronger than interactions among the other envelope glycoproteins.

Using the reverse genetics approach, the virulence determinants of EAV have been mapped to both nonstructural (nsp1, nsp2, nsp7, and nsp10) and structural proteins (GP2, GP4, GP5, and M). However, it appears that the major virulence determinants are located in the structural protein genes of the virus. The interaction among the GP2, GP3, GP4, GP5, and M envelope proteins plays a major role in determining the CD14+ monocyte tropism, while the tropism for CD3+ T lymphocytes is determined by the GP2, GP4, GP5, and M envelope proteins but not the GP3 protein. Using an *in vitro* cell culture model of persistent EAV infection, it has been demonstrated that combined amino acid substitutions in E, GP2, GP3, and GP4 proteins or a single amino acid substitution in the GP5 protein could establish persistent infection in HeLa cells.

Table 63.3. Molecular Properties of Roniviruses

Virus (Genome Size; bp)	Replicase Proteins ORFs	Replicase Proteins Size (aa)	Structural Proteins ORFs	Structural Proteins Protein Name	Structural Proteins Size (aa)
YHV	1a	4074	2	N	146
(26 652–26 673)	1ab	6692	3	gp116	1666[a]
				gp64	
				p20	
			4	Polypeptide	20
GAV	1a	4060	2	N	144
(26 253)	1ab	6706	3	gp116	1640[a]
				gp64	
				p20	
			4	Polypeptide	83

Molecular data are based on the following GenBank sequences: YHV (YHV1992)—FJ848673 and GAV (NC_010306).
[a]Polyprotein encoded by ORF3.

However, no specific viral proteins involved in establishment in persistent infection in the stallion reproductive tract yet have been identified. Using reverse genetics, the major virulence determinants of PRRSV were mapped to nsp3–nsp8 and ORF5, whereas other minor virulence determinants have also been identified in nsp1–nsp3, nsp10–nsp12, and ORF2. Thus, the virulence determinants of EAV and PRRSV appear to be very complex and involve multiple genes encoding both envelope and nonstructural proteins (multigenic).

FIGURE 63.3. *Comparison of the putative neutralization determinants located in the N-terminal ectodomain of the GP5 proteins of EAV, PRRSV, and SHFV, and GP7 of SHFV. Conserved (black circles) and nonconserved (dark gray circles) glycosylation sites as well as putative major neutralization sites (brown boxes) and nonneutralization epitopes (hatched box) are depicted. Recently identified third putative glycosylation site in some strains of EAV is depicted in open gray circles. (Modified with permission from Balasuriya and MacLachlan 2004.)*

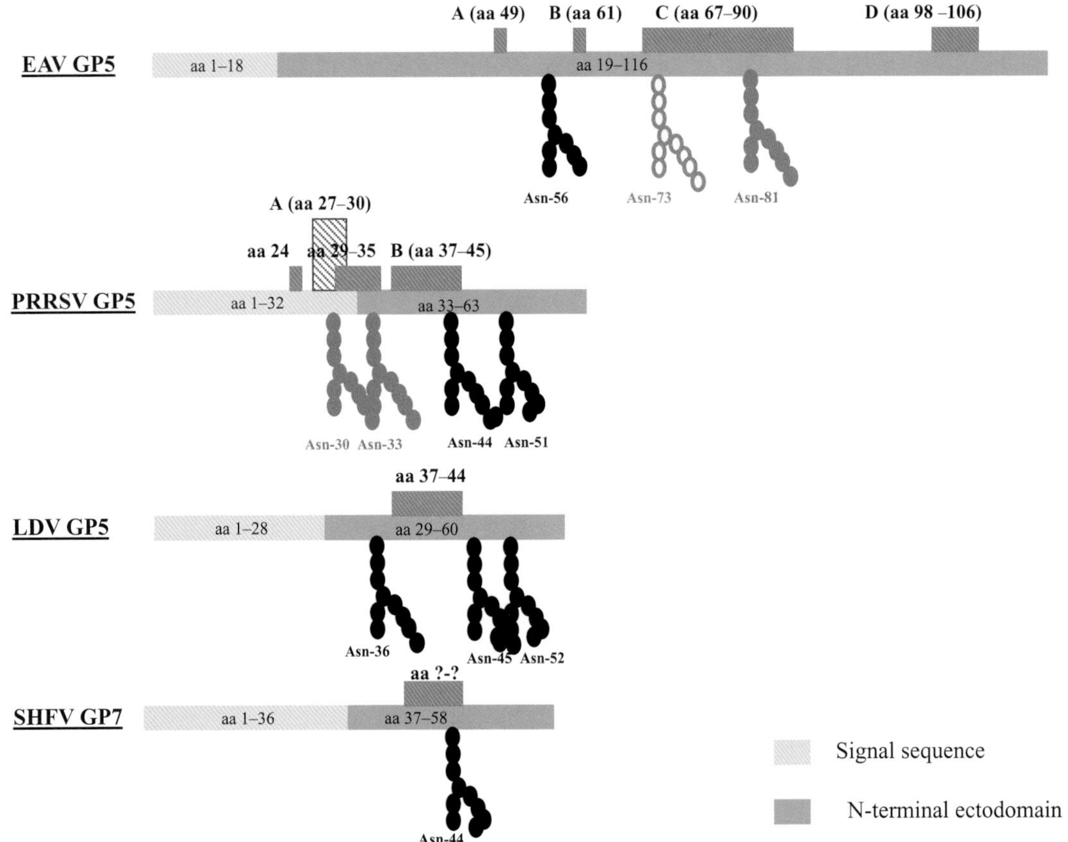

The structural proteins of SHFV are not well characterized. However, in contrast to other arteriviruses, the SHFV genome contains four additional ORFs due to the duplication of ORF2a, ORF2a2, ORF3, and ORF4 (identified as ORF2b, ORF4a, ORF5, and ORF6, respectively; Table 63.2 and Figure 63.2A). ORF2b, ORF4a, ORF5, and ORF6 are predicted to encode four additional duplicated proteins (E′, GP2′, GP3′, and GP4′). ORF2a2 and ORF4a of SHFV encode two proteins that are homologous to the E protein of other arteriviruses. However, unlike the E protein, E′ is not predicted to be myristylated. The E proteins of other arteriviruses have been shown to be fatty acid-acylated, ion channel proteins that function in the uncoating process during virus entry. The SHFV GP7a protein and GP7 major envelope glycoprotein are the counterparts of GP5a and GP5 proteins of other arteriviruses (Table 63.2). The GP7 protein has structural features common to other arteriviruses and is predicted to express the major neutralization epitopes of the virus (Figure 63.3).

Arteriviruses primarily replicate in the macrophages of their natural hosts. EAV can infect horses, donkeys, mules, and zebras, and replicates primarily in macrophages and endothelial cells; but it also replicates in selected epithelia, mesothelium, and smooth muscle cells of the tunica media of smaller arteries, venules, and the myometrium. Unlike other arteriviruses, EAV replicates in a variety of primary cultures, including equine pulmonary artery endothelial cells, horse kidney, rabbit kidney, and hamster kidney cells. It also replicates in cell lines such as baby hamster kidney (BHK-21), rabbit kidney-13 (RK-13), African green monkey kidney (VERO), rhesus monkey kidney (LLC-MK2), hamster lung (HmLu), SV-40-transformed equine ovary, and canine hepatitis virus-transformed hamster tumor cells (HS and HT-7). PRRSV primarily infects pigs, but recently, chickens and ducks that were exposed to PRRSV in drinking water shed the virus in their feces, suggesting that they are susceptible to infection with the virus. American PRRSV (type 2) isolates replicate in porcine alveolar macrophages (PAM), CRL-11171 and an African green monkey cell line (MA-104), and derivatives thereof (CL2621 or MARC-145). Most, if not all, European PRRSV (type 1) isolates replicate best or exclusively in PAMs. However, European PRRSV isolates have been adapted to grow in the CL2621 cell line. Vaccine strains of PRRSV replicate much more efficiently (100–1000 times) in derivatives of monkey kidney cell lines than in PAMs. LDV primarily replicates in primary cultures of mouse macrophages from 1- to 2-week-old mice and other mouse macrophage cell lines, but not other cell lines. SHFV infects and replicates in primary cultures of peritoneal macrophages from rhesus and patas monkeys and also replicates in the MA-104 cell line.

Similar to other enveloped viruses, arteriviruses bind to cell surface receptor(s) using their envelope proteins, which mediate the process of cell attachment and membrane fusion with the host cell membrane (Figure 63.4). Except for PRRSV, the specific cellular receptors for other arteriviruses have not been identified yet. Potential cellular molecules involved in PRRSV virus attachment and internalization have recently been identified. These include CD163 (a member of the macrophage scavenger receptor family), sialoadhesin (a macrophage-restricted surface molecule), and heparan sulfate glycosaminoglycans. It has been shown that GP4 and GP2 of PRRSV interact with the CD163 molecule and play a critical role in viral attachment. For EAV it has been demonstrated that heparan sulfate may play a critical role in cellular attachment. It has been shown that interaction among all minor (GP2, GP3, and GP4) and major (GP5 and M) envelope proteins of EAV plays a major role in determining the CD14+ monocyte tropism, while the tropism for CD3+ T lymphocytes was determined by GP2, GP4, GP5, and M envelope proteins but not the GP3 protein. EAV and other arteriviruses appear to enter susceptible cells by a low-pH-dependent endocytic pathway. Following uncoating of the viral genome, arterivirus replication starts with the translation of the two large replicase polyprotein genes (ORF1a and ORF1b) located in the 5′ three quarters of the genome through a ribosomal frameshifting (Figure 63.5). These two replicase polyproteins are processed into 13 or 14 cleavage products or "nonstructural proteins" (nsps) and a variety of processing intermediates by three viral proteases (Figure 63.5). Both the 5′-leader sequence (5′-UTR) and transcription regulatory sequences (TRSs) located upstream of each ORF play a critical role in genome replication and transcription of viral proteins. The TRSs are short-conserved sequence elements (5′-UCAAC-3′) that determine a base-pairing interaction between positive and nascent minus-strand RNA and are essential for leader–body joining. Arterivirus replication occurs in the cytoplasm of the infected cells, and host cell membranes are modified into typical vesicular double-membrane vesicles that are thought to carry the viral replication/transcription complex. However, some of the viral proteins (nsp1 and N) are translocated to the nucleus during viral replication. The viral structural protein-encoding genes are overlapping and located in the 3′ one fourth of the genome (Figure 63.2). These structural protein genes are expressed from a 3′-co-terminal nested set of subgenomic mRNAs (sgmRNAs). All sgmRNAs have a common 5′-leader sequence derived from the 5′-UTR of the viral genome. The arterivirus replication and transcription are processed through different minus-strand intermediates (Figure 63.6): a full-length minus-strand template is used for replication, while subgenome-sized minus strands produced during a process of discontinuous RNA synthesis are used to synthesize sgmRNAs. The initiation of full-length minus-strand RNA (or antigenome) synthesis, which is also used as a template for new genome RNA replication, occurs after recognition of RNA signals near the 3′ end of the viral genome by the RNA-dependent RNA polymerase (RdRp) complex. For production of new genomic RNA, recognition of signals present close to the 3′ end of the antigenome is used. The N protein encapsidates the newly synthesized viral genomic RNA, and arteriviruses acquire their envelope during budding through the endoplasmic reticulum and/or the Golgi complex. After budding, progeny virus particles are transported in intracellular vesicles to the plasma membrane for release.

Genus *Ronivirus*

Roniviruses are enveloped, bacilliform (40–60 nm × 150–200 nm) virions with rounded ends (Figure 63.1C and D).

FIGURE 63.4. *Schematic overview of EAV life cycle. DMV, double-membrane vesicle; ER, endoplasmic reticulum; ERGIC, ER-Golgi intermediate compartment; NC, nucleocapsid.*

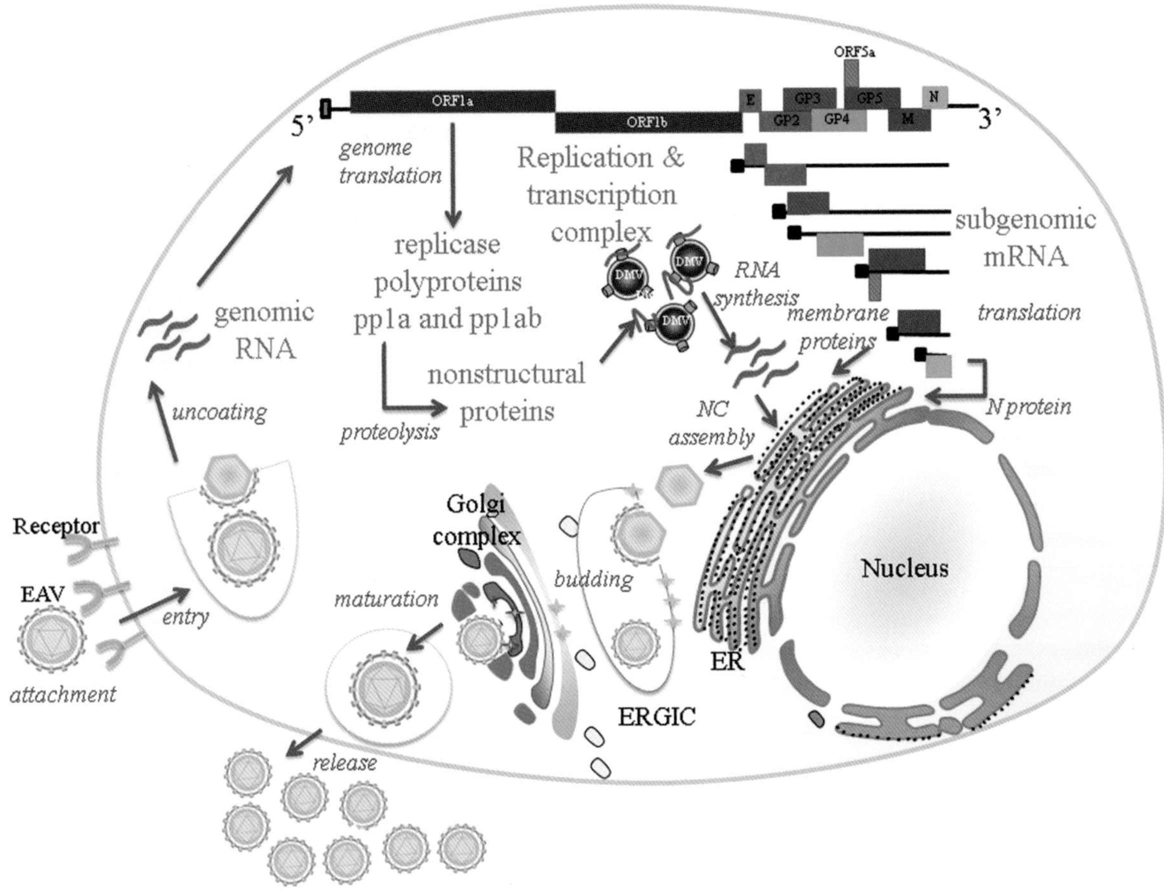

FIGURE 63.5. *Schematic presentation of arterivirus genome expression. The 5′-leader sequence (blue box) and the body TRSs (pink boxes) located upstream of each gene are indicated. Translation of E and GP2 genes, as well as ORF5a and GP5 genes occurs by leaky scanning of the 5′-proximal end of sgmRNA2 and sgmRNA5. The processing of EAV replicase polyprotein 1ab is shown on the left hand bottom corner of the figure. The predicted PCPβ and CP cleavage sites are indicated by green and blue arrows, respectively. The 3CLSP (SP) cleavage sites are indicated by black arrowheads. The genes encoding structural proteins are depicted in various colors. PCP, papain-like cysteine protease; CP, cysteine protease; 3CLSP (SP), 3-chymotrypsin-like serine protease; ZF, predicted zinc finger; Hel, helicase; Ne, NendoU; nsp, nonstructural protein.*

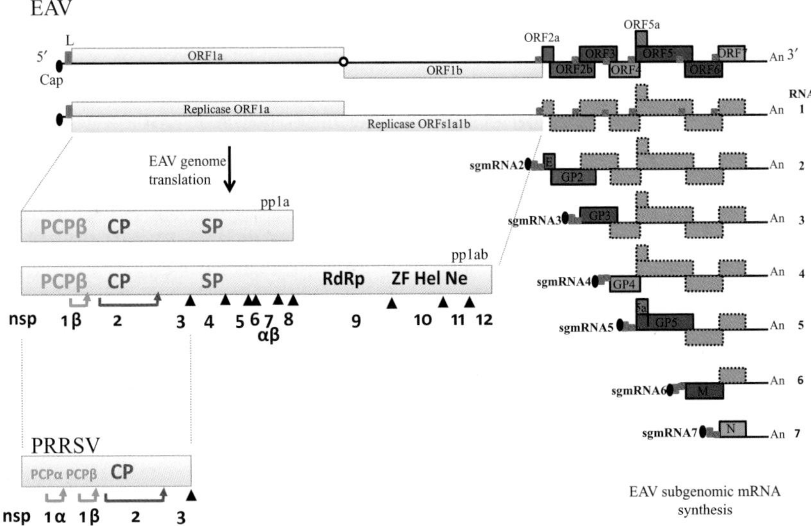

FIGURE 63.6. *Illustration of arterivirus replication (genome synthesis; top panel) and transcription (sgmRNA synthesis; bottom panel) based on "discontinuous extension of minus-strand RNA model." Replication mode—the RdRp produces a full-length minus-strand RNA (antigenome) that serves as the template for synthesis of new genomic RNA. Transcription mode—the minus-strand RNA synthesis is proposed to be discontinuous and regulated by TRSs. The antibody TRS serves as a "jump" signal of the nascent minus strand to leader TRS located at the 5′ end of the plus-stranded full-length genome. Subsequently, the nascent minus strand, with an antibody TRS at its 3′ end, would be redirected to the 5′-proximal region of the genomic template by a base-pairing interaction with the TRS at the 3′ end of the leader (+L). After the addition of the antileader (−L) to the nascent minus strands, the subgenome-length-minus strands would then serve as templates for sgmRNA synthesis. (Adapted from Pasternak* et al. *2006, and modified from Balasuriya and Snijder 2008 with permission.)*

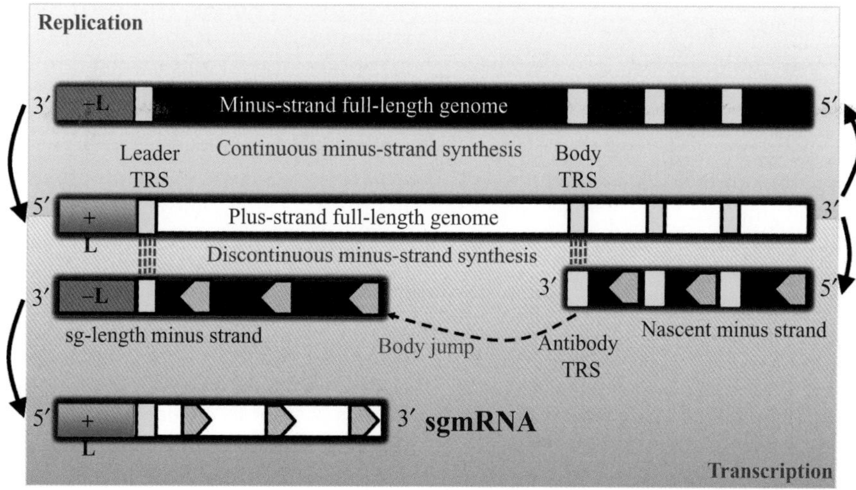

The nucleocapsid has helical symmetry and is comprised of coiled filament of 16–30 nm diameter. The nucleocapsid is surrounded by the envelope, which has diffuse projections (approximately 8 nm thick and 11 nm in length) extending from the surface. The most economically important and well-studied roniviruses include the YHV and GAV of black tiger shrimp. YHV virions have a buoyant density of 1.18–1.20 g/ml in sucrose. Like other nidoviruses, the ronivirus genome is a positive-sense, single-strand RNA molecule of 26.2–26.6 kb that contains a 5′-cap structure and a 3′-polyadenylated tail, and includes 5 open reading frames (5′-ORF1a–ORF1b–ORF2–ORF3–ORF4–polyA-3′; Figure 63.2B). YHV can remain infectious for at least 72 hr in seawater, and the virus can be effectively disinfected with 30 ppm calcium hypochlorite.

Like the other members of the order Nidovirales, these viruses encode two large replicase polyproteins (pp) from their genomic RNA: ORF1a (pp1a) and ORF1ab fusion product (pp1ab). The pp1a and pp1ab are processed into a number of nsps, which include viral proteases, RdRp, helicase, and other conserved enzymic domains. Full-length genomic RNA (RNA1) and two sgmRNAs (sgmRNA2 and sgmRNA3) are produced during replication. Similar to arteriviruses, viral structural protein genes are expressed from the two nested sets of 3′-coterminal sgmRNAs (sgmRNA2 and sgmRNA3). Unlike the other nidoviruses, the N protein of okaviruses is encoded by ORF2, which resides immediately downstream of the 5′-terminal ORF1a/ab replicase gene (Table 63.3). The ORF3 encodes a polyprotein that is cleaved to produce two envelope glycoproteins (gp116 and gp64) and an approximately 25 kDa N-terminal triple-membrane-spanning protein of unknown function. The ORF4-encoded polypeptide may be expressed in infected cells at extremely low level, but its function is unknown.

Arteriviruses

Equine Arteritis Virus

Disease. There is only one known serotype of EAV; however, field strains differ in their virulence and neutralization phenotype. Phylogenetic analysis based on ORF5 segregates EAV strains into North American and European lineages with the European lineage further subdivided into two subgroups. EAV is the causative agent of equine viral arteritis (EVA) in horses, a respiratory and reproductive disease that occurs throughout the world. The clinical signs displayed by EAV-infected horses depend on a variety of factors including the genetics, age and physical condition of the horse(s), challenge dose and route of infection, strain of virus, and environmental conditions. The vast majority of EAV infections are inapparent (or subclinical), but acutely infected animals may develop a wide range of clinical signs including pyrexia, depression, anorexia, dependent edema (scrotum, ventral trunk, and limbs), stiffness of gait, conjunctivitis, lacrimation and swelling around the eyes (periorbital and supraorbital edema), respiratory distress, urticaria, and leukopenia. The incubation period of 3–14 days (usually 6–8 days following venereal exposure) is followed by pyrexia of up to 41 °C that may persist for 2–9 days. The virus causes abortion in pregnant mares, and abortion rates during natural outbreaks of EVA can vary from 10 to 60% of infected mares. EAV-induced abortions can occur at any time between 3 and 10 months of gestation. EAV infection can cause a severe fulminating interstitial pneumonia in neonatal foals, and a progressive pneumoenteric syndrome in older foals. A high proportion of acutely infected stallions (10–70%) become persistently infected and shed the virus in semen; however, there is no evidence of any analogous persistent infection of mares, geldings, or foals. The virus persists in the ampulla of the male reproductive tract, and the establishment and maintenance of the carrier state in stallions is testosterone dependent.

Host–Virus Relationship

Distribution, Reservoir, and Transmission. EAV is distributed throughout the world, although the seroprevalence of EAV infection varies between countries and horses of different breeds and age in the same country. In the United States, about 70–90% of adult Standardbred horses are seropositive for EAV, as compared to only 1–3% of the Thoroughbred population. Similarly, a high percentage of European Warmblood horses are seropositive for EAV. Seroprevalence to EAV increases with age, indicating that horses may be repeatedly exposed to the virus as they age. Persistently infected carrier stallions function as the natural reservoir of EAV and disseminate the virus to susceptible mares at breeding (Figure 63.7). The two principal modes of EAV transmission are horizontal transmission by aerosolization of infectious respiratory tract secretions from acutely infected horses and venereal transmission during natural or artificial insemination with infective semen from persistently infected stallions. Recently, it has been demonstrated that the virus can also be transmitted during embryo transfer from mares inseminated with infective semen. EAV can also be transmitted through indirect contact with fomites or personnel. Congenital infection results from transplacental transmission (vertical transmission) of the virus when pregnant mares are infected late in gestation.

Pathogenesis and Pathology. Most information on the pathogenesis of EAV infection is derived from experimental studies in horses inoculated intranasally with various strains of EAV. It is to be stressed that with the notable exception of fetal and neonatal infections, EAV infection of horses is very seldom fatal. The numerous publications describing lesions caused by the highly virulent horse-adapted virulent Bucyrus strain of EAV reflect a severe fatal infection that is not representative of the disease caused by field strains of the virus. Most of the field strains of EAV cause only mild to moderate clinical disease in infected horses; however, some strains of EAV can cause severe disease. Initial multiplication of the virus takes place in the alveolar macrophages in the lung after respiratory infection, and the virus soon appears in the regional lymph nodes, especially the bronchial nodes. Within 3 days the virus is present in virtually all organs and tissues (viremia), where it replicates in macrophages and endothelial cells. The clinical manifestations of EVA reflect endothelial cell injury and increased vascular permeability. *In vitro* and *in vivo* studies have demonstrated increased transcription of genes encoding proinflammatory mediators—interleukin (IL)-1β, IL-6, IL-8, and tumor necrosis factor

FIGURE 63.7. *Transmission of EAV, depicting the central role of the carrier stallion in maintenance and spread of the virus.*

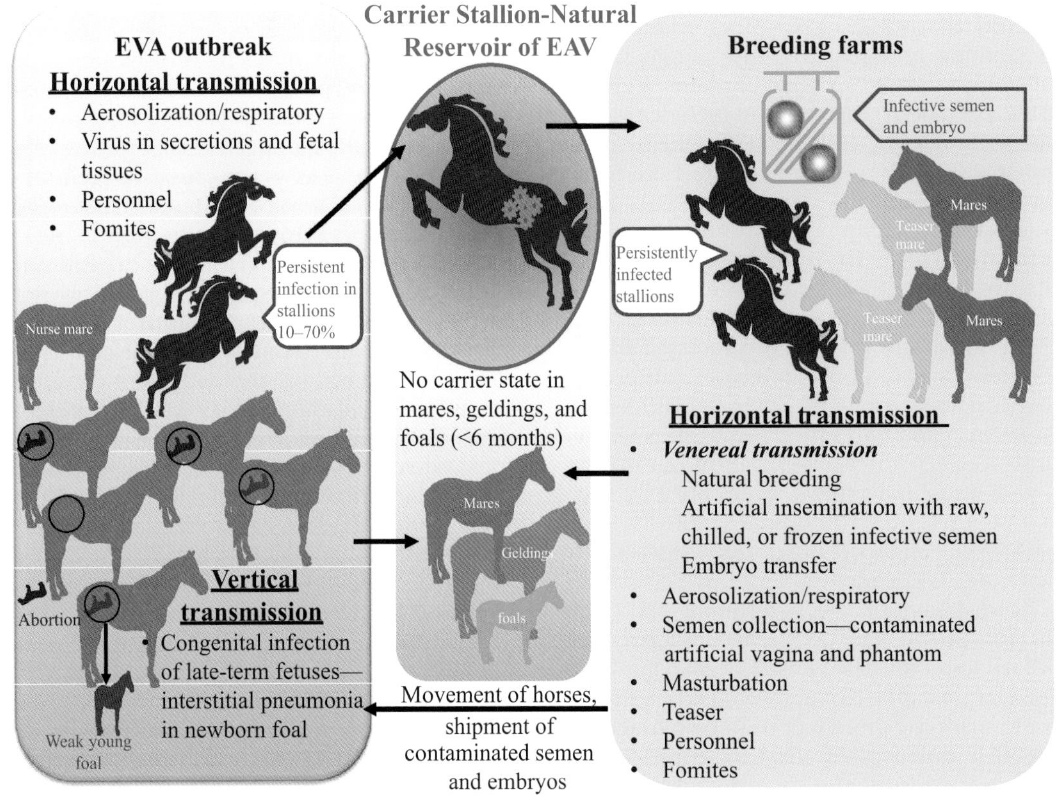

(TNF)-α—following EAV infection suggesting that these cytokine mediators are critical in determining the outcome of infection and severity of the disease. Furthermore, recent studies have demonstrated that clinical outcome of EAV infection is determined by host genetic factors. Specifically, based on the *in vitro* susceptibility of CD3+ T lymphocytes to EAV infection, horses were divided into susceptible and resistant groups. Subsequently, a genome-wide association study identified a common, genetically dominant haplotype, associated with the *in vitro* susceptible phenotype in the region of equine chromosome 11 (ECA11; 49572804-49643932). Experimental inoculation with EAV into horses with *in vitro* CD3+ susceptibility or resistance showed a significant difference between the two groups of horses in terms of proinflammatory and immunomodulatory cytokine mRNA expression and evidence of increased clinical signs in horses possessing the *in vitro* CD3+ T cell-resistant phenotype. These studies provided a direct evidence for a correlation between variation in host genotype and phenotypic differences in terms of the extent of viral replication, presence, and severity of clinical signs and cytokine gene expression caused by infection with EAV.

EAV infection of pregnant mares can result in the abortion of fetuses, which are usually partially autolyzed at the time of expulsion. Aborted fetuses may exhibit interlobular pulmonary edema, pleural and pericardial effusion, and petechial and ecchymotic hemorrhages on the serosal and mucosal surfaces of the small intestine. Neonatal foals occasionally develop a very severe, acute interstitial pneumonia. The characteristic histologic feature of EVA is a severe necrotizing panvasculitis of small vessels. Affected muscular arteries show foci of intimal, subintimal, and medial necrosis, with edema and infiltration of lymphocytes and neutrophils. Prominent vascular lesions are also seen in the placenta, brain, liver, and spleen of the aborted fetuses. Lungs of affected neonatal foals have severe interstitial pneumonia.

Host Response to Infection. Animals that recover from EAV infection or those that are vaccinated with either inactivated or attenuated strains of EAV develop neutralizing antibodies and are resistant to subsequent challenge with EAV. Neutralizing antibodies are detected within 1–2 weeks following exposure to the virus, reach maximum titers from 2 to 4 months, and persist for 3 years or more. With the exception of persistently infected stallions, EAV is eliminated from the tissues of infected horses by 28 days after the exposure. Foals born to immune mares are protected against clinical EVA by passive transfer of neutralizing antibodies in their colostrum. Neutralizing antibodies appear a few hours after colostrum feeding, peak at 1 week of age, and gradually decline to extinction from 2 to 7 months of age. The serologic response of horses to the individual structural and nonstructural proteins of EAV varies significantly. Immunoblotting studies have confirmed that infected horses respond to a number of viral structural proteins (GP5, M, and N) and that sera from horses other than carrier stallions most consistently recognized the conserved carboxy-terminal region of the M protein. Similarly, sera from horses experimentally or persistently infected with EAV strongly reacted with nsp2, nsp4, nsp5, and nsp12. However, horses vaccinated with the current modified live virus vaccine did not react with nsp5 and reacted weakly with nsp4. The innate immune response to EAV infection is not fully characterized, but studies have shown that the virus inhibits type I interferon (IFN) production in infected cells. Recent studies have demonstrated that nsp1, nsp2, and nsp11 are capable of inhibiting type I IFN activity. Of these three nsps, nsp1 has the strongest inhibitory effect by inhibiting IFN synthesis. The failure to induce type I IFN in EAV-infected cells may allow the virus to subvert the equine innate immune response. There is very little work done on the equine cellular immune response to EAV infection, and the specific viral protein that is targeted by the cytotoxic T lymphocyte response of EAV-infected horses remains to be thoroughly characterized.

Laboratory Diagnosis. It is to be stressed that EVA is subclinical or mild in horses, and that other, more important, viral respiratory infections clinically resemble EVA. Confirmation of a diagnosis of EVA is currently based on virus isolation (VI) and/or serological demonstration of rising neutralizing antibody titers (fourfold or greater) in paired serum samples taken at a 21- to 28-day interval using the virus neutralization test (VNT). The VNT is the principal serological assay used to detect evidence of EAV infection by most laboratories around the world, and it continues to be the current World Organization for Animal Health (OIE) prescribed standard test for EVA (gold standard). Several laboratories have developed and evaluated enzyme-linked immunosorbent assays (ELISAs) to detect antibodies to EAV using whole virus, synthetic peptides, or recombinant viral proteins (e.g., GP5, M, and N) as antigens. Various studies have shown that the source of antigen as well as the sera evaluated can markedly influence the results obtained with EAV protein-specific ELISAs and competitive ELISA. However, none of these ELISAs or recently described microsphere immunoassay (Luminex) has yet been shown to be of equivalent sensitivity and specificity to the VNT.

EAV can be isolated from nasal swabs or anticoagulated blood collected from adult horses with signs of EVA, or the tissues of aborted equine fetuses (lung, spleen, lymph nodes, and placenta). Carrier stallions are first identified by serological tests as they are always seropositive, and persistent infection is confirmed by VI from semen in cell culture, by test breeding using seronegative mares (and monitoring these for seroconversion to EAV after breeding), or by reverse transcription polymerase chain reaction (RT-PCR)—standard RT-PCR or real-time RT-PCR (rRT-PCR)—to identify viral nucleic acid in semen. Identification of the carrier stallion is of critical epidemiological importance in the prevention and control of EAV infection. VI is currently the OIE-approved gold standard for the detection of EAV in semen and is the prescribed test for international trade. However, it has been demonstrated that at least one of the rRT-PCR assays described in literature has equal to or higher sensitivity than VI for the detection of EAV nucleic acid in semen samples. Histopathologic examination coupled with immunohistochemical staining is also useful for diagnosis of abortion in particular, as are standard RT-PCR or rRT-PCR assays.

Treatment and Control. Currently there are no means available for eliminating the carrier state in stallions persistently infected with EAV other than surgical castration. There is no specific treatment for horses infected with EAV. However, there are preliminary data to support that GnRH (gonadotropin-releasing hormone) vaccines or antagonists can temporarily limit the shedding of the virus in the semen of carrier stallions. Furthermore, peptide-conjugated phosphorodiamidate morpholino oligomer (PPMO) targeting the genomic 5′-terminus of EAV has been capable of curing HeLa cells persistently infected with EAV under *in vitro* conditions. The PPMO-cured HeLa cells were free of infectious virus, viral antigens, and EAV nucleic acid as measured by plaque assay, indirect immunofluorescence assay, and rRT-PCR, respectively. While these findings demonstrate that PPMOs can be used to eliminate persistent EAV infection in cell culture, the efficacy of PPMO against EAV *in vivo* remains to be addressed.

There are currently two commercial vaccines that are widely used for protective immunization of horses against EAV infection: a live attenuated—modified live virus (MLV)—and an inactivated (killed). The MLV vaccine is administered intramuscularly to horses, but this vaccine is not recommended for use in pregnant mares, especially during the last 2 months of gestation, or in foals less than 6 weeks of age. It is recommended that foals be vaccinated at 6 months of age. Colts should be vaccinated prior to the onset of puberty as this prevents them from becoming persistently infected carriers. Thus, protective immunization of prepubertal colts is central to control of the spread of EAV infection. Experimental EAV vaccines have also been developed recently using recombinant DNA technology, but none of them have made to the market.

Outbreaks of EVA can be prevented by the identification of persistently infected stallions and the institution of management practices to prevent the introduction of EAV-infected horses. Carrier stallions should be kept physically isolated and bred only to mares that are seropositive from previous natural exposure or vaccination. Mares should be kept isolated from other seronegative horses after being bred by carrier stallions.

Porcine Reproductive and Respiratory Syndrome Virus

Disease. The European—type 1, prototype LV—and American—type 2, prototype VR-2332 virus—isolates of PRRSV represent genetically and antigenically distinct groups of the same virus. Both viruses are associated with outbreaks of similar reproductive and respiratory disease in pigs although there is only 55–70% nucleotide identity in the various genes of viruses of the two types. Recent phylogenetic analysis based on ORF5 sequences from GenBank has identified three subtypes of type 1 PRRSV circulating around the world. Subtype I includes PRRSV strains from Western European countries, Thailand, and the United States. Subtype II includes PRRSV strains form Eastern European countries (Lithuania, Russia, and some strains from Belarus), and subtype III includes strains only from Belarus. The subtype I is further subdivided into 12 clades (A–L). Clade A includes the LV that was first isolated in the Netherlands in 1990, as well as other PRRSV strains from many Western European countries, some strains from the United States and Thailand. Type 1 PRRSVs have been introduced into five non-European countries in North America (the United States and Canada) and Asia (Thailand, China, and South Korea). Similar phylogenetic analysis of type 2 PRRSV strains has identified nine lineages. Seven of the nine lineages have most of the PRRSV strains isolated in North America, whereas two lineages (3 and 4) contained strains only isolated from Asia. Numerous Asian isolates of PRRSV were found within the seven North American lineages (1, 2, and 5–9) indicating the introduction of North American strains to Asian countries.

Clinical signs of porcine reproductive and respiratory syndrome (PRRS) are extremely variable and influenced by strains of the virus, immune status of the herd, and management practices. Low-virulence strains of PRRSV may result in widespread infection of swine with minimal occurrence of disease, whereas highly virulent strains can cause severe clinical disease in susceptible herds. All ages of pigs are susceptible to infection with PRRSV in immunologically naive herds. Acute PRRSV infection of susceptible pigs is characterized by anorexia, fever (39–41 °C), dyspnea, and lethargy. Affected swine are lymphopenic, and exhibit transient cutaneous hyperemia or cyanosis of extremities that is most visible on the ears, snouts, mammary glands, and vulvas. Transplacental transmission of PRRSV occurs most efficiently in the third trimester of pregnancy (usually after 100 days of gestation), and the abortion rate in affected sows can range from 10 to 50%. Sow mortality is considerably lower. Affected litters contain a variable mixture of normal pigs, weak small pigs, stillborn pigs, and partially or completely mummified fetuses (so-called SMEDI; stillbirth, mummification, embryonic death, and infertility). Infected sows can also exhibit nervous signs such as ataxia and circling. PRRSV-infected boars may continue to shed viruses in their semen for prolonged periods of time.

In 2006, a highly virulent strain of PRRSV emerged in China (also designated as porcine high fever disease) and spread into other countries in Asia. The pigs infected with this highly virulent strain of PRRSV developed prolonged high fever (41–42 °C), severe respiratory signs, red discoloration of the body, blue ears associated with high mortality (20–100%), and morbidity (50–100%). The full-length genomic sequence analysis of the virus revealed two distinct deletions in the nonstructural protein 2 (nsp2) in comparison to all previously reported North American genotype PRRSVs. The whole-genome-based phylogenetic analysis of Chinese PRRSV strains and representative North American and European strains suggests that the newly emerged highly virulent virus has evolved from a Chinese strain that circulated in 1996 (PRRSV CH-1a).

Host–Virus Relationship

Distribution, Reservoir, and Transmission. PRRSV appears to be endemic in virtually all swine-producing countries of the world and PRRS has now emerged as the most prevalent swine disease in the world. The original source of the virus and the circumstances under which it was introduced into the domestic swine population are unknown. The PRRSV has been demonstrated in samples collected from wild boars in Europe and North America by RT-PCR. Transmission of PRRSV usually occurs by close contact between infected and uninfected animals. Swine are susceptible to PRRSV by a number of routes of exposure, including oral, intranasal, vaginal, intramuscular, and intraperitoneal. PRRSV is shed in respiratory tract secretions, saliva, semen, mammary secretions, urine, and feces of infected animals. Susceptible pigs are naturally infected by inhalation of infectious aerosols or ingestion of PRRSV-contaminated food (horizontal transmission). Congenital infection results from transplacental transmission (vertical transmission) of the virus. Transmission of PRRSV to females has been demonstrated during breeding with semen from persistently infected carrier boars. PRRSV can also be transmitted through indirect contact with fomites or personnel, and some pigs harbor the virus in their tonsils long after the virus is cleared from other tissues. There is evidence that flies and mosquitoes might serve as mechanical vectors of PRRSV. PRRSV could establish a chronic, persistent infection in lymph nodes (e.g., inguinal and sternal), tonsils, and the male reproductive tract. The virus has been isolated from tonsils and lymph nodes of pigs for up to 157 days postinfection (DPI). Low-level replication of the virus occurs in the lymphoid tissues, and thus, the shedding of PRRSV in oropharyngeal secretions is considered to be long lasting. PRRSV has been detected in semen samples of experimentally infected boars for variable periods from 4 to 92 DPI. The longest period of time where PRRSV nucleic acid in semen has been detected by RT-nested PCR is up to 92 DPI. However, by using VI and swine bioassay, it has been only possible to detect the virus in semen samples lasting from 4 to 42 DPI. The presence of PRRSV in semen of infected boars could be either due to virus replication and shedding from the reproductive tract (epididymis and bulbourethral glands) or direct dissemination (via monocytes and macrophages) from tissues other than those of the reproductive tract. Shedding of the virus in semen is of particularly concern because of the widespread use of artificial insemination in swine breeding.

Pathogenesis and Pathology. PRRSV replicates in macrophages and dendritic cells, especially those in the lungs and lymphoid tissues. Viremia occurs soon after infection, and can last for 1–2 weeks in mature animals and 8 weeks in young pigs. The duration of viremia is no longer than 28 DPI, but viral RNA has been detected in serum by RT-PCR up to 251 DPI. Gross lesions are usually observed in only a few organ systems (e.g., respiratory and lymphoid). Microscopic lesions of PRRS include diffuse interstitial pneumonia, myocarditis, vasculitis, and encephalitis. Lymphoid tissues exhibit lymphoid hyperplasia and follicular necrosis with mixed inflammatory cell infiltration. Clinical outbreaks of PRRSV can be complicated by bacterial pneumonia, septicemia, or enteritis.

The PRRSV primarily replicates in macrophages in lung and lymphoid tissues and to a lesser extent other tissues. The clinical outcome of PRRSV infection is highly variable, ranging from mild, subclinical infections to acute deaths of adult animals. The differences in clinical signs in infected pigs are attributed to numerous factors including host genetics, management practices, and virulence phenotype of the infecting PRRSV strain. The clinical signs and pathological lesions due to PRRSV are caused by a number of mechanisms. These include the apoptosis of PRRSV-infected macrophages and surrounding cells (indirect apoptosis), induction of proinflammatory and immunomodulatory cytokine production (IL-1, IL-6, IL-10, IL-12, TNF-α, and IFN-γ), polyclonal B cell activation and decrease in bacterial phagocytosis, and killing by macrophages leading to increase in bacterial respiratory disease and septicemia. Recently, it has been demonstrated that PRRSV infection modifies the porcine innate immune response and alters disease outcome in pigs coinfected with other respiratory viral pathogens such as porcine respiratory coronavirus. Variation in genetic resistance/susceptibility to PRRS has been reported among different breeds of pigs. The breeds that show more resistance to PRRS have increased cell-mediated immune response with the increased number of IFN-γ-secreting cells. Similarly, reduced or delayed PRRSV replication in some pig breeds was associated with high level of TNF-α and IL-8 mRNA expression. In addition, specific swine major histocompatibility complex—swine leukocyte antigen class I, II, and III (SLA I, II, and III)—alleles influence the susceptibility/resistance to PRRS, and studies have shown that SLA class I and II alleles regulate the level of circulating virus and antiviral immune responses in pigs.

Host Response to Infection. The humoral immune response to PRRSV varies significantly between pigs, and there are reports that suggest that protective immunity is strain specific with some degree of heterologous protection against other strains of PRRSV. It has been shown that passive transfer of PRRSV antibodies fully protected pregnant sows against challenge with virulent PRRSV. Piglets born to immune sows acquire anti-PRRSV antibodies by ingestion of colostrum, and these maternal antibodies persist in piglets up to 6–8 weeks of age. Pigs infected with PRRSV also develop antibodies to the GP3, GP4, and the M and N proteins, as well as nonstructural proteins (e.g., nsp1, nsp2, and nsp7), and multiple antigenic sites on these proteins have been described. Pigs infected with PRRSV produce a variety of virus-specific antibodies; virus-specific IgM appears by 5–7 days after infection and IgG by 7–14 days. ELISA antibody titers peak by 5–6 weeks after infection and persist thereafter. However, PRRSV-neutralizing antibodies appear slowly, usually between 4 and 5 weeks postinfection, and do not peak until approximately 10 weeks after infection. The appearance of neutralizing antibodies is associated with the clearance of PRRSV from the lungs of infected pigs. Despite the significant role that neutralizing antibodies seem to play in protection, their effectiveness might be limited against heterologous PRRSV strains. The neutralization determinants (epitopes) of PRRSV have not been fully characterized although different viral envelope proteins, including GP2, GP3, GP4, GP5, and M protein, have been identified as inducers of neutralizing antibodies using different techniques. However, specific neutralization epitopes have been identified only in GP3 and GP4 of European PRRSV strains and in GP5 of both North American and European PRRSV strains (Figure 63.3).

The T cell (CD4+ and CD8+)-mediated immune response is delayed in pigs infected with PRRSV, and IFN-γ-producing T cells appear between 4 and 12 weeks after infection. IL-12, one of the key modulators of T_{H1}-type cellular response, produced at a lower level following PRRSV infection and along with the increased levels of IL-10 may be capable of shifting the immune response toward a less effective T_{H2} response. The porcine T cell response appears to be directed against GP2, GP3, GP4, GP5, M, and N proteins of the virus, and the M protein may express some of the important T cell epitopes targeted by the cell-mediated immune response to PRRSV. Thus, the M protein is the most potent inducer of T cell proliferation. Two distinct regions on GP5 of the North American PRRSV appear to contain immunodominant T cell epitopes: amino acids 117–131 and 149–163. How conserved the T cell epitopes are or whether they could provide cross-protection against different PRRSV strains is yet to be determined.

In recent years, the innate immune response to PRRSV infection has been extensively studied, and these studies have shown that the virus attenuates the innate immune response by blocking the IFN-α production by the infected cells (e.g., macrophages) and evades the antiviral cytokine response. As a result of diminished innate immune response, adaptive immune responses are compromised, leading to weak cell-mediated responses, the delayed appearance of the neutralizing antibodies leading to prolonged viremia and persistent infection of the pigs. However, virus strain differences and cell-type differences in respect to response to PRRSV-mediated type I IFN-suppression have been reported. Recent studies have shown that four of the twelve nsps have strong to moderate inhibitory effects (nsp1 > nsp2 > nsp11 > nsp4) on type I IFN production in infected cells. These proteins inhibit both type I IFN induction and signaling pathways. Furthermore, a recent study has also shown that immunocompetent fetuses infected with PRRSV could initiate an antiviral response by increased expression of cytokines associated with inflammatory and immunomodulatory (T_{H1} and T_{H2}) cytokines. Interestingly, the PRRSV has developed strategies to subvert the innate, humoral, and cell-mediated immunity responses of pigs, which make the development of vaccine(s) against PRRS extremely difficult (Table 63.4).

Laboratory Diagnosis. Diagnosis of PRRSV may be complicated by the fact that many infections are inapparent, but PRRS should be considered when there are clinical signs of respiratory disease associated with reproductive failure in a herd. PRRSV antibodies are detected by using a variety of serological assays, including ELISA, microsphere immunoassay (Luminex), immunofluorescence assay, immunoperoxidase monolayer assay, and serum virus neutralization assay. Serological examination of acute and convalescent pig sera may provide evidence of seroconversion. VI from clinical specimens such as bronchioalveolar lavage fluid, lung, lymph node, buffy coat, and serum can be done in PAM, MA104, and its derivatives and CRL-11171 cell lines, although different strains or isolates of PRRSV vary in their ability to replicate in different cell types. Various PCR assays (e.g., standard RT-PCR, RT-nested PCR, and rRT-PCR) have been developed to detect viral nucleic acid in blood, semen, tissue homogenates, pulmonary lavage fluid, oropharyngeal scrapings, oral fluid, and other clinical specimens. These assays are highly specific and sensitive and give a rapid diagnostic turnaround time as compared to the VI in cell culture. While VI amplifies infectious virus, PCR detects viral RNA in clinical specimens. Currently, there are several rRT-PCR assays for the diagnosis of PRRSV and discriminating between European and North American PRRSV strains.

Treatment and Control. Both modified live attenuated (MLV) and killed vaccines are available for prevention of PRRSV infection in pigs. They can be used to immunize sows or weanling piglets; however, there is considerable variation in the relative safety and efficacy of MLV vaccines. MLV vaccines induce long-lasting protection as compared to killed vaccines, but do not completely prevent reinfection with wild-type virus and subsequent virus transmission. Furthermore, there have been reports of underattenuation and reversion of MLV vaccine strains to a more virulent types that can be spread from vaccinated to unvaccinated swine. The MLV vaccines are used to reduce disease occurrence and severity, as well as duration of viremia and virus shedding. The killed vaccines are used for vaccinating sows and gilts to reduce reproductive losses caused by PRRSV. There are no specific treatments for PRRS in pigs. Although a PPMO targeting a highly conserved sequence in the 5′-terminal region of the PRRSV genome that inhibits virus replication in culture has been used as a candidate for experimental treatment of young pigs. Prevention and control programs have been developed to eradicate the virus from infected herds. The objective of PRRSV prevention programs is to stop the introduction of either the virus into negative herds or new strains into PRRSV-infected herds. Implementation of strict biosecurity and herd closure measures whereby the herd is closed to new introductions for a period during which the resident virus dies out has been effective to control PRRSV infection from sow herds.

Lactate Dehydrogenase-Elevating Virus

The murine arterivirus LDV was first isolated from tumor-bearing laboratory mice with elevated levels of plasma lactate dehydrogenase (LDH) enzyme activity, but was later found to be endogenous in house mouse populations (*Mus musculus domesticus*) in several countries, although the worldwide incidence not known. LDV causes lifelong asymptomatic, persistent infections in mice that can only be recognized by elevated levels of plasma LDH. Attempts to infect *Peromyscus* mice, rats, guinea pigs, and rabbits with LDV have been unsuccessful. LDV replicates in permissive macrophages in the spleen, lymph nodes, thymus, and liver of infected mice. The subpopulation of macrophages that are permissive to LDV infection are also responsible for the normal clearance of the LDH enzyme from circulation. The continuous destruction of these macrophages by LDV leads to elevated levels of LDH in blood, thus the name of the virus. The persistent infection that characterizes LDV infection of mice is maintained by replication

Table 63.4. Immune Evasion Mechanisms of PRRSV

Viral Strategies	Mechanism of Immune Evasion	Viral Proteins Involved	Consequences
Evasion of Innate Immune Response			
Downregulation of IFN-α production pathway and interference with IFN-α-signaling pathway	Block dsRNA-induced IRF-3 and IFN promoter activation Inhibition of STAT1, STAT2, and ISG3 in IFN-signaling pathways Inhibition of ISG15-dependent RIG-I and JAK1 pathways Interfering with NF-κB-signaling pathway Inhibition of IRF3 phosphorylation and nuclear translocation	Nsp1 Nsp1 Nsp2 Nsp2 Nsp11	Decreased innate immune response Minimal IFN-α response in infected lung macrophages Delayed humoral and cell-mediated immune responses
Reduction in NK cell activity	Reduction in NK cell-mediated cytotoxic function	?	Failure to kill virus-infected cells and decreased IFN-γ production leading to decreased innate immune response
Interference with antigen presentation by dendritic cells and macrophages	Apoptosis of infected dendritic and macrophage cells, downregulation of CD11b/c, CD14, CD80/86, SLA class I, and SLA class II	?	Downregulation of antigen presentation and induction of IL-10 and downregulation of inflammatory cytokine production and T cells
Induction of IL-10 and suppression of IL-12	Direct targeting of IL-10 promoter by the N protein	N	Suppression of T cell responses leading to decreased IFN-γ production
Evasion of Adaptive Immune Response			
Genetic and antigenic variation	Viral quasispecies due to high error rate of viral RdRp and lack of proofreading capability Intragenic recombination Variation in other B cell epitopes Variation of T cell epitopes	GP3[a], GP4[a], and GP5[b] Nsp2, GP3, and GP5 Nsp2 Nsp2, GP2, GP3, and GP5	Lack of cross-protection due to variation in neutralization epitopes(NEs) Persistence of the virus Lack of conserved B cell epitopes Lack of conserved T cell epitopes
Glycan shielding of neutralizing epitopes	Masking of neutralizing epitopes	GP5	Delayed neutralizing antibody response, decreased sensitivity of the virus to neutralization, and persistence of the virus
"Decoy" epitope	Masking of neutralizing epitopes	GP5	Delayed neutralizing antibody response and persistence of the virus
Interference with T cell response	Induction of regulatory T cells (Treg; CD4+ CD25+ Foxp3+)	?	Delayed T cell response

[a]Variation in NEs of PRRSV-EU strains only.
[b]Variation in NEs of PRRSV-EU and PRRSV-NA strains.
?, not known.

of LDV in new permissive macrophages that are continuously regenerated from apparently nonpermissive precursor cells. Other than the elevated LDH level and subtle changes in host immunity, persistent LDV infection of mice is generally asymptomatic and infection of laboratory mice is now very uncommon.

Anti-LDV antibodies begin to appear 4–5 days postinfection and peak at 3–4 weeks. Antibodies that neutralize LDV appear in mice only after 4 weeks postinfection, and these antibodies are directed against the GP5 protein of the virus. The replication of LDV in macrophages allows it to avoid host defense mechanisms, although the precise mechanism of immune evasion and persistent infection is still unclear. It has been shown that most virus stocks contain both neuropathogenic (LDV-C and LDV-v) and nonneuropathogenic (LDV-P and LDV-vx) variants. LDV-P and LDV-vx variants establish persistent infection in mice by resisting neutralization due to the presence of large N-linked polygalactosaminoglycan chains on the short N-terminal ectodomain of the GP5 (VP-3P envelope glycoprotein according to old nomenclature; Figure 63.3). In addition to carrying the neutralization determinants, the N-terminal ectodomain of LDV, GP5 is also involved in host cell receptor binding. Neuropathogenic LDV-C and LDV-v variants lack two N-terminal N-glycosylation sites on their GP5 (Asn-36 and Asn-45), which permits them to interact with an alternative receptor on motor neurons and also enhances their immunogenicity and sensitivity to neutralization. Therefore, neuropathogenic variants are strongly suppressed in immunocompetent mice because of their sensitivity to neutralization, and at the same time, the non-neuropathogenic, neutralizing antibody-resistant variants predominate in persistently infected mice. The infection of mice of certain strains (C58, AKR, PL/J, and C3H/FgBoy) by neurovirulent strains of LDV can lead to fatal age-dependent poliomyelitis (ADPM). ADPM develops only in aged mice that become spontaneously immunosuppressed at 6–12 months of age or in younger mice that were experimentally immunosuppressed.

LDV successfully evades host immune response in a number of ways, thereby establishing lifelong persistent infection in mice. LDV infection modulates a variety of immune responses through a number of direct and indirect effects, including depression of cellular immunity, cytokine perturbations, and macrophage function. Thus, modulation of the immune response is the major concern for adventitious infection of laboratory mice with LDV. Natural killer (NK) cells mediate minimal control of the virus in infected mice. Infection elicits a strong and specific antiviral immune response, but serum antibody and T cell responses are not elicited in time to clear the high titers of replicating virus during the acute stage of infection, largely because the virus replicates so rapidly within the first few hours following infection. The major factor in reducing virus titers in plasma during the early phase of infection is exhaustion of the target cell population (macrophages), rather than any virus-specific immune response. Cytotoxic T cells disappear during persistent infection, apparently through clonal exhaustion. In addition, there is inhibition of IL-4 production with suppression of helper T cells. The virus isolated during early infection is efficiently neutralized, whereas the virus isolated from persistently infected mice is neutralization resistant, suggesting selection for neutralization-escape variants within the quasispecies population (see earlier). Infection of immunocompetent mice triggers polyclonal B cell activation, with enhanced specific and nonspecific IgG2a-restricted antibody responses. In infected mice, viremia occurs in the form of infectious virus–IgG complexes.

LDV transmission between mice is relatively inefficient, despite the lifelong viremia that occurs in infected mice and the secretion of the virus in urine, feces, and saliva. Feces contain high titers of the virus, and thus coprophagic behavior of mice probably plays an important role in transmission of the virus. LDV transmission from mother to offspring through the placenta or via breast milk is highly efficient if the mother is immunologically naïve. However, transmission via these routes from persistently infected mothers is rare because anti-LDV antibodies block transplacental transmission of the virus and its release into milk. Generally horizontal transmission of LDV between mice is restricted by mucosal barriers although horizontal transmission of LDV does occur among laboratory mice that fight and bite one another. The sexual transmission of LDV among mice has not been demonstrated.

LDV can only be quantitated by an end-point dilution assay in mice, which is based on the increase in plasma LDH activity that accompanies LDV infection in mice. The presence of LDV in mice or in other materials is readily detected by injecting plasma, tissue homogenates, or other materials (e.g., transplantable mouse tumors) into groups of two to three mice and assaying their plasma LDH activity 4–5 days later. Transplantable mouse tumors can be readily freed of LDV by a 3-week *in vitro* propagation or passage in a host animal other than mice.

Simian Hemorrhagic Fever Virus

Simian hemorrhagic fever virus (SHFV) was first isolated from rhesus macaques suffering from hemorrhagic fever, in primate research centers in both the Soviet Union and the United States. African monkeys of three genera—African green monkey (*Ceropithecus aethiops*), patas (*Erythrocebus patas*), and baboon (*Papio anuibus*)—are persistently infected in the wild population with the SHFV, and they do not exhibit any clinical signs of disease. Accidental transmission of SHFV from African monkeys to any of three species of Asian macaque monkeys (*Macaca mulatta*, *Macaca arctoides*, and *Macaca fascicularis*) results in a generally fatal hemorrhagic fever. Clinical signs of simian hemorrhagic fever (SHF) in macaques include anorexia, fever, cyanosis, skin petechia and hemorrhages, nosebleeds, facial edema, bloody diarrhea, dehydration, adipsia, and proteinuria. Death generally occurs 5–25 days after the onset of clinical signs, and mortality approaches 100% in macaques. The high lethality observed in macaque monkeys may be due to an extreme sensitivity of their macrophages to cytocidal infection by SHFV. Infection of captive patas monkeys with SHFV from persistently infected patas monkeys results in persistent infection without any clinical signs. However, infection of captive patas monkeys with SHFV from diseased macaque monkeys results in transient mild disease, indicating the selection of more virulent variants during epizootics in macaque monkeys. The humoral immune response against SHFV varies with the species of monkeys and the infecting virus strain. More virulent strains of SHFV induce neutralizing antibodies in patas monkeys 7 days after experimental infection. However, only low levels of anti-SHFV antibodies are found in many persistently infected patas monkeys. Neutralizing antibodies against one strain of SHFV do not completely neutralize other strains, indicating that there is variation in the neutralization determinants of individual strains of SHFV. Based on the hydrophobicity, membrane topology and putative N-linked glycosylation sites of GP7 encoded by ORF7 of SHFV (homologous to GP5 encoded by ORF5 of other arteriviruses), GP7 is predicted to contain the neutralization determinants of the virus (Figure 63.3).

The prevalence and incidence of SHFV infection among African monkeys in endemic areas of Africa is not known, but the incidence of persistent subclinical infections in wild patas monkeys appears to be high. The method of transmission of SHFV among African monkeys in the wild is unclear. Infection most likely occurs through wounds and biting, but sexual transmission has not been ruled out. SHFV is not transmitted transplacentally from persistently infected mothers to their offspring. Several epizootics of SHF in captive macaque colonies have originated from accidental mechanical transmission of SHFV from asymptomatic, persistently infected African monkeys. Once illness becomes apparent in the macaque colony, the SHFV spreads rapidly throughout the colony, most likely by direct contact and aerosols. There are no vaccines to prevent SHFV infection in monkeys.

Persistently infected monkeys can be identified by the presence of SHFV that replicates in primary cultures of peritoneal macrophages from rhesus and patas monkeys. The most sensitive method for detection of persistent infection in monkeys is experimental inoculation of macaque monkeys, and there are currently no molecular diagnostic assays for detection of SHFV. Indirect immunofluorescent assay, ELISA, and neutralization assays are available for serological diagnosis of SHFV infection. However, these assays are not reliable because of the low level of anti-SHFV antibodies found in many persistently infected monkeys. Accidental transmission of SHFV from persistently infected African monkeys to macaque monkeys in primate centers can be minimized by strict adherence to proper sanitary conditions and animal care practices.

Roniviruses

Yellow-Head Virus and Gill-Associated Virus. Yellow-head disease (YHD) virus was first detected in 1990 in black tiger shrimp (*P. monodon*) farmed in Central Thailand, and since then the YHV has spread into Southeast Asia and the Indo-Pacific region. In 1993, a virus morphologically identical to YHV was detected in wild and farmed *P. monodon* in Australia, and was given the name lymphoid organ virus (LOV) in relation to the lesions in the lymphoid organs. Subsequently, in 1995 and 1996, an apparent pathogenic form of this virus was detected in high levels in the gills of moribund, farmed *P. monodon* displaying YHD-like histopathological lesions and named as the gill-associated virus (GAV). It is now evident that LOV is same as GAV and causes the mild and/or chronic form of infection in *P. monodon*a, and the GAV has become the accepted name for both of these viruses. Furthermore, limited sequence comparisons have indicated that LOV and GAV are minor variants of the same virus, and YHV is a distinct but closely related variant (topotype). Recently, phylogenetic analysis based on ORF1b sequence of 57 viruses has identified existence of at least six genetic lineages (genotypes 1–6) of YHV. YHV and GAV belong to genotypes 1 and 2, respectively, and cause clinical disease in black tiger shrimp. In contrast, virus strains belonging to genotypes 3–6 have been detected exclusively as low-level infections in apparently healthy shrimp.

YHV is a major pathogen of farmed *P. monodon* shrimp and is listed by the OIE as causing a notifiable disease in shrimp. YHV and GAV are transmitted horizontally via several routes, including exposure to free water-borne virus during cohabitation and cannibalism of infected carcasses. There is no direct evidence of transmission of YHV vertically, but there is substantial evidence of vertical transmission of GAV in wild and farmed *P. monodon* in East Coast of Australia. Under experimental conditions, YHV appears to be more virulent than GAV and causes 100% mortality within 3–4 days of infection in *P. monodon*. In contrast, with GAV the mortality occurs 7–14 days postinfection, and similarly, farm outbreaks are presented as a chronic disease involving progressive appearance of relatively low numbers of moribund shrimp. Shrimp with YHD show pale or bleached appearance of the body with a yellowish discoloration of the cephalothorax due to yellowing of the hepatopancreas (HP). The HP of infected shrimp is swollen and soft compared to that of normal shrimp. The tissue distribution and histopathology seen in YHD infections are very similar and include necrosis of gill lamellae, HP, lymphoid organ, and heart. Histologically, GAV differs from YHV in that the lesions are limited to the gills and the lymphoid organ. Moreover, intensely basophilic inclusions found in the lymphoid organ of YHV-infected shrimp are not as evident in GAV-infected shrimps.

The diagnosis of GAV and YHV is achieved by routine hematoxylin and eosin histopathological examination and transmission electron microscopy (TEM). The diagnosis can be further confirmed by *in situ* hybridization with virus-specific probe and immunohistochemical staining with polyclonal rabbit antiserum or Mabs to either of these viruses. A nitrocellulose enzyme assay using rabbit polyclonal antibodies and a Western immunoblotting assay using Mabs have been described for the detection of YHV in gill tissues and hemolymph samples of *P. monodon*. Recently, several RT-PCR and rRT-PCR assays have been developed for the detection of GAV and YHV in samples. The Western immunoblotting assay is highly specific and is recommended by the OIE as a confirmatory diagnostic test for YHV infection in combination with *in situ* nucleic acid hybridization, TEM, and RT-PCR. The control of YHV and GAV in *P. monodon* is mainly achieved by adapting a variety of management strategies, including virus exclusion or prevention through the use of specific pathogen-free and/or specific pathogen-resistant shrimp breeding stocks.

References

Balasuriya UB and MacLachlan NJ (2004) The immune response to equine arteritis virus: potential lessons for other arteriviruses. *Vet Immunol Immunopathol*, **102**, 107–129.

Balasuriya UB and Snijder EJ (2008) Arterivirus, in *Animal Viruses: Molecular Biology* (eds TC Mettenleiter and F Sobrino), Caister Academic Press, Norwich, United Kingdom, pp. 97–148.

Brinton-Darnell M and Plagemann PG (1975) Structure and chemical-physical characteristics of lactate dehydrogenase-elevating virus and its RNA. *J Virol*, **16** (2), 420–433.

Gorbalenya AE, Enjuanes L, Ziebuhr J, and Snijder EJ (2006) Nidovirales: evolving the largest RNA virus genome. *Virus Res*, **117**, 17–37.

Gravell M, London WT, Rodriguez M *et al.* (1980) Simian haemorrhagic fever (SHF): new virus isolate from a chronically infected patas monkey. *J Gen Virol*, **51**, 99–106.

Pasternak AO, Spaan WJ, and Snijder EJ (2006) Nidovirus transcription: how to make sense... ? *J Gen Virol*, **87**, 1403–1421.

Snijder EJ, Siddell SG, and Gorbalenya AE (2005) The order Nidovirales, in *Topley and Wilson's Microbiology and Microbial Infections*, 10th edn (eds BWJ Mahy and V ter Meulen), Edward Arnold, London.

Spilman MS, Welbon C, Nelson E, and Dokland T (2009) Cryo-electron tomography of porcine reproductive and respiratory syndrome virus: organization of the nucleocapsid. *J Gen Virol*, **90**, 527–535.

Zhang S and Bonami JR (2007) A roni-like virus associated with mortalities of the freshwater crab, *Eriocheir sinensis* Milne Edwards, cultured in China, exhibiting "sighs disease" and black gill syndrome. *J Fish Dis*, **30** (3), 181–186.

Further Reading

Balasuriya UBR (2012) Equine viral arteritis, in *Infectious Diseases of the Horse*, 3rd edn (eds D Sellon and M Long), Saunders Elsevier.

Balasuriya UBR and Snijder EJ (2007) Arteriviruses, in *Animal Viruses: Molecular Biology* (eds TC Mettenleiter and FS Caister), Academic Press, Chapter 3, pp. 97–148.

de Groot RJ, Cowley JA, Enjuanes L *et al.* (2012) Order Nidovirales, in *Virus Taxonomy, Ninth Report of the International Committee on Taxonomy of Viruses* (eds AMQ King, MJ Adams, EB Carters, and EJ Lefkowitz), Elsevier Academic Press, London, pp. 785–795.

Enjuanes L, Gorbalenya AE, de Groot RJ *et al.* (2008) Nidovirales, in *Encyclopedia of Virology* (eds BWJ Mahy and MHV Regenmortel), Elsevier, Oxford, pp. 419–430.

Faaberg KS, Balasuriya, UBR, Brinton MA *et al.* (2012) Family Arteriviridae, in *Virus Taxonomy, Ninth Report of the International Committee on Taxonomy of Viruses* (eds AMQ King, MJ Adams, EB Carters, and EJ Lefkowitz), Elsevier Academic Press, London, pp. 796–805.

Gorbalenya AE, Enjuanes L, Ziebuhr J, and Snijder EJ (2006). Nidovirales: Evolving the largest RNA virus genome. *Virus Res*, **117**, 17–37.

Lunney JK and Rowland RRR (2010) Progress in porcine respiratory and reproductive syndrome virus biology and control. *Virus Res*, **154**, 1–224.

Perlman S, Gallagher T, and Snijder EJ (eds) (2008). *Nidoviruses*, ASM Press, Washington, DC.

Siddell SG, Ziebuhr J, and Snijder EJ (2005) Coronaviruses, toroviruses and arteriviruses, in *Topley and Wilson's Microbiology and Microbial Infections* (eds BWJ Mahy and V ter Meulen), Hodder Arnold, London, pp. 823–856.

Snijder EJ and Spann WJM (2007) Arteriviridae, in *Fields Virology*, 5th edn (eds DM Knipe and PM Howley), Lippincott Williams & Wilkins, Philadelphia, PA, pp. 1337–1355.

64 Reoviridae

D. Scott McVey, William Wilson, and Barbara Drolet

Viruses in the Reoviridae family infect a wide range of species, including mammals, fish and shellfish, insects, and plants. All of the viruses in this family have a segmented genome of double-stranded RNA (dsRNA), and the number of individual genome segments varies between genera. The family is grouped into nine genera: *Orthoreovirus, Orbivirus, Rotavirus, Aquareovirus, Coltivirus, Oryzavirus, Cypovirus, Phytoreovirus,* and *Fijivirus*. The latter four genera are confined to insects, plants, or both. The *Coltivirus* genus includes Colorado tick fever virus, which is a tick-transmitted human pathogen. Orthoreoviruses and rotaviruses (Figure 64.1— a rotavirus) infect a wide variety of vertebrate species. The host range of orbiviruses—includes both vertebrates and invertebrates, with bluetongue virus (BTV) serving as the prototype. The *Aquareovirus* host range includes fish and shellfish, with golden shiner virus serving as the prototype. Table 64.1 includes a list of genera and species that are important in veterinary medicine.

Orthoreoviruses

Mammalian Orthoreoviruses

Disease. Reoviruses (genus *Orthoreovirus*) have been isolated from the respiratory and/or gastrointestinal tract of many animal species, including nonhuman primates, rodents, horses, cattle, sheep, swine, cats, and dogs. Reoviruses are usually isolated from healthy animals, thus their designation as "respiratory enteric orphan" viruses because they typically are not associated with any disease. However, reoviruses are sometimes isolated from animals with mild respiratory and/or enteric disease, and reovirus infection of infant (neonatal) mice can cause severe systemic disease. Experimental infection of kittens with reovirus serotype 3 has caused conjunctivitis, photophobia, gingivitis, serous lacrimation, and nasal discharge. All three serotypes of reovirus have been isolated from sheep, and experimental infections with serotype 1 have been reported to cause enteritis and pneumonia.

Etiologic Agent

Physical, Chemical, and Antigenic Properties. There are three serotypes (1, 2, and 3) and many strains of mammalian reoviruses. Strains of reovirus that vary in virulence have been identified by sequence analysis of individual viral genes and proteins. Mammalian reoviruses all possess a genome of ten distinct segments of dsRNA. The genome segments are of different sizes (grouped as large, medium, and small). Each encodes a single protein except the S1 gene, which includes two distinct open reading frames. The complete reovirus particle has no envelope and exhibits icosahedral morphology with a diameter of approximately 85 nm. The reovirus particle consists of eight structural proteins arranged into inner and outer protein capsids (coats). The inner protein core contains the viral RNA-dependent RNA polymerase (transcriptase), as well as other enzymes that mediate mRNA synthesis and capping, helicase activity, and other functions that are necessary for virus replication. The predominant outer coat protein, sigma 1, is the primary determinant of virus serotype and hemagglutination and also is the cell attachment protein. Enzymatic digestion of the outer capsid protein sigma 3 from intact reovirus particles generates infectious subviral particles, and removal of the outer capsid proteins sigma 1, sigma 3, and mu 1 generates core particles. All three particles are important in the lifecycle of reovirus replication. Genetic diversity of strains of reovirus occurs through accumulation of mutations within individual viral genes (genetic drift) and by the exchange of entire genome segments (reassortment) between viruses during mixed infections with more than one reovirus strain or serotype.

Resistance to Physical and Chemical Agents. Reoviruses are stable at low temperatures (4 °C to room temperature) and are resistant to high temperature (55 °C) for short periods of time. Reoviruses are also resistant to detergents, many disinfectants, and stable over a wide pH range (pH 2–9). They are inactivated by exposure to 95% ethanol and sodium hypochlorite (bleach).

Veterinary Microbiology, Third Edition. Edited by D. Scott McVey, Melissa Kennedy and M.M. Chengappa.

FIGURE 64.1. *Negatively stained preparations of porcine rotavirus, with coronaviruses on the lower right side of the figure. (Courtesy of Dr Richard Hesse, Kansas State University.)*

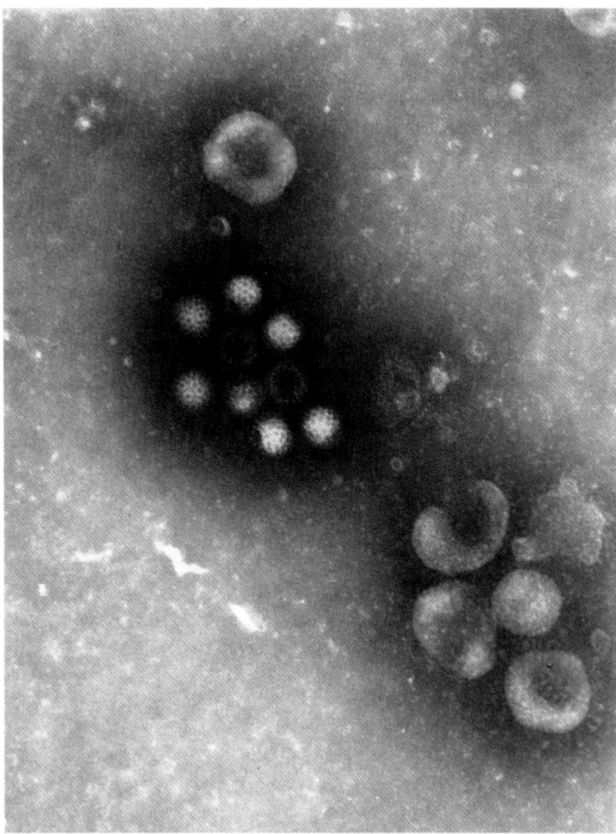

Distribution, Reservoir, and Transmission. Mammalian reoviruses have a wide geographic distribution and are commonly present in river water, untreated sewage, and stagnant water, likely reflecting fecal contamination by infected animals and/or humans. The mode of transmission is apparently by direct contact or exposure to materials contaminated by virus-infected feces (oro-fecal) and/or respiratory discharge. Reoviruses infect most mammals and they replicate in a variety of cell cultures.

Table 64.1. Genera Within the Reoviradae that Include Viruses Relevant to Veterinary Medicine

Genus	Serogroup	Minimum Number of Serotypes
Orthoreovirus	Mammalian	3
	Avian	11
Orbivirus	Bluetongue	26
	Epizootic hemorrhagic disease	8 (possibly 9)
	African horse sickness	9
	Equine encephalosis	7
	Palyam	11
Rotavirus	5 major groups	Uncertain
Aquareovirus	Not designated	Uncertain

Pathogenesis and Pathology. In murine studies, reoviruses have infected either intestinal or respiratory epithelial cells after oro-fecal enteric or aerosol respiratory infection, respectively. Initial virus replication occurs in regional lymphoid tissues after reovirus infection of either the gastrointestinal (Peyer's patches) or respiratory (bronchus-associated lymphoid tissues) tracts. The virus sometimes gains entry to the systemic circulation in infected neonatal mice, leading to pancreatitis, myocarditis, myositis, encephalomyletitis, or hepatitis, with the specific disease process and pathogenesis reflecting the properties of the individual infecting strain of reovirus as well as the age and resistance of the infected mouse. Reoviruses can cause encephalitis and hepatitis in primates.

Host Response to Infection. Both respiratory and enteric infection of mice with mammalian reoviruses results in induction of humoral and cellular immune responses, natural killer cells, as well as interferons and other cytokines, all of which are potentially important in terminating infection.

Laboratory Diagnosis. Reovirus infections can be diagnosed by virus isolation or detection, and by serology. Virus can be isolated from tissues and from rectal, nasal, and throat swabs by cell culture techniques, although blind passage may be required before cytopathic effect (CPE) becomes visible. Virus isolates can be serotyped by either hemagglutination inhibition (HI) or virus neutralization (VN) testing with serotype-specific antisera. Reoviruses can be identified in tissues or cell culture by immunofluorescent antibody staining (FA) or immunohistochemistry (IHC). Serologic testing is done using paired sera and VN or enzyme-linked immunosorbent assay (ELISA).

Treatment and Control. Since reovirus infection in mammals is usually mild, treatment is not required. No vaccines or control measures have been described and are unlikely to be developed in the future unless reoviruses are determined to be of greater importance as animal pathogens.

Avian Orthoreoviruses

Disease. Avian reoviruses (genus *Orthoreovirus*) are of economic significance to the poultry industry. Systemic reovirus infections of poultry can cause a variety of clinical syndromes, including gastroenteritis, hepatitis, myocarditis and pericarditis, pneumonia, and failure to thrive. Acute reovirus infections also lead to increased mortality and carcass condemnations in affected flocks, as well as poor growth and food conversion efficiency (stunting syndrome). Arthritis and tenosynovitis are common in birds that survive acute reovirus infection; reoviruses are a major cause of avian arthritis, and this disease occurs principally in broiler chickens and, less often, in layer birds and turkeys.

Etiologic Agent

Physical, Chemical, and Antigenic Properties. The avian reoviruses largely resemble their mammalian counterparts but differ in that they produce cell fusion in cell cultures (syncitia), lack hemagglutinating activity, and are typically unable to grow in mammalian cell lines. Avian and mammalian reoviruses exhibit varying degrees of antigenic relatedness. At least 11 serotypes of avian reovirus have been described, and strains of avian reoviruses vary significantly in their virulence. All share common antigens as determined by agar gel immunodiffusion (AGID) and complement fixation (CF).

Infectivity for Other Species and Culture Systems. Avian reoviruses replicate in embryonated chicken eggs, primary avian cell cultures, and, once adapted, certain established mammalian cell lines.

Distribution, Reservoir, and Transmission. Avian reoviruses are prevalent worldwide in chickens, turkeys, and other avian species. Avian reoviruses persist in nature through environmental contamination and by continued transmission of the virus from infected birds, including those persistently infected with the virus, to susceptible birds. Transmission occurs both horizontally and vertically. Horizontal transmission is predominantly by the oro-fecal route and occurs through both direct and indirect contact. Vertical transmission has been demonstrated following oral, tracheal, and nasal inoculation of breeder chickens.

Pathogenesis and Pathology. Infection with avian reoviruses is usually inapparent, and the occurrence of disease reflects the age of the bird at infection (young birds are predisposed), the virulence of the infecting virus strain, and the route of exposure. Reovirus-induced arthritis is initially characterized by acute inflammation within affected joints that progresses to pannus formation with erosion of articular cartilage; thus, reovirus-induced arthritis in chickens somewhat mimics human rheumatoid arthritis. Gross lesions in affected chickens often also include extensive swelling of the digital flexor and metatarsal extensor tendons that can lead to chronic hardening and fusion of the tendon sheaths.

Host Response to Infection. Antibody responses to avian reoviruses have been demonstrated by AGID, CF, and VN tests. The mechanism or mechanisms responsible for protective immunity are poorly defined, and variable degrees of cross-strain protection have been reported.

Laboratory Diagnosis. Reovirus-induced avian arthritis must be differentiated from arthritis and synovitis caused by other viruses and bacteria. A definitive diagnosis requires demonstration of reovirus infection by direct FA staining of tissues (tendon sheaths), virus isolation, or serology.

Treatment and Control. There is no treatment for avian viral arthritis, and the infection is best controlled by proper management procedures and vaccination with either attenuated or killed viruses.

Orbiviruses

Orbiviruses are important pathogens of livestock. Fourteen serogroups have been described and five are of real or potential veterinary significance: (1) BTV, (2) epizootic hemorrhagic disease virus (EHDV), (3) Palyam virus, (4) African horse sickness virus (AHSV), and (5) equine encephalosis virus (EEV). Like mammalian reoviruses (orthoreoviruses), orbiviruses have a double capsid structure, possess a segmented dsRNA genome (10 segments), and replicate in the cytoplasm of infected cells. Orbiviruses are distinguished from orthoreoviruses and rotaviruses because they replicate in both insects and mammals, and by the fact that they are not enteric pathogens of vertebrates. Orbiviruses replicate within the midgut epithelium of the hematophagous (blood sucking) insects that transmit these viruses. Progeny viruses are released and infect several secondary organs including salivary glands facilitating transmission to susceptible mammalian hosts.

Bluetongue Virus

Disease. Bluetongue (BT) is an arthropod-transmitted virus disease of domestic and wild ruminant species caused by BTV. BT occurs most commonly in sheep (sore-muzzle, catarrhal fever) and certain species of wildlife, particularly white-tailed deer. BT in sheep and deer is characterized by congestion, hemorrhage, and ulceration of the mucous membranes of the mouth, nose, and upper gastrointestinal tract. Other characteristic lesions include hyperemia of the coronary band and necrosis of both cardiac and skeletal muscles. BTV infection of sheep and deer is sometimes fatal, with terminal occurrence of disseminated intravascular coagulation. Sheep that survive severe bouts of BT are frequently emaciated, weak, and lame, and have a protracted convalescence during which they are susceptible to secondary infections. Breaks may occur in the wool fiber of convalescent sheep. Cattle are commonly infected with BTV in endemic areas, but clinical disease is extremely uncommon for most serotypes. Vaccine strains of BTV, and those propagated in cell culture, can cross the placenta of pregnant sheep and cattle to infect the developing fetus, leading to fetal death, abortion, stillbirths, or teratogenic defects in progeny.

The major economic impact of BT is that it is a reportable disease by almost all regulatory authorities, along with foot-and-mouth disease and at least fourteen other diseases that are considered to have major adverse economic and societal ramifications. As a consequence, the international movement of ruminants and their germplasm from BTV-endemic countries is regulated and controlled. BTV recently was recognized as a potential pathogen of carnivores. Inadvertent infection of pregnant dogs with a BTV-contaminated vaccine caused abortion and death. Serologic evidence of BTV infection has also been demonstrated in African carnivores.

Etiologic Agent

Physical, Chemical, and Antigenic Properties. The genome of BTV and other orbiviruses includes 10 segments of dsRNA, each of which encodes at least one protein (Table 64.2). The BTV particle is composed of seven structural proteins, two of which form the outer protein capsid, two form the outer layer of the inner core that surround the remaining three inner core proteins. The outer capsid protein, VP2, contains the serotype-specific epitopes recognized by neutralizing and hemagglutination-inhibiting antibodies (see Figure 64.5). The other outer capsid protein, VP5, contributes to the conformation of the neutralizing epitopes on VP2. Four nonstructural (NS) proteins also occur in BTV-infected cells, with NS-1 forming cytoplasmic macrotubular structures that are characteristic of orbivirus-infected cells. The inner core protein VP7 contains epitopes that are common to all serotypes and strains of BTV, which is the basis of group-specific serological assays such as AGID and competitive ELISA (cELISA).

There is considerable heterogeneity within the BTV serogroup, with 26 distinct virus serotypes, each with potentially distinct biological properties. This genetic diversity has arisen as a consequence of both genetic drift of individual gene segments, as well as the reassortment of gene segments during mixed infections of either insect or ruminant hosts with more than one BTV serotype or strain. Interestingly, recent sequence and phylogenetic analyses have shown that prolonged co-evolution of BTV with the different species of vector insects that occur in various regions of the world has resulted in strains of BTV that are unique to each region, so-called virus topotypes.

Infectivity for Other Species and Culture Systems. BTV commonly infects domestic (sheep, cattle, and goats) and wild (deer, antelope, wild sheep species, etc.) ruminants. The viruses can be adapted to grow in suckling mice, embryonated chick eggs (ECEs), and a variety of mammalian and insect cell cultures. Replication of BTV is facilitated by incubation temperatures of 37 °C in mammalian cultures, 33.5 °C in ECEs, and 27–30 °C in insect cultures.

Table 64.2. Molecular Constituents of Orbiviruses

Gene	Encoded Protein	Role
1	VP1	RNA polymerase; minor component of viral core particle
2	VP2	Receptor binding; serotype determination; component of outer capsid
3	VP3	Interacts with genomic RNA; structural component of viral core particle
4	VP4	RNA capping enzymes; minor component viral core particle
5	VP5	Structural interactions with VP2; component of outer capsid
6	NS1	Virus tubules; not a virion component
7	VP7	Group antigen; structural component of viral core particle
8	NS2	Binds RNA; virus inclusion bodies; nonstructural
9	VP6	Helicase; binds RNA; minor component of viral core particle
10	NS3/3A	Virus egress from infected cells; nonstructural
	NS4	Virus egress from infected cells; nonstructural

Resistance to Physical and Chemical Agents. Similar to Reoviruses, orbiviruses are stable at low temperatures (4 °C to room temperature) and are resistant to high temperature (55 °C) for short periods of time. They are inactivated by exposure to 95% ethanol, sodium hypochlorite (bleach), and some quaternary ammonium disinfectants (such as Roccal ROCCAL®-D Plus).

Distribution, Reservoir, and Transmission. BTV has been isolated from ruminants in all continents except Antarctica. Infection occurs throughout tropical, subtropical, and temperate regions of the world, coincident with the distribution of susceptible ruminants and competent vector insects (*Culicoides* spp.). The virus is not contagious between ruminants; rather, infection occurs only following the bites of BTV-infected *Culicoides* insects. Subclinical and/or asymptomatic BTV infection of ruminants occurs throughout endemic regions of the world. Outbreaks of BT occur only sporadically, within the vectors' ranges allowing incursions of BTV into immunologically naive populations of ruminants.

Vector *Culicoides* insects become persistently infected with BTV after feeding on a viremic ruminant (Figure 64.2). These hematophagous insects are true biologic vectors of BTV. They obtain the virus from blood feeding on an infected animal and then transmit virus to other ruminants after an extrinsic incubation period of 4–20 days. During this period, the virus infects and disseminates from the midgut of the insect to its salivary glands. Replication of BTV within the insect vector is dependent on ambient temperature; thus, increased replication of BTV in vector insects occurs at higher temperatures, but the increased temperature can shorten the lifespan of these insects. Transmission of BTV can occur year-round in climates that permit insect (*Culicoides*) activity in all seasons,

FIGURE 64.2. *Midges acquiring a blood meal. (Photograph courtesy of the USDA ARS Arthropod-Borne Animal Diseases Research Unit, Manhattan, KS.)*

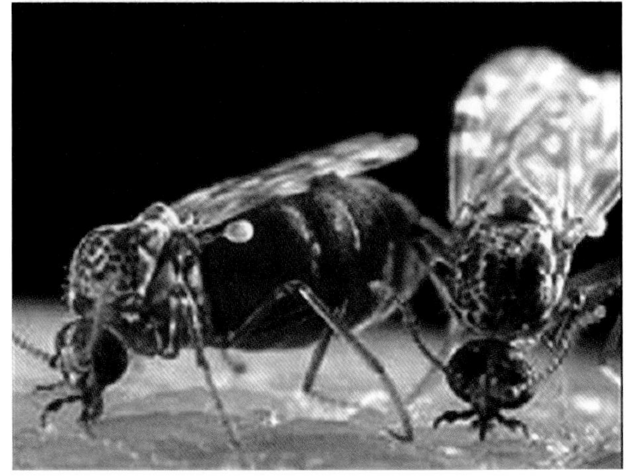

with the virus persisting in a perpetual vector-ruminant cycle of infection. In contrast, transmission of BTV is highly seasonal in regions of the world at the northern and southern extremities of the vectors' range (approximately latitudes of 35°S and 45°N). In these areas, BTV transmission typically occurs only in the late summer and fall when vector populations peak and when ambient temperatures are highest (likely reflecting the influence of temperature-dependent virogenesis). The traditional global range of BTV has recently expanded into Mediterranean Europe after the northern spread of competent vectors, perhaps as a consequence of global warming.

Pathogenesis and Pathology. For most BTV serotypes, sheep and some species of deer are very susceptible, whereas cattle infections are typically subclinical. The pathogenesis of BTV infection appears to be similar in all ruminant species. The virus multiplies initially in the lymph node(s) draining the site of infection, and viremia occurs as early as 3 days later with a subsequent febrile response. Upon systemic distribution, virus replicates in mononuclear phagocytic cells and the endothelium of small blood vessels resulting in vascular injury, thrombosis, and infarction of the affected tissues including the upper gastrointestinal and respiratory tracts, coronary bands, heart, and skeletal muscle. Disseminated intravascular coagulation likely contributes to the vascular injury, hemorrhage, and tissue infarction that are characteristic of severe cases of BT in sheep and deer.

Viremia in BTV-infected ruminants is highly cell associated. Virus initially is associated with all blood cell types, and titers of virus in each cell fraction reflect the proportion of each cell type in blood; thus, BTV initially is most associated with platelets and erythrocytes, and less so leukocytes. Late in the course of infection, however, virus appears to be exclusively associated with erythrocytes. It is this association that facilitates both prolonged infection of ruminants as well as infection of the hematophagous *Culicoides* insect vectors that feed upon them. BTV infection of ruminants can be prolonged (up to approximately 60 days); however, with the exception of one unconfirmed report, persistent BTV infection of ruminants does not occur.

The gross lesions of BT include facial edema and hyperemia, with or without hemorrhage (petechial and ecchymotic) of the oral and nasal mucosa, skin, and coronary band. Ulcerations and erosions also may occur in and around the mouth, especially on the hard palate. Hemorrhages at the base of the pulmonary artery are very characteristic of severe cases of BT. Petechial hemorrhages may also occur in the myocardium, pericardium, skeletal musculature, and the tissues of the upper gastrointestinal tract (Figure 64.3 A, B, C, and D).

FIGURE 64.3. *Sheep with bluetongue disease demonstrating depression (A), dyspnea (B), and typical cyanosis of the tongue (B) and coronary band (C), and ulceration and hemorrhage from the nasal cavity mucosa (D). (Photographs courtesy of the USDA ARS and Timothy J. Graham DVM Arthropod-Borne Animal Diseases Research Umnit Unit, Manhattan, KS.)*

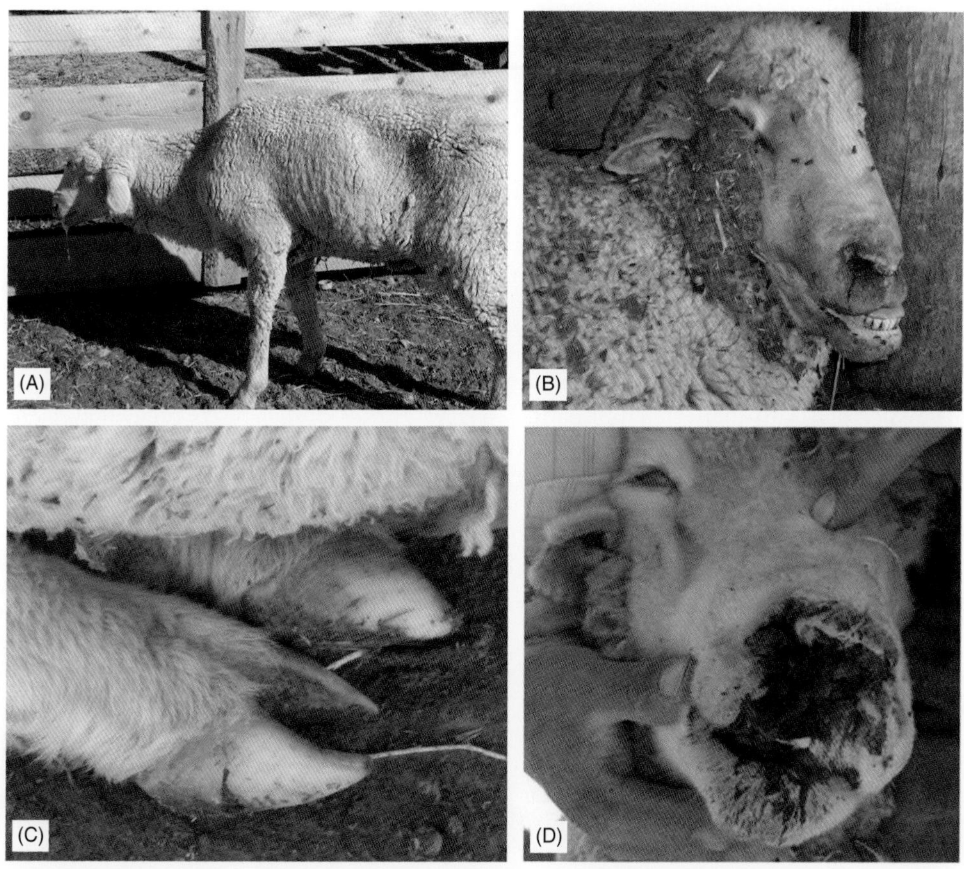

Host Response to Infection. BTV-infected ruminants develop both humoral and cellular immune responses. Virus-neutralizing (serotype-specific) and nonneutralizing (group-specific) antibodies develop 7–14 days after infection. However, virus can coexist in blood with high titers of neutralizing antibody for several weeks because of the intimate association of BTV with the cell membrane of infected erythrocytes. Limited degrees of cross-serotype viral neutralization may occur following infection of an animal with a single BTV serotype and subsequent exposures to additional serotypes can generate production of a set of broadly cross-reactive neutralizing antibodies. However, immunization of sheep and cattle primarily provides homologous, serotype-specific protection.

Laboratory Diagnosis. Initial diagnosis of BT in sheep and deer is based on the characteristic clinical signs of affected animals in known BTV-endemic areas. BT typically occurs in the late summer and fall. Confirmation of the diagnosis requires virologic testing, usually by either polymerase chain reaction (PCR) assay or by virus isolation using inoculation of susceptible sheep, ECEs, suckling mice, or cell cultures. The cell cultures most often used include Vero and BHK; multiple blind passages are often required before CPE is observed. Upon adaptation to cell culture, virus can be identified by fluorescent antibody staining or VN assay. BTV is very commonly detected in the blood of healthy ruminants in endemic areas, especially if sensitive nested PCR assays are used because these can detect BTV nucleic acid for up to 200 or more days after infection. Thus, the mere demonstration of virus or nucleic acid in the blood of ruminants certainly is not proof of disease causality.

Serologic diagnosis can be performed using tests for group-specific (AGID, CF, ELISA, IFA) or type-specific (viral neutralization, HI) antibodies. Paired serum samples are required to demonstrate seroconversion or an increase in titer. A single serological test is often meaningless because a high proportion of ruminants are seropositive in BTV-endemic areas, and the vast majority of these animals never experience obvious clinical disease following BTV infection.

Treatment and Control. There is no specific treatment for BT, although stress appears to exacerbate clinical disease. Furthermore, transmission of BTV to unaffected ruminants can be prevented by moving animals indoors (if feasible) where insect vectors are not present. Vaccination of sheep with attenuated strains of BTV has been practiced for many years in South Africa and North America; the South African vaccine incorporates fifteen different BTV serotypes, and requires vaccination on three different occasions. Potential disadvantages of live attenuated virus vaccines include reversion to virulence and their ability to be transmitted in nature. Furthermore, live attenuated virus vaccines potentially can reassort their genome segments with field strains of BTV to create novel variant viruses. Finally, live attenuated vaccine strains of BTV have been repeatedly shown to be able to cross the placenta to cause fetal death or injury, whereas field strains of the virus typically cannot. The exception to this was the recent BTV serotype 8 outbreak in Europe. Recombinant baculovirus-expressed virus-like particles and canary pox expressing VP2 antigens have recently been developed as experimental BTV vaccine candidates, avoiding some of the retained virulence problems inherent to live attenuated virus vaccines.

Epizootic Hemorrhagic Disease and Ibaraki Viruses

Epizootic hemorrhagic disease (EHD) is an arthropod-transmitted virus disease of wild ruminants caused by EHDV. EHDV is an important cause of disease and mortality in white-tailed deer in North America and, to a lesser extent, pronghorn antelope and bighorn sheep. EHDV infection of domestic ruminants is common in endemic areas, and EHDV may be an important pathogen of domestic livestock, especially associated with severe outbreaks in deer. A notable exception is Ibaraki disease of cattle in Japan and Korea; the causative agent, Ibaraki virus, is closely related to EHDV serotype 2. EHDV shares many features with BTV, and EHD of white-tailed deer closely resembles fulminant BT with hyperemia, hemorrhage and ulceration of the upper gastrointestinal tract, necrosis of cardiac and skeletal muscle, and terminal disseminated intravascular coagulation with widespread bleeding (Figure 64.4 A and B). Additional features of Ibaraki disease in cattle include marked dysphagia as a consequence of necrosis of muscles of the larynx, pharynx, esophagus, and tongue.

Like BTV, EHDV infection occurs throughout tropical and temperate regions of the world, and EHDV infection of ruminants has been described in Africa, Asia, and the Americas. EHDV closely resembles BTV in terms of its epidemiology, including dissemination by *Culicoides* insect vectors, pathogenesis of infection in ruminants, replication strategy, molecular structure, and methods of diagnosis. There is some discrepancy over the currently recognized eight serotypes of EHDV. It has been proposed that Ibaraki virus be classified as EHDV serotype 2 resulting in nine serotypes.

FIGURE 64.4. *Enzootic hemorrhagic disease. (A) Photograph taken of a white-tailed deer that died 9 days after experimental infection with EHDV showing edema and congestion of the conjunctiva. (B) Photograph taken of a white-tailed deer that died 7 days after experimental infection with EHDV showing severe congestion and hemorrhage of the tracheal mucosa. (Photographs courtesy of Dr Mark Ruder of the USDA ARS Arthropod-Borne Animal Diseases Research Unit, Manhattan, KS.) (A reprinted with permission, Ruder (2012).*

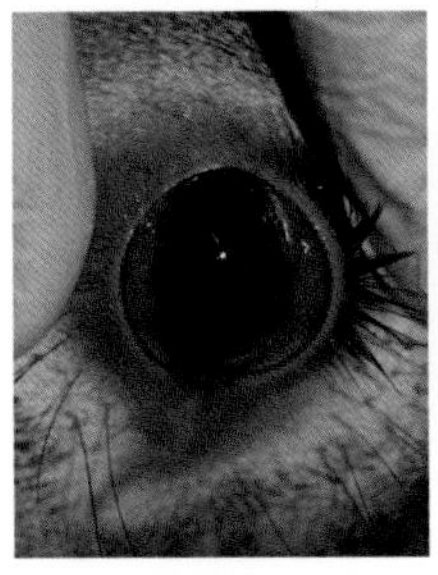

(A)

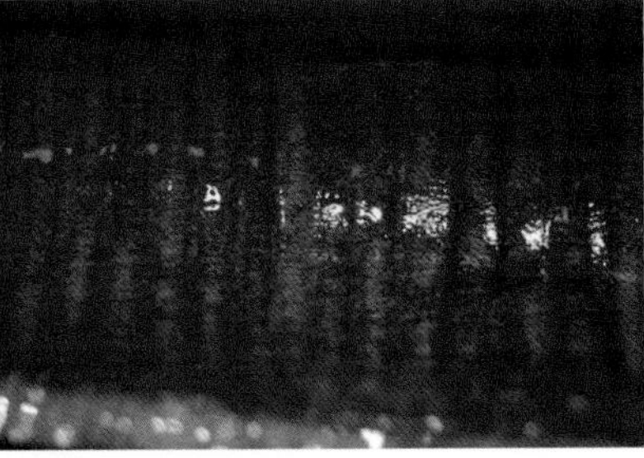

(B)

Others have proposed (based on genetic sequences and serology data) that there are only seven serotypes with type 3 proposed to be a type 1. With the exception of Ibaraki virus vaccines and autogenous vaccines, vaccines are not widely available for EHDV.

Palyam Virus

Palyam viruses are insect-transmitted orbiviruses that cause abortion and teratogenesis among cattle in Africa, Asia, and Australia. Fetuses that survive infection with Palyam viruses prior to mid-gestation may develop brain malformations, including hydranencephaly and/or false porencephaly. Like the other orbiviruses of veterinary importance, Palyam viruses are disseminated by *Culicoides*-insect vectors. There are 11 serotypes of Palyam viruses. The pathogenesis and teratogenic effects of Chuzan (Kasaba) virus infection of fetal cattle have been especially well described.

African Horse Sickness Virus

Disease. African horse sickness (AHS) is an arthropod-transmitted Orbivirus disease of equids, including horses, mules, and donkeys. The causative agent, AHSV, is zoonotic, although fatal infection of humans is rare. Fatal AHSV infection of dogs also has been described. AHS of horses varies greatly in severity, depending on the infecting strain of virus and the susceptibility of the infected horse. There are several distinct forms of AHS, including (1) a peripheral form characterized by edema of the head; (2) a central form characterized by pulmonary edema, high fever, severe depression, coughing, discharge of fluid from the nostrils, and rapid death of many affected horses; (3) an intermediate form that is characterized by fever, edema of the head and subcutis (supraorbital edema is highly characteristic), and significant mortality of affected horses; and (4) horse sickness fever, which is a febrile disease with a more benign course.

Etiologic Agent

Physical, Chemical, and Antigenic Properties. The causative agent of AHS belongs to a distinct serogroup within the genus *Orbivirus*. Nine serotypes of AHSV have been identified by cross-neutralization studies in mice. All types share common group-specific antigens.

Infectivity for Other Species and Culture Systems. AHSV infections have been documented in horses, donkeys, mules, zebras, goats, dogs, and large African carnivores such as lions. Disease has been described in horses and dogs. The virus can be propagated in suckling mice and adapted to grow in ECEs and cell cultures (Vero and BHK).

Distribution, Reservoir, and Transmission. AHS occurs throughout southern Africa, with periodic epizootics in northern Africa, the Middle East, Asia (the Indian subcontinent), and, on occasion in the past, Mediterranean Europe (the Iberian Peninsula). AHS is not contagious; rather, the virus is transmitted only by *Culicoides* insects that serve as true biologic vectors. Like BT, AHS occurs most commonly in the late summer and fall in endemic areas, and the distribution of AHSV is dependent on the presence of competent insect vectors and ambient temperatures that facilitate temperature-dependent virogenesis within these vectors. Zebras have been implicated as potential mammalian reservoirs of AHSV in southern Africa, because AHSV infection is asymptomatic in zebras and AHSV viremia is more prolonged in zebras than in horses. Dogs may become infected with AHSV by eating infected horse meat, and serological surveys have shown that antibodies to AHSV are common among large wild carnivores in southern Africa.

Pathogenesis and Pathology. The incubation period of AHS is generally less than 7 days following the bite of an AHSV-infected *Culicoides* insect. The incubation period is shortest in horses infected with virulent strains of AHSV, and mortality in susceptible horses infected with highly virulent AHSV can reach 95%. AHSV replicates in mononuclear cells of the lymph nodes, spleen, thymus, and pharyngeal mucosa, and in vascular endothelium. The lesions of AHS result from vascular injury to small blood vessels, although it is uncertain whether the vascular injury that characterizes AHS is a result only of direct virus-mediated endothelial injury or if vasoactive mediators released from AHSV-infected mononuclear phagocytic cells also contribute. The severe central form of AHS is characterized by pulmonary edema, hydrothorax, and hydropericardium, with epicardial and endocardial hemorrhages. Subcutaneous edema can be extensive in horses that suffer a more protracted form of the disease.

Host Response to Infection. All serotypes of AHSV share common group antigens and induce development of antibodies that may be recognized by CF, AGID, and indirect FA. Viral neutralizing antibodies also develop following infection; these are predominantly serotype-specific, but some cross-neutralization activity has been observed.

Laboratory Diagnosis. Field diagnosis of AHS, especially in nonendemic areas, should be supported by viral isolation or serology to distinguish other infections that can produce similar clinical signs. PCR tests are available. The presence of virus also can be rapidly identified in tissue specimens using an AHSV-specific capture ELISA. Virus isolation is a slower but accurate method of virus detection. Intracerebral inoculation of suckling mice with blood or tissue suspension is a very sensitive method of isolating AHSV, although time-consuming serial passage may be required for viral adaptation. Cell cultures are not as efficient in isolating virus as mouse or horse inoculation. Virus can be identified by VN, HI, or FA.

Serologic diagnosis requires paired serum samples for demonstrating seroconversion or an increase in antibody titer. Assays routinely used for such purposes include competitive ELISA and CF, which are group-specific tests and detect antibodies to AHSV regardless of the infecting virus serotype, and VN assay, which is very sensitive but serotype specific.

Treatment and Control. No specific treatment of AHS is available. Hyperimmune horse serum confers transient protection. Stabling of horses in insect-secure facilities is assumed to reduce exposure of animals to the *Culicoides* vector. Annual vaccination of horses with attenuated virus vaccines that include the nine recognized serotypes of AHSV is widely practiced in southern Africa, and to control incursions of AHSV into Europe. There are several potential problems inherent in the use of multivalent modified live AHSV vaccines, including lack of protection against all serotypes of the virus, reversion to virulence of vaccine strains of virus, acquisition and dissemination of vaccine viruses by vector insects, and reassortment of gene segments between different virus strains/serotypes during mixed infections.

Equine Encephalosis Virus

EEV has been isolated from horses with hepatic lipidosis and vague neurologic signs, but its importance as a primary pathogen is uncertain. The virus has also been isolated from aborted fetuses. Serologic studies have shown that EEV infection is very widespread and common among horses in southern Africa. The seven recognized serotypes of EEV share common group antigens and closely resemble AHS viruses. The epidemiology of EEV infection is also like that of AHSV, with transmission by *Culicoides* insects.

Rotaviruses

Disease

Rotaviruses cause enteritis and diarrhea in many mammalian species (including humans) and birds. *Rotavirus* infections are an important cause of diarrhea in young farm animals, including calves, lambs, foals, and piglets. The virus infects mature absorptive cells at the tips of the intestinal villi with resulting malabsorption, maldigestion, and diarrhea. The clinical severity of the infection depends on factors such as the age and susceptibility of the affected animal, the virulence of the infecting strain of *Rotavirus,* and the presence of other enteropathogenic organisms.

Table 64.3. Serotype and Genotype Determinants among Rotaviruses

A–E (possible F and G) Group Typing	PCR or RNA Fingerprinting – VP6
G genotypes P genotypes	PCR – VP7 PCR – VP4

Etiologic Agent

Physical, Chemical, and Antigenic Properties. Rotaviruses represent a distinct genus within the family Reoviridae. The viruses are nonenveloped, contain a segmented (11 segments) dsRNA genome, and exhibit a double-shelled capsid morphology with an overall diameter of the mature virion of approximately 100 nm (see Fig 64.2). At least 13 different rotavirus proteins have been identified, with 2 of the 11 gene segments encoding two distinct proteins. Of these 13 proteins, 7 are structural virion components (including enzymes) and 6 are NS proteins that are produced in *Rotavirus*-infected cells but that are not incorporated into virions.

The rotaviruses currently are organized into five major groups (A–E), with two possible additional species (F, G). Many distinct strains and/or serotypes of *Rotavirus* occur within each group (Table 64.3). Rotaviruses within each group share common antigens, can reassort their genome segments during mixed infections, have considerable sequence homology of conserved viral genes, and tend to infect the same species of animals. Neutralizing antibodies are induced by the outer capsid proteins VP7 and VP4 (Figure 64.5), whereas VP6 expresses determinants common to each rotavirus group and subgroup.

FIGURE 64.5. *Diagram demonstrating the structure of a rotavirus, demonstrating outer capsid and the inner core particle. (From Fayquet (2005). Copyright @ Elsevier (2005), with permission.)*

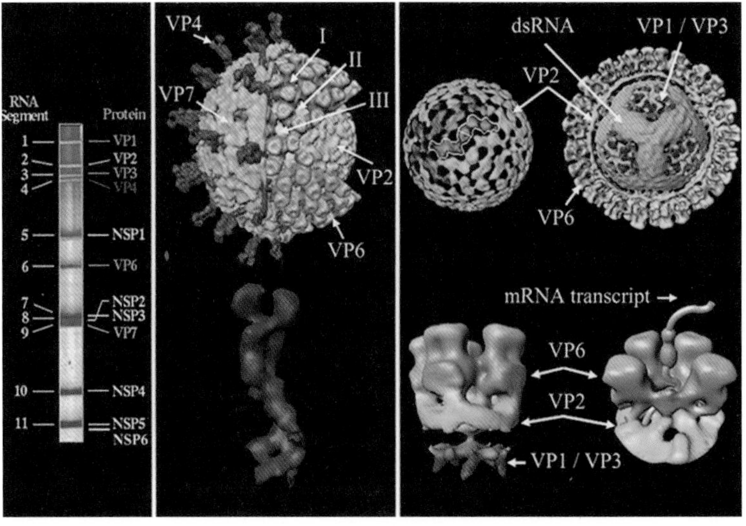

Infectivity for Other Species and Culture Systems. Although rotaviruses obtained from one species can sometimes infect other species, strains of *Rotavirus* are largely species specific in their tropism. Rotaviruses are difficult to propagate in cell culture. A major advance in the propagation of rotaviruses was the discovery that low concentrations of trypsin are required to initiate virus infection and replication in cell culture. Trypsin cleaves the viral outer coat protein, VP3, to facilitate infection of cell cultures, and once adapted rotaviruses grow well in cell culture. The most common cell lines used are kidney epithelial cells, especially the rhesus monkey kidney cell line, MA104.

Distribution, Reservoir, and Transmission. Rotaviruses are distributed worldwide and occur in many different animal species. High titers of virus are excreted in the feces of infected animals, and the virus is very stable in the environment if associated with feces. Transmission to other animals occurs by ingestion of virus, following either direct or indirect oro-fecal transmission.

Pathogenesis and Pathology. The pathogenesis of *Rotavirus* infection is similar regardless of the animal species affected. After oral infection, the virus infects the mature adsorptive epithelial cells that line the apical (lumenal) aspects of the intestinal villi. The infection progresses from the upper to the lower portions of the small intestine, and in some species, to the colon. Destruction of these mature villus enterocytes leads to villus atrophy, and the mature absorptive cells that line the villi are replaced by more immature cells from the intestinal crypts, leading to maldigestion, small intestinal malabsorption, and diarrhea. Interestingly, the NSP4 protein of rotavirus alone can induce intestinal hypersecretion from crypt cells, suggesting that both malabsorption and hypersecretion of fluid and electrolytes contribute to the diarrhea of rotaviral enteritis. The disease is worst in young animals and can rapidly lead to fatal acidosis, dehydration, and hypovolemic shock.

Animals that die of Rotavirus enteritis are dehydrated and have very liquid intestinal contents. Diarrhea is fluid and yellow/white (the so-called white scours), which frequently stains the perineum of affected animals. Histologic lesions include villus atrophy with loss of mature absorptive cells covering the villi, and hyperplasia of the immature cells within the intestinal crypts.

Host Response to Infection. Animals infected with *Rotavirus* develop local and systemic humoral immune responses that can be identified by various serologic techniques. Viral-neutralizing antibody is serotype-specific and directed at VP4 and VP7. The Rotavirus ELISA detects antibodies to group and subgroup determinants. Local immunity within the bowel is very important in preventing severe rotaviral enteritis in young animals; thus, ingestion of colostrum with high titers of *Rotavirus*-neutralizing antibody provides temporary immunity against disease in neonates.

Laboratory Diagnosis. Diagnosis of *Rotavirus*-induced diarrhea requires identification of the virus in feces or in tissues obtained at necropsy. Electron microscopy (EM), immune EM, and indirect fluorescent antibody (IFA) staining of feces and/or intestinal tissue sections all facilitate direct visualization of virus or viral antigens, but *Rotavirus* in feces is most easily detected by antigen-capture ELISA. The ELISA is very sensitive and, depending on the capture antibody used, can distinguish different types. Direct examination of the dsRNA genome of rotaviruses in the feces of animals can be done by polyacrylamide gel electrophoresis, which also identifies the specific group of *Rotavirus* that is present. PCR assays also are available.

Virus isolation is usually done on MA104 cells in the presence of low concentrations of trypsin. Avian rotaviruses are isolated on primary chicken embryo liver and kidney cells.

Serologic diagnosis can be done by ELISA or VN assays; however, the utility of data obtained usually is uncertain because of the widespread distribution of rotavirus infection, which means that a high proportion of animals are seropositive regardless of disease status.

Treatment and Control. Treatment of clinically ill animals is guided by disease severity, and treatment of severe cases involves replacement fluid therapy to treat dehydration and acidosis, minimization of environmental stress, and treatment of secondary infections.

Control is often difficult because of the stability of the virus in feces leading to long-term environmental contamination. Although often challenging to implement, stringent sanitation practices can minimize exposure. Vaccine strategies are best directed at the dams of suckling neonates to ensure that high titers of antibody are present in the colostrum and milk of these animals.

Aquareoviruses

Aquareoviruses are morphologically and physicochemically similar to orthoreoviruses, but have 11 segments of dsRNA. Seven of the 12 proteins (genome segment 11 encodes two proteins) are structural, with VP7 representing the major capsid protein. Six genotypes (A–F) have been proposed for *Aquareovirus*. Viruses in this genus infect both fish and shellfish, causing necrosis in the parenchymal organs of infected fish and high mortality in fish hatcheries. Aquareoviruses replicate in fish or shellfish cell lines at 16 °C and can induce syncytia formation.

References

Ruder MG, Howerth EW, Stallknecht DE *et al.* (2012). Vector competence of Culicoides sonorensis (Diptera: Ceratopogonidae) for epizootic hemorrhagic disease virus serotype 7. *Parasites and Vectors*, **5**, 236, 1–8.

Fayquet CM, Mayo MA, Maniloff J (eds) *et al.* (2005) *Virus Taxonomy: Eighth Report of the International Committee on Taxonomy of Viruses*. Elsevier, San Diego, CA, p. 485.

Further Reading

Lazarow PB (2011) Viruses exploiting peroxisomes. *Curr Opin Microbiol*, **14** (4), 458–469. Epub August 6, 2011.

Savini G, Afonso A, Mellor P *et al.* (2011) Epizootic hemorrhagic disease. *Res Vet Sci*, **91** (1), 1–17. Epub June 12, 2011.

Maclachlan NJ. (2011) Bluetongue: history, global epidemiology, and pathogenesis. *Prev Vet Med*, **102** (2), 107–111. Epub May 12, 2011.

Falconi C, López-Olvera JR, and Gortázar C. (2011) BTV infection in wild ruminants, with emphasis on red deer: a review. *Vet Microbiol*, **151** (3–4), 209–219. Epub February 23, 2011.

McDonald SM and Patton JT. (2011) Assortment and packaging of the segmented rotavirus genome. *Trends Microbiol*, **19** (3), 136–144. Epub December 31, 2010.

Depaquit J, Grandadam M, Fouque F *et al.* (2010) Arthropod-borne viruses transmitted by Phlebotomine sandflies in Europe: a review. *Euro Surveill*, **15** (10), 195–207.

Randolph SE and Rogers DJ. (2010) The arrival, establishment and spread of exotic diseases: patterns and predictions. *Nat Rev Microbiol*, **8** (5), 361–371. Epub April 7, 2010.

Tate JE, Patel MM, Steele AD *et al.* (2010) Global impact of rotavirus vaccines. *Expert Rev Vaccines*, **9** (4), 395–407.

Maclachlan NJ and Guthrie AJ. (2010) Re-emergence of bluetongue, African horse sickness, and other orbivirus diseases. *Vet Res*, **41** (6), 35. Epub January 27, 2010.

Birnaviridae

MELISSA KENNEDY

The family Birnaviridae includes three genera: *Avibirnavirus* (infects poultry), *Aquabirnavirus* (infects fish), and *Entomobirnavirus* (infects insects). Infectious bursal disease virus (IBDV; genus *Avibirnavirus*) is the best studied. Infectious pancreatic necrosis virus (IPNV; genus *Aquabirnavirus*) is a significant pathogen of salmonid fish.

Infectious Bursal Disease

Disease

Infectious bursal disease (IBD), also known as Gumboro disease after the town in Delaware (North America) where it was first identified, is an economically important virus disease of young chickens. The IBD virus replicates in immature B lymphocytes in the bursa of Fabricius (BF), leading to reduced immunologic responsiveness. The virus can cause relatively high mortality in chickens 3–6 weeks of age, and profound immunosuppression in birds infected earlier in life. The clinical disease in birds over 3 weeks of age is characterized by soiled vent feathers (birds often peck at their own vents), diarrhea, depression, anorexia, trembling, severe prostration, dehydration, and eventual death. In the United States, economic losses are typically due not so much to bird death but rather to reduced weight gain and carcass condemnation due to hemorrhages in skeletal muscle. Highly virulent strains of IBD virus that cause high mortality in affected flocks have become increasingly important in Europe and other regions of the world. While these strains, referred to as very virulent IBD (vvIBD) are antigenically similar to the classical strains, they can infect chicks in the face of maternal immunity previously protective against the classical strains. Infection of birds less than 3 weeks of age results in economically devastating inapparent infection. Such birds are extensively immunocompromised and exhibit increased susceptibility to a variety of other infectious diseases. Further more, affected birds respond poorly to vaccination.

Etiologic Agent

Physical, Chemical, and Antigenic Properties. IBDV particles are nonenveloped with icosahedral symmetry (60 nm in diameter). The genome includes two segments of double-stranded RNA (dsRNA), designated A and B, that encode five proteins. Segment A has two open reading frames and encodes a nonstructural protein (VP5) as well as a polyprotein that is cleaved into two structural proteins (VP2, VP3) and the viral protease (VP4). Gene segment B encodes the viral RNA-dependent RNA polymerase (VP1). There are two serotypes of IBDV and marked antigenic and genetic variation within each type. Strains of IBDV serotype 1 cause disease in chickens throughout the world, while serotype 2 strains, which primarily infect turkeys, neither cause disease nor protect against serotype 1.

Resistance to Physical and Chemical Agents. IBDV is extremely stable and resists inactivation following acid treatment (stable at pH 3), lipid solvents, various disinfectants, and heat (survives 60 °C for 30 min).

Infectivity for Other Species and Culture Systems. IBDV principally affects chickens, although turkeys, ducks, and some other species of domestic and wild birds can also be infected with the virus. The virus can be propagated in embryonating chicken eggs, with subsequent embryo mortality, as well as in a variety of avian cell cultures.

Host–Virus Relationship

Distribution, Reservoir, and Transmission. IBD occurs worldwide in intensive poultry-raising areas. The virus persists in nature because of its stability. The virus has reportedly persisted in poultry houses, following depopulation, for more than 100 days. There is no evidence of a true carrier state in birds.

Transmission of IBDV occurs by ingestion of virus from feces or feces-contaminated fomites, feed, and water.

Pathogenesis and Pathology. Initial replication of IBDV occurs in the intestinal tract within hours of ingestion of the virus, from where it disseminates to numerous tissues, including the BF. Other lymphoid organs such as thymus, spleen, and tonsils may also be affected, and disseminated lymphoid atrophy is especially characteristic of birds infected with very virulent strains of IBDV.

The striking age-dependent nature of the response of chickens to IBDV likely reflects the maturation of the BF

Veterinary Microbiology, Third Edition. Edited by D. Scott McVey, Melissa Kennedy and M.M. Chengappa.

at the time of infection. Specifically, birds are most susceptible to IBD from 3 to 6 weeks of age, whereas bursectomized birds of the same age do not develop disease. Birds older than 6 weeks also do not develop severe disease, nor do those infected prior to 3 weeks of age. The impaired immunologic responsiveness that occurs in chicks infected early in life has been attributed to bursal injury, which results in failure to seed B lymphocytes to peripheral lymphoid organs and diminished humoral immunity. Cellular immunity is also reduced in IBDV-infected young chicks.

Gross lesions may include dehydration, darkened pectoral muscles, and hemorrhages in the pectoral and leg muscles. The appearance of the BF is dependent on the state of disease. The BF initially becomes enlarged due to edema and hyperemia, but this rapidly is followed by progressive atrophy that is marked by approximately 8 days after infection. Bursal necrosis and hemorrhage are characteristic of advanced disease.

Histologically, the epithelial surfaces of the BF have multiple erosions, and there is extensive necrosis of lymphocytes within lymphoid follicles so that these become depleted of lymphocytes. Edema and infiltration of heterophils occur initially in the affected BF, followed by formation of cystic cavities bound by columnar epithelial cells and lymphoid depletion. Pathology in other lymphoid organs is less severe and recovery more rapid, except in birds infected with very virulent strains of IBDV.

Host Response to Infection. Following infection, birds develop a humoral immune response that is measured by viral neutralization, agar gel immunodiffusion, and enzyme-linked immunosorbent assay tests. In birds that recover, the BF may become repopulated with B lymphocytes. While T lymphocytes are required for protection against IBD and viral clearance, they can cause bursal damage and slow recovery through cytokines and cytotoxic responses. Adult birds transfer maternal antibody to developing embryos, and if present in sufficient titer, the antibody lends protection to the hatched chick for variable periods of time.

Laboratory Diagnosis

Field diagnosis can usually be made based upon the characteristic clinical signs and high morbidity and rapid recovery of most affected birds. Atrophy of the cloacal bursa is characteristic of inapparent IBDV infection in young chicks. Definitive diagnosis of IBD can be carried out by direct fluorescent antibody (FA) staining of sectioned tissues or viral isolation from the bursa and spleen. Isolation can be made by inoculation of embryonated chicken eggs or cell cultures. Serology is also useful for diagnostic purposes. Types and subtypes of IBDVs can only be distinguished through neutralization assays. Increasingly, molecular diagnostic assays using reverse-transcription polymerase chain reaction (RT-PCR) are being utilized for IBD diagnosis, as well as strain characterization.

Treatment and Control

No treatment has been described for affected birds. Control of the disease may be facilitated by proper sanitation practices. Vaccination programs are widely used to control IBD. Immunization of breeder flocks is done to facilitate passive transfer of immunity to chicks. Vaccination of chicks is also practiced, but to be effective, levels of maternal antibody must be low at the time of vaccination. Both attenuated and killed virus vaccines are available.

Infectious Pancreatic Necrosis

IPNV is the cause of a highly contagious and fatal disease of salmonid fish (trout and salmon) that is increasingly important to the aquaculture industry worldwide. The disease is not only severe in fish that are less than 6 months old but also occurs in older fish following stresses such as that associated with relocation from fresh to salt water. Affected fingerlings appear dark in color and swim with a rotating action (whirling). Petechial hemorrhages may be present in the abdominal viscera of affected fish, along with necrosis of the pancreas. The virus also affects commercially raised yellowtails with high mortality and is classically referred to as viral ascites due to accumulation of fluid in the abdomen (ascites) and associated abdominal distension. Eels can be infected with resulting clinical disease. Fish that survive infection with IPNV become carriers and serve as a source of infection to other fish, especially under hatchery conditions. The virus is very stable in the environment. The virus can be identified in the tissues of affected or carrier fish by virus isolation in fish cell cultures or RT-PCR techniques. Up to 10 serotypes of IPNV have been described, with the neutralizing epitopes being mapped to VP2. Efforts to develop effective vaccines are complicated by the multiple serotypes of IPNV and the difficulty in immunizing very young fish that are especially susceptible to the virus. Control is based on husbandry efforts that maximize hygiene and sanitation and minimize crowding, stress, and introduction of infected replacement stock and/or eggs. Vigorous identification and culling of carrier fish is advocated as a method of controlling the disease.

Further Reading

Muller H, Islam MR, and Raue R (2003) Research on infectious bursal disease—the past, the present and the future. *Vet Microbiol*, **97** (1-2), 153–165.

Essbauer S and Ahne W (2001) Viruses of lower vertebrates. *J Vet Med*, **48**, 403–475.

Retroviridae

FREDERICK J. FULLER

Retroviruses (family Retroviridae) are enveloped, single-stranded RNA viruses that replicate through a DNA intermediate (provirus) using an RNA-dependent DNA polymerase (reverse transcriptase (RT)). This large and diverse family includes members that are oncogenic, are associated with a variety of immune system disorders, and cause degenerative and neurologic syndromes.

Classification

The family Retroviridae (Latin *retro*, meaning reverse) is classified into two subfamilies, the Orthoretrovirinae and Spumaretrovirinae, and seven genera (Table 66.1). Classification is based on genome structure and nucleic acid sequence, in addition to older classification criteria based on morphology, serology, biochemical features, and the species of animal from which the retrovirus was isolated.

The genus *Lentivirus* (Latin *lenti*, meaning slow) includes the human immunodeficiency viruses (HIV) as well as many important animal retroviruses. Lentiviruses are most often associated with chronic immune dysfunction and neurologic diseases. The members of the genus *Spumavirus* (Latin *spuma*, meaning foam) are nononcogenic viruses found in spontaneously degenerating cell cultures, causing the formation of multinucleated vacuolated (foamy) giant cells. No diseases have been directly associated with spumaviruses in humans or animals. The remaining retrovirus genera are termed the oncornaviruses (Greek *onkos*, meaning tumor) or the RNA tumor viruses because of their ability to induce neoplasia, although they are now known to cause other kinds of diseases as well. These genera are the ***Alpharetrovirus*** (e.g., avian leukosis virus), ***Betaretrovirus*** (e.g., mouse mammary tumor virus), ***Gammaretrovirus*** (e.g., feline leukemia virus (FeLV)), ***Deltaretrovirus*** (e.g., bovine leukemia virus (BLV)), and ***Epsilonretrovirus*** (e.g., walleye dermal sarcoma virus (WDSV)).

Several additional features need to be considered in the classification and description of the Retroviridae. Exogenous retroviruses spread horizontally (or vertically but nongenetically) from animal to animal, similar to the mechanism of transmission of other kinds of viruses. In contrast, endogenous retroviruses are transmitted genetically. The endogenous retroviruses persist as integrated DNA proviruses that are passed from generation to generation through the DNA in the gametes of the host animal species. Thus, the endogenous proviral genome occurs in each cell of the animal. Many vertebrates possess such endogenous retroviral DNA sequences. These endogenous retroviruses are usually not pathogenic for their host animals and are often not expressed. When replication of endogenous viruses does occur in the host cell of origin, it is usually restricted. Cells from animal species other than the host species are sometimes unrestricted, however, and can support the replication of the retrovirus in an exogenous manner. The endogenous mode of transmission occurs in many of the oncornaviruses, but is not known to occur in the lentiviruses or the spumaviruses. Endogenous retroviruses may play important roles in protection from related exogenous retroviruses. Endogenous retroviruses account for a substantial portion of the genetic information of every animal species (about 8% of the human genome). Recent evidence suggests that endogenous retroviruses can play a critical role in ovine placental morphogenesis.

Some members of the oncornaviruses are also classified by their interaction with cells of different species. **Ecotropic** strains replicate only in cells from animal species of origin and **xenotropic** strains replicate only in cells of other species. **Amphotropic** strains replicate in both. Most of the endogenous retroviruses are also xenotropic.

The morphology of retroviruses in transmission electron micrograph is also useful in classification (Figure 66.1). The size range of retrovirus particles is from 80 nm to 130 nm. Type A particles occur only inside cells and consist of a ring-shaped nucleoid surrounded by a membrane. B-type virions have an eccentric core and C-type virions a central core. D-type virions have a morphology intermediate between B and C virions with an elongated, dense core. The core of lentiviruses has a shape that resembles an ice-cream cone with a flat base.

General Features of Retroviruses

Many of the features of retroviruses are known in great detail because of the extensive work done on the

Veterinary Microbiology, Third Edition. Edited by D. Scott McVey, Melissa Kennedy and M.M. Chengappa.

Table 66.1. Classification of Retroviruses Indicating the Two Subfamilies and Seven Genera with a Few Virus Examples in Each Genus. The Oncogenic Retroviruses Include the First Five Genera of the Orthoretrovirinae Subfamily

Subfamily	Genus	Virus Examples
Orthoretrovirinae	*Alpharetrovirus* (Oncogenic)	Avian leukosis virus Avian erythroblastosis virus Avian myeloblastosis virus Avian myelocytomatosis virus Rous sarcoma virus
	Betaretrovirus (Oncogenic)	Mouse mammary tumor virus Simian type D retrovirus (simian AIDS-related virus) Ovine pulmonary adenocarcinoma virus (Jaagsiekte) Squirrel monkey retrovirus
	Gammaretrovirus (Oncogenic)	Murine leukemia virus Feline leukemia virus Porcine type C oncovirus Feline sarcoma viruses Murine sarcoma virus Woolly monkey sarcoma virus Avian reticulendotheliosis virus
	Deltaretrovirus (Oncogenic)	Bovine leukemia virus Human T-lymphotropic viruses 1 & 2 Simian T-lymphotropic virus
	Epsilonretrovirus (Oncogenic)	Walleye dermal sarcoma virus Walleye epidermal hyperplasia virus
	Lentivirus	Visna/maedi virus (ovine progressive pneumonia) Caprine arthritis encephalitis virus Equine infectious anemia virus Bovine immunodeficiency virus Feline immunodeficiency virus Primate lentiviruses (HIV 1&2, SIV)
Spumaretrovirinae	*Spumavirus*	Human spumavirus Simian foam virus Bovine syncytial virus Feline syncytial virus

oncornaviruses in cancer research and the lentiviruses in acquired immunodeficiency syndrome (AIDS) research. The members of the family Retroviridae share many common features in their composition, organization, and life cycle, although the details of individual retroviruses vary.

Components of Retroviruses

A typical retrovirus virion is composed of 2% nucleic acid (RNA), 60% protein, 35% lipid, and 3% (or more) carbohydrate. Its buoyant density is 1.16–1.18 g/ml.

Retroviral Lipids. Retroviral lipids are mainly phospholipid and occur in the virion envelope. They form a bilayered structure similar to the outer cell membrane from which the retrovirus envelope is derived.

Retroviral Nucleic Acid

Retroviral RNA. Retroviral particles contain RNA as their genetic material. This genomic RNA is present in each viral particle as a dimer of two linear, single-stranded, positive-sense copies that are noncovalently joined near their 5′ ends (Figure 66.2). Hence, the virion is diploid. The genomic RNA has a sedimentation size of 60 to 70S in neutral sucrose gradients. Upon denaturation, each RNA copy has a sedimentation coefficient of 38S. The molecular weight of monomer RNA determined by electrophoresis in polyacrylamide gels is approximately 2 to 5×10^6 daltons, or about 7 to 11×10^3 bases. Host cell transfer RNA (tRNA) is associated with genomic RNA near the 3′ terminus and serves as a primer for the synthesis of DNA by the reverse polymerase. The type of tRNA packaged in the virion is useful in the classification of retroviruses. The 3′ terminus of each RNA monomer has a poly (A) tract. The 5′ terminus has a methylated nucleotide cap.

Proviral DNA. Within a cell the retroviral RNA genome is reverse transcribed into a DNA copy, and it is the proviral DNA form that serves as the intracellular retroviral genome. The retroviral DNA is several hundred bases longer than the retroviral RNA genome due to duplication of repeated and unique terminal sequences present in the RNA genome during the reverse transcription process. These sequences form the long terminal repeats (LTR) that flank the genes in the retroviral DNA (see Figure 66.2B). The proviral DNA is covalently integrated in the DNA of the infected host cell. This integration is facilitated by a viral enzyme,

FIGURE 66.1. *Transmission electron photomicrographs of budding and mature virions of feline immunodeficiency virus (A, B); feline leukemia virus (C, D); feline syncytium-forming virus (E, F); human immunodeficiency virus (G, H); simian immunodeficiency virus (I, J); and visna-maedi virus (K, L). Uranyl acetate and lead citrate stain. (Reproduced with Permission from Yamamoto et al., 1998.))*

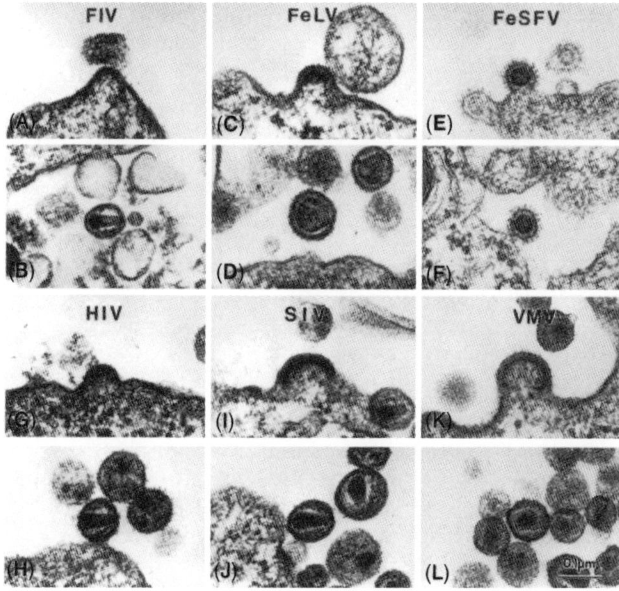

appropriately termed integrase, which is encoded in the polymerase open reading frame.

Retroviral Nucleic Acid Structure and Sequence. The sequence of structural genes of retroviruses, from the 5′ end to the 3′ end of genomic RNA, is Gag-Pol-Env. Some retroviruses such as the lentiviruses, spumaviruses, and deltaretroviruses have additional genes (tax and rex) that regulate expression of the retroviral genome and other accessory functions (see Figure 66.3). Highly oncogenic retroviruses often have an oncogene in place of a portion of the Pol and/or Env gene.

FIGURE 66.2. *The nucleic acid forms of a retrovirus. Retroviral RNA structure (A); retroviral DNA (Proviral DNA) after reverse transcription (B).*

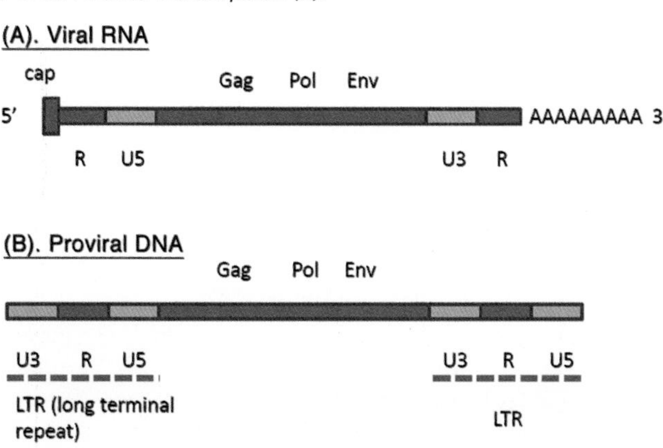

Retroviral Proteins

Retroviral Structural Proteins. Retroviral structural proteins are encoded by the Gag gene and the Env gene (Figure 66.4). Gag (group-specific antigen) proteins form the core of the virus and consist of three major proteins. The nucleocapsid (NC) is a small protein (about 5–10 kd) that interacts with retroviral RNA. The capsid (CA) protein (about 25 kd) forms the major structural element of the retroviral core. The matrix (MA) protein (about 15 kd) serves to join the retroviral core with the retroviral envelope. In some retroviruses, there are additional small core proteins.

The Env (envelope) gene is responsible for the synthesis of two glycoproteins that are noncovalently linked. These two glycoproteins form trimeric multimers in some retroviruses. The glycoprotein outside of the retrovirus (SU, surface) is a knob-like glycoprotein (about 100 kd) that is responsible for binding the retrovirus to its cellular receptor during infection. The other glycoprotein (TM, transmembrane) is a spike-like structure (about 50 kd) that attaches the SU protein to the retroviral envelope.

Retroviral Enzymes. The Pol gene encodes several proteins with enzymatic activities that are important for the replication of retroviruses. These enzymatic proteins are found within the retroviral particle, but in a much lower molar concentration than the retroviral structural proteins.

The RT enzyme is responsible for the production of the retroviral DNA genome from the retroviral RNA genome. To accomplish this, RT possesses several catalytic functions, including an RNA-dependent DNA polymerase and an **RNase H** activity. RT requires the presence of a divalent cation to function, and the type of divalent cation (magnesium or manganese) that a particular retrovirus requires is useful in retroviral classification. The measurement of RT activity is one of the principal laboratory methods for the detection and assay of retroviruses.

The Pol gene also encodes other enzymes. The retroviral **protease** (PR) mediates cleavage of Gag and Pol polyproteins during retroviral assembly and maturation. The protease of the Human Immunodeficiency virus has been an important target of antiretroviral drugs. The retroviral **integrase** (IN) functions to covalently link the retroviral DNA into the host cell's DNA as an integrated provirus. Some retroviruses also encode a **deoxyuridine triphosphatase** (dUTP) enzyme that is required for virus replication in nondividing cells.

Other Retroviral Proteins. For many members of the Retro viridae, only the proteins encoded by the Gag, Pol, and Env genes are present. Other retroviruses (Deltaretrovirus, Epsilonretrovirus, Lentivirus, and Spumavirus) contain additional genes whose products serve functions such as controlling the level of provirus transcription, facilitating transport of retroviral mRNA, enhancing retroviral replication in specific cell types, and interfering with host immunity.

FIGURE 66.3. *The proviral DNA structures of some retroviruses. All retroviruses encode the gag, pro, pol, and env genes. In addition, some groups of retroviruses encode additional genes that can be of cellular origin (V-Onc) or viral genes like tax, orfa (Viral Cyclin), and orfb (Rank1) that can play a role in oncogenesis. Note that a complex lentivirus like the human immunodeficiency virus has six additional genes beyond gag, pro, pol, and env.*

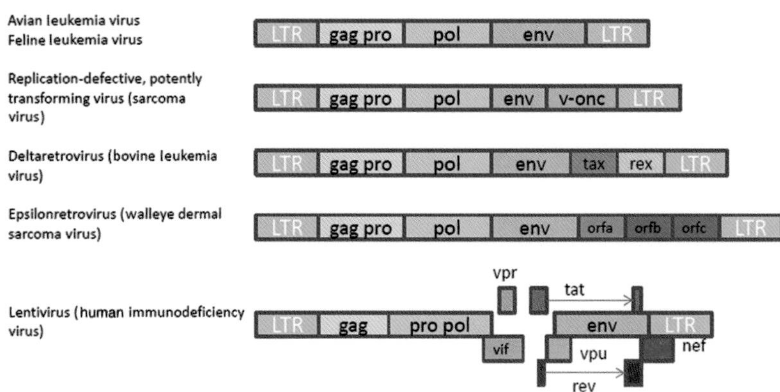

Retroviral Replication

A general scheme of retroviral replication is shown in Figure 66.5. A retroviral particle binds to a specific receptor on the surface of a target cell via the SU protein. The retrovirus penetrates the cell and the retroviral core undergoes specific structural changes. The retroviral RNA within the modified core is reverse transcribed by RT using the associated tRNA primer, first to an RNA/DNA hybrid form, then to a linear double-stranded DNA form with long terminal repeats. The newly made retroviral DNA is still associated with some viral core proteins and enzyme activities in a structure termed the integration complex. In some retroviruses, infection must occur within dividing cells so that

FIGURE 66.4. *Schematic drawing of a retrovirus particle including the common structural features. Note the two copies of viral RNA per particle and the transfer RNA that functions to prime viral RNA synthesis with reverse transcriptase. Particles are approximately 100 nm in diameter.*

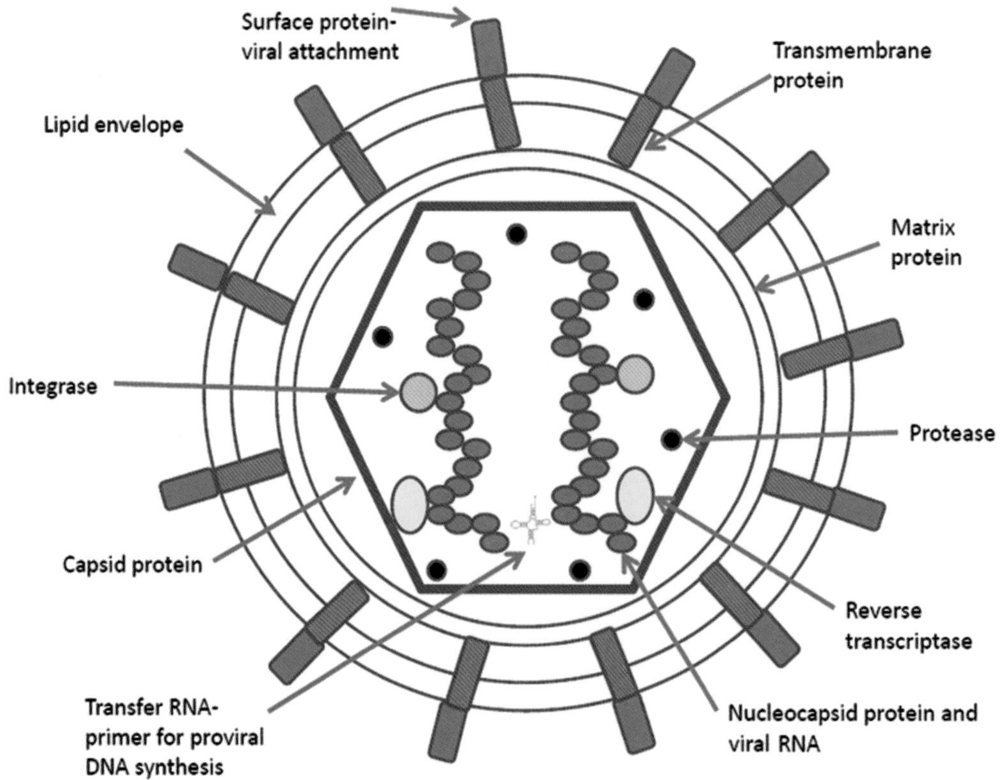

FIGURE 66.5. *Overall replication strategy for a retrovirus. Viral DNA synthesis is accomplished by the viral enzyme reverse transcriptase upon uncoating in the cell cytoplasm. Viral DNA must be integrated into cellular DNA for the cellular enzyme DNA-dependent RNA transcriptase (PolII) to make full-length viral genomic RNA as well as subgenomic viral messenger RNAs.*

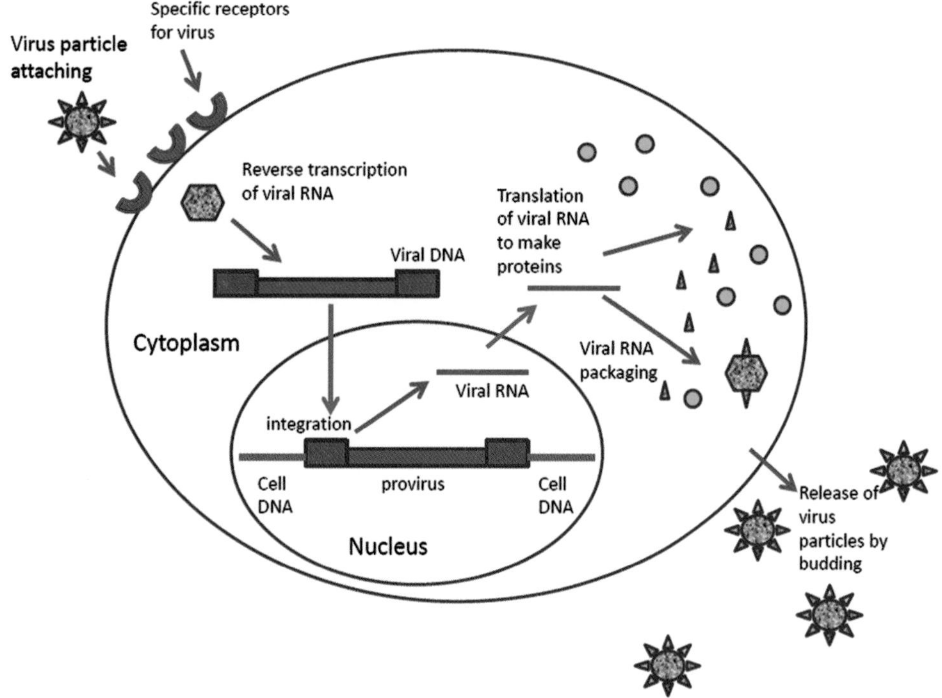

the integration complex can access the host DNA, while in other retroviruses the integration complex is actively transported into the nucleus of the cell, allowing such retroviruses to replicate in nondividing or terminally differentiated cells.

The retroviral DNA is integrated into the host cell's DNA by the activity of the IN enzyme. The integration of retroviruses is not at a specific site within the cellular DNA, rather integration can occur at many sites. The integrated DNA provirus behaves very much as a eukaryotic gene. It may be transcribed into mRNA and genomic RNA using host cell enzymes to produce more virus or it may remain latent for long periods of time and replicate when the cellular DNA is replicated by the cell.

New retroviral particles are produced by budding from cellular membranes. Immature retroviral Gag polyprotein and genomic RNA assemble and acquire envelopes as they exit infected cells by budding through the plasma membranes into which retroviral SU and TM envelope proteins have been inserted.

In the final step, the PR cleaves the Gag polyprotein into the mature structural proteins of matrix, capsid, and nucleocapsid.

Immunologic Characteristics of Retroviruses

Retroviral proteins possess various types of antigenic sites. Type-specific antigens that define the serologic subgroups are associated with the envelope glycoproteins. Group-specific antigens are shared by related viruses and, in general, are associated with the virion core proteins. There are also interspecies antigens that are shared by otherwise unrelated viruses derived from different host species. RT is also antigenic and contains type-, group-, and interspecies-specific determinants.

Oncogenic Viruses and Oncogenes

Oncogenic viruses can produce inappropriate cell growths in the tissues of susceptible hosts. Cancers are malignant tumors that are characterized by loss of normal cellular controls resulting in unregulated growth and ability to invade adjacent tissues and to metastasize to other parts of the body. Cancers are classified by their tissue of origin: sarcomas are malignant tumors of connective tissue (mesenchyme); carcinomas are malignant tumors of epithelial origin.

The ability of oncogenic viruses to cause cancers under either natural or experimental conditions has been the subject of intense study for almost a century and this work has made significant contributions to the understanding of viruses, neoplasia, and cell biology. The fundamental discovery in the field is that oncogenic viruses cause cancer via genes they carry or activate. These genes are termed oncogenes.

Oncogenesis by Retroviruses

There are several mechanisms by which retroviruses are associated with cancer. Highly oncogenic or acutely transforming retroviruses cause cancer rapidly and efficiently, often within days or weeks of infection. Such retroviruses are rare in natural animal populations, but are used extensively in the laboratory for the study of cancer. Rous sarcoma virus (RSV) of chickens, which was discovered in 1910, is the prototype highly oncogenic retrovirus.

In highly oncogenic retroviruses, all or part of an oncogene exists in the viral genome, usually in place of viral genes. This retroviral oncogene is responsible for the ability of a highly oncogenic retrovirus to cause oncogenic transformation of a cell. There are more than 20 different retroviral oncogenes known. Each of these has a corresponding gene that can be found in the genome of normal cells. The normal gene that corresponds to a viral oncogene is termed a c-oncogene or proto-oncogene, and the viral version is called a v-oncogene. In a normal cellular environment, the gene products of proto-oncogenes usually have some function in growth regulatory pathways, such as protein kinases, growth factors or their receptors, GTP binding proteins, or transcriptional activation factors. When they are part of a retroviral genome, these proto-oncogenes are under the control of the retroviral LTR rather than being regulated by normal cellular mechanisms, and are often expressed at high levels. The v-oncogene may also be truncated, contain point mutations, or be fused with another retroviral gene. This aberrant expression of mutant protein can lead to abnormal growth of the infected cell and the beginning of progression to neoplasia.

For example, in RSV, the src oncogene is responsible for sarcomatous transformation. The v-src gene was originally acquired from the normal c-src cellular proto-oncogene when illegitimate recombination (a rare event) occurred between retroviral and the cellular genomic sequences for c-src. The c-src gene product is a 60 kd protein that has protein kinase activity and is located near the inner surface of the plasma membrane. The kinase activity is part of an intricate cellular signal transduction pathway that mediates cell growth. Other examples of v-oncogenes with c-oncogene counterparts in normal cells are found in other acute transforming retroviruses, for example, myb (avian myeloblastosis virus), erb (avian erythroblastosis virus), myc (avian myelocytomatosis virus), and ras (mouse sarcoma virus).

Highly oncogenic retroviruses are usually defective. The reason they are defective is that they lack their full complement of Gag-Pol-Env genes because the v-oncogene takes the place of a portion of the retroviral genome. In order to replicate, these defective retroviruses require a replication-competent helper virus to supply the missing gene products. The helper retrovirus is usually a closely related retrovirus that is not defective and contains the usual Gag-Pol-Env complement of genes. Since the defective, highly oncogenic virus is packaged into a virion composed of the envelope proteins of the helper virus, the host range of the highly oncogenic virus is dependent upon the helper virus. In nature, the generation of a defective, highly oncogenic sarcoma virus will most likely cause multiclonal tumors in that host within days or weeks, resulting in the death of that host. It would be rare that this highly oncogenic virus would be transmitted to another animal. The presence of the genome of one retrovirus with the protein components of another virus is termed a pseudotype.

Weakly oncogenic (nonacutely transforming) retroviruses cause neoplasia less rapidly and much less efficiently than do highly oncogenic retroviruses. Such viruses exist in domestic animals. Weakly oncogenic retroviruses do not carry a v-oncogene and do not require a helper virus. However, examination of the tumors produced by the weakly oncogenic viruses usually shows a clonal proliferation of cells with a retroviral genome near a cellular oncogene. For example, avian leukosis virus is often integrated near or in the c-myc gene. The mechanism by which weakly oncogenic retroviruses cause cancer is known as insertional or cis-activational oncogenesis. During retroviral replication, proviral DNA is inserted into many random locations in the host genome. Occasionally the integration of the provirus occurs close to a cellular proto-oncogene. This can sometimes produce inappropriate transcription of the oncogene, either by read-through from the retroviral promoter, or by enhancer activity by the retroviral LTR. Integration of the provirus near a proto-oncogene tends to be a very rare event and, therefore, occurs much less frequently and at much lower efficiency than when the retrovirus carries its own oncogene. The tumors are clonal in origin because, although many cells are infected, only one rare cell has undergone insertional oncogenesis and progresses to a tumor. The level of virus replication is directly correlated to the incidence of tumor formation. The more virus replication that occurs in the host, the more likely a rare integration event near a proto-oncogene will occur. In addition, the inappropriate activation of a proto-oncogene is just one event in a multifactorial process that leads to cancer.

A third mechanism of retroviral oncogenesis occurs in the bovine leukemia virus-human T lymphotropic virus genus of Retroviridae. These viruses have a regulatory gene called tax in addition to Gag, Pol, and Env. The protein product of tax functions as a transactivator to upregulate retroviral transcription by binding to specific DNA sequences in the LTR of the retrovirus. Under some circumstances, the Tax protein can sometimes also bind to transcriptional activator sequences in cellular genes and may disrupt regulatory pathways of the infected cell. Unlike insertional oncogenesis, the integrated provirus is not necessarily adjacent to a proto-oncogene, since it is the Tax protein that produces the oncogene activation (in trans), rather than the retroviral DNA itself. Like insertional oncogenesis, the transactivation of a proto-oncogene is just one event in a multifactorial process that leads to cancer.

Oncogenesis by DNA Viruses

Many of the DNA viruses, including the adenoviruses, papovaviruses (polyoma, papilloma), herpesviruses, hepadnaviruses, and poxviruses, have oncogenic potential. In contrast to highly oncogenic retroviruses, the v-oncogenes of DNA viruses are not cellular derivatives but are true viral genes. The normal function of these viral genes is to activate cellular pathways for DNA replication. This activation is required for DNA viruses to multiply in resting cells that lack the enzymes and materials the virus needs for its own DNA replication. The mechanism of neoplastic transformation by oncogenic DNA virus is that the viral genes that activate cellular DNA replication are functional, but the genes for viral production for some reason are not. This causes the infected cell to get inappropriate activation signals without the subsequent viral production that destroys the cell. The result is inappropriate cell activation and division and is one of the initial steps that can lead to the development of a cancer. Like the weakly oncogenic retroviruses, insertion and transactivation mechanisms are also known for DNA viruses.

Avian Leukosis/Sarcoma Complex-Alpharetrovirus

Disease

The avian leukosis/sarcoma complex of viruses (ALSVs) induces a wide variety of diseases in chickens. These have been of great economic importance to the poultry industry, as well as being important research tools for the understanding of cancer. These diseases include lymphoid leukosis, erythroblastosis, myeloblastosis, myelocytomatoses, sarcomas, osteopetrosis, hemangiomas, and nephroblastoma. The signs of disease produced by the ALSVs are not specific, and differential diagnosis requires careful his-to-path-ologic examination and laboratory testing.

In lymphoid leukosis, the most common and economically important disease caused by ALSVs, the comb may be pale, shriveled, and occasionally cyanotic. Inappetence, emaciation, and weakness occur frequently. Enlargement of the liver, bursa of Fabricius, kidneys, and the nodular nature of the tumors can sometimes be detected on palpation.

ALSV also causes sporadic cases of lymphoid tumors, such as erythroblastosis, myeloblastosis, and myelocytomatoses. Clinical signs of these diseases include lethargy, general weakness, and pallor or cyanosis of the comb. In more advanced disease, weakness, emaciation, diarrhea, and occasionally profuse hemorrhage from feather follicles are observed.

Osteopetrosis, in which the long bones of the limbs are commonly affected, is also caused by ALSV. Thickening of the diaphyseal or metaphyseal region can be detected by inspection or palpation. Affected chickens are usually stunted, pale, and walk with a stilted gait or limp.

Reticuloendotheliosis virus (REV) is a retrovirus found in chickens and turkeys that is unrelated to the viruses of the *Alpharetrovirus* genus (leukosis/sarcoma group). REV is actually classified in the genus *Gammaretrovirus* based on nucleic acid homology and biochemical properties. REV causes neoplastic disease and nonneoplastic runting in several species of poultry.

Etiologic Agent

Classification. ALSVs are classified into five subgroups, A–E, on the basis of differences in their viral envelope glycoprotein antigens that determine virus-serum neutralization properties and viral interference patterns with members of the same or different subgroups. Subgroup E viruses include ubiquitous endogenous leukemia viruses of low pathogenicity. Additional subgroups (F, G, H, I) comprise retroviruses from pheasants, quail, and partridges and have antigenic properties and host ranges distinct from that of the viruses in subgroups A–E.

It is important to note that many of the highly oncogenic avian alpharetroviruses (type C) that are used in research studies are defective and require a helper virus to replicate. These viruses are packaged as pseudotypes using the envelope proteins of a helper virus. They, therefore, take on the interference and neutralization properties of their helper virus.

Physical, Chemical, and Antigenic Properties. In size, shape, and ultrastructural characteristics, viruses of the avian leukosis/sarcoma complex are alpharetroviruses (type C) and are indistinguishable from one another. ALSVs within a subgroup cross-neutralize to varying extents. Viruses of different subgroups do not cross-neutralize except for partial cross-neutralization between subgroups B and D.

Resistance to Physical and Chemical Agents. The infectivity of ALSVs is abolished by treatment with lipid solvents such as ether or detergents (sodium dodecyl sulfate). These viruses are rapidly inactivated at higher temperatures, whereas viruses of this group can be preserved for long periods at temperatures below 26 °C. The stability of viruses of this group changes little between pH 5 and pH 9. Outside this range, however, inactivation rates are markedly increased.

Infectivity for Other Species and Culture Systems. ALSVs occur in chickens and have also been isolated from pheasants, quail, and partridges. More distantly related retro viruses occur in turkeys. Experimentally, some of the ALSVs have a wide host range, especially RSV. Some strains of RSV induce neoplasms in other species of birds and even mammals, including monkeys, although only very young or immunologically tolerant animals are generally susceptible.

The avian oncornaviruses, like many retroviruses, are not cytocidal for the cells in which they replicate. In chicken embryo fibroblast cell culture, RSV and other highly oncogenic members of the ALSV group induce rapid transformation of cells characterized by alterations in cell growth properties and cell morphology. These cells proliferate to produce discrete colonies or foci of transformed cells within a few days. The number of transformed foci is inversely proportional to the viral dilution and can be used as a gauge of viral concentration. Various strains of sarcoma virus can induce transformation in mouse, rat, and hamster embryo fibroblasts, as well as in chickens.

Although members of the weakly oncogenic ALSV group induce neoplastic disease, they produce no obvious cytopathic effects or detectable levels of transformation in chicken fibroblast culture. Their presence is assessed by an immunofluorescence focus assay with type-specific chicken antisera or by their ability to induce resistance to transformation by RSV. This resistance occurs when the glycoproteins (attachment sites) of an identical or related virus block the cell receptors for the superinfecting virus. Stocks of leukosis virus originally detected by interference with RSV are referred to as resistance-inducing factor strains.

FIGURE 66.6. *Transmission of avian leukosis virus (ALV). Horizontal transmission of ALV (adult to adult) to a susceptible adult bird typically results in a short-term viremia and the development of immunity and cessation of the viremia. These infections rarely result in the development of lymphoid leucosis. In ovo transmission (hen-to-chick) transmission is the primary concern. The chick will hatch with immune tolerance to the virus and a chronic viremia. Continuous virus replication in the bird can commonly result in the development of lymphoid leucosis. Endogenous avian retroviruses are transmitted genetically via egg and/or sperm. Gene expression of endogenous viruses are typically low (or no expression) and rarely result in disease.*

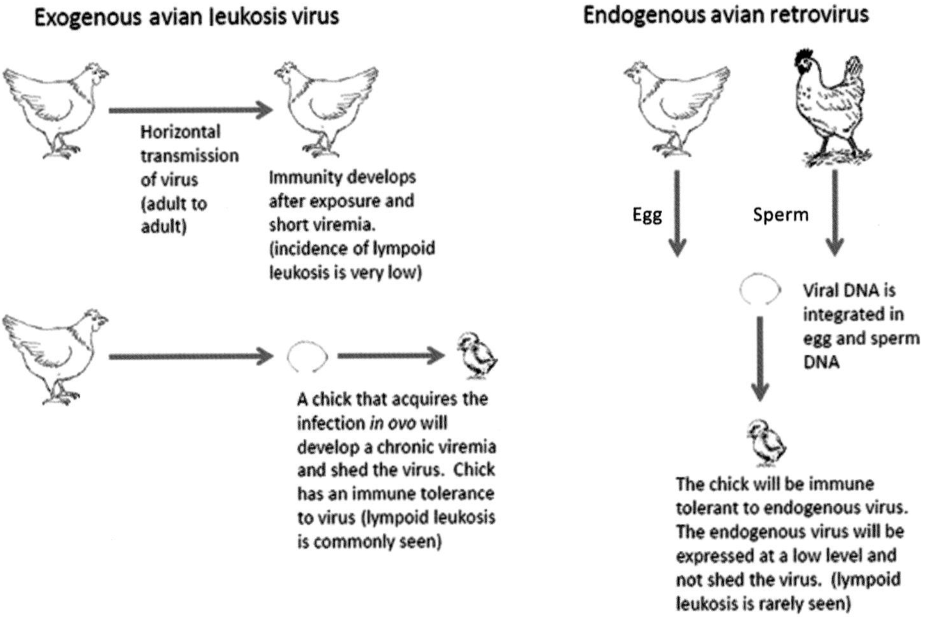

Host–Virus Relationship

Distribution, Reservoir, and Transmission. ALSVs occur naturally in chickens and most flocks of chickens worldwide harbor various strains of ALSV, except for those derived from specific pathogen-free birds. Even in infected flocks, the frequency of lymphoid tumors is typically low and mortality is usually 2% or less, although sometimes losses can be much higher. The reservoir host for ALSV is the infected chicken.

Transmission can be either vertical (from hen through egg) or horizontal. Vertically infected chicks are immunologically tolerant to the virus and fail to produce neutralizing antibodies, and remain viremic for life (Figure 66.6). Horizontal infection is through infected saliva and feces and is characterized by transitory viremia followed by the development of antibodies. Tumors are more frequent in vertical than horizontal infections.

Endogenous leukosis viruses, such as those of subgroup E, are usually transmitted genetically in the germ cells in the form of a DNA provirus. Many of these endogenous ALSVs are defective, but some (RAV-O) are released in an infectious form and can be transmitted horizontally, although most chickens are genetically resistant to infection.

Pathogenesis and Pathology. ALSVs induce a wide variety of neoplasms. The pathogenesis of infection of birds with ALSVs depends on whether the particular ALSV in question carries an oncogene or not. ALSVs containing a v-oncogene are highly oncogenic retroviruses, transform cells in culture, are usually defective, and are most often products of the research laboratory and occur only sporadically in nature, if at all. ALSV strains that contain a particular v-oncogene usually cause a rapid and relatively reproducible type of neoplastic disease in a high percentage of infected chickens.

In contrast, naturally occurring ALSVs are weakly oncogenic, cause disease by insertional oncogenesis, do not transform cells at detectable levels in culture, are usually not defective, and are naturally transmitted. The oncogenic spectrum of non-oncogene-containing strains of ALSVs tends to overlap, so that a given strain of ALSV can induce many kinds of tumors depending on other factors, such as the amount of virus, age, and genotype of chicken, and route of infection. This is consistent with the concept of insertional oncogenesis for these viruses in which the ALSV infects and replicates in a variety of cell types, but in order to produce neoplastic transformation, it must integrate near an appropriate cellular proto-oncogene.

Under natural conditions, the most common disease caused by ALSV is lymphoid leukosis. Transformation of lymphocytes occurs in the bursa of Fabricius, usually at a few months after infection. These early ALSV-induced lesions sometimes regress, while others enlarge and eventually spread to other visceral organs. Grossly visible neoplasms are of variable size and organ distribution, almost always involve the liver (a synonym for lymphoid leukosis is big liver disease), spleen, and bursa of Fabricius. Individual neoplasms are soft, smooth, and glistening and are usually miliary or diffuse, but may be nodular, or a combination of these forms. These neoplastic masses are composed of large B lymphocytes that express surface immunoglobulin. There are often no consistent or significant hematologic changes in circulating blood, and frank lymphoblastic leukemia is rare. Fully developed lymphoid leukosis occurs in birds at about 4 months of age and older.

Erythroblastosis occurs sporadically in ALSV-infected chicken flocks. The liver and spleen are enlarged by a diffuse infiltration of proliferating erythroblasts, and the bone marrow is effaced by the same cells. Affected chickens become anemic and thrombocytopenic. Blood smears show an erythroblastic leukemia. Induction of erythroblastosis by naturally occurring, slowly transforming ALSV involves activation of the cellular oncogene c-erbB by insertional oncogenesis. Highly oncogenic, laboratory strains of ALSV carry the v-form of this oncogene and are termed avian erythroblastosis virus (AEV). Some strains of AEV can kill chickens by erythroblastosis within a week after experimental infection.

Myeloblastosis is relatively uncommon under natural conditions and tends to occur in adult chickens. The target organ in this disease is bone marrow, and the first neoplastic alteration is in the form of multiple foci of proliferating myeloblasts, which is followed by leukemia and invasion of other organs, especially liver, kidney, and spleen. Microscopic examination reveals massive intravascular and extravascular accumulations of myeloblasts with variable proportions of promyelocytes. The v-myb gene is carried by the highly oncogenic avian myeloblastosis virus strains. These laboratory strains produce mortality a few weeks after experimental infection.

Myelocytomatosis is another form of leukosis that occurs sporadically in chickens. In this disease, tumors characteristically occur on the surface of bones in association with the periosteum and near cartilage, and at the costochondral junctions, posterior sternum, and cartilaginous bones of the mandible and nares. They consist of compact masses of uniform myelocytes. Earliest changes occur in bone marrow in which there is crowding of intersinusoidal spaces by myelocytes, destruction of sinusoid walls, and eventual overgrowth of the bone marrow. Tumors may crowd through the bone and extend through the periosteum. The v-myc oncogene is carried by the highly oncogenic avian myelocytomatosis virus.

Various benign and malignant connective tissue tumors occur sporadically in ALSV-infected chickens. There are a number of laboratory strains of avian sarcoma virus (ASV), the most famous of which is RSV. ASVs induce sarcomas (tumors of connective tissue), including fibrosarcoma and fibroma; myxosarcoma and myxoma; histiocytic sarcoma, osteoma, and osteogenic sarcoma; and chondrosarcoma. These highly oncogenic ASVs carry an oncogene such as src (in RSV), fps, ros, or yes.

Infection with ALSV is important in its own right. ALSV-infected chickens (compared with specific pathogen-free chickens) exhibit poor growth and egg production even in the absence of tumor formation. The pathogenesis of subclinical ALSV infection of birds is poorly understood.

Host Response to Infection. Chickens exposed to ALSV virus fall into four classes: (1) no viremia, no antibodies; (2) no viremia, antibody; (3) viremia, antibody; and (4) viremia, no antibody. Category 1 includes birds that are genetically resistant. Most exposed chickens are included in category 2, and antibody persists throughout the life of these birds and is passed via the yolk to progeny chicks. The passive immunity provided by such antibodies generally lasts for 3–4 weeks. In addition to the neutralizing antibodies directed against the envelope proteins, antibodies are produced to the internal group-specific antigens (Gag proteins), which are nonneutralizing and not protective. Although virus-neutralizing antibodies restrict the amount of virus, they have little direct effect on growth of the virus-induced neoplasms. Few chickens occur in the third category, which may represent chickens that are in the process of clearing an acute infection with ALSV. Most chickens in category 4 acquire ALSV vertically when in the egg and are immunologically tolerant to the virus. Hens in category 4 transmit virus to a high proportion of their progeny through the egg.

Since there are multiple subgroups (A–D) that commonly occur in chicken flocks and are not cross-neutralized by antibody, the status of a chicken for one subgroup of ALSV is independent of other viral subgroups.

Laboratory Diagnosis

ALSV can usually be isolated from plasma, serum, tumor tissue, and albumin, or from the embryo of infected eggs. Since ALSV is generally not cytopathogenic, complement fixation, fluorescent antibody, or radioimmunoassay (RIA) tests must be used to detect and identify the viruses in cell culture. An ELISA test is used for direct detection of virus in egg albumen or vaginal swabs. These tests have been used directly on test material (egg albumin) or indirectly on the cell cultures used for viral isolation. All tests require a source of chicken embryos free from endogenous ALSV.

Another means of identifying virus is based on phenotypic mixing of viruses. Chicken fibroblasts that are transformed with envelope-defective strains of RSV are nonproducers (NP) of infectious RSV. Superinfection of NP cultures by another ALSV acting as a helper virus results in production of infectious RSV, which produces transformed foci on susceptible chicken embryo fibroblasts.

Treatment and Control

Attempts to produce effective vaccines have been largely unsuccessful. Congenitally infected chicks are most likely to develop neoplasms and shed the virus are immunologically tolerant to ALSV and cannot be immunized.

It is possible to eradicate ALSV from chickens by establishing breeder flocks that are free of exogenous ALSVs. Hens are selected that are negative for ALSV antigens in their eggs. The fertile eggs laid by the selected hens are hatched and the chicks reared in isolation in small groups. The birds without leukosis virus antigen or antibody are used as the breeders for a leukosis virus-free flock. The flock must then be maintained in isolation from untested chickens.

Ovine Pulmonary Adenocarcinoma Virus (Jaagsiekte)— *Betaretrovirus* Genus

Disease

Ovine pulmonary adenocarcinoma or Jaagsiekte (Afrikaner name for "panting sickness") is an invariably fatal respiratory neoplastic disease that progresses slowly. It is worldwide in distribution (except Australia, New Zealand and Iceland) and affects primarily sheep and infrequently found in goats.

Etiologic Agent

Ovine pulmonary adenocarcinoma virus is a betaretrovirus. The envelope protein of this exogenous virus appears to be alone sufficient to induce cell transformation and no evidence of viral oncogene expression has been demonstrated.

Physical, Chemical, and Antigenic Properties. The lack of a cell culture system to replicate the virus has hampered efforts to characterize the virus particles. Genomic sequencing of virus from infected sheep lung exudates has revealed a genomic organization and homology most like that of the betaretroviruses including mouse mammary tumor and simian type D (Mason-Pfizer monkey virus (MPMV)) viruses. Antibodies to the capsid protein simian type D and mouse mammary tumor virus will react with Jaagsiekte capsid protein.

Infectivity for Other Species and Culture Systems. Sheep are the primary hosts for this virus. Goats can be infected but are less susceptible to both infection and development of disease than sheep. It has not been possible to grow the virus in cell cultures.

Host–Virus Relationship

Distribution, Reservoir, and Transmission. The disease is endemic worldwide (except Australia, New Zealand, and Iceland) and the incidence varies from 1% to 20% depending on the country (uncommon in the United States). It is frequently seen coincident with the ovine lentivirus. Virus can be transmitted via respiratory droplets.

Pathogenesis and Pathology. The virus has a tropism for type 2 pneumocytes and bronchial cells (nonciliated) that express the cellular receptor hyaluronidase 2. Tumors that develop from proliferation of these two cell types eventually compromise lung function and death results from asphyxia or secondary bacterial infection (frequently pasteurellosis) of the lower respiratory track resulting in pneumonia. Secretion of substantial quantities of surfactant (produced by type 2 pneumocytes) and copious lung fluids is a characteristic of this disease. Metastatic spread of the lung tumors can occur to regional lymph nodes and on rare occasions to cardiac or muscle tissues.

Host Response to Infection. There is a closely related endogenous betaretrovirus in the genome of sheep and goats. These endogenous retroviruses may play a role in protection from exogenous ovine retroviruses in ovine evolution. These endogenous retroviruses are expressed in the placenta and have been shown to be required for normal development of the placenta. As a consequence, no antibodies are developed to an infection with the exogenous virus. This is one of the explanations for this being an invariably fatal disease.

Laboratory Diagnosis

Serologic tests do allow identification of sheep or goats infected with exogenous virus; therefore, pcr-based tests for viral nucleic acid in lung exudates (where endogenous virus is not expressed) or ELISA for viral antigens can be used diagnostically.

Treatment and Control

There is no treatment that has proven effective for this disease. Iceland was able to eradicate the disease in the early 1950s by identification and severe depopulation measures. There is an age-related resistance and by raising lambs under strict isolation conditions along with culling of infected sheep and exposed cohorts, eradication was successful.

Simian Type D Retrovirus—*Betaretrovirus* Genus

Disease

Simian type D retrovirus causes a fatal immunosuppressive disease in monkeys. Infected animals show an initial generalized lymphadenopathy and splenomegaly accompanied by fever, weight loss, diarrhea, anemia, lymphopenia, granulocytopenia, and thrombocytopenia. Profoundly immunosuppressed animals develop diseases caused by opportunistic pathogens, the most common of which is disseminated cytomegalovirus infection.

Etiologic Agent

Classification. Primate retroviruses are represented in four distinct genera: (1) *Betaretrovirus* genus, which includes the simian type D retrovirus (SRV); (2) the *Deltaretrovirus* genus, which includes the simian T-lymphotropic viruses (STLV) and human T-lymphotropic viruses (HTLV); (3) the primate lentiviruses, which include the HIV types 1 and 2 (HIV-1 and HIV-2) and the simian immunodeficiency viruses (SIV); and (4) the simian and human spumaviruses. Although SRV is in a separate genus from the primate lentiviruses (HIV and SIV) that cause acquired immunodeficiency in humans (AIDS) and simians (SAIDS), many aspects of the immunodeficiency and associated opportunistic infections are similar.

The MPMV was the original SRV to be isolated.

Physical, Chemical, and Antigenic Properties. SRV is a type D retrovirus (*Betaretrovirus* genus). The type D viruses are characterized by the formation of cytoplasmic type A precursor core particles. Mature type D viruses are pleomorphic in shape, spheroid, enveloped, and 80–100 nm in diameter. The NC is isometric to spherical with an asymmetric, spherical nucleoid.

The RT of SRV has a preference for Mg^{2+} and uses $tRNA^{Lys}$ as a primer for negative-strand DNA reverse transcription.

SRV consists of at least five serotypes based on neutralization properties of the envelope.

Infectivity for Other Species and Culture Systems. SRV infects several species of monkeys. Serologic surveys have shown no conclusive evidence of SRV infection in animal handlers who work with monkeys.

SRV isolates replicate in both T and B lymphocytes as well as in macrophages. Various human and monkey cell lines of T and B lymphocyte, macrophage, and fibroblast origin support the growth of SRV. SRV induces syncytia in Raji cells, which can be used as a method to quantitate the virus.

A human counterpart of SRV—a human type D retrovirus—has been reported. The distribution and clinical significance of this virus remains to be determined, as does its relationship to SRV.

Host–Virus Relationship

Distribution, Reservoir, and Transmission. SRV is indigenous and widespread in Asian macaques but does not naturally infect African monkey species. In one study, about 25% of captive macaques in United States primate centers were seropositive; however, the prevalence varies widely based on the location and the species studied.

SRV is transmitted primarily in the saliva by biting. Mortality has been estimated to be 30–50%, and often occurs at an early age. Inapparent carriers that are viremic but antibody negative may be an important reservoir for SRV.

Pathogenesis and Pathology. SRV infects both T and B lymphocytes *in vivo* and causes a profound depletion of both of these kinds of lymphocytes leading to fatal immunosuppressive disease. The absolute lymphocyte count decreases but the CD4/CD8 ratio remains relatively stable. In the lymph nodes, there is a depletion of lymphocytes and an absence of plasma cells. SRV also infects macrophages, but not granulocytes.

Host Response to Infection. Some infected monkeys die acutely 7–20 weeks after experimental inoculation, whereas some remain persistently infected, and some develop neutralizing antibody and become nonviremic and remain healthy.

Laboratory Diagnosis

Serologic screening methods include ELISA and Western immunoblotting. Because infected monkeys may be seronegative, however, it is necessary to include virus isolation as part of the screening process. Techniques based on antigen capture and polymerase chain reaction (PCR) have also been developed.

Treatment and Control

It is important to establish and maintain specific retrovirus-free breeding colonies, both for animal health as well as improving the quality of nonhuman primates used in biomedical research and, potentially in the future, transplantation. A serial test and removal program can eliminate SRV infection in group-housed monkeys.

Vaccines against SRV have demonstrated effectiveness under experimental conditions.

Feline Leukemia/Sarcoma Virus—Gammaretrovirus

Disease

The FeLV causes a variety of important diseases of cats. The most significant consequence of persistent FeLV infection is severe immunosuppression that results in the development of opportunistic secondary infections. Clinical syndromes produced by FeLV infection in cats also include tumors of the hemolymphatic system (lymphoma, leukemia), refractory anemia, ulceration of the oral cavity, a feline panleukopenia-like syndrome, FeLV-induced neurologic syndrome, and immune-complex glomerulonephritis.

Lymphoma (lymphosarcoma) is the most common neoplasm in cats, although only about 70% of all lymphomas in cats are caused by FeLV infection. Multicentric lymphosarcoma that affects a variety of tissues (including liver, gastrointestinal tract, kidneys, spleen, bone marrow, and central nervous system (CNS)) is the most common tumor in FeLV-infected cats, whereas thymic and alimentary (gastrointestinal) forms predominate in uninfected cats. Young cats with lymphoma tend to be infected with FeLV, whereas older cats with lymphoma tend not to be. Cats with lymphoma typically present with weight loss, often accompanied by any combination of respiratory difficulty, diarrhea, vomiting, and constipation. FeLV can also cause abnormal proliferation of erythroid and myeloid cells, resulting in a variety of myeloproliferative disorders including leukemias.

Transmissible fibrosarcoma in cats is associated with infection by feline sarcoma virus (FeSV) and typically occurs in young cats. The more common fibrosarcomas that occur in older cats are not associated with FeSV. The FeSV-induced fibrosarcomas tend to be poorly differentiated and more invasive than non–FeSV-induced tumors.

Etiologic Agent

Classification. Three subgroups of exogenous FeLV (A, B, and C) are distinguished by viral interference tests and antibody neutralization tests. These two properties are associated with the envelope glycoprotein.

FeSVs are replication defective, highly oncogenic (acute transforming) viruses that have acquired an oncogene through recombination of the FeLV genome with one of several cellular oncogenes. FeSVs are thought to develop de novo in FeLV-infected cats and not to be naturally transmitted from cat to cat.

Cats also have endogenous feline retroviruses such as RD-114 that are transmitted genetically. Multiple copies of the RD-114 provirus are found in all cat cells. These endogenous viruses are not associated with any known feline disease.

Physical, Chemical, and Antigenic Properties. Morphologically, the feline retroviruses are typical mammalian type C retroviruses of the *Gammaretrovirus* genus. FeLV is composed of two envelope proteins, gp70 (SU) and p15E (TM), and three Gag proteins, p10 (NC), p15 (MA), and p27 (CA). The Gag proteins are produced in great excess in infected cells and are useful in laboratory diagnosis of FeLV infection of cats.

Resistance to Physical and Chemical Agents. Like most enveloped viruses, FeLV is sensitive to inactivation by lipid solvents and detergents. FeLV is rapidly inactivated at 56 °C, but only minimal inactivation occurs at 37 °C for up to 48 h in culture medium. The virus is rapidly inactivated by drying.

Infectivity for Other Species and Culture Systems. FeLV-A replicates exclusively in cat cells, whereas FeLV-B and FeLV-C replicate in a variety of cell types, including human cells. The host range specificity of FeLV is associated with the envelope glycoprotein, gp70. No relationship has been shown between FeLV and human disease, and there is no evidence that FeLV disease is transmissible to humans.

Since the much rarer sarcoma virus, FeSV, is defective, the host range of this virus is dependent upon the helper leukemia virus that supplies the protein for its envelope. Most experimental studies have been conducted with the FeSV (FeLV-B) pseudotype. FeSV can transform fibroblasts from nonfeline species, including dog, mouse, guinea pig, rat, mink, sheep, monkey, rabbit, and human. FeSV has been found to be oncogenic in many of the animal species tested, although inoculation of fetal or newborn animals is generally required to show oncogenesis of FeSV in species other than cats.

Host–Virus Relationship

Distribution, Reservoir, and Transmission. FeLV infection of cats occurs throughout the world, and the cat is the only known reservoir of the virus. About 2% of the cats in the United States are seropositive, indicating either past or current infection, and some 50% of these seropositive cats are positive for FeLV antigens by immunofluorescent antibody test (IFA) of their peripheral blood leukocytes, indicating current infection. FeLV-A occurs in infected cats either alone (50%) or in combination with FeLV-B or FeLV-C.

FeLV is excreted in saliva and tears and possibly the urine. Transmission appears to occur during close contact via biting or licking (grooming). It is possible that infection may occur via contaminated feeding dishes. Prolonged, extensive cat-to-cat contact is required for efficient spread. In environments with multiple cats, the presence of one infected cat greatly increases the risk of infection for other cats. FeLV is also transmitted congenitally, and most kittens exposed in utero or before 8 weeks of age become persistently viremic.

Pathogenesis and Pathology. Upon penetrating the oral, ocular, or nasal membranes, the FeLV replicates in lymphocytes in the local lymph nodes of the head and neck. Acute FeLV disease, manifested by fever, lymphadenopathy, and malaise, develops 2–4 weeks after infection; however, these signs are seldom conspicuous. In about one-half of infected cats, the animals recover quickly and become FeLV antibody positive, FeLV antigen negative. Some of these cats have probably cleared the virus and the virus remains latent in others. The long-term significance of latent FeLV infection has not been determined, and FeLV-viremia may be reactivated under conditions of stress or corticosteroid therapy in some of these cats.

In cats that do not mount an adequate immune response, the FeLV replicates in the rapidly dividing cells of the bone marrow. These cats are persistently infected with FeLV and are positive for FeLV antigen by the IFA test in peripheral blood leukocytes. The cycle of infection is complete after viral replication in epithelial cells of the salivary glands, where infectious FeLV is shed in the saliva.

The time from the onset of viremia to the appearance of the later signs of FeLV infection is termed the induction period. This period ranges from months to years, with an average of about 2 years. Most persistently viremic cats die within 3.5 years of infection. Persistently infected cats often develop leukopenia, immune deficiency, and secondary opportunistic infections. FeLV-induced immune deficiency must be distinguished from that induced by feline immunodeficiency virus (FIV), which is a different retrovirus.

Host Response to Infection. About half of FeLV-infected cats produce protective amounts of neutralizing antibodies to the major envelope glycoproteins while FeLV is confined to cells of the local lymph nodes, and the virus is eliminated or remains latent. These cats do not become persistently infected with FeLV, and usually live out a normal life span. The response to FeLV infection depends on the age of the cat, the dose of virus received, and probably other genetic and virologic factors. Kittens tend to respond poorly and, as a result, are predisposed to persistent FeLV infection.

Laboratory Diagnosis

Because some cats are able to clear a FeLV infection, and many cats have been vaccinated against FeLV, tests for antibody to FeLV are of limited utility. The most useful tests for FeLV diagnosis detect FeLV antigens. An enzyme-linked immunosorbent assay (ELISA) is available for FeLV antigens in serum or saliva and is especially useful as a rapid screening method. An immunofluorescence antibody test (IFA) is used to detect FeLV antigens inside of infected cells, which is evidence that the virus is replicating in the bone marrow and that the cat is persistently viremic.

Treatment and Control

Vaccines against FeLV are available, although their efficacy under field conditions is controversial. Current FeLV vaccines either contain the inactivated ("killed") whole virus or a subunit protein preparation of the virus. Kittens should be vaccinated twice starting at 9–10 weeks of age, with the second dose of the vaccine given 3–4 weeks later, and with annual booster vaccinations. Eight-five percent of cats under 12 weeks of age, if exposed, become persistently infected, but cats over 6 months of age have only a 10–15% chance of becoming persistently infected if exposed. Use of FeLV vaccines is thus potentially most beneficial in young cats.

FeLV infection in catteries can be controlled by test and removal procedures and can be combined with FeLV vaccination, since vaccination will not interfere with the laboratory detection of FeLV antigen in infected cats.

A diagnosis of FeLV infection does not necessarily dictate euthanasia, since a FeLV-positive healthy cat may live for years. Because the cat is probably shedding virus that could infect other cats; however, precautions to reduce the chance of spreading the virus and contact with opportunistic pathogens should be instituted.

Bovine Leukemia Virus—Deltaretrovirus

Disease

BLV is a cause of lymphoma (lymphosarcoma; lymphoreticular neoplasia) in older cattle—so-called enzootic bovine leukosis (EBL), which occurs very sporadically in BLV-infected cattle. Cattle with EBL are usually older than 3 years, with the peak of tumor incidence between 5 and 8 years. Affected cattle typically are afebrile with nonpainful enlargement of peripheral lymph nodes (lymphadenopathy). Depending on the involvement of different organs, affected cattle can exhibit signs of gastrointestinal dysfunction, paralysis, exophthalmos, and cardiac dysfunction. Neoplastic lymphocytes can invade the blood to cause lymphoid leukemia in some affected cattle. The forms of lymphomas that occur in calves (less than 6 months of age) and juvenile cattle (6–18 months of age) are not associated with BLV infection.

Etiologic Agent

Classification. Because of its genome structure, nucleotide sequence, and size and amino acid sequence of the structural and nonstructural viral proteins, BLV has recently been grouped in a genus (*Deltaretrovirus*) with the HTLV-I and HTLV-II, and the closely related STLV. These viruses can induce diseases with similar pathologies, characterized by low viremia, long latency period, and a lack of preferred proviral integration sites in the tumors (i.e., the provirus is not necessarily found near an oncogene).

Physical, Chemical, and Antigenic Properties. Morphologically, BLV resembles other type C retroviruses. Antibody to gp51 is neutralizing.

Resistance to Physical and Chemical Agents. The infectivity of BLV is abolished by lipid solvents, periodate, phenol, trypsin, and formaldehyde. Infectivity is rapidly destroyed at 56 °C but can be retained for prolonged periods at less than 50 °C. Pasteurization destroys the infectivity of this virus, which is of interest because infected lymphocytes are found in the milk of infected dairy cattle.

Infectivity for Other Species and Culture Systems. BLV has been shown to be infectious for several animal species other than cattle, including sheep, goats, and pigs. Under natural conditions, the oncogenic potential of BLV appears to be expressed only in cattle and sheep. Since there are no significant antigenic or genetic differences between bovine and ovine isolates, the agent designated ovine leukemia virus is regarded as BLV infecting a heterologous host.

BLV replicates in cell culture from a wide variety of species, including bovine, human, simian, canine, ca-prine, and equine cells. Although BLV replicates in human cells, humans are not known to be infected. Seroepidemic studies among high-risk humans (veterinarians, farmers, animal keepers, and slaughterhouse personnel) revealed no infections, and BLV has not been associated with human neoplasms.

Host–Virus Relationship

Distribution, Reservoir, and Transmission. The geographic distribution of BLV is worldwide. The reservoir is infected cattle. Disease is directly related to BLV prevalence, which can vary widely but is highest in intensive dairy areas (up to 50% or even higher). In addition to production losses associated with BLV infection of cattle, additional losses result from exportation restrictions by foreign countries that halt export of BLV-positive cattle or semen from infected bulls.

BLV is transmitted horizontally under conditions of close contact, and most commonly occurs when heifers are introduced into the milking herd. The virus is highly cell-associated, and transmission is by blood or tissue containing lymphocytes between animals, by trauma, contaminated veterinary equipment, or other less defined routes. Transmission of BLV can occur through the skin and the reproductive, alimentary and reproductive tracts, and is easily transmitted to susceptible calves or sheep by as few as 2500 lymphocytes from infected animals. Experimental transmission has also been accomplished with milk and colostrum, both of which contain lymphocytes, but this route is likely unimportant. In utero transmission of BLV has been documented, but occurs infrequently. The transmission of BLV by hematophagous flies and ticks has been demonstrated experimentally; however, field observations do not support a major role for such vectors. BLV-infected cattle with virus-induced persistent lymphocytosis are major reservoirs of the virus and pose the greatest risk for transmission.

Pathogenesis and Pathology. Most BLV infections are asymptomatic. There is a brief viremia soon after infection of susceptible cattle, followed by a long incubation period when the virus remains quiescent as provirus that is randomly integrated into the genome of infected cells. Only a low percentage of BLV-infected animals ever develop lymphoma, suggesting that the incubation period for induction of neoplasia is longer than the lifespan of many infected animals. Some cattle develop only a transient viremia without seroconversion, and after 3–4 months virus can no longer be isolated, whereas others develop persistent lymphocytosis within months or years after infection.

Neoplasms in cattle with EBL typically involve any combination of internal and superficial lymph nodes, heart, abomasum, intestines, kidneys, uterus, liver, spleen, epidural space of the lumbar spinal cord, and retrobulbar fat (of the eye). Distribution of the tumor is unpredictable, but blood is often not involved. Both T lymphocytes and B lymphocytes can be infected with BLV, but the tumors are composed only of proliferating B lymphocytes.

Host Response to Infection. Most BLV-infected cattle develop antibodies to BLV structural proteins. A greater response is usually detected to the glycosylated proteins gp51 and gp30 than to the internal proteins p24, p15, p12, and p10 and to the RT. Whereas most infected cattle develop high titers of virus-specific antibodies, some remain persistently seronegative.

Antibodies to BLV are also detected in the milk and colostrum and are partially protective against infection of calves. Antibodies do not provide protection against tumor development in infected animals, however, and do not prevent the spread of infectious BLV by carriers.

Laboratory Diagnosis

A variety of serologic tests (agar gel immunodiffusion (AGID), immunofluorescence, and ELISA) that detect BLV-specific antibody can be used. The animal usually becomes seropositive 4–12 weeks after viral exposure. BLV induces syncytia in target cells.

Treatment and Control

Infection, once established, appears to be lifelong in infected cattle. There is no treatment for lymphoma or BLV infection in cattle. BLV can be eliminated from a herd by repeated serologic testing and immediate removal of positive animals.

Walleye Dermal Sarcoma Virus—*Epsilonretrovirus* Genus

Disease

Proliferative skin lesions in walleye fish were first reported from Oneida Lake in New York State in the late 1960s. Since then these diseases have been reported in the United States and Canada. Retroviruses from two proliferative skin lesions in walleye (*Sander vitreus*), walleye dermal sarcoma (WDS) and walleye epidermal hyperplasia (WEH), have been isolated and demonstrated to be responsible. About 10% of walleyes can be affected with WEH and up to 27% with WDS yearly in Oneida Lake. One of the most fascinating aspects of these proliferative diseases is its seasonal nature. Young walleye will present with the lesions in late fall and winter and the lesions will spontaneously regress in the spring. Lesions are rarely observed in the summer months.

Etiologic Agent

The epsilonretroviruses include three fish retroviruses: WDSV and walleye epidermal hyperplasia viruses type 1 and type 2 (WEHV-1, WEHV-2). There are two additional viruses, which may be added to this group upon completion of their genome sequences, perch epidermal hyperplasia virus types 1 and 2. The exogenous piscine retroviruses, snakehead retrovirus and salmon swim bladder sarcoma-associated virus (SSSV), have not yet been assigned to a specific genus.

Physical, Chemical, and Antigenic Properties. WDSV was originally cloned from tumor DNA in 1990 and found to be 12.7 kb in length. Sequence analysis identified, in addition to gag, pro, pol and env, three open reading frames, designated orf a, orf b and orf c, that encode viral accessory proteins related to cellular cyclin (orfa), RACK1 (orfb) and a proapoptotic (orfc) protein.

Infectivity for Other Species and Culture Systems. Dermal sarcoma can be experimentally transmitted to several perch species, sauger (*Stizostedion canadense*) and yellow perch (*Perca flavescens*).

Host–Virus Relationship

Distribution, Reservoir, and Transmission. The virus and host have developed a delicate balance that allows significant transmission of the virus with minimal mortality in the host species. Tumors develop in the fall and winter months with minimal virus replication and when water temperatures warm in the spring, virus replication greatly increases in the tumor cells resulting in significant shedding of virus during spawning (highest fish densities) and regression of the tumors. Young fish are more susceptible to the virus and development of tumors. Evidence indicates that one season of tumor development and regression provides immunity into adulthood.

Pathogenesis and Pathology. The lesions are cutaneous mesenchymal neoplasms that are found on any portion of the fish, arise from the superficial surface of the scales and range in size from 0.1–1.0 cm in diameter (see Figure 66.7). If extensive, individual skin tumors can merge to form large neoplasms with lymphocytic infiltrates. The tumors consist of nodular masses of fibroblasts on the epidermis. The tumors are not encapsulated and frequently become ulcerated when regressing. The ulceration during regression occurs at a time of maximal virus shedding. Spread of the tumor below the dermis is only occasionally observed. The timing of the entire process is elegant since maximal virus shedding occurs in the spring at a time of maximal fish-to-fish contact. The virus induces both the

FIGURE 66.7. *Dermal sarcomas on a yearling walleye. (Image courtesy of P.R. Bowser, Cornell University.)*

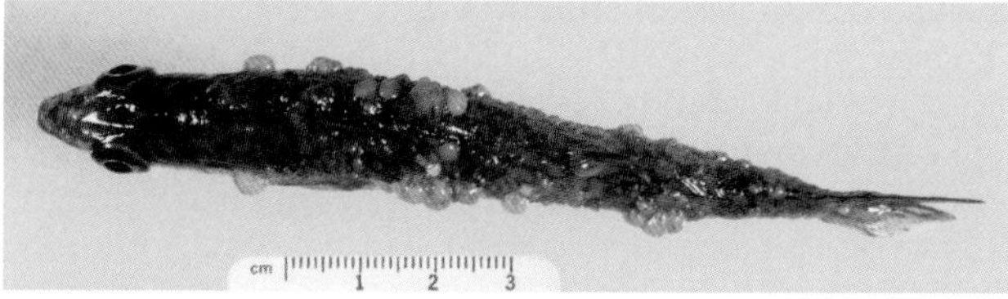

proliferation of virus-infected cells (fall and winter) as well as the regression of those cells (spring) for maximal virus production. The orfa (viral cyclin) and orfb (RACK1-like) proteins are expressed during cellular proliferation consistent with the concept that these proteins induce that proliferation during times of low viral gene expression. The orfc protein is a proapoptic protein that is expressed only during periods of high virus expression and replication consistent with tumor regression.

Host Response to Infection. This is an infection and disease of mostly young walleye. Evidence indicates that infection, development of tumors and regression of tumors is a once in a lifetime event. This suggests that host immunity develops as a result of this cycle. Inflammatory responses at lesional sites are occasionally observed.

Laboratory Diagnosis

Gross lesions along with histopathologic observation can be utilized. The spontaneous regression upon the arrival of warmer temperatures is also an indicator of this disease.

Treatment and Control

No treatment or control measures have been applied to this viral disease. Theoretically, isolation of fish with dermal lesions from unaffected fish during the winter months when there is little virus shedding that occurs through the spring when tumors regress (high virus shedding) should prevent the transmission that occurs in the spring months. Recovered fish should no longer have the capacity to harbor and transmit virus.

Visna/Maedi/Progressive Pneumonia Viruses and Caprine Arthritis Encephalitis Virus—*Lentivirus* Genus

Disease

These viruses cause several different diseases that involve the lungs, joints, mammary glands, and CNS of affected sheep and goats. Initial signs of visna are subtle and insidious, consisting of a slight aberration of gait, especially of the hindquarters; trembling of the lips, unnatural tilting of the head; and in rare instances, blindness. The signs progress to paresis or even total paralysis. Fever is absent. Unattended animals die of inanition, hence the name visna, which means "wasting" in Icelandic. Signs of visna typically occur in sheep over 2 years of age, and the clinical course is protracted.

Maedi and progressive pneumonia viruses cause a similar chronic pneumonia in infected sheep. Early manifestations include progressive loss of condition accompanied by dyspnea. Eventually, breathing requires the use of accessory muscles and is accompanied by rhythmic jerks of the head. There is sometimes a dry cough, but no nasal discharge. The clinical phase is protracted, although affected animals often die from secondary bacterial pneumonia.

Caprine arthritis-encephalitis virus (CAEV) induces several disease syndromes in domestic goats, including chronic progressive arthritis, mastitis, and occasionally interstitial pneumonia in older goats, and an acute paralytic syndrome in kids that is characterized by hind limb ataxia, weakness, and paralysis.

Etiologic Agent

Classification. The agent of visna/maedi/progressive pneumonia and the closely related organism of CAEV are lentiviruses. The name designations are largely historical and refer to the site of virus isolation or the predominant pathology in an individual animal. Ovine progressive pneumonia virus is synonymous with maedi virus.

Physical, Chemical, and Antigenic Properties. The virion is composed of four structural proteins designated gp135, p30, p16, and p14. Minor structural proteins include a RT, integrase, and dUTPase. Neutralization tests have shown that variations in virus strains occur during infection in individual animals. If an animal is inoculated with plaque-purified virus, many months later viruses can be isolated that are not neutralized by antiserum that neutralizes the original inoculum strain. Both the inoculum strain and the variant strains can be isolated simultaneously, indicating that new strains do not replace parental virus. With time, neutralizing antibodies are produced to the new strains.

The RT of these viruses has a preference for Mg^{2+} and uses $tRNA^{Lys}$ as a primer for negative-strand DNA reverse transcription.

Visna/maedi/progressive pneumonia virus and CAEV show extensive cross-reaction by immunodiffusion assays involving the major structural protein.

Resistance to Physical and Chemical Agents. Lentiviruses are relatively resistant to ultraviolet irradiation. Infectivity is abolished by lipid solvents, periodate, phenol, trypsin, ribonuclease, formaldehyde, and low pH (less than 4.2). Infectivity is relatively stable at 0–4 °C in the presence of serum, but infectivity is rapidly destroyed at 56 °C.

Infectivity for Other Species and Culture Systems. Visna and ovine progressive pneumonia have been described only in sheep and goats. Some breeds of sheep appear to be more susceptible, especially Icelandic sheep, which are highly inbred. The visna virus infects cells derived from many vertebrate species but replicates efficiently only in sheep cells. Unadapted virus isolates replicate best in macrophage cultures.

Host–Virus Relationship

Distribution, Reservoir, and Transmission. These viruses cause disease in sheep and goats throughout much of the world. The frequency of infection varies widely based on control programs, but can range to greater than 75% in some flocks in the United States. Infected sheep serve as the reservoir.

Transmission is via respiratory exudates and aerosol. Virus is excreted in the milk, and lambs raised on infected ewes are infected at a young age. Infection rates are increased by practices that pool milk. Intrauterine transmission is infrequent.

Pathogenesis and Pathology. The ovine lentiviruses infect cells of the monocyte–macrophage system. Visna is a chronic and progressive encephalomyelitis characterized by multifocal areas of chronic inflammation with accompanying demyelination. The process begins immediately beneath the ependyma bordering the ventricles, but spreads throughout the brain and spinal cord.

The lungs of sheep with progressive pneumonia are markedly expanded, with as much as a two- or threefold increase in lung weight. The histopathologic changes include thickening of the interalveolar septa as a result of infiltration of lymphocytes, monocytes, and macrophages. The thickening may be so pronounced as to obliterate the alveoli. Lymphoid accumulations with the formation of follicles and germinal centers are scattered throughout the lung parenchyma.

Some adult sheep infected with ovine lentiviruses develop chronic arthritis and/or mastitis.

Caprine arthritis encephalitis virus (CAEV) causes a peculiar motor spinal dysfunction in goat kids at 2–4 months of age. The lesions in affected goats resemble those of visna. Goats that survive infection with CAEV as kids often develop progressive, chronic arthritis, mastitis, and, occasionally, interstitial pneumonia that resembles ovine progressive pneumonia.

Host Response to Infection. Most lentivirus infections of ruminants are subclinical, likely because of the prolonged incubation period of the diseases these viruses induce. Lesions in all of these diseases include chronic, ongoing inflammation; thus, the lesions themselves likely result in part from the host's immune response.

In experimental infections, complement-fixing antibodies appear a few weeks after inoculation, rise to a maximum within 2 months, and remain constant throughout the course of disease. Neutralizing antibodies appear later, reach a maximum at about 1 year, and then remain constant. However, the virus persists despite a vigorous humoral immune response, possibly because most infected cells are not producing viral antigens and are, therefore, undetectable by the immune surveillance mechanisms.

Laboratory Diagnosis

In its early stages, visna is difficult to distinguish from other CNS diseases; however, the progressive protracted course, the absence of fever, and the pleocytosis in the cerebrospinal fluid (CSF) are all characteristic of visna. Tremor of the head, grinding of teeth, and intense itching are more characteristic of scrapie than visna.

Virus can be isolated from CNS, lung, spleen, peripheral blood leukocytes, and CSF, but because of the limited viral replication can be difficult. Group-specific tests that detect antibodies that appear early and are maintained throughout the disease are preferred over serum neutralization for serologic diagnosis. Neutralization tests are of less value in diagnosis because they become positive much later in disease and are strain specific. Thus, serologic tests such as AGID are now used to identify lentivirus-infected sheep and goats.

Treatment and Control

No effective vaccine currently exists and no useful therapeutic agents are available. Control of these viruses and their diseases is by serologic testing and the elimination of infected animals. Visna and maedi were eliminated from Iceland as the result of an eradication program.

Equine Infectious Anemia Virus—*Lentivirus* Genus

Disease

Equine infectious anemia virus (EIAV) can cause severe anemia in horses, but the clinical presentation of EIA is highly variable. In the acute form, signs develop suddenly 7–21 days postinfection. Signs can include fever, anorexia, thrombocytopenia, and severe anemia. There may also be profuse sweating and a serous discharge from the nose. Such attacks often last for 3–5 days, after which the animal appears to recover. Horses in the early acute stage of the disease are seronegative for EIA.

Subacute disease often follows the acute infection after a convalescence of 2–4 weeks. Acute signs are repeated along with weakness, edema, petechiae, lethargy, depression, anemia, and ataxia. The animal again appears to recover and the cycle may then recur.

Chronic EIA is the classical presentation of so-called swamp fever, which resembles the subacute form but is milder and seldom leads to death. The cycle of fever, weight loss, anorexia, and clinical signs can recur six or more times. Each episode usually lasts 3–5 days, and the interval between cycles is irregular (weeks to months). The frequency and severity usually decrease after 6–8 episodes, usually within the first year. Most horses are then without clinical signs but carry the virus for the remainder of their lives. EIA can be induced by stress or immunosuppressive drugs.

EIAV infection in horses generally results in clinical signs that are inapparent, subclinical, or mild. These horses remain asymptomatic but have antibody to the virus and are lifelong carriers of the virus. Asymptomatic but chronically viremic (low viral load) animals have been observed for periods in excess of 18 years.

Etiologic Agent

Classification. EIAV is a Lentivirus, and was the first animal disease to be identified as caused by a filterable virus (1904).

Physical, Chemical, and Antigenic Properties. EIAV is composed of two envelope-encoded glycoproteins (gp 90 = SU and gp 45 = TM) and four major nonglycosylated proteins (p26 = CA, p15 = MA, p11 = NC, and p9). The p26 is the major core protein and demonstrates group specificity, while the envelope-associated glycoproteins demonstrate hemagglutination activity and are type specific.

The EIAV genome is highly mutable. When the virus is placed under selective pressure by the host immune system, individual nucleotide substitutions (mutations) produce novel antigenic variants of the gp 45 and gp 90 envelope proteins. It is thought that these antigenic variants cause EIA's characteristic episodic recurrence. In cell culture (where there is no immune selection), antigenic types remain stable and neutralizable by serum antibodies from the horse from which the virus was isolated. When introduced into a new horse, these same strains produce new antigenic viral variants that no longer are neutralized by the original antibodies.

Resistance to Physical and Chemical Agents. EIAV is readily inactivated by common disinfectants that contain detergents. The virus is also inactivated by sodium hydroxide, sodium hypochlorite, most organic solvents, and chlorhexidine. EIAV heated in horse serum at 58 °C for 30 min shows no infectivity for horses. However, at 25 °C, EIAV remains infectious on hypodermic needles for 96 h.

Infectivity for Other Species and Culture Systems. Horses, ponies, donkeys, and mules are susceptible to infection by EIAV. There is only one report of human infection, and no cases of EIA-like disease have been identified. Attempts to propagate the virus in lambs, mice, hamsters, guinea pigs, and rabbits have failed. Primary isolates of EIAV can be propagated only in equine leukocyte cultures, where it grows in cells of the monocyte/macrophage lineage. Laboratory strains of EIAV can be propagated in a variety of cell lines from several species, including human fetal lung fibroblasts. These laboratory strains display significant sequence differences from primary isolates, particularly in the U3 region of the LTR.

Host–Virus Relationship

Distribution, Reservoir, and Transmission. The distribution of EIAV is worldwide but is most prevalent in warm climates. Infection rates vary widely but the disease is increasingly rare in countries such as the United States. Horses, donkeys, and mules are the only known reservoirs and natural hosts of the virus.

Mechanical inoculation of blood is considered the major mode of EIAV transmission. EIAV is naturally transmitted by hematophagous insects, especially deer and stable flies. EIAV does not replicate in the insect cells, but flies can transmit the virus by simple mechanical transfer of infected blood. The transmission of EIAV via blood can also be through contaminated needles; thus it is important not to share needles or use unsterilized needles in veterinary procedures. Viral transmission to the nursing foal from a carrier mare is well documented. EIAV can also be transmitted in utero but this is probably rare.

Pathogenesis and Pathology. Acute EIA is related to massive viral replication. Anemia reflects reduced life span of red blood cells (RBCs) as a consequence of hemolysis and erythrophagocytosis by activated macrophages. A decrease in complement levels and the presence of complement-coated erythrocytes have been observed in EIAV-infected horses. Decreased erythropoiesis levels and perturbations in iron metabolism also contribute to anemia in chronic cases.

Lesions of EIA reflect the duration and severity of infection and disease, and can include widespread hemorrhage and necrosis of lymphatic tissues, anemia, edema, and emaciation. Microscopic lesions include activation of the mononuclear phagocytic system in all lymphoid tissues, activation of Kupffer cells, and hemosiderin deposition in many organs. Immune complex-mediated glomerulonephritis and hepatic centrolobular necrosis are common, the latter as a consequence of severe, acute-onset anemia. Granulomatous ependymitis, meningitis, choroiditis, subependymal encephalitis, and hydrocephalus are associated with ataxia.

Host Response to Infection. Horses infected with EIAV develop persisting antibody titers within 45 days. Most animals become ELISA-positive within 12 days and AGID-positive within 24 days of infection.

Laboratory Diagnosis

Laboratory diagnosis depends on the detection of specific antibody using an AGID test (Coggins test). More sensitive ELISA tests are also now available.

Treatment and Control

No specific treatments are available. Supportive therapy is the most important factor in recovery.

Affected animals should be either euthanized because the virus is contagious or physically isolated. Spread of EIAV can be reduced by control of stable flies and mosquitoes. Repeated use of hypodermic needles and transfusions from untested donors must be avoided.

Infected stallions should not be bred to seronegative mares, although the reverse need not be true. Uninfected foals can usually be obtained from positive mares and positive stallions if they are isolated from the infected mare and her milk.

A vaccine against EIAV is used in some countries (Cuba, China) but probably does not provide broad protection against all variants of EIAV.

Bovine Immunodeficiency Virus—*Lentivirus* Genus

Disease

Despite its provocative name, the significance of bovine immunodeficiency virus (BIV) as a cause of immune dysregulation and chronic inflammation in cattle is uncertain. Unsubstantiated reports implicate BIV as a cause of lethargy, mastitis, pneumonia, lymphadenopathy, and chronic dermatitis, but these reports are viewed with increasing skepticism. A closely related virus, Jembrana disease virus, has been described in Bali cattle (*Bos javanicus* in Indonesia). Disease symptoms in these cattle consist of fever, anorexia, lymphadenopathy and occasionally death.

Etiologic Agent

Classification. BIV is a lentivirus that is not closely related to any other known lentivirus.

Physical, Chemical, and Antigenic Properties. The morphology and physical properties of BIV closely resemble those of other lentiviruses. BIV has an SU glycoprotein of 100 kd and a TM glycoprotein of 45 kd, and Gag proteins, MA, CA, and NC, of 16, 26, and 7 kd, respectively. BIV also produces several nonstructural proteins. The RT of BIV has a preference for Mg2+.

Infectivity for Other Species and Culture Systems. Experimental infection of rabbits and sheep with BIV is possible, but these animals do not develop disease. BIV can be cultured in cells from a variety of species, including bovine, rabbit, and canine, but not primates or humans.

Host–Virus Relationship

Distribution, Reservoir, and Transmission. The distribution of BIV is probably worldwide. In the United States, the prevalence of BIV infection is low but may be much higher in individual herds. Herds infected with BIV are often also infected with BLV.

Pathogenesis and Pathology. Cells of the monocyte/macrophage support replication of BIV in infected cattle.

Host Response to Infection. BIV infection in cattle results in a strong host antibody response. However, like most other lentiviruses, BIV induces a chronic lifelong infection. The vast majority of infections are subclinical.

Laboratory Diagnosis

Infected cattle can be detected by serologic tests for antibodies to BIV. BIV isolation from blood can also be used to detect infected animals.

Treatment and Control. There is no vaccine or treatment for BIV infection. The importance of BIV infection as a pathogen of cattle remains most uncertain.

Feline Immunodeficiency Virus—*Lentivirus* Genus

Disease

Feline immunodeficiency virus (FIV) infection of cats produces acute fever and lymphadenopathy, followed by an asymptomatic carrier phase. In some cats, FIV infection causes profound immunodeficiency leading to secondary chronic infections. FIV infection of cats shares common features with AIDS of humans and FIV infection of cats has become an important animal model for AIDS research.

Etiologic Agent

Classification. FIV is a lentivirus that is not closely related to any other known lentivirus.

Physical, Chemical, and Antigenic Properties. The morphology and physical properties of FIV closely resemble those of other lentiviruses. FIV has an SU glycoprotein of 95kd and a TM glycoprotein of 41 kd, and Gag proteins, MA, CA, and NC, of 16, 27, and 10 kd, respectively. FIV also codes for several nonstructural proteins. The RT of FIV has a preference for Mg^{2+}.

Resistance to Physical and Chemical Agents. FIV is inactivated by appropriate concentrations of disinfectants such as chlorine, quaternary ammonium compounds, phenolic compounds, and alcohol. It survives at 60 °C for only a few minutes.

Infectivity for Other Species and Culture Systems. FIV infects domestic cats, although there is serologic evidence that FIV-like viruses infect wild Felidae in Africa (lions, cheetahs) and the Americas (puma, bobcats, jaguars). FIV isolates replicate in primary cultures of feline mononuclear cultures stimulated to divide with mitogen and supplemented with interleukin-2 (IL-2; T cell growth factor). Some isolates of FIV are also able to replicate in established feline cell lines. FIV does not replicate in nonfeline cell lines. There is no link between FIV and any human disease, including AIDS.

Host–Virus Relationship

Distribution, Reservoir, and Transmission. FIV is endemic in cats throughout the world, although the virus is not as contagious as FeLV. FIV is shed in saliva, and the most important route of transmission is probably through bites. Free-roaming male cats, which are most likely to fight, are most frequently infected with FIV. The virus is not efficiently spread by casual, nonaggressive contact among cats. Sexual contact probably is also not a primary means of spreading FIV. Transmission from an infected queen to her kittens can occur.

Cats remain infected with FIV for life, although the majority of FIV infections are clinically silent.

Dual infection of FIV and FeLV is not uncommon, and cats infected with both FIV and FeLV appear to have a more severe disease course.

Pathogenesis and Pathology. There are no definitive gross or histologic changes in the tissues of FIV-infected cats, even in more advanced stages of disease. Following initial infection, the virus replicates in regional lymph nodes, and then spreads to lymph nodes throughout the body, sometimes resulting in a transient generalized lymphadenopathy. Most infections are asymptomatic, whereas lymphoid depletion and immune suppression occur in some cats that are then susceptible to secondary opportunistic infections. FIV appears to infect both CD4 and CD8 lymphocytes, as well as macrophages *in vivo*. Many cats manifest an absolute decrease in the number of CD4 lymphocytes with an inversion of the CD4/CD8 ratio.

Host Response to Infection. Infected cats typically respond with vigorous humoral (antibody) and cell-mediated immune responses. These responses appear to be sufficient to limit the initial acute phase of the disease. Like most lentiviruses, however, FIV is never eliminated. It probably produces various degrees of subclinical immune dysfunction in the majority and clinically significant immunodeficiency and associated secondary infections in a minority, of infected cats.

Laboratory Diagnosis

FIV infection is most easily diagnosed by detecting antibodies in the blood. Antibody to FIV can be detected using ELISA tests, Western immunoblotting, and indirect fluorescent antibody (IFA). The Snap® Test (Idexx) or ELISA is often used as a first screening test, followed by Western blot as a confirmatory test. FIV infection can also be diagnosed by virus isolation and PCR to detect FIV nucleic acid.

Young kittens may be antibody positive (and thus have a positive test result) without actually being infected with FIV due to passive transfer of FIV antibodies from their mother.

Treatment and Control

Treatment of FIV-associated disease is largely supportive. Secondary and opportunistic infections are treated with appropriate antimicrobial therapy. Control of FIV infection is by avoiding contact with stray cats and avoiding cat fights. A vaccine is available that has been shown to provide some protection from infection.

Simian Immunodeficiency Virus—*Lentivirus* Genus

Disease

The SIV comprises a number of lentiviruses indigenous in many simian species living in the wild in Africa. In their natural African simian hosts, these viruses apparently cause little or no disease. In contrast, the Asian macaques, which are not infected with SIV in the wild, are susceptible to a fatal immunosuppressive syndrome called SAIDS when infected by some strains of SIV.

SIV-infected Asian macaques often develop a transient skin rash soon after infection. Lymph nodes and spleen may be initially enlarged. The architecture of lymph nodes becomes disrupted and eventually atrophies. The main clinical features of SAIDS in Asian macaques are wasting and persistent diarrhea. Opportunistic infections occur and often persist in the immunocompromised monkey. Virtually all Asian macaques infected with pathogenic SIV strains develop fatal SAIDS within 2 months to 3 years.

The fatal immunodeficiency disease caused by SIV in Asian macaques is the major animal model for AIDS in humans. Further, an awareness of the biology of SIV is important for the occupational health of animal caretakers, technicians, and veterinarians who handle monkeys, as well as use of primates in biomedical research and medicine. Artificially generated simian/human immunodeficiency virus (SHIV) strains of virus have been constructed that contain HIV-derived envelope genes with SIV-derived genomes that have been used extensively in the laboratory for studying immunity and pathogenesis to HIV envelope proteins in a nonhuman primate model system.

Etiologic Agent

Classification. The primate lentiviruses exist as a broad continuum. For example, the prototype SIV isolate from Asian macaques (designated SIVmac) is only about 50% related to HIV-1, but is 75% related to HIV-2 based on nucleic acid sequence. Other SIV isolates from chimpanzees (SIVcpz) are much more closely related to HIV-1 than to HIV-2. Further, some SIV isolates from other African primate species are even closer to HIV-2 than is SIVmac. Many isolates of SIV and HIV have been made and their nucleic acids sequenced and classified in phylogenetic trees of sequence relatedness in an effort to understand the origin of AIDS and the diversity and epidemiologic potentials of the primate lentiviruses.

Physical, Chemical, and Antigenic Properties. The morphology and physical properties of SIV closely resemble those of other lentiviruses. SIV has an SU glycoprotein of 120 kd and a TM glycoprotein of 32 kd, and Gag - proteins, MA, CA, and NC of 16, 28, and 8 kd, respectively. SIV also codes for several nonstructural proteins that - function in regulation of viral expression and accessory functions.

The RT of SIV has a preference for Mg^{2+} and uses $tRNA^{Lys}$ as a primer for negative-strand DNA reverse transcription.

On the basis of seroepidemiologic data, as many as 30 distinct SIV strains may be harbored in their African monkey hosts. The prototype SIVmac strain is antigenically more closely related to HIV-2 than to HIV-1, in agreement with the sequence homology overall. SIV isolated from chimpanzees, SIVcpz, however, is more closely related to HIV-1 than to other SIV types.

Infectivity for Other Species and Culture Systems. SIV isolates replicate in primate (including human) lymphocyte cultures in stimulated cells that have a CD4 receptor. SIV isolates do not replicate in nonprimate cells. Cross-species transmission of SIV to humans is possible and SIV has infected humans in laboratory accidents. HIV is able to infect chimpanzees, although it is not highly pathogenic.

Host–Virus Relationship

Distribution, Reservoir, and Transmission. SIV is carried as an apparently harmless infection in its natural hosts, species of African nonhuman primates (Cercopithecus, including African green monkeys, and Cercocebus, including sooty mangabeys). The prevalence of infection in both zoos and in the wild is variable, but can be over 50%. In Asian macaques, in which the SIV is not found in nature, SIV produces a fatal immunodeficiency disease that has many features in common with AIDS.

Transmission of SIV is by biting and also by poor veterinary practices or intentionally by experimental protocol. Mother-to-infant and sexual transmission is thought to occur rather inefficiently in nature.

Pathogenesis and Pathology. Asian macaques in the initial stages of illness tend to have hyperplastic lymphoid tissues, whereas lymphoid depletion characterizes later stages of the disease. The types of lesions vary greatly depending on the presence of secondary infections and the stage of disease. SIV persists in both Asian macaques and its natural hosts despite a strong humoral and cellular immune response; however, fatal immunosuppression soon occurs in infected macaques. Neutralization escape mutants arise and become the dominant phenotype. The kinetics of viral infection and alteration of CD4 lymphocytes parallel those observed in human HIV-1 infection and provide reliable markers for disease progression.

Host Response to Infection. Infected monkeys generally respond with vigorous antibody responses and cell-mediated immune responses. These responses appear to be sufficient to limit the initial acute phase of SIV infection. Like most lentiviruses, however, SIV is never eliminated in either its natural host or in Asian macaques.

Laboratory Diagnosis

SIV infection is most easily diagnosed by detecting antibodies in the blood. Antibody to SIV can be detected using indirect fluorescent antibody, Western blots, and ELISA tests. SIV infection can also be diagnosed by virus isolation, detection of viral antigen, and PCR to detect SIV nucleic acid.

Treatment and Control

Experimental vaccines and therapies are being evaluated as part of the current massive efforts in AIDS research and development. To date, the more effective approaches have involved the use of nef (accessory gene) deleted live viruses. These have provided the best efficacy for resisting challenge with virulent viruses in adult macaques. However, use of nef deleted live viruses in juvenile macaques has resulted in the development of some disease, likely due to the ability to partially restore some nef function(s). Further studies hope to capitalize on the efficacy of these deleted live virus vaccines and minimize the potential of reversion to virulence.

Reference

Yamamoto JK, Sparger E, Ho EW *et al.* (1988) Pathogenesis of experimentally induced feline immunodeficiency virus infection in cats. *Am J Vet Res*, **49**, 1246.

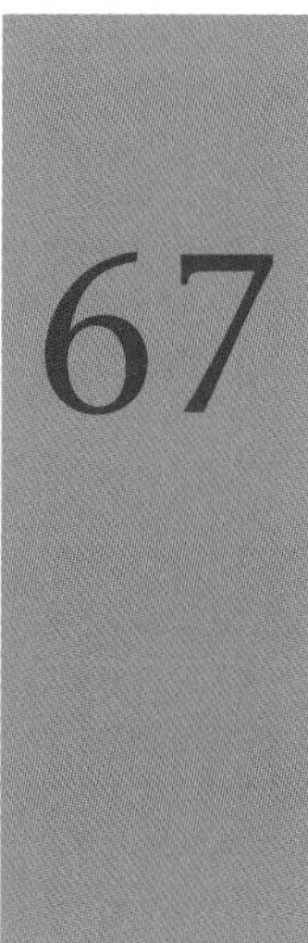

67 Transmissible Spongiform Encephalopathies

DONGSEOB TARK AND JUERGEN A. RICHT

Transmissible spongiform encephalopathy (TSE) is the collective term given to a unique group of progressive, uniformly fatal, degenerative, central nervous system (CNS) diseases of humans and animals that share a similar pattern of clinical disease, neuropathology, pathogenesis, and etiology. While human TSEs are inherited (15%), sporadic (80%), and infectious (5%), most animal TSEs are infectious diseases that can be transmitted to susceptible hosts. For many years the identification of the infectious cause remained elusive, but Stanley Prusiner postulated in 1982 that an abnormal host protein called a prion (derived from "proteinaceous infectious particles"; abbreviated as PrP^{Res}, PrP^{Sc}, PrP^{BSE}, or PrP^{CWD}) was the infectious agent and that propagation of this protein was a post-translational event, not requiring nucleic acid or genetic material. Prusiner's "protein-only" hypothesis suggests that an abnormal prion protein (PrP^{Sc} as a misfolded scrapie form of the normal prion protein) is able to induce the conversion of the cellular prion protein (PrP^{C}) to the abnormal PrP^{Sc}; this mechanism can explain both the heritable and infectious disease presentations of the TSEs. Since his initial proposal, a large body of research work by Prusiner and others has been published that supports his original hypothesis and Prusiner received the Nobel Prize for his work in 1997. The concept of the prion as an infectious agent is now widely accepted, and a few believe that genetic material associated with the prion agent still may be found. Counterhypotheses include: (i) the virion hypothesis, which suggests that the infectious organism has a small central core of nucleic acid protected and/or surrounded by protein; and (ii) some sort of unconventional virus or bacteria that have been proposed as critical factors related to pathogenesis and propagation of the TSE pathogen. Given the vast amount of research work supporting the prion hypothesis, and the apparent lack of data supporting the other hypotheses, the remainder of this discussion is based on the premise that the prion is the infectious etiology for this group of diseases.

TSEs generally have a limited host range. So far, human TSEs have been exclusively found in humans (excluding experimental studies). They include two forms of Creutzfeldt–Jakob disease (CJD), Gerstmann–Sträussler—Scheinker syndrome (GSS), fatal familial insomnia, Kuru, and variant CJD (vCJD), which is the exception because of its relationship with bovine spongiform encephalopathy (BSE). Some of these human TSEs (familial CJD, GSS, and fatal familial insomnia) are inherited, while sporadic CJD occurs spontaneously at a rate of one per million population per year. The animal TSEs are considered to be mainly infectious and, with the notable exception of BSE, they have a narrow host range. The animal TSEs and their respective natural hosts include scrapie in sheep and goats, BSE in cattle and other species (exotic ungulate encephalopathy in exotic ungulates, feline spongiform encephalopathy in felids, and vCJD in humans), transmissible mink encephalopathy in mink, and chronic wasting disease in deer, elk, and moose. While there are many similarities shared by all TSE diseases, there are also salient differences in the behavior of the various TSEs, most notably related to their tissue distribution within hosts, their means of transmission, and very importantly the zoonotic potential of BSE. Additionally, atypical prions have been reported in scrapie and BSE. Interestingly, atypical scrapie ("Nor98" or "Nor98-like" scrapie) cases were detected in sheep having classical scrapie-resistant genotypes. There have been three types of BSE agents characterized so far: (i) classical; (ii) high molecular weight or H-type; and (iii) low molecular weight or L-type BSE. Atypical BSE and scrapie agents may be spontaneously occurring or genetic forms of prions.

Original chapter written by Drs. Barr and Zee.

Scrapie Disease

Scrapie (referred to as "classical scrapie") is the prototype of the prion diseases and is a chronic, progressive, and

Veterinary Microbiology, Third Edition. Edited by D. Scott McVey, Melissa Kennedy and M.M. Chengappa.

uniformly fatal degenerative CNS disease that occurs naturally in only sheep and goats. There is no evidence to indicate that scrapie is a zoonosis. Classical scrapie can be differentiated from atypical scrapie. The unusual scrapie form was first detected in Norwegian sheep in 1998 and was designated Nor98 scrapie. Thereafter, Nor98-like strains of scrapie or "atypical scrapie" were reported in most of the European countries, as well as in North America.

Scrapie is endemic and occurs throughout the world including Europe, North America, Asia, and Africa with a few exceptions (e.g., Australia and New Zealand). Interestingly, atypical scrapie was detected in Australia and New Zealand. Scrapie prevalence, based on current detection methodology, is low with less than 0.05% in endemic countries. Scrapie is caused by an abnormal prion protein designated PrP^{Sc} (prion protein, scrapie). Within the world's sheep population, there is a varying degree of susceptibility and resistance to classical scrapie following exposure to PrP^{Sc}. The reasons for this diversity in disease susceptibility are complex and poorly understood, although sheep breed and genotype, as well as the infecting PrP^{Sc} strain, likely all play some role. For scrapie and atypical scrapie, the genotype of individual sheep at codons 136, 141, 154, and 171 within the prion protein sequence is a major factor in determining the degree of disease susceptibility and/or resistance. Codons 136 and 171 are critical for classical scrapie, whereas codon 141 of the PrP gene is closely related with susceptibility to atypical scrapie. Like all TSEs, scrapie has a rather long incubation period from infection to the onset of clinical signs, ranging roughly from 18 to 60 months. The progression of clinical signs is directly correlated with the progressive accumulation and spread of PrP^{Sc} throughout the CNS, and is accompanied by a unique pattern of degenerative and vacuolar lesions in the CNS that is shared by all TSEs. Many cases of atypical/Nor98 scrapie have been identified during active surveillance of culled or fallen stock and even clinically normal sheep at slaughter. Atypical scrapie is frequently diagnosed in sheep without neurological findings and pruritus, which is different from classic scrapie; however, ataxia was reported in several cases. In the majority of cases, atypical scrapie has been detected as a single case in herd tested. Therefore, atypical scrapie is considered to be a low-contagious or noncontagious prion disease under natural conditions.

Scrapie is spread by direct contact with infected sheep, probably through oral infection (i.e., ingestion) of PrP^{Sc}. It is also possible that natural infection could occur infrequently through scarified mucous membranes. Scrapie can be experimentally transmitted by inoculation, including transmission through large volume blood transfusions from infected sheep. This suggests that there is a low level of PrP^{Sc} in the blood of scrapie-infected sheep. Indeed, PrP^{Sc} was detected in leukocytes from sheep, clinically infected with scrapie using protein misfolding cyclic amplification (PMCA). A recent study also shows that scrapie infectivity is associated with various blood components such as peripheral blood mononuclear cells, B cells, platelets, and plasma cells of classical scrapie-infected sheep.

Natural contact transmission occurs most frequently when naive sheep or goats are exposed to infected ewes shedding PrP^{Sc} at, or soon after, lambing, and this transmission likely results from the expulsion of PrP^{Sc}-infected placenta and/or contaminated fetal/uterine fluids. There is as yet no clear evidence of true vertical transmission (either true genetic transmission or in utero transmission). Lambs appear to be more susceptible to infection than adults. Epidemiologic studies suggest that indirect transmission of scrapie also occurs through exposure to contaminated environments where scrapie-infected sheep have previously been kept. For example, on a previously scrapie-infected farm in Iceland, scrapie was diagnosed in lambs about 2 years after restocking. This farm had not been disinfected after the culling of scrapie-infected sheep 16 years earlier. This means that infectious scrapie agent could persist for a long time in the environment. This likely occurs more often where there has been previous high-density confinement of scrapie-infected animals and especially where previous lambing has taken place. One study suggests that scrapie can be transmitted via hay mites in contaminated environments.

The clinical signs of scrapie are progressive and consist of one or more of the following CNS signs: behavioral changes, locomotor problems (incoordination, paresis, proprioceptive limb deficits, and hypermetria), mild head or neck tremors, hyperesthesia, and pruritus, often resulting in patchy wool loss from rubbing or biting. Behavioral changes include withdrawal from the flock, nervousness, or aggression. Classical scrapie-infected sheep also progressively lose body condition. A classic behavior often used to aid in clinical diagnosis of scrapie consists of upward extension of the head and neck with an accompanying licking, nibbling motion, or teeth grinding in response to rubbing the sheep's rump region. However, it should be emphasized that the particular clinical signs seen in any individual infected animal are highly variable. On the contrary, the majority of the atypical scrapie cases including Nor98-like scrapie have been found through an active surveillance in clinically asymptomatic sheep and fallen stock. Generally, atypical scrapie-infected sheep showed ataxia, poor body condition, but no pruritus or loss of wool in most of the reported cases.

Etiologic Agent

It is generally accepted that the etiology of scrapie is a prion, an abnormal isoform of a normal host protein of sheep called PrP^{Sc}. PrP^{Sc} is very similar in its size and shares high homology in its amino acid sequence and similarity in its biochemical and physicochemical properties to abnormal prion proteins responsible for other TSEs. Much of the following expanded discussion of PrP^{Sc} (and scrapie) also holds true for other abnormal prions and the respective disease they cause. In the following discussion, the abbreviation PrP^{Res} (referring to "resistant" PrP) is used to reference all abnormal prion proteins as a group, and PrP^{Sc} to reference the specific abnormal prions causing scrapie.

Prion Origin, Structure, and Biochemistry

PrP^{Res} is derived from normal cellular proteins ("cellular prion protein" or PrP^{C}) that are found in multiple tissues of all mammalian species. They are cell membrane-associated proteins attached via a glycosyl phosphatidylinositol anchor. PrP^{C} is a 35–36 kDa protein that is especially abundant in the CNS (approximately 50 times more than in other tissues) within neurons and glial cells. It also occurs in cells of the mononuclear phagocytic system (macrophages, dendritic cells, and follicular dendritic cells). The precise function of PrP^{C} is uncertain. Possible functions include aspects of copper metabolism, interactions with the extracellular matrix, olfactory discrimination, and apoptosis and signal transduction. PrP^{C} does not cause disease. PrP^{Res} is identical in amino acid sequence and length to PrP^{C} of the host species, where they have replicated and differ only in their secondary and tertiary spatial conformation from their originating PrP^{C}. The tertiary conformational change in PrP^{Res} is the putative basis for transformation into an infectious pathogen that propagates and spreads within host tissues to cause disease. PrP^{Res} has a protease-resistant core (27–30 kDa; approximately 142 amino acids) designated PrP27-30, which has been found in brains from humans and animals with prion diseases. This smaller portion of the PrP^{Res} also retains infectivity. The PrP^{C} is derived from a single copy gene in humans and animals, the prion protein gene (PRNP or Prnp gene). While the precise nature of the structural changes between PrP^{C} and PrP^{Res} is still not determined, the central feature thought to be responsible for the physicochemical and infectious transformation of PrP^{Res} is a change in the portion of the alpha-helical and coil structure of PrP^{C} to a larger percentage of rigid beta-pleated sheets in PrP^{Res} (the percentage of beta-pleated sheets increases significantly with the transformation to PrP^{Res}). Once in a susceptible host, the propagation of new PrP^{Res} occurs by a post-translational event that does not involve DNA or RNA, whereby existent host PrP^{C} is transformed to PrP^{Res}. Experimental evidence suggests that the PrP^{Res} actually serves as a physical template for the conversion of PrP^{C} when the latter interacts with the PrP^{Res} template. The process also appears to require the presence of a second species-specific host protein ("X") that binds to PrP^{C} and facilitates the transformation to new PrP^{Res}. Once completed, the new PrP^{Res} can then serve as a new template for further propagation of PrP^{Res}. In the case of inherited TSEs of humans, mutations or insertions in the human Prnp gene are postulated to cause the resultant altered PrP^{C} to spontaneously convert to PrP^{Res}, which then can act as a template for the conversion of PrP^{C}.

Biochemically, PrP^{C} is labile and can be inactivated relatively easily by a variety of methods, such as enzyme digestion and heat. In contrast, PrP^{Res} is very resistant to inactivation with enzymes, heat, ultraviolet light, ionizing radiation, acids, bases, certain autoclaving procedures, formalin fixation, and disinfectants. Because of the high resistance of PrP^{Res} to destruction or inactivation, effective procedures to inactivate PrP^{Res} are rather limited; they include steam autoclaving at 134–138 °C for a minimum of 18 min, alkaline hydrolysis, incineration, Environ LpH, and exposure to 2N NaOH or 2% sodium hypochlorite for 1 h at room temperature. This resistance to destruction and inactivation explains the potential longevity of PrP^{Res} in the environment. It also allows for transmission of the TSEs even through contaminated feeds that are cooked or processed, as well as transmission through the use of inadequately autoclaved and contaminated surgical instruments, or via human/veterinary biologicals derived from tissues or fluids harvested from infected animals/humans.

Host–Prion Relationship

The host–prion relationships for scrapie and other TSEs are complex, as expected with a disease caused by an infectious agent that actually represents a conformational modification of the host PrP^{C}.

PRNP Polymorphisms

The susceptibility of sheep to scrapie following PrP^{Sc} exposure appears to be controlled by the sheep PRNP genotype, the strain of the scrapie PrP^{Sc} to which it is exposed, and other poorly understood factors such as sheep breed. One major factor that affects both the incubation period and the susceptibility of sheep to classical scrapie is the sheep's genetic makeup at codons 136, 154, and 171 of the PrP gene. At codon 136, valine (V) is associated with higher susceptibility than alanine (A). At codon 154, histidine (H) is linked with higher susceptibility than arginine (R), and at codon 171, glutamine (Q) and histidine (H) are associated with susceptibility and arginine (R) with resistance. Of the possible polymorphic combinations at these three codons, only five have been found frequent in nature, including $A_{136}R_{154}R_{171}$, $A_{136}R_{154}Q_{171}$, $A_{136}H_{154}Q_{171}$, $A_{136}R_{154}H_{171}$, and $V_{136}R_{154}Q_{171}$. Codon 171 appears to be the most significant in determining sheep susceptibility or resistance, while codon 136 is next in importance and codon 154 seems to be less of a factor. In particular the Q/Q polymorphism at codon 171 is linked with a high degree of susceptibility for classical scrapie, while Q/R and R/R polymorphisms at codon 171 are associated with resistance to classical scrapie. In North America, scrapie is diagnosed most commonly in sheep with the Q/Q polymorphism at codon 171. Classical scrapie has only been very rarely diagnosed in Suffolk sheep with the Q/R polymorphism at codon 171, and only one scrapie-positive Suffolk sheep has ever been diagnosed with the R/R polymorphism at codon 171. Further data suggest that when scrapie sheep are found with the Q/R polymorphism at codon 171, these sheep also are more likely to have the A/V polymorphism at codon 136. In North America, the United States Department of Agriculture (USDA), National Scrapie Eradication Program has used these genetic susceptibility patterns to establish criteria for removal or restricted movement of scrapie-exposed sheep. The criteria are based first on determining the PRNP polymorphism of the positively diagnosed scrapie-infected sheep. This helps establish information on the potential strain of scrapie present. Once the scrapie-infected PRNP genotype pattern is known, criteria are established for removal or restriction of remaining sheep in the flock with susceptible PRNP polymorphisms, as a means for disease eradication. These criteria are lengthy and complex, but salient features include the following: If positive-scrapie sheep are Q/Q at codon 171, all remaining Q/Q sheep in the flock are removed or under restricted movement. In rare instances where scrapie is diagnosed in a Q/R sheep, it has been found almost entirely in sheep with A/V_{136} and Q/R_{171} polymorphisms. Therefore, if scrapie infections are detected in Q/R_{171} sheep, then all Q/R_{171} sheep, in addition to the Q/Q_{171} sheep, are targeted for removal or placed under restricted movement. If an RR_{171} sheep is found to be positive, the whole flock will be removed.

Sheep heterozygous or homozygous for VRQ or ARQ are highly susceptible to classical scrapie. The PrP genotype of sheep with atypical scrapie is mainly AHQ and/or $AF_{141}RQ$, phenylalanine (F) at position 141 instead of leucine (L). Therefore, F_{141} and H_{154} alleles seem to be associated with increased susceptibility to atypical scrapie.

PrP genetic polymorphisms are also documented in goats, although there is much less known regarding the impact of specific polymorphisms on susceptibility/resistance of goats to scrapie.

Prion Strains

Data from various animal studies indicate that strains of prions can exist within a single prion disease. Different strains of scrapie are reported. The data supporting different PrP^{Sc} strains initially came from two observations: experimental inoculation of different PrP^{Sc} isolates into susceptible hosts resulted in variable incubation times, and the brain lesions induced by these isolates also differed in both distribution and severity. Additionally, biochemical PrP^{Sc} typing is now available, which is based on the degree of proteinase K (PK) resistance, the ratios of PrP^{Res} glycoforms and the site of PK cleavage. The European Food Safety Authority (EFSA) summarized the criteria to define TSEs in small ruminants (classical scrapie, atypical scrapie, and BSE in small ruminants) as presented in Table 67.1.

The strain of prion, which seems to be enciphered in the conformation of PrP^{Sc}, imprints its conformation on the recruited PrP^C. This hypothesis infers that each strain has a unique tertiary structure, but also suggests that the effect each strain has on a host is dependent to some degree on the PrP^C amino acid sequence of the host, which is dictated by the host genome, and which takes part in determining the final conformational structure of the PrP^{Res}.

Scrapie Disease Pathogenesis

The pathogenesis of scrapie includes the following: PrP^{Sc} is first detected in follicular dendritic cells and macrophages within the tonsils and gut-associated lymphoid tissues (GALT; especially ileal Peyer's Patches) after oral exposure of genetically susceptible sheep. PrP^{Sc} multiplies at these sites and then spreads through the lymph vascular system to peripheral lymph tissues, including the spleen, and numerous lymph nodes where it is detected next. PrP^{Sc} may be detected at this time in the retropharyngeal lymph nodes and in lymph follicles of the third eyelids of sheep. PrP^{Sc} is also found in spinal ganglia of the autonomic nervous system, the adjacent thoracic spinal cord, and in the dorsal vagal nucleus of the vagus nerve within the caudal brain stem. The early CNS invasion with prions likely occurs through invasion of nerve endings within the lymph follicles of the ileum or elsewhere in the gastrointestinal tract, and they travel through these nerves of the autonomic nervous system or the vagus nerve to the thoracic cord and vagal nucleus of the brain stem, respectively. Once within the CNS, the PrP^{Sc} multiplies and spreads. The increased PrP^{Sc} production within the CNS is directly related to the progressive development of CNS degenerative lesions and the onset of clinical signs.

There is no humoral or cellular immune response to the PrP^{Sc} because the protein is identical in its amino acid sequence to the host PrP^C and therefore considered a self-antigen. Thus, there is no serum antibody test to allow for antemortem detection of exposure. Lesions associated with scrapie or any other TSE are found only within the CNS (aside from secondary lesions such as hair loss). These lesions are bilateral in distribution and mainly associated with the gray matter areas. They consist of three basic changes: (i) spongiform change, which refers to vacuolation within the neuropil of gray matter that represents

Table 67.1. Classification of TSEs in Small Ruminants According to EFSA

	Experimental Methods		
TSE Type	"Stringent" Western Blot	"Mild Proteinase K" Western Blot	Immunohistochemistry and Histopathology
Classical scrapie	Three PrP^{Res} bands (range of 16–30 kDa) reacting with both N-terminal and core-specific antibodies	Same as left	Vacuolation in gray matter and/or immunolabeling in the medulla involving the DMNV[a]
Atypical scrapie/Nor98	Negative or different band pattern (range of 10–35 kDa) from other TSEs	Multiple PrP^{Res} band pattern including an unglycosylated band at <15 kDa	Immunostaining in the cerebellum is greater than in the brain stem DMNV at the level of the obex is not staining Distribution of PrP^{Sc} deposition restrictively in the cerebellum, substantia nigra, thalamus, and basal nuclei
BSE in small ruminants	Three PrP^{Res} bands reacting with core-specific antibodies but not or weak reacting with anti-N-terminus-specific antibodies Molecular mass of unglycosylated PrP^{Res} band lower than that of classical scrapie	Same as left	Vacuolation in grey matter and/or immunolabeling in the medulla involving the DMNV.

Adapted from the EFSA Opinion on Atypical TSEs in Small Ruminants.
[a] DMNV, dorsal motor nucleus of the vagus.

intracytoplasmic vacuolation of nerve processes; (ii) neuronal degeneration/loss, which includes intracytoplasmic vacuolation of neurons, shrunken, dark, angular neurons, rare necrotic neurons, and neuronal loss; and (iii) astrocytosis or the hypertrophy and hyperplasia of astrocytes within the gray matter (see Chapter 72). The lesions occur first in the caudal brain stem and progress from there to other regions of the brain stem, cerebellum, and cerebral cortex. PrP^{Sc} can be illustrated even prior to detection of CNS lesions by the use of immunohistochemistry (IHC).

The PrP^{Sc} deposits around and within neurons and glial cells within the neuropil. In atypical/Nor98-like scrapie, the PrP^{Sc} detection sites mainly include the cerebellum, substantia nigra, thalamus, and basal nuclei but exclude the brain stem and the dorsal motor nucleus of the vagus (DMNV) at the level of the obex, which are primary target sites for the diagnosis of classical scrapie. There is also no obvious vacuolation in brain stem neuroanatomical sites that are generally affected in classical scrapie. Recent studies in pregnant scrapie-infected sheep indicate that fetal genetic susceptibility plays a major role regarding both maternal transmission of infection to the fetus and the potential spread of scrapie within a flock. The results indicate that in utero fetal infection does not occur in infected ewes. However, the fetal membranes can become infected with PrP^{Sc} during gestation, serving as a source for shedding of PrP^{Sc} into the environment both at and for some time after lambing. Whether the placenta becomes infected is controlled by the PrP genotype of the fetus. As an example, PrP^{Sc} was found in the placenta of infected ewes when the fetal genotype was QQ at codon 171 but was not detected in the placenta if the fetus was a resistant QR genotype at codon 171. At lambing, placental PrP^{Sc} is a high-risk source for infection, and very young lambs with susceptible genetic polymorphisms are at the highest risk for infection. The reason for this increased susceptibility of young animals is unknown, but it is theorized that the more developed GALT in young animals (which atrophies in older animals) may be responsible for this.

Cross-species Barriers

For most TSEs, the susceptible host species range is rather limited. The barrier limiting cross-species transmission is termed the cross-species barrier. Experimentally, these cross-species barriers can often be overcome, albeit with some difficulty. The factors used to promote transmission across these barriers are direct intracerebral inoculation of the candidate PrP^{Res} into a different host species and multiple serial passages of infected CNS tissue through the new species. The exact basis for the species barrier is poorly understood and probably very complex, but contributing factors known to affect the species barrier include the following:

1. The degree of homology in the PrP^{C} amino acid sequence of the donor and recipient: The genetically determined host PrP^{C} amino acid sequence is important as it is thought to have a direct effect on the ability of PrP^{C} to refold in a manner that mimics the PrP^{Res} tertiary conformation.
2. The strain of prion: As mentioned previously, this is enciphered in the conformation of the PrP^{Res}.
3. As a side note, evidence now suggests that the process of experimentally adapting the candidate PrP^{Res} across the species barrier in most cases creates modifications of the original PrP^{Res}, and thus essentially creates a new strain of PrP^{Res}.

Subclinical Carriers of Infection

There is some experimental evidence to suggest that, under certain circumstances, and with PrP^{Res} from certain TSEs, PrP^{Res} infections can result in subclinical carriers that do not develop disease. In addition, it may be very difficult to detect the PrP^{Res} in these carriers except by bioassay. As an example, experimental infection across the species barriers in rodents may require multiple serial passages through that rodent species. In such instances following initial inoculation of the resistant host, the PrP^{Res} may not be detected, and the host may live its entire life without contracting a TSE. However, when brain material from such a host is subsequently serially passed through the same species, a TSE disease may eventually result as the cross-species barrier adaptation results. Recently, it was demonstrated that lymphoid tissue was more permissive than brain in cross-species transmissions using transgenic mice, indicating that lymphoid tissue could harbor prions that do not replicate in the CNS.

Laboratory Diagnosis

Several diagnostic tests for prion disease have been developed for specific detection of PrP^{Res} in tissues. These tests rely on the use of polyclonal or monoclonal antibodies to the PrP protein. Since these antibodies cannot differentiate between PrP^{C} and PrP^{Res}, the test methodologies utilize the biochemical differences between PrP^{C} and PrP^{Res} to first destroy PrP^{C} using digestion or denaturing procedures (i.e., proteinase K or formic acid treatment, and/or denaturation by autoclaving), leaving only PrP^{Res} with its intact antigenic epitopes. This group of tests, which includes IHC, Western blot (WB), and enzyme-linked immunosorbent assay (ELISA) methodologies, has been utilized successfully for detection of PrP^{Res} in a variety of TSE diseases. It should be noted that atypical scrapie PrP^{sc} is more sensitive to proteinase K than classical scrapie, and OIE therefore recommends to use a reduced concentration of the proteinase K enzyme in order to detect atypical scrapie by the WB method. Furthermore, the selection of the brain region used in the confirmatory test is critical to detect atypical scrapie because brain stems might be negative in the majority of atypical/Nor98 scrapie cases; however, atypical scrapie has been detected in the obex of some animals.

PrP^{Sc} can be detected antemortem by IHC in the third eyelid or in rectal biopsies. The biopsy consists of a small aggregate of the lymphoid follicles that can be visualized and excised on the inner surface of the third eyelid. A negative test result does not completely ensure that the animal is scrapie free for the following reasons: the animal may be in the early incubation stages of infection, or represent one of the small percentage of clinically affected sheep where

PrP^{Sc} is not present/detected in lymph tissue prior to CNS infection; or there may not be sufficient lymphoid tissue present (this seems to occur more in very aged animals and possibly in some sheep breeds more than others).

PMCA is a new method that can exponentially amplify PrP^{Sc} *in vitro* using normal cellular host PrP (PrP^C) or recombinant prion protein ($rPrP^C$) as the amplification substrate. The principle of PMCA is similar to the polymerase chain reaction, which is used to amplify DNA, but it uses PrP^C or $rPrP^C$ instead of dNTPs, primers, and Taq polymerase. PMCA consists of alternating steps of incubation at 37 °C and sonication. The incubation step allows the conversion of PrP^C into PrP^{Sc} and produces de novo PrP^{Sc} resulting in expansion of PrP^{Sc} in the presence of excess PrP^C. The newly aggregated PrP^{Sc} is dissociated into smaller units during the subsequent sonication step. The incubation and sonication steps are repeated, and the quantity of de novo formed PrP^{Sc} depends on the number of PMCA cycles (incubation and sonication) carried out. The PMCA technique is now automated and optimized, and it has been shown that serial PMCA is able to detect PrP^{Sc} in blood of scrapie-infected hamsters; similar data were obtained in sheep with preclinical and clinical scrapie infection. Another rapid ultrasensitive prion detection test is the quaking-induced conversion (QuIC) reaction test, which enables amplification of prion-seeded amyloid fibrils through alternate incubation and shaking (instead of sonication in PMCA). PMCA and QuIC are able to detect subfemtogram levels of PrP^{Sc} in cerebral spinal fluid (CSF), brain homogenate, and blood from scrapie-infected animals. PMCA and QuIC technology may be useful future diagnostic tools for ante- and post-mortem diagnosis of prion diseases.

The postmortem diagnosis in clinically affected animals is often made by histopathologic evaluation of the brain (see Chapter 72). The extent of the lesions, and therefore the accuracy in diagnosis through routine histology, is directly related to the severity of the clinical disease at the time of death.

Treatment and Control

There is no treatment available for scrapie, so the disease is handled by prevention, control, or eradication. In North America, there is a federally regulated program to eradicate the disease, which includes the following:

1. A Scrapie Flock Certification Program monitors flock disease status over an extended period with the goal of assigning status to flocks with no evidence of scrapie. The program has requirements for individual animal identification, record keeping, reporting, and restrictions on flock additions to ensure scrapie is not introduced into flocks free from detectable scrapie.
2. The eradication of scrapie is sought through disease surveillance, and diagnosis, identification of infected/exposed flocks, elimination of positive or susceptible/exposed animals, and monitoring of sheep movement to control potential spread of scrapie and to allow for successful trace-back from positively diagnosed animals to their flocks of origin.

Within an individual flock, determination of the flock status and strict limitations on the addition of new animals are the best means for prevention and control. Initial determination of the flock status can best be obtained through the Scrapie Flock Certification Program. Maintenance of a disease-free flock is achieved by maintaining a closed flock, particularly a closed ewe flock. If new introductions are to be made, care should be taken to ensure that new additions come from flocks with disease-free status as can best be determined (often difficult). Third eyelid testing of animals over 14 months of age can be considered in making this assessment but is not foolproof. Genotype testing to select for new additions with resistant genotypes is also useful, although research has not eliminated the possibility of a resistant genotype carrier animal. The feeding of ruminant meat and bonemeal to ruminants is prohibited in many countries including the United States.

Bovine Spongiform Encephalopathy Disease

Bovine spongiform encephalopathy (BSE or "mad cow disease") is a chronic, progressive, and uniformly fatal degenerative CNS disease that occurs naturally in cattle, exotic ungulates, and domestic and exotic felids, and is the likely cause of vCJD, a rather newly recognized TSE in humans. BSE emerged as a newly recognized TSE in England in 1986. The incidence of BSE in cattle rapidly increased, largely in dairy cattle throughout the United Kingdom over the next few years. Shortly thereafter, additional new TSE diseases were then recognized in both captive exotic ungulates and felids from zoos in England, and also in domestic cats in the United Kingdom. Experimental studies and characterization of the PrP^{Res} from this latter group of prion diseases established that PrP^{BSE} was the cause, indicating that BSE, unlike other TSEs, had an unusually wide susceptible host range. Significantly, vCJD also emerged in a small number of young human patients in England at the same time. Unlike sporadic CJD, vCJD occurs in humans at a much younger age and has a different time course, electroencephalogram (EEG) pattern, and pattern of clinical CNS signs. Sheep, pigs, primates (macaques), marmosets, lemurs, and mice are experimentally susceptible to BSE infection, although natural occurrence of disease has not been described in these species, except that BSE-like cases in goats have been confirmed or suspected recently. Sheep are susceptible experimentally to oral inoculation with BSE, which raises substantial concerns as to how it would be differentiated from scrapie. Because of the association with vCJD, BSE is considered a major threat to public health, which is the basis for national eradication programs in all countries where it exists, and extensive national surveillance and prevention programs in countries where the disease does not.

Following the widespread detection of BSE in the United Kingdom, cases of BSE occurred in other countries through the export of infected meat and bone meal (MBM), infected live animals, and possibly other infected animal products. As of November 2011, a total of 25 countries (OIE data) had reported cases of BSE. These include several countries in Europe, as well as Japan, Israel, the United States, and Canada.

Epidemiologic analyses strongly suggest that the primary mode of natural BSE transmission is through the ingestion of contaminated MBM-containing infected offal. Horizontal transmission from animal to animal does not occur to any significant extent. Young cattle appear more susceptible to infection than adults, and there is an increased risk for BSE among calves born from BSE-affected cows, suggesting a low level of maternally associated transmission. However, the mechanism responsible for this increased calf risk is unknown (i.e., what role does direct cow-to-calf maternal infection vs. genetic predisposition vs. feed-borne exposure play?). There is no strong evidence to suggest transmission from a contaminated environment, although the occurrence of a small number of new BSE cases in the United Kingdom following the enforced animal protein feed ban in animals born after August 1, 1996, is disconcerting.

The initial source of the infected material responsible for the emergence of BSE in the United Kingdom may never be known. Three theories have been offered to explain the emergence of BSE: (i) BSE arose from the feeding of MBM containing sheep offal contaminated with scrapie to cattle; (ii) BSE arose from a single spontaneous or genetic case of BSE in a cow that was then rendered and fed as contaminated MBM to other cattle; or (iii) BSE arose from animal feed imported from the Indian subcontinent and contaminated with human remains suffering from human prion diseases. Epidemiologic evidence suggests that a change in the rendering process in England in the late 1970s may have allowed for increased survival of PrP^{Res}, regardless of the source (offal from infected sheep, bovine, or other species), increasing exposure of cattle to this PrP^{Res}. Epidemiologic data supporting scrapie as the initial source for BSE include the following: the sheep population increased significantly in the 1980s, when BSE likely emerged, possibly increasing the prevalence of endemic scrapie in the United Kingdom; and MBM was a cheap feed source listed for dairy calf starter feeds. However, it is difficult to explain by these point source theories (whether it arose initially from scrapie-infected sheep or a BSE-infected cow) how BSE simultaneously emerged at multiple sites in the United Kingdom, unless this single source was widely distributed. Once BSE infections were established in the cattle population, transmission could be easily amplified by repeated recycling of BSE-infected bovine tissue into MBM fed to cattle. BSE soon reached epidemic proportions in the United Kingdom. The epidemic peaked in 1992–1993 with 37 280 cases diagnosed in 1992. Disease eradication and prevention programs that were established (see Section "Treatment and Control," below) have been successful in greatly reducing the numbers of cases. Transmission of BSE to felids and exotic ungulates is thought to have occurred through feeding of infected animal protein, and although the source for vCJD (human) is unclear, ingestion of contaminated bovine products is considered the most likely source.

BSE has a long incubation period with a mean incubation period of 4–5 years. Clinical signs include a loss of condition or weight loss, coupled with one more CNS signs that include behavioral changes (apprehension, fear, easily startled, and depression), hyperesthesia, hyperreflexia, muscle fasciculations, tremors, myoclonus, ataxia, hypermetria, pruritus, and autonomic dysfunctions (reduced rumination and bradycardia).

Etiologic Agent

BSE is caused by the PrP^{BSE} prion with physicochemical properties common to all abnormal prions. The different phenotypes of human and animal TSE agents can be biochemically differentiated by the degree of glycosylation and the molecular mass of the PrP^{Res} fragments in WB analysis. In recent years, atypical forms of BSE have been reported in European countries, North America, and Japan. There are two atypical BSEs, called L-type and H-type, which can be biochemically differentiated from classical BSE. The L-type BSE is characterized by a slightly lower molecular mass of unglycosylated PrP^{Res} compared to classical BSE, whereas the H-type BSE shows a slightly higher molecular mass of unglycosylated PrP^{Res} when compared to classical BSE. The majority of atypical BSEs have been detected through active national surveillance of slaughtered animals (e.g., healthy, sick, emergency slaughter, downer, and fallen cattle as recommended by the OIE guidelines). In general, these atypical BSEs do not have distinct clinical signs as described for classical BSE. Importantly, about 85% of atypical BSE cases were reported in cattle more than 10 years of age. In active surveillance for BSE in France during 2001–2007, the estimated incidence of atypical BSE—H-type and L-type—was 0.41 and 0.35 per million adult cattle tested, but 1.9 and 1.7 in cattle more than 8 years of age, respectively. This frequency is similar to that of sporadic CJD, which is about 1 case per million inhabitants per year. On the basis of these results, the origin of atypical BSE cases is unknown, but they may represent spontaneously occurring TSE forms.

Another study on atypical BSE cases revealed an E211K (glutamic acid, E to lysine, K) polymorphism at position 211 within the bovine PRNP in an animal with H-type BSE; the E211K bovine germline polymorphism is similar to E200K of humans, which is a known pathological mutation in humans with a high incidence of inherited CJD.

So far, there are no detectable differences in age susceptibility or incubation periods reported for various cattle breeds. PrP^{BSE} has not been found in sheep and only in goats, although the potential risk of BSE-infected sheep is recognized.

Host–Prion Relationship

While polymorphisms in the PrP gene of cattle have been rarely identified, so far there is no evidence suggesting these polymorphisms have a significant effect on disease susceptibility except for the E211K polymorphism. However, it has been reported that two 23- and 12-bp insertion/deletion polymorphisms of the putative promoter region and intron 1 within bovine Prnp are associated with BSE susceptibility in cattle because these regions modulate Prnp expression levels. Unlike scrapie, PrP^{BSE} is not readily detected in lymphoid tissues prior to the onset of CNS infectivity and clinical disease. PrP^{BSE} has been detected only in the CNS (brain and spinal cord), peripheral nervous system, and retina of naturally infected cattle. Experimental studies indicate that it does track through lymph tissues, but it is detected inconsistently and in relatively small amounts as compared to scrapie. The following is a brief summary of experimental studies in cattle.

Following oral inoculation of cattle, PrP^{BSE} is first detected in lymphoid follicles of the distal ileum at 6 months postinoculation (PI). It can occasionally be found in the ileum at later PI dates. It has also been detected in the tonsil between 6 and 14 months PI. It is first detected in the CNS and dorsal root ganglia at 32 months PI, followed by trigeminal ganglia at 36 months PI. PrP^{BSE} has not been detected in retropharyngeal, mesenteric, or popliteal lymph nodes of naturally infected cattle. Within the CNS, it progressively accumulates and is associated with degenerative CNS lesions that are generally similar to other TSEs. As with other TSEs, there is no immunologic response to the PrP^{BSE} by the host.

Laboratory Diagnosis

There is no antemortem test currently available for the diagnosis of BSE. Postmortem diagnostic tests on the brain are available that are similar to those for scrapie (IHC, ELISA, and WB tests on CNS specifically obex, not lymphoid tissue). These tests are used in BSE-infected countries as part of their national surveillance and eradication programs. Routine histopathology of the brain of clinically affected animals will show lesions compatible with BSE, but confirmation of the diagnosis requires confirmatory testing by IHC or WB. In the United States, a national surveillance program for BSE is conducted by the Animal Plant Health Inspection Service (APHIS) of the USDA. Targeted surveillance samples include field cases of cattle exhibiting neurologic disease, cattle condemned at slaughter for neurologic reasons, rabies-negative cattle submitted to public health laboratories, neurologic cases submitted to veterinary diagnostic laboratories and teaching hospitals, cattle that are "nonambulatory" ("downers"), and cattle dying on farms.

Treatment and Control

There is no treatment for BSE. Countries with confirmed BSE cases are attempting to eradicate it, and countries where it is not present institute preventative/surveillance programs to prevent its occurrence. In the United Kingdom, a series of key regulatory measures were taken by the government to stop the food-borne transmission of BSE. These measures, coupled with detection, diagnosis, and eradication programs, have proven to be very successful in stemming the epidemic and drastically reducing the number of bovine cases. The first of these measures was a ban on the use of MBM in ruminant feed in July 1988. This was followed in September 1990 by a further ban on the use of specified bovine offal in feedstuffs of any species including humans; these were bovine tissues thought to harbor the highest concentration of infectious material (also known as "specified risk material") including skull, brain, trigeminal ganglia, eyes, tonsils, spinal cord, dorsal root ganglia, and the distal ileum of the small intestine. The list may vary depending on safety guidelines or regulations of different countries. While these measures resulted in a significant reduction in new cases, evidence suggested that new feed-borne cases continued in animals, and in March 1996, the feed ban was extended to a total ban on the use of mammalian proteins in feed produced for any farm animals.

BSE-like cases have been recently reported in goats. The pathogenesis of BSE in small ruminants is distinct from bovine BSE. Experimentally, BSE infectivity on sheep is detected in nervous and also in various lymphoreticular tissues, the latter in contrast to bovine BSE. Therefore, it is necessary to improve surveillance of small ruminants to prevent the BSE-like agent from entering the human food chain through food products of small ruminants.

Chronic Wasting Disease

Chronic Wasting Disease (CWD) is a fatal, chronic, progressive, degenerative CNS disease of mule deer (*Odocoileus hemionus*), white-tailed deer (*Odocoileus virginianus*), moose (*Alces alces shirasi*), and elk (*Cervus elaphus nelsoni*) found primarily in North America. There are no reported human TSE cases associated with CWD. CWD was first diagnosed in mule deer in 1967 and identified in 1978 as a TSE through the examination of brains of affected deer by Dr Elizabeth Williams. The disease was subsequently recognized as an endemic disease in deer and elk in an area that encompassed portions of Colorado, Wyoming, and Nebraska. The range and incidence of the disease began to increase after 1990. The reasons for this sudden spread are not clear, but both unique features of the disease and the husbandry of captive cervids likely contributed. CWD can spread horizontally via direct contact transmission, in distinct contrast to BSE where contact transmission does not appear to occur. The horizontal transmission of CWD appears to be very efficient. Infectious CWD agents have been detected in saliva, blood, urine, velvet, and feces. These findings suggest that environmental contamination with infectious body fluids such as saliva, urine, or feces plays an important role in horizontal transmission of CWD in both free-ranging and captive herds. Modeling studies suggest that horizontal transmission through shedding of PrP^{CWD} probably begins even before the onset of clinical signs in infected cervids. CWD spreads from infected to uninfected cervids when comingled in confined surroundings. In addition to direct contact transmission, indirect transmission from contaminated pastures or paddocks occurs, and this indirect transmission appears to be more efficient than is reported with scrapie. This relative ease of both direct and indirect contact transmissions likely explains the very high prevalence of CWD in some infected captive herds (>90% of mule deer over a 2-year period in one herd). The prevalence of CWD in free-ranging cervids from endemic areas can also be high (up to 30%).

Aside from the relative ease of transmission, geographical spread of the disease has most likely also been facilitated through transportation of infected deer and elk between farms. In North America (as of March 2012), the disease had been detected in free-ranging deer and elk in Colorado, Wyoming, Nebraska, Wisconsin, South

Dakota, North Dakota, New Mexico, Illinois, Kansas, Maryland, Minnesota, New York, Utah, Virginia, West Virginia, and Saskatchewan, Canada, and in farmed cervids in South Dakota, Nebraska, Colorado, Oklahoma, Kansas, Minnesota, Montana, Wisconsin, New York, Wyoming, Michigan, and the Canadian provinces of Alberta and Saskatchewan. CWD-infected free-ranging moose have been identified in Colorado and Wyoming. CWD has also been diagnosed in farmed cervids exported to the Republic of Korea.

Maternal transmission may occur, but there is no direct evidence so far. In the wild, it is possible that transmission might also occur from decay of CWD-infected carcasses, with release of the PrP^{CWD} into the environment. Experimental CWD infections have been documented in cattle, sheep, and goats, but only following intracerebral inoculation. There appears to be a substantial species barrier between these host species and infection with PrP^{CWD}. Natural transmission from deer or elk to these species has not been documented. There is no evidence of experimental transmission to cattle by either direct contact or oral inoculation more than 5 years following exposure.

Based on examination of natural cases, CWD is thought to have a minimum incubation period of 16–17 months, which is an appreciably shorter incubation period than either scrapie or BSE. The clinical signs in deer or elk with CWD include loss of body condition and one or more of the following CNS abnormalities: behavioral changes (changes in interactions with handlers, walking patterns, depression, and lowered head and ears), polydipsia, polyuria, increased salivation or drooling, incoordination, ataxia, head tremors, wide-based stance, and hyperexcitability. However, because clinical signs may not be observed in free-ranging deer, the salient findings at necropsy may include loss of condition and death due to aspiration pneumonia, possibly due to dysphagia, hypersalivation, or difficulties in swallowing.

Etiology

CWD is caused by the PrP^{CWD} prion, which has physicochemical properties similar to other abnormal prions. The origin of PrP^{CWD} will probably never be known, but might include a spontaneous PrP^{CWD} formation in a cervid or cross-species adaptation from scrapie-infected sheep or contaminated feedstuff. Several reports suggested the possible existence of different CWD strains similar to sheep scrapie. When ferrets were inoculated with two CWD isolates, the results showed different strain-like features such as different clinical courses, survival times, pathological lesions, and biochemical properties. In addition, two distinct CWD strains were identified in CWD-infected material using cervidized transgenic mice. These two CWD strains have different incubation times and neuropathological profiles, although they show similar biochemical properties.

Host–Prion Relationship

There are species-specific polymorphisms that affect susceptibility to CWD infection. It has been shown that the amino acids located at position 96 and 225 in deer PrP and 132 in elk PrP are associated with susceptibility to CWD infection. In free-ranging mule deer from Wyoming and Colorado, deer with an S225S (serine, S) genotype had a 30 times greater probability of CWD infection than deer with an S225F (S/phenylalanine, F) genotype. In white-tailed deer, it was suggested that a G96S (G, glycine, and S, serine) polymorphism might be associated with reduced susceptibility to CWD, but not with resistance to CWD, since CWD was detected in some G96S animals. Elk PrP is polymorphic at codon 132 (methionine, M/leucine, L), which corresponds to the polymorphic locus at human PrP codon 129 (M/valine, V). The codon 129 polymorphism in humans is related with susceptibility to CJD including vCJD. In transgenic mice and elk experiments, L 132 polymorphism seems to be associated with less susceptibility to CWD when compared to M132.

Like scrapie, PrP^{CWD} is readily detectable in lymphoid tissues throughout the body of infected deer and elk, and the pathogenesis of tissue distribution shares many similarities to scrapie. Following oral exposure, PrP^{CWD} is detected first in lymphoid tissues (GALT and the retropharyngeal lymph node) prior to detection in the brain. Experimentally, it has been found in the Peyer's patches of the ileum, ileocecal lymph node, tonsil, and retropharyngeal lymph node by 42 days after infection. It is first detected in the brain within the dorsal nucleus of the vagus nerve located in the caudal brain stem (obex), similar to scrapie. In one study, PrP^{CWD} was first detected in the obex 3 months following first detection in the GALT. Lesions specific for CWD are confined to the CNS and are similar in overall nature to other TSEs.

Laboratory Diagnosis

There is no validated antemortem diagnostic test for CWD. Several potential antemortem diagnostic techniques have been developed for surveillance and managing of CWD such as tonsil and rectal biopsies. Tonsil biopsy has been evaluated to detect preclinical CWD in deer, but this technique is not easy to apply in the field. Recently, another antemortem diagnostic test using rectoanal mucosa-associated lymphoid tissue has been evaluated in captive elk during clinical as well as preclinical stage. This method could detect subclinically CWD-infected elk, a diagnosis confirmed by postmortem tests.

Postmortem diagnostic tests available are similar to those used for scrapie and BSE, and some of the monoclonal antibodies used for detection of scrapie or BSE in the United States are also utilized for detection of PrP^{CWD} (Figure 67.1). PMCA has been developed to amplify and detect low concentrations of PrP^{Res} from CWD-infected tissue and body fluids. This highly sensitive method might have a good chance to detect asymptomatic animals in early stages of prion infection. A presumptive diagnosis can also be made based on routine histopathology in clinically affected animals if sufficient CNS lesion development has occurred. Confirmation of the diagnosis through additional tests as described for scrapie and BSE confirms the diagnosis.

FIGURE 67.1. *Obex from white-tailed deer (O. virginianus)—the entire DMNV is bright red with minimal spillover into the adjacent neurological tissue. IHC for PrP^{CWD} demonstrates the presence of the pathogenic prion in the brain. (Courtesy of Dr Mark Hall and Dr Aaron Lehmkuhl at the USDA APHIS National Veterinary Services Laboratory, Ames, Iowa, USA.)*

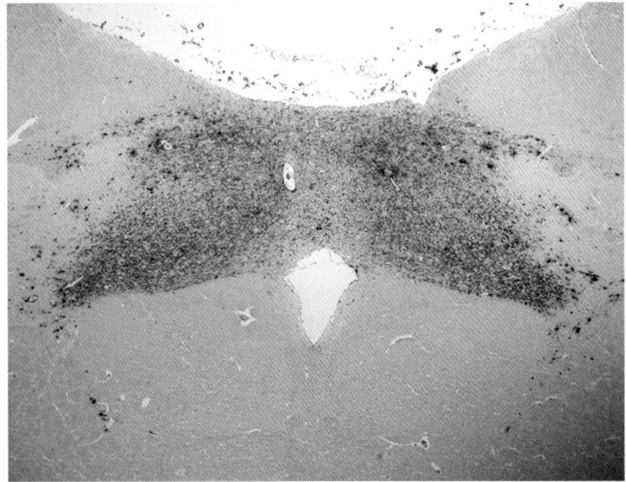

Treatment and Control

There is no treatment for CWD. Efforts to control or eradicate CWD are complicated because of the long incubation period, the resistance of the etiologic agent to disinfection procedures, the absence of reliable antemortem diagnostic tests, and the various potential routes of transmission including animal-to-animal contact and environmental contamination. Quarantine and depopulation of affected herds are primary means for control in farmed facilities. Even with depopulation of infected farmed facilities, there is "concern" to risk of reinfection following placement of new uninfected stock due to possible environmental contamination. There are also concerns for spread from infected farmed to adjacent free-ranging populations across fence lines or, conversely, from endemic-free populations to farmed facilities. An active, efficient surveillance program is therefore recommended in farmed facilities, not only to identify and remove infected animals but also to prevent movement of infected animals to other farmed facilities. Management of free-ranging populations is even more problematic. Current management involves active surveillance to determine prevalence, coupled with reduction of prevalence through targeted culling in endemic areas. Human-facilitated relocation, or feeding of free-ranging cervids, is banned in endemic areas. Selective culling of clinical animals by itself has not significantly affected prevalence in endemic areas. A program of localized population reduction in Colorado has been instituted, but the effectiveness of this program has yet to be determined. It is thought that an aggressive program of selective culling or general population reduction may be effective in regions where new cases of free-ranging infection are detected early, and prior to the establishment of endemic infections in populations. The potential for transport of hunter-killed infected carcasses to uninfected areas and subsequent contamination of these new environments via discarded infected offal also represents a significant concern for potential spread of CWD to new regions. There is a USDA program currently in place to eradicate CWD from farmed elk operations in the United States.

Further Reading

Hörnlimann B, Riesner, D, and Kretzschmar, H (2007) *Prions in Humans and Animals*, Walter De Gruyter.

Tatzelt, J (2011) *Prion Proteins*, Springer Publications.

PART IV

Clinical Applications

Circulatory System and Lymphoid Tissues

Douglas E. Hostetler

The circulatory system includes the blood vascular and lymphatic systems. The blood vascular system is composed of the heart, arteries, capillaries, veins, and components of blood itself. Infections involving the pericardial sac, which encloses the heart, are also included in this chapter. The lymphatic system includes lymphatic capillaries, afferent lymphatic vessels that drain interstitial fluid and cells from tissues, lymph nodes, and efferent lymphatics that recirculate lymph and cells (primarily lymphocytes) from lymph nodes to the blood vascular system. Because of the functional association with and cellular trafficking through the circulatory system, infections involving other lymphoid tissues (spleen, bone marrow, and thymus) are included in this chapter. Mucosa-associated lymphoid tissues, although less organized, are included with other lymphoid tissues. The role of mucosa-associated lymphoid tissues in immune surveillance and as potential entry sites for some pathogens into the host is specifically discussed in those chapters on systems where they are found or chapters covering specific agents involved.

While functionally similar, there are anatomic differences in the organization of lymphoid tissues of animals and birds. Birds possess a bursa of Fabricius, a lymphoepithelial organ, which is dorsal to and communicates with the cloaca. It is a primary lymphoid organ serving as the main site of B lymphocyte differentiation. For the most part, poultry do not have lymph nodes but rather rely on cecal tonsils, Peyer's patches, and Meckel's diverticulum in the intestines; lymphoid follicles in various organs; the spleen; and a special paranasal concentration of lymphoid tissue (Harderian gland) for secondary immune functions.

Antimicrobial Properties

Phagocytic cells in the spleen and liver provide the primary defense for the vascular system by removing potential pathogens from circulation. Depending on the location in the vascular system and severity of injury caused directly by an infectious agent or its toxin or as a result of the subsequent inflammatory response, ability to repair damage is variable. Cardiac muscle has little regenerative capability following infectious processes that result in myocardial cell death. Such injury leads to scar formation. Injuries to small vessels that destroy endothelial cells can result in thrombus formation in those vessels. Unaffected vascular endothelial cells at the periphery of the lesion are able to proliferate and reendothelialize those areas that affected vessels supplied.

The lymphoid tissue plays a major role in defense of the body from infection. It is central to the development of the animal's immune system (primary lymphoid tissues) and plays an ongoing role in immune surveillance and defense. Details on mechanisms of immune defense provided by lymphoid tissues are covered in Chapter 2. Because of the surveillance role it plays, lymphoid tissue is exposed to numerous potentially pathogenic microbes, which if not contained may involve the lymphoid tissue in the disease process or cause a systemic infection.

Transient and Persistent Microbes

As a rule, the circulatory system and lymphoid tissues are not recognized to have a normal microbial flora. Transient bacteremias do occur, often as a result of traumatic or invasive events (e.g., dental extractions, endoscopic procedures of the digestive tract, and urethral catheterization) or subsequent to treatments that compromise mucosal barriers (e.g., chemotherapy and radiation therapy). This allows normal mucosal inhabitants to enter the bloodstream. Chronic conditions, such as severe gingival disease, that compromise the normal host barriers may also lead to spontaneous bacteremia. In some instances, no predisposing event or condition is recognized to account for a bacteremic episode. The resulting bacteremia is usually transient, lasting only a short period of time (<30 min) before removal by phagocytes in the liver and spleen.

Not all microorganisms appear to be removed that rapidly and may persist in the vascular system for longer periods. For example, a persistent but subclinical bacteremia with *Bartonella* spp. occurs in some cats. Bacteremias can serve as a source of microorganisms for serious infections of the circulatory system (e.g., infectious endocarditis and bacterial sepsis).

Veterinary Microbiology, Third Edition. Edited by D. Scott McVey, Melissa Kennedy and M.M. Chengappa.

Microscopic and molecular-based studies suggest that the bloodstream may in fact be colonized with specific microbes rather than just being periodically exposed to organisms through transient bacteremias, and that these "residents" persist in the blood in a benign fashion. However, evidence that a true normal microbial flora of the bloodstream exists remains to be conclusively demonstrated.

Some viruses, particularly retroviruses, persistently infect cells in the lymphoid tissue and blood for the life of the animal.

Infections

Access of microbial pathogens to the circulatory system occurs through a number of mechanisms, including direct inoculation into the blood (e.g., insect bites, contaminated needles, and blood transfusions) or by spread from initial site of infection via the vascular system or the lymphatics draining that site.

Microbial agents that enter via the lymphatic system may be eliminated or, at least, arrested at regional lymph nodes, or, if they avoid containment at the lymph nodes, they spread to the bloodstream and can disseminate to other sites in the body. The circulatory system, therefore, provides a means for delivery of many microbial agents from their site of entry to their ultimate target organ(s) in the body. Depending on the agent involved, the circulatory system itself may or may not be affected. For many viral infections, a viremia is the primary means of dissemination in the host but is often a clinically inapparent event. Similarly, some bacteria and fungi in animals reach their primary or secondary target organs via the circulatory system without obvious or major clinical signs of circulatory system involvement.

The focus of this chapter is on infections in which the circulatory system and/or lymphoid tissues are one of the primary sites affected in the infectious process. In addition to specific lesions or clinical signs directly related to the circulatory system and/or lymphoid tissues, many of these agents also cause systemic, nonspecific signs that include fever, anorexia, depression, prostration, and weight loss. Some infections of the blood vascular system present as rapidly fatal infections with few or no premonitory signs (e.g., anthrax and blackleg). Some of the most common and/or important infectious agents affecting the circulatory system and lymphoid tissues of domestic animals and poultry are listed in Tables 68.1, 68.2, 68.3, 68.4, 68.5, 68.6, and 68.7. Specific chapters on each of these pathogens should be referred to for more details on pathogenesis, spectrum of clinical signs, and the diseases they cause.

Bacterial Sepsis

Bacterial sepsis and septic shock are characterized by vascular collapse and multiorgan failure. In addition to the signs specifically related to altered organ perfusion, clinical signs of sepsis include fever, tachypnea, and hypothermia. The most common agents involved in sepsis are gram-negative bacteria belonging to the family Enterobacteriaceae, although other gram-negative pathogens (e.g., *Pseudomonas aeruginosa*, members of the family Pasteurellaceae) and gram-positive cocci (e.g., staphylococci and streptococci) also cause sepsis and septic shock. Sepsis frequently occurs in neonates, and is especially important in production animals, horses, and poultry. In veterinary me-dicine, the increasing level of intensive care-afforded animals with debilitating conditions has increased the risk for acquiring nosocomial infections and thus the potential for bacterial sepsis to develop in those patients.

Central to the development of septic shock is lipopolysaccharide in gram-negative organisms or other major cell wall components in gram-positive organisms (e.g., peptidoglycan and lipoteichoic acid). These pathogen-associated molecules bind to receptor signaling complexes on monocytes and macrophages. Toll-like receptors, transmembrane signal transducing coreceptors, play a central role in this process. Exposure of cells to

Table 68.1. Common and/or Important Infectious Agents of Circulatory System and Lymphoid Tissues of Dogs

Agent	Disease	Circulatory/Lymphoid-Associated Findings
Viruses		
Canine adenovirus 1	Infectious canine hepatitis	Disseminated intravascular coagulopathy, oral petechial hemorrhages, lymphadenopathy
Canine distemper virus	Canine distemper	Leukopenia, myocarditis in neonates
Canine herpesvirus 1	Canine herpesvirus disease	Generalized ecchymotic hemorrhages in neonatal puppies, lymphoid necrosis
Canine parvovirus	Canine parvovirus disease	Leukopenia, lymphoid necrosis, myocarditis
Bacteria		
Bartonella[a] spp.	Infectious valvular endocarditis	Heart murmur, valvular endocarditis
Borrelia burgdorferi	Canine Lyme borreliosis	Cardiac arrhythmias, myocarditis
Ehrlichia canis[b]	Canine ehrlichiosis	Anemia, bleeding tendencies, limb edema, lymphadenopathy, splenomegaly
Erysipelothrix spp.	Infectious valvular endocarditis	Heart murmur, emboli formation, valvular endocarditis
Leptospira spp.	Leptospirosis	Generalized hemorrhages, icterus, septicemia
Neorickettsia helminthoeca	Salmon poisoning	Lymphadenopathy, splenomegaly
Rickettsia rickettsii	Rocky Mountain spotted fever	Edema, hemorrhages, lymphadenopathy, myocarditis, vascular obstruction

[a]Includes *B. vinsonii* ssp. *berkhoffi* and *B. clarridgeiae*.
[b]Other *Ehrlichia* spp. cause clinical signs related to anemia, leukopenia, and thrombocytopenia.

Table 68.2. Common and/or Important Infectious Agents of Circulatory System and Lymphoid Tissues of Cats

Agent	Disease	Circulatory/Lymphoid-Associated Findings
Viruses		
Feline immunodeficiency virus	Feline immunodeficiency	Anemia, leukopenia, lymphadenopathy, secondary infections
Feline infectious peritonitis virus	Feline infectious peritonitis	Immune complex vasculitis/perivasculitis, lymphadenopathy, pericardial effusion
Feline leukemia virus	Feline leukemia	Anemia, lymphoid depletion, lymphosarcoma, myeloproliferative disease, secondary infections
Feline panleukopenia virus	Feline panleukopenia	Leukopenia, mesenteric lymphadenopathy
Feline sarcoma virus	Feline sarcoma	Fibrosarcomas
Bacteria		
Mycoplasma haemofelis	Feline infectious peritonitis	Anemia, icterus, splenomegaly
Francisella tularensis	Tularemia	Leukopenia, mesenteric lymphadenopathy
Streptococcus canis	Cat strangles	Cervical lymphadenitis, lymph node abscesses
Yersinia pestis	Plague	Cervical/submandibular lymphadenitis, lymph node abscesses, septicemia

Table 68.3. Common and/or Important Infectious Agents of Circulatory System and Lymphoid Tissues of Horses

Agent	Disease	Circulatory/Lymphoid-Associated Findings
Viruses		
African horse sickness virus	African horse sickness	Vasculitis with pulmonary, subcutaneous, and eyelid edema
Equine infectious anemia virus	Equine infectious anemia	Anemia, hemorrhages, icterus, splenomegaly
Equine viral arteritis virus	Equine viral arteritis	Edema, hemorrhages, leukopenia, vessel infarction
Venezuelan equine encephalitis virus	Venezuelan equine encephalitis	Cellular depletion of lymph nodes, spleen, and bone marrow
Bacteria		
Actinomyces spp.	Actinomycosis	Mandibular lymph node abscesses
Anaplasma phagocytophila	Equine ehrlichiosis	Anemia, edema of the legs, hemorrhages
Agents of neonatal septicemia[a]	Neonatal septicemia	Septicemia, hypotension, organ failure
Burkholderia mallei[b]	Farcy, glanders	Lymphangitis, lymphadenitis, splenic abscesses
Corynebacterium pseudotuberculosis	Ulcerative lymphangitis	Lymphangitis
Neorickettsia risticii	Potomac horse fever	Leukopenia, mesenteric lymphadenopathy
Streptococcus equi ssp. *equi*	Strangles purpura hemorrhagica	Immune-complex vasculitis, edema
Fungi		
Histoplasma farciminosum	Epizootic lymphangitis	Lymphangitis, regional lymphadenitis
Sporothrix schenckii	Sporotrichosis	Lymphangitis

[a]Includes *Actinobacillus equuli, Escherichia coli, Salmonella, Streptococcus equi* ssp. *zooepidemicus.*
[b]Classified as a foreign animal disease agent in the United States.

Table 68.4. Common and/or Important Infectious Agents of Circulatory System and Lymphoid Tissues of Cattle

Agent	Disease	Circulatory/Lymphoid-Associated Findings
Viruses		
Alcelaphine herpesvirus 1[a]	Malignant catarrhal fever	Hemorrhages, leukopenia, lymphoid proliferation, lymphadenopathy
Bovine leukemia virus	Bovine leukemia	Lymphosarcoma
Ovine herpesvirus 2	Malignant catarrhal fever	Hemorrhages, leukopenia, lymphoid proliferation, lymphadenopathy
Rift Valley fever virus[a]	Rift Valley fever	Splenomegaly, widespread hemorrhages
Rinderpest[a]	Rinderpest	Leukopenia, destruction of lymphoid organs
Bacteria		
Anaplasma marginale	Anaplasmosis	Anemia, icterus, splenomegaly
Arcanobacterium pyogenes	Traumatic reticulopericarditis	Pericarditis (often polymicrobial)
	Infectious valvular endocarditis	Heart murmur, heart failure, valvular endocarditis
Bacillus anthracis	Anthrax	Edema, septicemia, splenomegaly, bleeding from orifices
Clostridium chauvoei	Blackleg	Myocarditis, pericarditis
Clostridium haemolyticum	Bacillary hemoglobinuria	Icterus, intravascular hemolysis, hemorrhages
Ehrlichia ruminantium[a]	African heartwater disease	Edema, hemorrhages, hydropericardium, splenomegaly
Leptospira spp.	Leptospirosis	Anemia, icterus, intravascular hemolysis
Mycobacterium avium ssp. *paratuberculosis*	Johne's disease	Granulomatous lymphangitis of mesenteric lymph vessels
Mycobacterium bovis	Bovine tuberculosis	Granulomatous tracheobronchial/mediastinal lymphadenitis
Pasteurella multocida serotypes B : 2 or E : 2[a]	Hemorrhagic septicemia	Edema, hemorrhages, hemorrhagic lymphadenopathy
Salmonella spp.[b]	Salmonellosis	Septicemia, splenomegaly

[a]Classified as a foreign animal disease in the United States.
[b]Common serotypes include *Dublin* and *Typhimurium*.

Table 68.5. Common and/or Important Infectious Agents of Circulatory System and Lymphoid Tissues of Goats and Sheep

Agent	Disease	Circulatory/Lymphoid-Associated Findings
Viruses		
Bluetongue virus	Bluetongue	Edema of head and neck, hemorrhages, hyperemia
Peste des petits virus[a]	Peste des petits	Generalized lymphadenopathy, leukopenia, splenomegaly
Rift Valley fever virus[a]	Rift Valley fever	Splenomegaly, widespread hemorrhages
Rinderpest virus[a]	Rinderpest	Leukopenia, destruction of lymphoid organs
Bacteria		
Anaplasma ovis	Anaplasmosis	Anemia
Bacillus anthracis	Anthrax	Edema, septicemia, splenomegaly, bleeding from orifices
Corynebacterium pseudotuberculosis	Caseous lymphadenitis	Lymphadenitis, lymph node abscesses
Mycoplasma haemovis	Eperythrozoonosis	Anemia
Mannheimia haemolytica (S)	Septicemic pasteurellosis	Hemorrhagic septicemia in lambs
Mycoplasma mycoides ssp. *mycoides* (G) (large colony type)	Septicemic mycoplasmosis	Septicemia, pericarditis
Pasteurella trehalosi (G)	Septicemic pasteurellosis	Hemorrhagic septicemia in kids
Staphylococcus aureus	Tick pyemia of lambs	Lymphadenopathy, septicemia

G, goats; S, sheep.
[a]Classified as a foreign animal disease in the United States.

Table 68.6. Common and/or Important Infectious Agents of Circulatory System and Lymphoid Tissues of Pigs

Agent	Disease	Circulatory/Lymphoid-Associated Findings
Viruses		
African swine fever virus[a]	African swine fever	Generalized edema/hemorrhages/infarctions, hemorrhagic lymph nodes, pericarditis, skin cyanosis, splenomegaly
Encephalomyocarditis virus	Encephalomyocarditis	Hydropericardium, myocarditis, pericarditis
Hog cholera[a]	Hog cholera, classical swine fever	Generalized hemorrhages/infarctions, hemorrhagic lymph nodes, lymphoid depletions, skin cyanosis, splenic infarcts
Lelystad virus	Porcine reproductive and respiratory syndrome	Secondary infections due to macrophage depletion
Porcine circovirus 2	Postweaning multisystemic wasting syndrome	Lymphadenopathy, myocarditis, poor growth
Bacteria		
Bacillus anthracis	Anthrax	Pharyngeal lymphadenopathy and edema, septicemia
Burkholderia pseudomallei[a]	Melioidosis	Lymph node and splenic abscesses
Erysipelothrix rhusiopathiae	Erysipelas	Hemorrhages, splenomegaly, skin cyanosis, infectious valvular endocarditis
Escherichia coli	Septicemia	Septicemia in unweaned pigs, skin cyanosis, congested organs, lymphadenopathy
Escherichia coli (Shiga-like toxin positive)	Edema disease	Edema in subcutaneous tissue/stomach mucosa due to vasculitis
Haemophilus parasuis	Glasser's disease	Pericarditis, septicemia
Mycobacterium avium[b]	Swine mycobacteriosis	Granulomatous cervical, pharyngeal, and mesenteric lymphadenitis
Mycoplasma spp.[c]	Mycoplasma polyserositis	Pericarditis with other serositides
Mycoplasma haemosuis	Porcine eperythrozoonosis	Anemia, icterus, splenomegaly
Salmonella[d]	Salmonellosis	Lymphadenopathy, skin cyanosis, septicemia, splenomegaly
Streptococcus porcinus	Jowl abscess	Cervical lymphadenitis
Streptococcus suis	Streptococcal septicemia	Pericarditis, septicemia

[a]Classified as a foreign animal disease agent in the United States.
[b]Proposed that swine strains of *Mycobacterium avium* be included in the ssp. *hominissuis*. Other mycobacterial species involved include *M. kansasii*, *M. xenopi*, and *M. fortuitum*. *Rhodococcus equi* is also occasionally involved.
[c]Includes *Mycoplasma hyopneumoniae*, *M. hyorhinis*, and *M. hyosynoviae*.
[d]Most common serotypes are Choleraesuis var. Kunzendorf and Typhimurium.

Table 68.7. Common and/or Important Infectious Agents of Circulatory System and Lymphoid Tissues of Poultry

Agent	Disease	Circulatory/Lymphoid-Associated Findings
Viruses		
Avian influenza virus H5 or H7[a] (highly pathogenic)	Avian influenza, fowl plague	Generalized hemorrhages; edema of head, wattles, and comb; lymphoid necrosis; myocarditis
Avian leucosis viruses (C)	Lymphoid leucosis	Anemia, hemangiomas, lymphoid tumors, sarcomas
Chicken anemia virus	Chicken anemia	Anemia, hemorrhages, hydropericardium, hypoplasia of lymphoid, and hemopoietic tissues
Exotic Newcastle disease virus[a]	Exotic Newcastle disease	Generalized hemorrhages (especially intestinal), edema
Infectious bursal disease virus (C)	Infectious bursal disease, Gumboro disease	Enlarged/hemorrhagic (especially intestinal) edema
Marek's disease virus (C)	Marek's disease	Lymphoid tumors of heart, bursa, thymus, spleen
Reticuloendotheliosis virus (T)	Reticuloendotheliosis	Lymphoreticular neoplasia, lymphomas
Turkey adenovirus 2 (T)	Hemorrhagic enteritis of turkeys	Immunosuppression, intestinal hemorrhage, splenomegaly
Bacteria		
Borrelia anserine	Avian spirochetosis	Anemia, hemorrhages, splenomegaly
Chlamydophila psittaci (T)[b]	Ornithosis, chlamydiosis	Pericarditis, splenomegaly, fibrin exudates
Erysipelothrix rhusiopathiae	Erysipelas	Generalized hemorrhages, pericarditis, septicemia
Escherichia coli	Colisepticemia	Pericarditis, omphalitis, septicemia, splenomegaly
Mycobacterium avium	Avian tuberculosis	Splenic granulomas
Pasteurella multocida	Fowl cholera	Generalized hemorrhages, pericarditis, septicemia
Salmonella[b]	Salmonellosis[c]	Myocarditis, omphalitis, pericarditis, splenitis

C, chicken; T, turkey.
[a]Classified as a foreign animal disease agent in the United States.
[b]Includes serovars Pullorum, Gallinarum, and Typhimurium.
[c]Includes pullorum disease, fowl typhoid, and parathyroid.

these microbial products results in a dysregulation of the immune response and the production of excessive levels of proinflammatory cytokines (tumor necrosis factor-α, interleukin 1, and interleukin 6), which are largely responsible for the systemic effects observed in sepsis. Toll-like receptors are also found on endothelial cells lining blood vessels.

Some gram-positive organisms produce superantigens that nonspecifically activate large populations of T lymphocytes to produce excessive amounts of proinflammatory cytokines. Coagulation abnormalities, specifically disseminated intravascular coagulation, can also be a consequence of sepsis.

During a bacterial septicemia, rarely are organisms present in high enough numbers to be detected by direct microscopic examination. Some bacteria are, however, present in large enough numbers in the blood during the terminal stages of disease to be detected in direct smears. *Bacillus anthracis*, the etiologic agent of anthrax, causes an overwhelming septicemia, predominately in ruminants, and results in large numbers of organisms being found in the blood just prior to death. *Pasteurella multocida*, the agent of fowl cholera, and *Borrelia anserina*, the agent of avian spirochetosis, can also be found in large numbers in the blood of affected birds.

Infections Involving the Heart and Pericardium

The major infectious processes of the heart are infectious valvular endocarditis (usually bacterial) and myocarditis (bacterial or viral). Infections of the pericardium occur either as a result of a systemic infection, from a focus within the heart (e.g., endocarditis), or by extension of an infectious process from adjacent tissues (e.g., pleuropulmonary infections or traumatic reticulopericarditis).

Infectious Valvular Endocarditis

Valvular endocarditis results from bacteria from another site in the body seeding one of the heart valves. Preexisting injury or functional abnormality of the heart valve allows for platelet and fibrin deposition. These deposits provide sites for attachment for bacteria that are present in the circulation, often as a result of one of the mechanisms of transient bacteremia previously described. Attachment to the heart valve is mediated through a number of bacterial surface adhesins that include surface glucans and fibronectin-binding proteins. Exposed extracellular matrix on the valve may also serve as a receptor favoring bacteria expressing fibrinogen or laminin-binding proteins. A preexisting heart valve lesion is not an absolute requirement for infectious valvular endocarditis to develop. Other cardiac abnormalities (e.g., subaortic stenosis in dogs) or invasive vascular procedures, including catheterization, also predispose to heart valve infections. Sequelae to valvular endocarditis include embolization, multiorgan infarction, and sudden death.

Bacteria involved in infectious endocarditis are predominantly, but not exclusively, gram-positive organisms and include streptococci, enterococci, staphylococci, *Corynebacterium*, and *Arcanobacterium* spp. The genus *Erysipelothrix* is specifically associated with valvular endocarditis in some animals (swine, dogs, and poultry). When gram-negative organisms are involved, they are usually members of the families Enterobacteriaceae and Pseudomonadaceae. *Bartonella*, another gram-negative organism, is increasingly being recognized as a cause of infectious valvular endocarditis in dogs.

Myocarditis

Myocarditis, an inflammation of the heart muscle, is usually the result of systemic infection with foci of infection in the heart. Damage occurs directly to myocytes or to vascular endothelial vessels supplying heart muscle. The mechanisms of injury to the heart muscle vary and include (i) direct toxic action of an agent on myocytes, (ii) effects of circulating toxic products, or (iii) immune-mediated mechanisms. A wide variety of infectious agents have potential to cause myocarditis. Some common microbial agents specifically associated with myocarditis in animals include canine parvovirus, encephalomyocarditis virus in pigs, *Clostridium chauvoei* in cattle, and *Listeria monocytogenes* in ruminants and poultry.

Infections Involving the Pericardium

Hydropericardium or pericardial effusion, a serous fluid accumulation in the pericardial cavity, in conjunction with other systemic signs is a characteristic of certain infectious diseases (e.g., heartwater in cattle, African horse sickness, and chicken anemia virus infection) and is the result of vascular damage. Fluid accumulations in the pericardial sac also result from damage due to immune-complex deposition in vessels (e.g., feline infectious peritonitis).

Pericarditis denotes an inflammation of the pericardium. Like myocarditis, a number of viral and bacterial agents can be involved. Pericarditis is often part of a systemic infection involving other serosal surfaces and cavities (e.g., Glasser's disease in pigs and *Mycoplasma* septicemia in goats).

The most common traumatic pericardial infection is traumatic reticulopericarditis (hardware disease) in cattle. This is most often associated with the extension of an ingested linear metallic object (e.g., wire and nail) through the reticulum and diaphragm into the pericardial sac. It provides bacteria the necessary access to the pericardial space in order for infection to establish. Such infections are usually polymicrobial, with *Arcanobacterium pyogenes* and *Fusobacterium necrophorum* frequently involved. The clinical signs associated with pericarditis in cattle are those of right-sided heart failure, decreased production, exercise intolerance, tachycardia secondary to decreased cardiac output, jugular distension (Figure 68.1), jugular pulses, and submandibular edema. Muffled heart sounds may also be present. There may also be a murmur characterized as a "washing machine" murmur if there is a gas fluid interface within the pericardial sac.

FIGURE 68.1. *The right jugular furrow of a Holstein cow in right-sided congestive heart failure exhibiting jugular distension. The right-sided congestive heart failure is due to pericardial effusion, in this case, secondary to traumatic reticulopericarditis.*

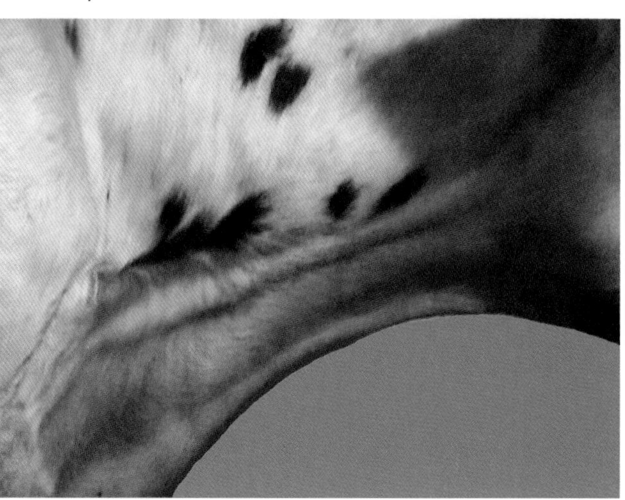

Infections Affecting Blood Vessels

In general, the endothelium of blood vessels plays an interactive role in most inflammatory reactions through endothelial–leukocyte interaction, procoagulation activity, and release of mediators (cytokines and chemokines). Microbes that specifically infect endothelial cells of small vessels and capillaries can cause necrosis with increased vascular permeability resulting from direct vascular endothelial injury by an agent or its toxin (e.g., Shiga-like toxin) or by immune-complex deposition and an ensuing inflammatory response. Disruption of the endothelial barrier leads to edema and/or hemorrhages in affected organs. Clinical signs depend on the agent and vascular site(s) in the body primarily affected (e.g., African horse sickness and the pulmonary vasculature with an ensuing pulmonary edema). Central nervous system signs in dogs as a result of bleeding into the brain are attributed to *Rickettsia rickettsii*, the Rocky Mountain spotted fever agent, and the vascular damage it causes. Similarly, damage to the integrity of vessels walls due to immune-complex deposition in feline infectious peritonitis in cats results in the fluid accumulations in serosal cavities, as is found in the "wet form" of the disease. In addition to severe hepatic necrosis, Rift Valley fever virus causes massive generalized endothelial damage resulting in widespread hemorrhages. Loss of endothelial anticoagulant activity and platelet activation may cause thrombosis of blood vessels and infarction in some systemic infections, ultimately leading to tissue necrosis at the affected site (e.g., skin lesions of erysipelas in swine). Details on the pathogenesis of these and other infectious diseases that affect the blood vasculature and associated pathology are covered in greater detail in chapters on the specific agent or system(s) involved.

Omphalitis, an inflammation of the umbilicus of neonates, deserves special attention. Both the umbilical arteries and veins can be involved. It is especially important in farm animals and horses. The bacteria responsible are either of enteric origin, inhabitants of mucosal surfaces, or environmental contaminants (e.g., *Actinobacillus* spp.,

FIGURE 68.2. *Multiple liver abscesses secondary to an ascending umbilical vein infection in a 3-month-old Gelbvieh heifer.*

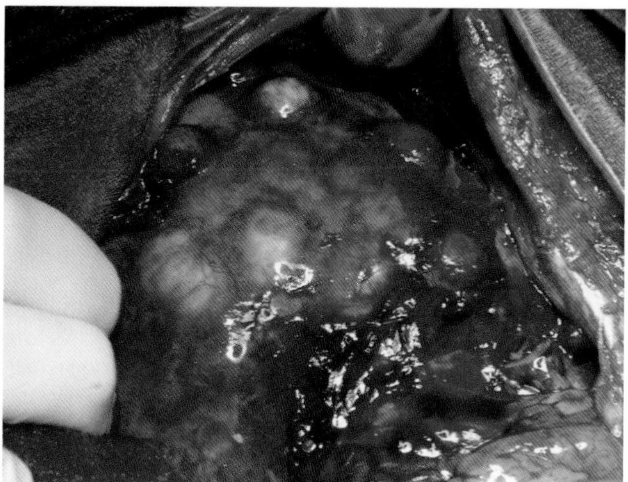

FIGURE 68.3. A. marginale *in blood from an ox stained with Wright's stain. (Courtesy of Dr Bruce Brodersen.)*

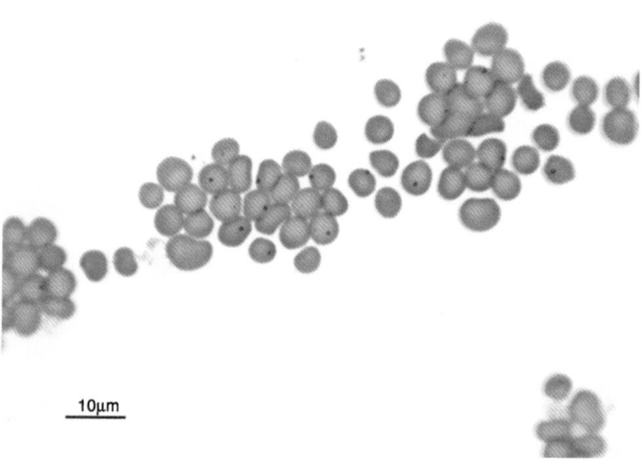

A. pyogenes, *Escherichia coli*, and streptococci). Umbilical infections can lead to local abscess development or, sometimes, serve as a site for establishment of *Clostridium tetani* and the development of tetanus. When omphalophlebitis, an inflammation of the umbilical vein, becomes infected, the infection can extend along the remnants of the fetal circulation to involve the liver (Figure 68.2).

A septicemia may also develop from umbilical infections (navel ill), which can lead to infections elsewhere in the body, including polyarthritis and meningitis. Failure of passive transfer is a common predisposing factor in these cases. In poultry, yolk sac infection and omphalitis are also a serious problem. A variety of organisms are involved, *E. coli*, *Salmonella*, and *Pseudomonas* being prominent etiologic agents.

Infections Involving Red Blood Cells

Anemia is a common finding in many infectious processes. A number of mechanisms lead to anemia and include suppression of erythropoiesis, sequestration of red blood cells (RBCs), antibody-mediated hemolysis, erythrophagocytosis, direct lysis of RBCs, and alterations in RBC membranes that decrease overall lifespan.

Anaplasma marginale specifically infects RBCs in cattle (Figure 68.3). Infections elicit an immune response that results in removal of both infected and uninfected RBCs and may lead to a packed cell volume as low as 6%.

Chicken anemia virus disease and FeLV infections in cats are causes of anemia due, at least in part, to decreased erythropoiesis. The bacterial hemoparasite, *Mycoplasma haemofelis*, causes anemia in cats by multiple mechanisms including RBC sequestration and antibody-mediated hemolysis. Immune-mediated hemolytic anemia is also important in FeLV infections and canine ehrlichiosis. Immune-mediated hemolysis can be the result of (i) presence of microbial antigens on the RBCs, (ii) cross-reactions between antigens of normal RBC proteins and an infectious agent, or (iii) exposure of usually unexposed RBC antigens during the infectious process. Intravascular hemolysis resulting in anemia can be the result of action of certain bacterial toxins (e.g., phospholipase C). *Leptospira* spp. and *Clostridium hemolyticum* are notable agents that destroy RBCs by this mechanism. Anemia in these cases is often accompanied by hemoglobinuria.

Infections Involving White Blood Cells

A number of viruses affect cells of the myeloid and lymphoid series. Venezuelan equine encephalitis virus is a prominent example of a virus that destroys hemopoietic and lymphoreticular cells, leading to cellular depletion in bone marrow, lymph nodes, and the spleen. Many viral infections that target cells in these series predispose animals to secondary infections consequent to the immunosuppressive effects that occur. One of the main targets of infectious bursal disease virus in chickens is the cloacal bursa, which is initially enlarged and edematous but eventually becomes atrophied. The resulting B lymphocyte deficiency leads to secondary infections. Feline leukemia virus, feline immunodeficiency virus in cats, and porcine circovirus in pigs similarly make animals more susceptible to secondary infections through immunosuppressive effects. These effects can be long-term; however, other viral infections (e.g., distemper virus, hog cholera virus, parvoviruses, and bovine viral diarrhea virus) cause temporary leukopenias and the immunosuppressive effect is short-term.

Bacterial agents may also infect white blood cells. Certain members of the genera *Anaplasma*, *Ehrlichia*, and *Neorickettsia* are pathogens of cells belonging to the myeloid or megakaryocyte series. Fungal agents are not commonly associated with infections of the myeloid or lymphoid cell series. However, the systemic fungal agent *Histoplasma capsulatum* specifically infects macrophages and, therefore, histoplasmosis is considered a disease of the monocyte-macrophage system.

Infections of Lymph Nodes, Lymphatics, and Other Lymphoid Tissues

Lymph nodes play a major role in filtering primary sites of infection via the lymphatic vessels and, therefore, act as principal sites for containment of potential pathogens. Many viral infections are dispersed to other parts of the body (target organs) by this route.

Lymphadenitis, an inflammation of the lymph node, can occur in a single lymph node or multiple lymph nodes draining a common region (regional lymphadenitis) or manifest as a generalized lymphadenitis in systemic infections. Depending on the agents involved, the inflammatory response can be nonsuppurative, suppurative, necrotizing, or granulomatous. In some cases, depending on the agent and the host response, lymph node abscessation occurs. Microbial agents causing lymph node abscesses are usually but not exclusively bacterial or fungal. Particular organisms consistently associated with lymph node abscesses include *Corynebacterium pseudotuberculosis* in sheep and goats (caseous lymphadenitis) and *Streptococcus equi* ssp. *equi* in horses (strangles). Although less common now, *Streptococcus porcinus* was an important cause of cervical lymph node abscesses in swine (jowl abscesses). *Yersinia pestis* should always be considered when mandibular lymph node abscesses (often bilateral) are detected in cats from geographic regions where plague is endemic. *Francisella tularensis* causes lymphadenopathy with abscessation in cats, along with generalized signs of infection. *Streptococcus canis* also causes purulent inflammation of lymph nodes on the head and neck in cats. Outbreaks, presumably via oral transmission, have been described in cats kept in colonies.

Generalized or regional lymphadenitis is encountered with the systemic mycotic infections (blastomycosis, coccidioidomycosis, cryptococcosis, and histoplasmosis) and typically results in a caseous-type necrosis in the affected lymph node.

Lymphangitis is an acute or chronic inflammation of the lymphatic channels that results when infections are not contained locally. Infections usually involve subcutaneous lymphatics. Lymphangitis is not common in animals, but when it occurs the etiologic agents are most often bacterial or fungal. Parasitic agents should also be considered as causes of lymphangitis in animals but are not within the scope of this book. Inflammation of the lymphatic walls can result in lymphatic obstruction and persistent lymphedema in sites drained by the affected lymphatics. Lymphatic vessels may be swollen (corded), with sporadic discharging abscesses occurring along the lymphatic tracts. Lymphangitis is most commonly recognized in horses. *Sporothrix schenckii*, a dimorphic fungus, and *C. pseudotuberculosis* are classical causes of equine lymphangitis. Although considered foreign animal disease agents in the United States, *Burkholderia mallei* (agent of glanders) and *Histoplasma farciminosum* (agent of epizootic lymphangitis) should also be considered as potential causes of lymphangitis in horses in countries where these agents are found. *Mycobacterium avium* ssp. *paratuberculosis*, the agent of Johne's disease in ruminants, causes a granulomatous lymphangitis in the mesentery of the intestines in conjunction with granulomatous enteritis.

The spleen plays an active role in antigen trapping as well as removal of defective erythrocytes. Splenitis commonly occurs as a consequence of generalized infections due to acute congestion and/or reactive hyperplasia. Salmonella septicemia is a common cause of splenomegaly in many animals. In cattle, anthrax and anaplasmosis should also be considered. In pigs, African swine fever and erysipelas, along with *Salmonella*, are potential agents to consider when splenomegaly is detected.

The thymus is an uncommon site for infections in animals. Viruses that infected T lymphocytes (e.g., feline leukemia virus and feline immunodeficiency virus) cause thymic atrophy. A lymphohistiocytic thymusitis with depletion of cortical thymocytes is a major pathologic feature in epizootic bovine abortion, a disease limited to the western United States. The suspected etiologic agent is a deltaproteobacterium spread by the *Ornithodoros coriaceus* tick.

Neoplasias of the Hemopoietic and Lymphoid Tissues with Infectious Etiologies

Various viral-induced neoplasias involving hemopoietic and lymphatic tissues occur in animals. Marek's disease virus, a herpesvirus, causes a lymphoproliferative disease that predominately affects nervous tissues but also causes lymphoid tumors in a number of other tissues including the heart, bursa, thymus, and spleen. A number of animal retroviruses exist and are able to integrate proviral v-onc genes into host cellular DNA. The ability of

FIGURE 68.4. *An extradural mass at the lumbar intumescence in an 8-year-old Angus cow. Bovine leukemia virus infection, a retrovirus, can lead to adult-onset multicentric BLV (Bovine leukosis virus)-associated lymphosarcoma.*

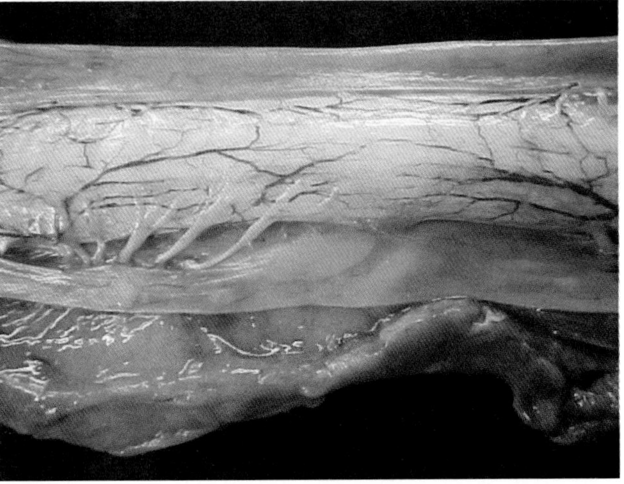

feline leukemia virus to infect different hemopoietic cells accounts for the variety of disorders of the hemopoietic system seen in infected cats. In addition, solid neoplasias including lymphosarcoma (e.g., thymic lymphosarcoma) can occur. The bovine leukemia virus, also a retrovirus, causes lymphosarcoma that can involve a number of organs including heart, kidney, spleen, lymph nodes, and brain (Figure 68.4). Avian retroviruses of the leukosis/sarcoma group cause various neoplasias of hemopoietic origin (erythroblastosis, myeloblastosis, and myelocytomatosis), as well as lymphoid leukosis and endothelial tumors (hemangiomas). Viruses of reticuloendotheliosis group cause lymphoid leukosis and reticu-loendotheliosis in turkeys.

Digestive System and Associated Organs

DOUGLAS E. HOSTETLER

The primary function of the digestive system is to process food in order to provide nutrition for the body. This is performed by a series of complex physical, secretory, and absorptive processes. An in-depth description of all of the varied and interactive functions of the digestive system is well beyond the scope of this chapter. Because the digestive system in its simplest term represents an open tube to the environment, the opportunity for exposure of the digestive system to potential pathogens is great.

The anatomy of the digestive system varies markedly among different animals. In carnivorous animals, it includes the oral cavity, esophagus, stomach, and small and large intestines. The digestive system of herbivores is substantially different from carnivores both anatomically and functionally. Among the herbivorous animals there is also great variation in the digestive system makeup depending on the digestive mechanisms employed (e.g., rumination and cecal digestion). In poultry, further specialization of the digestive system is seen by the presence of a crop (a diverticulum of the esophagus for storage of food) and the division of the stomach into a glandular stomach (proventriculus) and muscular stomach (ventriculus or gizzard). Some of these anatomic differences selectively predispose to specific infectious processes. Infectious diseases of the accessory organs of the digestive system are also covered in this chapter and include common diseases of the hepatobiliary system and pancreas.

Antimicrobial Properties of the Digestive System

There are a number of anatomic, physiologic, and immunologic mechanisms in place to protect the digestive system from infection by potentially pathogenic microbes. Following are the major protective features of the digestive system.

Original chapter written by the late Dr. Richard L. Walker.

Gastric Acidity

Acid production in the stomach provides a major protective barrier against pathogens reaching distal sites in the digestive system. The normal acidic environment in the stomach effectively inactivates some viruses and kills most enteric bacteria. Its importance is evident in humans by the increased risk for enteric infections observed in individuals with achlorhydria or in individuals when stomach acid has been neutralized.

Peristalsis

Peristaltic activity in the digestive system is a mechanism, whereby nonadhering microorganisms are swept distally. In the small intestine, peristaltic activity plays a major role in host defense. The occurrence of disease is a function of a large enough number (relative infective dose) of pathogens being in contact with the enterocytes long enough to adhere and establish an infection. The most important regulator of the size of this population is peristaltic activity, since there are few other regulators such as those that exist in the large bowel (Eh, fatty acids, and pH). Peristalsis also has an indirect protective role by maintaining distribution and numbers of the normal bacterial flora.

Mucus and Mucosal Integrity

The mucus layer and the integrity of mucosal surface are important factors in providing a barrier to infection in the digestive system, as well as to systemic infections that originate through the digestive system. The mucus barrier, composed of mucin glycoproteins secreted by goblet cells, binds organisms, thereby blocking interaction with underlying epithelial cells and, along with peristalsis, promotes their removal. The monolayer of epithelial cells lining the digestive system provides an additional barrier to entry by luminal organisms. Intestinal enterocytes are zippered together by intercellular junctional complexes. Damage to intestinal epithelium allows for intercellular translocation of potentially pathogenic microbes. Some microbes are

Veterinary Microbiology, Third Edition. Edited by D. Scott McVey, Melissa Kennedy and M.M. Chengappa.

able to translocate across intestinal mucosa by intracellular means.

Bacterial Interference

Once the normal flora is established, it gives an animal a very potent defense against microorganisms that might cause disease, if they establish. An example of the effectiveness of this "colonization resistance" is the exclusion of Salmonella from the intestinal tract of poultry by "cocktails" containing normal flora microorganisms. Disrupting colonization resistance puts the animal at risk by exposing receptors on potential target cells and eliminating a mechanism for regulating the population size of facultative organisms, including species or strains with pathogenic potential. Products of normal bacterial flora, especially the anaerobes that make up the majority of the oral and colonic flora, are important in controlling pathogen establishment (see Section "Microbial Flora of the Digestive System"). The newborn animal is particularly susceptible to enteric disease because, besides being immunologically naive, it is devoid of established flora. The most vulnerable area is the mid-jejunum and distal ileum.

Immune Defense

Passive protection is afforded in the neonate by colostrum. Immunoglobulins in colostrum, specific for antigenic determinants on adhesins used by pathogens for attachment, combine with these structures to block attachment of the pathogen to its target cell. Failure of passive transfer and thus the absence of these protective immunoglobulins is one of the major factors leading to the increased susceptiblity of neonates to enteric infections.

The active immune defense mechanisms in the digestive system rely on patrolling phagocytes and humoral and cell-mediated immunity. There is a normal background of neutrophils, macrophages, plasma cells, and lymphocytes found in the lamina propria indicating a continuous surveillance activity. When stimulated by potential pathogens, inflammatory mediators and chemotactic agents are produced and result in an influx of additional inflammatory cells. As part of the body's mucosal immune system, the gut-associated lymphoid tissue (GALT) is composed of lymphoid tissue in Peyer's patches and lymphocytes in the lamina propria. The microfold (M) cells overlying follicles of Peyer's patch play a role in antigen sampling for the immune system but may also provide a portal of entry for some pathogens. The benefits of GALT and antigen sampling in the digestive system are not just local but rather benefit the entire host through the common mucosal immune system. Secretory IgA and associated secretory component, which provides resistance to luminal degradation, has a role in osponization and neutralizing. Specific IgM antibodies are also involved.

Commensal bacteria play an important role in the development of the mucosal immune system of the gastrointestinal tract by promoting lymphoid follicle development; however, the immune system responds more vigorously to pathogenic organisms than it does to commensal organisms. This is possibly due to the closer attachment of pathogens to mucosal cells or that commensal organisms, being more permanent residents, temper the immune response directed toward them by blocking proinflammatory responses. Inappropriate inflammatory response to normal commensal bacteria is hypothesized to be an underlying cause for inflammatory bowel disease in humans.

In parts of the digestive tract, the normal flora is integral to maintaining an active innate host surveillance system. In the mouth, for instance, the periodontal microbiota stimulates the formation of an interleukin-8 (IL-8) gradient that promotes migration of neutrophils to bacterial/epithelial interfaces. Thus, these commensal microbial communities in the oral cavity provide for an active surveillance in the gingival sulci against potential oral pathogens.

As an associated organ of the digestive system, the liver plays a major role in removal of pathogens from the bloodstream. This innate host defense is accomplished by a complex neutrophil-Kupffer cell (resident liver macrophage) interaction.

Other Antimicrobial Products

Saliva, along with providing an important flushing effect, contains a number of potential antimicrobial agents, including antibodies, complement, lysozyme, lactoferrin, peroxidases, and defensins. In the intestines, bile salts and antimicrobial peptides contribute to limiting and influencing the microbial makeup. Both alpha and beta defensins are produced by cells of the intestinal tract (e.g., Paneth cells). Lactoferrin and peroxidase from the pancreas may also affect bacterial growth in the intestine. In addition to the antibodies in colostrum, the presence of other factors such as lactoferrin and lysozyme provide additional protection for the digestive system in neonates.

Microbial Flora of the Digestive System

A microbial flora that is part of a complex ecosystem inhabits the digestive tract. In addition to its role in protection against the establishment of pathogens, the normal flora plays an important role in physiological health of the host through functions that include promoting functional intestinal villi formation, synthesis of nutrients (e.g., vitamin K and water soluble vitamins (ruminants)), and contributing to the establishment of a functional intestinal mucus consistency by degradation of the secreted glycoproteins.

Establishment

The result of interactions between host and microbe is an ecosystem comprised of many thousands of niches, each inhabited by the species or strains of microbes most aptly suited to that location, to the exclusion of others. The host contributes to the establishment of a normal flora by furnishing receptors for adhesins on the surface of prospective niche dwellers. The niche dweller is the one that has successfully competed for that particular site.

The fetus is microbiologically sterile as it starts down the birth canal. Microorganisms are acquired from the birth canal and, after birth, from the environment. The immediate environment of the newborn is populated with microorganisms excreted by the dam and other animals. These microbes are ingested, compete for niches, and with time become established as part of the normal flora. During the first days to months after birth, the flora is in a state of flux due to the interplay between the various microbes, the niches of the host, and the changing diet. Diet influences the nutritional environment at the level of the niche, which in turn influences the kinds of microbes that will successfully compete for these nutrients. Throughout its life the host's normal flora is influenced by a number of other factors (e.g., aging of the host) and adapts accordingly.

Members of the normal flora establish themselves in a particular niche utilizing various bacterial and host properties in the process. A powerful way for bacteria to secure a particular niche against other species is to secrete antibiotic-like substances such as bacteriocins (cationic membrane-active compounds that form pores in the target cells) and microcins (similar to bacteriocins but smaller than 10 kDa and active against gram-negative microorganisms). Both of these substances are significant, especially in the communities living in the oral cavity. Microcins probably play a significant role in regulating the population composition in the gastrointestinal portion of the digestive system. The role of bacteriocins in this region is less clear.

An important mechanism for regulating population size and ensuring niche security is fatty acid excretion by obligate anaerobes. In the gingival sulcus, dental plaque, and the large bowel, the obligate anaerobes in this manner play a central role in regulating the size and composition of the normal facultative flora, the members of which may include potential pathogens. Under the conditions of the bowel (low Eh (<500 mv) and pH of 5–6), butyric, acetic, and lactic acids are extremely toxic to facultative anaerobes, especially members of the family *Enterobacteriaceae*. Another way for bacteria to compete successfully is to acquire nutrients more successfully than competitors.

Disruption

Antimicrobial drugs are the single most efficient agents at decreasing colonization resistance. Most antimicrobial agents affect the microbial flora of the oral cavity by depleting the number of streptococci that inhabit the surface of the cheeks and tongue. As a result, these areas are usually repopulated with resistant (to the antimicrobial agent being administered) members of the family *Enterobacteriaceae* within 24–48 h. Resistant members of the environmental flora are also found. Members of the genus *Pseudomonas* are notorious examples of this group.

Antimicrobials also affect the members of the obligate anaerobic communities that inhabit the gingival sulcus and dental plaque in the mouth and the large bowel. Overgrowth of various members of the family *Enterobacteriaceae* results because of decreases in levels of fatty acids. Colonization by potential pathogens (e.g., *Salmonella* spp.) is enhanced by antibiotics affecting obligate anaerobes living in the bowel.

Composition

Bacterial species as well as some protozoal and fungal species constitute the bulk of the microflora in the alimentary canal of animals. The overwhelming majority of the normal flora is obligate anaerobic bacteria (up to 99.9%). Viruses are typically only transient residents of the alimentary canal.

The microbial flora of the mouth is roughly uniform among domestic mammals. No information is available for fowl. The description that follows is general and applies to carnivores and herbivores. The buccal surface, tongue, and teeth (plaque) are inhabited by facultative and obligate aerobes. These include streptococci (alpha and nonhemolytic), members of the family *Pasteurellaceae*, *Actino-myces* spp., enterics (*Escherichia coli* being the most common), *Neisseria* spp., CDC group EF-4 ("eugonic fermenter"), and *Simonsiella* (a unique oral commensal that forms characteristic monoseriate filaments). The flora of the gingival sulcus is composed almost entirely of obligate anaerobes, the most common genera being *Bacteroides*, *Fusobacterium*, *Peptostreptococcus*, *Porphyromonas*, and *Prevotella*. Saliva contains a mixture of facultative and obligate species of anaerobes and aerobes. The esophagus does not possess a normal flora but is contaminated with organisms found in saliva.

In ruminants, rumen flora is composed of a complex microbial community that includes bacteria (eubacteria and archaea), fungi, and protozoa. The rumen flora is in a delicately balanced symbiotic relationship with the host that is necessary to maintain rumen health for its proper fermentative function. The bulk of the flora are obligate anaerobes, with *Prevotella* spp. and *Butyrivibrio* spp. being among the most common genera found. Also included are bacteria (*Ruminococcus*, *Fibrobacter*) specifically required for digestion of cellulose-rich forages. Disruptions in the normal rumen flora can lead to serious metabolic and physiological problems (see Section "Infections of the Stomach, Ruminant Forestomach, and Abomasum"). The flora of the rest of the alimentary canal varies substantially among different animals, as is shown in Tables 69.1, 69.2, 69.3, 69.4, and 69.5.

Digestive system–associated organs (liver, gall bladder, and pancreas) are not generally considered to have a normal flora but may be transiently seeded as a result of asymptomatic bacteremia. Clostridial spores are readily found in the liver of many animals but remain dormant unless tissue oxygen tension becomes low enough to allow spores to germinate and vegetative cells to proliferate.

Infections of the Digestive System and Associated Organs

Infections of the digestive system and associated organs are important in all domestic animals. Some digestive system pathogens (e.g., enterotoxigenic *E. coli*, rotaviruses) are specific for a particular animal family, while others

Table 69.1. Microbial Flora of the Chicken

	Number of Viable Microorganisms/Gram of Contents[a]					
	Stomach		Small Intestine			
	Crop	Gizzard	Upper	Lower	Cecum	Feces
Total	6	6	8–9	8–9	8–9	8–9
Anaerobes	3	5–6	<2	<2	8–9	7–8
Enterbacteriaceae[b]	6	<2	1–2	1–3	5–6	6–7
Streptococci/Enterococci	2	<2	4	3–5	6–7	6–7
Lactobacillus	5–6	2–3	8–9	8–9	8–9	8–9

[a]Expressed as $\log_{10}$ of the number of organisms cultured.
[b]Mainly *E. coli.*

affect a wide variety of animals (e.g., *Salmonella enterica* serovar Typhimurium). In addition to differences in animal susceptibility—age, immune status, and genetic susceptibility—individuals within a species may also predispose to infection by specific pathogens. Some of the most common and/or important pathogens of the digestive system of major domestic animals and poultry are listed in Tables 69.6, 69.7, 69.8, 69.9, 69.10, 69.11, and 69.12.

Infections of the Oral Cavity

The oral cavity of animals is susceptible to infection by a various endogenous (usually bacterial or fungal) and exogenous microbes (usually viral). Viral pathogens are often contagious and may, therefore, affect large populations of animals at a time. Infections from endogenous microbes tend to involve one or a limited number of animals.

Table 69.2. Microbial Flora of the Bovine

	Number of Viable Microorganisms/Gram of Contents[a]				
		Small Intestine			
	Abomasum	Upper	Lower	Cecum	Feces
Total	6–8	>7	6–7	8–9	9
Anaerobes	7–8	NA[c]	5–6	8–9	6–9
Enterbacteriaceae[b]	3–4	>7	5–6	4–5	5–6
Streptococci/Enterococci	6–7	2–3	3–4	4–5	4–5
Yeasts	2–3	–	<3	2	–

[a]Expressed as $\log_{10}$ of the number of organisms cultured.
[b]Mainly *E. coli.*
[c]Not available.

Table 69.3. Microbial Flora of the Horse

	Number of Viable Microorganisms/Gram of Contents[a]				
		Small Intestine			
	Stomach	Upper	Lower	Cecum	Feces
Total	6–8	NA[c]	6–7	8–9	8–9
Anaerobes	3–5	3–4	4–6	3–4	3–5
Enterbacteriaceae[b]	6–7	5–6	5–6	6–7	5–6
Streptococci/Enterococci	–	–	–	–	<3
Yeasts	6–8	NA[c]	6–7	8–9	8–9

[a]Expressed as $\log_{10}$of the number of organisms cultured.
[b]Mainly *E. coli.*
[c]Not available.

Table 69.4. Microbial Flora of the Pig

	Number of Viable Microorganisms/Gram of Contents[a]				
		Small Intestine			
	Stomach	Upper	Lower	Cecum	Feces
Total	3–8	3–7	4–8	4–11	10–11
Anaerobes	7–8	6–7	7–8	7–11	10–11
Enterbacteriaceae[b]	3–5	3–4	4–5	6–9	6–9
Streptococci/Enterococci	4–6	4–5	6–7	7–10	7–10
Yeasts	4–5	4	4	4	4
Spiral Organisms	NA[c]	NA[c]	NA[c]	NA[c]	8

[a]Expressed as $\log_{10}$ of the number of organisms cultured.
[b]Mainly *E. coli*.
[c]Not available.

Table 69.5. Microbial Flora of the Dog

	Number of Viable Microorganisms/Gram of Contents[a]				
		Small Intestine			
	Stomach	Upper	Lower	Cecum	Feces
Total	>6	>6	>7	>8	10–11
Anaerobes	1–2	>5	4–5	>8	10–11
Enterbacteriaceae[b]	1–5	2–4	4–6	7–8	7–8
Streptococci/Enterococci	1–6	5–6	5–7	8–9	9–10
Spiral Organisms (relative amounts)	1+	1+	1+	4+	0

[a]Expressed as $\log_{10}$ of the number of organisms cultured.
[b]Mainly *E. coli*.

Table 69.6. Common and/or Important Infectious Agents of the Digestive System of Dogs

Agent	Major Clinical Manifestations (Common Disease Name)	Age Group(s) Commonly Affected
Viruses		
Canine adenovirus 1	Diarrhea, jaundice, vomiting	Typically less than 6 months
Canine coronavirus	Diarrhea, vomiting	Any age, typically in puppies
Canine distemper virus	Diarrhea, vomiting, dental enamel hypoplasia (distemper)	Any age, most susceptible at 4–6 months
Canine oral papillomavirus	Oral cavity warts (oral papillomatosis)	Typically less than 1 year
Canine parvovirus	Diarrhea, vomiting	Any age, most susceptible at 2–4 months
Bacteria		
Campylobacter jejuni/coli.	Diarrhea with or without blood	Any age, typically less than 6 months
Leptospira spp.[a]	Hepatitis, vomiting (leptospirosis)	Any age
Neorickettsia helminthoeca	Diarrhea, vomiting (salmon poisoning)	Any age
Salmonella spp.	Diarrhea, vomiting	Any age, young and old most susceptible
Fungi		
Histoplasma capsulatum	Diarrhea with or without blood, oral ulcers, weight loss (histoplasmosis)	Any age, typically less than 4 years
Algae		
Prototheca spp.	Bloody Diarrhea (protothecosis)	Any age

[a]Includes *Leptospira* serovars *canicola*, *grippotyphosa*, and *icterohemorrhagiae*.

Table 69.7. Common and/or Important Infectious Agents of the Digestive System of Cats

Agent	Major Clinical Manifestations (Common Disease Name)	Age Group(s) Commonly Affected
Viruses		
Feline calicivirus	Ulcerative stomatitis	Typically less than 1 year of age
Feline immunodeficiency virus	Secondary gingivitis/stomatitis, diarrhea	Any age
Feline infectious peritonitis virus	Ileal or colonic granulomas with vomiting or constipation	Any age, typically less than 2 years of age
Feline leukemia virus	Secondary gingivitis/stomatitis, diarrhea, vomiting/diarrhea due to alimentary lymphoma	Any age
Feline panleukopenia virus	Diarrhea, vomiting	Any age, typically kittens 2–12 months of age
Feline rotavirus	Diarrhea	1–8 weeks of age
Bacteria		
Campylobacter jejuni/coli	Diarrhea	Any age, typically less than 6 months
Salmonella spp.	Diarrhea	Any age, young and old most susceptible

Table 69.8. Common and/or Important Infectious Agents of the Digestive System of Horses

Agent	Major Clinical Manifestations (Common Disease Name)	Age Group(s) Commonly Affected
Viruses		
Equine rotavirus	Diarrhea	1–8 weeks of age
Vesicular stomatitis virus	Oral ulcers/vesicles	Any age
Bacteria		
Clostridium perfringens (Types A, B, C)	Bloody diarrhea (hemorrhagic enterocolitis)	Less than 1 week of age
Clostridium difficile	Diarrhea	Adults and foals less than 2 weeks
Clostridium piliforme	Diarrhea, hepatitis, sudden death (Tyzzer's disease)	1–8 weeks of age
Neorickettsia risticii	Diarrhea (Potomac horse fever)	Typically in adult animals
Rhodococcus equi	Diarrhea, mesenteric lymphadenitis	2–6 months of age
Salmonella spp.[a]	Diarrhea	Any age

[a]Common serotypes include *Salmonella* serotypes Typhimurium, Anatum, and Agona.

Table 69.9. Common and/or Important Infectious Agents of the Digestive System of Cattle

Agent	Major Clinical Manifestations (Common Disease Name)	Age Group(s) Commonly Affected
Viruses		
Alcelaphine herpesvirus-1[a]	Oral ulcers (Malignant catarrhal fever)	Any age
Bovine coronavirus	Diarrhea	1–4 weeks of age
Bovine papular stomatitis virus	Oral ulcers	Less than 6 months of age
Bovine rotavirus	Diarrhea	1–3 weeks of age
Bovine viral diarrhea virus	Oral/esophageal ulcers, diarrhea	Any age
Ovine herpesvirus-2	Oral ulcers (Malignant catarrhal fever)	Any age
Rinderpest virus[a]	Oral ulcers, diarrhea, (rinderpest)	Any age
Vesicular viruses[b]	Vesicles/ulcers on tongue, oral mucosa	Any age
Bacteria		
Actinobacillus lignieresii	Oral pyogranulomas (wooden tongue)	Adult animals
Actinomyces bovis	Granulomas of mandible or maxilla (lumpy jaw)	Adult animals
Arcanobacterium pyogenes	Liver abscesses, weight loss	Adult animals
Clostridium haemolyticum (*C. novyi* type D)	Hepatic necrosis, sudden death, (bacillary hemoglobinuria, red water disease)	Any age
Clostridium perfringens (types B, C)	Bloody diarrhea (hemorrhagic enterocolitis)	Less than 2 weeks of age
E. coli-enterotoxigenic[c]	Diarrhea (ETEC diarrhea)	Less than 1 week of age
E. coli-attaching and effacing	Diarrhea (AEEC diarrhea)	Calves
Fusobacterium necrophorum	Liver abscesses, weight loss	Adult animals
	Necrotic lesions of oral cavity (necrotic stomatitis)	Calves
Mycobacterium avium ssp. *Paratuberculosis*	Diarrhea, weight loss (Johne's disease)	2 years of age
Salmonella spp.[d]	Cholecystitis, diarrhea with or without blood (salmonellosis)	Any age, calves 2 weeks to 2 months most susceptible
Yersinia pseudotuberculosis	Diarrhea, weight loss	Calves, adults
Fungi		
Agents of mycotic rumenitis[e]	Decreased appetite and weight loss (mycotic rumenitis)	Ruminating animals

[a]Considered a foreign animal disease in the United States.
[b]Includes foot and mouth[a] and vesicular stomatitis virus.
[c]Includes fimbrial types K99 (also designated F5) and F41.
[d]Common serotypes include *Salmonella* serotypes Dublin, Montevideo, Newport, and Typhimurium.
[e]Includes *Absidia, Aspergillus, Mucor,* and *Rhizopus* species.

Table 69.10. Common and/or Important Infectious Agents of the Digestive System of Goats and Sheep

Agent	Major Clinical Manifestations (Common Disease Name)	Age Group(s) Commonly Affected
Viruses		
Bluetongue virus (S)	Cyanosis of mucous membranes, oral ulcers	Any age
Nairobi sheep disease virus[a] (S)	Bloody diarrhea	Any age
Peste des petits virus[a]	Diarrhea, necrotic stomatitis	Any age
Rotavirus	Diarrhea	Typically 1–8 weeks of age
Rift Valley fever virus[a]	Hepatic necrosis, diarrhea	Any age
Rinderpest virus[a]	Oral ulcers, diarrhea, (rinderpest)	Any age
Vesicular viruses[b]	Vesicles/ulcers on tongue, oral mucosa	Any age
Bacteria		
Clostridium haemolyticum (S)	Hepatic necrosis, sudden death, (bacillary hemoglobinuria, red water disease)	Any age, usually adults
Clostridium novyi—type B	Hepatic necrosis, sudden death, (infectious necrotic hepatitis, Black disease)	Any age, usually adults
Clostridium perfringens (type B)	Bloody diarrhea (lamb dysentery)	Less than 2 weeks of age
Clostridium perfringens (type C)	Bloody diarrhea (necrotic enteritis)	Less than 1 weeks of age
Clostridium perfringens (type D)	Diarrhea, sudden death (entertoxemia)	Rapidly growing animals
Clostridium septicum (S)	Hemorrhagic abomasitis (braxy)	Usually young animals
E. coli-enterotoxigenic[c]	Diarrhea (ETEC diarrhea)	Less than 1 week of age
Mycobacterium avium ssp. *Paratuberculosis*	Diarrhea, weight loss (Johne's disease)	2 years of age
Salmonella spp.	Cholecystitis, diarrhea with or without blood (salmonellosis)	All ages affected

G, goats; S, sheep.
[a]Considered a foreign animal disease in the United States.
[b]Includes foot and mouth[a] and vesicular stomatitis virus.
[c]Includes fimbrial types K99 (also designated F5) and F41.

Table 69.11. Common and/or Important Infectious Agents of the Digestive System of Pigs

Agent	Major Clinical Manifestations (Common Disease Name)	Age Group(s) Commonly Affected
Viruses		
African swine fever virus[a]	Diarrhea, vomiting (African swine fever)	Any age
Hemagglutinating encephalomyelitis virus	Vomiting (vomiting and wasting disease)	Up to 3 weeks of age
Hog cholera virus[a]	Diarrhea, vomiting (classical swine fever)	Any age
Porcine circovirus type 2	Diarrhea, icterus	Nursery and growing pigs
Porcine epidemic diarrhea virus	Diarrhea, vomiting	Typically postweaning piglets
Swine rotavirus	Diarrhea	1–8 weeks of age
Transmissible gastroenteritis virus	Diarrhea and vomiting, (transmissible gastroenteritis)	All ages, most severe in piglets
Vesicular viruses[b]	Vesicles/ulcers in oral cavity	Any age
Bacteria		
Brachyspira hyodysenteriae	Bloody diarrhea (swine dysentery)	Growers and finishers
Brachyspira pilosicoli	Diarrhea (colonic spirochetosis)	Weaners, growers, and finishers
Clostridium perfringens (type A)	Diarrhea	Sucklings, weaners, and growers
Clostridium perfringens (type C)	Bloody diarrhea (necrotic enteritis)	Typically less than 1 week of age
E. coli-attaching and effacing	Diarrhea	1–8 weeks of age
E. coli-enterotoxigenic[c]	Diarrhea (ETEC diarrhea)	1 day to 8 weeks of age
E. coli-Shiga-like toxin positive	Diarrhea, edema of stomach wall (edema disease)	Typically recent postweaning
Fusobacterium necrophorum	Necrotic ulcers in oral cavity (oral necrobacilosis)	1–3 weeks of age
Lawsonii intracellularis	Diarrhea (intestinal adenomatosis)	6–20 weeks of age
	Bloody diarrhea (proliferative hemorrhagic enteropathy)	Finishers, breeders
Salmonella spp.[d]	Diarrhea with or without blood, rectal strictures	Typically postweaning

[a]Considered a foreign animal disease in the United States.
[b]Includes foot and mouth[a], vesicular stomatitis, swine vesicular disease[a], and vesicular exanthema of swine viruses.
[c]Includes fimbrial types K88, K99, 987P (also designated F4, F5, and F6, respectively) and F41. F18 is associated with postweaning diarrhea and edema disease.
[d]Usual serovars are Typhimurium var Copenhagen or Choleraesuis var kunzendorf.

Table 69.12. Common and/or Important Infectious Agents of the Digestive System of Poultry

Agent	Major Clinical Manifestations (Common Disease Name)	Age Group(s) Commonly Affected
Viruses		
Hemorrhagic enteritis virus (T)	Bloody droppings	4–9 weeks of age
Avian rotavirus	Watery droppings	Up to 5 weeks of age
Turkey coronavirus (T)	Watery droppings, weight loss, (blue comb disease)	Any age, typically 1–6 weeks
Exotic Newcastle disease virus[a]	Stomatitis, esophagitis, necrohemorrhagic enteritis	Any age
Bacteria		
Borrelia anserina	Greenish diarrhea (avian spirochetosis)	Any age
Chlamydophila psittaci (T)	Green gelatinous droppings, hepatitis (ornithosis)	Any age
Clostridium colinum	Watery droppings, liver necrosis (ulcerative enteritis)	3–12 weeks of age
Clostridium perfringens (types A and C)	Diarrhea, sudden death (necrotic enteritis)	2–16 weeks of age
Salmonella serotype Pullorum[b]	Diarrhea, liver necrosis	Typically less than 3 weeks
Salmonella serotype Gallinarum[b]	Diarrhea, liver necrosis	More common in adult birds
Fungi		
Candida albicans	Diphtheritic membrane on crop, esophagus, and mouth (thrush, sour crop)	Young birds more susceptible

C, Chickens; T, Turkeys.
[a]Considered a foreign animal disease in the United States.
[b]Other *Salmonella* serotypes (paratyphoid infections) are usually asymptomatic except in very young birds (<2 weeks of age).

A number of viruses cause diseases of the oral cavity. The viruses that cause the vesicular stomatides variously affect ruminants, horses, and swine. Included in this group are foot-and-mouth disease virus (picornavirus), vesicular stomatitis virus (rhabdovirus), swine vesicular disease virus (enterovirus), and vesicular exanthema of swine virus (calicivirus—now believed to be extinct). These are contagious viruses. Lesions initially present as vesicles that eventually rupture and leave painful ulcers in oral mucosa. The coronary band and heel junctions of the digits may also be involved, causing moderate to severe lameness. The exotic nature of some of the vesicular viruses makes them of substantial economic importance in countries free of these diseases. Other viruses are important causes of erosive stomatitis and include bovine viral diarrhea virus in cattle, feline calicivirus, rinderpest virus in sheep and cattle, bluetongue virus in sheep, and the malignant catarrhal fever viruses in cattle. Periodically, orbiviral infections adapted to one species (e.g., epizootic hemorrhagic disease (EHD) of white-tailed deer) will infect cattle and cause signs resembling other vesicular diseases (Figure 69.1).

Clinical signs and pathogenesis of infections are described in detail in specific chapters related to these viruses. Other common viral infections of the oral cavity are bovine papular stomatitis, which causes papules on various structures throughout the oral cavity and canine oral papillomatosis, which in turn presents with cauliflower-like growths (papillomas) that can be widespread throughout the oral cavity.

Bacterial causes of oral infections typically originate endogenously from normal oral flora. Infections such as actinobacillosis (woody tongue) and actinomycosis (lumpy jaw) (Figure 69.2) in cattle are initiated by some preceding trauma that breaches the normal mucosal barrier and allows the introduction of *Actinobacillus lignieresii* and *Actinomyces bovis*, respectively.

Gingival and periodontal diseases are more common problems in dogs and cats than other animals. Multiple bacterial species, predominately gram-negative anaerobes, are involved. Spirochetes also make up a large percent of the bacterial population found in gingivitis and periodontal diseases, but their role in disease pathogenesis is unclear. In cats secondary bacterial gingivitis can be the result of underlying immunosuppressive viral infections (FeLV, FIV).

Mycotic oral infections are uncommon in most animals. Oral candidiasis (thrush) caused by Candida species (usually *C. albicans*) is the most common mycotic oral infection encountered. Prior antibiotic treatment, stressful conditions or debilitating diseases that disrupt normal oral flora all predispose to infection. It occurs in all animals but with varying frequency. Candidiasis is especially common in poultry, where it frequently also involves other

FIGURE 69.1. *The photograph depicts erosion of the oral mucosa of an Angus-cross cow infected the orbivius of epizootic hemorrhagic disease of white-tailed deer (EHD).*

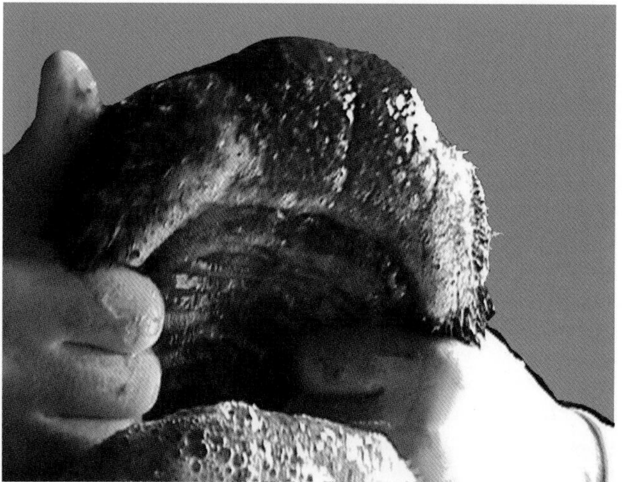

FIGURE 69.2. *The photograph depicts a sagittal section of the mandible of an aged crossbred cow infected with Actinomyces bovis. Multiple abscesses and "sulfur" granules are observed within the proliferative mass of bone.*

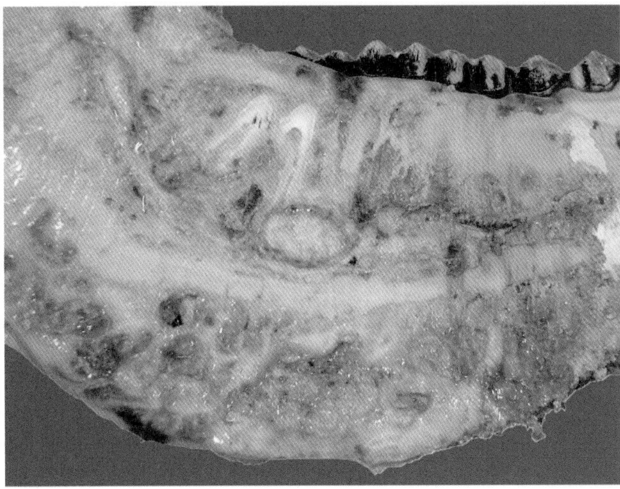

parts of the digestive system. Lesions in the mouth appear as ulcer-like plaques. In dogs, oral granulomas as a result of disseminated *Histoplasma capsulatum* infections, one of the systemic mycoses, occur with enough frequency to be worth noting. Other fungal infections of the oral cavity are rare.

Infections of the Esophagus

Infections of the esophagus are relatively uncommon, probably due to the rapid passage of material through the esophagus and the tough stratified squamous epithelium that lines it. Some viral infections, typically as part of a systemic infection, cause esophageal erosions or ulcers. Most notable among these are bovine viral diarrhea virus in cattle and exotic Newcastle disease virus in poultry. Mucocutaneous candidiasis in birds most commonly involves the crop (sour crop, crop mycosis) but can also involve the esophagus proper and proventriculus. A pseudomembrane composed of necrotic material overlying mucosal surfaces is the typical presentation.

Infections of the Stomach, Ruminant Forestomach, and Abomasum

Because its contractile nature causes relatively rapid transit of ingested material, as well as its mucus coating and acidic environment, the stomach does not provide a very hospitable environment for pathogens. Recently, much attention has been paid to *Helicobacter* species, an organism that has adapted to live in the stomach, as the cause of gastritis and gastric ulcers in humans. Many *Helicobacter* species have been identified in animals; however, their role in disease remains to be clearly established, in part due to their frequent colonization of clinically normal animals. In sheep, a severe hemorrhagic abomasitis (braxy) caused by *Clostridium septicum* occurs and is related to particular feed types. A *Sarcina*-like organism has been associated with abomasal tympany in lambs and goats.

In ruminants, damage to mucosal surface of the forestomach or disruption in the rumen flora can lead to serious and potentially fatal consequences. In dairy cattle, if integrity of the reticulum is penetrated by foreign linear objects such as ingested wire (hardware disease), peritonitis and pericarditis may develop. These infections are polymicrobial with *Arcanobacterium pyogenes* and *Fuso-bacterium necrophorum* commonly involved.

Sudden dietary changes to carbohydrate-rich feeds, which are easily fermentable, lead to a decrease in rumen pH. The lower pH kills acid-sensitive rumen flora and damages rumen mucosa. Bacterial rumenitis may develop and can serve as a source of organisms for embolic hepatitis that eventually result in liver abscessation. Common agents recovered from liver abscesses are the familiar abscess producers of ruminants, *A. pyogenes* and *F. necrophorum*. Mycotic rumenitis also develops subsequent to ruminal acidosis or prior antibiotic treatment that has disrupted rumen flora. The fungal agents involved in mycotic rumenitis are often angioinvasive, causing a severe vasculitis, which leads to further tissue necrosis. The zygomycetes (*Mucor, Rhizopus,* and *Absidia*) and *Aspergillus* spp. are the fungi most frequently involved. Mycotic rumenitis may also serve as a source for hematogenous dissemination of fungal elements leading to mycotic abortion.

Infections of the Small and Large Intestines

Microbial infections of the small and large intestines affect all domestic animals. Effective vaccination against many of the major viral enteric pathogens (e.g., parvoviruses and distemper virus) in dogs and cats has substantially decreased the incidence of contagious enteric diseases in companion animals. Holding dogs and cats in close confinement, such as in kennels, shows, and animal shelters, increases the risk for contracting contagious enteric diseases.

Intestinal infections of both bacterial and viral origin remain of great clinical and economic significance in horses, production animals, and poultry due to intensive rearing conditions, management factors (e.g., failure to insure adequate passive transfer or proper manure management), and the absence of effective vaccines against some of the major pathogens. Host age susceptibility exists for some enteric pathogens (e.g., *Clostridium perfringens* type C, enterotoxigenic *E. coli,* and rotavirus). Neonates, in general, are the most susceptible.

The major clinical manifestations of microbial infections of the intestinal tract are diarrhea and vomiting. Vomiting often occurs in enteric infections in small animals and swine as part of the enteric defense response and is regulated by the vomition center in the brain. Diarrhea is defined as increase in frequency, fluidity, or volume of feces due to an increase in water content. Insults to the intestines that cause increased secretion or decreased absorption can result in diarrhea. Severity, duration, and characteristics (watery, bloody, etc.) of diarrhea differ depending on the agent involved. Whether diarrhea is actually a benefit to the host, pathogen, or both is unclear. Diarrhea not only serves the host as means to eliminate a buildup of pathogens but also serves the pathogen by providing a means for dissemination and, thereby, maximizes potential for the pathogen to infect other hosts.

Viral infections involving the small and large intestines may be limited to the digestive tract (e.g., rotaviruses and coronaviruses) or be part of a multisystem infectious process (e.g., African swine fever virus, canine distemper virus, and parvoviruses). Intestinal viral infections may be acquired directly via the oral route or as a result of a viremia with localization to intestinal epithelial cells. Some viruses acquired by the oral route are acid resistant, which allows their passage through the stomach, while others are acid-sensitive but can be protected by the buffering action and fats in milk or in feedstuffs with a rapid gastric transit time. Attachment to intestinal epithelial cell receptors (e.g., sialic acid-containing oligosaccharides) via viral attachment proteins is the initial step in establishing infection. This is followed by uptake of the virus into the cell, often through receptor-mediated endocytosis, and replication within the cell. Subsequent destruction of epithelial cells resulting in loss of absorption and resorption capacity and disruption in osmotic equilibrium is manifest by diarrhea. Rotavirus and coronavirus are common causes of viral enteritis in many animals and affect predominantly villus epithelial cells. The time course from exposure to manifestation of clinical signs is usually short. Other viruses affect crypt epithelial cells (e.g., Rinderpest virus in sheep and canine parvovirus) and cause more severe tissue damage. The spectrum of clinical signs and details on pathogenesis associated with specific viral agents that affect the intestines of domestic animals are found in the specific chapters on those agents.

Bacteria are also major pathogens of the small and large intestines. To produce disease in the intestinal tract, potentially pathogenic bacteria must first adhere to target cells. If the target cell is part of a niche occupied by normal flora, the microorganisms will encounter "colonization resistance," which they must overcome before adhering. Adherence results from the interaction (selective adsorption) of microbial surface structures (adhesins) with receptors on target cells. Adhesins are considered virulence factors because most pathogens cannot produce disease without first adhering to a target cell. Fimbrial adhesins are protein in nature and protrude from the surface of the bacterial cell. They are responsible for adherence of some bacteria to carbohydrate moieties that are part of glycoproteins on the surface of host cells. The most commonly found fimbriae (type 1 fimbriae) on the surface of gram-negative bacteria have affinity for mannose-containing glycoproteins on the surface of cells. Bacteria expressing type 1 fimbriae, when mixed with red blood cells, agglutinate these cells; this agglutination is inhibited by mannose (mannose-sensitive). Intestinal epithelial cells display structures that serve as receptors for fimbriae expressed by enteropathogenic strains of bacteria.

Other structures on the surface of bacterial cells influence how the bacterium will interact with host cells. These structures are carbohydrates and influence the interaction by rendering the surface of the bacterial cell relatively hydrophilic. This hydrophilic property imparts a repulsive force relative to the host cell surface, since the host cell surface is somewhat hydrophobic. On the other hand, protein receptors on the surface of some host cells have affinity for these surface carbohydrates. The outcome of the latter interaction is adhesion.

FIGURE 69.3. *The photomicrograph depicts a section of jejunum from an 11-day-old piglet infected with enterotoxigenic Escherichia coli (ETEC). Immunohistochemistry was used to demonstrate the bacteria that are adherent to the enterocytes. Rabbit anti-O8 was used as the primary antiserum. Alkaline phosphatase-labeled goat anti-rabbit serum and fast red were subsequently used in the staining procedures. Bar = 20 μm. (Courtesy of Dr Rod Moxley.)*

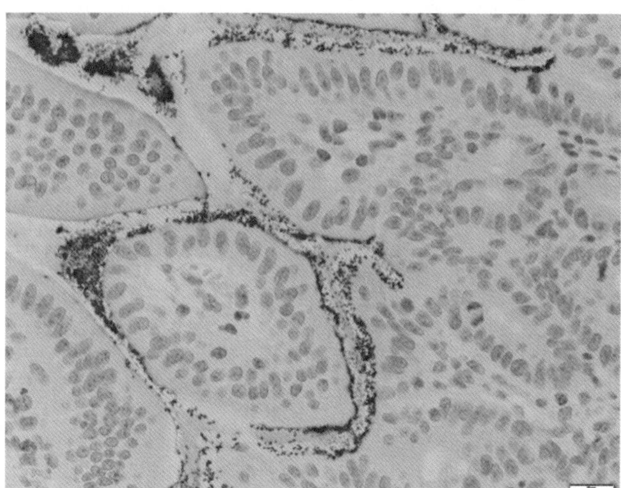

After adherence, the pathogen may produce disease by (1) secretion of an exotoxin, resulting, for example, in disruption of fluid and electrolyte regulation of the target cell; (2) invasion of the target cell, causing its death, usually by the action of a toxin (a cytotoxin); or (3) invasion of the target cell and the lymphatics, resulting in a systemic infection. The mechanisms by which the host is affected by different bacterial enteric pathogens are varied and complex. In some cases, as in the enterotoxigenic *E. coli*, the diarrhea is solely a result of the production of enterotoxin and little to no pathology is observed (Figure 69.3).

Other pathogens (e.g., *Salmonella*) use complex communication systems to translocate effector proteins into host cells (e.g., type III secretion systems) as well as produce both enterotoxic and cytotoxic effects. Still other pathogens, such as *Mycobacterium avium* ssp. *paratuberculosis*, exert their effect on the intestinal tract by translocating through mucosal epithelial cells and existing in macrophages in the lamina propria and regional lymph nodes. A granulomatous enteritis results, however, the severity of the lesion does not necessarily correlate with the severity of clinical signs. Specific details on the mechanism of pathogenesis and resulting pathology of the important bacterial pathogens of the intestines of domestic animals are covered in the respective chapters on each agent.

Organisms known to be pathogens of the intestinal tract in certain animals may be found as normal flora in others. Their role in causing disease in some animals, if any, remains to be established. As an example, *Campylobacter jejuni* is the most common cause of diarrhea in humans and is commonly found in the intestinal tract of companion and domestic animals—but its ability to cause disease in some animals is unclear. There is a high carriage rate of *C. jejuni* in chickens with no apparent adverse effects on birds greater than 2 weeks of age.

Various factors predispose or make more likely that an enteric pathogen will establish and cause disease. The importance of antimicrobials on the disruption of normal flora and in allowing pathogens to establish has already been discussed. Other factors that create stress for the host will also result in changes in the intestinal flora, mainly resulting in a drop in the anaerobic component. The level of coliform bacteria will be higher after a decrease in concentration of fatty acids produced by anaerobic flora. The actual reason for the decrease in the number of obligate anaerobes is not known. In addition to these changes, the amount of fibronectin (a glycoprotein) coating epithelial cells in the oral cavity decreases. Since this glycoprotein possesses receptors for gram-positive species in the oral cavity, decrease in this population occurs with a corresponding increase in gram-negative species, especially members of the family Enterobacteriaceae.

Fungal infections of the intestines are not common. Of those encountered, granulomatous enteritis in dogs caused by *H. capsulatum* is among the most common. *Pythium insidiosum*, an oomycete, causes granulomas in the submucosa or muscularis layer of the small intestine (and sometimes stomach) in dogs, and it is manifest by vomiting, diarrhea, and weight loss. Rare algal infections caused by *Prototheca* species result in an intractable diarrhea as part of a more generalized process (usually with ocular involvement) in dogs.

Infections of Digestive System-Associated Organs

Infections of the liver occur through a number of routes and include the (1) portal vein, (2) hepatic artery, (3) ascension through the biliary system, and (4) contiguous spread from adjacent infectious processes (e.g., reticulitis).

The liver may be a target for a number of viruses, often as part of a systemic infection. Liver damage can occur by infection of endothelial cells (e.g., canine adenovirus 1), causing vascular stasis and hypoxia as well as through infection of parenchymal cells resulting in hepatocellular necrosis.

A number of bacterial genera and species can affect the liver. Clostridial species are among the most important. Clostridial spores of *C. haemolyticum* (*C. novyi* type D) and *C. novyi* type B, the agents of bacillary hemoglobinuria and infectious necrotic hepatitis, respectively, are present in the liver of cattle and sheep. They germinate when local liver necrosis results subsequent to immature fluke migration or when some other event damages the liver (e.g., liver biopsies). Upon germination under this anaerobic environment, a number of cytolytic toxins are produced that further damage the liver. The agent of Tyzzer's disease, *Clostridium piliforme*, causes a rare but acute and highly fatal infection in a number of animals. It is most important in laboratory animals. Foals are most commonly affected among domestic animals. Characteristic spindle-shaped bacilli are found in the liver along the edge of areas of hepatic necrosis. *Clostridium colinum* causes hepatic necrosis along with ulcerative lesions in the intestines of chickens and turkeys (ulcerative enteritis).

Certain serovars of *Leptospira* will cause a nonspecific reactive hepatitis. Severity of the lesions can vary from severe chronic hepatitis to mild diffuse hepatocellular vacuolation. Often renal involvement also occurs.

As already mentioned, rumenitis provides a source of bacteria through the portal system that can result in liver abscesses. Miliary liver abscesses, most commonly in ruminants, results from hematogenous seeding by a number of different bacteria. Common agents include *Yersinia pseudotuberculosis* and *Rhodococcus equi*. In poultry, liver granulomas are periodically reported to be caused by a gram-positive anaerobic rod, *Eubacterium tortuosum*, and are thought to be of intestinal origin.

The gall bladder infections can be viral (e.g., canine infectious hepatitis virus and Rift Valley fever virus in sheep) and bacterial (e.g., *Salmonella enterica* serotype *Dublin* in calves) in etiology. Infections of the pancreas are rarely reported in domestic animals.

Diseases of the Digestive System of Unknown but Suspected Infectious Etiology

It is not uncommon for the cause of diarrhea in domestic animals to go undiagnosed. There are a number of important conditions of the digestive tract of domestic animals that are believed to be infectious in origin; however, no specific agent has been conclusively demonstrated to be the cause. In some cases, multiple agents are likely involved and/or some interplay between host and environment is necessary for clinical signs to develop. Some major diseases of suspected infectious etiology, but where the specific agent(s) has not been conclusively identified, include poult enteritis mortality syndrome in turkeys, colitis X in horses (possibly caused by a Clostridial infection), hemorrhagic gastroenteritis in dogs, winter dysentery in cattle (possibly caused by bovine corona- virus), and hemorrhagic jejunal syndrome in dairy cattle (suspected to be caused by *Clostridium perfringens* type A).

70 Integumentary System

DOUGLAS E. HOSTETLER

The integument is the largest organ of the body. It plays a major role in temperature regulation, sensory perception, and protection against fluid loss, and provides a barrier from external insults, including potentially pathogenic microorganisms. It is composed of epidermis, dermis, subcutis, hair follicles, and glandular structures. Glandular structures include sweat and sebaceous glands as well as specialized structures such as anal sacs. Hair type and density vary on the body according to functional need, including sensory, thermoregulatory, and protective functions. Birds have evolved feathers, probably originating from scales, in place of hair. Footpads, horns, hooves, nails, and beaks are all specialized keratinized structures of the integumentary system.

The epidermis is in continual contact with the surrounding environment and provides a home for a resident flora. The outer layer of the epidermis, keratinized stratum corneum, is held together by lipid cement, and together they form the major physical barrier of the skin. Epidermal thickness varies among animals, among breeds, and at different sites on individual animals. The dermis, through collagen and elastic fibers, provides tensile strength and elasticity to the integumentary system and also varies substantially in thickness throughout the body. The hypodermis provides additional flexibility along with insulation through adipose tissue.

The external ear canal is included in this chapter because the external surface is covered with skin (pinna) or epithelium and glandular structures (external auditory meatus). Overall, the lesions found in otitis externa are similar to those found in skin infections, and some of the important pathogens responsible for otitis externa are the same ones that cause infections elsewhere on the skin.

The mammary gland, although technically not part of the integumentary system, is also included in this chapter because of its direct communication with the skin. Mammary gland pathogens, some of which are resident or transient flora of the skin, primarily enter through the streak canal of the teat. The teat sphincter and a keratin plug produced by epithelial cells lining the teat canal provide the primary physical barrier for the mammary gland.

Original chapter written by the late Dr. Richard L. Walker.

Antimicrobial Properties of the Skin

The skin provides a less favorable environment for microbial growth than do mucous membranes of the alimentary, respiratory, and urogenital systems owing to properties presented in the following sections.

Dryness

The normal dryness of the skin surface limits the ability of many microbes to survive and establish. Conditions that interfere with the normal evaporative process cause proliferation of resident and transient skin flora through increased moisture retention and changes in temperature, pH, and CO_2 tension. Excessive folding of the skin in certain animal breeds and obese individuals is a prime example of an anatomic condition that increases hydration and temperature of the stratum corneum, providing a more hospitable environment for bacterial proliferation.

Desquamation

Continuous shedding of superficial skin layers eliminates transient organisms. Resident flora numbers are also reduced but are promptly replenished from the residual population.

Secretions and Excretions

Holocrine sebaceous glands secrete lipids, including long-chain fatty acids, many of which inhibit bacteria. They and the apocrine sweat glands contribute to an intercellular seal in superficial epidermal layers, limiting microbial access. Apocrine and eccrine sweat glands excrete lactate, propionate, acetate, caprylate, and high concentrations of sodium chloride. Interferon, lysozyme, transferrin, and all classes of immunoglobulins are also present. Keratinocytes synthesize the antimicrobial peptides—cathelicidins and beta-defensins. All these substances contribute to the self-sterilizing action of the skin—that is, its resistance to colonization by transient microorganisms.

Veterinary Microbiology, Third Edition. Edited by D. Scott McVey, Melissa Kennedy and M.M. Chengappa.

Microbial Interactions

Resident bacteria exclude intruders by excreting inhibitory metabolites (e.g., volatile fatty acids) and bacteriocins, and by occupying available niches.

Immune System

A skin immune system responds to local antigenic stimuli, including microbial ones, and comprises cell types corresponding functionally to those operating on mucosal surfaces. Langerhans cells, an antigen-presenting cell, and intraepithelial T lymphocytes are prominent constituents of the system. Keratinocytes participate in immune defense by producing immune-modulating substances. The interaction between these cells constitutes the skin-associated lymphoid tissue. Complement, cytokines, and immunoglobulins are found in the emulsion layer of the skin and are important to overall integumentary immunocompetence.

Microbial Flora of the Skin

The microbial flora of the skin plays an important role in defense and is probably acquired at birth from the dam. These microorganisms are limited to the superficial epidermal layers, where intercellular cohesion is relaxed prior to desquamation, and to the distal portions of gland ducts and hair follicles. The microbial flora exists predominately in microcolonies, rather than being evenly distributed over the skin. Bacterial adhesion, through lipoteichoic acids in gram-positive cocci, is critical to the establishment and persistence of resident flora. Keratinization defects, as found in seborrhea, provide additional attachment sites and allow for increased numbers of resident flora, as well as changes in overall flora makeup.

Bacteria and yeast variably colonize sites on the skin of animals. The greatest numbers are found in moist, protected areas such as the axilla, inguinal region, interdigital spaces, and ear canals. Their concentration is lower than on colonized mucous membranes, rarely exceeding $10^5/cm^2$ and, in some areas, $10^2/cm^2$.

Gram-positive organisms predominate among resident flora. Among the gram-positives, coagulase-negative staphylococci constitute the majority. Certain strains of coagulase-positive staphylococci are also considered to be resident organisms in some animals. Facultatively anaerobic diphtheroids (*Corynebacterium* and *Propionibacterium* spp.) are consistently present, as are *Micrococcus* spp. and viridans streptococci. Of gram-negatives, only *Acinetobacter* spp. are considered a major part of the resident flora. The main fungal resident is a lipophilic yeast, *Malassezia*, which resides on the skin and in the external ear canal. Viruses are not generally considered part of the normal skin flora. Viral agents that directly infect the skin are maintained in animal populations by persistently infected individuals but are also capable of surviving for extended periods in the environment, which can serve as an alternate source for infecting other animals.

Various transient microbial flora can be encountered. Beta-hemolytic streptococci (generally Lancefield group G) on cat or dog skin are usually associated with abnormal conditions. Members of the family *Enterobacteriaceae*, particularly *Escherichia coli* and *Proteus mirabilis*, and enterococci are common transients. The feet of farm animals carry fecal bacteria, some of which participate in foot infections, most notably *Fusobacterium necrophorum* and *Prevotella melaninogenica*. The agent of ovine footrot, *Dichelobacter nodosus*, although hardly a normal commensal, is limited to epidermal tissues.

Transient fungal flora of the skin represent contaminants of airborne or soil origin. Many genera can be isolated from the skin. Common transient fungal genera found on the skin include *Aspergillus*, *Chrysosporium*, *Cladosporium*, *Penicillium*, and *Scopulariopsis*.

Sterilization of the skin is impossible due to the physical inaccessibility to much of the skin flora. Thorough cleansing of shaved skin with soap and water, followed by soaking with 70% alcohol, will remove 95% of the flora. More than 99% removal of skin flora is claimed for repeated povidone iodine applications and rinses with chlorhexidine (0.5%) in alcohol. Following such treatment there is rapid repopulation, usually by the same organisms.

Infections of the Skin

Susceptibility of skin to infection is inversely related to thickness and compactness of the stratum corneum. Specific animal breeds, because of anatomic conformations, physiologic factors, or genetic factors, are more predisposed to skin infections than others.

Integumentary infections are often secondary, requiring a disruption in the host's innate defense mechanisms. Factors such as trauma, excessive moisture, irritants, insect or animal bites, and burns are all predisposing causes for skin infections to develop. Underlying diseases, including preexisting skin conditions and immunological disorders also predispose to secondary skin infections. Deep dermal and subcutaneous infections typically require some form of traumatic implantation that allows for the introduction of microbial pathogens that would otherwise not persist on the external epidermal layer.

Systemic infections sometimes involve the integumentary system. Agents with trophism for vascular endothelium or epithelial cells can cause focal or generalized lesions in the skin.

Viral Infections of the Skin

A number of viruses gain entry to the host via the skin, either through abrasions, insect or animal bites or by exposure to contaminated equipment (e.g., needles and harnesses). Some of these viruses simply use the integumentary system as a route for entry into the host and cause either systemic infections or have primary targets that are organs or systems other than the skin (e.g., rabies virus). Details on mechanisms used for entry, replication, and spread via the integumentary system for specific viruses are covered in chapters on those individual viruses.

For some viruses the skin is the primary site of infection or is one of the principal sites where clinical signs manifest. The papillomaviruses and poxviruses are prominent viral pathogens of the integumentary system in animals. The papillomaviruses are introduced through skin abrasions and infect epithelial cells. Infected epithelial cells become hyperplastic. Hyperkeratosis is the result. The lesions (papillomas) are typically raised and filiform, and may be pedunculated. The papillomaviruses are fairly host-specific, although bovine papillomaviruses 1 and 2 are associated with equine sarcoids.

Members of the family Poxviridae also affect a number of animals and birds. Many viruses in this family have a limited host range, although some are zoonotic. Transfer occurs through contact with skin lesions, scabs from infected animals, or mechanically by biting insects. The parapox virus that causes sore-mouth in sheep and the fowlpox virus in poultry can be transmitted by respiratory droplets, as well as by direct contact with lesion material or contaminated equipment. Depending on the virus involved, clinical disease can be mild to severe. Generalized signs include fever and anorexia. The skin lesions are typically papulonodular and become pustular or proliferative, eventually resulting in the production of scabs that leave scars.

Cutaneous manifestations are part of the overall clinical presentation of some generalized or multisystem viral infections. Viruses that cause vesicular diseases (foot-and-mouth disease, swine vesicular disease, vesicular exanthema of swine, and vesicular stomatitis viruses) produce vesicles that variably affect the teats, coronary bands, and interdigital areas of the skin. The vesicles readily rupture leaving ulcerative lesions that may become secondarily infected with bacteria. In addition to the lymphoreticular and neurological lesions it produces, the Marek's disease virus of chickens causes nodules to develop in the feather follicles and uses feather follicle dander as a primary means of spreading virus to other birds. Canine distemper virus causes nasal and footpad hyperkeratosis in dogs as a late clinical manifestation.

Bacterial Infections of the Skin

Bacteria associated with skin infections primarily originate from the environment or direct or indirect contact with carrier animals, or are resident flora of the skin, oral cavity, genital tract, or lower digestive tract of the affected animal. Bacterial skin infections are classified as superficial pyodermas (e.g., impetigo and superficial bacterial folliculitis) or deep pyodermas (e.g., folliculitis, furunculosis, cellulitis, and subcutaneous abscesses). Coagulase-positive staphylococci (e.g., *Staphylococcus aureus*, *S. intermedius*, and *S. hyicus*) are the primary agents of superficial pyodermas. They produce a myriad of enzymes and toxins that contribute to the disease process. Along with cell wall components, some of these microbial products have potent chemotactic effects that account for the pyogenic inflammatory response observed in staphylococcocal infections. *S. hyicus*, the cause of greasy pig disease, produces an exfoliative toxin that specifically causes separation of intraepidermal layers resulting in focal erosions in the epidermis. In neonatal pigs, this generalized epidermitis is associated with substantial mortality.

Dermatophilus congolensis, an actinomycete, also causes a superficial dermatitis, most often in horses and ruminants. Infection stimulates an intense inflammatory response that is characterized by alternating waves of inflammatory cells followed by newly generated epidermis. In contrast to the abundance of products produced by coagulase-positive staphylococci, few virulence factors are recognized in *Dermatophilus*. It produces an extracellular serine protease that may contribute to the overall disease process; however, environmental factors are key to the development of disease. Persistent wetting of the skin or insect bites are needed for *Dermatophilus* to initially invade the epidermis. Once invasion occurs, an inflammatory reaction is induced, which results in profuse cellular exudation. If predisposing conditions remain to promote invasion of newly generated epidermis, the infection/inflammatory cycle repeats, giving rise to the characteristic histopathology; otherwise, the infection resolves.

Deep bacterial pyodermas involve the dermis and sometimes the subcutaneous tissue. Injury or trauma almost always precedes the development of deep pyodermas. In some cases, deep skin infections occur as a result of the extension of a superficial pyoderma. Again, coagulase-positive staphylococci are frequently involved, although other bacteria may be secondarily involved. Furunculosis (inflammation of the dermis and subcutis) and folliculitis (inflammation of the hair follicle) are most commonly recognized in dogs but also occur with some frequency in horses, goats, and sheep.

Subcutaneous abscesses are typically the result of a bite wound or penetrating foreign body. The bacteria introduced usually represent members of the oral flora and cause an accumulation of purulent exudate in the dermis and subcutaneous tissue. Subcutaneous abscesses most commonly occur in cats and most frequently involve *Pasteurella multocida* and obligate anaerobic bacteria. Subcutaneous abscesses are also common in ruminants, with *Arcanobacterium pyogenes* frequently being recovered. *Corynebacterium pseudotuberculosis* causes subcutaneous abscesses in sheep and horses. In cattle, *C. pseudotuberculosis* infections manifest as an ulcerative dermatitis rather than forming abscesses.

Cellulitis is a loose purulent inflammation of the subcutaneous tissue. It is generally poorly contained and extends rapidly along tissue planes from the site of initiation. A variety of bacterial agents cause cellulitis. Among the most serious forms of cellulitis is the anaerobic cellulitis caused by one of a number of histotoxic clostridial species. Under anaerobic environments these species produce potent and highly destructive toxins. Horses, ruminants, swine, and poultry are most commonly affected by clostridial cellulitis. Infections have a high fatality rate, even in the face of aggressive treatment. An *E. coli*-associated cellulitis in broiler chickens is an especially economically important disease for the poultry industry, accounting for a substantial percentage of condemnations at slaughter plants. *S. aureus* causes an acute cellulitis in horses that spreads rapidly and causes necrosis of the overlying skin. Thoroughbred racehorses are most commonly affected.

Other bacterial infections of the skin include mycobacterial granulomas. Cats are most commonly affected by these organisms, although infections also occur in swine, cattle, and dogs. The saprophytic mycobacteria responsible are introduced by some trauma. If they establish, infections are characterized by chronic, nonhealing wounds with draining fistulas. A specific entity in young cats referred to as feline leprosy is caused by *Mycobacterium lepraemurium* and presents as cutaneous nodules of the head and extremities that sometimes ulcerate. A regional lymphadenopathy is often present. A second, more generalized form of the disease caused by an unidentified mycobacterium has been described in older cats. Pyogranulomatous dermatitis caused by *Actinomyces* spp. occurs in dogs (*A. viscosus* or *A. hordeovulneris* associated with plant awns) and cattle (*A. bovis*). Draining tracts and the presence of yellow granules composed of bacterial colonies, sometimes surrounded by a homogenous eosinophilic material, are found in the draining material.

Some bacterial skin infections involve two or more bacteria working in concert. In contagious ovine footrot, *F. necrophorum* causes an interdigital dermatitis in macerated skin, which allows *D. nodosus* to establish by fimbrial attachment and proliferate. Production of a number of serine and basic proteases by *D. nodosus* results in an undermining of the sole and, thereby, allows for additional opportunistic bacteria to invade, further aggravating the condition.

A substantial integumentary component is part of certain systemic bacterial infections. The urticarial plaques and diffuse erythematous lesions in the skin of swine, resulting from cutaneous infarctions, are characteristic of erysipelas. The effects on vascular endothelium of bacterial toxins or hypersensitivity reactions to bacterial antigens may also manifest in the skin. Subcutaneous swelling of the eyelids, lips, and forehead occur in edema disease in pigs, caused by Shiga-like toxin producing strains of *E. coli*. The dependent edema resulting from the vasculitis that occurs in *purpura* hemorrhagica in horses is a sequelae to infection with *Streptococcus equi* ssp. *equi*.

Fungal Infections of the Skin

Fungal infections of the skin are classified as superficial cutaneous mycoses or subcutaneous mycoses. In addition, fungal agents that cause systemic mycoses (*Blastomyces dermatitidis*, *Coccidioides immitis*, *Cryptococcus neoformans*, and *Histoplasma capsulatum*) cause pyogranulomatous lesions in the integumentary system subsequent to disseminated infection.

The most important of the superficial mycotic infections is dermatophytosis or ringworm. It denotes a specialized dermatomycosis caused by fungi that specifically attack keratinized structures. These fungi (*Microsporum* spp. and *Trichophyton* spp.) produce enzymes (keratinases) that digest keratin and infect growing hair and stratum corneum (Figure 70.1). Lesions are inflamed, crusty, or scaly and often circular to oval in shape due to the centripetal progression of the lesion. Affected hair is brittle, leaving areas of alopecia. Dermatophytes are not always pathogens and can represent transient flora of the skin (usually geophilic

FIGURE 70.1. *Photomicrograph of a section of a skin biopsy stained with PAS depicting hair colonized by fungal hyphae (arrow) and spores (arrowhead). (Courtesy of Dr Bruce Brodersen.)*

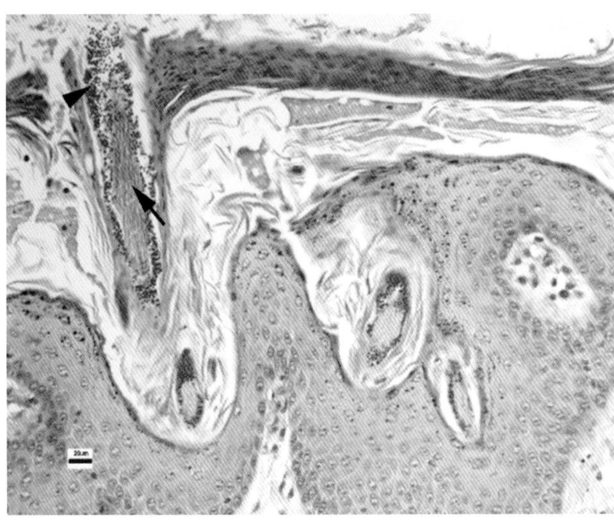

dermatophytes) or be carried inapparently (zoophilic dermatophytes).

Malassezia, a lipid-dependent yeast, is the other main fungal agent involved in superficial mycotic infections of the skin. It causes an erythematous, scaly lesion. Since it can be found in low numbers on normal skin, clinical relevance of its isolation must be decided based on clinical signs.

Abnormal environmental conditions can overwhelm the host defense mechanisms and lead to opportunistic mycotic infections of the skin. Skin biopsies and cultures are sometimes helpful in the identification these unusual dermatologic pathogens, as in the case of the *Prototheca* spp. dermatitis, diagnosed in the skin biopsy of the bat in Figure 70.2.

FIGURE 70.2. *Photomicrograph of a section of a skin biopsy stained with H&E demonstrating numerous protothecal sporangia in the dermis. (Courtesy of Dr Alan Doster.)*

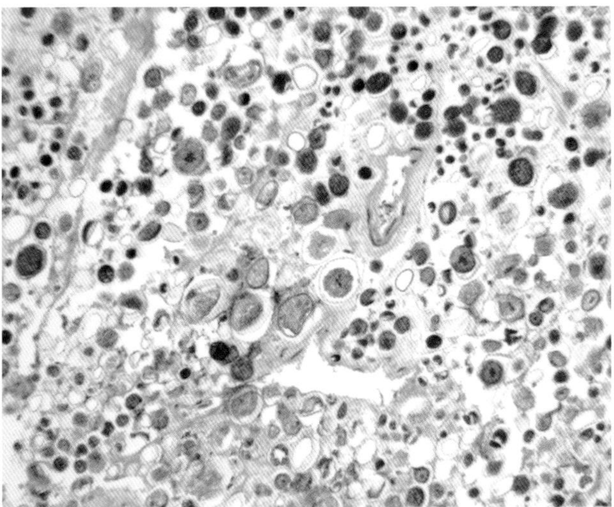

Table 70.1. Common and/or Important Infectious Agents of the Integumentary System of Dogs

Agent	Major Clinical Manifestations (Common Disease Name)
Viruses	
Canine distemper virus	Nasal and footpad hyperkeratosis (distemper)
Canine papillomavirus	Cutaneous papillomas (canine papillomatosis)
Bacteria	
Actinomyces viscosus, A. hordeovulneris	Draining tracts, subcutaneous abscess
Brucella canis	Scrotal dermatitis
Staphylococcus intermedius[a]	Cellulitis, folliculitis, furunculosis, impetigo
Fungi	
Malassezia pachydermatis	Exfoliative dermatitis
Microsporum canis, M. gypseum, Trichophyton mentagrophytes	Circular, scaly, crusty, alopectic skin lesions (dermatophytosis, ringworm)
Pythium insidiosum	Ulcerative and pyogranulomatous skin lesions (cutaneous pythiosis)
Systemic mycotic agents[b]	Papules, nodules, abscess, draining tracts

[a]Other coagulase-positive *Staphylococcus* sp. involved in pyoderma include *S. aureus* and *S. schleiferi* ssp. *coagulans*.
[b]Includes *Blastomyces dermatitidis, Coccidioides immitis, Cryptococcus neoformans*, and *Histoplasma capsulatum*.

The subcutaneous mycoses involve the dermis and subcutaneous tissues and may be localized lesions or spread via the lymphatics. Most of the fungal agents involved are from an environmental source (e.g., soil and plant material) and gain entry by traumatic introduction. A number of different subcutaneous mycotic infections are recognized and classified by their gross and histopathologic characteristics. These different conditions include chromoblastomycosis, phaeohyphomycosis, and eumycotic mycetoma. They are described in more detail in Chapter 46. More than one fungal agent may be responsible for each of these conditions. For example, eumycotic mycetomas—which are characterized by (1) localized swelling at the infection site (tumefaction), (2) draining sinus tracts, and (3) the presence of granules or grains composed of colonies of the causative agent—are caused by more than 14 species of dematiaceous (pigmented) fungi and more than 9 species of hyaline (colorless) fungi. They produce dark- and white-grained mycetomas, respectively.

Sporotrichosis is a subcutaneous mycosis caused by the dimorphic fungus, *Sporothrix schenckii*. Lesions of sporotrichosis are ulcerative nodules or recurrent draining tracts in the skin. Infections may also involve the lymphatics causing a lymphangitis, in addition to the skin lesions. Cats, horses, and dogs are most commonly affected.

Cutaneous pythiosis is caused by an oomycete, *Pythium insidiosum*, and therefore is not a true fungal infection. It is found in swamps and ponds, and the disease is associated with exposure to those environments. Skin infections are characterized by firm or spongy, ulcerated lesions that often have draining fistulous tracts. Necrotic masses of tissue (kunkers) may be found in the lesion. Although uncommon, horses and dogs are most frequently affected. An additional genus, *Lagenidium*, has also been reported to be involved in such lesions.

When one of the systemic mycotic agents involves the integumentary system, the lesions are typically ulcerative nodules that may develop draining tracts. These

Table 70.2. Common and/or Important Infectious Agents of the Integumentary System of Cats

Agent	Major Clinical Manifestations (Common Disease Name)
Viruses	
Cowpox virus[a]	Macules, papules, nodules (cowpox virus infection)
Feline sarcoma virus	Cutaneous and subcutaneous nodules
Bacteria	
Mycobacterium spp.[b]	Chronic nodular dermatitis, draining tracts, panniculitis (atypical mybacteriosis)
Mycobacterium lepraemurium	Noduloulcerative skin lesions with lymphadenopathy (feline leprosy)
Obligate anaerobic bacteria[c]	Subcutaneous abscesses
Pasteurella multocida	Subcutaneous abscesses
Fungi	
Cryptococcus neoformans	Draining tracts, nodules, ulcers (crytococcosis)
Microsporum canis	Alopecia annulare skin lesions (dermatophytosis, ringworm), pseudomycetoma
Sporothrix schenckii	Draining tracts, ulcerative nodules (sporotrichosis)

[a]Not seen in the United States.
[b]Includes *M. fortuitum, M. chelonei, M. xenopi*, and *M. phlei*.
[c]Includes *Peptostreptococcus* spp., *Fusobacterium* spp., *Porphyromonas* spp., and *Clostridium* spp.

Table 70.3. Common and/or Important Infectious Agents of the Integumentary System of Horses

Agent	
Viruses	
Bovine papillomaviruses 1&2	Verrucous, fibroplastic or flat and thickened skin lesions (equine sarcoid)
Equine papillomavirus	Cutaneous papillomas of lips and nose (equine papillomatosis)
Equine viral arteritis virus	Edema of distal limbs, scrotum, and ventrum
Vesicular stomatitis virus	Vesicules/ulcers on coronary band
Bacteria	
Bacillus anthracis	Diffuse subcutaneous and dermal edema (anthrax)
Burkholderia mallei[a]	Subcutaneous nodules that ulcerate, lymphangitis (farcy)
Clostridium perfringens[b]	Cellulitis
Corynebacterium pseudotuberculosis	Pectoral (pigeon breast) or inguinal abscesses, lymphangitis (ulcerative lymphangitis)
Dermatophilus congolensis	Exudative dermatitis (dermatophilosis, rain rot)
Rhodococcus equi	Cutaneous abscesses, cellulitis
Staphylococcus aureus[c]	Cellulitis, folliculitis, furunculosis
Fungi	
Histoplasma farciminosum[a]	Nodules of head, neck, and leg; lymphangitis (histoplasmosis farciminosi)
Pythium insidiosum	Ulcerative pyogranulomatous lesions (cutaneous pythiosis, swamp cancer)
Sporothrix schenckii	Ulcerative nodules on legs, lymphangitis (sporotrichosis)
Trichophyton equinum, T. mentagrophytes, M. equinum	Crusty skin lesions; hair loss often involving head, shoulders, and back (dermatophytosis, ringworm)

[a]Considered a foreign animal disease agent in the United States.
[b]Other clostridial species include *C. septicum, C. sordellii,* and *C. sporogenes.*
[c]Other coagulase-positive species affecting horses include *S. intermedius* and *S. hyicus* ssp. *hyicus.*

pyogranulomatous skin lesions may be the initial clinical manifestation of an infection even though organisms responsible for the skin lesions almost always originate from disseminated respiratory tract infections.

Common and/or important agents of the integumentary system of domestic animals and poultry are listed in Tables 70.1, 70.2, 70.3, 70.4, 70.5, 70.6, and 70.7.

Otitis Externa

Otitis externa in dogs is one of the most common dermatological problems encountered. There is a direct relation between ear conformation and otitis externa, with pendulous-eared dogs being predisposed to infection. The L-shaped configuration of the external meatus is a further

Table 70.4. Common and/or Important Infectious Agents of the Integumentary System of Cattle

Agent	
Viruses	
Bovine herpesvirus 2	Mammary vesicles and ulcers (bovine mammillitis)
Bovine papillomavirus	Cutaneous papillomas (bovine papillomatosis, warts)
Lumpy skin disease virus[a]	Generalized or local papules and nodules that ulcerate (lumpy skin disease)
Pseudocowpox virus	Mammary vesicles, papules, and scabs (pseudocowpox)
Pseudorabies virus	Uncontrolled pruritis (pseudorabies)
Vesicular viruses[b]	Vesicles and ulcers on coronary band and interdigital areas
Bacteria	
Actinobacillus lignieresii	Head and neck abscess, draining fistulas
Actinomyces bovis	Draining tracts, subcutaneous abscesses(actinomycosis, lumpy jaw)
Arcanobacterium pyogenes	Subcutaneous abscesses
Clostridium septicum	Cellulitis (malignant edema)
Corynebacterium pseudotuberculosis	Ulcerative dermatitis
Dermatophilus congolensis	Exudate epidermitis (dermatophilosis)
Fusobacterium necrophoruml[c], *Prevotella melaninogenicus*[c]	Interdigital dermatitis, cellulitis (interdigital necrobacillosis, footrot)
Salmonella Dublin	Gangrene of distal extremities, ears, and tail due to terminal endarteritis
Fungi	
Trichophyton verrucosum	Round to oval, crusty skin lesions with alopecia (dermatophytosis, ringworm)

[a]Considered a foreign animal disease agent in the United States.
[b]Includes foot-and-mouth disease virus[a] and vesicular stomatitis virus.
[c]Agents act synergistically.

Table 70.5. Common and/or Important Infectious Agents of the Integumentary System of Sheep/Goats

Agent	Major Clinical Manifestations (Common Disease Name)
Prions	
Scrapie prion	Pruritus, excoriations, self-mutilation (scraple)
Viruses	
Bluetongue virus	Erythema, edema of ears and muzzle, coronitis (bluetongue)
Goat pox, sheep pox viruses[a]	Papules, vesicles, pustules (goat pox, sheep pox)
Parapoxvirus	Crusting proliferative muco9cutaneous lesions, teat lesions (contagious ecthyma, soremouth)
Vesicular viruses[b]	Vesicles and ulcers on teats, coronary bands, and interdigital areas
Bacteria	
Clostridium novyi	Edema of the head, neck, and thorax (big head in rams)
Corynebacterium pseudotuberculosis	Skin abscesses (caseous lymphadenitis)
Dermatophilus congolensis	Exudative dermatitis (dermatophilosis, lumpy wool disease, strawberry footrot)
Dichelobacter nodosus/ Fusobacterium necrophorum[c]	Interdigital dermatitis, underrunning of the sole (contagious footrot)
Staphylococcus aureus[d]	Pustular dermatitis of face, udder, teats and ventral abdomen (staphylococcal dermatitis)
Fungi	
Trichophyton verrucosum, T. mentagrophytes	Crusting, circular skin lesions with alopecia (dermatophytosis, ringworm, club lamb fungus)

[a]Considered a foreign animal disease agent in the United States.
[b]Includes foot-and-mouth disease virus[a] and vesicular stomatitis virus.
[c]Agents act synergistically.
[d]*Staphylococcus aureus* ssp. *anaerobius* is associated with subcutaneous abscesses in sheep.

complicating factor because it limits aeration and drainage. An abundance of lipid-rich earwax and heavy ear canal hair additionally contribute to development of otitis externa. A breed predilection (e.g., cocker spaniels) for development of otitis externa is also evident.

The agents of canine otitis externa are endogenous in origin and are not thought to play the initiating role in the disease process, but rather act as opportunists once other factors are in place. Infections are frequently polymicrobial. Commonly recovered agents from canine otitis externa are listed in Table 70.8.

Table 70.7. Common and/or Important Infectious Agents of the Integumentary System of Poultry

Agent	Major Clinical Manifestations (Common Disease Name)
Viruses	
Fowlpox	Papules and nodules of beak, comb, and wattles (avian pox)

Table 70.6. Common and/or Important Infectious Agents of the Integumentary System of Pigs

Agent	Major Clinical Manifestations (Common Disease Name)
Viruses	
African swine fever virus[a]	Reddish-purple discoloration of skin (African swine fever)
Hog Cholera virus[a]	Erythema, purple discoloration of skin, necrosis of ears and tail (hog cholera)
Swinepox virus	Macules, papules, pustules (swinepox)
Vesicular viruses[b]	Vesicles and ulcers on coronary band and interdigital areas
Bacteria	
Bacillus anthracis	Diffuse subcutaneous and dermal edema of neck and thorax (anthrax)
Erysipelothrix rhusiopathiae	Congested raised skin lesions, rhomboidal-shaped necrotic skin lesions (erysipelas)
Escherichia coli (Shiga-like toxin positive)	Subcutaneous edema of lips and eyelids (edema disease)
Salmonella choleraesuis	Reddish-purple discoloration of the skin
Streptococcus equi ssp. *zooepidemicus, S. dysgalactiae* ssp. *equisimilus*	Pustular dermatitis, subcutaneous abscesses
Staphylococcus hyicus	Generalized exudative dermatitis (exudative epidermitis, greasy pig disease)
Fungi	
Microsporum nanum, Trichophyton spp.	Reddish circular skin lesions with crusting at periphery (dermatophytosis, ringworm)

[a]Considered a foreign animal disease agent in the United States.
[b]Includes foot-and-mouth,[a] vesicular stomatitis virus, swine vesicular disease, and vesicular exanthema of swine viruses.

Table 70.8. Common Agents of Canine Otitis Externa and Key Organism Characteristics

	Typical Colonies On		Ancillary Tests		
Agent	Blood Agar (24–48 h)	MacConkey Agar	Gram Stain	Oxidase	Catalase
Staphylococcus intermediate	White or off-white, often with double-zone hemolysis	No Growth	Positive cocci	NA	Positive
Staphylococcus schleiferi ssp. *coagulans*	White, hemolytic	No Growth	Positive cocci	NA	Positive
Proteus mirabilis	Swarms, no discrete colonies	Colorless	Negative rods	Negative	NA
Pseudomonas aeruginosa	Gray to greenish, fruity odor, hemolytic	Colorless, sometime pigment detected	Negative rods	Positive	NA
Streptococcus canis	Gray to greenish, fruity odor, hemolytic	No growth	Positive cocci	NA	Negative
Escherichia coli	Smooth, gray, some strains are hemolytic	Pink to red with red haze	Negative rods	Negative	NA
Klebsiella pneumonia	Mucoid, whitish-gray	Mucoid, pink without red haze	Negative rods	Negative	NA
Malassezia[a]	No growth or tiny colonies	No growth	Variable staining, budding yeast	NA	NA

NA, not applicable.
[a]May require prolonged incubation. Best recovery on Sabouraud's dextrose agar at 37 °C under microaerophilic conditions.

Mastitis

Mastitis, an inflammation of the mammary gland, occurs in all animal species. It is most common in dairy cattle and is of greatest economic significance to the dairy industry. For mastitis to develop, the innate physical barriers must be breached. Once that occurs, both innate immunity (lactoferrin, complement, resident immune cells) and specific immunity play a role in preventing microbial pathogens from establishing. If a pathogen does establish in the mammary gland, chemotactic gradients formed by inflammatory cytokines and chemokines result in rapid recruitment on inflammatory cells in an effort to control the infection. Most of the clinical signs associated with mastitis are a consequence of the inflammatory response.

Bacteria are the main infectious agents of mastitis, although viruses are important mammary pathogens in some animals (Maedi-visna, sheep; CAE, goats). Fungi (e.g., *Candida*, *Aspergillus*, and *Pseudallescheria*) and an achlorophyllous algae, *Prototheca*, are rare causes of mastitis in cattle but can occasionally cause herd outbreaks.

Table 70.9. Agents of Bovine Mastitis

Agent[a]	Frequency	Specific Features
Arcanobacterium pyogenes	Occasional	Associated with teat injury or cannula/dilator use, poor treatment response
Clostridium perfringens	Rare	Causes gangrenous mastitis
Coagulase-negative Staphylococcus spp.	Frequent	Source is skin, many infections transient
Escherichia coli	Frequent	Environmental source, acute infections, may cause systemic illness
Klebsiella pneumoniae	Occasional	Severe mastitis, associated with sawdust/wood shaving bedding
Mycoplasma spp.[b,c]	Frequent	Cow is source, spread by milking, destructive mastitis, cow not usually systemically ill, can be eradicated
Mycobacterium spp.	Rare	Spread by contaminated treatment equipment or materials
Nocardia spp.	Rare	Spread by contaminated treatment equipment or materials
Pasteurella multocida	Rare	Sporadic infections, suggests cross-contamination during treatment
Prototheca spp.	Rare	Achloric algae, associated with poor environmental hygiene, not treatable
Staphylococcus aureus[b]	Frequent	Source is infected udder, spread by milking, rare cause of gangrenous mastitis, can be eradicated
Streptococcus agalactiae[b]	Occasional	Causes high bulk tank somatic cell count, can be eradicated
S. dysgalactiae ssp. *dysgalactiae*	Frequent	Bovine origin, survives in environment
Streptococcus uberis	Frequent	Found on bovine skin and environment

[a]Also consider *Corynebacterium bovis*, *Serratia*, *Bacillus*, *Pseudomonas*, and various other *Enterobacteriaceae*.
[b]Contagious pathogens.
[c]Most common species recovered are *M. bovis*, *M. californicum*, and *M. canadense*

Different organisms predominate as mastitis pathogens depending on the animal involved. Coliforms (dogs, swine), *S. aureus* (sheep, goats), beta-hemolytic streptococci (horses), *Mannheimia haemolytica* (sheep), and *Mycoplasma* species (sheep, goats) are the most commonly encountered bacteria.

The agents associated with mastitis in cattle are extensive and are classified as either "contagious" pathogens where the mammary gland is the source or as "environmental" pathogens when they originate from transient skin flora or environmental reservoirs. Cow age, parity, stage of lactation, milking operation management methods, and environmental sanitation control (housing and bedding) are underlying factors in most cases of mastitis. Common agents of bovine mastitis are listed in Table 70.9.

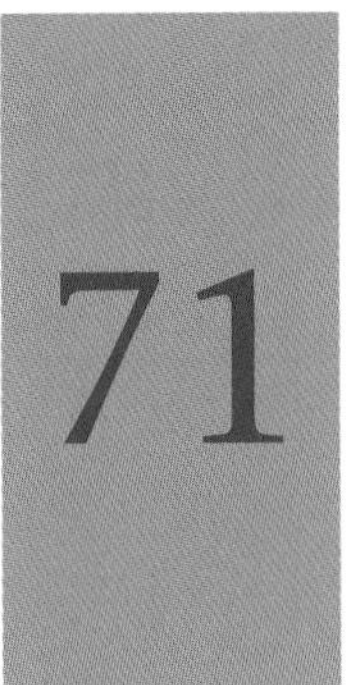

71 Musculoskeletal System

Douglas E. Hostetler

The musculoskeletal system provides a structural framework for the body, protects vital organs, and provides the capacity for locomotion. It is composed of the axial and appendicular skeleton and associated ligaments, muscles, and tendons. Joint spaces and bursas and their synovial membranes are included in this system.

The musculoskeletal system does not have a normal flora per se, although seeding from transient bacteremias or "trafficking" through supposed sterile sites may occur. Bacterial spores (*Clostridium* sp.) may be found dormant in muscle, particularly in ruminants, subsequent to entry through the digestive tract and hematogenous distribution.

Antimicrobial Defenses of the Musculoskeletal System

The antimicrobial defenses of the musculoskeletal system predominately rely on the circulating immune defenses.

Normal healthy bone is considered fairly resistant to infection. Even direct inoculation of bone with pathogenic bacteria does not usually lead to infection unless predisposing factors are present. Bone undergoes constant remodeling, and injured/infected bone can be resorbed and replaced with new bone.

Muscle has a rich blood supply and, therefore, benefits from its intimate association with circulating innate immune defenses. Skeletal muscle also has great ability to regenerate necrotic muscle segments resulting from inflammatory/infectious processes.

In synovial membrane-lined sites (synovial joints, bursas, and tendon sheaths), the synovium is composed of a thin cellular surface layer of predominately macrophages and fibroblast-like synoviocytes and an underlying rich vascular layer. Production of proinflammatory cytokines by cells at these sites (chondrocytes, synoviocytes, and synovial macrophages) promotes a strong inflammatory response in the face of infection. The rich blood supply to synovial membranes not only predisposes to localization of microbial agents but also allows for rapid recruitment of vascular immune defenses. While the inflammatory response is important for controlling infection, it can also lead to degradative changes to articular cartilage in synovial joints by stimulating production of catabolic metalloproteinases and inhibiting synthesis of collagen and proteoglycans. As inflammation resolves, fibrosis may lead to decreased functionality.

Infections of the Musculoskeletal System

Infections of the musculoskeletal system are initiated by introduction of microbial agents through (i) direct inoculation from traumatic or iatrogenic events, (ii) extension of infectious processes from contiguous focuses, or (iii) hematogenous seeding from distantly infected sites or during septicemia. Within the musculoskeletal system sites of traumatic injury, areas of active growth with increased vascularity or sites with specific vascular features (e.g., discontinuous epithelium in capillaries in vertebral end plates and metaphyses) are predisposed to infection. Viral, bacterial, and fungal agents can be involved. Parasite infections of muscle are also important but are not within the context of this book. As a rule, bacteria are the most common microbial agents involved among the three groups of agents discussed here. Specific bacterial factors are important for infection to develop. Adherence factors (e.g., fibrinogen or fibronectin-binding proteins), toxins that promote inflammatory response and tissue damage (e.g., superantigens and cytotoxins), and factors that aid in evasion of the immune system (e.g., capsules and protein A)—all provide an advantage to establishment and persistence.

The major infectious processes in the musculoskeletal system are (i) infections of bone including vertebral body and associated intervertebral disk infections; (ii) infections involving articular surfaces or bursas including their synovial membranes; and (iii) infections of skeletal muscle, tendons, and surrounding fascia. These infectious processes do not necessarily occur as distinct entities (e.g., infection of metaphyseal bone and associated joint infections in neonatal septicemia in some animals). Diseases of neurologic origin that affect muscle activity as a result of inhibition of neurotransmitter release (tetanus and botulism) are covered in Chapter 72. Microbial agents causing cellulitis may overlap with musculoskeletal infections and are also covered in Chapter 69. Common and/or

Veterinary Microbiology, Third Edition. Edited by D. Scott McVey, Melissa Kennedy and M.M. Chengappa.

Table 71.1. Common and/or Important Infectious Agents of the Musculoskeletal System of Dogs and Cats

Agent	Major Clinical Manifestations (Common Disease Name)
Viruses	
Feline syncytium-forming virus (C)	Arthritis
Bacteria	
Actinomyces spp.[a]	Diskospondylitis, osteomyelitis
β-Hemolytic *Streptococcus* spp. (D)	Arthritis, diskospondylitis, myositis, necrotizing fasciitis
Borrelia burgdorferi (D)	Arthritis (Lyme disease)
Brucella canis (D)	Diskospondylitis, osteomyelitis
Leptospira spp.	Polymyositis
Obligate anaerobes[b]	Myositis
Pasteurella multocida (C)	Myositis
Staphylococcus intermedius	Arthritis, diskospondylitis, myositis, osteomyelitis
Fungi	
Aspergillus spp. (D)	Diskospondylitis, osteomyelitis
Blastomyces dermatitidis (D)	Osteomyelitis
Coccidioides immitis (D)	Osteomyelitis

C, cats; D, dogs.
[a]Includes *A. viscosus* and *A. hordeovulneris.*
[b]Includes *Fusobacterium, Bacteroides, Porphyromonas,* and *Peptostreptococcus.*

important agents associated with musculoskeletal infections of domestic animals and poultry are listed in Tables 71.1, 71.2, 71.3, 71.4, 71.5, and 71.6.

Infections of Bone (Including Vertebral Body and Intervertebral Disk Infections)

Osteitis is an inflammation of the bone. Osteomyelitis and periostitis denote involvement of the medullary cavity and periosteum, respectively. Osteomyelitis can be further divided into hematogenous or posttraumatic osteomyelitis. Most bone infections are bacterial in nature. While a variety of bacteria can cause bone infections, a select number of them predominate within animal groups. In companion animals and poultry, coagulase-positive *Staphylococcus* species (*S. intermedius*, *S. aureus*, and *S. hyicus*) are frequently involved. Other organisms encountered include enterics (*Escherichia coli* and *Proteus* spp.) and obligate anaerobes. In horses, the agents most commonly isolated from osteomyelitis in neonates are *Actinobacillus equuli* ssp. *equuli*, *E. coli*, *Streptococcus equi* ssp. *zooepidemicus*, and *Salmonella*, while coagulase-positive staphylococci predominate in adults. In ruminants and pigs, *Arcanobacterium pyogenes* and *Salmonella* are major causes of osteomyelitis.

Table 71.2. Common and/or Important Infectious Agents of the Musculoskeletal System of Horses

Agent	Major Clinical Manifestations (Common Disease Name)
Bacteria	
Actinobacillus equuli ssp. *equuli*	Arthritis, osteomyelitis (joint ill)
Brucella abortus	Atlantal or supraspinous bursitis (poll evil/fistulous withers), osteomyelitis
Escherichia coli	Arthritis, osteomyelitis (joint ill)
Histotoxic *Clostridium* spp.[a]	Myositis (clostridial myositis)
Salmonella spp.	Arthritis, osteomyelitis (joint ill)
Staphylococcus aureus	Myositis
Streptococcus equi ssp. *equi*	Atlantal or supraspinous bursitis (poll evil/fistulous withers), osteomyelitis, myositis, tenosynovitis
Streptococcus equi ssp. *zooepidemicus*	Arthritis, osteomyelitis (joint ill)

[a]Includes *C. perfringens, C. sordellii,* and *C. septicum.*

Table 71.3. Common and/or Important Infectious Agents of the Musculoskeletal System of Cattle

Agent	Major Clinical Manifestations (Common Disease Name)
Bacteria	
Actinobacillus lignieresii	Myositis
Actinomyces bovis	Osteomyelitis (lumpy jaw)
Arcanobacterium pyogenes	Arthritis, diskospondylitis, fasciitis, myositis, osteomyelitis
Clostridium chauvoei	Myositis (blackleg)
Escherichia coli	Arthritis, osteomyelitis
Fusobacterium necrophorum	Arthritis, diskospondylitis, osteomyelitis
Histotoxic *Clostridium* spp.[a]	Myositis (malignant edema)
Mycoplasma spp.[b]	Arthritis, bursitis, tenosynovitis
Salmonella spp.	Arthritis, osteomyelitis

[a]Includes *C. perfringens, C. novyi, C. septicum,* and *C. sordellii.*
[b]Includes *M. bovis, M. californicum, M. alkalescens,* and *M. arginine.*

Table 71.4. Common and/or Important Infectious Agents of the Musculoskeletal System of Sheep and Goats

Agent	Major Clinical Manifestations (Common Disease Name)
Viruses	
Bluetongue virus (S)	Muscle infarction
Caprine arthritis-encephalitis virus (G)	Arthritis
Bacteria	
Arcanobacterium pyogenes (S)	Diskospondylitis, myositis
Chlamydophila percorum	Arthritis
Corynebacterium pseudotuberculosis	Myositis
Erysipelothrix rhusiopathiae (S)	Arthritis (erysipelas)
Histotoxic *Clostridium* spp.[a]	Myositis
Mycoplasma spp. (G)[b]	Arthritis, tenosynovitis

S, sheep; G, goats.
[a]Includes *C. perfringens, C. novyi, C. septicum,* and *C. sordellii.*
[b]Includes *M. mycoides* ssp. *mycoides* (large colony type), *M. capricolum* ssp. *capricolum,* and *M. putrefaciens.*

Table 71.5. Common and/or Important Infectious Agents of the Musculoskeletal System of Pigs

Agent	Major Clinical Manifestations (Common Disease Name)
Bacteria	
Arcanobacterium pyogenes	Arthritis, osteomyelitis
β-Hemolytic *Streptococcus* spp.	Arthritis
Brucella suis	Arthritis, diskospondylitis (brucellosis)
Clostridium septicum	Myositis (malignant edema)
Erysipelothrix rhusiopathiae	Arthritis, diskospondylitis (erysipelas)
Haemophilus parasuis	Arthritis (Glasser's disease)
Mycoplasma hyorhinis	Arthritis
Mycoplasma hyosynoviae	Arthritis
Pasteurella multocida	Atrophy of nasal turbinate bones (atrophic rhinitis)
Streptococcus suis (type 2)	Arthritis

Others of note in production animals are *E. coli* and *Fusobacterium necrophorum*.

The microvasculature (discontinuous epithelium and lack of basement membrane) and possibly the slow blood flow through capillaries in areas of active growth favor the establishment of infections (hematogenous osteomyelitis). Macrophages associated with vascular endothelium are the main defense in these areas. Infections also occur in areas of bone with poor or interrupted vascular supply from trauma (posttraumatic osteomyelitis) or when adjacent tissue infections result in ischemic injury. If the medullary as well as periosteal vascular supply to bone becomes compromised during an infectious process, a sequestration of necrotic bone may result. In some cases, persistent drainage from sinus tracts develops. Under these conditions, bacteria are better able to establish and more difficult to eliminate because they become inaccessible to immune defenses and refractory to antibiotic treatment. Host cellular products, and perhaps some bacterial products, stimulate monocytes and fibroblast to produce osteolytic cytokines and stimulate osteoclastic activity, causing greater separation of living from dead bone.

Table 71.6. Common and/or Important Infectious Agents of the Musculoskeletal System of Poultry

Agent	Major Clinical Manifestations (Common Disease Name)
Viruses	
Reovirus	Arthritis, bursitis, tenosynovitis
Bacteria	
Arcanobacterium pyogenes (T)	Osteomyelitis
Erysipelothrix rhusiopathiae (T)	Arthritis (erysipelas)
Escherichia coli	Arthritis, bursitis, osteomyelitis, tenosynovitis
Mycoplasma meleagridis (T)	Bowing of tibiotarsal bone, cervical vertebrae deformation
Mycoplasma synoviae	Arthritis, bursitis, tenosynovitis (infectious synovitis)
Staphylococcus aureus, S. hyicus	Arthritis, bursitis, osteomyelitis, tenosynovitis

T, turkeys.

Use of synthetic material in reconstructive or replacement surgeries (e.g., hip replacements) may also disrupt the innate resistance of bone to infection by providing an avascular surface and protection from immune defenses. Bone cement used in some replacement surgeries may itself inhibit phagocytosis and complement activity. Host fibronectin deposited on implant material allows for bacterial attachment, which is followed by production of exopolysaccharides (glycocalyx) by bacteria. Along with host products, the glycocalyx forms biofilms that provide bacteria protection from host defenses and killing by antibiotics.

Bite wounds, penetrating foreign bodies, orthopedic surgical procedures, and traumatic injuries are possible initiating events for development of osteomyelitis in companion animals. The long bones are most commonly affected.

In production animals, hematogenous osteomyelitis is a frequent event. Hematogenous osteomyelitis in neonatal ruminants is associated with failure of passive transfer. Infections begin at the metaphysis or the epiphysis beneath articular cartilage and often occur in conjunction with or subsequent to infectious synovitis. In neonatal infections, vessels that cross the growth plates are important for spreading infection to the metaphysis from joints. Epiphyseal osteomyelitis in conjunction with arthritis in calves is commonly caused by *Salmonella* serovar *Dublin*. *A. pyogenes* osteomyelitis in older calves and adults more commonly begins on the metaphyseal side of the growth plate. *A. pyogenes* also causes a hematogenous vertebral osteomyelitis in pigs associated with tail biting or foot lesions. Commercial turkeys develop focal areas of osteomyelitis caused by *S. aureus* or *E. coli*. The proximal tibiotarsus and proximal femur are most often affected, and infections are associated with a green discoloration of the liver in adolescent male turkeys (turkey green-liver osteomyelitis complex). Hematogenous osteomyelitis is uncommon in dogs and cats.

Posttraumatic osteomyelitis is also common in production animals, usually in adults. In cattle a chronic pyogranulomatous inflammation involving the mandible ("lumpy jaw") or maxilla is caused by *Actinomyces bovis* (see Figure 69.2).

Viral agents rarely cause inflammatory bone disease. Distemper virus in dogs may damage osteoblasts and cause growth retardation. Canine hepatitis virus can cause metaphyseal hemorrhage and necrosis.

Fungal bone infections occur but at a low frequency. Fungal osteomyelitis is usually the result of dissemination from another site, most often the lung. Many of the systemic mycotic agents are capable of causing fungal osteomyelitis. *Coccidioides immitis* is notable for disseminating to the appendicular skeleton in dogs. Disseminated *Blastomyces dermatitidis* infections in dogs can involve the bones in up to 30% of the cases with vertebrae, and long bones are most commonly affected.

Diskospondylitis, an inflammatory process of the intervertebral disk and adjacent vertebrae, is a particularly common site for bone infections to occur. It usually begins at the vertebral end plates. The discontinuous capillary epithelium and slow-flowing venous channels predispose this area to bacterial seeding. Diskospondylitis is most common in dogs and ruminants and often results via hematogenous dissemination. The L7–S1 region is a commonly affected site in the dog, but any vertebral body can be affected. *Staphylococcus intermedius* is the most common agent identified.

Vertebral infections of T13–L3 in the dog are associated with migration of foreign bodies (e.g., plant awns). *Actinomyces* spp. are the usual agents involved. Diskospondylitis associated with *Brucella* species deserves particular attention. The persistent bacteremia that occurs with some *Brucella* species predisposes to infection at extragenital sites, and *Brucella* should always be considered as a potential agent in diskospondylitis in dogs (*B. canis*) and pigs (*B. suis*). Calves with diskospondylitis caused by hematogenous dissemination of either *A. pyogenes* or *F. necrophorum* present with paresis or paralysis.

German shepherd dogs are particularly prone to developing diskospondylitis and osteomyelitis of fungal origin caused by *Aspergillus* spp. *Aspergillus terreus* and *A. deflectus* are the most common species recovered.

Infections Involving Articular Surfaces, Bursas, and Synovial Membranes

Arthritis denotes an inflammatory process of a joint space. Most joint infections are bacterial, but viral and fungal infections do occur. Monoarticular infections typically arise from direct inoculation or spread from a contiguous site (e.g., distal interphalangeal joint infection in cattle following sole abscessation) (Figure 71.1).

FIGURE 71.1. *A swollen lateral digit of a bull with septic arthritis of the distal interphalangeal joint secondary to extension of an infected pododermatitis circumscripta lesion (sole ulcer).*

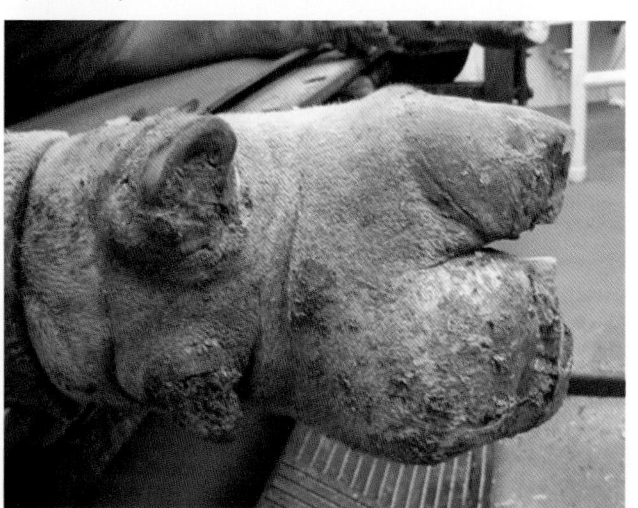

FIGURE 71.2. *A swollen left carpal joint from a calf with septic arthritis secondary to, failure of passive transfer, an umbilical infection, and septicemia.*

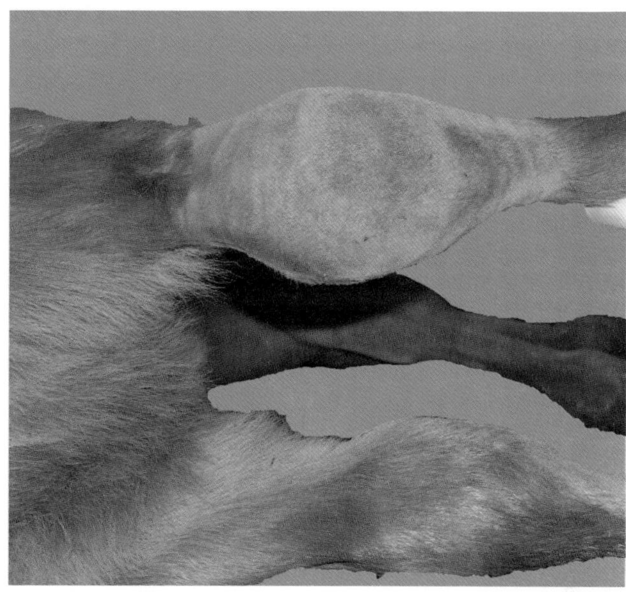

Hematogenous infections frequently result in polyarthropathies. In neonates, the umbilicus or gastrointestinal tract are common entry points. Arthritis is a common sequela to septicemia, especially in young animals and especially where there is failure of passive transfer (Figure 71.2). In adult animals, joint abnormalities, immunosuppressive diseases, infections at other sites in the body, intra-articular injections, surgery, and joint prostheses all predispose to joint infections.

Infection of the joint usually begins in synovial tissue, in part, because of the rich vascular supply and lack of basement membrane. Infection results in expression of a cascade of inflammatory mediators (tumor necrosis factor, interleukin 1, interleukin 6, and nitric oxide) that result in increased blood flow to the area, increased capillary permeability, and an influx of inflammatory cells. The agent involved dictates the type and intensity of inflammatory response. Synovitis in unchecked infections results in increased synovial fluid containing cellular exudates that subsequently progresses to involve the articular surfaces. Alone or in combination, bacterial products, products resulting from the inflammatory response, and proteases already present or produced by cells in the joint damage articular cartilage. Once damaged, the articular cartilage has limited capacity for repair.

Current evidence suggests that when viable bacteria are no longer detectable in cases of septic arthritis, the inflammatory response continues and further destruction to articular cartilage ensues. This is likely due to residual bacterial products such as peptidoglycan–polysaccharide complexes that continue to promote an inflammatory response. Even bacterial DNA, specifically unmethylated CpG motifs, appears to stimulate a variety of cell types to produce proinflammatory cytokines leading to further tissue destruction. Joint functionality may be further affected by fibrosis that results during resolution of the inflammatory process. In some cases ankylosis of the joint occurs.

Postinfective arthritis, which is associated with microbial fragments localizing in the joint during a septicemia but without microbial replication in the joint itself, is less well recognized in veterinary medicine than it is in human medicine. When it occurs, joint damage results solely from immune mechanisms.

Morphologic variants of bacteria have also been associated with joint infections. Bacterial L-forms, which are wall-less bacteria, which have "turned off" the genes responsible for cell wall synthesis, and small colony variants of bacteria, which have decreased growth rates presumably due to defective respiratory metabolism, have been associated with persistent joint infections.

In species where transphyseal vessels provide a direct connection between the metaphyses and the epiphyseal cartilage (e.g., ruminants and horses), both acute osteomyelitis and joint infections are common. This is also true when metaphyseal bone is included within the joint capsule. Sometimes synovitis represents only one of a number of clinical manifestations of systemic infectious processes (e.g., polyserositis in pigs caused by *Mycoplasma hyorhinis* or *Haemophilus parasuis*).

Bacterial arthritis is uncommon in companion animals. When it occurs, coagulase-positive *Staphylococcus* species and *Streptococcus* species are the most common agents involved. Infections result from direct inoculation from trauma or surgery. The canine stifle joint appears particularly predisposed to postsurgical infections. Recurrent lameness, sometimes involving multiple joints, is associated with a chronic and progressive arthritis due to *Borrelia burgdorferi*, the Lyme disease agent.

Arthritis is common in production animals and horses, and a variety of organisms can be involved. In neonates, *Salmonella* and *E. coli* are the main agents. Mycoplasma arthritis in ruminants is also an important entity in feedlot cattle and dairy calves. In addition to arthritis, which usually involves carpal and hock joints, tenosynovitis and bursitis occur. *Mycoplasma bovis* is the usual species recovered. In goats, mycoplasma arthritis affects both kids and adults. *Mycoplasma mycoides* ssp. *mycoides* (large colony type) and *M. capricolum* ssp. *capricolum* are principal species isolated. Mycoplasma arthritis is also important in pigs. Chlamydial joint infections (*Chlamydophila percorum*) are commonly recognized in goats and sheep ("stiff lamb disease"). Infections can present in conjunction with conjunctivitis. The chlamydial species involved is different from the species associated with goat and sheep abortions. In horses, joint infections in neonates are caused by organisms also associated with neonatal osteomyelitis and include *E. coli*, *Salmonella*, *Actinobacillus*, and *Streptococcus* spp. In adult horses, *Staphylococcus* or *Streptococcus* spp. are usually involved.

Bursitis refers to an inflammation of the synovial lined bursas and can be affected in a manner similar to synovial membranes in joints. Of specific importance are *Brucella abortus* and *S. aureus* infections of the atlantal and supraspinous bursas in horses. These infections may spread to involved spinous processes of adjacent vertebrae.

Although bacteria are responsible for most cases of infectious arthritis, viral agents are sometimes involved. Feline syncytium-forming virus infections cause both proliferative and erosive forms of joint involvement in cats. Caprine arthritis-encephalitis virus is of substantial importance in goats causing a hyperplastic polysynovitis, usually in goats older than 12 months. Avian reovirus causes arthritis and tenosynovitis in turkeys and chickens. The digital flexor and metatarsal extensor tendons and hock joints are most commonly affected. The stability of the virus, potential for horizontal and vertical transmission, and high-density rearing practices used today make it a potentially serious flock problem.

Infections of Skeletal Muscle, Tendons, and Fascia

Infections of skeletal muscles are uncommon. While viral and fungal agents occasionally cause muscle infections, bacteria again are the most frequent of the three groups involved. Myositis can be in the form of a localized abscess, granuloma, or diffuse inflammatory process that spreads along fascial planes. Preceding events include trauma, injections, bite wounds, or a contiguous infectious process (e.g., cellulitis, subcutaneous abscess, and osteomyelitis). Pyogenic bacteria cause localized abscesses (e.g., *Pasteurella multocida* in cats). Granulomatous and pyogranulomatous myositis is associated with bacterial species known to evoke granulomatous pyogranulomatous inflammatory responses (e.g., *Mycobacterium bovis*, *Actinomyces* spp., *Actinobacillus lignieresii*). Clostridial myositis is typically a more diffuse infectious process and spreads rapidly along fascial planes. It is the most severe and aggressive form of the infectious myositides due to the production of potent histotoxins. Myositis may occur subsequent to or in conjunction with clostridial cellulitis. Most animal species are affected; however, clostridial myositis is most common in ruminants and horses. Clostridial agents usually reach affected sites by direct penetration (e.g., penetrating wound and injections) or, in the case of *Clostridium chauvoei*, the agent of blackleg, are already present in muscle as dormant spores. When tissue becomes devitalized, producing

FIGURE 71.3. *Necrotic and emphysematous muscle due to* C. chauvoei *infection. (Courtesy of Dr Bruce Brodersen.)*

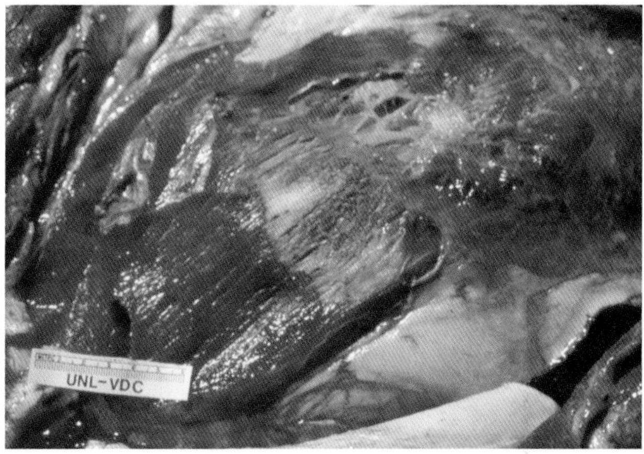

an anaerobic environment, the spores germinate and vegetative cells proliferate. Numerous cytotoxic exotoxins produced by these clostridial species contribute coagulative muscle necrosis (Figure 71.3).

Hemolytic *Streptococcus* spp. have been associated with severe necrotizing fasciitis in dogs. In horses, immune complex vasculitis is the supposed mechanism by which muscle damage due to vessel infarction and hemorrhage results post-*S. equi* ssp. *equi* infections.

Tendon sheaths have an inner synovial membrane and may become infected as a result of hematogenous dissemination, trauma (e.g., bite wounds), treatments (e.g., sheath injections in horses), or spread from a contiguous focus. Tenosynovitis is especially important in horses, most commonly involving digital tendons. Infections typically result from a wound with a variety of bacteria being involved or subsequent to sheath injection, where *S. aureus* is usually the cause.

Nervous System

DOUGLAS E. HOSTETLER

The nervous system is divided into the central and peripheral nervous systems. The central nervous system includes the brain and spinal cord, the cerebrospinal fluid that bathes it, and the meningeal layers that cover it. The peripheral nervous system is comprised of nerves that arise from the central nervous system (cranial or spinal nerves) and innervate muscles or effector organs. The peripheral nervous system is further divided into somatic sensory and autonomic divisions.

Nervous system infections most commonly involve the central nervous system. In some cases, peripheral nerves are the targeted site for infectious or immunological processes or microbial toxin action, or serve as the site for entry of infectious agents or toxic products that act on the central nervous system. The nervous system does not have a normal microbial flora. Some viruses (e.g., herpesviruses and distemper virus) can cause latent infections, and in some cases viruses integrate into the host genome as proviruses (e.g., visna virus).

Antimicrobial Defenses

Sensitivity of the nervous system to injury makes exclusion of microbial pathogens or their toxins of paramount importance. Anatomic and immunological defenses are the primary defense mechanisms available; the following sections present these defenses.

Anatomic Defenses

The skull and vertebrae provide rigid coverings that protect the brain and spinal cord from traumatic or penetrating injuries that might lead to introduction of microbial pathogens. The meningeal layers (pia, arachnoid, and dura) provide further anatomic barriers that act to contain or prevent infectious processes from progressing into the nervous system parenchyma.

The blood–brain barrier provides the major anatomical separation between the nervous system parenchyma and components of the vascular system. It protects the central nervous system from agents disseminated via the bloodstream from other sites in the body. Central to the blood-brain barrier are the capillary endothelial cells, which form tight intercellular junctions that prevent movement of blood constituents into the central nervous system. Movement of substances across the endothelial cells is further controlled by specialized carrier transport systems. Astrocyte processes and pericytes, a subclass of microglial cells, which surround capillaries and an extracellular matrix, contribute to the overall makeup of the blood–brain barrier. Not all areas are protected by the blood–brain barrier (e.g., pituitary and choroid plexus). The secretory selectivity of choroid plexus epithelial cells and ependymal cells contributes to a barrier between the blood and cerebrospinal fluid. Nerves of the peripheral nervous system are protected from inflammatory reactions and immune responses by a blood nerve barrier, although it is not as restrictive as the blood–brain barrier.

Immunological Defenses

Much of our knowledge of immune defense of the nervous system is based on studics in rodents and humans. The central nervous system has long been considered an immunologically privileged site because it lacks an organized lymphatic system for antigen delivery to lymph nodes and normally has greatly reduced expression of major histocompatibility complex determinants. Current evidence indicates that the nervous system has a much more advanced immunological defense system than was previously thought. Antigens from the cerebrospinal fluid are able to access lymph nodes (cervical) by lymphatic drain-age along cranial nerves. Major histocompatibility antigens are expressed by cells in the central nervous system parenchyma (e.g., astrocytes and microglial cells) under proper conditions. The blood–brain barrier contributes to the relative immune privilege of the healthy central nervous system by excluding entry of large molecules from the blood and by restricting immune cell entry. This restriction is not absolute and, although few immune cells are normally found, both activated and naive T lymphocytes can penetrate the blood–brain barrier and are present in the absence of inflammation, suggesting a “patrolling” function. While an active immune system is in place, it is geared to provide a degree of protection and yet minimize innocent bystander damage. This is meant to avoid inflammatory responses that lead to profound or

Veterinary Microbiology, Third Edition. Edited by D. Scott McVey, Melissa Kennedy and M.M. Chengappa.

irreversible disturbances in neuronal function. Local inflammatory responses are regulated by immunosuppressive mechanisms. Subclasses of glial cells express cytokines (e.g., interleukin 6 and transforming growth factor $\beta 2$) that help restrict the inflammatory response. An ability to induce T lymphocyte apoptosis is also present.

The central nervous system possesses certain innate immune capabilities. Complement plays an essential role in innate immune defense. Both neuronal cells and astrocytes have ability to produce complement components. A number of nervous system pathogens will induce complement component synthesis (e.g., exotic Newcastle disease virus and *Listeria monocytogenes*), which plays a direct role both in pathogen killing by membrane attack complex formation and in recruitment of leukocytes. Uncontrolled complement activation, resulting from progressing infectious processes, contributes to pathology when host cell membrane complement inhibitors are overwhelmed.

Various cell types are also critical to central nervous system defense. Microglia cells are myeloid bone marrow-derived cells. When activated, they produce various chemokines and cytokines, act as macrophages, and potentially have a role in antigen presentation. Dendritic cells, which are potent antigen-presenting cells, have also been demonstrated in the brain. Astrocytes have been shown to be involved in antigen presentation and chemokine/cytokine production. In the face of an inflammatory response, astrocytes become activated and can form glial scars to insulate damaged areas of the brain parenchyma. Nerve cells, themselves, are capable of producing certain cytokines (interferon γ).

During infectious processes, migration of inflammatory cells from the vascular system to affected sites is important for controlling progressing infectious processes. Inflammatory cell migration is mediated, as elsewhere in the body, through production of chemokines and expression of adhesion ligands (selectins and integrins).

Infections of the Nervous System

For microbial pathogens to affect the nervous system, they or their products must reach the nervous system (route of infection), be able to penetrate or interrupt anatomic barriers, and establish and persist by evading or subverting immune defenses. Clinical signs resulting from infection depend on whether and where the infection is localized, what agent is involved, and the type and degree of inflammatory response induced. Most nervous system infectious processes have a rapid progression, requiring timely intervention. Most infections involve the brain or meninges; however, other areas can be involved concomitantly or serve as the principal targeted site. The decreased frequency of spinal cord involvement is most likely due to reduced blood flow to the spinal cord rather than some greater inherent resistance to infection than the brain. In some cases, the major or sole clinical manifestation is related to spinal cord lesions. For example, equine herpesvirus 1 infections may result in immune complex-related vasculitis causing necrosis that affects both the brain and the spinal cord. Lesions in the spinal cord are sometimes the source for the predominant clinical signs. Peripheral nerve involvement is less frequent but is the site for important neurological diseases (e.g., Marek's disease in chickens).

The presence or growth of a microbial agent in the nervous system is not necessary for signs to develop. Microbial toxins ingested or produced at another site in the host (e.g., *Clostridium perfringens* ε-toxin, botulinum toxin, and tetanus toxin) and immune-mediated events affecting vessels supplying the central nervous system (e.g., feline infectious peritonitis virus and equine herpesvirus 1) are responsible for important nervous system diseases.

The role of infectious agents in autoimmune diseases is still poorly understood. In humans, cross-reacting pathogens and host antigens results in molecular mimicry and has been associated with certain nervous system diseases. Notable is the mimicry between lipopolysaccharide structures of selected serotypes of *Campylobacter jejuni* and gangliosides (e.g., GM1 and GD1a) of motor neurons. This is thought to account for the association between antecedent *Campylobacter* infections and some cases of Guillain–Barré syndrome, an acute demyelinating poly-neuropathy, in humans. Some cases of acute canine polyradiculoneuritis (coonhound paralysis) may similarly be associated with immune reactions to viral or bacterial infections.

Some of the most common and/or important microbial agents associated with nervous system infections in domestic animals and poultry are listed in Tables 72.1, 72.2, 72.3, 72.4, 72.5, 72.6, and 72.7.

Routes of Infection

The hematogenous route is the most common route of entry for microbial pathogens. Other important routes include retrograde movement within neurons or extension of the infectious processes from contiguous sites. Some pathogens appear capable of using more than one of these routes (e.g., *Listeria*).

Hematogenous Route. Systemic infections or infectious processes that involve multiple organ systems typically reach the nervous system by this route. Infection occurs when pathogens enter through vessels of the choroid plexus, meninges, or parenchyma, or from septic emboli that lodge in vessels and result in direct damage to vascular endothelial cells. Some viruses are able to cross the blood–brain barrier themselves or are carried across in infected immune cells, while others directly infect the endothelium of capillaries or cells of the choroid plexus or ependyma.

Studies with *Escherichia coli* show that (i) a high degree of bacteremia, (ii) invasion of brain microvascular endothelial cells, (iii) host cell actin cytoskeletal rearrangement, and (iv) specific signaling mechanisms promote translocation of *E. coli* across the blood–brain barrier. Different bacteria use different signaling mechanisms. Cytokines produced by astrocytes and microglial cells and nitric oxides from inflammatory cells in response to insults contribute to disruption of vascular barrier and further loss of ability to exclude entry of pathogens.

Table 72.1. Common and/or Important Infectious Agents of the Nervous System of Dogs

Agent	Disease(s)	Neurologic Signs
Viruses		
Canine adenovirus 1	Infectious canine hepatitis	Seizures
Canine distemper virus	Canine distemper	Ataxia, seizures
Canine herpesvirus	Canine herpesvirus disease	Depression, opisthotonus, seizures
Pseudorabies virus	Pseudorabies	Intense pruritus, seizures
Rabies virus	Rabies	Temperature change, aggressive behavior, paralysis
Bacteria		
Agents of otitis externa[a]	Otitis media and interna	Vestibular dysfunction
Ehrlichia canis	Ehrlichiosis	Ataxia, cerebellar and vestibular dysfunction, seizures
Clostridium botulinum	Botulism	Flaccid paralysis, paresis
Clostridium tetani	Tetanus	Opisthotonus, seizures, tremors
Rickettsia rickettsii	Rocky Mountain spotted fever	Ataxia, depression, seizures, vestibular dysfunctions
Fungi		
Cryptococcus neoformans	Cryptococcosis	Ataxia, head tilt, paresis, seizures

[a]Includes *E. coli*, *Proteus* spp., *Pseudomonas* spp., and *Streptococcus* spp.

Table 72.2. Common and/or Important Infectious Agents of the Nervous System of Cats

Agent	Disease(s)	Neurologic Signs
Prions		
BSE prion[a]	Feline spongiform encephalopathy	Ataxia, behavioral changes, muscular tremors
Viruses		
Feline panleukopenia virus	Cerebellar hypoplasia	Ataxia
Feline immunodeficiency virus[b]	Feline acquired immunodeficiency syndrome	Aggressive or psychotic behavior, seizures
Feline infectious peritonitis virus	Feline infectious peritonitis	Ataxia, paresis, seizures
Feline leukemia virus	Epidural lymphoma	Posterior paresis
	Feline leukemia	Abnormal vocalization, hyperesthesia, paresis
Pseudorabies virus	Pseudorabies	Hyperexcitability, paralysis, paresis
Rabies virus	Rabies	Aggressive behavior, paralysis
Fungi		
Cryptococcus neoformans	Cryptococcosis	Ataxia, paresis, cranial nerve deficits, seizures

[a]Classified as a foreign animal disease in the United States.
[b]Congenital infection.

Table 72.3. Common and/or Important Infectious Agents of the Nervous System of Horses

Agent	Disease(s)	Neurologic Signs
Viruses		
Equine encephalomyelitis viruses (WEE, EEE, VEE[a])	Equine encephalomyelitides	Ataxia, drowsiness, head pressing, paralysis
Equine herpesvirus 1	Myeloencephalitis	Ataxia, tetra- or paraplegia
Rabies virus	Rabies	Ascending paralysis, ataxia, depression, vocalization
West Nile virus	West Nile encephalitis	Ataxia, muscle tremor, paresis, seizures, somnolence
Bacteria		
Clostridium botulinum[b]	Botulism	Flaccid paralysis, muscle fasciculation, paresis
Clostridium tetani	Tetanus	Muscle spasms, prolapsed third eyelid, rigid "saw-horse" stance, seizures
Streptococcus equi ssp. *equi*	Brain abscess, meningitis	Ataxia, depression, seizures, vestibular dysfunctions
	Guttural pouch infection	Dysphagia, head shaking
Fungi		
Aspergillus fumigatus	Guttural pouch mycosis	Dysphagia, head shaking

[a]Classified as a foreign animal disease agent in the United States.
[b]Most commonly types B and C.

Table 72.4. Common and/or Important Infectious Agents of the Nervous System of Cattle

Agent	Disease(s)	Neurologic Signs
Prions		
BSE prion[a]	Bovine spongiform encephalopathy	Aggressive or apprehensive behavior, ataxia, ear twitching
Viruses		
Akabane virus[a,b]	Hydranencephaly, neurogenic arthrogryposis (Akabane disease)	Sensory and motor deficits at birth
Alcelaphine herpesvirus 1[a]	Malignant catarrhal fever (wildebeest)	Ataxia, head pressing, paralysis, tremors, seizures
Bovine viral diarrhea virus[b]	Cerebellar hypoplasia	Head tremors, incoordination
Infectious bovine rhinotracheitis	Bovine herpesvirus-1 encephalitis	Ataxia, hyperexcitability, tremors
Ovine herpesvirus 2	Malignant catarrhal fever (sheep)	Ataxia, head pressing, paralysis, tremors, seizures
Pseudorabies virus	Pseudorabies	Intense pruritus, salivation, seizures, vocalization
Rabies virus	Rabies	Ataxia, paralysis
Bacteria		
Arcanobacterium pyogenes	Brain/pituitary abscess	Ataxia, blindness, depression, facial paralysis
Histophilus somni	Thromboembolic meningoencephalitis, otitis media and interna	Ataxia, blindness, opisthotonus, stupor
Clostridium botulinum[c]	Botulism	Flaccid paralysis, loss of tongue withdrawal and palpebral reflex, muscle fasciculation, paresis
Clostridium tetani	Tetanus	Opisthotonus, seizures, tremors
Escherichia coli	Meningitis	Blindness, head pressing, seizures, somnolence
Fusobacterium necrophorum	Brain/pituitary abscess	Ataxia, blindness, depression, facial paralysis
Listeria monocytogenes	Listeriosis	Ataxia, circling, facial paralysis, head tilt
Mycoplasma bovis	Otitis media and interna	Ataxia, droopy ear, head tilt
Pasteurella multocida	Otitis media and interna	Ataxia, droopy ear, head tilt

[a]Classified as a foreign animal disease agent in the United States.
[b]Congenital infection.
[c]Most commonly types B, C, and D.

Table 72.5. Common and/or Important Infectious Agents of the Nervous System of Sheep and Goats

Agent	Disease(s)	Neurologic Signs
Prions		
Scrapie prion	Scrapie	Ataxia, exaggerated nibbling reflex, intense pruritus, muscle tremors
Viruses		
Akabane virus[a,b]	Hydranencephaly, neurogenic arthrogryposis (Akabane disease)	Sensory and motor deficits at birth
Bluetongue virus[a]	Cerebellar hypoplasia, hydranencephaly	Blindness at birth, inability to walk
Border disease virus[a]	Hypomyelinogenesis	Ataxia, tremors
Caprine arthritis-encephalitis virus	Caprine arthritis-encephalitis	Paralysis, paresis, tremors
Louping ill virus[b]	Louping ill	Ataxia, head pressing, paralysis, tremors, seizures
Rabies virus	Rabies	Ataxia, constipation, paralysis
Visna virus (S)	Visna	Abnormal gait, ataxia, paralysis, paresis
Bacteria		
Arcanobacterium pyogenes	Brain/pituitary abscess	Ataxia, blindness, head pressing, head tilt
Clostridium botulinum	Botulism	Ataxia, flaccid paralysis
Clostridium perfringens type D	Focal symmetrical encephalomalacia	Coma, depression, head pressing, opisthotonus
Clostridium tetani	Tetanus	Opisthotonus, seizures, tremors
Escherichia coli	Meningitis	Blindness head pressing, seizures, somnolence
Listeria monocytogenes	Listeriosis	Ataxia, circling, facial paralysis, head tilt

S, sheep.
[a]Congenital infection.
[b]Classified as a foreign animal disease agent in the United States.

Table 72.6. Common and/or Important Infectious Agents of the Nervous System of Pigs

Agent	Disease(s)	Neurologic Signs
Viruses		
Hemagglutinating encephalomyelitis virus	Vomiting and wasting disease	Sensory and motor deficits at birth
Encephalomyocarditis virus	Encephalomyocarditis	Blindness at birth, inability to walk
Porcine enterovirus 1	Porcine polioencephalomalacia (Talfan/Teschen)	Ataxia, tremors
Hog cholera virus[a,b]	Cerebellar hypoplasia	Paralysis, paresis, tremors
Nipah virus[a]	Nonsuppurative meningitis	Ataxia, head pressing, paralysis, tremors, seizures
Pseudorabies virus	Pseudorabies	
Rabies virus	Rabies	Ataxia, constipation, paralysis
Bacteria		
Clostridium tetani	Tetanus	Opisthotonus, muscle rigidity, seizures, stiff gait, tremors
Escherichia coli (Shiga toxin-positive)	Edema disease	Ataxia, edema of face, paralysis, stiffness
Haemophilus parasuis	Meningitis (Glasser's disease)	Ataxia, paddling, tremors
Listeria monocytogenes	Listeriosis	Ataxia, hyperexcitability, trembling
Streptococcus suis (type 2)	Meningitis	Ataxia, depression, paralysis, seizures, tremors

[a]Classified as a foreign animal disease agent in the United States.
[b]Congenital infections cause congenital tremors in piglets.

Retrograde Movement within Neurons. Some infections result when an agent infects peripheral nerves and moves in a retrograde fashion to reach the central nervous system (e.g., rabies virus, pseudorabies virus). Binding to specific cell receptors is necessary for entry. For example, rabies viruses use nicotinic acetylcholine and low-affinity nerve growth factor receptors to attach and penetrate cells. In some cases cell-to-cell junctions, including synaptic junctions, are crossed. Some herpesviruses latently infect sensory ganglia and are later activated and may extend into the central nervous system. Tetanus toxin moves in a retrograde fashion in the peripheral nerves to reach the central nervous system.

Extension of Infectious Process from Contiguous Sites. Parenchymal or meningeal infections may result from extension of infectious processes involving paranasal sinuses, tooth roots, or the middle ear (e.g., otitis media and interna in calves). Infections of the epidural and subdural spaces usually result by direct invasion of pathogens subsequent to trauma or surgery (e.g., tail-docking in sheep). Bacterial infections of vertebrae or intervertebral disks can involve the spinal cord by direct extension or as a result of pressure from epidural abscessation.

Infections of the Central Nervous System

Once a pathogen establishes, injury results from either direct cytotoxic effects by the pathogen or due to the inflammatory response directed at the pathogen, or a combination of both. Clinical signs associated with infections are varied and typically progressive. Specific clinical signs may aid in localizing the infections to the meninges (nuchal rigidity and depressed mental status), cerebrum (circling, behavioral changes, and seizures), brain stem

Table 72.7. Common and/or Important Infectious Agents of the Nervous System of Poultry

Agent	Disease(s)	Neurologic Signs
Viruses		
Avian encephalomyelitis virus	Avian encephalomyelitis	Ataxia, paralysis, tremors
Avian influenza virus[a]	Avian influenza	Ataxia, depression
Eastern equine encephalitis virus (T)	Eastern equine encephalitis	Ataxia, depression, paralysis
Exotic Newcastle disease virus[a]	Exotic Newcastle disease	Depression, paresis, torticollis, tremors
Marek's disease virus (C)	Marek's disease	Ataxia, leg or wing paresis/paralysis
Bacteria		
Clostridium botulinum[b]	Botulism (limberneck)	Flaccid paralysis, inability to support head
Listeria monocytogenes	Listeriosis	Ataxia, paralysis, seizures
Salmonella enterica ssp. *arizonae* (T)	Meningitis/encephalitis (arizonosis)	Ataxia, paralysis, seizures
Fungi		
Aspergillus fumigatus	Mycotic encephalitis	Loss of equilibrium, torticollis
Ochroconis gallopavum[c]	Mycotic encephalitis	Loss of equilibrium, torticollis

C, chickens; T, turkeys.
[a]Classified as a foreign animal disease agent in the United States.
[b]Most commonly type C.
[c]*Dactylaria gallopava* is the obsolete name for this organism.

(cranial nerve deficits and head tilt), cerebellum (ataxia and tremors), or spinal cord (tetra- or paraplegia).

Mechanism of Central Nervous System Injury

Vascular Damage. Damage to blood vessels may be the initiating factor in disease. Microbial toxins can cause vasogenic cerebral edema through effects on the blood–brain barrier and resultant leakage of proteins into extracellular spaces. This is the proposed mechanism of action of *C. perfringens* type D ε-toxin, which produces a focal symmetrical encephalomalacia, especially involving the thalamus, hippocampus, and midbrain in sheep and the Shiga-like toxin of toxigenic *E. coli* strains associated with edema disease in swine. Viral effects on the vascular system include immune-mediated vasculitis and perivascular inflammation (e.g., feline infectious peritonitis, equine herpesvirus 1). Rickettsial agents (*Ehrlichia* and *Rickettsia*) induce endothelial damage and vasculitis that lead to bleeding in the brain. Thrombosis of vessels may cause malacia of brain parenchyma (e.g., *Histophilus somni* in calves, *Salmonella enterica* ssp. *arizonae* in turkeys). Septic emboli may result in brain abscesses.

Injury to Brain Parenchyma or Meninges. Injury to cells in the central nervous system is by direct action of the pathogen or from the resulting inflammatory response. The inflammatory response can be suppurative, nonsuppurative, granulomatous, or some combination of these and is predominately influenced by the agent involved. Inflammatory processes of the brain parenchyma (encephalitis), meninges (meningitis), or spinal cord (myelitis) occur - independently or in combination. Disorders in myelin formation result in some cases (e.g., distemper and visna). Movement of infectious agents may occur within the cerebrospinal fluid or interstitium, or within different cell types.

Viral Infections. Viruses with neurotrophic properties affect all animal species (see Tables 72.1, 72.2, 72.3, 72.4, 72.5, 72.6, and 72.7). Some viruses specifically affect the nervous system (e.g., rabies virus in all species and pseudorabies virus in most species), and other viruses involve the nervous system as part of a multisystem disease process (e.g., malignant catarrhal fever virus in cattle, exotic Newcastle disease virus in poultry, and distemper virus in dogs). Viruses usually reach the central nervous system via the bloodstream, often as the result of a secondary viremia. Entry is via one of the methods described previously (see Section “Routes of Infection). Effects on specific cell types in the nervous system are either due to direct viral cytocidal effects or damage resulting from the ensuing inflammatory response. Gliosis, perivascular cuffing, and neuronal degeneration typically characterize viral encephalitis. Viral infections in the central nervous system only rarely serve as the primary mechanism for transmission between hosts. Typically transmission relies on infection at other sites in the body.

Some viral infections in the dam affect the fetal nervous system and lead to developmental problems, including cerebellar hypoplasia (bovine viral diarrhea virus and panleukopenia virus), hydranencephaly (bluetongue virus), and hypomyelinogenesis (Border disease virus).

Bacterial Infections. Bacterial meningitis in dogs and cats is relatively uncommon and often associated with primary infections at other sites (e.g., urinary tract infection and endocarditis). Involvement of the nervous system may also arise from local extension of infectious processes (e.g., ear infections, tooth root abscesses, and sinus infections). Organisms involved are usually endogenous and include aerobes (*Staphylococcus*, *Streptococcus*, *Pasteurella*, and *Actinomyces*) and anaerobes (*Bacteroides*, *Porphyromonas*, *Fusobacterium*, and *Peptostreptococcus*).

Bacterial meningitis is more common in neonates, with horses and production animals most commonly affected. In these animals, the etiology agent is often an enteric organism (e.g., *E. coli*) and is associated with failure of passive transfer of maternal immunoglobulins. *Haemophilus*, *Pasteurella*, *Salmonella*, and *Streptococcus* are other genera encountered with some frequency in bacterial meningitis. Prolonged bacteremia and the total bacterial numbers appear directly related to the likelihood that the blood–brain barrier will be crossed. In bacterial meningitis, a fibrinopurulent response typically results.

Brain abscesses are also more common in horses and ruminants than in companion animals and develop as a result of bacteremia, trauma (direct implantation), or spread from a contiguous site. *Streptococcus equi* ssp. *equi* is the most common cause of brain abscesses in horses, a form of the so-called bastard strangles, and is related to a bacteremic event subsequent to rhinopharyngitis and lymph node abscessation (strangles). Brain abscesses in cattle are also associated with primary extraneural infections (e.g., hardware disease). The pituitary gland is an especially common site in ruminants, possibly due to the anatomy and close association of the rete mirabilis with the pituitary gland. Common ruminant pyogenic agents (*Arcanobacterium pyogenes* and *Fusobacterium necrophorum*) are the usual suspects in these cases. Infections involving vertebrae and intervertebral disks, especially in dogs, ruminants, and swine, may involve the spinal cord and manifest as posterior paralysis/paresis. Some bacterial species exhibit a greater degree of neurotropism than others (e.g., *Listeria* in ruminants and *H. somni* in beef cattle). Lesions associated with *Listeria* encephalitis typically are in the form of microabscesses in the brain stem (pons and medulla oblongata) and are almost pathognomonic for *Listeria* encephalitis. Histophilosis results in thrombotic meningoencephalitis (formerly TEME) (Figure 72.1).

As already mentioned, bacterial toxins rather than the agent itself may be responsible for clinical signs and pathology. Some bacterial toxins directly affect the vasculature of the central nervous system (e.g., ε-toxin of *C. perfringens* in enterotoxemia and Shiga-like toxin of *E. coli* in edema disease). On the other hand, tetanospasmin (tetanus toxin), the toxin produced by *Clostridium tetani*, binds to peripheral nerves and travels to the central nervous system where it blocks the release of inhibitory neurotransmitters from presynaptic inhibitory motor nerve endings. Clinical signs of tetanus in cattle commonly include a stiff gait, failure to eructate, limb extensor rigidity, raised tail head, and tetany

FIGURE 72.1. *Foci of necrosis with hemorrhage in cerebrum due to* H. somni *infection. Thrombosed meningeal blood vessels with suppurative inflammation in the meninges and neuropil are present (inset). (Courtesy of Dr Bruce Brodersen.)*

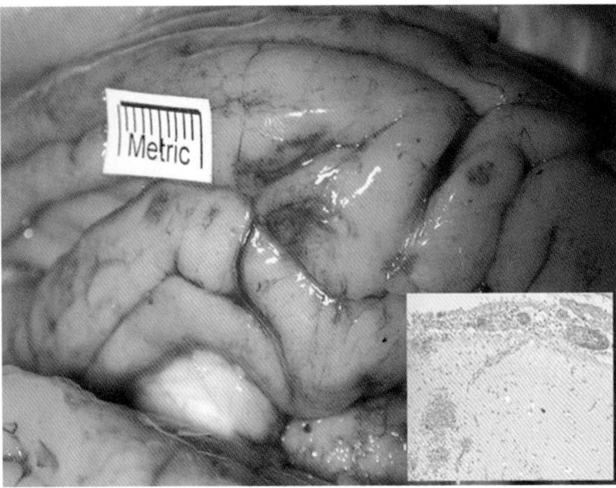

FIGURE 72.2. *A recently fresh, adult crossbred cow presented with clinical signs consistent with tetanus. Note the mouthful of long-stemmed grass that she is unable to masticate or swallow. She has a "saw-horse" stance, her tail is elevated, and her nictitating membrane is partially prolapsed.*

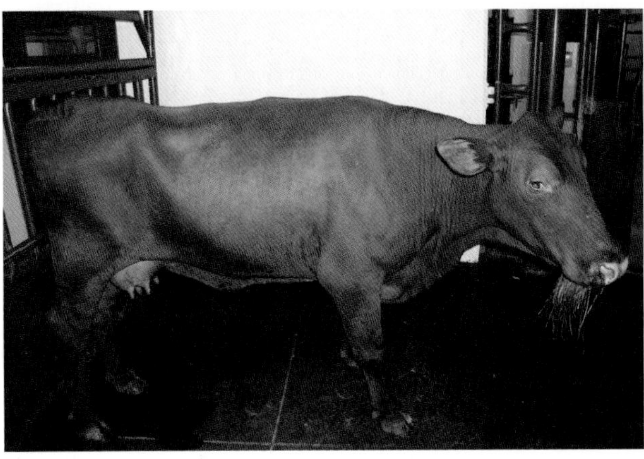

of facial muscles. Passive prolapse of the nictitating membrane may occur due to spasm of the retractor muscles of the ocular globe. Spasm of the masseter muscles may produce the classic sign of "lockjaw." (Figure 72.2)

Fungal Infections. As a general rule, fungal infections of the central nervous system are infrequent. When they occur, the inflammatory response is typically granulomatous. Most of the systemic mycotic agents (*Blastomyces*, *Coccidioides*, *Cryptococcus*, and *Histoplasma*) have the potential to be involved in nervous system disease, but this usually occurs secondarily and late in the course of the infection. Most fungal infections result from hematogenous dissemination. *Cryptococcus neoformans* is the most common fungus encountered in nervous system disease and most commonly affects dogs and cats. It produces a number of virulence factors, including a large polysaccharide capsule, which allows it to persist. Evidence suggests that it uses monocytes and endothelial cells to cross the blood–brain barrier. Granulomatous encephalitis with focal caseonecrotic lesions caused by *Aspergillus* sp. has been described in poultry. Outbreaks of mycotic encephalitis in poultry flocks caused by a thermophilic fungus, *Ochroconis gallopavum* (*Dactylaria gallopava*—obsolete name), have also been reported.

Prion Diseases. Transmissible spongiform encephalopathies or prion diseases—bovine spongiform encephalopathy (BSE), scrapie, and feline spongiform encephalopathy—are rare but important nervous system diseases because they are largely untreatable, may cross species barriers, and can have substantial economic impact because of public health concerns. An abnormal conformer of normally present prion protein (PrP^{c}) designated PrP^{Res} (for "resistant" PrP) is believed to cause conversion of normal PrP^{c} into the pathological isoform. Acquired principally through ingestion of PrP^{Res}-contaminated material (e.g., meat and bonemeal in BSE and possibly infected placenta or feces in scrapie), prions are able to pass from the digestive tract and are potentially amplified in the lymphoreticular system before moving up the peripheral nervous system to the brain. The accumulation of PrP^{Res} is responsible for the pathology (neuronal intracellular spongiosis) associated with transmissible spongiform encephalopathies.

Infections of the Peripheral Nervous System

As noted previously, the peripheral nervous system is less frequently involved in infectious processes than the central nervous system; however, some important diseases specifically or predominantly involve the peripheral nervous system. The toxin of *Clostridium botulinum* affects peripheral nerves, specifically components of the synaptic vesicle docking and fusion complex at peripheral motor nerve terminals. This blocks the release of acetylcholine resulting in the flaccid paralysis characteristic of the disease. Involvement of peripheral nerves, usually sciatic and brachial nerve plexuses, is a characteristic feature of Marek's disease virus. Grossly enlarged nerves with both inflammatory and neoplastic histologic characteristics, as well as myelin degeneration, are found. Mycotic and bacterial infections of the guttural pouch of horses may involve the glossopharyngeal and vagus nerves, resulting in swallowing difficulties or laryngeal hemiplegia.

Ocular Infections

Douglas E. Hostetler

The primary function of the eye is vision. Factors that affect vision impact overall animal well-being. In this chapter, the ocular system includes the eyelids, lacrimal apparatus, conjunctiva, the eye itself, and the surrounding fascia. The eye includes the cornea, sclera, lens, uveal tract, retina, optic nerve, and aqueous and vitreous chambers. The major sites for infectious ocular disease to develop are the conjunctiva, cornea, and uveal tract.

Antimicrobial Properties of the Eye

Considering the frequent exposure to environmental elements, the eye is remarkably resistant to infection. Mechanical, anatomical, antimicrobial, and immunological factors all play roles in protecting the eye from infection. The following sections detail these specific factors.

Mechanical and Anatomic Factors

The eyelids, including the cilia, and blink (menace) and corneal reflexes provide a barrier to external insults that may traumatize the eye and predispose to infection by endogenous or exogenous microbes. Intact conjunctiva and cornea epithelium provide additional barriers to infection. Precorneal tear film, a complex multilayered fluid, continuously coats exposed surfaces of the eye without impairing vision. The tear film has a number of functions including lubrication, retarding evaporation, and nutrient transport. Meibomian and lacrimal glands, the conjunctiva, and cornea all contribute to the composition of the tear film. Tears provide overall protection for the eye surface through the uniform coating effect and by mechanically rinsing the eye of noxious materials and microbes.

Protection for internal structures of the eye comes from tight junctions of endothelial and epithelial cells that form the blood-aqueous and blood-retinal barriers. The blood aqueous barrier is formed by ciliary epithelial cells between capillaries in the ciliary stroma and aqueous fluid in the posterior chamber of the eye. The blood-retinal barrier is composed of tight junctions of endothelial cells of retinal capillaries and cells of the pigmented retinal epithelium. These barriers afford protection to intraocular structures of the eye from microbes of hematogenous origin. When microbes from systemic infections do involve intraocular sites, it is these areas where infection typically initiates. Breakdown of blood-ocular barriers is largely the result of inflammatory processes that disrupt tight junctions.

Antimicrobial Factors

In addition to serving as an interface to ameliorate the effects of external stimuli, tears contain nonspecific antimicrobial substances that include the following:

1. *Lactoferrin*: Lactoferrin is a substantial protein component of tears (up to 25%). By binding free iron, lactoferrin makes this essential enzyme component unavailable to bacteria, thereby limiting bacterial growth. In addition, lactoferrin may have a role in enhancing natural killer cell function and inhibiting formation of C3 convertase.
2. *Lysozyme*: Tears are rich in lysozyme (up to 40% of tear protein). The enzymatic action of lysozyme on the glycan chain of the peptidoglycan of bacterial cell walls provides nonspecific protection from exogenous and resident bacteria. Variation in lysozyme concentration occurs among different animals and may, in part, account for variation in susceptibility of different animals to external ocular infections. Decrease in the lysozyme concentration in tears correlates with increased ocular infections.
3. *Antimicrobial peptides*: Broad-spectrum cationic antimicrobial peptides are innately produced by ocular surface tissues. These peptides act as natural antibiotics through interactions with bacterial cell surfaces. They may also play a role in signaling that activates host cell processes involved in immune defense. Antimicrobial peptides can be detected in the conjunctiva, cornea, and tears.

Immunological Factors

The conjunctiva is part of the common mucosal immune system, which includes gastrointestinal, respiratory, urogenital, and mammary mucosa. It is unclear if

Original chapter written by the late Dr. Richard L. Walker.

Veterinary Microbiology, Third Edition. Edited by D. Scott McVey, Melissa Kennedy and M.M. Chengappa.

antigen-presenting capabilities exist in the conjunctiva or lacrimal gland lymphoid tissue. It is plausible that ocular immunization occurs by passage of antigen through the nasal lacrimal duct to gut-associated lymphoid tissue or bronchial-associated lymphoid tissue sites. Plasma cells in the lacrimal glands are derived by clonal expansion and differentiation of IgA committed B lymphocytes that localize in the lacrimal gland. IgA is produced, which in turn combines with secretory component. Secretory IgA is resistant to proteolytic enzymes in tears and constitutes the major immunoglobulin in tears. Its role in microbial defense includes preventing bacterial attachment and neutralization of viruses. A functional complement system is also present in tears.

Because of its rich vascular supply, an aggressive inflammatory response, predominately composed of neutrophils, occurs in the conjunctiva. The cornea, due to its avascular nature, is suppressed or delayed in its inflammatory response.

The intraocular immune response is programmed to prevent an overexuberant response that may irreparably damage intraocular structures and ultimately vision. Subsets of T lymphocytes that cause substantial bystander injury are suppressed, and the immune response is more localized.

Competitive Inhibition Effect of Microbial Flora

It is possible that the normal flora, as elsewhere in the body, plays a protective role in the ocular system by inhibiting establishment of more pathogenic species.

Microbial Flora of the Eye

A normal conjunctival flora is present but varies by animal, breed, geography, housing conditions, and time of year. The most commonly recovered flora are gram-positive organisms and include staphylococci, micrococci, streptococci, diphtheroids, and *Bacillus* spp. Less frequently nonenteric, gram-negative bacteria are isolated and include predominately *Moraxella*, *Neisseria*, and *Pseudomonas* species. In ruminants, *Moraxella* species may be the predominant bacterial type in normal eyes. *Mycoplasma* species are also found as conjunctival flora in some animals. Few studies have been done to actually quantitate the relative numbers of each of the different species that constitute normal flora. Not all conjunctival specimens from normal animals yield microbial growth, indicating that the conjunctiva is not heavily populated by normal flora. Internal structures of the eye are normally sterile.

Ocular Infections

Ocular infections can be primary infections or part of multisystem infectious processes (e.g., upper respiratory tract infections). The organisms involved are often contagious and may affect populations of animals rather than individuals. In other cases, ocular infections are secondary to insults that comprise the integrity and innate defenses of the eye. Compromising factors in these cases include decreased tear production, excess ultraviolet radiation, immunosuppressing diseases, trauma or penetrating injuries, anatomic defects (e.g., entropions), or surgical interventions. In such situations, normally benign ocular or other endogenous flora can cause serious infections once they gain entry to unprotected sites. A number of systemic infectious diseases also include ocular manifestations as a consequence of dissemination from the initial focus of infection.

Depending on the microbial agent involved, the agent's tissue trophism, route of exposure, and the host's ability to contain infection, ocular infections may or may not be limited to specific parts of the eye. The inflammatory process can and frequently does involve structures in the eye adjacent to the site of initial infection or, especially in uncontrolled infections, becomes widespread to involve intraocular cavities and surrounding structures (endophthalmitis, panophthalmitis). Route of exposure of the eye to infectious agents is through surface contact with endogenous or exogenous microbes or via the blood stream or lymphatic system and, perhaps, by extension from nervous tissues.

Common and/or important infectious agents of the ocular system in domestic mammals and poultry are listed in Tables 73.1, 73.2, 73.3, 73.4, 73.5, 73.6 and 73.7.

Infectious processes of the eye frequently include those presented in the following sections.

Eyelid and Lacrimal Apparatus Infections

Bacteria are the most common cause of infections of eyelid margins (blepharitis) and lacrimal glands. The source

Table 73.1. Common and/or Important Infectious Agents of the Ocular System of Dogs

Agent	Major Clinical Manifestations (Common Disease Name)
Viruses	
Canine adenovirus 1	Corneal edema, immune-complex uveitis, keratitis (blue eye)
Canine distemper virus	Chorioretinitis, conjunctivitis, optic neuritis (distemper)
Canine papillomavirus	Papillomas of eyelids and conjunctiva
Bacteria	
Beta-hemolytic streptococci	Conjunctivitis, dacryocystitis
Brucella canis	Anterior uveitis, endophthalmitis
Coagulase-positive staphylococci	Blepharitis, conjunctivitis, dacryocystitis
Ehrlichia spp.	Anterior uveitis, conjunctival hyperemia, chorioretinitis
Leptospira spp.	Anterior uveitis
Rickettsia rickettsii	Anterior uveitis, chorioretinitis, conjunctival hyperemia, retinal hemorrhage
Fungi	
Blastomyces dermatitidis	Anterior uveitis, chorioretinitis, endophthalmitis
Cryptococcus neoformans	Chorioretinitis, optic neuritis
Algae	
Prototheca spp.	Anterior uveitis, chorioretinitis

Table 73.2. Common and/or Important Infectious Agents of the Ocular System of Cats

Agent	Major Clinical Manifestations (Common Disease Name)
Viruses	
Feline herpesvirus 1	Conjunctivitis, corneal ulcer, stromal keratitis (feline viral rhinotracheitis)
Feline immunodeficiency virus	Anterior uveitis, chorioretinitis
Feline infectious peritonitis virus	Anterior uveitis, chorioretinitis, keratic precipitates, keratitis (feline infectious peritonitis)
Feline leukemia virus	Anterior uveitis, uveal lymphosarcoma, retinal hemorrhage
Feline panleukopenia virus	Retinal degeneration, retinal dysplasia (feline panleukopenia—in utero infection)
Bacteria	
Chlamydophila felis	Conjunctivitis (feline pneumonitis)
Mycoplasma felis[a]	Conjunctivitis
Fungi	
Cryptococcus neoformans	Chorioretinitis, optic neuritis (cryptococcosis)

[a]Role as an ocular pathogen is uncertain.

for bacteria is endogenous, with staphylococci and streptococci being the most common agents. In dogs, a purulent blepharitis occurs in conjunction with juvenile pyoderma. Dermatophyte infections may extend to involve eyelids.

Conjunctival Infections

Infections of the conjunctiva induce an inflammatory response characterized by hyperemia, chemosis, and cellular exudate. Conjunctivitis occurs both as a local infection (e.g., *Chlamydophila* infections in cats) or as part of a systemic disease (e.g., distemper in dogs).

Viral-induced conjunctivitis (e.g., alphaherpesviruses conjunctivitis) often occurs in conjunction with upper respiratory or digestive tract infections when virus specifically attaches to and replicates in surface epithelial cells. Cytopathic effects caused by viruses and induction of an inflammatory response account for clinical signs observed. Conjunctival infections may spread to or concurrently involve the cornea (keratoconjunctivitis).

Table 73.3. Common and/or Important Infectious Agents of the Ocular System of Horses

Agent	Major Clinical Manifestations (Common Disease Name)
Viruses	
African Horse Sickness virus[a]	Conjunctivitis, eyelid and periorbital edema
Equine arteritis virus	Conjunctivitis, periorbital edema
Equine herpesvirus 2	Conjunctivitis, keratitis
Equine influenza virus	Conjunctivitis
Bacteria	
Leptospira spp.	Panuveitis (equine recurrent uveitis)
Pseudomonas aeruginosa	Keratitis, corneal ulcer
Fungi	
Aspergillus spp.	Keratitis, corneal ulcer
Fusarium spp.	Keratitis, corneal ulcer

[a]Classified as a foreign animal disease agent in the United States.

Table 73.4. Common and/or Important Infectious Agents of the Ocular System of Cattle

Agent	Major Clinical Manifestations (Common Disease Name)
Viruses	
Alcelaphine herpesvirus 1[a]	Anterior uveitis, conjunctivitis, corneal edema, eyelid edema, keratitis (malignant catarrhal fever)
Bovine herpesvirus 1	Conjunctivitis, corneal edema/opacity (infectious bovine rhinotracheitis)
Bovine papillomavirus	Papillomas of eyelid and conjunctiva
Bovine viral diarrhea virus	Cataracts, retinal atrophy, optic neuritis (bovine virus diarrhea-in utero infection)
Ovine herpesvirus 2	Anterior uveitis, conjunctivitis, corneal edema, eyelid edema, keratitis (malignant catarrhal fever)
Bacteria	
Arcanobacterium pyogenes	Orbital cellulitis
Histophilus somni[b]	Retinal hemorrhages, retinitis (thromboembolic meningoencephalitis
Listeria monocytogenes	Conjunctivitis, keratitis, uveitis
Moraxella bovis	Conjunctivitis, keratitis, corneal ulcer, panophthalmitis (infectious bovine keratoconjunctivitis or pinkeye)
Mycoplasma bovoculi	Conjunctivitis

[a]Classified as a foreign animal disease agent in the United States
[b]"Haemophilus somnus" is the obsolete name for this organism.

Table 73.5. Common and/or Important Infectious Agents of the Ocular System of Sheep and Goats

Agent	Major Clinical Manifestations (Common Disease Name)
Prions	
Scrapie prion	Retinal Detachment
Bacteria	
Chlamydophila pecorum[a]	Conjunctivitis keratitis
Listeria monocytogenes	Conjunctivitis keratitis, uveitis
Moraxella spp. *Branhamella ovis*[a]	Conjunctivitis keratitis
Mycoplasma conjunctivae	Conjunctivitis keratitis (infectious keratoconjunctivitis)

[a]Role as an ocular pathogen is uncertain.

Table 73.6. Common and/or Important Infectious Agents of the Ocular System of Pigs

Agent	Major Clinical Manifestations (Common Disease Name)
Viruses	
African swine fever virus[a]	Conjunctivitis (African swine fever)
Classical swine fever virus[a]	Conjunctivitis (Classical swine fever, hog cholera)
Porcine rubelavirus	Corneal opacity/edema, keratitis (blue eye disease)
Pseudorabies virus	Conjunctivitis, keratitis
Swine influenza virus	Conjunctivitis
Bacteria	
Chlamydia suis	Conjunctivitis
Escherichia coli (Shiga toxin positive)	Palpebral edema (edema disease)
Pasteurella multocida	Conjunctivitis, nasolacrimal duct occlusion (atrophic rhinitis

[a] Classified as a foreign animal disease agent in the United States.

Bacterial infections of the conjunctiva may begin in the conjunctiva or may result from extension of eyelid or lacrimal gland infections. *Chlamydia/Chlamydophila* conjunctivitis occurs in a number of animal species and can be a primary conjunctivitis or, in addition, involve other sites. Bacterial conjunctivitis may develop secondary to primary viral conjunctival infections. As with viral conjunctivitis, concurrent corneal involvement may occur. Fungal infections of the conjunctiva are rare.

Table 73.7. Common and/or Important Infectious Agents of the Ocular System of Poultry

Agent	Major Clinical Manifestations (Common Disease Name)
Viruses	
Avian encephalomyelitis virus (C)	Cataracts, uveitis
Infectious laryngotracheitis virus	Conjunctivitis, keratitis
Marek's disease virus (C)	Loss of iris pigmentation, panuveitis
Newcastle disease virus[a]	Conjunctival edema, hemorrhage
Bacteria	
Bordetella avium (T)	Conjunctivitis
Chlamydophila psittaci	Conjunctivitis
Escherichia coli	Conjunctivitis, endophthalmitis
Haemophilus paragallinarum	Conjunctivitis, periorbital edema
Mycoplasma gallisepticum	Conjunctivitis
Pasteurella multocida	Conjunctivitis, eyelid edema, orbital cellulitis
Salmonella spp.[b]	Endophthalmitis
Fungi	
Aspergillus spp.	Endophthalmitis, keratitis

C, Chicken; T, Turkey.
[a]Classified as a foreign animal disease agent in the United States.
[b]Includes *Salmonella arizonae.*

Corneal Infections

Corneal inflammation (keratitis) with or without loss of the epithelium and part of the stroma (corneal ulcer) is a common condition in most animals. Keratitis can begin externally on the epithelial surface or internally at the level of the endothelium. Because it is avascular, the initial inflammatory response in the cornea results from migration of neutrophils from the conjunctiva or limbic sclera. In chronic disease the cornea becomes vascularized and directly participates in the inflammatory response.

Among the most common causes of viral keratitis are members of the herpesviruses. Cats and cattle are most frequently affected. In some herpesvirus infections, recurrence sometimes results from reactivation of latent infections in sensory ganglia (e.g., trigeminal ganglia) following stress.

Primary bacterial keratitis is rare. However, once the cornea is breached a number of bacterial species will readily establish and spread to involve the corneal stroma. These opportunistic bacteria include staphylococci, streptococci, and *Pseudomonas* species. Damage to the cornea due to bacterial toxins and enzymes (e.g., proteolytic enzymes of *Pseudomonas*) is further exacerbated by enzymes from recruited neutrophils (e.g., collagenases and elastases). *Pseudomonas aeruginosa* can be an especially virulent corneal pathogen once it is established and is associated with so-called melting ulcers but still requires a break in the corneal epithelial barrier in order to establish. *Moraxella* bovis is one of the few bacteria in veterinary medicine that cause a primary bacterial keratitis. It produces specific virulence factors including adhesins (fimbria) for adherence to epithelial cells and toxins that cause necrosis of epithelial cells (Figure 73.1).

Mycotic keratitis (keratomycosis) is of greatest significance in horses. Exposure of the eye to plant material often introduces the fungus, although some studies have found various fungi on the conjunctiva from normal equine eyes. These most likely represent transient flora as a result of

FIGURE 73.1. *The photograph depicts a calf with a deep corneal ulcer attributable to infectious bovine keratoconjunctivitis caused by a* Moraxella bovis *infection.*

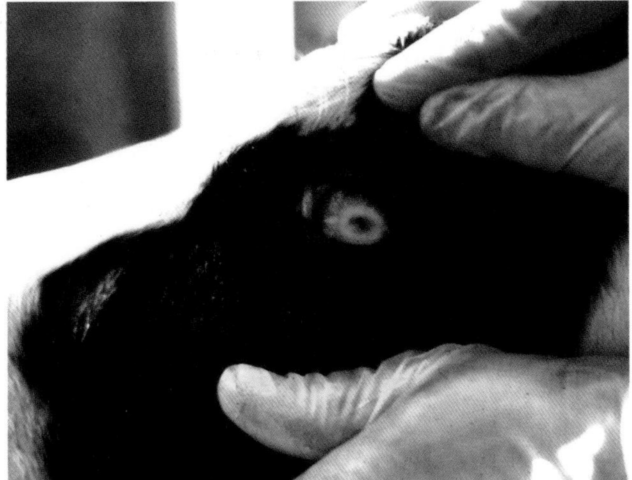

random environmental exposure. The intact corneal epithelium provides an excellent barrier to fungal infections, thus requiring trauma to the corneal epithelial as a preceding event to the development of keratomycosis. Corticosteroid use enhances the likelihood of fungal infections of the equine cornea and exacerbates the condition once present. Typically, mycotic infections of the cornea do not have a concurrent conjunctivitis.

Intraocular Infections

Intraocular infections are frequently the consequence of a systemic infection with exogenous organisms that localize in the uveal tract (iris, ciliary body, choroid). The infection may initiate and/or predominate at a particular site in the uveal tract; however, involvement of other sites in the tract is common. At some level, at least histologically, widespread involvement of the uveal tract occurs in most infections. Uveitis can be divided on the basis of the anatomic site most prominently involved in the inflammatory process (e.g., anterior uveitis) and whether adjacent sites are also involved (e.g., chorioretinitis). In intraocular infections, extension to other parts of the eye occurs due to proximity of other structures (e.g., retinal involvement), the fluid nature inside the eye, and the open communication between intraocular chambers. Depending on the agent, stage of the inflammatory response and even the animal involved, the inflammatory response in the uveal tract can be suppurative, lymphoplasmacytic, granulomatous, or some combination of these responses.

The pathogenesis of viral-induced uveitis is either by direct infection of the uveal tract and subsequent inflammatory response or through deposition of immune complexes resulting in immune-mediated type III hypersensitivity reactions. Likewise, bacterial uveitis occurs subsequent to bacterial (e.g., *Brucella*) localization to the uveal tract or in some cases from immune complex deposition (e.g., *Leptospira*). Nonspecific bacterial uveitis can result subsequent to other preexisting bacterial conditions (e.g., gingivitis and prostatitis). All of the systemic mycoses agents (*Blastomyces*, *Histoplasma*, *Coccidioides*, and *Cryptococcus*) have the capability of causing a panuveitis. Most present clinically as a chorioretinitis, with dogs and cats predominately affected. In dogs, *Prototheca*, an achlorophyllous alga, causes a granulomatous chorioretinitis in conjunction with other systemic manifestations (e.g., bloody diarrhea and paresis).

Congenital defects of ocular structures in utero infections, usually viral in origin, occur in some animal species. Bovine viral diarrhea virus infections in pregnant cows have been linked to retinal atrophy and cataracts in calves. Panleukopenia in cats is associated with dysplastic ocular development in kittens.

Infections of the Orbit

Infections in the orbit can be the result of a foreign body, penetrating wound from the oral cavity or hematogenous dissemination. Purulent infections in the form of orbital cellulitis and retrobulbar abscesses most often result. All animal species can develop orbital infections, although most occur in dogs and cats. The etiology is usually a mixture of bacterial agents, often including *Pasteurella* species.

74 Respiratory System

Douglas E. Hostetler

The primary function of the respiratory system is gaseous exchange. The structure of the respiratory tract is such that noxious substances, particulate material, and microbial pathogens are prevented from entering and compromising the distal portions of respiratory tract where gaseous exchange occurs. Innate protective properties are present at all levels of the respiratory tract.

In most vertebrates, the respiratory system is composed of the nasal cavity, sinuses, larynx, pharynx, trachea, bronchi and bronchioles, and lungs. In birds, the respiratory system is more complex and markedly different from other vertebrates. Most notably, birds possess large, subcutaneous, infraorbital sinuses that communicate with the nasal cavity and are especially predisposed to infection—in part, because of poor drainage. The lungs of birds are fairly rigid compared with other vertebrates. Air sacs are present that communicate with the lungs and are located in the coelom and medullary cavity of some bones.

Antimicrobial Properties of the Respiratory System

The act of breathing exposes the respiratory tract to airborne microorganisms, including potentially pathogenic ones. Resident microorganisms are present in most upper parts of the tract, while various defense mechanisms operate to exclude or eliminate them from other sites.

Different protective mechanisms operate in the nasopharyngeal, tracheobronchial, and pulmonary portions of the respiratory tract. Aerodynamic filtration operates through different forces at these levels in depositing variously sized airborne particles. Inertial forces deposit larger particles (>5 μm in diameter) in the nasopharyngeal and upper tracheobronchial sections through impaction. In small bronchi and beyond, where air velocity is reduced, gravity acts to sediment particles 5 to 10 μm in size. In the smallest bronchioles and alveoli, particles measuring less than 1 μm gain contact with membranes through Brownian movement.

Original chapter written by the late Dr. Richard L. Walker.

The mucus lining covering airway epithelium contains numerous substances with antimicrobial properties or that provide protective effects. Lysozyme, which is selectively bactericidal by its action on peptidoglycan, is present in varying quantities throughout the respiratory tract. Broad-spectrum antimicrobial peptides, beta-defensins, produced by ciliated epithelial cells are active against viruses, bacteria, and fungi. Their expression is increased upon exposure to microbial components (e.g., lipopolysaccharide). The antimicrobial reactive nitrogen species, nitric oxide, is also produced by ciliated epithelial cells, primarily by inducible nitric oxide synthetase (iNOS). Bacterial products modulate the expression of iNOS. Nitric oxide plays an important role as a biological mediator in the regulation of host defense and inflammation, producing both pro- and anti-inflammatory effects. Also present in the mucus are immunoglobulins and interferon and lactoferrin, which by binding iron, makes it unavailable to most bacteria. Alpha-1 antitrypsin, an enzyme inhibitor that reduces the destructive effect of inflammatory reactions, plays a protective role.

Nasopharyngeal Compartment

Protective mechanisms in the nasopharyngeal compartment include vibrissae (guard hairs) around the nostrils of some animals that arrest the largest inhaled particles (15 μm in diameter) and the nasal conchae. The nasal conchal arrangement creates a turbulent airflow that increases the chances that particles will impact mucosal surfaces. Once impinged on the mucus-lined nasal turbinates or the nasopharyngeal wall, they encounter mucociliary action (see Section "Mucociliary Apparatus") and are transported to the caudal pharynx to be swallowed and eliminated via the digestive tract.

In the humid, warm nasal passages, particles swell through hydration, becoming more likely to impinge on a mucous membrane. Warming of air in the nasal passages also benefits cold-sensitive clearance mechanisms in the lower tract. Pharyngeal lymphoid tissues act in the filtration of microorganisms and initiation of the immune responses as a constituent of the mucosa-associated lymphoid tissue.

The resident flora provides colonization resistance as well as production of antibacterial substances. The

Veterinary Microbiology, Third Edition. Edited by D. Scott McVey, Melissa Kennedy and M.M. Chengappa.

sneeze reflex aids in clearing infectious particles from this area.

Tracheobronchial Compartment

The tracheobronchial compartment includes the larynx, trachea, bronchi, and bronchioles. Closure of the glottis during swallowing protects this area from contamination. Coughing removes gross accumulations of fluid. The tracheobronchial compartment is lined by mucociliary epithelium, which traps particles and transports them cranially to the pharynx (see section "Mucociliary Apparatus"). Deposition of particles on airway membranes is favored by bronchial branching due to directional airflow changes.

Bronchiolar-associated lymphoid tissue (BALT) is distributed along the airways and is concentrated at bronchial bifurcations, which corresponds to sites where the greatest trapping of inhaled particles occurs. BALT includes both cellular and humoral immune responses. Epithelial cells mediate the active transport of IgA from the lamina propria to the airway lumen.

Pulmonary Compartment

Clearance mechanisms of the pulmonary compartment (alveoli) consist of pulmonary alveolar macrophages (PAMs), neutrophils, and monocytes recruited from the blood. Particles are disposed of by phagocytosis. Susceptible microorganisms are killed and digested. Phagocytes migrate to sites where mucociliary transport occurs or via the lymphatics to remove other engulfed particles. The same protective substances as in tracheobronchial secretions operate at the pulmonary level, supplemented by those derived from alveolar macrophages.

Mechanisms

Overall, the mucociliary apparatus and PAMs constitute the main clearance mechanisms of the respiratory tract and are described in greater detail in the following sections.

Mucociliary Apparatus

The mucociliary apparatus is composed of ciliated and secretory cells. Ciliated cells are pseudostratified in the nasal and cranial tracheobronchial portions of the tract, simple columnar in the smaller bronchi, and simple cuboidal in the smallest bronchioles. The cilia, some 250 per cell, measuring 5.0 × 0.3 μm, resemble eukaryotic flagella and beat up to 1000 times a minute. The density of ciliated cells decreases gradually from the proximal to distal bronchioles. Alterations in cilia activity or deciliation of the epithelial cells hinder clearance activity and promote invasion by opportunistic pathogens. In addition, loss of ciliated epithelial cell function results in decreased production of antimicrobial substances and cytokines that mediate the inflammatory response.

The secretory components of the mucociliary apparatus are goblet cells, interspersed with ciliated cells, and, in the nose, trachea, and larger bronchi, submucosal serous and mucous glands. Serous fluid bathes the cilia, while a viscid mucus layer engages their tips. Mucus is propelled, along with particles trapped in it, caudally in the nasopharynx and cranially in the tracheobronchial compartment toward the pharynx by cilia beating at a rate of up to 20 mm/min. The particle clearance rate is fastest in the trachea and slowest in the smallest airways, where goblet cells are absent, mucus is sparse, and cilia beat more slowly—an arrangement that prevents logjams in the large airways. The trachea (e.g., cat) can be cleared within an hour, and all airways within a day.

Mucociliary clearance is inhibited by temperature extremes, respiratory viruses, some bacteria (e.g., *Bordetella*), dryness, general anesthetics, dust, noxious gases (sulfur dioxide, carbon dioxide, ammonia, tobacco smoke), and hypoxia. Mucus production through disruption of goblet cell integrity increases in response to irritant exposure.

Pulmonary Alveolar Macrophage

The PAM is a monocyte adapted to the lung environment and is located in the alveolar space. It is recruited from the blood when needed. The pulmonary alveolar macrophage is a pleomorphic cell, 20–40 μm in diameter, with many lysosomal granules containing numerous bioactive substances. Also produced by PAMs are mediator substances—complement components, interleukin 1, and tumor necrosis factor—which enable additional cellular and humoral defenses to be mobilized. Complement and IgG receptors on PAMs enhance its phagocytic capability. PAMs are motile and usually exist in the alveolus less than a week. Energy is obtained mainly by oxidative phosphorylation. The absence of ciliated epithelial cells and mucus-producing cells in the alveolus requires that PAMs remove particles that reach the alveoli.

Particles ingested by PAMs—other than susceptible bacteria killed upon ingestion—are removed via the mucociliary escalator or via interstitial centripetal or centrifugal lymphatics. The centripetal route leads directly to the hilar lymph nodes and may require 2 weeks. The centrifugal route goes via the pleura and may take months. Agents that cannot be removed are sequestered by inflammatory processes (abscesses, granulomas).

PAM activities are inhibited by sulfur dioxide, ozone, nitrogen oxides, and respiratory viruses. Bacterial leukotoxins and hemolysins destroy PAMs and are major virulence factors produced by some important bacterial respiratory pathogens (e.g., *Mannheimia haemolytica* in cattle and *Actinobacillus pleuropneumoniae* in swine).

Microbial Flora

The density and constituency of the microbial flora of the respiratory tract varies among animals and within the respiratory tract itself. The resident flora are limited to the nasal cavity and pharynx where a highly diverse flora can be found. For example, more than 30 different gram-positive bacterial species alone can be recovered from the nasal conchae and tonsils of unweaned and weaned piglets. Overall, the nasal flora consistently includes viridans streptococci and coagulase-negative staphylococci along with potential pathogens that vary with the animal host. Although not usually considered a respiratory tract pathogen, coagulase-positive staphylococci can colonize the nose and be carried at a high rate in some populations. There they serve as a source for infections elsewhere in the body (e.g., integumentary infections). Some of the resident flora of the upper respiratory tract and oropharynx represent major respiratory bacterial pathogens (e.g., members of the *Pasteurellaceae* and *Streptococcus* and *Mycoplasma* species) if they are able to establish in lower parts of the tract. Many potentially pathogenic mycoplasmas are normal residents of the upper respiratory tract of the host they affect or are carried there by persistently infected individuals. They play a prominent role as pathogens at most levels in the respiratory tract, contributing to "respiratory disease complexes," or under the proper circumstances are by themselves significant pathogens.

As with the digestive tract, the resident flora of the respiratory system confers colonization resistance that is reduced by antibiotic treatment and environmental changes that alter its composition.

Nonresident organisms include both potential pathogens and harmless transients. Transient flora are comprised of microbes that enter during the breathing process and, therefore, reflect the environment in which the animal is maintained. Environmental factors, such as dry, dusty environments or confined environments where ventilation is poor, increase the microbial load and types of transient flora an animal is exposed to. It is not uncommon to isolate *Escherichia coli* and other enteric bacteria from the upper respiratory tract as transient flora. The significance of their presence in the nasopharynx is difficult to assess without corresponding clinical and pathologic information.

The larynx, trachea, bronchi, and lungs lack a resident flora. However, the lower portion of the respiratory tract is continually being exposed to microbes that are present in the upper portion. In the uncompromised respiratory tract, these organisms are quickly removed by the natural host defense mechanisms. Fluid from the distal tract may contain up to 10^3 bacteria/ml in normal animals (e.g., cats).

Infections of the Respiratory System

Respiratory tract infections are of substantial importance in all animals. Some of the most common and/or important agents responsible for respiratory tract diseases in major domestic animals and poultry are listed in Tables 74.1, 74.2, 74.3, 74.4, 74.5, 74.6, and 74.7. Agent characteristics, route of infection, host susceptibility, and host immune response determine the location(s) in the respiratory tract affected, severity of the infection, and associated pathology. Pathogens of the respiratory tract covered in this chapter include viral, bacterial, and fungal agents, as well as one aquatic protistan parasite, *Rhinosporidium*.

Potential respiratory viral pathogens belong to a range of families (e.g., *Adenoviridae*, *Caliciviridae*, *Coronaviridae*, *Herpesviridae*, *Paramyxoviridae*, and *Orthomyxoviridae*). The

Table 74.1. Common and/or Important Infectious Agents of the Respiratory System of Dogs

Agent	Major Clinical Manifestations (Common Disease Name)
Viruses	
Canine adenovirus 2	Nasal discharge, tracheobronchitis (kennel cough syndrome) bronchointerstitial pneumonia
Canine distemper virus	Nasopharyngitis, laryngitis, bronchitis, bronchointerstitial pneumonia (distemper)
Canine parainfluenza virus 2	Nasal discharge, tracheobronchitis (canine kennel cough syndrome)
Bacteria	
Actinomyces spp.	Pyogranulomatous pneumonia, pleuritis
Bordetella bronchiseptica	Tracheobronchitis (infectious tracheobronchitis, kennel cough), bronchopneumonia
Escherichia coli	Bronchopneumonia
Nocardia spp.	Pyogranulomatous pleuritis
Obligate anaerobes[a]	Bronchopneumonia
Pasteurella multocida	Bronchopneumonia
Fungi	
Agents of systemic mycoses[b]	Granulomatous pneumonia
Aspergillus fumigatus	Rhinitis, sinusitis (nasal aspergillosis)
Cryptococcus neoformans	Granulomatous nasal masses (cryptococcosis)
Protist	
Rhinosporidium seeberi	Nasal granulomas (rare)

[a]Includes *Bacteroides, Peptostreptococcus, Fusobacterium,* and *Porphyromonas* species.
[b]Includes *Blastomyces dermatitidis, Coccidioides immitis, Cryptococcus neoformans,* and *Histoplasma capsulatum.*

Table 74.2. Common and/or Important Infectious Agents of the Respiratory System of Cats

Agent	Major Clinical Manifestations (Common Disease Name)
Viruses	
Feline calicivirus	Rhinitis, interstitial pneumonia, tracheitis (feline calicivirus disease)
Feline herpesvirus 1	Rhinotracheitis (feline viral rhinotracheitis)
Feline infectious peritonitis virus	Pleural effusion, pyogranulomatous pleuritis
Bacteria	
Bordetella bronchiseptica	Tracheobronchitis, bronchopneumonia (feline bordetellosis)
Chlamydophila felis	Pneumonia (feline pneumonitis), rhinitis
Obligate anaerobic bacteria	Pleural empyema (pyothorax)
Pasteurella multocida	Pleural empyema (pyothorax)
Fungi	
Cryptococcus neoformans	Rhinitis, granulomatous nasal masses, sinusitis, pneumonia

Table 74.3. Common and/or Important Infectious Agents of the Respiratory System of Horses

Agent	Major Clinical Manifestations (Common Disease Name)
Viruses	
African Horse Sickness virus[a]	Pulmonary edema (African horse sickness)
Equine adenovirus 1	Bronchiolitis, interstitial pneumonia (equine adenovirus disease)
Equine herpesvirus 1	Rhinitis, pneumonitis (equine rhinopneumonitis)
Equine herpesvirus 4	Rhinitis, pneumonitis
Equine influenza virus	Rhinitis, tracheobronchitis, interstitial pneumonia (equine influenza)
Equine viral arteritis virus	Rhinitis, interstitial pneumonia
Hendra virus[a]	Pulmonary edema with respiratory distress
Bacteria	
Actinobacillus equuli ssp. *haemolytica*	Bronchopneumonia, pleuritis
Burkholderia mallei[a]	Rhinitis, pyogranulomatous nasal nodules (glanders)
Burkholderia pseudomallei[a]	Abscesses in nasal mucosa, embolic pneumonia, pulmonary abscesses
Escherichia coli	Bronchopneumonia, pleuritis
Mycoplasma felis	Pleuritis
Obligate anaerobes[b]	Bronchopneumonia, pleuritis
Rhodococcus equi	Pyogranulomatous pneumonia
Streptococcus equi ssp. *equi*	Guttural pouch empyema, rhinopharyngitis, retropharyngeal lymph nodes abscesses (strangles), sinusitis
Streptococcus equi ssp. *zooepidemicus*	Bronchopneumonia, pleuritis, sinusitis
Fungi	
Aspergillus species	Guttural pouch mycosis
Protist	
Rhinosporidium seeberi	Nasal granulomas (rare)

[a]Considered a foreign animal disease agent in the United States.
[b]Includes Fusobacterium, Peptostreptococcus, and Prevotella.

Table 74.4. Common and/or Important Infectious Agents of the Respiratory System of Cattle

Agent	Major Clinical Manifestations (Common Disease Name)
Viruses	
Bovine herpesvirus 1	Rhinotracheitis (infectious bovine rhinotracheitis)
Bovine respiratory coronavirus	Interstitial pneumonia
Bovine respiratory syncytial virus	Interstitial pneumonia (bovine respiratory syncytial virus disease)
Parainfluenza virus 3	Rhinitis, interstitial pneumonia (parainfluenza virus 3 infection)
Bacteria	
Arcanobacterium pyogenes	Embolic pneumonia, lung abscesses
Fusobacterium necrophorum	Necrotic laryngitis (calf diphtheria)
Histophilus somni[a]	Bronchopneumonia, otitis media
Mannheimia haemolytica	Bronchopneumonia (enzootic pneumonia, shipping fever)
Mycobacterium bovis	Granulomatous pneumonia, pleuritis (bovine tuberculosis)
Mycoplasma bovis	Bronchopneumonia, otitis media
Mycoplasma dispar	Pneumonia-alveolitis
Mycoplasma mycoides ssp. *mycoides-small colony type*[b]	Bronchopneumonia, pleuritis (contagious bovine pleuropneumonia)
Pasteurella multocida	Bronchopneumonia (enzootic pneumonia, shipping fever), otitis media
Salmonella Dublin	Interstitial pneumonia
Fungi	
Mortierella wolfii	Embolic pneumonia

[a]"Haemophilus somnus" is the obsolete name of this organism.
[b]Considered a foreign animal disease agent in the United States.

majority of the bacterial respiratory tract pathogens belong to the family *Pasteurellaceae* or to the genera *Bordetella*, *Mycoplasma*, and *Streptococcus*. Some important respiratory tract pathogens are associated with specific, well-defined clinical entities (e.g., *Rhodococcus equi* and pyogranulomatous pneumonia in foals). Under the proper conditions, a number of opportunistic bacteria (e.g., *Actinomyces* spp., members of the family *Enterobacteriaceae*, obligate anaerobes) from the oral cavity and lower digestive tract can cause or contribute to respiratory disease (e.g., aspiration pneumonia). Fungal agents of the respiratory tract are predominately the agents of systemic mycoses (*Blastomyces dermatitidis*, *Coccidioides immitis*, *Cryptococcus neoformans*, and *Histoplasma capsulatum*) and *Aspergillus* spp. Individual chapters on particular respiratory tract pathogens should be consulted for details on pathogenesis and pathology specific to a particular agent.

Many infectious respiratory diseases are multifactorial, requiring environmental, host, and agent factors to be in play. Respiratory infections commonly involve sequential infection with different pathogens (e.g., viral pneumonia leading to secondary bacterial pneumonia). Respiratory tract infections can initiate either by the aerogenous or hematogenous route. A factor predisposing to infection of hematogenous origin, especially in cats, pigs, and ruminants, is the role played by pulmonary intravascular macrophages in removing blood-borne pathogens.

Infections of the Nasopharyngeal Compartment

The major infectious diseases of the nasopharyngeal compartment are rhinitis and sinusitis, which can occur independently or concomitantly. Rhinitis is an inflammation of the nasal mucosa. Common signs of rhinitis are sneezing and nasal discharges of varying composition. The characteristic of the exudate in rhinitis is the result of serous or mucus secretions, alterations in vascular permeability (fibrinogen deposition), and influx and type of inflammatory cells.

Viral rhinitis can be caused by a number of viruses (e.g., herpesviruses, adenoviruses, and influenza viruses) and occurs, to some degree, in most animals. In general, ciliated

Table 74.5. Common and/or Important Infectious Agents of the Respiratory System of Sheep and Goats

Agent	Major Clinical Manifestations (Common Disease Name)
Viruses	
Caprine arthritis/encephalitis virus (G)	Interstitial pneumonia
Jaagsiekte sheep retrovirus (S)	Interstitial pneumonia, pulmonary carcinoma (ovine pulmonary adenocarcinoma)
Maedi/visna virus (S)	Interstitial pneumonia (ovine progressive pneumonia, maedi)
Parainfluenza virus 3	Interstitial pneumonia
Bacteria	
Arcanobacterium pyogenes	Pulmonary abscesses, traumatic pharyngitis
Fusobacterium necrophorum	Necrotic laryngitis, traumatic pharyngitis
Mannheimia haemolytica	Bronchopneumonia, pleuritis (pneumonic pasteurellosis)
Mycoplasma capricolum ssp. *capripneumoniae* (G)[a]	Bronchopneumonia, pleuritis (contagious caprine pleuropneumonia)
Mycoplasma mycoides ssp. mycoides-large colony type (G)	Pneumonia, pleuritis
Mycoplasma ovipneumoniae (S)	Interstitial pneumonia (ovine nonprogressive pneumonia)
Pasteurella trehalosi	Bronchopneumonia

S, sheep; G, goats.
[a]Considered a foreign animal disease agent in the United States.

Table 74.6. Common and/or Important Infectious Agents of the Respiratory System of Pigs

Agent	Major Clinical Manifestations (Common Disease Name)
Viruses	
Lelystad virus	Interstitial pneumonia (porcine reproductive and respiratory syndrome)
Nipah virus[a]	Alveolitis, bronchointerstitial pneumonia
Porcine herpesvirus 1	Rhinopharyngitis, tracheitis (pseudorabies, Aujeszky's disease)
Porcine herpesvirus 2	Rhinitis (inclusion body rhinitis)
Swine influenza virus	Rhinitis, tracheobronchitis, bronchointerstitial pneumonia (swine influenza)
Bacteria	
Actinobacillus pleuropneumoniae	Bronchopneumonia, pleuritis (porcine pleuropneumonia)
Bordetella bronchiseptica[b]	Rhinitis (atrophic rhinitis), bronchopneumonia
Fusobacterium necrophorum	Necrotic nasal cellulitis (necrotic rhinitis, bull nose)
Haemophilus parasuis	Bronchopneumonia, polyserositis (Glasser's disease)
Mycoplasma hyopneumoniae	Bronchopneumonia (enzootic pneumonia)
Mycoplasma hyorhinis	Polyserositis
Pasteurella multocida[b]	Rhinitis (atrophic rhinitis), bronchopneumonia
Salmonella species	Bronchointerstitial pneumonia
Streptococcus suis	Bronchopneumonia, pleuritis, embolic pneumonia

[a]Considered a foreign animal disease agent in the United States.
[b]*B. bronchiseptica* and *P. multocida* sometimes act synergistically.

epithelial cells are infected, sloughed, and subsequently replaced. Clinical signs reflect the associated inflammatory response. Secondary bacterial infections can be a complication of a primary viral rhinitis (e.g., rhinotracheitis virus and calicivirus infections in cats predispose to bacterial rhinitis and sinusitis). Latently infected animals that periodically shed virus (e.g., infectious bovine rhinotracheitis virus) are a common source for infections in naive animals.

Bacterial infections of the nasopharyngeal compartment, while not as frequent as viral infections, are still significant. Notable among these are atrophic rhinitis in pigs, contagious rhinopharyngitis (strangles) in horses, and sinus infections in poultry (see discussion on sinusitis, 2nd paragraph following). In atrophic rhinitis in pigs, the dermonecrotic toxin of *Pasteurella multocida* (type D) induces osteolysis of nasal turbinates and distortion of the nasal cavity (Figure 74.1). To a lesser extent, the dermonecrotic toxin of *Bordetella bronchiseptica* is also involved. Pigs present with sneezing and a clear to cloudy nasal discharge. The disease can be a mild, nonprogressive, or more active, progressive form. Reduced weight gain, poor feed conversion, and increased susceptibility to other respiratory infections are the main consequences of atrophic rhinitis.

Streptococcus equi ssp. *equi*, the cause of contagious rhinopharyngitis (strangles) in horses, typically also involves submandibular and/or retropharyngeal lymph nodes. The resulting intense inflammatory response produces a thick, bilateral, purulent nasal discharge. Strangles is considered highly contagious. Serious consequences can result from strangles infections including guttural pouch empyema (see discussion below on sites that communicate with the upper respiratory tract), "bastard strangles," and purpura hemorrhagica.

Sinusitis is an inflammation of one of the nasal sinuses. It can result from extension of a nasal cavity infection into sinuses or be related to other problems of the oral-nasal cavities (e.g., extension of infection from an infected tooth). It is an occasional occurrence in most animals. Agents involved are typically resident flora of the nasal cavity or those involved in rhinitis.

In poultry, sinusitis is an especially common problem that has major economic consequences due to the contagious nature of some of the agents involved and potential for large numbers of birds to be affected. A number of microbial agents can infect the sinuses of birds, and typically sinusitis is found in conjunction with clinical signs in other areas of the respiratory system (e.g., Gallid herpesvirus 1 in chickens, avian influenza viruses). *Mycoplasma*

Table 74.7. Common and/or Important Infectious Agents of the Respiratory System of Poultry

Agent	Major Clinical Manifestations (Common Disease Name)
Viruses	
Avian infectious bronchitis virus (C)	Air sacculitis, tracheobronchitis (avian infectious bronchitis)
Avian influenza virus	Air sacculitis, sinusitis, tracheitis (avian influenza)
Avian paramyxovirus 1[a]	Hemorrhagic tracheitis (exotic Newcastle disease)
Avian pneumovirus	Rhinotracheitis, sinusitis (turkey rhinotracheitis), periorbital and infraorbital sinus swelling in chickens (swollen head syndrome)
Avian poxvirus	Diphtheritic lesions of nares, pharynx, larynx and trachea (pox-diphtheritic form)
Gallid herpesvirus 1 (C)	Laryngotracheitis (infectious laryngotracheitis)
Bacteria	
Bordetella avium	Rhinotracheitis, sinusitis (bordetellosis turkey coryza)
Escherichia coli	Colisepticemia, secondary pneumonia
Haemophilus paragallinarum (C)	Rhinitis, sinusitis (fowl coryza)
Mycoplasma gallisepticum	Air sacculitis (chronic respiratory disease), rhinitis, sinusitis (infectious sinusitis) (T)
Mycoplasma synoviae	Air sacculitis, sinusitis
Ornithobacterium rhinotracheale	Air sacculitis, bronchopneumonia, sinusitis
Pasteurella multocida	Air sacculitis, pneumonia
Fungi	
Aspergillus fumigatus	Tracheitis, air sacculitis, pneumonia (brooder pneumonia)

C, chickens only; T, Turkeys.
[a]Considered a foreign animal disease agent in the United States.

gallisepticum in turkeys (infectious sinusitis) and *Haemophilus paragallinarum* in chickens (fowl coryza) are among the most economically important causes of sinusitis in poultry. Poor growth performance and decreased egg production are among the main reasons for economic losses.

Sinusitis in cattle can occur following dehorning if foreign material enters the open frontal sinuses during the healing process and overwhelms the clearance mechanisms.

FIGURE 74.1. *Severe turbinate atrophy due to* Bordetella bronchiseptica *and toxigenic* Pasteurella multocida *type D infection. Center is normal. (Courtesy Dr Bruce Brodersen.)*

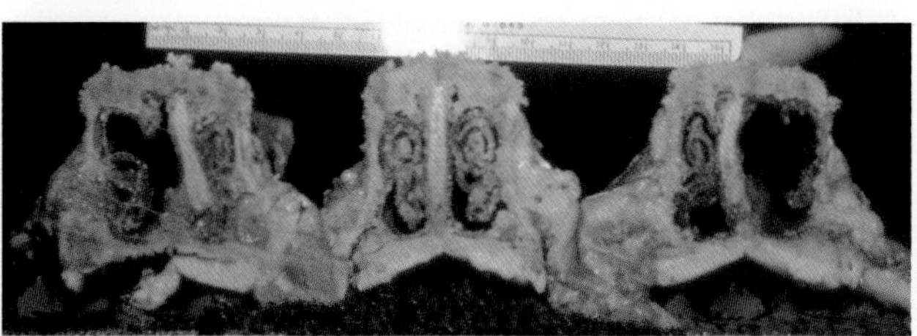

Fungal infections of the nasopharyngeal compartment are infrequent and when they occur they evoke a granulomatous inflammatory response. *Aspergillus* rhinitis and sinusitis in dogs and nasal cryptococcosis in cats are among the most important fungal infections of the nasal cavity.

Rhinosporidium seeberi, a protist in the class *Mesomycetozoea*, is a rare cause of granulomatous nasal masses containing large spherules and endospores of *Rhinosporidium*. Grossly the nasal lesions resemble multilobed granular polyps. Although any animal including poultry can be infected, most cases are reported in dogs and horses. Infections are associated with exposure to freshwater ponds, lakes, or rivers.

Sites that communicate with the upper respiratory tract may be affected by the direct extension of an infectious process in the nasopharyngeal compartment or become infected independent of other nasopharyngeal disease by residents of the nasopharyngeal compartment. Guttural pouch empyema in horses, caused by *S. equi* ssp. *equi*, develops as a sequel to primary rhinopharyngitis or rupture of an abscessed retropharyngeal lymph node (strangles). Unilateral nasal discharge, especially when the head is down, is a common way for guttural pouch infections to present. Incomplete drainage from the guttural pouch, scarring of the pharyngeal opening, and development of concretions (chondroids) on the floor of the guttural pouch interfere with resolution of the infection. Fungal infections also occur in the guttural pouch of horses (guttural pouch mycosis), typically involving the dorsal wall of the medial compartment. *Aspergillus* species (especially *A. nidulans*) are the most common etiologic agents. The initiating factor(s) for guttural pouch mycosis has not been clearly elucidated. When guttural pouch infections involve neural or vascular structures, serious (dysphagia, laryngeal hemiplegia, and Horner's syndrome due to nerve injury) or even fatal (rupture of the internal carotid artery) consequences may result.

Otitis media in calves is commonly caused by respiratory pathogens (e.g., *Mycoplasma bovis*, *Pasteurella multocida*, and *Histophilus somni*) harbored as residents of the upper respiratory tract. The likely route of infection is via the auditory tube into the middle ear. Calves present with a head tilt, *nystagmus*, and droopy ear(s) (Figure 74.2). The tympanic bullae are typically partially or completely filled with caseous debris and serosanguineous fluid. In some cases, the disease progresses and results in otitis interna and meningitis, where calves may exhibit severe neurologic signs. Other species of animals are similarly but less commonly affected.

Infections of the Tracheobronchial Compartment

The major diseases of the tracheobronchial compartment are laryngitis, tracheitis, and bronchitis. Viral and bacterial agents are the primary causes of infectious diseases of the tracheobronchial compartment. *Aspergillus* infections in poultry can, however, involve the trachea and bronchi.

Viral infections of the trachea and bronchi (e.g., equine influenza, infectious bovine rhinotracheitis, and infectious laryngotracheitis in chickens) damage respiratory

FIGURE 74.2. *The photograph depicts a Holstein calf with a head tilt secondary to otitis media-interna.* Mycoplasma bovis *was cultured from this calf's inner ear.*

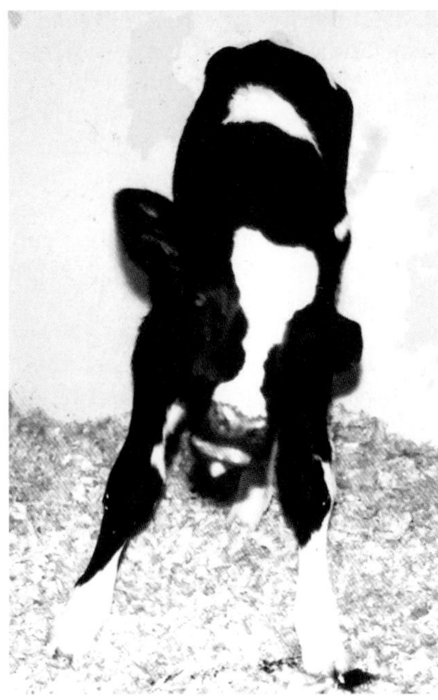

epithelial cells and interrupt the mucociliary apparatus. Tracheal lesions caused by many different viruses may not have particularly distinguishing features; however, inclusions in some infections assist in identifying the particular virus involved (e.g., infectious laryngotracheitis in chickens and avian pox viruses). Viral tracheitis is often sufficiently destructive to predispose to secondary bacterial infections.

Necrotic laryngitis in young feedlot cattle is one of the most common bacterial laryngeal diseases (Figure 74.3). *Fusobacterium necrophorum*, the etiologic agent, establishes in preexisting contact ulcers found on the laryngeal mucosa, which are suspected to originate from some preceding trauma (e.g., reflex coughing). Once established, *F. necrophorum* causes a severe necrotic laryngitis that can be fatal if untreated. Other ruminants are affected but less frequently.

FIGURE 74.3. *Necrotic laryngitis in a calf. Fibrinonecrotic diphtheric membrane is covering the arytenoid cartilages and anterior trachea. (Courtesy of Dr Alan Doster.)*

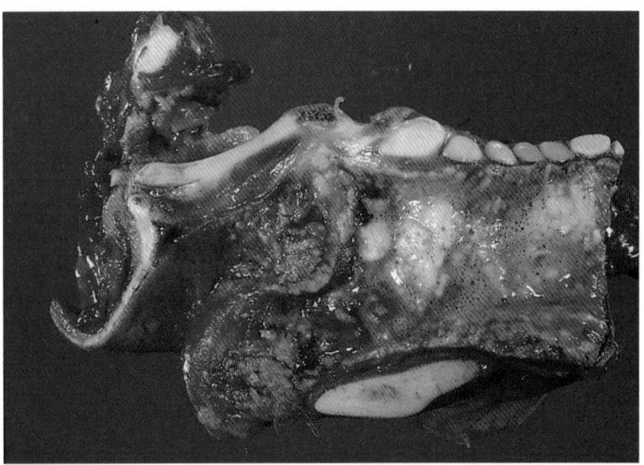

In dogs, the kennel cough syndrome, an infectious tracheobronchitis, involves multiple potential etiologic agents, sometimes working in concert. Kennel cough in dogs is considered contagious and is associated with dogs maintained in confined, close-contact environments (e.g., kennels and animal shelters). Viral agents include canine adenovirus 2 and parainfluenza virus 2. *Mycoplasma* species have been implicated, but their involvement is unproven. The bacterium, *B. bronchiseptica*, is also associated with the kennel cough syndrome. It is considered a primary pathogen of the respiratory tract because of its ability to adhere to ciliated epithelial cells and affect epithelial cell functions. Infections involving *B. bronchiseptica* tend to be more productive than those caused by viral agents. Evidence is growing that *B. bronchiseptica* is also a significant respiratory pathogen in cats.

In poultry, *Bordetella avium* is a common cause of upper respiratory infections (rhinitis, sinusitis, and tracheitis) in turkeys and to a lesser extent in chickens. Sneezing is the most common sign, along with an oculonasal discharge. After colonization, damage to ciliated respiratory epithelial cells and ciliostatic effects occur. Collapse of the trachea due to softening of tracheal rings may also result. Infections with *B. avium* predispose birds to other infections, such as colibacillosis.

Some microorganisms that affect the tracheobronchial compartment concurrently involve other parts of the respiratory system (e.g., feline viral rhinotracheitis, infectious bovine rhinotracheitis, and *B. avium* in turkeys). Additionally, systemic infections may involve epithelial cells in the tracheobronchial compartment (e.g., fibrinohemorrhagic tracheitis in exotic Newcastle disease in poultry), along with sites in the host outside the respiratory system.

Infections of the Pulmonary Compartment

The major infectious disease of the pulmonary compartment is pneumonia. Pneumonia can be classified morphologically as a(n) bronchopneumonia, interstitial pneumonia, granulomatous pneumonia, embolic pneumonia, or a mixture of these types. The agent, route of infection, and immune response determine the type of pneumonia that develops. Viruses, bacteria, and fungi are all potentially important pathogens of the pulmonary compartment. Chapters on specific pathogens should be consulted for details on pathogenesis and pathology associated with that particular agent.

Infections of the pulmonary compartment often require a preceding event(s) that impairs the innate antimicrobial factors. Confined housing environment, ammonia buildup (noxious gas), and transportation stress would typify the type of factors that sufficiently impair defenses and allow pathogens that would otherwise be rapidly cleared by innate host defense mechanisms to establish in the lower respiratory tract.

Some of the same viruses found in the upper respiratory tract cause mild lower respiratory tract disease (e.g., parainfluenza virus and adenoviruses). Serologic evidence indicates that a large percent of populations are inapparently or subclinically infected by these organisms. Other viruses are substantial pathogens of the pulmonary compartment in their own right, sometimes causing fatal infections (e.g., African Horse Sickness virus and Hendra virus). Viral respiratory pathogens in animals with the potential to be transmitted from animal to humans (e.g., influenza viruses, Hendra virus, and Nipah virus) are of substantial public health concern.

While some bacterial pathogens are considered primary pathogens of the pulmonary compartment (e.g., *R. equi* in horses and *A. pleuropneumoniae* in pigs), viral infections often precede bacterial infections and create an environment that allows bacteria to establish by damaging the mucociliary escalator system or altering the immune response by impairing phagocytic function. Once predisposing factors are in play, it is not uncommon to find multiple bacterial pathogens involved in lower respiratory tract infections.

The bovine respiratory disease complex is an example of the complex and, as yet, incompletely understood interactions of environmental factors along with specific infectious agents and host response. It constitutes one of the most economically significant disease complexes of cattle. Environmental or management-related stresses (weather and transportation) and/or viral infections (e.g., adenovirus, bovine respiratory syncytial virus, infectious bovine rhinotracheitis virus, and parainfluenza virus 3) are believed to alter respiratory tract epithelium and innate defenses. Possible immunosuppressive effects related to bovine viral diarrhea virus may also contribute to increasing susceptibility to bacterial infections. These factors allow one of the primary bacterial agents in bovine respiratory disease complex, *M haemolytica*, to establish in the pulmonary compartment. Armed with a number of virulence factors, *M. haemolytica* is able to engage the host defenses. Endotoxin activates pulmonary intravascular macrophages, neutrophils, and lymphocytes, and precipitates an inflammatory response that ultimately determines the degree of pulmonary injury and whether the pathogen is contained. In addition, leukotoxin from *M. haemolytica* destroys phagocytic cells and, at lower concentrations, further enhances the inflammatory response (Figure 74.4).

If pulmonary defenses are compromised sufficiently, more opportunistic bacterial pathogens are established and further aggravate the condition. It is common to recover *Arcanobacterium pyogenes*, a major abscess-former of ruminants, from more chronic bovine respiratory disease complex lesions (Figure 74.5).

The systemic mycoses (coccidioidomycosis, cryptococcosis, blastomycosis, and histoplasmosis), for the most part, begin in the lower respiratory tract causing a granulomatous pneumonia and an associated lymphadenopathy. Severity of respiratory infection varies based on individual animal immune status, breed, and animal species. Dogs, horses, and cats most commonly develop clinical disease. Inability of the animal to contain these infections to the respiratory tract leads to disseminated infections involving other systems in the body. Other than the systemic mycoses, fungal pneumonias are not common in animals. The exception is aspergillosis in poultry where pneumonia, often with concurrent tracheitis and air sacculitis, is a major respiratory tract disease. This is a disease of substantial economic significance to the poultry industry, especially the turkey industry. Closed environments that allow for increased concentration of aerosolized asexual reproductive structures (conidia) and/or moldy feeds are common predisposing factors. Growth in aerated air sacs, bronchi, and trachea permit the production of large numbers of conidia that are not typically produced in solid tissues.

FIGURE 74.4. *Bronchopneumonia in a calf caused by* Mannheimia haemolytica. *Cranioventral lung lobes are predominantly involved. (Courtesy Dr Alan Doster.)*

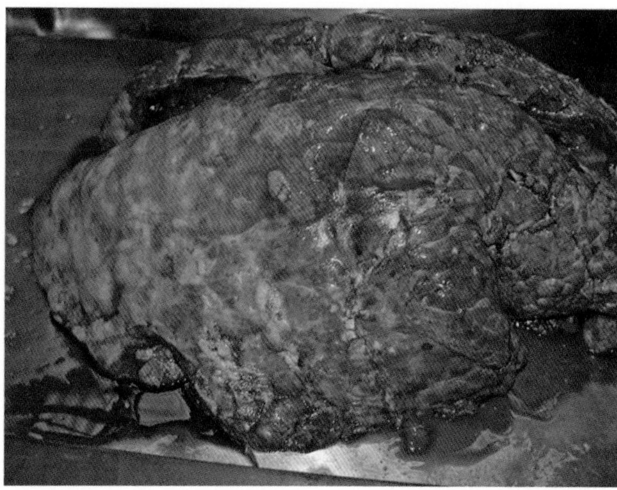

FIGURE 74.5. *Chronic bronchopneumonia in a calf. This calf had abscesses in the cranioventral lung lobes consistent with* Arcanobacterium pyogenes.

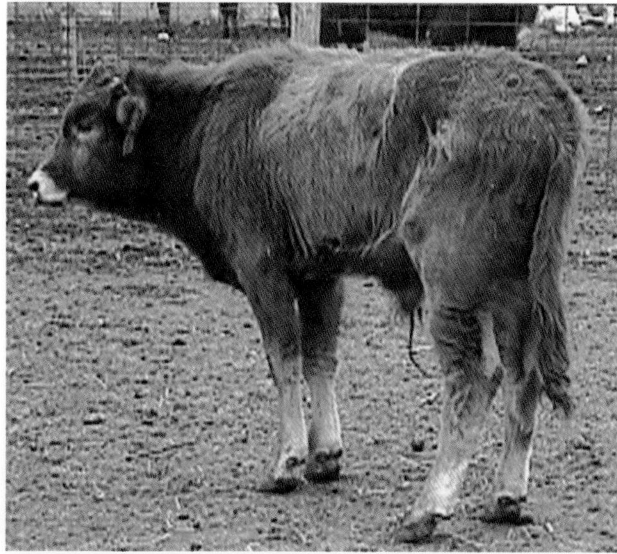

Aspiration pneumonias in most cases are polymicrobial in nature, and bacteria are usually the microbial agents involved. Aspiration pneumonia in animals results when impaired airway protection allows fluids or material to enter the lower respiratory tract, initially causing a chemical pneumonia. Common events leading to aspiration pneumonia are improper treatment procedures (e.g., drenching and improper stomach tubing), bottle or bucket feeding of young animals, poor sucking reflexes, nasopharyngeal tube feeding, choke, or aspiration of gastric or rumen fluids that might occur during the anesthesia recovery period. In newborns, aspiration of meconium may also lead to aspiration pneumonia. The bacteria most frequently involved in aspiration pneumonia typically reflect organisms found in the upper respiratory or digestive tracts and include *E. coli*, *Bordetella*, *Klebsiella*, *Pasteurella*, *Pseudomonas*, *Streptococcus*, and obligate anaerobes (*Fusobacterium*, *Peptostreptococcus*, *Prevotella*, and *Porphyromonas*).

75 Urogenital System

DOUGLAS E. HOSTETLER

The urinary and genital tracts are included together in this chapter because of their anatomical proximity, shared structures (urethra in males), and some overlapping disease processes. Common and/or important urogenital tract agents of domestic animals and poultry are listed in Tables 75.1, 75.2, 75.3, 75.4, 75.5, 75.6, and 75.7.

Urinary Tract

The urinary tract has a number of important functions, including elimination of metabolic wastes, acid–base regulation, maintenance of the extracellular potassium ion concentration, and endocrine functions (vitamin D conversion and production of erythropoietin and renin). The mammalian urinary system includes the kidneys, ureters, bladder, and urethra. The functional filtration unit of the kidney is the nephron, which includes the glomerulus, proximal and distal tubules, loop of Henle, and collecting duct. In birds, the urinary tract differs from mammals. Kidneys are divided into lobes. A bladder is absent and ureters enter the cloaca, medial to the deferent duct in the male and dorsal to the oviduct in the female. Urine, concentrated as a slurry, is voided with feces.

Antimicrobial Defenses

Because it is primarily an excretory system, the urinary tract is not subject to massive microbial exposure but has developed specific antimicrobial defenses to counter occasional exposure to potential pathogens. Protective features include the following:

Washout by Urine. The flow of urine, its direction, diluting effect, and frequent periodic removal discourages the establishment of microorganisms in the normally sterile portions of the tract, that is, the kidneys, ureters, bladder, and proximal male urethra. Urine retention is correlated with increased urinary tract infections (UTI).

Bacterial Interference. Colonization of the distal urethra by normal flora may block attachment sites for colonization of the lower urinary tract by potentially pathogenic organisms.

Glycoprotein Slime Layer. Mucin covering the epithelium may inhibit bacterial adhesion.

Epithelial Desquamation. Exfoliating epithelial cells promote shedding of uropathogens.

Local and Systemic Immune Defenses. Cysteine-rich antimicrobial peptides play a role in inhibiting bacteria from establishing. Immune response to UTIs has been studied mostly in humans and laboratory animals. Studies indicate that serum and urinary antibody titers tend to be low in cystitis and asymptomatic infections and high in pyelonephritis. Secretory immunoglobulin A (sIgA) tends to be most prominent in urine, but IgG and IgM antibodies also occur regularly. Serum IgA, IgG, IgM, and sIgA antibodies are produced in renal infections. The protective function of these antibodies is unclear. The ability to readily mobilize leukocytes promotes rapid clearance of uropathogens from the urinary system.

Antimicrobial Properties of Urine. Urine itself has properties that may play a role in limiting bacterial growth and include the following:

High Osmolality. Urine osmolality (1000 mOsm/kg) reduces growth, particularly of rod-shaped bacteria. It may, however, depress leukocyte activity and preserve bacteria with cell walls damaged by immune reactions or antibiotic therapy. Combined with high concentrations of ammonia, which is anticomplementary, urine osmolality may contribute to the susceptibility of the renal medulla to infection.

Urine pH. While extremes in pH discourage multiplication of some bacteria, ranges bactericidal to common urinary tract pathogens are unlikely to be reached.

Urine Constituents. Urea imparts to urine an unexplained bacteriostatic effect, which is diminished by removal of urea from urine and enhanced by dietary supplementation. Methionine and hippuric and ascorbic acids produce an antibacterial effect largely by acidifying the urine. Urinary ammonium nitrogen also has antibacterial properties.

Veterinary Microbiology, Third Edition. Edited by D. Scott McVey, Melissa Kennedy and M.M. Chengappa.

Table 75.1. Common and/or Important Infectious Agents of the Urogenital System of Dogs

Agent	Major Clinical Manifestations (Common Disease Name)
Viruses	
Canine adenovirus 1	Immune-complex glomerulonephritis (infectious canine hepatitis)
Canine herpesvirus	Abortion, balanoposthitis, infertility in females
Bacteria	
Brucella canis	Abortion, epididymitis (canine brucellosis)
Escherichia coli	Cystitis, epididymitis, orchitis, prostatitis, pyometra, vaginitis
Leptospira spp.	Interstitial nephritis, renal failure (leptospirosis)
Other agents of UTI (see Table 75.8)	Cystitis

Normal Flora

For most of the urinary tract there is no resident flora. The distal urethra does have a resident flora and is colonized by bacteria that are generally not associated with UTI. The flora is predominantly gram-positive and includes coagulase-negative *Staphylococcus* spp., *Streptococcus* spp., *Corynebacterium* spp., and *Enterococcus* spp., but varies according to animal, housing, and hygiene. Small numbers of bacteria may enter the bladder via the urethra, especially in the female, but are normally removed during urination. The significance of asymptomatic bacteriuria is unclear; however, when detected, investigation into potential underlying diseases is warranted.

Certain viruses that persistently infect tubular epithelial cells, although not normal flora, may cause a prolonged viruria (e.g., equine rhinitis A virus and arenaviruses).

Diseases

Host Factors. A number of host factors can predispose an animal to UTIs:

Animal Susceptibility. UTIs are most common and of greatest significance in dogs. In cats, idiopathic lower urinary tract disorders are frequently encountered. Viral,

Table 75.2. Common and/or Important Infectious Agents of the Urogenital System of Cats

Agent	Major Clinical Manifestations (Common Disease Name)
Viruses	
Feline infectious peritonitis virus	Immune-mediated pyogranulomas of kidney
Feline leukemia virus	Immune-complex glomerulonephritis, fetal absorption, abortion, renal lymphoma
Feline panleukopenia virus	Abortion, congenital abnormalities (panleukopenia)
Feline rhinotracheitis virus	Abortion

Table 75.3. Common and/or Important Infectious Agents of the Urogenital System of Horses

Agent	Major Clinical Manifestations (Common Disease Name)
Viruses	
Equine herpesvirus 1	Abortion (equine viral rhinopneumonitis)
Equine herpesvirus 3	Vesicles/erosions on external genitalia
Equine infectious anemia	Immune-complex glomerulonephritis
Equine viral arteritis virus	Abortion (equine viral arteritis)
Bacteria	
Actinobacillus equuli ssp. *equuli*	Glomerulonephritis (sleepy foal disease)
Escherichia coli	Abortion
Leptospira spp.	Abortion
Pseudomonas aeruginosa	Pyometra
Staphylococcus aureus	Postcastration spermatic cord infection (scirrhous cord)
Streptococcus equi ssp. *zooepidemicus*	Abortion, endometritis
Taylorella equigenitalis[a]	Cervicitis, endometritis (contagious equine metritis)
Fungi	
Aspergillus spp.	Abortion
Candida spp.	Endometritis

[a]Considered a foreign animal disease agent in the United States.

nutritional, and metabolic factors have been implicated in the etiology, particularly of obstructive forms. However, bacterial involvement in feline urinary tract disease is uncommon. Infections, particularly cystitis and pyelonephritis, are important in cattle and swine. UTIs are less common in goats, sheep, poultry, and horses.

Anatomic and Physiologic Factors. Interference with the free flow of urine and with complete emptying of the bladder predisposes to UTI. This can be due to tumors, polyps, calculi, anatomic anomalies (e.g., ectopic ureters and patent urachus), and neural defects. Vesicoureteral reflux, the reentry of urine into the ureters during urination, causes bladder urine to reach the renal pelvis, possibly carrying bacteria into a susceptible area. Reflux is aggravated (perhaps initiated) by infection and complicates existing infections by increasing the likelihood of renal involvement.

Other Host Factors. Other host factors include endocrine disturbances such as diabetes mellitus and hyperadrenocorticism (Cushing's disease). Long-term use of corticosteroids appears to predispose dogs to UTI.

Routes of Infection. The primary means by which uropathogens reach the urinary tract are the ascending and hematogenous routes. The ascending route via the urethra is most common. The presence of potential pathogens near the urethral orifice and the usual localization of infection in the bladder point to the urethral orifice as the portal of entry of bacteria to the urinary tract. Pyelonephritis is a

Table 75.4. Common and/or Important Infectious Agents of the Urogenital System of Cattle

Agent	Major Clinical Manifestations (Common Disease Name)
Viruses	
Bovine papillomavirus	Penile and vaginal fibropapillomas
Bovine viral diarrhea virus	Abortion, congenital abnormalities
Infectious bovine rhinotracheitis virus	Abortion, infectious pustular vulvovaginitis, balanoposthitis
Rift Valley fever virus[a]	Abortion (Rift Valley fever)
Bacteria	
Arcanobacterium pyogenes	Abortion, metritis, pyometra, seminal vesiculitis
Brucella abortus	Abortion, epididymitis, orchitis, seminal vesiculitis
Campylobacter fetus ssp. *venerealis*	Early embryonic death (bovine venereal campylobacteriosis, vibriosis)
Corynebacterium renale group	Pyelonephritis
Epizootic bovine abortion agent (unidentified)	Abortion (foothill abortion)
Escherichia coli	Interstitial nephritis (white-spotted kidney disease), pyelonephritis, pyometra
Fusobacterium necrophorum, other anaerobes	Postparturient metritis
Leptospira spp.	Abortion
Listeria monocytogenes, L. ivanovii	Abortion
Mycoplasma spp., *Ureaplasma* spp.	Granular vulvitis
Fungi	
Aspergillus spp.	Abortion
Mortierella wolfii	Abortion

[a]Considered a foreign animal disease agent in the United States.

consequence of retrograde extension of infection from the bladder.

Infection of the urinary tract via the hematogenous route occurs secondary to bacteremia/viremia and primarily affects the kidney, causing glomerulonephritis or interstitial nephritis. It occurs less commonly than lower UTIs, probably due to the high resistance of the renal cortex, where infection begins. Young animals are especially at risk because of the greater likelihood for septicemia to occur in that age group.

Glomerulonephritis and Interstitial Nephritis. Glomerulonephritis is an inflammation of the glomerulus due to localization of an infectious agent in the glomerulus and ensuing inflammatory response or from deposition of immune complexes. Viral glomerulonephritis is the result of selected viruses (e.g., infectious canine hepatitis virus, equine arteritis virus, and nephrotoxic infectious bronchitis virus in chickens) replicating in glomerular capillary endothelial cells, usually as a consequence of a systemic viral infection. In bacterial glomerulonephritis, bacteria from a septicemia/bacteremia settle in the glomerulus (e.g., *Actinobacillus equuli* ssp. *equuli* in foals).

Table 75.5. Common and/or Important Infectious Agents of the Urogenital System of Sheep and Goats

Agent	Major Clinical Manifestations (Common Disease Name)
Viruses	
Akabane virus[a]	Abortion, dystocia due to arthrogryposis of fetus
Bluetongue virus (S)	Abortion, congenital abnormalities (bluetongue)
Border disease and bovine viral diarrhea viruses	Congenital abnormalities, stillbirths (Border disease, hairy shaker disease)
Cache Valley virus	Abortion, congenital abnormalities
Rift Valley fever virus[a]	Abortion
Bacteria	
Actinobacillus seminis (S)	Epididymitis
Brucella abortus, B. melitensis[a]	Abortion, orchitis
Brucella ovis (S)	Epididymitis, rare abortions
Campylobacter fetus ssp. *fetus*	Abortion
Campylobacter jejuni	Abortion
Chlamydophila abortus	Abortion (enzootic abortion of ewes)
Corynebacterium renale group	Balanoposthitis (ulcerative posthitis, pizzle rot), pyelonephritis
Coxiella burnetii	Abortion (Q-fever)
Histophilus somni[b] (S)	Epididymitis
Leptospira spp.	Abortion
Listeria monocytogenes, L. ivanovii	Abortion
Salmonella spp.	Abortion, metritis

S, sheep predominately.
[a]Considered a foreign animal disease agent in the United States.
[b]*H. ovis* is the obsolete name.

Table 75.6. Common and/or Important Infectious Agents of the Urogenital System of Pigs

Agent	Major Clinical Manifestations (Common Disease Name)
Viruses	
African swine fever virus[a]	Abortion, immune-complex glomerulonephritis (African swine fever)
Classical swine fever virus[a]	Abortion, embryonic death, immune-complex glomerulonephritis (classical swine fever, hog cholera)
Lelystad virus	Abortion (porcine reproductive and respiratory syndrome)
Pseudorabies virus	Abortion (pseudorabies)
Swine parvovirus	Embryonic death, mummification
Bacteria	
Actinobaculum suis	Cystitis, pyelonephritis, ureteritis
Brucella suis	Abortion, orchitis
Escherichia coli	Vaginitis (discharging sows)
Leptospira spp.	Abortion (leptospirosis)

[a]Considered a foreign animal disease agent in the United States.

Table 75.7. Common and/or Important Infectious Agents of the Urogenital System of Poultry

Agent	Major Clinical Manifestations (Common Disease Name)
Viruses	
Avian adenovirus (C)	Soft-shelled or shell-less eggs (egg drop syndrome)
Avian encephalomyelitis virus	Decreased egg production
Avian influenza virus	Decreased egg production, oophoritis
Avian leukosis virus (C)	Nephroblastoma, renal carcinoma
Avian pneumovirus	Decreased egg production
Infectious bronchitis virus (C)	Decreased egg production, decreased hatchability, nephritis (infectious bronchitis-nephrotoxic strains)
Newcastle disease virus[a]	Decreased egg production
Bacteria	
Escherichia coli (C)	Salpingitis
Gallibacterium anatis (C)[b]	Oophoritis, salpingitis
Haemophilus paragallinarum (C)	Decreased egg production (infectious coryza)
Mycoplasma gallisepticum	Decreased egg production, salpingitis
Mycoplasma iowae (T)	Reduced hatchability, increased embryo mortality
Salmonella pullorum	Oophoritis, salpingitis (pullorum disease)
Salmonella gallinarum	Oophoritis, salpingitis (fowl typhoid)
Salmonella enteritidis (phage type 4)	Oophoritis, salpingitis

C, chickens predominately; T, turkeys predominately.
[a]Considered a foreign animal disease agent in the United States.
[b]Includes organisms previously identified as *Actinobacillus salpingitidis*, *Pasteurella haemolytica*-like, or *Pasteurella haemolytica–Actinobacillus salpingitidis* complex.

The ensuing inflammatory response is typically suppurative. The result is an embolic nephritis (Figure 75.1).

In some hematogenous infections, the renal tubules rather than the glomeruli are the primary target. Interstitial nephritis is commonly seen with *Escherichia coli* septicemia in neonatal ruminants (white-spotted kidney) (Figure 75.2) and leptospirosis in a number of different animals.

Deposition of immune complexes in the glomeruli in the case of persistent viral infections (e.g., infectious canine hepatitis, equine infectious anemia, and feline infectious peritonitis), specific bacterial infections (e.g., *Borrelia* spp.), or chronic bacterial infections at other sites in the body may result in immune-complex glomerulonephritis.

Cystitis. Bacterial cystitis (inflammation of the urinary bladder), especially in dogs, is the most common UTI encountered by veterinarians. The ability of bacteria to adhere to epithelium is considered a prerequisite to establishment of cystitis. The infection may begin with colonization of the urethral orifice by a potential pathogen that subsequently reaches the bladder through multiplication, extension along the epithelial surface, or migration through active motility or random movement. The resulting infection, after further multiplication, is marked by bacteriuria. Pyuria and low-grade proteinuria may be present. Inflammation is triggered by the interaction of lipopolysaccharide (gram-negative bacteria) or muramyl dipeptides (gram-positive bacteria) with transitional cells of the bladder that secrete proinflammatory mediators, which attract polymorphonuclear neutrophil leukocytes. Signs, when present, include dysuria or urinary frequency or urgency. There may be hematuria and incontinence. Common agents implicated in canine UTIs and characteristic features are summarized in Table 75.8.

FIGURE 75.1. *Embolic nephritis in a foal caused by* A. equuli *ssp.* equuli. *(Courtesy of Dr Alan Doster.)*

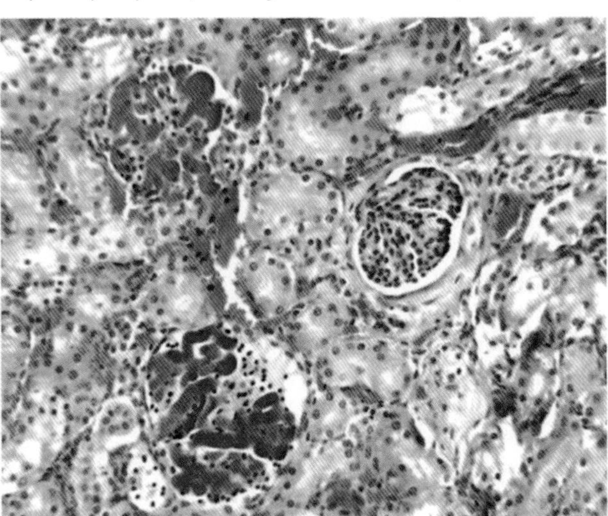

Pyelonephritis. The most serious complication of lower UTI is pyelonephritis, which is caused by an ascending infection via the ureters. Pyelonephritis is essentially an inflammation of the renal pelvis and renal parenchyma. Once bacteria reach the renal pelvis, they are hard to

FIGURE 75.2. *White-spotted kidney in a neonatal ruminant associated with interstitial nephritis secondary to* E. coli *septicemia. (Courtesy of Dr Alan Doster.)*

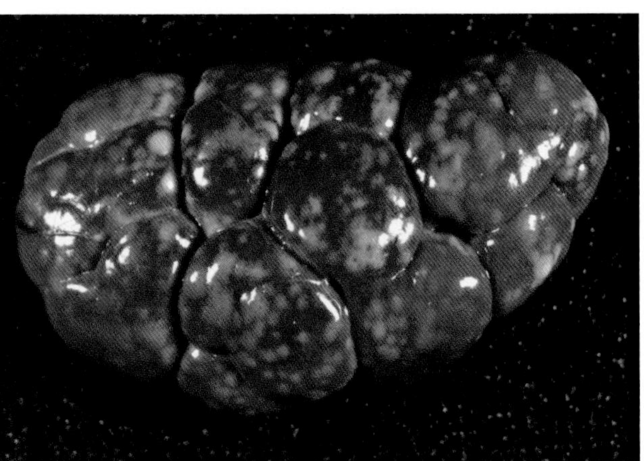

Table 75.8. Leading Bacterial Causes of UTIs in Dogs

Species	Prevalence (%)	Typical Colonies		Confirmatory Tests		
		Blood Agar	MacConkey Agar	Gram Stain	Oxidase	Catalase
Escherichia coli	42–46	Smooth gray; often hemolytic	Red discrete, surrounded by red haze	Negative rods	Negative	NA
Enterococcus	11–14	Very small (<1 mm)	No growth	Positive cocci	NA	Negative
Coagulase-positive *Staphylococcus*	12	White or off-white (often hemolytic)	No growth	Positive cocci	NA	Positive
Proteus mirabilis	6–12	Swarms; no discrete colonies	Colorless	Negative rods	Negative	NA
Klebsiella	8–12	Large, wet mucoid, whitish-gray	Pink, slimy coalescing; not surrounded by red haze	Negative rods	Negative	NA
Pseudomonas	<5	Gray to greenish-gray; fruity or ammonia odor; often hemolytic	Colorless, surrounded by blue-green pigment	Negative rods	Positive	NA

NA, not applicable.

eliminate due to the poor vascular supply and inhibitory effects of urine osmolarity and ammonia on immune defenses, as mentioned previously. Signs of pyelonephritis are vague. Fever is transient even during the acute phase. Pain in the thoracolumbar area is not specific unless directly associated with kidney palpation. Urinalysis may reveal lowered specific gravity and casts. In advanced cases, blood urea nitrogen is elevated. *E. coli* is the most common cause of pyelonephritis in animals. Other bacterial agents that cause cystitis have the potential to cause pyelonephritis, if they reach the renal pelvis.

Diphtheroid bacteria, belonging to the *Corynebacterium renale* group, are specifically associated with pyelonephritis in cattle. They colonize the lower genital tract and pass between animals by direct and indirect contact. Many clinical cases are probably endogenous. The process is an ascending UTI, beginning with cystitis, which proceeds to ureteritis and pyelonephritis. An anaerobic diphtheroid, *Actinobaculum suis*, causes UTI of sows. Like bovine pyelonephritis, the disease is apparently an ascending infection caused by a urealytic diphtheroid agent, limited to females and often related to breeding operations, pregnancy, and parturition.

Uroliths and UTIs. Uroliths of dogs are predominantly (70%) the result of infection and consist of struvite or apatite, or various combinations, and are often referred to as triple phosphate stones. Urease-producing bacteria are implicated—in dogs, chiefly coagulase-positive staphylococci, and to a lesser extent *Proteus mirabilis*. Inhibition of urease activity by urea analogs (e.g., acetohydroxamic acid) can suppress infectious stone formation. Uroliths in ruminants are related to nutritional factors rather that infectious ones.

Virulence Factors of Bacterial Uropathogens

Bacteria capable of initiating UTI require virulence determinants, the most firmly established of which are adhesins (e.g., the pyelonephritis-associated pilus, Pap). Fimbrial attachment of *E. coli* to surface slime glycoproteins by type 1 (mannose-sensitive) pili is probably of less significance than that mediated by several mannose-resistant adhesins, one of which is Pap, which attach to cell membrane glycolipids. *E. coli* isolates from different animals appear to maintain the same Pap alleles. Mannose-resistant adhesins occur commonly in uropathogenic *E. coli*, but irregularly in other strains. Other properties associated with uropathogenic *E. coli* include resistance to serum bactericidal action; hemolytic activity; and possession of certain O-antigens, iron-scavenging proteins, and bacteriocins. These properties are rare in random *E. coli* strains, suggesting that agents of UTIs represent a select subpopulation within their species.

Pili-mediated attachment to urothelium and urea hydrolysis are considered critical virulence factors in pathogenesis of the *C. renale* group infections. Urea breakdown with production of ammonia initiates an inflammatory process, high alkalinity in urine (pH 9.0), and suppression of antibacterial defenses, possibly through complement inactivation by ammonia.

Miscellaneous Urinary Tract-Associated Infectious Processes

Fungi are rarely involved in UTIs. Fungal hyphae can be detected in the urine of dogs with disseminated *Aspergillus* infections. Mycotic cystitis is rarely identified. The yeast *Candida albicans* is sometimes isolated from the urine of dogs with diabetes mellitus.

Kidney tumors are associated with infections with the avian leukosis/sarcoma complex of viruses. Renal lymphoma is associated with feline leukemia virus infections in cats.

Genital Tract

The primary function of the genital tract is reproduction. The genital tract in mammals includes the ovaries, oviducts, uterus, cervix, vagina, and external genitalia in females and the testes, ductus deferens, accessory sex organs, penis, and prepuce in males. In poultry, the genital tract differs substantially from mammals. In males the testes are internal and, lacking accessory sex glands and a distinct copulatory organ, the ductus deferens parallels the ureter into the cloaca. Females typically have only a single functional ovary (left) and oviduct with the shell gland (uterus), which empties into the cloaca.

Antimicrobial Defenses

Antimicrobial defenses are in place at all levels of the genital tract and include the following:

Anatomic Defenses. Stratified squamous epithelium in the vagina and vulva provides for resistance to infection. The cervix provides a physical barrier to infections of the upper genital tract, especially during pregnancy. The long urethra in males provides a barrier to retrograde infections.

Hormonal Defenses. Hormones play a part in protecting the genital tract from disease. Estrogens increase the blood supply to the vagina and uterus, the number of polymorphonuclear neutrophil leukocytes in the cervix and uterus, and the myeloperoxidase activity of phagocytic cells in the tract. These activities are important because the vagina and perhaps the uterus may become contaminated with potentially harmful agents during coitus.

Immune Defenses. The immune system of the genital tract appears to be similar in structure and function to other mucosal surfaces. There are lymphoid follicles in the submucosa from the cervix caudally. These follicles supply cells that will ultimately secrete IgA. IgG and IgM will be found in this area as well, but these isotypes probably arrive through transudation. In the uterus, IgG, IgM, and some sIgA are found. In the prepuce, mainly sIgA is found; it is probably secreted by the accessory glands or locally from cells arising from the lymphoid follicles in this area. The defensive potential of these antibodies depends upon the isotype. Antibodies of the IgA isotype make particles more hydrophilic, thereby negating any surface attraction an organism might have for usually hydrophobic host cell surfaces as well as sterically hindering attachment. IgG and IgM, on the other hand, will opsonize, trigger the complement cascade, and sterically hinder attachment. All immunoglobulins, if specific for epitopes comprising flagella, immobilize bacteria that use motility as a way to ascend the tract from the more caudal regions.

Normal Flora

Lower portions of the genital tract in all animals possess a normal flora. The flora varies by animal and within an individual is dynamic over time. Factors including age, parity, and hormones affect flora makeup. The actual microbial flora of the genital tract is likely to be more complex than presently recognized because optimal culture methods for highly fastidious organisms have not always been employed in past studies on normal flora prevalence. Population density of individual flora members is less well understood, yet it is probably equally or more important than the particular flora makeup in the overall ecology and stability of the microbial population of the genital tract.

In general, the female genital tract possesses a resident microbial flora caudal to the external cervical os. The uterus is normally sterile or transiently contaminated with small numbers of microorganisms. The vagina contains a flora that is mainly composed of species of obligate anaerobic bacteria, including both gram-negative and gram-positive species. The aerobic and facultative anaerobic organisms, about one-tenth the number of obligate anaerobes, include gram-positive and gram-negative species, as well as *Mycoplasma* and *Ureaplasma*.

As is the case with other mucosal surfaces, the flora should be thought of as protective insofar as other, perhaps more pathogenic, strains are excluded through colonization resistance. Mechanisms for exclusion include blocking attachment, efficient use of available substrates, and production of antimicrobial substances. In a more practical sense, the normal or transient flora does include some species that will contaminate the uterus should it become compromised. Some examples include *Streptococcus equi* ssp. *zooepidemicus* in mares with endometritis, *Arcanobacterium pyogenes* along with *Fusobacterium necrophorum* in cows with pyometra, and *E. coli* in bitches with pyometra. All of the organisms mentioned here are part of the normal or transient vaginal flora of the affected animals. The potential for these organisms to cause disease does not simply result from their presence but requires a critical level of replicative dominance over other flora before disease can occur. If the normal flora is disturbed, as during antibiotic treatment of bacterial endometritis in the mare, the vagina will be repopulated with other, more resistant, strains, which may ultimately infect the uterus if the underlying compromising condition goes uncorrected.

The resident flora of the external genitalia includes commensal anaerobes, which are largely gram-negative, nonspore formers; *Mycoplasma* spp.; α-hemolytic and β-hemolytic streptococci; lactobacilli; *Haemophilus* spp. (particularly *H. haemoglobinophilus* in dogs); corynebacteria; propionibacteria; and coagulase-negative staphylococci. *Taylorella equigenitalis*, a venereally transmitted pathogen of mares, may be carried inapparently in the clitoral fossa.

The prepuce and the distal urethra of the male genital tract possess a resident flora that plays a role similar to that played by the flora in the vagina. The origin of organisms responsible for bacterial disease in these areas is almost always endogenous. Some venereally transmitted organisms reside in the prepuce (e.g., *Campylobacter fetus* ssp. *venerealis* in cattle and *T. equigenitalis* in stallions) causing no adverse effects at these sites. The preputial cavity, including the preputial diverticulum of swine, is home for agents of pyelonephritis in cattle (*C. renale* group) and swine (*A. suis*).

Diseases

Host and Environmental Factors. For disease to occur in the genital tract frequently, some predisposing host and environmental factors must be in place and include the following:

Anatomic Factors. Vulvar conformation of mares is a well-known predisposing factor to infection of the vagina and uterus. The more horizontally positioned the vulva, the greater the tendency for fecal contamination of the vagina to occur. Urine pooling in the vagina predisposes to cervicitis and endometritis. Phimosis in males can lead to nonspecific inflammation and infection of the prepuce and penis.

Hormonal Factors. Hormones play a role in making the genital tract more susceptible to disease. In general, under the influence of progesterone, the uterus is more prone to infection. Neutrophil activity in the genital tract is suppressed under the influence of progesterone, including decreased migration and phagocytic ability. At least in bitches, during the luteal phase, receptors for *E. coli* are expressed. Colonization by *E. coli* expressing appropriate adhesins allows for establishment and can ultimately lead to development of pyometra. Whether the same occurs in other species is unknown.

Other Factors. Trauma that may occur during parturition can compromise integrity of the epithelial barrier leading to infection. Dystocias and retained fetal membranes increase chances for postparturient infections. Nutritional factors sometimes influence genital tract disease development. For example, posthitis in sheep occurs typically in animals on rich legume pastures that are high in proteins, which increase urea excretion, and estrogens. This leads to preputial swelling and urine retention in the sheath.

Infectious Processes. For most genital tract pathogens, the routes of exposure are venereal or by ingestion. Localization to the genital tract occurs by ascending or hematogenous routes. In some diseases, although venereally transmitted, pathogens localize to areas in the genital tract by a hematogenous means. Some genital tract pathogens reside in the digestive tract and become bloodborne to cause disease in the genital tract (e.g., *C. fetus* ssp. *fetus* in sheep).

Female Reproductive Tract. The most common infections of the female reproductive tract involve the vulva, vagina, cervix, and uterus. Vulvitis in cattle is associated with *Ureaplasma* and *Mycoplasma* spp., but a solid etiological link remains to be shown. Infectious bovine rhinotracheitis virus causes vulvovaginitis in cattle. Various coliforms, especially *E. coli*, cause vaginal-vulvar discharge in sows. Such infections are often related to hygiene and management practices. Vaginitis in dogs is most commonly associated with *Staphylococcus* spp, *Streptococcus* spp., or *E. coli*. In prepubertal females, vaginitis tends to resolve on its own as the dog matures. In older bitches, there is usually an underlying factor involved.

Uterine infections are typically related to breeding, pregnancy, or parturition, the nonpregnant uterus being fairly resistant to infection. During breeding or parturition when the cervix is open, infections of the uterus are most often ascending. Infections of the uterus can involve the endometrium (endometritis) or the entire wall of the uterus (metritis). Endometritis occurs in all animals but is most common and of greatest consequence in the horse. Inability of some horses with endometritis to resolve infections is in part due to defects in migration of neutrophils to the site of infection as well as decreased phagocytic ability of the neutrophils. *S. equi* ssp. *zooepidemicus* is the pathogen most commonly associated with endometritis in mares, although other organisms (enterics, other streptococci, *Pseudomonas*) can be involved.

If prior to resolution of a uterine infection the cervix closes and pus accumulates, a pyometra develops. Pyometras occur in all animals but are most frequent in dogs, cats, and cattle. Overall, *E. coli* is the organism most often associated with pyometra. A number of other organisms, including *Streptococcus* sp. and *Pseudomonas*, can also be involved. In cattle, *A. pyogenes* and obligately anaerobic bacteria are frequently found.

Fetus. Abortion, especially in farm animals and horses, is one of the most common and economically significant genital tract diseases. Abortion is essentially expulsion of the fetus before full development. A number of viral, bacterial, and fungal agents can trigger this process (see Tables 75.1, 75.2, 75.3, 75.4, 75.5, 75.6, and 75.7). During pregnancy, the placenta and/or fetus are infected predominately by the hematogenous route. Mares are an exception; bacterial and fungal placental infections most often originate through the cervical os.

A number of viruses can cause abortion in animals. The herpesviruses are prominent among the viruses involved and affect a number of different animals, most notably horses (equine herpesvirus 1). Viral-induced abortions result subsequent to fetal inflammatory lesions with necrosis, fetal anoxia, or endometrial lesions.

Bacteria responsible for abortion often cause a placentitis or placental edema. If the fetus becomes infected, typically large numbers of organisms are found in the fetal stomach fluid. In some bacterial abortions, lesions in the fetus may suggest the likely agent. As an example, the focal areas of hepatic necrosis in the fetus are suggestive of—however, not exclusive to—abortions in sheep caused by *C. fetus* ssp. *fetus* (Figure 75.3).

While most bacterial abortions occur in the last trimester, early fetal death and resorption occurs with some agents. In those cases, the infection presents clinically as an infertility problem (e.g., *C. fetus* ssp. *venerealis* in cattle).

Fungal abortions are most common in horses and cattle and typically are the result of a placentitis. The portal of entry in cattle is either the respiratory or gastrointestinal tract with subsequent hematogenous spread to the placenta. In horses, an ascending infection through the cervix is the most common route. Fetal lesions in cattle, if present, are for the most part limited to focal, hyperkeratotic lesions on the skin; in horses fetal lesions are uncommon. *Mortierella wolffi*, a zygomycete, causes a fulminating pneumonia with a high mortality rate in about 25% of affected cows as a result of a lung-uterus-lung infection cycle. Fungal elements absorbed from the uterus cause a fulminating embolic pneumonia in the cow that typically follows the abortion.

FIGURE 75.3. *Areas of acute hepatic coagulative necrosis in the liver of an aborted ovine fetus.* C. fetus *ssp.* fetus *was isolated. (Courtesy of Dr Alan Doster.)*

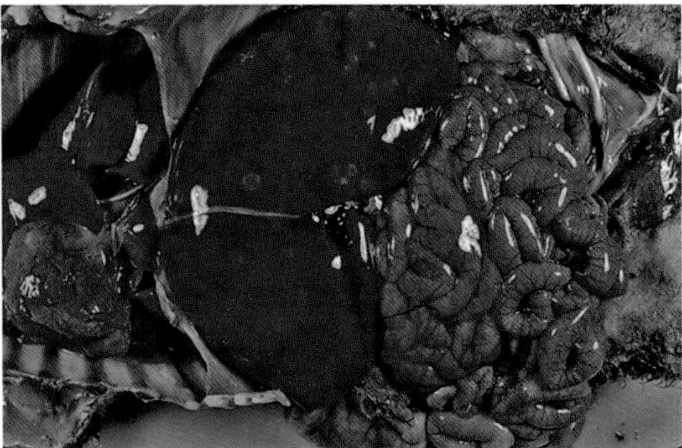

Some viral infections of the fetus result in congenital abnormalities. Factors influencing whether abnormalities develop are dependent on the stage of fetal development, immune competence of the fetus, and the particular viral strains responsible (e.g., feline panleukopenia virus; bovine viral diarrhea virus; and Akabane, Cache Valley, Border disease, and bluetongue viruses in sheep).

Details on the pathogenesis and pathology as it relates to individual abortifacient agents are found in specific chapters on those agents.

Male Reproductive Tract. In males, the predominant genital tract infections are orchitis, epididymitis, and infections of the accessory sex glands (prostatitis and seminal vesiculitis). Orchitis can develop by an ascending or hematogenous route. Occasionally periorchitis develops from descending peritonitis, which subsequently involves the testes. Epididymitis affects all animal species but is most common in rams. In younger rams, an ascending infection by age-dependent preputial residents—"*Actinobacillus seminis*," *Histophilus somni* ("*Histophilus ovis*" is the obsolete name)—is the rule. In adult rams, *Brucella ovis* is the main agent involved. It localizes to the epididymal ductules via the hematogenous route. Inflammation and extravasation of sperm lead to development of a spermatic granuloma.

Bacterial prostatitis most commonly occurs in dogs and is, in fact, the most common cause of prostatic disease in dogs. Infections are mostly ascending in origin and can be acute or chronic. Consequences include prostatic abscesses, which can rupture and cause peritonitis. Seminal vesiculitis occurs most commonly in bulls and is the most common cause for inflammatory cells detected during semen examination. Many potential agents have been implicated, with *A. pyogenes* the most frequently recovered.

Infections of the penis or prepuce can be transmitted from endogenous or exogenous sources. Various herpesviruses cause balanoposthitis in animals. Members of the *C. renale* group cause a necrotizing inflammation of the prepuce and adjacent tissues in wethers or rams. The disease develops in the presence of these urealytic agents in an area constantly irrigated with urine. Ammonia is thought to initiate the inflammatory process. A similar condition occurs occasionally in goats and bulls.

Genital Tract of Poultry. Infections of the oviduct (salpingitis) in poultry can be the result of an ascending infection from the cloaca or occur in conjunction with colibacillosis when the left abdominal air sac is involved. *E. coli* is the most common pathogen recovered. Although pullorum disease and fowl typhoid have become uncommon diseases in developed countries, oophoritis, salpingitis, and orchitis are all possible consequences of the septicemia associated with infections by *Salmonella* serovars *Pullorum* and *Gallinarum*, respectively.

Decreased egg production and/or hatchability can result from a number of systemic infections in poultry. A number of viruses (e.g., avian adenovirus, infectious bronchitis virus, and avian influenza virus) and bacteria (e.g., *Mycoplasma*, *Haemophilus paragallinarum*, and *Salmonella*) can affect overall egg production and hatchability. Some poultry pathogens (e.g., *Mycoplasma*, *Salmonella*) are transmitted vertically in eggs.

Index

Note: Page number followed by f and t indicate figure and table respectively.

Veterinary Microbiology, Third Edition. Edited by D. Scott McVey, Melissa Kennedy and M.M. Chengappa.